OPERATIVE

FOOT

SURGERY

JOHN S. GOULD, M.D.
Professor and Chairman
Department of Orthopaedic Surgery
Medical College of Wisconsin
Milwaukee, Wisconsin

Section Editors

FRANCESCA M. THOMPSON, M.D.   LAMAR L. FLEMING, M.D.
ANDREA CRACCHIOLO III, M.D.   GEORGE W. SIMONS, M.D.
ROBERT S. ADELAAR, M.D.   KEVIN P. BLACK, M.D.

W.B. SAUNDERS COMPANY
A Division of Harcourt Brace & Company
Philadelphia • London • Toronto • Montreal • Sydney • Tokyo

W.B. SAUNDERS COMPANY
A Division of
Harcourt Brace & Company

The Curtis Center
Independence Square West
Philadelphia, Pennsylvania 19106

Library of Congress Cataloging-in-Publication Data

Operative foot surgery / [edited by] John S. Gould.—1st ed.

    p.   cm.

ISBN 0–7216–3196–7

  1. Foot—Surgery.   I. Gould, John S.

[DNLM: 1. Foot—surgery.   WE 880 0615 1994]

RD563.065   1994

617.5′85059—dc20

DNLM/DLC   93–1960

OPERATIVE FOOT SURGERY   ISBN 0–7216–3196–7

Printed in the United States of America.

Last digit is the print number: 9   8   7   6   5   4   3   2   1

Dedication

To Edith Marion Spiller Gould and Nathaniel Gould, M.D.,
for their love, support, inspiration,
and model for the pursuit of excellence.

Contributors

ROBERT S. ADELAAR, M.D.
Professor of Surgery and Vice Chairman of Orthopedic Surgery, Medical College of Virginia, Richmond, Virginia; Chief, Section of Orthopedic Surgery, Medical College of Virginia, McGuire Veterans Hospital, Richmond, Virginia
Section Editor of Problems of the Adult Foot: Hindfoot and Miscellaneous; Surgical Treatment of Fractures of the Talus; Vertical Talus; Injuries of the Gastrocnemius-Soleus Complex

BENJAMIN A. ALMAN, M.D.
Instructor, Department of Orthopaedics, Tufts University School of Medicine, Boston, Massachusetts; Associate Staff, New England Medical Center Hospitals, Boston, Massachusetts
Metatarsus Adductus

ROBERT B. ANDERSON, M.D.
Chief, Foot and Ankle Service, Carolinas Medical Center, Charlotte, North Carolina; Presbyterian Orthopaedic Hospital; Charlotte Institute of Rehabilitation, Mercy Hospital
Sesamoiditis

DONALD E. BAXTER, M.D.
Clinical Professor of Orthopaedics, Baylor College of Medicine, Houston, Texas
Heel Pain Syndrome and Entrapment Neuropathies About the Foot and Ankle

KEVIN P. BLACK, M.D.
Associate Professor of Orthopaedics, Penn State College of Medicine, Penn State University Hospital–Milton S. Hershey Medical Center, Hershey, Pennsylvania
Section Editor of Foot and Ankle Injuries in Sports; Ankle Injuries in Sports; Bone and Joint Injuries of the Foot in Athletes

WALTHER BOHNE, M.D.
Associate Professor, Department of Orthopedic Surgery, New York Hospital–Cornell Medical Center, New York, New York; Attending Staff, Memorial Sloane Kettering and Hospital for Special Surgery, New York, New York
Regional Anesthesia for Foot Surgery

MICHAEL J. BRENNAN, M.D.
Assistant Clinical Professor of Orthopaedic Surgery, Medical College of Wisconsin, Milwaukee, Wisconsin; Orthopaedic Surgeon, Good Samaritan Hospital and St. Joseph's Hospital, Phoenix, Arizona
Metatarsal Fractures and Dislocations and Lisfranc's Fracture-Dislocations

JAMES W. BRODSKY, M.D.
Assistant Clinical Professor, Department of Orthopaedic Surgery, University of Texas Southwestern Medical School at Dallas, Dallas, Texas; Director, Diabetic and Orthopaedic Foot Clinic, Dallas Veterans Administration Hospital, Dallas, Texas; Attending Staff, Baylor University Medical Center, Dallas, Texas
Surgical Treatment and Reconstruction of the Diabetic Foot

DANIEL R. COOPERMAN, M.D.
Assistant Professor of Orthopedic Surgery, Case Western Reserve University, Cleveland, Ohio; Attending Physician, Rainbow Babies and Childrens Hospital and Metro Health Medical Center, Cleveland, Ohio
Peroneal Spastic Flatfoot

MICHAEL J. COUGHLIN, M.D.
Private Practice, Orthopaedic Surgery, St. Alphonsus Regional Medical Center, Boise, Idaho; Clinical Associate Professor of Surgery, Division of Orthopedics and Rehabilitation, Oregon Health Sciences University, Portland, Oregon
The Bunionette Deformity: Etiology and Treatment; The Pathophysiology and Treatment of the Juvenile Bunion

ANDREA CRACCHIOLO III, M.D.
Professor of Orthopaedic Surgery, UCLA School of Medicine, Los Angeles, California
Section Editor of Problems of the Adult Foot: Forefoot; Rheumatoid Arthritis of the Forefoot

CLIFFORD L. CRAIG, M.D.
Assistant Professor, Orthopaedic Surgery, Tufts University School of Medicine, Boston, Massachusetts; Orthopedic Surgeon, New England Medical Center, Boston, Massachusetts and Morton Hospital, Taunton, Massachusetts
Metatarsus Adductus

G. PAUL DeROSA, M.D.
Professor and Chairman, Department of Orthopaedic Surgery, Indiana University School of Medicine, Indianapolis, Indiana; Attending Physician, James Whitcomb Riley Hospital for Children, Indianapolis, Indiana
Flexible Flatfoot

DAVID M. DRVARIC, M.D.
Associate Professor, Section of Pediatric Orthopaedics, Department of Orthopaedics, Emory University School of Medicine, Atlanta, Georgia; Chief of Service, Department of Orthopaedics,

Grady Memorial Hospital, Atlanta, Georgia; Consultant, Henrietta Egleston Hospital for Children, Atlanta, Georgia
Cavus Foot

WILLIAM W. DZWIERZYNSKI, M.D.
Assistant Professor of Surgery, Department of Plastic and Reconstructive Surgery, Medical College of Wisconsin; Attending Surgeon, Froedtert Memorial Lutheran Hospital, Milwaukee, Wisconsin
Microsurgical Reconstruction of the Foot and Ankle

LAMAR L. FLEMING, M.D.
Professor and Chairman, Department of Orthopaedics, Emory University, Atlanta, Georgia
Section Editor of Trauma of the Adult Foot and Ankle

DAVID A. FRISCIA, M.D.
Assistant Clinical Professor, University of Southern California, Los Angeles, California; Active Staff, Eisenhower Medical Center, Rancho Mirage, California; Teaching Staff, Rancho Los Amigos Medical Center, Downey, California
Hallux Varus

JOHN S. GOULD, M.D.
Professor and Chairman, Department of Orthopaedic Surgery, Medical College of Wisconsin, Milwaukee, Wisconsin; Director, Department of Orthopaedic Surgery, Milwaukee County Medical Complex, Milwaukee, Wisconsin
Implant Arthroplasty of the Foot; Salvage of Failed Silicone Implants; Microsurgical Reconstruction of the Foot and Ankle; Metatarsal Fractures and Dislocations and Lisfranc's Fracture-Dislocations; Congenital Malformations of the Feet and Toes

SCOTT R. GREWE, M.D.
Clinical Instructor in Orthopedic Surgery, Oregon Health Sciences University, Portland, Oregon; Active Staff, Emanuel Hospital and Health Center, Providence Medical Center, and Good

Samaritan Hospital and Medical Center, Portland, Oregon; Attending Sports Medicine Physician, Shriners Hospital for Crippled Children, Portland, Oregon
Compartment Syndrome of the Foot

REGINALD L. HALL, M.D.
Assistant Professor, Division of Orthopaedic Surgery, Duke University Medical Center, Durham, North Carolina
Management of Foot Infections

WILLIAM G. HAMILTON, M.D.
Associate Clinical Professor of Orthopedic Surgery, Columbia University College of Physicians and Surgeons, New York, New York; Senior Orthopedic Attending Surgeon, St. Luke's–Roosevelt Hospital Center, New York, New York
Conditions Seen in Classical Ballet and Modern Dance

JOHN E. HANDELSMAN, M.D., F.R.C.S., M.Ch.(Orth.)
Chairman, Department of Orthopaedic Surgery and Director, Pediatric Orthopaedics, Schneider Children's Hospital, New York, New York; Professor of Orthopaedic Surgery, Albert Einstein College of Medicine, Yeshiva University, Bronx, New York
Angular Deformities of the Lesser Toes

MICHAEL M. HECKMAN, M.D.
Assistant Clinical Professor, Department of Orthopaedics, University of Texas Health Science Center at San Antonio, San Antonio, Texas; Chief of Orthopaedic Surgery, Spohn Hospital, Corpus Christi, Texas; Orthopaedic Surgeons and Sports Medicine Associates, Corpus Christi, Texas
Compartment Syndrome of the Foot

GEORGE B. HOLMES, JR., M.D.
Director of Foot and Ankle Surgery, University Orthopaedics, Chicago, Illinois; Assistant Professor of Orthopaedic Surgery, Rush Medical College, Chicago, Illinois; Attending Physician, Rush–Presbyterian–St. Luke's Medical Center, Chicago, Illinois
Hallux Rigidus; Nerve Compression Syndromes of the Foot and Ankle

HELEN M. HORSTMAN, M.D.
Associate Professor, Chief, Foot and Ankle Surgery, and Chief, Pediatric Orthopedic Surgery, Medical College of Pennsylvania, Philadelphia, Pennsylvania; Associate Surgeon, Children's Hospital of Philadelphia, Philadelphia, Pennsylvania
Neuromuscular Foot Deformities in Children

KENNETH A. JAFFE, M.D.
Assistant Professor, University of Alabama at Birmingham School of Medicine, Birmingham, Alabama; Attending Surgeon, University of Alabama Hospitals, Birmingham, Alabama
Foot Tumors

JEFFREY E. JOHNSON, M.D.
Associate Professor and Program Director, Foot Fellowship Program, Department of Orthopaedic Surgery, Medical College of Wisconsin, Milwaukee, Wisconsin; Assistant Professor, Milwaukee County Medical Complex, Milwaukee, Wisconsin; Consulting Staff, Children's Hospital of Wisconsin, Froedtert Memorial Lutheran Hospital, St. Michael's Hospital, St. Mary's Hospital, and St. Francis Hospital, Milwaukee, Wisconsin
Management of Foot Infections; Metatarsal Fractures and Dislocations and Lisfranc's Fracture-Dislocations; Late Reconstruction of Calcaneal Fracture Problems

KENNETH A. JOHNSON, M.D.
Professor of Orthopedic Surgery, Mayo Clinic, Scottsdale, Arizona; Head, Section of Foot and Ankle Surgery, Mayo Clinic, Scottsdale, Arizona
Hallux Varus

FRAZIER K. JONES
Orthopaedic Resident, University of Alabama Hospital, Birmingham, Alabama
Foot Tumors

ROBERT E. KETTLER, M.D.
Associate Professor, Medical College of Wisconsin, Milwaukee, Wisconsin; Acting Director of Clinical Anesthesia, Milwaukee County Medical Complex, Milwaukee, Wisconsin
Regional Anesthesia for Foot Surgery

NORMAN LICHT, M.D.
Active Staff, Munson Medical Center, Traverse City, Michigan; Associate, Paul Oliver Memorial Hospital, Frankfort, Michigan
Degenerative Problems of the Midtarsal Joints

ROGER A. MANN, M.D.
Director, Foot Fellowship Program; Director, Foot Surgery, Summit Medical Center, Oakland, California; Private Practice, Orthopaedic Surgery, Oakland, California
Hallux Valgus; Charcot-Marie-Tooth Disease

LELAND C. McCLUSKEY, M.D.
Staff Physician, Hughston Orthopaedic Clinic, Columbus, Georgia
Ankle Injuries in Sports

MICHAEL E. MILLER, M.D.
Clinical Associate Professor, Department of Orthopaedic Surgery, Emory University School of Medicine, Atlanta, Georgia; Director of Orthopaedic Surgery, Norwood Clinic/Carraway Hospital, Birmingham, Alabama
Fractures and Dislocations of the Ankle

MARK S. MIZEL, M.D.
Assistant Clinical Professor, Department of Orthopedics, Tufts University School of Medicine, Boston, Massachusetts; Director, Boston Foot and Ankle Center, New England Baptist Hospital, Boston, Massachusetts
Anatomy and Pathophysiology of the Lesser Toes

CLAUDE T. MOORMAN III, M.D.
Chief Resident, Division of Orthopaedic Surgery, Duke University Medical Center, Durham, North Carolina
The Rheumatoid Hindfoot

JAMES A. NUNLEY, M.D.
Professor of Surgery, Division of Orthopaedics and Attending Physician, Duke University Medical Center, Durham, North Carolina
The Rheumatoid Hindfoot

DROR PALEY, M.D., F.R.C.S.C.
Associate Professor, Chief, Pediatric Orthopedics, and Director, Maryland Center for Limb Lengthening, University of Maryland, Baltimore, Maryland; Attending Surgeon, Kernan Hospital and University of Maryland Hospital, Baltimore, Maryland
Fractures of the Calcaneus; Principles of Foot Deformity Correction: Ilizarov Technique

LANDRUS L. PFEFFINGER, M.D.
Assistant Clinical Professor, University of California at San Francisco, San Francisco, California; Active Staff, John Muir Hospital, Walnut Creek, California; Active Staff, Summit Hospital, Oakland, California; Active Staff, San Leandro Hospital, San Leandro, California; Courtesy Staff, San Ramon Regional Medical Center, San Ramon, California
Hemiplegic Disorders of the Foot

J. CHRISTOPHER REYNOLDS, M.D.
Director of the Foot Clinic, Brackenridge Hospital, Austin, Texas; Staff, Seton Medical Center, St. David's Medical Center, and Bailey Square Surgical Center, Austin, Texas
Morton's Neuroma—Interdigital Neuroma

MICHAEL D. ROOKS, M.D.
Associate Professor of Orthopaedics, Emory University School of Medicine, Atlanta, Georgia; Director, Microsurgical Research and Training Laboratory, Grady Memorial Hospital, Atlanta, Georgia; Orthopaedic and Hand Surgeon, Crawford Long Hospital of Emory University, Atlanta, Georgia; Consultant, Henrietta Egleston Hospital for Children, Atlanta, Georgia; Active Staff, Veterans Administration Medical Center, Decatur, Georgia
Tendon, Vascular, Nerve, and Skin Injuries

SALLY A. RUDICEL, M.D.
Associate Professor, Temple University, Philadelphia, Pennsylvania; Associate Chair, Department of Orthopaedics, Albert Einstein Medical Center, Philadelphia, Pennsylvania
Intractable Plantar Keratoses

CHARLES L. SALTZMAN, M.D.
Assistant Professor and Director of the Foot and Ankle Service, University of Iowa, Iowa City, Iowa
Hallux Varus

LEW C. SCHON, M.D.
Attending Orthopaedic Surgeon, Director, Dance Medicine Clinic, and Associate Director, Foot and Ankle Center, Union Memorial Hospital, Baltimore, Maryland
Heel Pain Syndrome and Entrapment Neuropathies About the Foot and Ankle

DAVID G. SCOTT, M.D.
Private Practice, Maryville Orthopaedic Center, Maryville, Tennessee; Staff Orthopaedic Surgeon, Blount Memorial Hospital, Maryville, Tennessee
Bone and Joint Injuries of the Foot in Athletes

MICHAEL J. SHEREFF, M.D.
Associate Professor, Medical College of Wisconsin, Milwaukee, Wisconsin; Director, Division of Foot and Ankle Surgery; Associate Attending Physician, Orthopaedic Foot and Ankle Center, St. Francis Hospital, Milwaukee, Wisconsin
Disorders of the Toenails

NAOMI N. SHIELDS, M.D., Major, USAF, MC
Chief, Orthopaedic Surgery Clinic, 377th Medical Group/SGHST, Kirtland Air Force Base, Albuquerque, New Mexico
Metatarsal Fractures and Dislocations and Lisfranc's Fracture-Dislocations

GEORGE W. SIMONS, M.D., M.S.O.S.
Professor, Department of Orthopedic Surgery and Medical Director, Human Motion Analysis Laboratory, Medical College of Wisconsin, Milwaukee, Wisconsin; Chief Senior Pediatric Orthopaedic Surgery Consultant, Children's Hospital of Wisconsin, Milwaukee, Wisconsin
Section Editor of Problems of the Pediatric Foot; Clubfoot

JUDITH W. SMITH, M.D.
Assistant Professor, Department of Orthopaedic Surgery, Emory University School of Medicine, Atlanta, Georgia; Attending Orthopaedist, Crawford Long Hospital of Emory University, and Grady Memorial Hospital, Atlanta, Georgia
Implant Arthroplasty of the Foot

JAMES B. STIEHL, M.D.
Associate Clinical Professor, Medical College of Wisconsin, Milwaukee, Wisconsin; Active Staff, Columbia Hospital, Milwaukee, Wisconsin
Late Reconstruction of Complex Ankle Fractures and Dislocations

JOHN G. THOMETZ, M.D.
Associate Professor, Medical College of Wisconsin, Milwaukee, Wisconsin; Chief, Pediatric Orthopedics, Children's Hospital of Wisconsin, Milwaukee, Wisconsin
Congenital Hallux Varus; Pediatric Ankle Fractures and Foot Fractures

FRANCESCA M. THOMPSON, MD.
Assistant Clinical Professor of Orthopaedic Surgery, Columbia University College of Physicians and Surgeons, New York, New York; Chief, Adult Orthopaedic Foot Clinic, St. Luke's–Roosevelt Hospital Center, New York, New York
Section Editor of Problems of the Adult Foot: Forefoot; Stabilization of the Second Metatarsophalangeal Joint

GEORGE H. THOMPSON, M.D.
Director of Pediatric Orthopaedics, Professor of Orthopaedic Surgery and Pediatrics, Case Western Reserve University, Cleveland, Ohio
Peroneal Spastic Flatfoot

SAUL G. TREVINO, M.D.
Associate Professor of Clinical Orthopaedic Surgery, Department of Orthopaedic Surgery, Baylor College of Medicine, Houston, Texas; Active Staff, Methodist Hospital, St. Luke's Episcopal Hospital, and Memorial Southwest Hospital, Houston, Texas; Provisional Staff, HCA Medical Center Hospital, Houston, Texas
Degenerative Problems of the Midtarsal Joints

RAY R. VALDEZ, M.D.
Active Staff, Memorial Southwest Hospital, Houston, Texas; Consultant, Memorial Geriatric Evaluation and Resource Center, Houston, Texas
Metatarsal Fractures and Dislocations and Lisfranc's Fracture-Dislocations

THOMAS E. WHITESIDES, Jr., M.D.
Professor of Orthopaedics, Emory University, Emory University Hospital, and Grady Memorial Hospital, Atlanta, Georgia
Compartment Syndrome of the Foot

SEYMOUR ZIMBLER, M.D.
Clinical Instructor of Orthopaedic Surgery, Harvard Medical School, Boston, Massachusetts; Clinical Professor of Orthopaedic Surgery, Tufts Medical School, Boston, Massachusetts; Visiting Orthopaedic Surgeon, Massachusetts General Hospital, Boston, Massachusetts
Metatarsus Adductus

Foreword

From the visions of a few,
An idea grew and grew.

And the American Orthopaedic Foot and Ankle Society was born in 1969, not much more than two decades ago.

In 1969, only a few names came to mind when surgery of the foot was discussed: Leleviere of France, and in the United States, Kite for his conservative cast treatment of clubfoot; Inman for his research; DuVries for his many original operations and textbook surgeries; Joplin for his sling operation for bunions; Lapidus with multiple surgical techniques; Milgram for his shoe and pad corrections; Kelikian for his bunion, hammer toe, and syndactyly operations; McBride for his bunion surgery; Kleiger for foot research; and Schwarz for pes planus work. However, most of these surgeons relied on their general orthopaedic trauma surgery to earn a living, and their footwork was an interesting sideline. In orthopaedic and surgical training programs, foot surgery was often the province of the junior resident.

Look at what has happened in approximately 20 short years! Gone are the days of hack, chop, and chip away. Then cover with shoes! Today, in this text, a brilliant array of well-trained foot and ankle surgeons comprehensively outline multiple procedures, most of which have been predicated on careful, documented research. The careful and constructive surgical treatment of trauma, hereditary disorders, and disease, from toenail to ankle, is presented in understandable prose and diagrams. Foot and ankle fellowships, 25 or more, are available throughout the country. Teaching is no longer only didactic: it now consists of visual and hands-on training. And surgery of the foot and ankle is fast becoming a most exact science. Footwear is now comfortable and lightweight, covering the foot, conforming to the foot, complementing the foot, and not compressing the foot. Certified pedorthists and trained shoe fitters are scattered throughout the country and available in ever-increasing numbers. They participate in our clinics and complement the fine work of our surgeons.

How has this materialized? Zero in on a small problem and solve it. Put all the small solutions together, and you have conquered a large problem. So, too, have in-depth study and research, and the careful, critical review of results, brought us this far. The present intense interest exhibited in exercise and health has increased the volume of our researchers and pushed us headlong onto the road to discovery and knowledge!

Little did our small band, who created the initial impetus, anticipate what could happen in so short a time. Those of us who have survived to see it happen can truly say:

God bless you all,
Who listened to the call,
And strove each day,
To create a better way.

NATHANIEL GOULD, M.D.

Preface

Over the centuries, physicians and surgeons have attempted to correct structural deformities of the foot and ankle brought on by injury and disease through the use of manipulations, splinting, and on occasion, operative intervention. In the 1800s, tenotomies performed by Stromeyer in Germany and Little in England were hailed as major advances in the management of clubfeet. In the twentieth century, Royal Whitman's talectomy for calcaneal deformity and the hindfoot arthrodeses of Hoke, Ryerson, and Lambrinudi have been significant surgical procedures for creating functional feet for patients inflicted with paralytic deformities and arthritis.

Today, a body of knowledge exists, much of which is or should be available to the modern foot and ankle surgeon. With the advent of true scientific inquiry, biomechanical research, gait analysis, peer review, and outcome studies, successful, well-conceived surgical procedures have emerged from the morass of empiric techniques and poorly designed and researched methodologies that plagued the efforts of the last generation of orthopaedic surgeons.

This text is intended for the use of residents in training, general orthopaedists, and the clinicians who focus their practice on foot and ankle problems. Nonoperative measures are cited, but the details of these treatments are not presented so that the allotted space can instead be used to describe surgical techniques, anticipated outcomes, possible problems, complications, and salvage methods. Historical reviews are intentionally limited; only current, sound alternatives to the author's preferred method are given, and essentially outdated procedures have been omitted.

The authors were chosen because of their known expertise in the areas on which they write, and their personal biases are acknowledged. The editorial board has attempted to guide the authors and to mold their respective sections to provide a fair "state-of-the-art" presentation for each area and condition.

The ultimate responsibility, however, for the completeness of the text and the minimization of inappropriate bias is mine, the editor's. It has been my honor and pleasure to work with the highly educated and skilled authors and section editors who made this work possible. I would also be remiss if I failed to acknowledge the talented copy editors, book editors, and artists who contributed so greatly to the continuity and consistency of style, which is often so difficult to achieve in a multiauthored book.

Finally, it is anticipated that bringing together the first major multiauthored compendium on operative technique for the foot and ankle will further establish the foot and ankle field as a fully recognized orthopaedic subspecialty.

JOHN S. GOULD, M.D.

Acknowledgments

The full support of my colleagues in the Department of Orthopaedic Surgery, particularly my coworkers in the Divisions of Foot Surgery, Pediatric Orthopaedics, and Sports Medicine, Drs. Jeffrey E. Johnson, Michael J. Shereff, C. Hugh Hickey, George W. Simons, John G. Thometz, Kevin P. Black, Gerald Harris (gait analysis), and Mr. Dennis Janisse (Pedorthics), have made it possible for the field of foot and ankle to emerge at the Medical College of Wisconsin and to have some influence on American orthopaedic education.

My editorial board, Drs. Francesca Thompson, Andrea Cracchiolo, Robert Adelaar, Lamar Fleming, George Simons, and Kevin Black, have done yeoman's work and remained steadfast friends and wonderful professional colleagues.

My mentor for life and constant friend, J. Leonard Goldner, M.D., James B. Duke Professor Emeritus at Duke, remains a continuing inspiration.

However, the unquestioned credit for any measure of success that I have achieved in my career and in the production of this work and for my efforts at achieving excellence must go to my mother, Edith Marion Spiller Gould, and to my father, Nathaniel Gould, M.D., the first acknowledged foot specialist and educator in our family.

Finally, great thanks and gratitude are due to my wife, friend, and confidant, Sheryl Hartford Gould, who has endured and encouraged my work.

JOHN S. GOULD, M.D.

Contents

PART I

PROBLEMS OF

THE ADULT FOOT:

FOREFOOT

Editors
FRANCESCA M. THOMPSON
ANDREA CRACCHIOLO III

1 Regional Anesthesia for Foot Surgery

WALTHER BOHNE
ROBERT E. KETTLER

The use of local anesthesia for foot surgery has become increasingly popular among foot surgeons for a variety of reasons and indications. Probably foremost among the reasons for its popularity is the very high rate of successful blocks and the low morbidity when local anesthesia is used by experienced practitioners. Additionally, surgeons are attracted to the benefits of the rapid turnover of surgical cases that occurs when this relatively easy technique is used. Medical contraindications are relatively uncommon.

The main limiting factors with regional anesthesia are the necessary tourniquet time and the need for additional anesthesia when distant donor sites are required for graft materials. Supplemental sedation and intravenous analgesia can prolong tourniquet use, and many procedures can be completed without the need for further tourniquet control.

Intravenous regional block for the lower extremity has few advocates, compared with its use in the upper. For more complex and longer procedures, regional anesthesia using the epidural route or general inhalation anesthesia is more appropriate.

PHARMACOLOGY

Lidocaine, mepivacaine, and bupivacaine are the preferred agents. A brief review of their pharmacology allows the practitioner to select them in a given clinical situation.

The systemic toxicity of local anesthetics is always a concern; however, this complication is relatively unlikely in regional anesthesia for foot surgery. Systemic toxicity is related to the serum level of local anesthetic, which is determined by the net effect of the rate of absorption and the rate of elimination. There is a paucity of information on the specific issue of local anesthetic pharmacokinetics in foot blocks; much of what has been established is from studies of epidural anesthesia, but this information can probably be extrapolated to foot block techniques.

The absorption of local anesthetics is related to several factors, but the total dose of drug injected and the site of injection are probably the most important. As the total dose of drug injected increases, the serum level of local anesthetic increases. Several investigators have studied the interaction of injectate concentration and volume and investigated whether one or the other is a more important determinant of serum level. The results of these investigations indicate that it is the total dose of drug that matters, so that large volumes of dilute anesthetic solutions result in the same serum levels as do small volumes of concentrated solutions, as long as the total dose of drug is the same. The site of injection affects the serum level of anesthetic because of the blood flow that the site receives: at sites with a higher blood flow, more absorption of the local anesthetic occurs. Also, any condition or adjunct that affects local blood flow affects local anesthetic absorption. For example, congestive heart failure or the use of vasoconstrictors in the anesthetic solution is associated with lower

3

serum levels of anesthetic. However, if the patient is hyperdynamic (as may be the case in chronic renal failure), serum levels are higher.

There are several means by which the increase in serum level related to absorption can be attenuated. The lung can function as a depot for local anesthetics and so serves as a buffer against the likelihood of toxicity. Local anesthetics bind to acid glycoproteins; consequently, factors affecting the serum levels of these proteins (e.g., smoking increases them and oral contraceptive agents decrease them) will affect levels of free local anesthetics and so affect the likelihood of toxicity. The local anesthetic agents that are esters (procaine, 2-chloroprocaine [Nesacaine MPF, Astra], and tetracaine) are metabolized relatively rapidly in the serum by plasma cholinesterase. However, the amides (lidocaine [Xylocaine, Astra], bupivacaine [Marcaine, Winthrop; Sensorcaine, Astra], mepivacaine [Carbocaine, Winthrop]) are metabolized in the liver and so have a relatively longer serum half-life. Liver disease can affect plasma cholinesterase production, but ester metabolism is usually not prolonged to a clinically significant degree. However, diseases affecting hepatic function can result in impaired metabolism of amide and can therefore lead to an increased chance of systemic toxicity. In general, the metabolites of either the esters or the amides (which are excreted in the urine) do not affect the likelihood of toxicity to an important degree.

Because so many interacting variables affect the likelihood of local anesthetic toxicity, it is difficult to make specific recommendations about dosage. Table 1–1 lists amounts that extensive experience by multiple anesthetic practitioners has shown to be safe.

As with all drug dosages, these amounts must be modified in individual clinical situations based on the practitioner's judgment and experience.

The issue of whether the combination of individual local anesthetic agents results in additive toxicity is a controversial one, but most experience seems to indicate that it does.

GENERAL PRINCIPLES

In general, the amounts of local anesthetic used for ankle, midtarsal, or digital blocks are less than those associated with a clinically important risk of systemic toxicity. Even if intravascular injection were to occur, the amount likely to be injected as a bolus is relatively small (e.g., 5 mL for each of the nerves in an ankle block), making systemic toxicity unlikely. The chance of intravascular injection can be reduced by aspiration prior to injection.

Some other general principles are worth mentioning before discussion of the individual blocks. Epinephrine should be avoided in digital and probably in midtarsal blocks to avoid digital ischemia secondary to vasospasm. Likewise, careful consideration should be given to the use of epinephrine for ankle blocks in patients with peripheral vascular disease. A field-of-infiltration technique of ankle block could provide satisfactory anesthesia of the foot; however, the infiltration of a large volume of solution could exert a tourniquet effect, so it is probably better to inject each nerve individually in performing an ankle block.

Tourniquets are often used to provide a bloodless surgical field. Midcalf tourniquets

	USUAL CONCENTRATION FOR FOOT ANESTHESIA (%)	MAXIMUM RECOMMENDED DOSE WITHOUT EPINEPHRINE (mg)	MAXIMUM RECOMMENDED DOSE WITH EPINEPHRINE (mg)	DURATION OF EFFECT WITHOUT EPINEPHRINE	DURATION OF EFFECT WITH EPINEPHRINE
AGENT					
Bupivacaine	0.25–0.5	150	200	400 min	24 hr is possible
2-Chloroprocaine	1	500	800	45 min	70 min
Lidocaine	1	400	500	60 min	120 min
Mepivacaine	1	400	500	60 min	120 min
Tetracaine	0.1–0.2	100	150	240 min	360 min

TABLE 1–1. SUGGESTED DOSES OF LOCAL ANESTHETICS IN FOOT ANESTHESIA

are usually well tolerated for relatively short procedures (about 30 minutes). Judicious sedation allows many patients to tolerate about 1 hour of tourniquet time. Circumferential subcutaneous infiltrations of the extremity proximal to the tourniquet have been recommended to facilitate tolerance of the tourniquet. Dilute anesthetic solutions (e.g., 0.5 percent lidocaine) are satisfactory for this purpose.

REGIONAL ANESTHESIA FOR DIGITAL, MIDTARSAL, AND ANKLE PROCEDURES

Digital Block of the Great Toe

For a digital block of the great toe, the injection should be at the level of the metatarsal diaphysis. The landmark is the first metatarsal diaphysis and the first web space (Fig. 1–1). The patient is supine, with the dorsum of the foot facing upward. After introduction of an intradermal wheal, using a 25-gauge needle, the injection is carried out from the dorsum along the tibial side of the metatarsal. The anesthetic is injected in a fan-like fashion dorsally and plantar on the medial side of the diaphysis; it is then redirected across the dorsum of the metatarsal into the first intermetatarsal space, where both superficial and deep injections are also carried out. At regular intervals, the surgeon should aspirate to ascertain that no local anesthetic is injected into blood vessels. Care should be taken to ensure that the plantar skin is not pierced by the needle. A more distal block into the first web should be effective to anesthetize branches of the superficial and deep peroneal nerves and the fibular hallucal digital nerve. With this technique, the great toe, including the first metatarsophalangeal joint, can be adequately anesthetized.

Digital Block of the Lesser Toes

The landmarks for digital block of the lesser toes are the neighboring web spaces and the diaphysis of the metatarsal of the involved ray. Intradermal wheals are raised over the intermetatarsal spaces at the level of the metatarsal neck. The injection is carried out on either side of the metatarsal from the dorsum; anes-

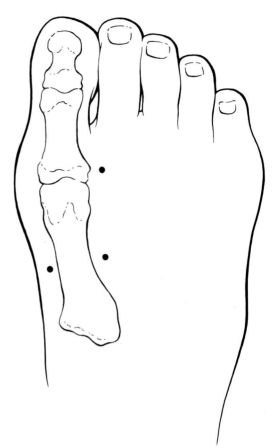

FIGURE 1–1. Injection points for local anesthetic block for the great toe.

thetic is first injected superficially and then deeply to block the branches of the superficial peroneal nerve (the sural nerve for the fifth toe) and the plantar digital nerves appropriately. Again, palpation on the sole of the foot should indicate to the surgeon the proper placement of anesthetic solution during the deep-injection phase. Further anesthetic can be added into the adjacent web spaces at the bifurcation of the common digital nerves if needed.

Digital Block of the Middle or Distal Phalanx of the Toe

The appropriate landmarks for blocks at the level of the middle or distal phalanx are the metatarsophalangeal joints. The anesthetic agent is injected through the dorsal skin both superficially and deeply to block the dorsal and plantar nerves. Small amounts of anesthetic, in the range of 5 mL on each side of the toe, should be adequate to avoid both a tourniquet effect and the possible creation of a local compartment syndrome.

Midtarsal Block

The midtarsal block for forefoot and multiple-toe surgery requires anesthetizing the superficial and deep peroneal nerves and the saphenous, sural, and medial and lateral plantar nerves. The dorsal nerves may be blocked in the subcutaneous plane. The deeper nerves (the medial and lateral plantar nerves and the deep peroneal nerve) require a subfascial injection. The ankle tourniquet delays absorption of the anesthetic agent and is well tolerated, and its use may be prolonged by additional intravenous sedation and analgesia.

Landmarks for the posterior tibial nerve branches are the tip of the medial malleolus and the pulse of the posterior tibial artery. The landmarks for the deep peroneal nerve are the distal edge of the extensor retinaculum and the pulse of the dorsalis pedis artery. With the patient in the supine position, the knee is flexed and the hip abducted. An intradermal wheal is raised over the pulse of the posterior tibial artery adjacent to the tip of the medial malleolus. Either a 25- or a 22-gauge needle is used. As the needle is advanced to either side of the posterior tibial vessels, aspiration is carried out before injection of the agent. The hip is then returned to the midline, and an intradermal wheal is raised over the pulse of the dorsalis pedis artery at the distal edge of the extensor retinaculum. Injection is carried out on either side of the artery to block the deep peroneal nerve. Aspiration is essential to prevent injection into the artery.

The branches of the superficial peroneal, saphenous, and sural nerves are anesthetized by a subcutaneous injection across the midtarsal region on the dorsum of the foot.

Ankle Block

To block essentially all the nerves of the foot, including the region of the heel, the posterior tibial nerve and its branches, the peroneal nerves, the sural nerve, and the terminal branches of the saphenous nerve must be blocked at the ankle level. The posterior tibial nerve lies in a sheath with the posterior tibial vessels. The posterior tibial artery is palpated behind the medial malleolus. The leg is flexed at the knee and abducted at the hip. The neurovascular bundle lies posterior to the posterior tibial and the flexor digitorum longus tendons (Fig. 1–2). A 1 1/2 inch long, 25- or 22-gauge needle is used. The skin wheal is raised with a 25-gauge needle. The nerve is deep to the vascular structures and is blocked by injection on either side of the pulse and deep to it. Again, it is essential to aspirate to avoid an intravascular injection. Although paresthesias may occur, indicating that the needle has come into contact with the nerve, the needle should be withdrawn slightly and redirected more anteriorly or posteriorly before injection to avoid an intraneural injection and possible neural damage. Some surgeons suggest that the injection be placed just behind the flexor digitorum longus tendon; the needle is advanced until it touches the medial tibia and is then withdrawn several millimeters, and the solution is injected.

The deep peroneal nerve is accessible just proximal to the ankle joint, where it lies on the anterior surface of the tibia (Fig. 1–3). It may run medial or lateral to the extensor hallucis longus tendon, but it always lies lateral to the anterior tibial tendon. The injection is placed lateral to the anterior tibial tendon and proximal to the tibial plafond over the extensor hallucis longus tendon. After the anterior aspect of the tibia is encountered, the needle is withdrawn 2 or 3 mm and the injection is performed. The injection is carried to either side of the great toe extensor. Aspiration is again important to avoid injecting into the anterior tibial artery. Through the same skin wheal, the anesthetic may be subcutaneously injected medially and laterally to block the superficial peroneal and saphenous nerves. The sural nerve, which lies in the subcutaneous tissue between the lateral malleolus and the lateral border of the Achilles tendon, is also easily anesthetized (Fig. 1–4).

COMPLICATIONS

The effect of intraneural injection would be prolonged paresthesias or potentially more serious damage due to pressure ischemia. Systemic toxicity may be due either to intravascular injection or to an overdose of the anesthetic agent. When a significant bolus of drug is injected intravascularly, convulsions may occur immediately. When an overdose occurs, a critical blood level of anesthetic agent must be reached before symptoms begin. This takes approximately 20 minutes. This phenomenon is heralded by the complaint of tinnitus, numbness around the mouth, headaches, facial twitching, and restlessness. These reactions may be followed by seizures and respiratory arrest. Hyperventilation with oxygen and other supportive measures are indicated. If the convulsions do not abate, intravenous diazepam (2.5 mg) may terminate them. If necessary, 50 to 100 mg of thiopental (Pentothal) may be used. If hypotension due to cardiovascular collapse occurs, intravenous fluids, the Trendelenburg position, and vasopressors should be used. Because digital and midtarsal blocks require a low dosage of anesthetic, systemic complications are exceedingly rare. Blocks at the ankle level are also very safe and are well tolerated. However, systemic monitoring by an anesthesiologist or a qualified anesthetist is important for appropriate patient comfort and safety.

CONCLUSIONS

Easy palpation of the landmarks of the foot and ankle, along with familiarity with the surface anatomy and the anatomic location of the nerves, makes regional anesthesia relatively easy, with low morbidity and few contraindications. In addition to the restraints listed in the introduction with regard to the planned surgical procedures, one must also consider allergic reactions to the agents and the reluctance of most children under the age of 16 to tolerate forms of injection anesthesia. For most other patients, including elderly and other high-risk persons, this method of anesthesia may be optimal.

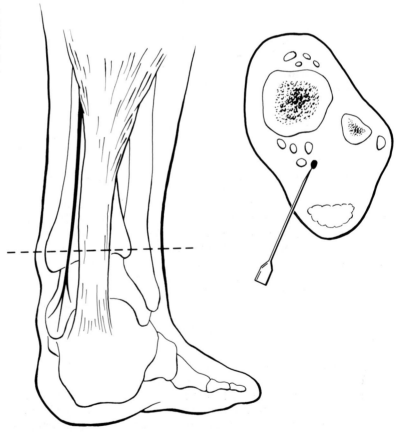

FIGURE 1–2. Block of the posterior tibial nerve. Note that it lies posterior to the posterior tibial and flexor digitorum tendons and to the posterior tibial artery and venous comitans. The flexor hallucis longus lies closer to the tibia.

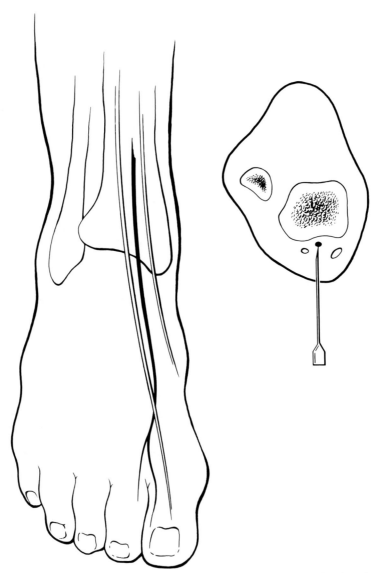

FIGURE 1–3. Block of the deep peroneal nerve proximal to the ankle joint. The nerve lies lateral to the anterior tibial tendon and medial to the extensor hallucis longus. Note the depth of the nerve. It is adjacent to the anterior tibial artery.

FIGURE 1–4. Block of the sural nerve behind the lateral malleolus and peroneal tendons in the subcutaneous tissue.

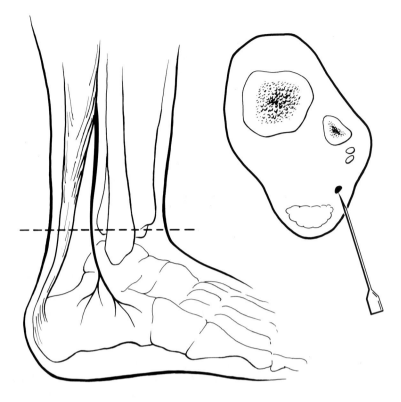

Suggested Readings

Local Anesthetic Pharmacology and Toxicology

1. Carpenter RL, Mackey DC: Local anesthetics. *In* Barash PG, Cullen BF, Stoelting RK (Eds): Clinical Anesthesia. Philadelphia, JB Lippincott, 1989, pp 371–403.
2. Covins BG: Pharmacology of local anesthetics. *In* Nunn JE, Utting JE, Brown BR Jr (Eds): General Anesthesia. London, Butterworths, 1989, pp 1036–1048.
3. Ritchie JM, Greene NM: Local anesthetics. *In* Gilman AG, Rull TW, Nies AS, Taylor P (Eds): Goodman and Gilman's The Pharmacological Basis of Therapeutics. New York, Pergamon Press, 1990, pp 311–331.

Nerve Block Technique

4. Lofstrum B: Nerve block at the ankle. *In* Eriksson E (Ed): Illustrated Handbook in Local Anesthesia. Copenhagen, I. Chr. Sorenson and Company AS, 1979, pp 112–115.
5. Mulroy MF: Peripheral nerve blockade. *In* Barash PG, Cullen BF, Stoelting RK (Eds): Clinical Anesthesia. Philadelphia, JB Lippincott, 1989, pp 371–403.
6. Thompson GE, Brown DL: The common nerve blocks. *In* Nunn JE, Utting JE, Brown BR Jr (Eds): General Anesthesia. London, Butterworths, 1989, pp 1049–1085.

2 *Hallux Valgus*

ROGER A. MANN

The hallux valgus deformity consists of lateral deviation of the proximal phalanx on the metatarsal head, associated with varying degrees of enlargement of the medial eminence, which is known as a bunion. At times, people have tended to consider all bunion deformities to be equal, whereas in reality, there are varying degrees of deformity as well as different types of deformities. For this reason, the physician must carefully evaluate the patient with a hallux valgus deformity, obtaining the patient's chief complaint and his or her expectations of the surgical procedure and performing a careful physical examination as well as a radiographic evaluation of the foot. This information is then used in the decision-making process involving the type of surgical procedure that would be most likely to yield a satisfactory result. One may no longer rely on a single procedure to correct all hallux valgus deformities but must consider an array of procedures, each one specifically designed to correct a specific problem.

PATIENT EVALUATION

The evaluation of the patient begins with a careful history of the patient's chief complaint, level of activities, occupation, sports involvement, and shoewear preference. It is also important to obtain the patient's expectation of what a surgical procedure will accomplish so that the patient will not be inadvertently misled.

Physical Examination

The physical examination should be carried out while the patient is standing as well as sitting. The overall posture of the foot should be observed, and careful evaluation is made of the range of motion of the ankle, subtalar, transverse tarsal, and metatarsophalangeal joints. The neurovascular status of the foot must also be carefully assessed. The plantar aspect of the foot is examined for abnormal callus formation, particularly beneath the second metatarsal head.

The motion of the first metatarsophalangeal joint is observed closely, along with the skin and the size of the medial eminence. The first metatarsal-cuneiform joint should be examined for hypermobility, which is present in about 3 to 5 percent of patients. Any deformities of the lesser toes, as well as the possibility of neuritic problems, should be carefully noted.

Radiographic Evaluation

Radiographic evaluation should include obtaining a weight-bearing, anteroposterior and lateral radiograph. The oblique radiograph is not weight bearing. The following measurements are useful in evaluating the foot with a hallux valgus deformity:

1. The degree of hallux valgus, which is the angle created by a line that bisects the proximal phalanx and the first metatarsal, is noted.
2. The intermetatarsal angle, which is the relationship between the lines bisecting the first and second metatarsal shafts, is observed.

10

3. The distal metatarsal articular angle, which measures the slope of the articular surface of the metatarsal head to the long axis of the metatarsal shaft, is evaluated.

4. It is noted whether the metatarsophalangeal joint is congruent or incongruent. A congruent metatarsophalangeal joint has no lateral subluxation of the proximal phalanx on the metatarsal head. An incongruent metatarsophalangeal joint has lateral subluxation of the proximal phalanx on the metatarsal head.

5. The configuration of the metatarsal-cuneiform joint should be examined for excessive medial deviation of the articulation.

6. The degree of arthrosis of the metatarsophalangeal joint, if any, should be noted.

7. The size of the medial eminence should be observed.

To simplify the decision-making process, I have found it useful to divide hallux valgus into three main classifications: (1) a congruent joint, (2) an incongruent joint, or (3) a joint with degenerative joint disease. As the algorithm in Figure 2–1 demonstrates, depending on the type of deformity as well as the magnitude of the deformity, one can select a procedure that will provide a satisfactory result for the patient.

I find it important to determine whether the hallux valgus deformity is congruent or incongruent because if a congruent joint is present, the relationship of the proximal phalanx to the metatarsal head must be maintained. If one were to attempt to change it, an incongruent surface relationship might be created. Conversely, if an incongruent, or subluxed, metatarsophalangeal joint is present, the proximal phalanx can be corrected onto the metatarsal head, giving rise to a satisfactory result, provided that the intermetatarsal angle will correct back into the normal range. If the intermetatarsal angle does not correct, then some type of an osteotomy probably should be carried out. If significant degenerative joint disease is present, a procedure must be carried out that addresses the problem. Attempting to realign a metatarsophalangeal joint in the face of significant arthrosis results in a painful, stiff joint. If the patient happens to be in the small group that has hypermobility of the metatarsal-cuneiform joint, one should consider a fusion of the first metatarsal-cuneiform joint along with a distal soft tissue correction.

SURGICAL PROCEDURES

This chapter is not designed to present all the various surgical procedures involving the great toe but, rather, describes those that are used most frequently.

The Akin Procedure

The Akin procedure[1] is an osteotomy at the base of the proximal phalanx and is used to correct a hallux valgus interphalangeus. If the metatarsophalangeal joint is congruent, the procedure may also be used along with excision of the medial eminence. If, however, there is an incongruent joint, the Akin procedure will probably not result in satisfactory correction.[6, 7] The procedure is also useful if there is residual hallux valgus deformity after previous surgery.

The main contraindication to the Akin procedure is the presence of any significant subluxation of the metatarsophalangeal joint.

Surgical Technique

1. A longitudinal skin incision is made over the medial aspect of the proximal phalanx and carried just proximal to the metatarsophalangeal joint. The incision is deepened down to the bone, exposing the proximal half of the proximal phalanx.

2. With the use of a power saw, a wedge whose apex is directed laterally is removed. This usually is 2 to 5 mm wide. The lateral cortex is left intact.

3. The osteotomy site is closed, and the alignment of the toe is carefully evaluated. Fixation can be with either an internal suture or an oblique pin.

4. If a medial eminence is present and is to be excised, the initial skin incision is made more proximal in order to expose the capsule of the metatarsophalangeal joint.

5. A vertical capsulotomy is carried out in order to expose the medial eminence. The medial eminence is excised in line with the medial aspect of the metatarsal shaft (Fig. 2–2).

6. The medial capsule is plicated.

7. The postoperative management is to maintain the toe in satisfactory alignment with a soft compression dressing, consisting of 2-inch Kling and 1/2-inch adhesive tape for 6 to

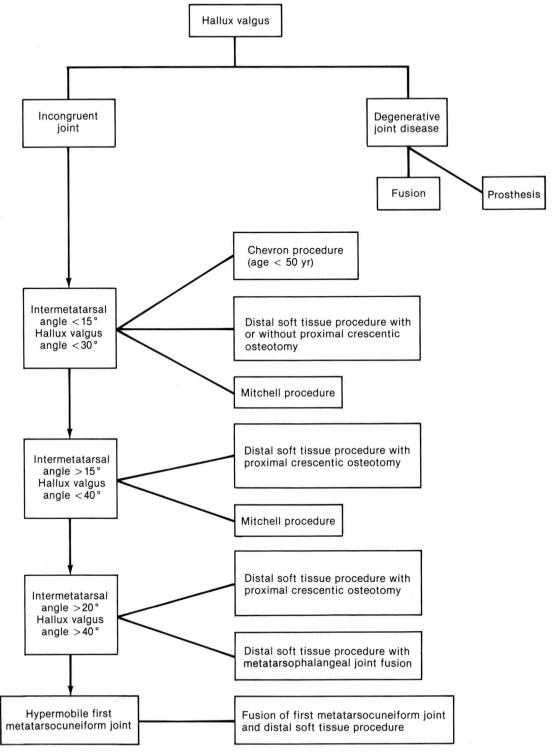

FIGURE 2–1. Algorithm for treatment of the patient with an incongruent joint. The procedure is based on the severity of the deformity. For degenerative joint disease, we recommend a fusion and rarely a prosthesis. (From Mann RA, Coughlin MJ: Surgery of the Foot and Ankle, 6th Ed. St. Louis, Mosby-Yearbook, 1993, p 199.)

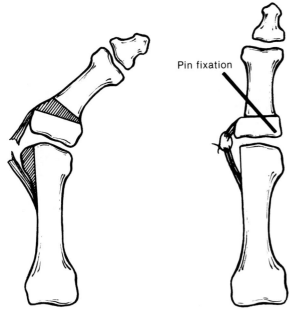

Pin fixation

FIGURE 2–2. The Akin procedure. The medial eminence is also excised. (Redrawn from Mann RA, Coughlin MJ: The Video Textbook of Foot and Ankle Surgery. Medical Video Productions, St. Louis, 1991, p 165.)

8 weeks. Once bony healing has occurred, the patient is permitted to walk without support.

Complications

A nonunion or malunion of the osteotomy site occurs infrequently. If the procedure is carried out in a case in which there is a significant hallux valgus deformity, correction of the deformity will not occur. One must also be careful when producing the osteotomy that an intra-articular fracture does not occur.

Chevron Procedure

The distal chevron procedure creates a metaphyseal osteotomy and displaces the fragment lateralward.[2, 3, 25] This produces some narrowing of the foot, and with plication of the medial capsule, some correction of the hallux valgus deformity can be achieved. If there is excessive lateral deviation of the metatarsal head, a medial closing wedge osteotomy may be added to the chevron procedure to help realign the articular surface in order to gain better correction.

The chevron procedure is used for the mild to moderate hallux valgus deformity in patients under the age of 50 in whom the hallux valgus angle is less than 30 degrees and the intermetatarsal angle is less than 12 degrees.[8] With a more severe deformity, this procedure may result in less than optimal correction.

Surgical Technique

1. A longitudinal incision centered over the medial aspect of the metatarsophalangeal joint is carried down to the joint capsule. Full-thickness dorsal and volar flaps are created to protect the dorsal medial and plantar medial cutaneous nerves to the great toe.

2. The medial joint capsule is opened. A vertically placed capsular incision starting 2 mm proximal to the base of the proximal phalanx and removing a 2- to 5-mm wedge of capsule more proximally is used. Soft tissue stripping, however, should be minimized.

3. The medial eminence is exposed and removed with an osteotome or power saw. The line of the osteotomy should be just medial to or at the sagittal sulcus and should be brought proximally to the base of the medial eminence, but it should not be in line with the metatarsal shaft. Removing the medial eminence in this manner leaves the maximum width of metatarsal head at the site where the osteotomy will be carried out (Fig. 2–3*A*).

4. A chevron-shaped osteotomy with limbs that form an angle of approximately 70 degrees is created. The apex of the osteotomy is at the center of the metatarsal head and is marked by drilling a 2-mm hole in the head. It is important that the plantar aspect of the osteotomy be carried out proximal to the joint capsule in order to avoid violating the articular cartilage on the plantar aspect of the metatarsal head (Fig. 2–3*B*).

5. The osteotomy site is gently freed and is displaced laterally for approximately 20 to 30 percent of the width of the shaft. The osteotomized bones are then fixed with a 0.045-inch Kirschner wire (Fig. 2–3*C*).

6. The medial prominence that was created by the lateral displacement of the metatarsal head is excised in line with the metatarsal shaft.

7. The capsular tissue is closed while the toe is held in satisfactory alignment.

8. When there is excessive lateral deviation of the metatarsal head, a modification of the chevron procedure can be performed in which

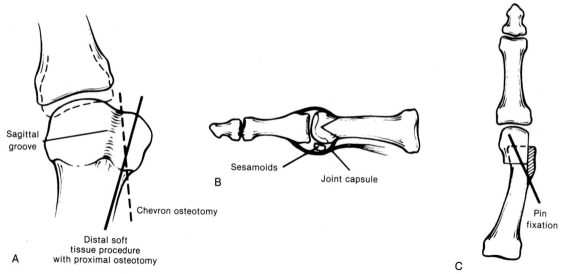

FIGURE 2–3. *(A),* Removal of the medial eminence. *(B),* Chevron osteotomy. *(C),* Postoperative management. (Redrawn from Mann RA, Coughlin MJ: The Video Textbook of Foot and Ankle Surgery. Medical Video Productions, St. Louis, 1991, p 164.)

slightly more bone is removed from the medial aspect of the chevron cut. This will permit rotation of the distal articular surface from its laterally placed position into better alignment with the metatarsal shaft.

9. The postoperative management involves applying a compression dressing consisting of 2-inch Kling and 1/2-inch adhesive tape, maintaining the toe in satisfactory alignment. The patient is permitted to walk in a postoperative shoe until the osteotomy is healed, at approximately 6 to 8 weeks. The pin is usually maintained across the osteotomy site for about 4 weeks.

Complications

The complication rate following a chevron procedure is low. Complications may include stiffness of the metatarsophalangeal joint; some shortening of the metatarsal, producing a transfer lesion beneath the second metatar-sal, and hallux varus, and avascular necrosis of varying degrees.[2, 8–10, 22] If the procedure is used on a deformity greater than that mentioned earlier in the indications, incomplete correction may result. In some cases an Akin procedure has been added to the chevron osteotomy in order to gain better correction of the more severe deformity, but this probably increases the possibility of developing an avascular necrosis or stiffness about the joint.

Distal Soft Tissue Procedure

The distal soft tissue procedure has evolved over a period of time from the Silver procedure,[24] as well as from the McBride procedure[19–21] and the DuVries modification of the McBride procedure.[5] It consists of attempting to rebalance the soft tissues about the metatarsophalangeal joint along with excision of the medial eminence.

The distal soft tissue procedure produces a satisfactory clinical result in the patient with a hallux valgus deformity of less than 30 degrees and an intermetatarsal angle of less than 15 degrees.[4, 17] Because the results of the procedure depend on whether the intermetatarsal angle will correct to 9 degrees or less, if a fixed intermetatarsal angle is present, a satisfactory result cannot routinely be achieved. For this reason, in patients with a hallux valgus deformity greater than that just described, a basal metatarsal osteotomy should probably be added to obtain full correction.

The procedure should not be carried out on a patient who has spasticity, either from cerebral palsy or from a head injury. The procedure is also contraindicated in a patient with significant arthrosis of the metatarsophalangeal joint.

Surgical Technique

1. The initial skin incision is made on the dorsal aspect of the foot in the first web space.

The incision is carried down in order to expose the adductor tendon.

2. The adductor tendon is detached from the lateral aspect of the fibular sesamoid and its insertion into the base of the proximal phalanx (Fig. 2–4 *A* and *B*).

3. The transverse metatarsal ligament is exposed as it passes from the second metatarsal into the fibular sesamoid, and it is then cut. Caution must be exercised when this ligament is cut because the nerve and blood vessels to the first web space pass immediately beneath it (Fig. 2–4*C* and *D*).

4. The lateral joint capsule is perforated and torn, bringing the toe into approximately 30 degrees of varus.

5. The next incision is made on the medial aspect of the first metatarsophalangeal joint in the midline. It is centered over the metatarsophalangeal joint and carried down to the joint capsule, creating full-thickness dorsal and plantar flaps.

6. The flaps are carefully dissected dorsally and plantarward in order to avoid damage to the dorsal medial and plantar medial cutaneous nerves to the great toe.

7. With the medial capsule exposed, a vertical capsulotomy is performed, starting ap-

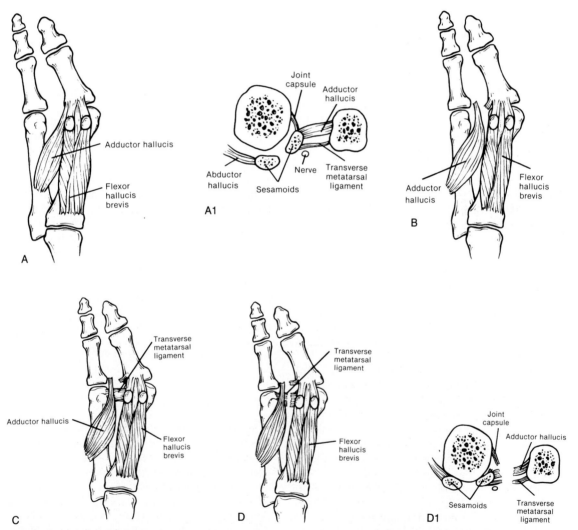

FIGURE 2–4. Distal soft tissue procedure. (*A* and *A1*), Preoperative view. (*B*), The adductor tendon is detached. (*C*), The exposed transverse metatarsal ligament. (*D* and *D1*), The transverse metatarsal ligament is incised.

Illustration continued on following page

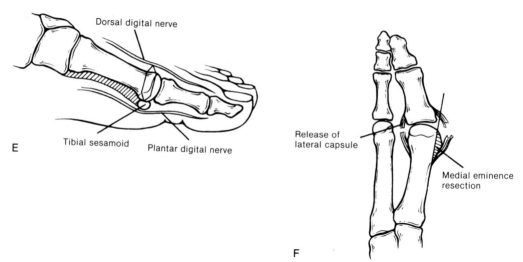

FIGURE 2–4 *Continued (E),* The incision on the medial aspect. *(F),* The medial eminence is removed. (Redrawn from Mann RA, Coughlin MJ: The Video Textbook of Foot and Ankle Surgery. Medical Video Productions, St. Louis, 1991, pp 161– 162.)

proximately 2 mm proximal to the base of the proximal phalanx. Moving 3 to 6 mm more proximally, depending on the severity of the deformity, a second cut is made in the capsule parallel to the first. The incisions are then brought together dorsally as an inverted V, approximately 1 cm medial to the extensor hallucis longus tendon. Plantarward, parallel incisions are brought together through the abductor hallucis tendon, ending at the medial side of the tibial sesamoid. An incision is then made along the dorsal medial aspect of the capsule so that it can be folded down in a plantar and proximal direction (Fig. 2–4E).

8. The medial eminence is then removed, starting 2 mm medial to the sagittal sulcus and in line with the medial aspect of the metatarsal shaft, and the edges are smoothed with a rongeur (Fig. 2–4F).

9. The soft tissue repair is now carried out by placing three sutures in the first web space, incorporating the capsular tissue on the lateral aspect of the first metatarsal, the adductor tendon, and the capsular tissue on the medial side of the second metatarsophalangeal joint. The foot is then squeezed in a mediolateral direction, and the sutures are tied.

10. The toe is held in satisfactory alignment, which means placing it into neutral position with respect to dorsiflexion and plantar flexion and in neutral to 2 or 3 degrees of varus, as well as supinating the toe so as to bring the sesamoids beneath the metatarsal head. Four

sutures are then placed in the medial capsule to hold it in satisfactory alignment.

11. The skin is closed in a routine manner, after which a compression dressing is applied for 24 hours. The patient is permitted to walk in a postoperative shoe.

12. The immediate postoperative dressing is removed, and a dressing consisting of 2-inch Kling and 1/2-inch adhesive tape is applied, binding the metatarsal heads together and creating a spica bandage, used to hold the toe in a derotated position to maintain the sesamoids beneath the metatarsal head and in proper varus-valgus alignment. This is reinforced with 1/2-inch adhesive tape. This dressing is changed weekly for 8 weeks, during which time the patient is allowed to walk in a post-operative shoe (Fig. 2–5).

Complications

Satisfactory realignment following a distal soft tissue procedure results if one uses the procedure in patients with a deformity less severe than that stated earlier. When one attempts to gain correction in patients with a more severe deformity, varying degrees of the deformity may recur. Hallux varus may occur; this is usually due to excessive excision of the medial eminence or overplication of the medial joint capsule.[4, 17] Leaving the fibular sesamoid

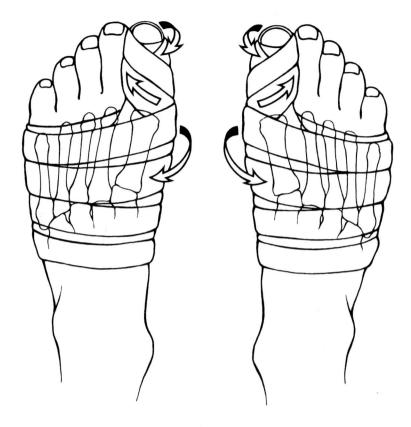

intact reduces the incidence of hallux varus to a minimal degree.

Distal Soft Tissue Procedure with Proximal Crescentic Osteotomy

The distal soft tissue procedure with a proximal crescentic osteotomy can be viewed as the natural extension of the distal soft tissue procedure previously described. It is added to the distal soft tissue procedure when the intermetatarsal angle cannot be brought back into satisfactory alignment. By adding the proximal osteotomy, one is able to correct hallux valgus deformities up to 40 to 50 degrees and obtain a reproducible result.[18] In treating the patient with a subluxed metatarsophalangeal joint, this procedure is used approximately 85 percent of the time. The procedure is contraindicated in the patient with a congruent joint and in one who has significant arthrosis of the metatarsophalangeal joint.

Surgical Technique

The distal soft tissue repair is carried out exactly as noted earlier. After having released the lateral joint structures, prepared the medial joint capsule, and removed the medial eminence, the operating surgeon must decide whether or not the intermetatarsal angle can be corrected.[15] The only reliable method I have been able to use is to apply lateral pressure on the metatarsal head (Fig. 2–6). One may thus determine whether there appears to be any fixed deformity between the first and second metatarsal shafts. If there is any tendency for the two metatarsals to spring apart after pressure is applied to the first metatarsal in a lateralward direction, a basal osteotomy should probably be carried out. If the first and second metatarsals literally sit next to each other, with no tendency to spring apart, an osteotomy is not necessary.

1. If an osteotomy is necessary, a third incision is made over the dorsal aspect of the base of the first metatarsal and carried down to the extensor tendon. The extensor tendon

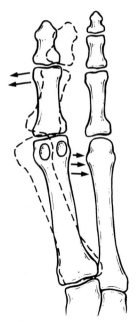

FIGURE 2–6. To determine whether an osteotomy is necessary, the first metatarsal head is pushed laterally. If there is any tendency for the metatarsal head to spring open, an osteotomy should be considered. (Redrawn from Mann RA, Coughlin MJ: The Video Textbook of Foot and Ankle Surgery. Medical Video Productions, St. Louis, 1991, p 166.)

is then retracted medially or laterally to expose the metatarsal shaft.

2. The metatarsal-cuneiform joint is identified, and the periosteum is stripped distal to the metatarsal-cuneiform joint over a distance of approximately 2 cm.

3. The osteotomy site is produced 1 cm distal to the metatarsal-cuneiform joint. The osteotomy is made with a crescentic or curved blade on an oscillating saw (Fig. 2–7).

4. The osteotomy site should not be perpendicular to the bottom of the foot or to the first metatarsal shaft; rather, it should be in a plane approximately halfway between these guidelines.

5. Fixation of the osteotomy site can be carried out by a screw placed from dorsal to plantar, by a single oblique pin, or by multiple pins. If a screw is used, which I prefer, a 3.5-mm drill bit is used to make a hole in the metatarsal before the osteotomy site is cut. The hole is made 1 cm distal to the osteotomy site, or approximately 2 cm distal to the metatarsal-cuneiform joint. It is drilled in a plane that is about 45 degrees to the metatarsal shaft, and it is advanced only about 5 mm into the bone.

6. The oscillating saw with the crescentic blade is then used to produce a basal osteotomy 1 cm distal to the metatarsal-cuneiform joint. The concavity of the cut is directed toward the heel. If the metatarsal shaft is too wide for the blade, it is imperative that the cut be brought out laterally, for the medial aspect of the osteotomy site can be finished easily with a small osteotome. Once the osteotomy has been completed, a small Freer elevator is used to ensure that all the soft tissue attachment is freed from around the osteotomy site so that it can be moved easily.

7. Three sutures are placed into the first web space, as previously described, between the capsules of the first and second metatarsophalangeal joints, incorporating the adductor tendon.

8. The osteotomy site is then corrected by placing a small Freer elevator on the proximal fragment of the metatarsal and displacing it as far medialward as possible. The distal portion of the metatarsal is then displaced lateralward so that there is a gliding motion at the osteotomy site, displacing the fragment lateralward 2 to 3 mm. After this has been achieved, the abnormal alignment between the first and second metatarsals will be corrected.

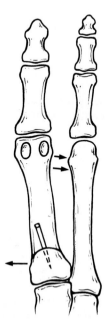

FIGURE 2–7. Osteotomy using a crescentic or curved blade. Note that the dome is convex distally to avoid overcorrection. (Redrawn from Mann RA, Coughlin MJ: The Video Textbook of Foot and Ankle Surgery. Medical Video Productions, St. Louis, 1991, p 167.)

9. The fixation of the osteotomy site using a screw is then completed by placing a centering device into the previously drilled hole and completing the hole with a 2.7-mm drill bit, after which a 26-mm long, 4.0-mm cancellous screw is inserted. This will give adequate fixation in most cases. If one wishes to use a pin for fixation, a 5/64-inch Steinmann pin can be placed obliquely across the osteotomy site to produce stability. Some surgeons have used several smaller Kirschner wires to obtain adequate fixation.

10. The medial joint capsule is plicated, as described previously, while the toe is held is satisfactory alignment.

11. A postoperative compression dressing is applied for approximately 18 to 24 hours. This dressing is then replaced by a dressing consisting of 2-inch Kling and 1/2-inch adhesive tape, as previously described. The patient is permitted to walk in a postoperative shoe. The dressing is changed weekly and maintained for 8 weeks. If a pin is used to fix the osteotomy site, it is usually removed after 4 weeks.

Results

The distal soft tissue procedure with a proximal osteotomy usually produces a satisfactory result in patients with a significant hallux valgus deformity.[15, 18] The main complication is hallux varus, which occurs in approximately 10 percent of patients, although it is usually less than 5 to 6 degrees, which is of little or no clinical significance. A more severe hallux varus deformity may occasionally occur if the osteotomy site is displaced too far laterally, translating the metatarsal head in a lateralward direction, or if too much of the medial eminence is removed.

Arthrodesis of the First Metatarsophalangeal Joint

An arthrodesis of the first metatarsophalangeal joint is indicated for a severe hallux valgus deformity, for degenerative or rheumatoid arthritis of the metatarsophalangeal joint, or as a salvage procedure for a deformed metatarsophalangeal joint resulting from previous surgery.[15] It should also be used for the patient who has a severe hallux valgus deformity and has had a stroke or head injury.

Surgical Technique

1. The skin incision is made over the dorsal aspect of the metatarsophalangeal joint, starting just proximal to the interphalangeal joint of the great toe and proceeding proximally for about 10 cm. It is deepened down to the extensor tendon, which is retracted medially or laterally.

2. By subperiosteal dissection, the metatarsal head is exposed, as is the base of the proximal phalanx.

3. With a sagittal microsaw, the distal portion of the metatarsal head is removed, creating a surface angled in slight dorsiflexion and valgus in relation to the metatarsal shaft.

4. The proximal phalanx is now held in correct alignment, which consists of placing it into approximately 15 degrees of valgus and 15 degrees of dorsiflexion in relation to the plantar aspect of the foot (30 degrees of dorsiflexion in relation to the first metatarsal shaft). A cut is made through the base of the proximal phalanx parallel to the first cut. After this has been achieved, the two pieces of bone are brought together, and the alignment is carefully checked. If the alignment is not satisfactory, it is corrected by recutting the metatarsal head (Fig. 2–8).

5. Once satisfactory alignment has been achieved, the joint is pinned with two crossed 0.045-inch Kirschner wires. When this has been achieved, good stability of the arthrodesis site can be obtained. Once again, the alignment is carefully observed.

6. Fixation of the arthrodesis site can then be carried out with a small fragment quarter tubular five- or six-hole plate placed on the dorsal aspect of the joint. Before the plate is placed on the bone, an interfragmentary screw is placed obliquely across the arthrodesis site to obtain compression of the bone surfaces. The plate is shaped and placed onto the dorsal aspect of the metatarsophalangeal joint, and it is secured using 4.0-mm cancellous screws. These screws are not designed specifically for the plate, but they can gain greater purchase into the bone.

7. Alternative methods of fixation include the use of two threaded 1/8-inch Steinmann pins if the bone stock is quite soft and screws and plates are not applicable.[15] In this situation, the pins are drilled out distally through the tip of the toe and then brought back proximally across the attempted arthrodesis site. These pins are left in place for approximately 12 weeks, until union occurs.

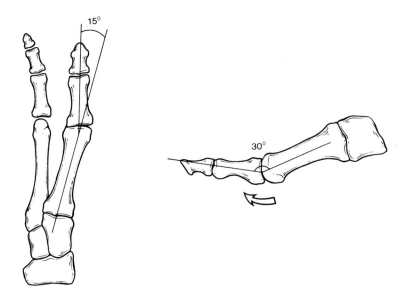

FIGURE 2–8. The proximal phalanx held in correct alignment. (Redrawn from Mann RA, Coughlin MJ: The Video Textbook of Foot and Ankle Surgery. Medical Video Productions, St. Louis, 1991, p 171.)

8. The postoperative regimen consists of allowing the patient to walk in a postoperative shoe until satisfactory union has occurred, which usually takes place in 10 to 12 weeks.

Results

After an arthrodesis, satisfactory union is achieved in about 95 percent of cases.[4, 15] The main problem that arises is malalignment of the metatarsophalangeal joint, but this can usually be avoided by careful operative planning. Degenerative changes of the interphalangeal joint may occur in approximately 25 to 40 percent of patients. Proper placement of the arthrodesis site reduces this risk significantly.

The Keller Procedure

The Keller procedure is a resection of the proximal portion of the proximal phalanx in order to decompress the metatarsophalangeal joint.[11, 12] It is used mainly as a salvage procedure, particularly in the older patient who is a poor ambulator. At times it is used in an older patient with slightly impaired vascularity in order to decompress the metatarsophalangeal joint to prevent recurrent ulcerations over the medial eminence. This procedure should not be carried out in a young, active individual.

Surgical Technique

1. The skin incision is made over the medial or dorsal medial aspect of the first metatarsophalangeal joint and carried down to the joint capsule. Full-thickness skin flaps should be created so that the dorsal and plantar volar nerves can be reflected without damage.

2. The base of the proximal phalanx is dissected free subperiosteally, and the medial eminence is exposed through a longitudinal incision made in line with the skin incision. The proximal third of the proximal phalanx is removed with a microsaw.

3. The medial eminence is removed in line with the metatarsal shaft (Fig. 2–9A).

4. The sesamoid sling is reapproximated to the base of the proximal phalanx, if possible, either through small drill holes in the base of the proximal phalanx or by reattaching it to the periosteum, which had been previously dissected off the proximal phalanx (Fig. 2–9B).

5. The medial capsule is then plicated and closed.

6. A 5/64-inch smooth Steinmann pin is placed longitudinally across the joint in order to maintain a space of about 5 mm between the base of the phalanx and the metatarsal head. The wound is closed in a routine manner.

7. A compression dressing is used for 18 to 24 hours, after which the patient is dressed in a snug compression dressing consisting of 2-inch Kling and 1/2-inch adhesive tape. The pin

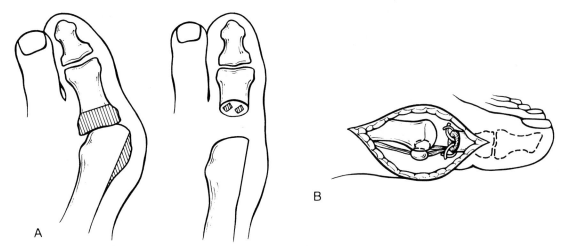

FIGURE 2–9. The Keller resection arthroplasty procedure. *(A)*, The medial eminence is removed. *(B)*, Reapproximation of the sesamoid sling. (Redrawn from Mann RA, Coughlin MJ: The Video Textbook of Foot and Ankle Surgery. Medical Video Productions, St. Louis, 1991, p 175.)

is left in place for approximately 3 weeks, after which active and passive range-of-motion exercise is begun. The patient ambulates in a postoperative shoe.

Results

This procedure, when used as a decompression procedure for a problem with ulceration, is usually quite successful. The major problem following a Keller procedure is that because of loss of adequate muscle attachment to the base of the proximal phalanx, the toe will tend to drift into dorsiflexion or valgus.[13, 23] As a result of loss of weight bearing by the great toe, frequently a transfer metatarsalgia will result. The procedure usually has a satisfactory result when performed for the indications listed.

References

1. Akin OF: The treatment of hallux valgus: A new operative procedure and its results. Med Sentinel 33:678, 1925.
2. Austin DW, Leventen EO: A new osteotomy for hallux valgus. Clin Orthop 157:25, 1981.
2a. Austin DW, Leventen EO: Scientific Exhibit of V-osteotomy of the First Metatarsal Head. Chicago, American Academy of Orthopaedic Surgery, 1968.
3. Corless JR: A modification of the Mitchell procedure. J Bone Joint Surg 55B:138, 1976.
4. Coughlin MJ: Arthrodesis of the first metatarsophalangeal joint with mini-fragment plate fixation. Orthopedics 13:1037–1044, 1990.
5. DuVries HL: Surgery of the Foot. St. Louis, CV Mosby, 1959.
6. Goldberg I, Bahar A, Yosipovichz Z: Late results after correction of hallux valgus deformity by basilar phalangeal osteotomy. J Bone Joint Surg 69A:64–67, 1987.
7. Haines RW, McDougall A: The anatomy of hallux valgus. J Bone Joint Surg 36B:262–293, 1954.
8. Hattrup SJ, Johnson KA: Chevron osteotomy: Analysis of factors in patient dissatisfaction. Foot Ankle 5:327–332, 1985.
9. Hirvensalo E, Bostman O, Tormaia P, et al: Chevron osteotomy fixed with absorbable polyglycolide pins. Foot Ankle 7:212, 1991.
10. Horne G, Tantzer T, Ford M: Chevron osteotomy for the treatment of hallux valgus. Clin Orthop 183:32–36, 1984.
11. Keller WL: Further observations on the surgical treatment of hallux valgus and bunions. N Y Med J 95:696, 1912.
12. Keller WL: The surgical treatment of bunions and hallux valgus. N Y Med J 95:696, 1912.
13. Love PR, Whynot AS, Farine I, et al: Keller arthroplasty: A prospective review. Foot Ankle 8:46–54, 1987.
14. Mann RA, Coughlin MJ: Hallux valgus: Etiology, anatomy, treatment and surgical considerations. Clin Orthop 157:31, 1981.
15. Mann RA, Coughlin MJ: Surgery of the Foot and Ankle, 6th Ed. St. Louis, Mosby-Yearbook, 1993, pp 167–276.
16. Mann RA, Oates JC: Arthrodesis of the first metatarsophalangeal joint. Foot Ankle 1:159, 1980.
17. Mann RA, Pfeffinger L: Hallux valgus repair: DuVries modified McBride procedure. Clin Orthop 272:213–218, 1991.
18. Mann RA, Rudicel S, Graves SC: Hallux valgus repair utilizing a distal soft tissue procedure and proximal metatarsal osteotomy: A long term followup. J Bone Joint Surg 74A:124–129, 1992.
19. McBride ED: The conservative operation for bunions. J Bone Joint Surg 10:735, 1928.

20. McBride ED: The conservative operation for "bunions": End results and refinements of technique. JAMA 105:1164, 1935.
21. McBride ED: Hallux valgus, bunion deformity: Its treatment in mild, moderate and severe stages. J Int Coll Surg 21:99, 1954.
22. Meier PJ, Kenzora JE: The risks and benefits of distal first metatarsal osteotomies. Foot Ankle 6:7–17, 1985.
23. Richardson EG: Keller resection arthroplasty. Orthopedics 13:1049–1053, 1990.
24. Silver D: The operative treatment of hallux valgus. J Bone Joint Surg 5:225, 1923.

3 *Hallux Rigidus*

GEORGE B. HOLMES, JR.

Hallux rigidus (hallux limitus) is representative of one of the degenerative joint diseases of the foot. This is a disorder of the first metatarsophalangeal joint that results in restricted motion and degenerative changes of the joint. Causative factors include improper shoewear, genetic or structural predispositions, metabolic disorders, and post-traumatic changes. Typically there is pain associated with limitation of dorsiflexion. Radiographic evaluation confirms degenerative joint changes. Treatment is based on both nonoperative and operative modalities.

PRESENTATION

Pain is the chief complaint of patients with hallux rigidus. The pain is primarily localized to the first metatarsophalangeal joint. There usually is no associated significant medial or lateral deviation of the great toe. Commonly, patients with hallux valgus have a decrease in pain when they walk barefoot. Patients with hallux rigidus, however, report more discomfort or no change in pain when walking barefoot. Pain is aggravated with walking and running and is decreased with rest. Patients tend to preferentially select a stiff-soled shoe rather than a more flexible-soled shoe. Female patients are unable to wear high-heeled shoes with ease. Patients may indicate an inability to comfortably stand on their toes.

Observation of the patient indicates an alteration in gait secondary to the decrease in dorsiflexion of the toes. Inspection of the foot reveals both soft tissue swelling and a bony prominence about the dorsum of the first meta-tarsophalangeal joint (Fig. 3–1). Palpation confirms dorsal soft tissue swelling and dorsal osteophytes. Dorsiflexion is significantly limited and is associated with pain. Plantar flexion can cause pain as result of traction of the extensor hallucis longus muscle over the dorsal osteophyte. On occasion, a positive Tinel sign can be elicited over the dorsal digital nerve as it courses over the dorsal medial osteophyte.

The radiographic evaluation includes anteroposterior and lateral weight-bearing views. The anteroposterior view demonstrates a flattened articular surface, narrowing of the joint space, and juxta-articular sclerotic changes (Fig. 3–2). Medial and lateral osteophytes are found on both the proximal and distal sides of the joint. The lateral view delineates the extent of the dorsal spur, which extends proximally from

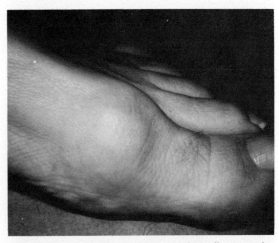

FIGURE 3–1. Dorsal osteophytes and swelling can be observed in this patient with hallux rigidus.

23

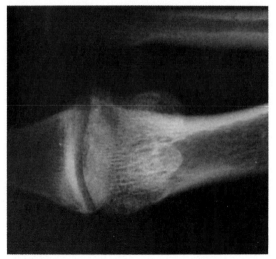

FIGURE 3–2. This patient has the classic findings of a flat joint, joint space narrowing, and subchondral sclerosis.

the distal aspect of the metatarsal head (Fig. 3–3). Also, there may be a free fragment owing to fracture of the large dorsal osteophyte. In some instances, there may be a second, smaller dorsal osteophyte originating from the proximal phalanx. Radionuclide scans, tomography, and magnetic resonance imaging are not necessary to confirm the diagnosis. However, it is helpful to compare views of the contralateral foot to determine the degree of degeneration in the affected joint. Patients frequently have bilateral symptoms, which necessitate radiographic studies of both feet.

PATHOPHYSIOLOGY

Typically, the patient who develops a hallux rigidus deformity has a flattened metatarsophalangeal joint rather than a more rounded joint. The flattening of the articular surfaces of the distal metatarsal and the proximal phalanx may lead to an abnormal distribution of forces. This factor, in turn, may accelerate degenerative changes at the joint. These changes are manifested by an increase in subchondral sclerosis and marginal osteophytes. Most commonly, these osteophytes are localized on the dorsal, medial, and lateral aspects of the joint.

CLASSIFICATION

Hallux rigidus has been previously classified as either acquired or congenital.[12] The congenital or juvenile form of hallux rigidus appears in the teen years. The chief complaints are exactly the same as those of any patient with hallux rigidus. Pain and swelling are localized to the first metatatarsophalangeal joint. Symptoms are aggravated by dorsiflexion of the great toe. Frequently, these young patients are involved in high-school or college sports activities such as football, basketball, gymnastics, or dance. Radiographic features differ slightly from those of acquired hallux rigidus in that often there is an osteochondritic defect noted in the metatarsal head.

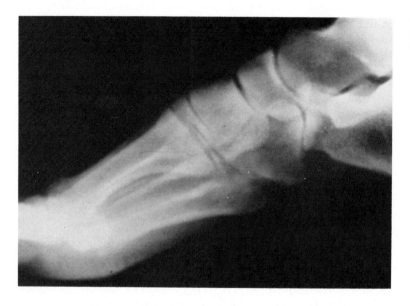

FIGURE 3–3. A large dorsal osteophyte is seen in this lateral view of a patient with hallux rigidus.

Most patients with hallux rigidus can be classified as having the acquired form. This type of hallux rigidus is either a result of trauma (acute and chronic) or a consequence of one of several of the arthritides. The traumatic insult can be acute. Typically, a traumatic insult becomes manifest as an intra-articular fracture or blunt soft tissue injury to the first metatarsophalangeal joint. Chronic trauma may be determined by a history of increased activity that imparts excessive stresses to the first metatarsophalangeal joint. Increased forces are chronically transmitted to the first metatarsophalangeal joint by high-heeled shoes, pointed-toe shoes, and shoes with a small or short toe box. It is reasonable to presume that acquired hallux rigidus, in large part, results from an interaction between trauma and various anatomic factors.

Acquired hallux rigidus has also been associated with arthritic processes such as infection, gout, rheumatoid arthritis, and psoriatic arthritis. Appropriate laboratory studies are mandatory to confirm the presence of these various conditions. Most certainly, anatomic factors and trauma play a contributory role in the development of hallux rigidus in association with these various arthritides.

TREATMENT

The conservative treatment of hallux rigidus is primarily directed toward the reduction of motion across the first metatarsophlangeal joint. This is achieved by modification of activity and shoewear. Patients should avoid extremes of dorsiflexion of the great toe such as occurs with deep squats. Women patients are encouraged to change from a high-heeled shoe to a low-heeled or flat shoe. Shoe modifications include the use of a wider toe box and a shoe with a steel shank and a rocker-bottom sole. These conservative measures are initially employed for both congenital and acquired hallux rigidus. Nonsteroidal anti-inflammatory agents are useful in augmenting the conservative approach.

There are two types of operative modalities for the treatment of hallux rigidus. First, there are techniques that enhance the mobility of the joint. This modality would include cheilectomy, the Moberg osteotomy, silicone implantation, and the Keller resectional arthroplasty. The second approach eliminates motion across the metatarsophalangeal joint. Viewed primarly as a salvage procedure, this approach involves an arthrodesis of the joint.

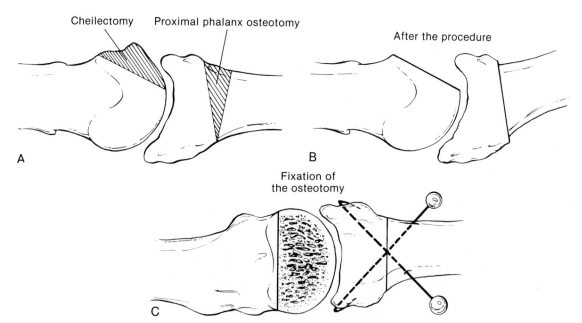

FIGURE 3–4. The Moberg proximal phalanx osteotomy. The small dorsal wedge is taken through the metaphyseal area. The medial cheilectomy incision is extended distally; the wedge is taken with a microsagittal saw or digital osteotome. Oblique Kirschner wire fixation from the medial and lateral proximal segment still allows early movement of the joint. The wedge taken is approximately 0.5 cm, and this changes the motion arc to allow more dorsiflexion.

The Moberg procedure is an operative alternative for adolescent patients who fail to respond to conservative treatment.[7] This procedure increases the range of motion of dorsiflexion by the resection of a dorsally based wedge of bone from the proximal aspect of the proximal phalanx (Fig. 3–4).

An operative option for acquired or adult hallux rigidus is cheilectomy.[6] The improvement of dorsiflexion is achieved by the removal of the osteophytes about the metatarsal head. The essential features of this technique are (1) a straight dorsal approach centered over the first metatarsophalangeal joint, with the extensor retinaculum entered medial to the extensor hallucis longus, (2) inspection of the joint for adequacy of the remaining articular cartilage, and (3) removal of the marginal dorsal, lateral, and medial osteophytes along with the dorsal one-quarter to one-third of the metatarsal head. A straight osteotome and rongeur are the basic instruments required for this resection (Fig. 3–5). Active range of motion is started about 2 weeks after surgery. The advantages of this procedure include a consistent

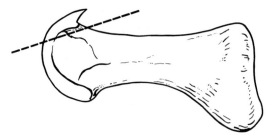

FIGURE 3–5. The dorsal osteophyte and a portion of the superior aspect of the articular cartilage are removed using a straight osteotome. Residual peripheral osteophytes on the margin of the metatarsal head and proximal phalanx are excised. Small defects on the articular surface may be excised to subchondral bone, which is also drilled to promote the formation of fibrocartilage. If the need for these additional steps is extensive, the likelihood of success with this procedure diminishes.

increase in the range of motion, high patient satisfaction, low complication rate, and low incidence of reoperative or secondary salvage procedures.

Two other procedures may be used for the enhancement of dorsiflexion of the great toe for hallux rigidus. A resectional arthroplasty

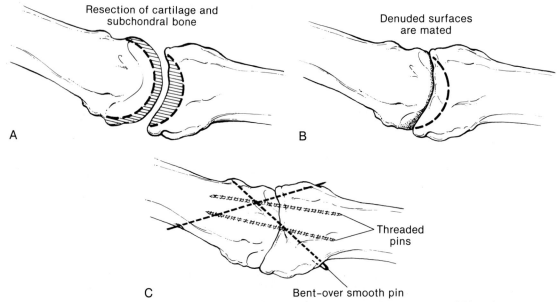

Resection of cartilage and subchondral bone

Denuded surfaces are mated

A

B

Threaded pins

C

Bent–over smooth pin

FIGURE 3–6. Arthrodesis of the first metatarsophalangeal joint. Although many techniques are available, I favor a cup-in-cone configuration to allow maximal bone contact and adjustment of the arthrodesis position. With a rongeur or power-driven concave reamer, the metatarsal head is reduced to a round cancellous ball of bone, which is fitted into a cup prepared in the proximal phalanx with a round or tear-shaped burr. A smooth 0.062-inch pin is driven across the arthrodesis site, and the position of the toe is checked (10 to 15 degrees of dorsiflexion from the plantar plane with 5 degrees of valgus). If necessary, the position is readjusted. Final fixation may be accomplished with a rosette of threaded 0.062-inch fixation pins; a screw and pins; or a dorsal plate. The editor prefers the single smooth pin and multiple threaded ones. Please note that in fusions of the metatarsophalangeal joint, the sesamoids are not excised. This may be done in rheumatoid arthritis.

such as the Keller procedure has been used, particularly in the more elderly, sedentary population. However, the problems of secondary hallux valgus or hallux rigidus deformity, cock-up toe deformity, weakened plantar flexion, and transfer metatarsalgia to the second metatarsal head must be strongly weighed before this procedure is selected.[2, 9, 11, 14] Another option is the use of a silicone implant. The disadvantages of this approach include the risk of late infection, implant fragmentation, implant loosening, silicone synovitis, and loss of bone stock for subsequent salvage procedures.[8, 10]

The various techniques of arthrodesis eliminate pain and joint motion by the establishment of fusion across the metatarsophalangeal joint.[1, 3–5, 13] These procedures are useful for severe, acquired hallux rigidus. Inspection of the joint should demonstrate extensive marginal osteophytes with sparse or absent articular cartilage. The essentials of the techniques of arthrodesis are (1) the removal of articular cartilage, (2) the creation of broad surfaces of cancellous bone at the metatarsophalangeal joint, and (3) the establishment of rigid fixation by means of pins, screws, or plates. The joint to undergo arthrodesis should be in 10 to 15 degrees of dorsiflexion to allow for a normal gait pattern. If these principles are followed, the various arthrodesis techniques are usually quite reliable in their elimination of pain (Fig. 3–6).[4, 5, 13] Complications include nonunion and improper dorsiflexion positioning of the arthrodesis.[1] Some techniques also impart the risk of developing arthritis at the interphalangeal joint of the great toe.

There are several techniques that may be used for the conservative and operative management of hallux rigidus. The successful employment of these various modalities demands the proper identification of the type and severity of the hallux rigidus. The goal remains the reduction or elimination of pain and the enhancement of patient mobility while minimizing the risk of complications or secondary salvage procedures.

References

1. Fitzgerald JAW: A review of long-term results of arthrodesis of the first metatarsophalangeal joint. J Bone Joint Surg 51(B):488–493, 1969.
2. Jordan HH, Brodsky AE: Keller operation for hallux valgus and hallux rigidus. An end result study. Arch Surg 62:586–596, 1951.
3. Lipscomb PR: Arthrodesis of the first metatarsophalangeal joint for severe bunions and hallux rigidus. Clin Orthop 142:48–54, 1979.
4. McKeever DC: Arthrodesis of the first metatarsophalangeal joint for hallux valgus, hallux rigidus, and metatarsus primus varus. J Bone Joint Surg 34(A):129–134, 1952.
5. Mann RA, Oates JC: Arthrodesis of the first metatarsophalangeal joint. Foot Ankle 1:159–166, 1980.
6. Mann RA, Clanton TO: Hallux rigidus: Treatment of cheilectomy. J Bone Joint Surg 70(A):400–405, 1988.
7. Moberg E: A simple operation for hallux rigidus. Clin Orthop 142:55–56, 1979.
8. Molster AO, Lunde OD, Rait M: Hallux rigidus treated with the Swanson Silastic hemi-joint prosthesis. Acta Orthop Scand 51:853–856, 1980.
9. Severin E: Removal of the base of the proximal phalanx in hallux rigidus. Acta Orthop Scand 18:77–87, 1949.
10. Shereff MJ, Jahss MH: Complications of Silastic implant arthroplasty in the hallux. Foot Ankle 1:95–101, 1980.
11. Stokes IAF, Hutton WC, Stott JRR, Lowe LW: Forces under the hallux valgus foot before and after surgery. Clin Orthop 142:64–72, 1979.
12. Thompson FM, Mann RA: Arthritides. *In* Mann RA (Ed): Surgery of the Foot. St. Louis, CV Mosby, 1986, pp 160–164.
13. Wilson CL: A method of fusion of the metatarsophalangeal joint of the great toe. J Bone Joint Surg 40(A):384–385, 1958.
14. Wrighton JD: A ten-year review of Keller's operation. Review of Keller's operation at The Princess Elizabeth Orthopaedic Hospital, Exeter. Clin Orthop 89:207–214, 1972.

4 *Hallux Varus*

KENNETH A. JOHNSON
CHARLES L. SALTZMAN
DAVID A. FRISCIA

A hallux varus deformity of the foot, in which the great toe deviates medially (negative hallux valgus angle), may be tolerated but is rarely satisfactory. In a shod society the toe will invariably chafe against the inside of the shoe and cause discomfort. This deformity has several interesting aspects anatomically and provides some insight into the exquisite musculotendinous balance about the first metatarsophalangeal joint. In addition, classifying the anatomic changes into appropriate categories allows a rational plan of treatment. Even more importantly, an understanding of this problem should enable the surgeon treating hallux valgus to decrease the occurrence of this unfortunate complication.

CLASSIFICATION

The *congenital* form of hallux varus is unusual, but individual case reports and small series have been described. By definition this deformity is present at birth. With asymmetrical growth and concomitant increased soft tissue tethering, the deformity may increase with age. The pediatrician or parent will commonly note the change in the great toe and refer the patient to the orthopaedic surgeon. Other congenital malformations may also be present.

Acquired hallux varus occurs as a complication of a systemic disease or of hallux valgus surgery. Probably the most common systemic disease is rheumatoid arthritis, but any of the collagen vascular diseases has the potential to cause this problem.

The vast majority of cases of hallux varus are secondary to hallux valgus surgery.[12, 15, 16, 25] A variation of the McBride bunionectomy is the usual culprit.[1, 10] Originally McBride advocated removal of the fibularward sesamoid as part of his hallux valgus realignment.[20, 21] However he later recommended that the sesamoid be retained to avoid this complication.[4, 22, 23] The number of cases he documented was quite small, and no statistical estimate of the occurrence of hallux varus can be gleaned from his articles. Mann,[19] an advocate of the McBride procedure, includes a crescentic first metatarsal base osteotomy with the distal soft tissue release. With this modification, there is a 12-percent incidence of hallux varus. Eight percent of these deformities were felt to be minor, leaving a 4-percent rate of symptomatically significant deformity. Since there is no buttress medial to the great toe, even a small degree of hallux varus has a propensity to increase with time. Other hallux valgus procedures may be iatrogenic causes of hallux varus, but this is unusual.

TYPE

For *congenital* hallux varus, the type is defined by the associated anatomic changes (Table 4–1), which may involve bone and soft tissue.[26] The type is thus somewhat descriptive for congenital hallux varus. Likewise, *acquired*

28

TABLE 4–1. HALLUX VARUS—CLASSIFICATION, TYPE, ANATOMIC CHANGES		
CLASSIFICATION	**TYPE**	**ANATOMIC CHANGES**
I. Congenital	Defined by associated anatomic changes	Abnormal bone and musculotendinous development, e.g., delta phalanx, phalangeal duplication, joint deformity, tight abductor hallucis tendon
II. Acquired		
1. Systemic disease	Defined by specific disease, e.g., rheumatoid arthritis	Joint destruction, capsular ligament loosening, tendon disruption, muscle spasm
2. Iatrogenic	A. MTP varus only	Asymmetric pull of flexor hallucis brevis (FHB) and abductor hallucis in an abduction-adduction plane (transverse); flexion moment on proximal phalanx retained
	B. MTP varus extension plus interphalangeal flexion	Asymmetric pull of FHB in transverse plane. The FHB action on the proximal phalanx is lost, allowing the proximal phalanx to dorsiflex at the MTP joint. A collapse deformity of the phalanges develops (intercalated segment) with flexion at the interphalangeal joint.

hallux varus can be classified according to the associated disease.

Acquired iatrogenic hallux varus, however, is typed according to the static positions of the metatarsophalangeal (MTP) and interphalangeal (IP) joints. Type II-2A is a pure hallux varus in which the MTP and IP joints are not flexed in the dorsoplantar (sagittal) plane. The other type (II-2B) of acquired iatrogenic hallux varus shows extension at the MTP joint of about 30 to 40 degrees and flexion of the IP joint to about 60 degrees (Fig. 4–1*A* and *B*). Because of this unusual configuration, it is sometimes called the "snake-in-the grass" deformity. This type is not only the most dramatic but unfortunately also the most common.

ANATOMIC CHANGES

In congenital hallux varus, physical examination along with radiographs will demonstrate the anatomic changes (see Table 4–1). Bone duplications and soft tissue contractures are evident and are important when planning surgical treatment.[30] Other studies such as arteriography will occasionally be used to clarify the vascular distribution.

With the acquired systemic hallux varus, the severity is variable (Fig. 4–2). Patients with rheumatoid arthritis are sometimes seen with hallux varus deformity of one foot and hallux valgus of the other. Undoubtedly, the course of the underlying disease causing joint destruction and soft tissue disease determines the pattern of great toe deformity.

The most consistent and understandable pattern develops with acquired iatrogenic hallux varus.[11, 25] Three aspects of hallux valgus surgery may contribute to hallux varus at the MTP joint: (1) excessive removal of the medial eminence, (2) unequal lateral release and medial plication to statically bind the MTP joint, and (3) ablation of the lateral attachment of the flexor hallucis brevis on the proximal phalanx.[3, 14] Each of these may be implicated to a variable extent in a specific patient. However, if extension at the MTP and flexion at the IP joints accompany the hallux varus (type II-2B), then disruption of the flexor hallucis brevis must have occurred (see Fig. 4–1*B*). Such a disruption can be caused not only by removal of the lateral sesamoid but also by release of the flexor hallucis brevis from the lateral base of the proximal phalanx while retaining the lateral sesamoid. Thus, maintaining the integrity of the lateral head of the flexor hallucis brevis is crucial in avoiding hallux varus. If the lateral head of the flexor hallucis brevis is excessively released, there is a tendency for "bowstringing" of the remaining tendons about the MTP joint as the great toe moves toward a varus position. If during removal of the medial eminence the medial groove for the tibialward sesamoid is destabilized, there will be a tendency for the tibial-

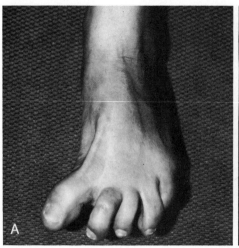
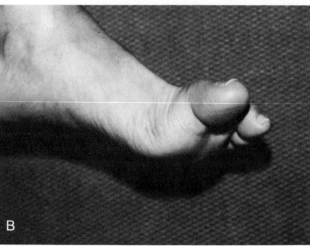

FIGURE 4–1. *(A)*, Anteroposterior view shows varus at the metatarsophalangeal joint and bowstringing of the extensor hallucis longus tendon. The lesser toes deviate toward the space vacated by the great toe. *(B)*, Medial view demonstrates extension at the metatarsophalangeal and flexion at the interphalangeal joints.

ward sesamoid to displace and rotate medially (Fig. 4–3). The medial head of the flexor hallucis brevis then becomes an abductor rather than a flexor in this new position, which tends to accentuate the deformity (Fig. 4–4*A* and *B*).

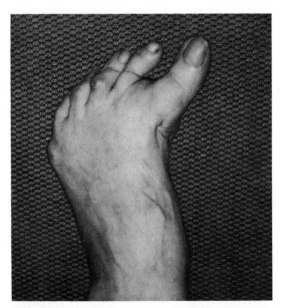

FIGURE 4–2. Severe hallux varus as a result of rheumatoid arthritis.

TREATMENT

An understanding of the classification, type, and anatomy of hallux varus will lead to its proper treatment.

Congenital Hallux Varus

The literature on treatment of congenital hallux varus is quite sparse, with no extensive series of cases. In general, treatment depends on the anatomic changes present,[9, 13, 18, 26, 27, 31] and most patients do well with appropriate soft tissue release and realignment. McElvenny used the extensor hallucis brevis to reinforce the lateral capsule of the MTP joint as well as to provide sling mechanisms for the extensor hallucis longus to prevent the bowstringing effect.[24] Farmer[7] described the technique of transferring a flap of skin and subcutaneous tissue from the first web space to the medial aspect of the first MTP joint along with syndactylization of the first web space. Transposition of tissue from the first web space (Farmer),[7] medial release of the joint capsule and abductor hallucis, syndactylization at the first web space, excision of supernumerary digits, lateral plication and reinforcement (McElvenny),[24] and osteotomies all may be

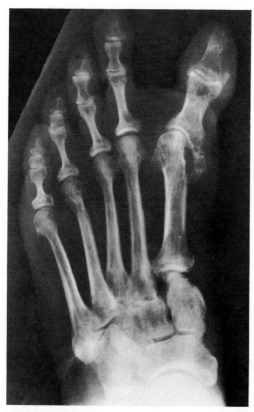

FIGURE 4–3. This radiograph shows the retained tibialward sesamoid bone rotated to the medial aspect of the first metatarsal head. In this position, the medial head of the flexor hallucis brevis is functioning as an abductor of the great toe.

used to some extent, depending on the specific anatomic changes in the individual case (also see Chapter 37).

Acquired Hallux Varus

For an acquired hallux varus secondary to systemic disease, treatment depends on the amount of deformity and the activity of the underlying systemic disease. Specifically, for rheumatoid arthritis, modifying the shoe to make room for the abnormal great toe position may be sufficient. Surgery is generally used only when there is involvement of the lesser MTP joints as well as the great toe. Thus some procedures, such as resection arthroplasty,[17, 25] are used at the lesser MTP joints. Generally, arthrodesis of the great toe can provide acceptable deformity correction and pain relief. In special circumstances, insertion of an MTP

double-stemmed silicone prosthesis may be appropriate, but only after the bone and tendon deformities have been corrected.[8] Rerouting of the extensor hallucis longus or other soft tissue procedures alone are unusual in systemic disease because of associated joint destruction and tendency for disease progression.

Iatrogenic hallux varus (type II-2A and B) provides the greatest reconstructive challenge. Many types of procedures have been suggested (Fig. 4–5A to H).[6, 28, 29] Usually, the MTP articulation will not show degeneration, so the surgical treatment involves realigning the distorted soft tissue.

In the unusual situation of acquired iatrogenic MTP varus only (type II-2A), a transfer of the abductor hallucis insertion from the plantar medial aspect of the proximal phalanx base to the plantar lateral aspect is indicated.[5, 11] This can be done by maintaining as much length of the abductor hallucis longus tendon as possible and then transferring it beneath the muscle mass of the flexor hallucis brevis and reattaching it to the lateral aspect of the proximal phalanx. Of course, a release of the medial capsular tissues and reefing of the lateral capsular tissues are done in conjunction with the abductor hallucis transfer.

The most common hallux varus deformity is the acquired iatrogenic type II-2B, in which the MTP joint is in extension and the IP joint in flexion. In this situation, it is appropriate to transfer the main unopposed extensor hallucis longus (EHL) deforming tendon (Fig. 4–6A to F) and place it in a reforming position on the plantar lateral aspect of the proximal phalanx.[15] Because the transfer of the EHL will leave the flexor hallucis longus (FHL) unopposed, it is necessary to perform an arthrodesis of the IP joint to prevent a flexion deformity. This also helps to correct the MTP extension by making the FHL act to flex the great toe at the MTP rather than the IP joint. In the extensor hallucis longus transfer, the L-shaped incision begins between the midportions of the first and second metatarsals (see Fig. 4–6A) and extends distally along the dorsolateral aspect of the great toe and then medially near the insertion of the extensor hallucis longus tendon. The extensor hallucis tendon is divided as far distally as possible; that is, to its insertion on the base of the distal phalanx. Care is taken to avoid disruption of the nail bed. The articular surfaces of the interphalangeal joint are

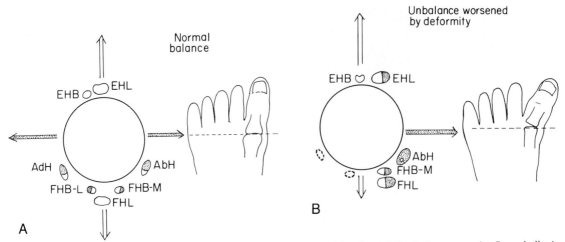

FIGURE 4–4. *(A),* Normal tendon arrangement about the first metatarsal head. *(B),* With hallux varus, the flexor hallucis brevis tendon displaces after the fibularward sesamoid bone has been removed. EHB, extensor hallucis brevis; EHL, extensor hallucis longus; AdH, adductor hallucis; AbH, abductor hallucis; FHB-L, flexor hallucis brevis lateral head; FHB-M, flexor hallucis brevis medial head; FHL, flexor hallucis longus.

removed and a 4.0 cancellous bone screw (see Fig. 4–6*B*) is used to fix the joint in extension.

A nonabsorbable back-and-forth suture is placed in the end of the extensor hallucis longus, and the tendon is freed of paratenon proximally to the region of the tarsometatarsal articulation. The tendon is passed under the intermetatarsal ligament between the heads of the first and second metatarsals and that ligament is used as a pulley. A prior surgical scar in this region has never interfered with use of the ligament as a suitable pulley. Passing the distal tendon of the extensor hallucis longus through a tunnel beneath this pulley brings it to the desired plantar and lateral aspect of the proximal phalanx of the great toe. A 9/64-inch (3.6-mm) drill hole is made dorsoventrally in the proximal phalanx to allow reattachment on the hallux of the extensor hallucis longus tendon after it is passed ventrodorsally (see Fig. 4–6*C* to *E*).

If necessary to position the toe correctly, a second incision may be made medial to the first MTP joint in order to release the capsular contractures and to reduce or excise a sesamoid that is displaced medially. Initially it was feared that resection of the dislocated sesamoid, which lies along the medial aspect of the head of the first metatarsal, might promote recurrence of the original hallux valgus, but this has not occurred. It is important to completely release the medial capsular structures and to excise the sesamoid if it is dislocated.

The realigned MTP position is held with a Kirschner wire across the joint for 6 weeks (see Fig. 4–6*F*). Postoperatively a compression dressing is used for 2 days, followed by application of a short non–weight-bearing cast (for 3 weeks) and then a short walking cast (for 3 more weeks). Removal of the Kirschner wire is followed by weight bearing and mobilization without a plaster cast.

Overcorrection of hallux varus back to hallux valgus has not been a problem, and a wide release medially is important. If necessary, skin grafting of the medial wound can be used to ensure that no medial tethering remains after EHL transfer. Continued use of the procedure confirms the reported experience with the first 15 toes that it is reliable and gives satisfactory results in most patients.[15]

It has been suggested that the EHL could be split and only the lateral portion transferred to the plantar lateral aspect of the proximal phalanx, but this is not reasonable since this requires the EHL to perform two actions simultaneously: extension of the IP joint and adduction of the MTP joint. The IP arthrodesis is necessary so that the FHL will act as a flexor at the MTP joint.

An arthrodesis at the MTP joint is the most reasonable treatment for hallux varus when MTP joint degenerative changes are present, when tendon scarring and decreased motion have occurred, or when the MTP joint is markedly subluxed or dislocated. The MTP

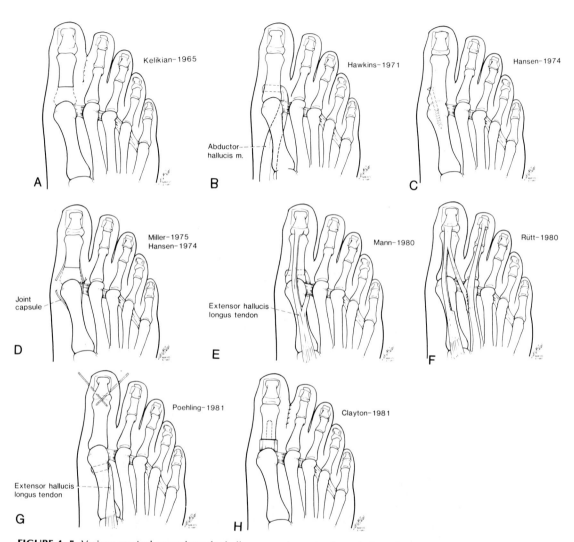

FIGURE 4–5. Various surgical procedures for hallux varus shown in chronologic order. (Courtesy of the Mayo Clinic.)

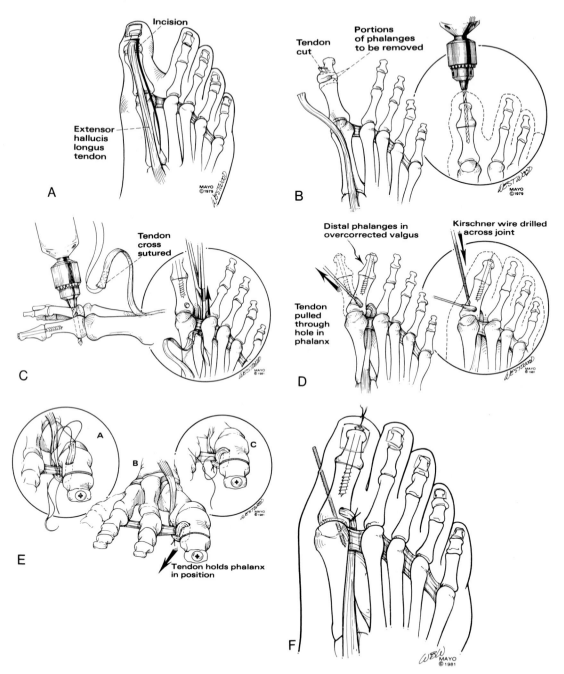

FIGURE 4–6. Surgical transfer of the extensor hallucis longus tendon from a deforming position to a corrective location. (Courtesy of the Mayo Clinic.)

arthrodesis is a useful procedure in providing proper toe alignment, but the loss of joint motion is a disadvantage.

References

1. Ahlbeck P: Operation av hallux valgus enligt McBride (abstract). Nordisk Med 77:166, 1967.
2. Baciu C, Sgarbura I: Quelques conclusion sur les resultats obtenus dans le traitement chirurgical de l'hallux valgus. Revue de 4,000 operations. Acta Orthop Belg 35:865–894, 1969.
3. Banks AS, Rush JA, Kalish SR: Surgical repair of hallux varus. J Am Podiatry Assoc 78:339–347, 1988.
4. Bateman JE: Pitfalls in forefoot surgery. Orthop Clin North Am 7:751–777, 1976.
5. Clark WD: Abductor hallucis tendon transfer for hallux varus. J Foot Surg 23:146–148, 1984.
6. DuVries HL: Acquired nontraumatic deformities of the foot. *In* Inman VT (Ed): Surgery of the Foot, 3rd Ed. St. Louis, CV Mosby, 1973, pp 223–226.
7. Farmer AW: Congenital hallux varus. Am J Surg 95:274–278, 1958.
8. Greenfogel SI, Glubo S, Werner J, et al: Hallux varus—surgical correction and review of literature. J Foot Surg 23:46–50, 1984.
9. Haas SL: An operation for the correction of hallux varus. J Bone Joint Surg 20:705–708, 1938.
10. Hansen CE: Hallux valgus treated by the McBride operation. A follow-up. Acta Orthop Scand 45:778–792, 1974.
11. Hawkins FB: Acquired hallux varus: Cause, prevention and correction. Clin Orthop 76:169–176, 1971.
12. Hawkins FB, Mitchell CL, Hedrick DW: Correction of hallux valgus by metatarsal osteotomy. J Bone Joint Surg 27:387–394, 1945.
13. Horwitz MT: Unusual hallux varus deformity and its surgical correction. J Bone Joint Surg 19:828–829, 1937.
14. Hunter WN, Wasiak GA: Traumatic hallux varus correction via split extensor tenodesis. J Foot Surg 23:321–325, 1984.
15. Johnson KA, Spiegl PV: Extensor hallucis longus transfer for hallux varus deformity. J Bone Joint Surg 66A:681–686, 1984.
16. Joplin RJ: Follow-up notes on articles previously published in the journal. Sling procedure for correction of splay foot, metatarsus primus varus, and hallux valgus. J Bone Joint Surg 46A:690–693, 1964.
17. Kelikian H: Hallux Valgus, Allied Deformities of the Forefoot, and Metatarsalgia. Philadelphia, WB Saunders, 1965, pp 433–435.
18. Kelikian H: The Hallux. *In* Jahss MH (Ed): Disorders of the Foot, Vol 1. Philadelphia, WB Saunders, 1982, pp 616–618.
19. Mann RA, personal communication, 1991.
20. McBride ED: A conservative operation for bunions. J Bone Joint Surg 10:735–739, 1928.
21. McBride ED: The conservative operation for "bunions." End results and refinements of technic. JAMA 105:1164–1168, 1935.
22. McBride ED: Hallux valgus, bunion deformity: Its treatment in mild, moderate and severe stages. J Int Coll Surg 21:99–105, 1954.
23. McBride ED: The McBride bunion hallux valgus operation: Refinements in the successive surgical steps of the operation. J Bone Joint Surg 49A:1675–1683, 1967.
24. McElvenny RT: Hallux varus. Q Bull Northwest Univ Med Sch 15:277–280, 1941.
25. Miller JW: Acquired hallux varus: A preventable and correctable disorder. J Bone Joint Surg 57A:183–188, 1975.
26. Mills JA, Menelaus MB: Hallux varus. J Bone Joint Surg 71B:437–440, 1989.
27. Mygind HB: Operativ behandling of hallux varus. Nord Med 26:914–916, 1953.
28. Poehling GG, DeTorre J: Hallux varus and hammertoe deformity. Orthop Trans 6:186, 1982.
29. Rütt A: Surgery of the lower leg and foot. *In* Hackenbroch M, Witt AN (Eds): Atlas of Orthopaedic Operations, Vol 2. Philadelphia, WB Saunders, 1980.
30. Sloane D: Congenital hallux varus. Operative correction. J Bone Joint Surg 17:209–211, 1935.
31. Thomson SA: Hallux varus and metatarsus varus. A five-year study (1954–1958). Clin Orthop 16:109–118, 1960.

5
Stabilization of the Second Metatarsophalangeal Joint

FRANCESCA M. THOMPSON

Patients often present with problems referable to the second metatarsophalangeal joint. Occasionally the third ray is involved as well. Although many investigators believe that these lesser toe problems originate from the influence of hallux valgus, this is not usually the case. More often, they appear to be due to repetitive stress, to a longer second metatarsal (Morton's foot), and to squeezing the forefoot in tight high-fashion shoewear, such that the soft tissue support on the plantar aspect of the second metatarsophalangeal joint becomes attenuated and stretched out, and develops abnormal motion; creates synovitis; and allows the development of distal contractures (e.g., at the proximal interphalangeal joint) as the soft tissue balance is lost around the ray. The prototype of this process is rheumatoid arthritis, in which intense synovitis invades the joint and destroys it, and rapid dislocation follows. This is not, however, the disorder addressed here, which is more subtle in onset.

IDIOPATHIC SYNOVITIS OF THE SECOND METATARSOPHALANGEAL JOINT

Patients can present with pain around the second metatarsophalangeal joint that arises from a synovitis that is not caused by infection, seropositive or seronegative arthritis, or acute trauma.[4] Typically, pain occurs under the second metatarsal head, with some soft tissue swelling of the metatarsophalangeal joint itself. Often there is a mild sausage-shaped swelling of the second toe itself, with mild contracture of the proximal interphalangeal joint and slight hammering of the second toe. As the process continues, the soft tissues stretch around the second metatarsophalangeal joint, so that the volar plate destabilizes and the joint becomes loose and starts to sublux dorsally as the patient toes off in gait. This abnormal motion aggravates the synovitis and pain. Radiographic evidence is somewhat skimpy; weight-bearing views show a reduced joint, but there may be some mild narrowing of the joint space or fuzziness in the articular space secondary to the mild dorsiflexion of the proximal phalanx. A technetium bone scan is likely to show increased uptake, but it is not selectively diagnostic and is therefore a low-yield procedure.

Conservative treatment should be directed to relieving pressure around the sore joint. Shoes with wider toe boxes, rocker-bottom–type soles, and felt metatarsal supports are all standard ways to decompress the area. In addition, decreased activity may help, such as decreasing mileage for runners and fewer sets for tennis players. A simple toe-retainer elastic device that slips over the base of the toe to attach to a thin foam pad under the metatarsal head can reduce the upward force of toe-off and perhaps prevent further stretching of the soft tissues. These methods should be used for at least 3 to 6 months unless the pain and disability progress inexorably and require operative intervention.

What this problem requires in its early stages, before the joint is grossly unstable, is a synovectomy. This procedure is accom-

Copyright Francesca M. Thompson, M.D.

36

plished through a transverse dorsal capsulotomy by way of a dorsal skin incision, which is usually placed just lateral to the extensor tendon or hockey sticked or zig-zagged over it (Fig. 5–1). The collateral ligaments need to be divided transversely as well; then, with sharp and rongeur dissection, the inflamed synovium is débrided. Attention should be directed to the possibility that the interdigital nerve may have adhered to the inflamed capsule, and if the nerve has developed a Morton's neuroma, it should be resected proximal to the deep intermetatarsal ligament (see Chapter 11 on neuroma resection via a dorsal approach). When the problem is handled in this early stage, usually enough residual stability remains, so that there is no need to pin the joint with a Kirschner wire (K-wire). This approach has been found to be successful at least two-thirds of the time.[4] Interestingly, the pathologic findings in these cases confirm the idiopathic etiology of the process: all that is found is abundant, lush synovium; chronic synovitis; no granulomas; no rheumatoid nodules; and no infection. Perhaps these cases represent the earliest presentation of the subluxating toe.

THE SUBLUXATING TOE

As soft tissue supports erode and stretch around the second metatarsophalangeal joint, the volar plate structures lose their integrity, and the toe itself seems to be held on a longer leash, such that it subluxes dorsally during motion of the joint, having lost its inferior restraints. This is a subtle finding on physical examination and must be determined with a specific provocative test of vertical stress.[6]

On physical examination of the foot, it is routine to check the range of motion of the metatarsophalangeal joints by rolling them up and down in their normal path of motion. This is not the vertical stress test. The examiner must grasp the head of the metatarsal firmly with the thumb and index finger of one hand and then grasp the base of the proximal phalanx with the thumb and index finger of the other hand. As one hand holds the metatarsal head down firmly, the other hand is raised in a straight, vertical direction, while holding the proximal phalanx horizontally. The idea is to see if the soft tissues inferiorly are loose enough to allow the proximal phalanx to be translated straight dorsally, rather than cocked

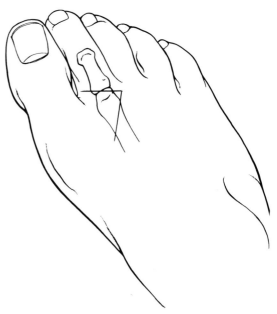

FIGURE 5–1. The dorsal approach to the metatarsophalangeal joint. A zig-zag incision provides access to both sides for division of the collateral ligaments without excessive retraction.

up in a dorsiflexed direction (Fig. 5–2). With experience, the examiner can grade the laxity encountered in this vertical stress test. Most often, the motion provoked elicits the pain the patient experiences in a way no other manipulation can. The examiner can also often feel the crepitation of the joint surfaces that are unstable. In addition, the examiner can classify the amount of dorsal displacement into grades 1, 2, and 3, which represent one-third to full uncovering of the metatarsal head, with the vertical stress test.

Initial conservative treatment of this problem is essentially similar to that described previously for synovitis. It is essential to attempt to strap the toe down to prevent further stretching of the soft tissues, particularly early in the disease process, when the vertical stress test results show grades at a 1 or 2 level. With continued strapping, it may be possible for the tissues to "scar in" and stabilize, in which case surgical intervention may not be required.

THE CROSSOVER TOE

The crossover toe is another variant on second toe instability.[1] Most of the patients in Coughlin's series were middle-aged (50 to 70

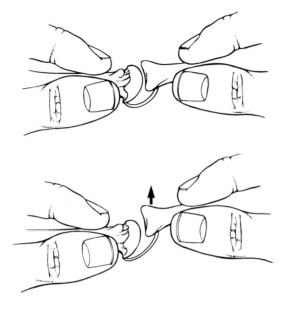

FIGURE 5–2. The vertical stress test for metatarsophalangeal subluxation. Note that this is *not* a test of dorsiflexion around the joint. The metatarsal head must be stabilized with one hand as the other hand exerts a straight vertical push while grasping the proximal phalanx. No vertical upward movement is a negative test result and indicates a normal volar plate (*top*). Upward vertical movement is a positive test result and indicates volar plate instability (*bottom*).

years old). Crossover toe can be insidious or abrupt in onset, with the second toe usually drifting medially and the patient experiencing pain in the lateral aspect of the second metatarsal head, in the area of the lateral collateral ligaments. On physical examination, the patient is tender to a varus stress directed against the lateral aspect of the second metatarsal head. In time, the inferior structures stretch out, and the toe starts to climb dorsally and to deviate more medially. It eventually comes to lie on top of the hallux, particularly when hallux valgus is a part of the patient's presentation, and this represents the full-blown crossover toe problem. When the problem is in this advanced stage, patients are most often distressed by crowding in the toe box of the shoe, with pain and pressure over the dorsum of the proximal interphalangeal joint, and women tend to be displeased by the cosmesis and the prominent dorsal bulge in their shoes.

Conservative management of this problem depends on the flexibility remaining at presentation. A reducible toe can be taped or strapped, whereas a rigidly elevated crossover

toe will have to be accommodated by an extra-depth toe box.

DISLOCATION OF THE SECOND METATARSOPHALANGEAL JOINT

The second metatarsophalangeal joint is the most commonly dislocated joint in the foot.[2] It is the end stage of the range of instabilities that have been discussed here, and it makes sense that a formerly located toe progresses in some way toward its final position of being bayoneted on the dorsum of the metatarsal head, with the proximal interphalangeal joint severely contracted and pressing upward into the toe box. Frequently there is painful callus under the uncovered metatarsal head. This condition is very often associated with hallux valgus, and correction of the hallux valgus is often required to allow room for reduction of the dislocated toe. Yet, at times, no hallux valgus is present, and the second joint dislocation is accompanied by a third joint dislocation as well.

Conservative management has fewer options because of toe stacking and difficulty in using ordinary shoewear. Extra-depth shoes with metatarsal felt supports to relieve metatarsal head pain, callus trimming, and molded Plastizote orthotics are the first line of defense; and in an elderly, low-demand patient with possible vascular compromise, conservative management is the preferred approach.

SURGICAL STABILIZATION OF THE SECOND METATARSOPHALANGEAL JOINT[3]

The goal of operative intervention in these variations of instability is to relieve pain by obtaining a reduced yet flexible joint. Ideally, vertical stress test results should be negative (see Fig. 5–2); the base of the proximal phalanx should articulate congruently with the metatarsal head; the tip of the toe should be able to touch the ground on weight bearing; and the metatarsophalangeal joint should be able to dorsiflex in its normal range at least as far as the hallux.

These goals are attained by analyzing the anatomic deformities in a stepwise fashion and by continuing the corrections until all deformities are reduced.

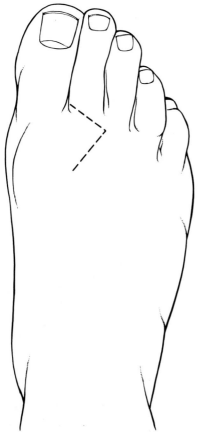

FIGURE 5–3. Operative stabilization of the second metatarsophalangeal joint; use a dorsal approach to release dorsal contractures. When the skin is very tight, a Z-plasty incision may be needed.

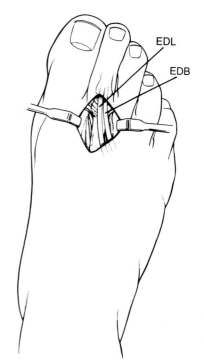

FIGURE 5–4. Note that the extensor digitorum brevis tendon (EDB) enters laterally; divide it. EDL, extensor digitorum longus tendon.

1. It is usually best to start with the contractures at the dorsum of the second metatarsophalangeal joint. Make a longitudinal or preferably a zig-zag incision over the extensor tendons (Fig. 5–3).

2. The short extensor enters laterally and may be divided (Fig. 5–4). The long extensor can be divided at this point or split longitudinally in a Z-plasty fashion for suture to appropriate length at the end of the correction (Fig. 5–5).

3. If the proximal phalanx is dorsiflexed, it is usually due to contracture at the dorsal capsule. Cut this transversely. Extend the cuts down to the collateral ligaments, which are generally contracted as well (Fig. 5–6).

4. Look inside the joint for synovitis and débride it.

5. Now manipulate the metatarsophalangeal joint with the vertical stress test. Is it stable? Is there a hammer toe?

6. If a hammer toe is present, it can be fixed by a resection arthroplasty, but the incision you make will depend on your decision to stabilize the laxity observed on the vertical

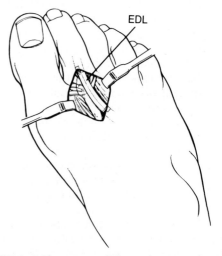

FIGURE 5–5. The extensor digitorum longus tendon (EDL) can be divided now or can be split longitudinally in a Z-plasty fashion for suture to an appropriate length at the end of the procedure (see Fig. 5–17).

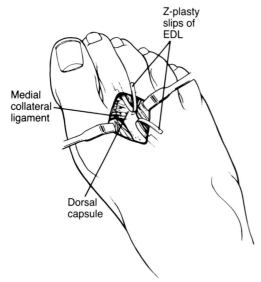

FIGURE 5–6. If the proximal phalanx is dorsiflexed, it is usually because of contracture at the dorsal capsule. Cut this transversely. Extend the cuts down through the collateral ligaments, which are generally contracted as well. EDL, extensor digitorum longus tendon.

stress test, perhaps with a flexor-to-extensor tendon transfer.

7. If you elect to perform a flexor-to-extensor transfer, make the incision on the plantar aspect of the toe first (Fig. 5–7). One choice is a transverse incision at the proximal volar crease of the toe, then a longitudinal incision along the tendon sheath of the flexor digitorum longus tendon along the proximal phalanx base, with another stab incision just distal to the distal interphalangeal joint, so that the flexor digitorum longus tendon is divided (Fig. 5–8) but the short flexor slips inserting onto the middle phalanx are preserved. Some surgeons like to make a longitudinal incision, either straight or zig-zagged along the plantar aspect of the toe, to make harvesting the flexor digitorum longus easier, but this incision is a large one to close at the end, and in combination with the exposure required dorsally on the same digit, may compromise healing.

8. Split the flexor digitorum longus tendon down its raphe (Fig. 5–9) and snap one tip with a straight hemostat and the other with a curved hemostat to differentiate the medial and lateral slips, in case they become twisted inadvertently during the course of the procedure (Fig. 5–10).

9. If the hammer toe needs to be resected because of a fixed flexion contracture, it should

be resected by the DuVries method, in which a dorsal ellipse of extensor retinaculum is removed over the head of the proximal phalanx (Fig. 5–11). The joint is then fully flexed, and the collateral ligaments are released sharply with a No. 6 blade until the entire head of the proximal phalanx is in the incision and can be removed transversely with a small bone cutter (Fig. 5–12).

10. The slips of the flexor digitorum longus must now be brought to the dorsal base of the toe. It may be necessary to extend the dorsal incision a bit distally and diagonally across the area where the tendon slips will be brought out dorsally. After this area has been exposed, it is vital that the track for passing the flexor digitorum longus tendon slips be placed directly on the periosteum of the phalanx, under the neurovascular structures. Usually it is easiest to pass an empty, small, curved hemostat from dorsal to plantar and then to grasp the flexor digitorum tendon slips on either side of the digit and pull each one up sequentially (Fig. 5–13).

11. After the tendons have been shifted (Fig. 5–14), the foot must be placed for optimal positioning of the tendon transfer. Place the ankle and foot plantigrade. Flex the toe about 20 degrees and suture the flexor digitorum slips to the extensor retinaculum (Fig. 5–

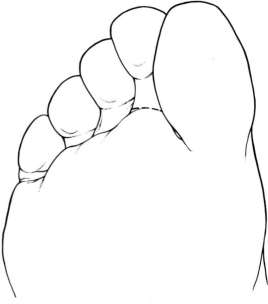

FIGURE 5–7. The flexor-to-extensor transfer requires a transverse skin incision at the proximal volar crease of the toe.

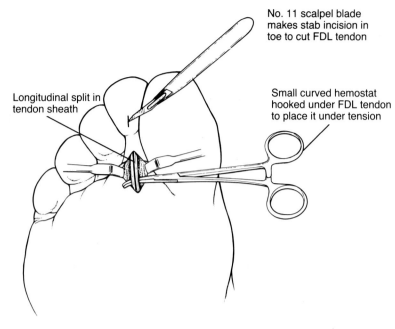

No. 11 scalpel blade makes stab incision in toe to cut FDL tendon

Longitudinal split in tendon sheath

Small curved hemostat hooked under FDL tendon to place it under tension

FIGURE 5–8. To harvest the flexor digitorum longus tendon (FDL), make a longitudinal split in the tendon sheath along the base of the proximal phalanx so that the tendon can be pulled into the wound with a small curved hemostat while the distal insertion is cut with a No. 11 blade stab wound into the distal pulp, avoiding transection of the flexor digitorum brevis tendons on the middle phalanx.

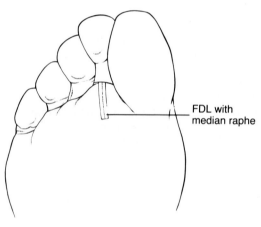

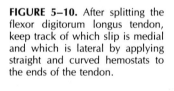

FDL with median raphe

FIGURE 5–9. Split the flexor digitorum longus tendon (FDL) along its raphe.

FIGURE 5–10. After splitting the flexor digitorum longus tendon, keep track of which slip is medial and which is lateral by applying straight and curved hemostats to the ends of the tendon.

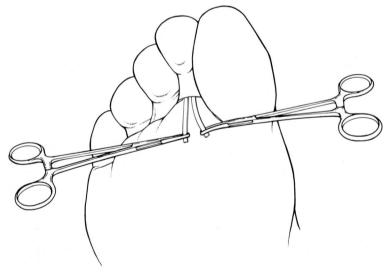

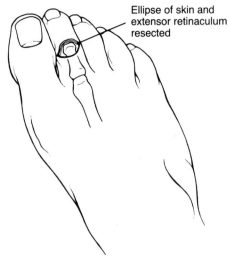

Ellipse of skin and
extensor retinaculum
resected

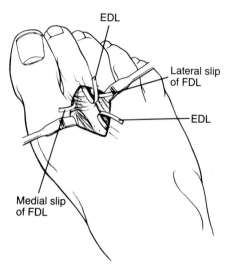

EDL

Lateral slip
of FDL

EDL

Medial slip
of FDL

FIGURE 5–11. If the hammer toe needs to be corrected because there is a fixed flexion contracture, it should be resected by the DuVries method (see Chapter 9). With this method, a dorsal ellipse of extensor retinaculum is removed over the head of the proximal phalanx, which is freed of soft tissue and removed transversely at the level of the distal diaphysis with a small bone cutter.

FIGURE 5–13. Going from dorsal to plantar, insert small curved hemostats closely against the bone to avoid trapping the neurovascular bundles and then bring the medial and lateral slips to the dorsum of the toe. EDL, extensor digitorum longus tendon; FDL, flexor digitorum longus tendon.

15) with colorless suture material, because the skin is thin and patients object to blue or black discoloration at the base of the toe. Although suturing the two slips to each other, rather

than to the extensor retinaculum, is a recognized method, some patients complain of a sense of a tight ring around the toe when this is done.

12. Now gently perform the vertical stress test. If the joint is stable, no further stabilization need be performed at this time. If there is a wildly positive result, you may need to reperform the flexor digitorum tendon slip fixation. If some relatively mild subluxation is present, it may be necessary to insert a K-wire across the metatarsophalangeal joint (Fig. 5–16). This is accomplished retrograde, by aiming the 0.062-inch K-wire into the articular

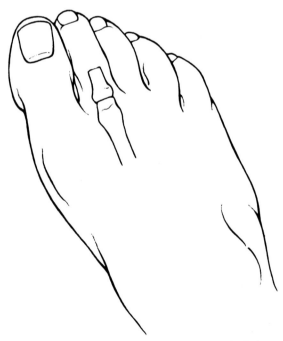

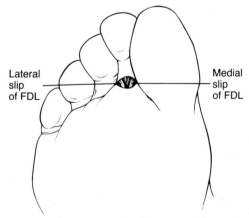

Lateral
slip
of FDL

Medial
slip
of FDL

FIGURE 5–12. The entire head of the proximal phalanx has been resected. It is important to resect all the metaphyseal bone to avoid recurrence.

FIGURE 5–14. The tendons have been passed from plantar to dorsal. FDL, flexor digitorum longus tendon.

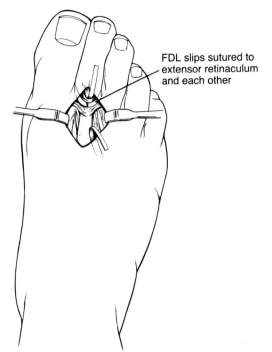

FIGURE 5–15. Hold the foot and ankle in a plantigrade position. Flex the toe about 20 degrees and suture the digitorum slips to the extensor retinaculum. FDL, flexor digitorum longus tendon.

surface of the base of the middle phalanx, out under the tip of the toenail, back down the shaft of the proximal phalanx, and then across the metatarsophalangeal joint into the metatarsal head and neck about 2 cm. The position of the toe should be slight plantar flexion and slight valgus, in keeping with the orientation of the other toes.

13. With the crossover toe deformity, stabilization requires rebalancing the loose lateral side and releasing the possibly contracted medial structures. Attempts can be made to suture the soft tissues to reef the lateral capsule. When the flexor digitorum longus tendon transfer is used, more pressure needs to be applied to the lateral slip to help in the rebalancing.

14. Dislocation of the metatarsophalangeal joint with bayoneting dorsally and dense plantar calluses requires more bony resection, as in the DuVries arthroplasty. After the soft tissue releases described previously have been performed, there may still be bony overlap that does not reduce after correction of the fixed hammer toe. In this case, the distal 2 mm of articular cartilage on the distal end of

the metatarsal head should be removed with a sharp osteotome and rounded with a rongeur. For the plantar callus, if the reduction of the dislocated proximal phalanx does not allow the second metatarsal head to reduce to the level of the others, the toe can then be plantarflexed 90 degrees and the plantar condyles can be removed. It is important to prevent the loss of the bony piece proximally by placing a skid under the metatarsal proximal to the resection. After the plantar condyle is osteotomized, it should be twisted to the side and removed from the area of the transected collateral ligaments.

15. After the DuVries arthroplasty, K-wire stabilization is required, as described earlier. What happens is that the previously contracted, shortened structures have been pulled out to some length and also shortened to some extent secondary to bony resection. It is imperative to observe the blood supply to the toe after release of the tourniquet. The operated toe is usually slow to lose its whiteness. Wait 15 minutes, and if color does not return to the toe, pull the K-wire.

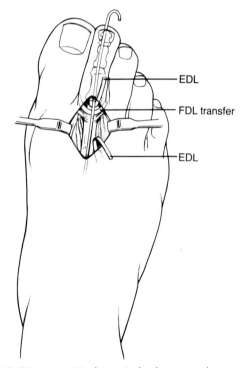

FIGURE 5–16. A Kirschner wire has been passed retrograde out of the middle phalanx and then back down the proximal phalanx and across the metatarsophalangeal joint. EDL, extensor digitorum longus tendon; FDL, flexor digitorum longus tendon.

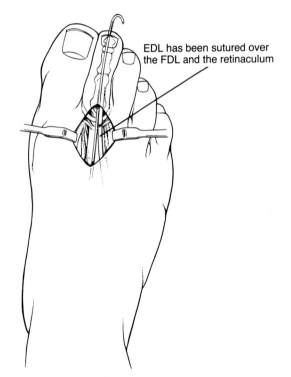

EDL has been sutured over the FDL and the retinaculum

FIGURE 5–17. The extensor digitorum longus tendon (EDL) has been sutured together at the appropriate length and tension. FDL, flexor digitorum longus tendon.

16. The extensor digitorum longus tendon is then repaired. Its length and tension are adjusted with the toe in the corrected position (Fig. 5–17).

POSTOPERATIVE MANAGEMENT

The patient is allowed to ambulate in a postoperative wooden-soled shoe with a bulky dressing. The postoperative dressing is changed in the first week. The foot is subsequently dressed with a 2-inch Kling dressing until the incisions heal, or as long as necessary to manage a concomitant hallux valgus correction.

The amount of time the K-wire is left in is evolving. Originally, it was left in 4 to 6 weeks, but this may lead to too much stiffness in dorsiflexion. The trend now is toward 2 to 3 weeks. After the pin is pulled, the proximal interphalangeal joint can be maintained in extension distally with adhesive taping but the metatarsophalangeal joint can be exercised by the patient into a dorsiflexed position. The goal is to achieve as much dorsiflexion in the second toe as in the hallux. Earlier motion seems to be important whether a soft tissue procedure only or the DuVries arthroplasty is done. Motion is controlled with a careful therapy program.

The patient also will need to manipulate the toe into plantar flexion as healing progresses so that the tip of the toe can be brought to touch the floor. Towel curling and "hanging ten" over a stair edge are useful methods for encouraging prehensile toe motion.

WHAT RESULTS SHOULD PATIENTS EXPECT?

Patients should expect improvement, but not perfection. A stable, flexible joint is the goal, and, it is hoped, patients will be closer to this goal at the end of recovery. However, patients must understand that they will not have a normal toe as it was before it was afflicted with synovitis, subluxation, crossing over, or dislocation. All of these events profoundly change the soft tissues, and the operative procedures described here are performed with the understanding that there will be loss of flexibility and motion.[5]

References

1. Coughlin MJ: Crossover second toe deformity. Foot Ankle 8:29–39, 1987.
2. DuVries HL: Dislocation of the toe. JAMA 160:728, 1956.
3. Mann RA, Coughlin MJ: Surgery of the Foot and Ankle, 6th Ed. St. Louis, CV Mosby, 1993.
4. Mann RA, Mizel MA: Monoarticular nontraumatic synovitis of the metatarsophalangeal joint: A new diagnosis. Foot Ankle 6:18–21, 1985.
5. Thompson FM, Deland JT: Flexor tendon transfer for metatarsophalangeal instability of the second toe: A critical review. American Orthopaedic Foot and Ankle Society Winter Meeting. Anaheim, CA, March 1991.
6. Thompson FM, Hamilton WG: Problems of the second metatarsophalangeal joint. Orthopedics 10:83–89, 1987.

6 *Sesamoiditis*

ROBERT B. ANDERSON

More than 50 percent of body weight is transmitted through the great toe complex, which includes the metatarsophalangeal joint and the tibial (medial) and fibular (lateral) sesamoid bones.[5] Disorders of the sesamoid bones can therefore occur with high-impact loading and repetitive stress. With consideration given to their plantar prominence and role in weight shift during gait, it is understandable why these relatively benign-appearing hallux sesamoid bones may contribute to significant patient disability.

ANATOMIC CONSIDERATIONS

The sesamoid bones derived their name from the ancient Greeks, who noted their resemblance to sesame seeds.[3] Although identified at multiple locations within the foot, the most constant of the sesamoid bones are those of the hallux metatarsophalangeal joint (Fig. 6–1). The larger and longer tibial sesamoid bone is slightly distal to the smaller and rounder fibular sesamoid bone. Both lie within the respective tendinous expansion of the medial and lateral heads of the flexor hallucis brevis muscle, and are held in close proximity to each other by an intersesamoidal ligament. The flexor hallucis longus tendon courses between the tibial and fibular sesamoid bones, plantar to the intersesamoidal ligament. The adductor hallucis and abductor hallucis tendons also contribute attachments to this plantar complex, developing a thick conjoined tendon inserting on the proximal phalanx distally.

Bipartite and multipartite tibial sesamoid bones occur in 10 to 33 percent of all feet. Multipartite sesamoids occur more frequently in females and are often bilateral. Partition and congenital absence of the fibular sesamoid bone is rare.[2]

The hallux sesamoid bones serve to dissipate impact forces to the first metatarsal head. In elevating the metatarsal head, they further increase the mechanical advantage of the flexor hallucis brevis tendon. Lastly, they provide protection for the flexor hallucis longus tendon and maintain the direction of its pull.

An unpaired sesamoid bone can arise at the hallux interphalangeal joint (see Fig. 6–1). This "subhallux sesamoid bone" occurs with a reported incidence of 5 to 58 percent, with a female predominance of 2.5:1. Bilateral involvement occurs in approximately 94 percent of this population.[1] The sesamoid bone lies within the plantar ligament of the interphalangeal joint and not within the substance of the flexor hallucis longus tendon. Typically, it is asymptomatic, and it may appear as an intractable plantar callus. In the diabetic patient, a mal perforans ulcer may occur secondary to the presence of this sesamoid bone.

CLASSIFICATION

A multiplicity of inflammatory disorders and acute injuries may occur within the hallux sesamoid bone. When one considers the repetitive forces transmitted through the metatarsophalangeal complex, as well as its delicately balanced and complex anatomic environment, this tendency for injuries is not surprising.

45

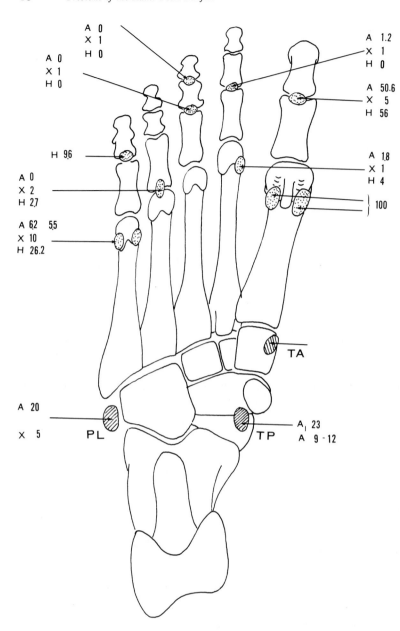

A 0
X 1
H 0

A 0
X 1
H 0

A 0
H 0

H 96

A 0
X 2
H 27

A 62   55
X 10
H 26.2

A 1.2
X 1
H 0

A 50.6
X 5
H 56

A 1.8
X 1
H 4

} 100

A 20

X 5

PL

TA

TP

A₁ 23
A 9 - 12

FIGURE 6–1. Sesamoids of the foot. Percentage of occurrence based on anatomic investigations (A), radiographic investigations (X), and histoembryologic investigations (H) in the literature. PL, os peroneum in the peroneus longus tendon in ossified form; TA, sesamoid in the tibialis anterior tendon; TP, sesamoid in the tibialis posterior tendon. (From Sarrafian SK: Anatomy of the Foot and Ankle: Descriptive, Topographic, Functional. Philadelphia, JB Lippincott, 1983, p 85.)

Sesamoiditis is a nonspecific term given to painful conditions that occur within the hallux sesamoid complex and that do not have accompanying radiographic changes. These conditions may include tendinitis of the flexor hallucis brevis or flexor hallucis longus, chondromalacia, or a synovitis of the metatarsophalangeal joint itself. These problems typically are related to inflammatory changes of repetitive stress and are not due to acute injury. Individuals with a rigid or cavus foot or with heel cord tightness are more often afflicted. Pain is elicited with direct palpation of the involved sesamoid bone. Symptoms can be reproduced with passive distal push of the sesamoid bone or passive dorsiflexion of the hallux itself. Rarely is erythema or swelling obvious to the examiner. Limited or painful range of motion of the metatarsophalangeal joint should raise suspicion of diffuse synovitis. Radiographs, including axial and oblique views of the sesamoid bone, are normal.

Osteochondritis is a rare condition of the sesamoid bone that occurs more frequently in young adult females and in the fibular sesamoid bone.[4] Although the clinical presentation is similar to that of sesamoiditis, progressive radiographic changes of sclerosis, fragmentation, and cyst formation do occur. Whether this condition represents a primary avascular event or is a late sequela to a stress phenomena or fracture is unknown.

Fractures of the sesamoid can occur from an acute event or may result insidiously from repetitive loading. As with most disorders of the sesamoid bone, the tibial sesamoid bone is more commonly injured because of its larger size and propensity to greater weight-bearing forces. Tenderness is demonstrable directly plantar to the involved sesamoid bone, and exacerbation of discomfort occurs with passive dorsiflexion of the hallux. A variable amount of swelling, erythema, and ecchymosis is present with acute fractures. Radiographs typically reveal a transverse fracture through the body of the sesamoid bone, although fractures occurring secondary to direct trauma may show variable comminution. An irregular contour to the fracture helps to differentiate it from a bipartite sesamoid bone, in which the contour of the bifurcation is smooth and is without sharp cortical edges. Nonunions of these fractures may occur and may remain symptomatic. Radiographic changes of cyst formation, fragmentation, and diastasis of the proximal and distal fragments have been reported.[5]

Hypertrophic changes within the sesamoid bone can occur and may appear with intra-articular or extra-articular involvement. The intra-articular variety is typically age related and may accompany diffuse arthritic conditions. The patient often presents with metatarsophalangeal joint pain and crepitance. Radiographs reveal osteophyte formation about the sesamoid bone and, in particular, from the distal pole. With the extra-articular condition, the bony hypertrophy will take the form of a plantar prominence, or "spur," which may result in an underlying intractable plantar keratosis. This particular disorder of the sesamoid bone can occur in either the tibial or the fibular sesamoid bone and is infrequently seen prior to the fifth decade of life.

Problems of the sesamoid bones are often difficult to distinguish from other problems of the hallux metatarsophalangeal joint. Although routine radiographs with sesamoid views for axial detail are important, ancillary studies are occasionally necessary. These studies may include a differential lidocaine block of the metatarsophalangeal joint to determine whether the symptoms are related to an intra-articular or extra-articular process. Although it is not diagnosis specific, a bone scan aids in identifying stress and traumatic fractures from bipartite sesamoid bones. Pinhole imaging is mandatory in localizing the uptake to the tibial or fibular sesamoid bone. Tomograms, in both anteroposterior and lateral planes, are helpful in obtaining fine detail of the sesamoid and are of particular value in assessing fracture union, tumors or cysts, and osteophyte formation. Computed tomography and magnetic resonance imaging have not been shown to be beneficial owing to the width of the imaging cuts. As improvements are made in the surface coils, magnetic resonance imaging may be of significant value, particularly in conditions without obvious radiographic abnormalities.

NONOPERATIVE TREATMENT

Other than for acute and stress fractures, the initial treatment for various sesamoid problems of the sesamoid bones is similar. Because weight bearing exacerbates the symptoms, a period of relative rest is in order. The hallux may be taped as it would for a turf toe condition, preventing painful dorsiflexion. Ice massage may be performed several times daily, and a course of nonsteroidal anti-inflammatory medications is recommended. Results of intra-articular cortisone injections are variable and run the risk of further ligament or tendon injury.

The most beneficial treatment, however, is shoe modification. Weight can be relieved from the symptomatic sesamoid with use of a semirigid orthosis. A well-molded medial longitudinal arch support with an extension under the lesser metatarsal heads achieves this goal. It is not recommended that the contact surface under the sesamoid bone be left free but rather filled with a viscoelastic polymer. A built-in J or C felt pad may be initially helpful, because this too alleviates some of the weight bearing in this region. However, this method often promotes further swelling and "window" edema within the surrounding tissue and complicates the current problem. The shoe itself may be modified with a lower heel, a more rigid sole, and a mild rocker bottom that aids in dissipating weight-bearing forces. A metatarsal bar may be applied to the sole in resistant cases.

For acute and stress fractures of the sesamoid bones, 4 to 6 weeks of immobilization in a short-leg walking cast is recommended. This cast should include a well-constructed platform that prevents hallux metatarsophalangeal joint motion. Thereafter, the sesamoid bone is provided with 6 weeks of protection using a semirigid orthosis with the goal of providing support proximal to the first metatarsal head and reducing the weight-bearing forces in the region of the fracture. Delayed union is considered at 4 months and nonunion at 6 months after the injury. Recalcitrant cases require surgical intervention.

In the event of an intractable plantar keratosis at either the metatarsophalangeal or interphalangeal level, appropriate padding or other weight-relieving appliances can be used. The diabetic patient must be observed closely because of the possibility of subsequent skin ulceration. In protracted cases involving the hallux sesamoid bone, shaving of the plantar spur can be considered. When hypertrophic changes of the sesamoid are more diffuse, sesamoidectomy may be necessary. For those recalcitrant cases at the interphalangeal joint that are secondary to a subhallux sesamoid bone, excision is recommended.

OPERATIVE TREATMENT

When an appropriate course of conservative therapy fails to relieve the symptoms and disability of a sesamoid condition, operative intervention is recommended. In most instances, sesamoidectomy is the procedure of choice. Although simple in theory, excision of the tibial or fibular sesamoid bone requires a thorough knowledge of the anatomy, appropriate anesthesia, and an adequate exposure of the surrounding soft tissue structures. In general, either sesamoid bone may be excised with reproducible good results. Excision of both sesamoid bones is avoided because of the risk of disrupting the distal insertion of the flexor hallucis brevis tendon, resulting in a cock-up deformity of the great toe.[4] Even with excision of a single sesamoid, meticulous repair of the defect is necessary to avoid imbalance of this ligamentous complex.

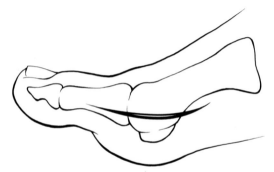

FIGURE 6–2. Skin incision placed slightly plantar to midline and centered at the eminence of the first metatarsal head.

Exposure of the Tibial Hallux Sesamoid Bone

A 5-cm skin incision extends from the metatarsal neck to the base of the proximal phalanx, maintaining a course slightly plantar to the midline (Fig. 6–2). The metatarsophalangeal joint capsule and abductor tendon are exposed with reflection of the plantar skin flap. Dissection of this skin flap plantarward is performed cautiously in order to avoid the plantar medial cutaneous nerve (Fig. 6–3).

In cases in which intra-articular exposure of the tibial sesamoid bone is required, a longitudinal incision divides the abductor tendon and the underlying capsule. Visualization of the sesamoid bone's articular surface and surrounding soft tissue structures is then easily achieved (Fig. 6–4).

When excision of the sesamoid is indicated, the bone can be "shelled out" using a Beaver blade or meniscotome. Dissection is performed directly on the bone in order to avoid creating an unmanageable defect within the plantar

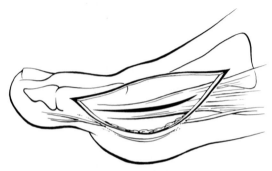

FIGURE 6–3. Capsule and abductor tendon identified. Plantar skin flap reflected, avoiding injury to the plantar medial cutaneous nerve.

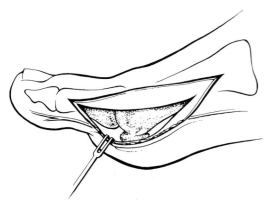

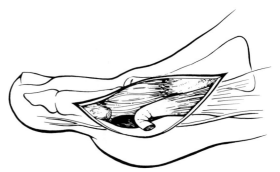

FIGURE 6–6. Transection and proximal mobilization of the abductor hallucis tendon for reconstruction of large defects following tibial hallux sesamoidectomy.

FIGURE 6–4. Intra-articular exposure of tibial sesamoid.

ligamentous complex, as well as to avoid injury to the adjacent flexor hallucis longus tendon.

Extra-articular exposure of the tibial sesamoid bone is facilitated best with upward traction applied to the plantar capsular flap using an Allis clamp (Fig. 6–5). Again, particular care is taken to avoid injuring the plantar medial cutaneous nerve. The sesamoid bone is palpated, and the overlying flexor hallucis brevis tendon and periosteum are incised longitudinally and are reflected.

Excision of the sesamoid bone may then be performed through this approach with the use of a Beaver blade. This exposure is also used for shaving of a plantar spur in cases of an intractable keratosis. Using an osteotome, the plantar half of the sesamoid bone may be resected, maintaining the integrity of the articular surface and the continuity of the ligamentous structure.

Following excision, the defect created within

this portion of the flexor hallucis brevis tendon is repaired primarily, typically with a 2–0 Vicryl suture. Primary repair should be performed with the hallux in a slightly plantar-flexed position. With comminuted fractures, fracture nonunions, and bipartite sesamoids, the defect can be large and may require reconstruction using the abductor hallucis tendon. The tendon is detached from its distal insertion on the capsule, is mobilized proximally to its musculotendinous junction, and is then redirected plantarward to the site of the defect (Fig. 6–6). No biomechanical problems have been encountered following this type of reconstruction.

Plantar Exposure of the Fibular Hallux Sesamoid

A 5-cm curvilinear plantar skin incision is fashioned just lateral to the large weight-bearing surface of the first metatarsal and medial to the palpable prominence of the second metatarsal head (Fig. 6–7).

The plantar lateral cutaneous nerve is identified in close approximation to the fibular sesamoid (Fig. 6–8). In conditions of an inflammatory nature, this nerve is often adherent to the overlying flexor hallucis brevis tendon. Mobilization of the nerve, and occasionally neurolysis, is indicated.

The flexor hallucis brevis muscle and periosteum overlying the sesamoid bone are divided longitudinally and are reflected. The sesamoid bone is excised, and because the defect is typically small, it can be managed with primary side-to-side closure. This closure is performed with the hallux in a slightly plan-

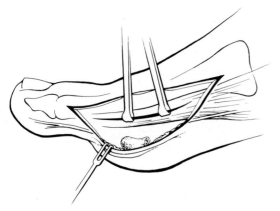

FIGURE 6–5. Extra-articular exposure of tibial sesamoid with flexor hallucis brevis tendon and periosteum reflected.

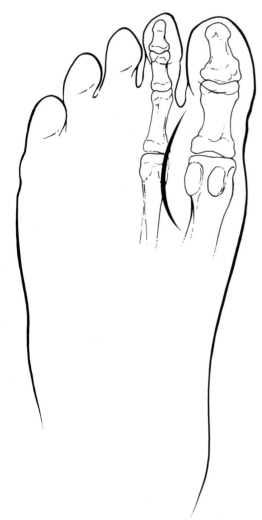

Dorsal Exposure of the Fibular Hallux Sesamoid

Dorsal exposure has limited applications in that it is indicated only if the fibular sesamoid has been displaced into the first web space. When this occurs, the sesamoid is rarely symptomatic.

A 4-cm longitudinal skin incision is made on the dorsum of the first web space and is extended proximally to the level of the metatarsal neck.

Blunt subcutaneous dissection is performed, and the first intermetatarsal space is enlarged with appropriate placement of a laminar spreader or neuroma retractor. The adductor tendon is identified and is partially detached

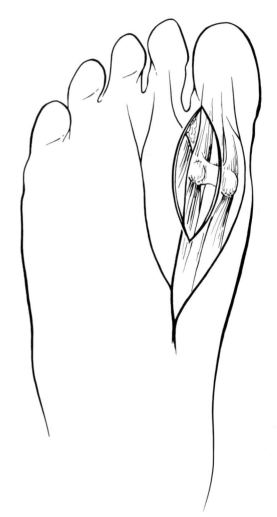

FIGURE 6–7. Curvilinear skin incision carefully positioned between weight-bearing surfaces of the first and second metatarsal heads.

tarflexed position. Proximal-to-distal closure of the defect and valgus posturing of the toe should be avoided for fear of disrupting the balance of the ligamentous complex about the metatarsophalangeal joint.

Although it is rarely symptomatic, a plantar spur of the fibular sesamoid bone is approached in a similar fashion. Shaving of the plantar half of this bony prominence is performed in the same manner as that described for the tibial sesamoid bone previously.

As with all plantar skin incisions, attention is given to meticulous reapproximation of the skin edges. Care is taken to avoid inversion or excessive eversion of the skin edge, which may result in painful or excessive scar formation.

FIGURE 6–8. Fibular sesamoid bone in close proximity to plantar lateral cutaneous nerve.

from its proximal insertion into the lateral joint capsule (Fig. 6–9).

The fibular sesamoid bone is identified, and the adductor tendon is detached from its lateral aspect. The sesamoid bone can then be secured with the use of a towel clip, and the remaining soft tissue attachments are transected. Dissection should be performed close to the bone surface in order to avoid injuring underlying neurovascular structures.

When most of the adductor tendon is detached during the sesamoid excision, reapproximation into the tissues on the base of the proximal phalanx is recommended.

Defects within the flexor hallucis brevis tendon created by excision of the sesamoid bone are very difficult to repair owing to limited exposure. Because the adductor and interosseous tendons are fairly mobile, closure of large defects may be performed with surrounding soft tissues.

Excision of the Subhallux Sesamoid

A 4-cm medial longitudinal skin incision is centered at the interphalangeal joint of the hallux.

Subcutaneous reflection of the skin flap plantarward identifies the flexor hallucis longus tendon. The tendon is divided longitudinally within its raphe, just proximal to its insertion into the distal phalanx. With careful reflection, the subhallux sesamoid bone is identified within the plantar ligament of this interphalangeal joint.

Excision is performed using a Beaver blade, with care taken to avoid transection of the flexor hallucis tendon. The tendon is subsequently reapproximated with an absorbable suture.

Author's Preferred Method

The surgical approach for excision of the tibial hallux sesamoid bone is fairly standard and options are few. The intra-articular approach is preferred because it provides direct assessment of the metatarsophalangeal joint as well as the sesamoid bone. A diffuse synovitis can be appreciated. With excision of the intra-articular sesamoid bone, one avoids the risk of injury to the plantar medial cutaneous nerve that is possible with an extra-articular expo-

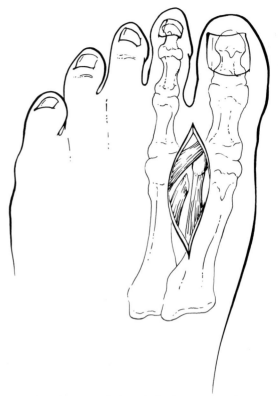

FIGURE 6–9. Approach through first intermetatarsal space. Sesamoid exposure following partial release of the adductor hallucis tendon.

sure. No matter which approach is used, meticulous repair of the resulting defect is recommended.

The selection of a surgical approach to the fibular hallux sesamoid bone is much more controversial. I have avoided the dorsal approach for two reasons. First, it involves significant dissection and release of the adductor tendon. Second, resulting defects are difficult to visualize and repair. This dorsal approach would be most useful when the sesamoid is laterally displaced into the first web space. However, this scenario is rarely symptomatic. In cases in which the fibular sesamoid bone remains reduced within the sulcus of the first metatarsal head, a plantar approach has been used with good success. It not only provides direct access to the sesamoid but avoids needless injury to a normal adductor tendon. This plantar approach is similarly recommended when preoperative evaluation elicits a positive Tinel sign or other evidence of possible injury to the plantar lateral cutaneous nerve. Not only may neurolysis be easily performed with this approach, but the nerve may be generously mobilized in a lateral direction, into the intermetatarsal space, thereby avoiding postoperative scar formation and weight-bearing forces. I have encountered no wound-healing problems with this plantar approach as long as the incision is placed between the prominences of the first and second metatarsal heads.

Postoperative Management

For all procedures involving the subhallux or hallux sesamoid bones, a similar postoperative regimen is followed. The skin incision is reapproximated with interrupted sutures, or subcuticular closure with Steri-Strips when off the weight-bearing surface. A compression dressing is applied, and the foot is placed into a plaster splint, protecting the hallux from dorsiflexion stress. Non–weight bearing is recommended for 2 weeks. The foot is then placed into a postoperative wooden shoe. It is preferred that this shoe have a mild rocker bottom for dissipation of weight-bearing forces. Ambulation is encouraged within this postoperative shoe for a period of 2 weeks. Thereafter, the patient progresses to unlimited activity in a shoe with a semirigid sole and mild rocker bottom. A well-constructed athletic shoe typically fills this requirement. In cases of sesamoidectomy in which large defects require reconstruction, the use of a short-leg cast immobilizing the hallux is recommended during this period. At 6 weeks after the operation, no restrictions are given to activity or shoewear. The patient may experience slight but permanent loss of motion within the metatarsophalangeal joint, particularly to dorsiflexion. Although this loss of motion is seldom disabling, it may prove frustrating to the professional athlete, particularly ballet dancers, and to those patients insistent upon the wear of high-heeled shoes. The patient should be well informed of this potential loss preoperatively.

Complications

Although complications following excision of the sesamoid bone are not common, they can occur when one fails to understand the intricacy of this plantar ligamentous complex. The sesmoid bones lie in delicate balance within a complex anatomic environment.

When this balance is disrupted, vector forces within the flexor hallucis brevis and flexor halllucis longus tendons can change. This change may lead to a progressive and permanent deformity.

As stated previously, clawing of the great toe can occur with disruption of the distal attachment of the flexor hallucis brevis tendon.[2,4] This deformity can result from excision of both the tibial and fibular sesamoid bones. The deformity may occur after simultaneous excision, or it may occur when an excision of a sesamoid bone follows another by even an interval of several years. Disability occurs not only from dorsal corns and damaging shoewear but also from loss of push-off strength as well. Salvage of this particular deformity typically requires an arthrodesis of the hallux metatarsophalangeal joint.

Hallux varus may occur following fibular sesamoidectomy and has been reported in previous reviews of the original McBride bunion procedure.[2,6] With disruption of the lateral head of the flexor hallucis brevis tendon, the medial head with its tibial hallux sesamoid bone rotates with the adjoining abductor hallucis tendon to a supinated position. The flexor hallucis longus tendon then shifts medially. It remains taut and may lead to a dynamic hallux varus with an intrinsic imbalance that may further result in clawing. This complication can be managed with an extensor hallucis longus tendon reconstruction and interphalangeal fusion as described by Johnson.[7]

In a similar situation, a mild preoperative hallux valgus may progress following excision of the tibial sesamoid bone. In an effort to avoid these hallux malalignments, it is imperative that the defect within the flexor hallucis brevis tendon following sesamoidectomy be meticulously repaired. The abductor or adductor hallucis tendon may be used for reconstruction if the defect is excessive. An adequate period of postoperative immobilization is then required for adequate ligamentous healing.

One of the more disabling complications that may result from sesamoid surgery is that of injury to the plantar cutaneous nerves. These nerves, and particularly the plantar medial cutaneous nerve, may be inadvertently transected or contused with overzealous retraction of the plantar skin flap, or may be caught in a closing suture. Painful weight bearing may ensue with hypesthesia in the distal hallux. A positive Tinel sign can be demonstrated, and the diagnosis is further substantiated with a selective lidocaine block. Should peripheral nerve blocks and desensitization exercises fail to provide adequate relief of the patient's symptoms, surgical re-exploration is recommended. The involved nerve is identified, transected at a more proximal level, and diverted into a non–weight-bearing area.

References

1. Berquist TH: Radiology of the Foot and Ankle. New York, Raven Press, 1989, pp 390–393.
2. Jahss MH: The sesamoids of the hallux. Clin Orthop 57:88–97, 1981.
3. Helal B: The great toe sesamoid bones: The lus or lost souls of Ushaia. Clin Orthop 157:82–87, 1981.
4. Mann RA: Surgery of the Foot. St. Louis, CV Mosby, 1986, pp 213–220.
5. McBryde AM, Anderson RB: Sesamoid foot problems in the athlete. Clin Sports Med 7:51–60, 1988.
6. Turner RS: Dynamic post-surgical hallux varus after lateral sesamoidectomy: Treatment and prevention. Orthopaedics 9:963–969, 1986.
7. Johnson KA, Spiegl PV: Extensor hallucis longus transfer for hallux varus deformity. J Bone Joint Surg 66A:681–686, 1984.

7 The Bunionette Deformity: Etiology and Treatment

MICHAEL J. COUGHLIN

The bunionette is characterized by a prominence of the lateral condyle of the fifth metatarsal head. Chronic irritation of the overlying bursa[9] and the development of a thickened callus on the plantar-lateral,[18] or the lateral aspect[20, 26] of the fifth metatarsal head may result from friction between the underlying

---

This chapter is an adaptation of material published in Mann RA, Coughlin MJ: Keratotic disorders of the plantar skin. *In* Mann RA, Coughlin MJ (Eds): Surgery of the Foot and Ankle, 6th Ed. St. Louis, Mosby–Year Book, 1993, pp 413–463. Reprinted with permission of the publisher.

bony abnormality and constricting footwear.[13] The fifth toe deviates in a medial direction at the metatarsophalangeal joint, and the magnitude of this measurement is termed the metatarsophalangeal-5 angle (Fig. 7–1). Kelikian[23] described the prominent lateral condyle of the fifth metatarsal bone as being "analogous to the medial eminence of the first metatarsal head" in a hallux valgus deformity. Although symptoms are often isolated to the metatarsal head region, it appears that several anatomic variations in the fifth metatarsal may lead to a symptomatic bunionette deformity.[13, 15, 26, 43] It is important to recognize the specific charac-

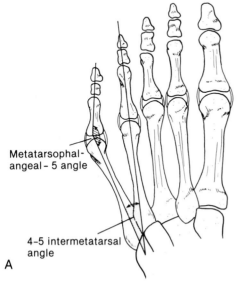
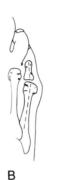
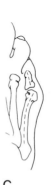
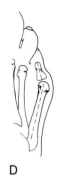

Metatarsophal-
angeal – 5 angle

4–5 intermetatarsal
angle

A
B
C
D

FIGURE 7–1. *(A),* The fifth metatarsophalangeal joint angle; the 4–5 intermetatarsal angle. *(B),* Bunionette due to a prominent fifth metatarsal condyle. *(C),* Angulation at the distal fifth metatarsal, causing prominence. *(D),* Splay or increased 4–5 metatarsal angulation, resulting in the bunionette deformity. *(A* and *C* from Mann RA, Coughlin MJ: The Video Textbook of Foot and Ankle Surgery. Medical Video Productions, St. Louis, 1991; *B* and *D* from Mann RA, Coughlin MJ: Surgery of the Foot and Ankle, 6th Ed. St. Louis, Mosby–Year Book, 1993, pp 442–443.)

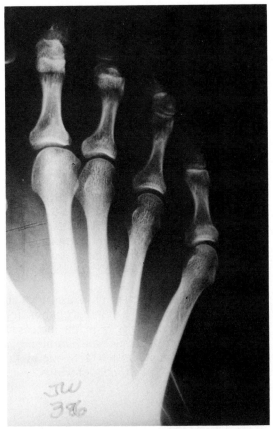

FIGURE 7–2. Splay or increased divergence of the entire fifth metatarsal. (From Mann RA, Coughlin MJ: Surgery of the Foot and Ankle, 6th Ed. St. Louis, Mosby–Year Book, 1993, p 442.)

teristics of this abnormality because it may significantly influence the choice of surgical correction.

A prominent fifth metatarsal head may be caused by divergence of the fourth and fifth metatarsals.[2, 11, 22, 26] The "4–5 intermetatarsal angle" defines the magnitude of this divergence (Fig. 7–2). It is quantified by measuring the angle of two lines that bisect the base and neck of the respective fourth and fifth metatarsal bones.[35] Fallat and Bucholz[15] reported that the 4–5 intermetatarsal angle averaged 6.2 degrees in normal subjects (range, 3 to 11 degrees). The 4–5 intermetatarsal angle averaged 9.6 degrees (range, 5 to 14 degrees) in patients with a symptomatic bunionette deformity. It is generally believed that an intermetatarsal angle greater than 8 degrees is abnormal, although a concurrent bunionette deformity may be asymptomatic and require no treatment. A prominence of the lateral condyle of the fifth metatarsal head can be

caused by lateral bowing in the diaphysis of the fifth metatarsal (Fig. 7–3).[6, 13–15, 31, 43] Although the proximal fourth and fifth metatarsals maintain a normal intermetatarsal alignment, a lateral diaphyseal angulation leads to prominence of the fibular condyle.[6, 14, 15, 31, 43]

An enlarged fifth metatarsal head (Fig. 7–4) may also be symptomatic.[6, 13, 15, 38] This may be due to actual hypertrophy of the lateral condyle. Fallat and Bucholz[15] and Throckmorton and Bradlee[39] found that with pes planus, the lateral plantar tubercle of the fifth metatarsal rotates to a more lateral position. Fallat and Bucholz[15] questioned whether or not hypertrophy of the fifth metatarsal head occurred. They hypothesized that with a pronated foot, the radiographic appearance of the fifth ray is comparable to that seen with "hypertrophy" of the fifth metatarsal head. The association of pes planus[15, 18, 20, 39] with bunionette formation supports this concept. Diebold and Bejjani[12] found that two-thirds of the patients in their series had significant cases of pes planus. Fallat and Bucholz[15] noted that with pes planus, the 4–5 intermetatarsal angle

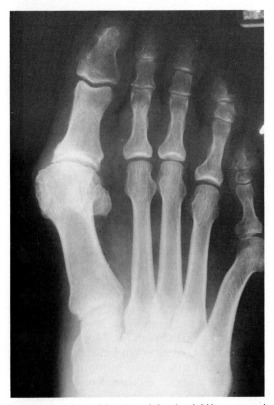

FIGURE 7–3. Lateral bowing of the distal fifth metatarsal. (From Mann RA, Coughlin MJ: Surgery of the Foot and Ankle, 6th Ed. St. Louis, Mosby–Year Book, 1993, p 443.)

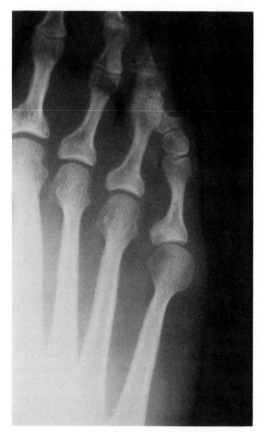

FIGURE 7–4. Enlargement or prominence of the fifth metatarsal condyle. (From Mann RA, Coughlin MJ: The Video Textbook of Foot and Ankle Surgery. Medical Video Productions, St. Louis, 1991.)

increased an average of 3 degrees. Regardless of whether the actual etiology is due to hypertrophy of the fifth metatarsal head or due to fifth metatarsal pronation, prominence of the fifth metatarsal lateral condyle can lead to painful symptoms without deviation or divergence of the fifth metatarsal bone.

Kitaoka and associates[25] reported that an increase in the 4–5 intermetatarsal angle was the most frequently associated metatarsal abnormality in patients with symptomatic bunionettes. Enlargement of the fifth metatarsal head and fifth metatarsal lateral deviation actually occurred in less than 10 percent of the symptomatic patients in their series.

Regardless of the underlying metatarsal anatomy and orientation of the fifth metatarsophalangeal joint, increased pressure develops over the fifth metatarsal head because of constricting footwear.[13, 37] The high frequency of occurrence of a bunionette deformity in the female population[26] is most likely due to the

predilection in this population for high fashion footwear. With time and chronic pressure, a thickened bursa and hypertrophic keratosis may develop, leading to a progressively symptomatic bunionette deformity.

PHYSICAL EXAMINATION

Physical findings may include an inflamed lateral bursa,[18, 38, 39] which may be associated with a lateral,[12] a plantar,[12, 18, 26] or combined plantar-lateral keratotic lesion.[12, 20] Diebold and Bejjani[12] reported that one-half of their patients had a pure lateral keratotic lesion, whereas one-third had a pure plantar lesion. The decision-making process regarding specific surgical repair for a symptomatic bunionette depends to a large extent on the location of the keratotic lesion.

Although a bunionette may occur as an isolated deformity,[12] it is not uncommon for a hallux valgus deformity with an increased 1–2 intermetatarsal angle and bunionette formation with an increased 4–5 intermetatarsal angle (a "splayfoot deformity") to occur.[3, 9, 11, 18, 22, 37]

CONSERVATIVE CARE

Symptoms are frequently aggravated by shoes that place pressure on a prominent fifth metatarsal head. Davies[9] stated that "rarely do these cases require active treatment other than provision of well-fitting shoes." The recognition that constricting footwear leads to pain and swelling over a bunionette has led to recommendation of roomy footwear as a means to relieve discomfort.[9, 11, 23, 26, 31, 38] Leach and Igou[26] and Mann[31] advocated padding the prominent fifth metatarsal, and Leach and Igou[26] also recommended shaving or paring of any prominent callus to relieve symptoms. Although conservative treatment is effective in a significant number of patients,* with the development of chronic soft tissue thickening and keratoses, surgical intervention may be necessary.

SURGICAL TREATMENT

A variety of operative approaches have been used to correct a bunionette deformity, includ-

_____

*See references 9, 11, 23, 26, 31, 33, and 38.

ing lateral condylectomy,[11, 13, 17, 28, 32, 38] metatarsal head resection,[23, 33] ray resection,[4] distal metatarsal osteotomy,* diaphyseal midshaft metatarsal osteotomy,[6, 16, 31, 41] and proximal metatarsal osteotomy.[3, 12, 15, 20, 29, 34] Although correction of the underlying pathology is necessary to prevent recurrence, preservation of the fifth metatarsophalangeal joint function is important. Postoperative complications such as recurrence,[23] transfer lesion formation,[22] subluxation, and dislocation[31] are not uncommon. Careful evaluation of the pathology and meticulous surgical technique may help to minimize the development of such complications.

Lateral Condylectomy

Resection of the lateral metatarsal condyle has been used to treat the symptomatic bunionette.† In the presence of an isolated prominent lateral fifth metatarsal condyle without lateral deviation of the fifth metatarsal shaft or a significant increase in the 4–5 intermetatarsal angle, a lateral condylectomy may be effective treatment.[31] Pronation of the fifth ray, or pes planus, is not necessarily a contraindication to lateral condylectomy if the prominent fifth metatarsal head is the only significant deformity present.

Technique

A lateral longitudinal incision is centered over the metatarsal head. Careful dissection is necessary to protect the dorsal and plantar sensory nerves of the fifth toe. The dissection is carried down directly to the capsule, and then the soft tissue is reflected off of the metatarsal head. The neurovascular bundles are protected in the dorsal and plantar soft tissue flaps. Various capsular incisions have been advocated with lateral condylectomy, however, an inverted L capsular incision allows adequate exposure (Fig. 7–5A). The capsule is released along the dorsal and proximal margins of the metatarsal head. A sagittal saw or small osteotome is used to resect the lateral condyle in a line parallel with the fifth metatarsal shaft (Fig. 7–5B). With distal traction placed on the fifth toe, the metatarsophalangeal joint is distracted and an intra-articular

medial capsular release is performed (Fig. 7–5C). The fifth toe is then realigned by reefing of the lateral capsule. Proximally, the capsule is repaired to the abductor digiti quinti muscle and metaphyseal periosteum (Fig. 7–5D). On the dorsal aspect, there is usually soft tissue with which to repair the capsule. On the dorsal proximal apex of the capsular release, there may be insufficient tissue present to reattach the capsule. Interrupted sutures may be secured through drill holes in the metaphysis of the fifth metatarsal bone in order to stabilize the repair.

Postoperatively, the toe is maintained in appropriate alignment in a gauze and tape dressing for 6 weeks. The patient ambulates in a wooden-soled shoe and, later, in an open-toed sandal.

Postoperative Complications

Unfortunately, although this procedure has been frequently recommended,* only anecdotal reports have been published. Postoperative complications include recurrence of the bunionette deformity (Fig. 7–5E and F),† subluxation and dislocation of the metatarsophalangeal joint,[20, 31, 37] and a poor weight-bearing pattern postoperatively following excessive resection.[26] Kaplan and colleagues[20] recommended meticulous repair of the abductor digiti quinti tendinous insertion and believed that this might diminish the incidence of later subluxation and dislocation of the metatarsophalangeal joint.

Preoperative radiographic evaluation of a bunionette deformity is very important. When divergence of the fifth metatarsal shaft occurs because of an increased 4–5 intermetatarsal angle or lateral deviation of the distal fifth metatarsal shaft, a condylectomy does not effectively correct the deformity. In the presence of a widened 4–5 intermetatarsal angle, a fifth metatarsal osteotomy is necessary.[29] The significant recurrence rate of a bunionette deformity following a lateral condylectomy is in large part due to the use of a condylectomy when the use of a metatarsal osteotomy is preferable. Kelikian[23] observed that a lateral condylectomy is at best "a temporizing measure like a simple exostectomy on the medial side of the foot; in time deformity will recur." When only an enlarged lateral condyle is

*See references 18, 19, 20, 22, 24, 26, and 37.
†See references 9, 11, 13, 17, 28, 31, 32, and 38.

*See references 9, 11, 13, 17, 28, 31, 33, and 38.
†See references 18, 23, 26, 28, 33, 37, and 43.

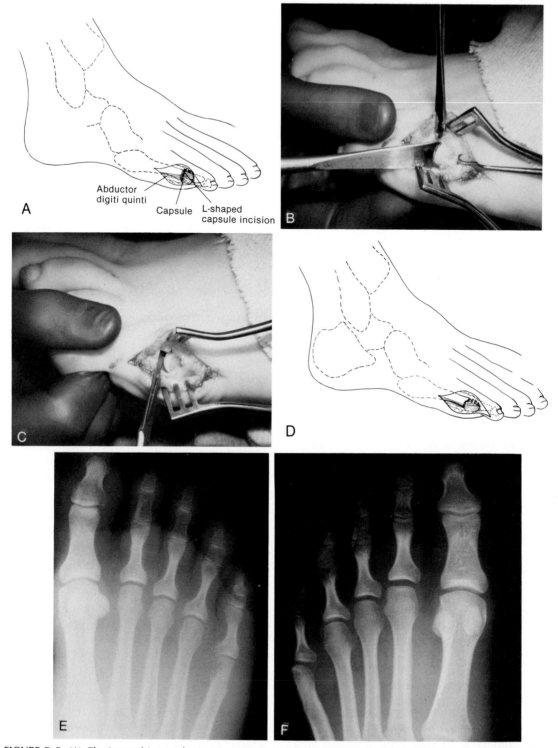

FIGURE 7–5. *(A),* The inverted L capsular incision. *(B),* Removal of the lateral condyle in line with the metatarsal shaft. *(C),* The intra-articular medial capsular release. *(D),* Capsular repair (see text). *(E),* An apparently well-corrected bunionette. *(F),* Recurrence of the bunionette with subluxation of the joint. *(A to D* from Mann RA, Coughlin MJ: The Video Textbook of Foot and Ankle Surgery. Medical Video Productions, St. Louis, 1991; *E* and *F* from Mann RA, Coughlin MJ: Surgery of the Foot and Ankle, 6th Ed. St. Louis, Mosby–Year Book, 1993, pp 447–448.)

present, a condylectomy may be an adequate repair.

Metatarsal Head Excision

Because of the high failure rate of lateral condylectomy in the treatment of the bunionette deformity, more extensive fifth metatarsal resection procedures have been advocated. Fifth metatarsal head resection[42] as well as resection of the fifth metatarsal head and a portion of the lateral base of the proximal phalanx[2] has been recommended. McKeever[33] resected the fifth metatarsal head and a portion of the metatarsal diaphysis, whereas Brown[4] resected the entire fifth ray and amputated the fifth toe. Kelikian[23] favored McKeever's technique but syndactylized the fourth and fifth toes.

Technique

A lateral longitudinal incision is centered directly over the lateral eminence. In the presence of ulceration beneath the fifth metatarsal head (i.e., diabetic trophic ulceration) in which

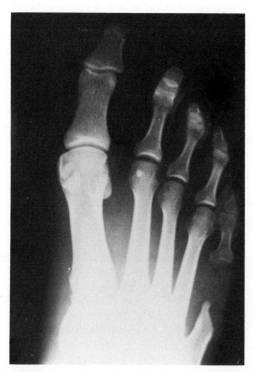

FIGURE 7–6. Resection of the fifth metatarsal head (see text). (Courtesy of Michael J. Coughlin, M.D.)

a fifth metatarsal head excision is contemplated, a dorsal incision may be used.

In rheumatoid arthritis, in which the resection of multiple metatarsal heads is contemplated, an incision may be placed in the fourth interspace to allow access to both the fourth and fifth metatarsal heads. In resecting the fifth metatarsal head, the capsule is released and the fifth metatarsal head is exposed. A small bone cutter is used to transect the fifth metatarsal shaft in the metaphyseal region, and a rongeur is used to bevel any sharp edges (Fig. 7–6). An intermedullary 0.045-inch Kirschner wire is used to align the metatarsal bone and the toe; however, in the presence of infection, hardware is contraindicated. The intramedullary wire is usually retained for 4 weeks postoperatively. The capsule and skin are loosely approximated and a gauze-and-tape dressing is applied for postoperative compression. The Kirschner wire is removed 4 to 6 weeks following surgery. Ambulation is allowed in a wooden-soled shoe, and following removal of internal fixation, the toe is taped in appropriate alignment for 4 to 6 weeks more.

Postoperative Complications

Metatarsal head resection may be associated with retraction of the fifth toe,[26] development of intractable plantar keratotic transfer lesions beneath the fourth metatarsal head,[26] and subluxation of the fifth toe.[20]

Ray resection and fifth metatarsal head excision are both salvage procedures that should be reserved for severe deformity, deformity with rheumatoid arthritis (in which several metatarsal head resections have been performed), intractable ulceration, and for the treatment of recurrent deformity that is complicated by significant soft tissue contracture. In general, it is preferable to use less radical procedures that maintain fifth toe function.

Fifth Metatarsal Osteotomy

An osteotomy of the fifth metatarsal may be used to correct deviation or lateral angulation of the fifth metatarsal. Davies[9] stated that it was "unnecessary and unsatisfactory" to perform a fifth metatarsal osteotomy. LeLievre,[29] on the other hand, recognized that an increased 4–5 intermetatarsal angle should be corrected as part of a bunionette repair.

Kelikian[23] cautioned that delayed healing may occur with a fifth metatarsal osteotomy; however the location of the osteotomy and the surgical technique performed has a profound effect on the ultimate success rate. Distal, midshaft diaphyseal, and proximal metatarsal osteotomies have been used in the treatment of the bunionette deformity.

Several types of distal fifth metatarsal osteotomies have been performed. Although it achieves less correction of a widened 4–5 intermetatarsal angle than a more proximal osteotomy, a distal metatarsal osteotomy achieves significantly more correction than a lateral condylectomy. Some types of distal osteotomies are relatively unstable, and this factor has led to a concern regarding postoperative recurrence of deformity,[22] loss of alignment,[20] and the possibility of the development of a transfer plantar keratotic lesion.

Midshaft diaphyseal osteotomy allows a greater degree of correction than has been reported with a distal metatarsal osteotomy. Osteotomies in this region do not appear to threaten the more tenuous proximal metatarsal vascular supply. When internally fixed, this procedure appears to offer a stable correction that has a minimal risk of transfer lesion development.[6]

A proximal fifth metatarsal osteotomy is inviting in that it achieves correction at the site of the deformity. Recent information[36] regarding the circulation to the proximal fifth metatarsal may make this choice less optimal.

Distal Metatarsal Osteotomy

The distal fifth metatarsal osteotomy was initially described by Hohmann.[19] Kaplan and associates[20] used a closing wedge distal metatarsal osteotomy that was internally fixed with a Kirschner wire. They recommended internal fixation in order to prevent rotation with resultant loss of correction of a distal metatarsal osteotomy. Haber and Kraft[18] recommended a distal crescentic osteotomy. They did not internally fix the osteotomy site and reported both delayed healing and excessive callus formation. Throckmorton and Bradlee[39] performed a transverse chevron osteotomy in the fifth metatarsal metaphysis. Although no internal fixation was used, they relied on the intrinsic stability of the chevron osteotomy to maintain alignment. They stressed that this

procedure was not effective in correcting a bunionette deformity with a plantar keratosis.

Sponsel[37] performed an oblique distal osteotomy and allowed the distal fragment to float without internal fixation. An 11-percent delayed union rate was reported.

Keating and coworkers[22] also performed a distal oblique osteotomy. They did not internally fix the osteotomy site. Transfer lesions developed in 75 percent of patients, and a 12-percent recurrence rate was reported. Keating and associates[22] attributed the development of transfer lesions and recurrent lesions to dorsiflexion and medial displacement of the capital fragment following this distal osteotomy. Their overall success rate was 56 percent. Diebold and Bejjani[12] cautioned that the results of distal fifth metatarsal osteotomies are often unsatisfactory because of the difficulty in achieving adequate fixation of the osteotomy in the metaphyseal region of the fifth metatarsal.

Although Sponsel[37] attempted a distal "Mitchell-type" osteotomy without success, Leach and Igou[26] performed a "reverse" Mitchell procedure on 11 feet. They reported an average preoperative 4–5 intermetatarsal angle of 11.7 degrees and a postoperative 4–5 intermetatarsal angle of 4.9 degrees, achieving a 6.8-degree correction of the intermetatarsal angle. No nonunions occurred.

Kitaoka and Leventen[24] performed a modified distal oblique osteotomy on 23 feet and in 16 patients. The 4–5 intermetatarsal angle was decreased from 13 to 8 degrees for a 5-degree correction. Measurement of the forefoot was noted to be diminished by 4 mm postoperatively. One nonunion was reported; however, 87 percent of patients reported good results postoperatively.

Technique

Distal Oblique Osteotomy

A lateral longitudinal incision is centered over the fifth metatarsal head. The dorsal and proximal capsule is detached using the L-type capsular release as previously described (see discussion under Lateral Condylectomy). The lateral condyle of the fifth metatarsal is exposed (see Fig. 7–5*A*), and the abductor digiti quinti is divided. A sagittal saw is used to resect the lateral eminence, and an oblique osteotomy of the neck of the metatarsal is performed (Fig. 7–7*A*) in a distal-lateral to

FIGURE 7–7. *(A)*, Bunionette prior to distal transverse osteotomy. *(B)*, Postoperative x-ray film of the distal transverse fifth metatarsal osteotomy. (From Mann RA, Coughlin MJ: Surgery of the Foot and Ankle, 6th Ed. St. Louis, Mosby–Year Book, 1993, p 454.)

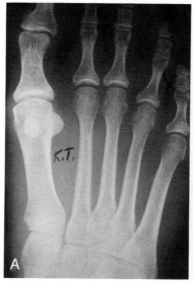
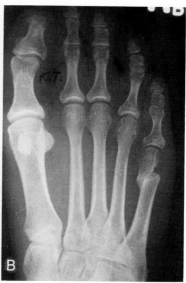

proximal-medial direction. The metaphyseal portion of the distal fragment is resected with a rongeur, and the capital fragment is then displaced in a medial direction. It is then impacted on the proximal fragment (Fig. 7–7B). No fixation was recommended for this technique. The foot is dressed in a gauze-and-tape dressing. The patient is allowed to ambulate in a postoperative shoe. The toe is taped in appropriate alignment for 4 weeks following the removal of the bandage.

Distal Chevron Procedure

Another method used to treat an enlarged fifth metatarsal head is resection of the prominent lateral condyle in combination with a chevron osteotomy.

A longitudinal lateral skin incision is centered over the metatarsal head. The dissection is carried down directly to the capsule, and this method helps to avoid injury to the superficial dorsal and plantar neurovascular bundles. The capsule is released with an inverted L-type incision along the dorsal and proximal margins (see Fig. 7–5A). Soft tissue stripping is minimized in order to avoid vascular compromise to the distal fifth metatarsal fragment. A sagittal saw is used to resect the lateral eminence in a line parallel with the fifth metatarsal shaft (see Fig. 7–5B). Two to three mm of the lateral eminence is removed. A small drill hole is centered in the midportion of the

fifth metatarsal head to mark the apex of the osteotomy, which is based proximally. Then a very thin sagittal saw is used to create a horizontal (medial to lateral direction) chevron osteotomy at an angle of approximately 60 degrees (Fig. 7–8A). It is important not to disrupt the fifth metatarsal medial capsular structures because release of the capsule may compromise metatarsal head vascularity and lead to subsequent avascular necrosis. The capital fragment is then displaced 3 mm in a medial direction and is impacted on to the proximal fragment (Fig. 7–8B). Although Kirschner wire fixation is optional, it is recommended if there is any tendency toward redisplacement or angulation at the osteotomy site (Fig. 7–8C and D).

The sagittal saw is then used to resect the metaphyseal flare that remains. The lateral capsule is repaired. Proximally, the capsular structures are sutured to the abductor digiti quinti muscle. Dorsally, the capsule is repaired to the dorsal periosteum. At the dorsal proximal aspect, there may not be enough tissue with which to repair the capsular structures. In this area, it may be necessary to secure the capsule through drill holes in the metaphysis if there is a paucity of tissue present.

Postoperative Complications

A distal fifth metatarsal osteotomy may be an effective means to reduce an enlarged fifth metatarsal head or a large lateral condyle.

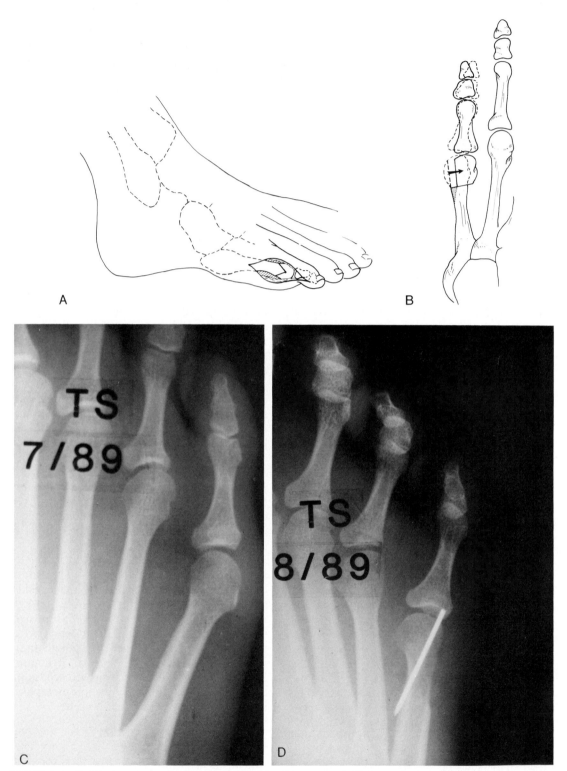

FIGURE 7–8. *(A),* Distal 60-degree chevron osteotomy of the fifth metatarsal. *(B),* 3-mm displacement of the distal segment. *(C),* Preoperative bunionette. *(D),* After chevron osteotomy. (Courtesy of Michael J. Coughlin, M.D.)

Although a lateral condylectomy may be used for a distal fifth metatarsal abnormality, the distal oblique osteotomy or the chevron osteotomy appears to afford more correction than a condylar resection alone. Potential complications such as malunion, displacement, or development of intractable plantar keratotic transfer lesions make the use either of a stable osteotomy or internal fixation preferable to the floating type of osteotomy described by Hohmann,[19] Keating and colleagues,[22] and Sponsel.[37] In the presence of a lateral keratosis, either an oblique osteotomy or a chevron osteotomy may provide an adequate correction. However, since a chevron-type osteotomy does not allow dorsal translation of the capital fragment, this procedure is less optimal in the presence of either a plantar or plantar-lateral keratosis. Some dorsal translation may be afforded by making the chevron cuts slightly in a plantar-to-dorsal direction so that the capital fragment is elevated.

Midshaft Diaphyseal Osteotomy

An osteotomy in the diaphyseal region has been employed infrequently to correct the bunionette deformity. Yancy[43] performed a double transverse closing wedge osteotomy in the diaphysis to correct a bunionette deformity with lateral angulation of the fifth metatarsal. Voutey[41] also performed a transverse osteotomy in the diaphysis but noted problems with rotation, angulation, and pseudoarthrosis. Gerbert and colleagues[16] performed a midshaft closing wedge osteotomy and achieved fixation with a circlage wire. They observed that for plantar and lateral keratotic lesions, a biplane osteotomy may be used to displace the distal fragment in a medial and dorsal direction. Unfortunately, no long-term follow-up in these series was reported. Mann[31] reported on an oblique fifth metatarsal diaphyseal osteotomy for the treatment of diffuse, large keratotic lesions on the plantar-lateral and plantar aspect of the fifth metatarsal head. He used an obliquely oriented osteotomy, which allowed a dorsal-medial translation of the metatarsal bone as the distal metatarsal fragment was rotated. He advocated fixation with either a wire loop, Kirschner wire, or small fragment screw. A fifth metatarsophalangeal joint realignment and lateral eminence resection was not included in this procedure. Although no

series were reported, one case of nonunion was noted. Coughlin[6] reported on a modification of this oblique diaphyseal osteotomy in which the lateral eminence was resected and a realignment of the fifth metatarsophalangeal joint was performed. Eleven patients underwent surgical correction, and all osteotomies united. The intermetatarsal angle was reduced from 9.13 degrees to 0.04 degrees, for an average correction in the intermetatarsal angle of 9 degrees. The metatarsophalangeal-5 angle, which averaged 17.6 degrees prior to surgery, was reduced to an average of 0 degrees postoperatively, for a 17-degree correction. No transfer lesions were reported.

Technique

A longitudinal incision is centered over the lateral aspect of the fifth metatarsal head. The incision extends from the base of the fifth metatarsal to the midportion of the proximal phalanx (Fig. 7–9A).[7] The dissection is carried down to the capsule in order to protect the dorsal and plantar cutaneous nerves. The abductor digiti quinti muscle is reflected off of the metatarsal diaphysis and retracted in a plantar direction. The fifth metatarsophalangeal joint capsule is released using the L-type capsular release previously described (see Fig. 7–5A). The lateral condyle of the fifth metatarsal is then resected using a very thin sagittal saw in a line parallel with the fifth metatarsal shaft (Fig. 5–7B). The fifth toe is grasped and distracted, and the medial fifth metatarsophalangeal capsule is then released in order to allow later realignment of the fifth toe. The diaphyseal osteotomy is performed with a very fine sagittal saw. In the presence of a lateral keratosis, the osteotomy is directed in a horizontal direction (Fig. 7–9B). Longitudinally, the osteotomy is directed from a plantar-distal to dorsal-proximal direction as described by Mann.[31] Prior to completion of the osteotomy, the distal fragment is drilled with a gliding hole and the proximal fragment is drilled with a fixation hole. The fixation hole is then tapped. The osteotomy is completed and the distal metatarsal is then rotated (Fig. 7–9C) until it is parallel with the fourth metatarsal shaft. A minifragment screw is then tightened to secure fixation (Fig. 7–9D and E). A second screw may be placed or a Kirschner wire added to re-enforce fixation. The abductor digiti quinti muscle is closed over the metatarsal shaft. The

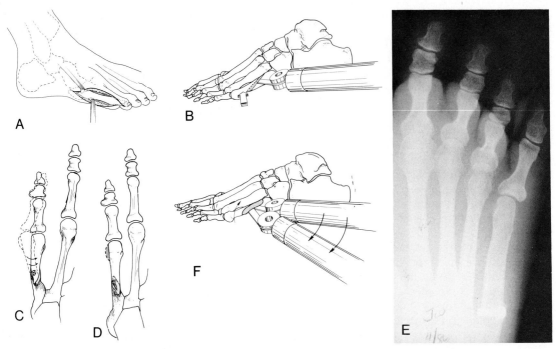

FIGURE 7–9. *(A)*, Exposure of the diaphyseal osteotomy. *(B)*, The diaphyseal osteotomy (see text). *(C)*, Alignment of the distal segment. Osteotomy of the lateral prominence is also carried out. *(D)*, Fixation is achieved with a minifragment screw. *(E)*, An x-ray film of the completed osteotomy. *(F)*, A cephalad-directed osteotomy to correct plantar alignment of the distal fragment. (*A* to *D* and *F* from Mann RA, Coughlin MJ: The Video Textbook of Foot and Ankle Surgery. Medical Video Productions, St. Louis, 1991; *E* from Mann RA, Coughlin MJ: Surgery of the Foot and Ankle, 6th Ed. St. Louis, Mosby–Year Book, 1993, p 458.)

L-shaped lateral capsular flap is repaired (as previously described), realigning the metatarsophalangeal joint. A gauze-and-tape dressing is applied and changed on a weekly basis. The patient is seen weekly for 6 weeks. The patient is allowed to ambulate in a wooden-soled shoe; however, casting may be employed for an unreliable patient.

In the presence of a plantar-lateral or plantar keratosis, an oblique osteotomy may still be used. However, the direction is altered. The sawblade is directed in a slightly cephalad direction in order to have an elevating effect on the distal fragment when this fragment is rotated (Fig. 7–9F). (The diagram demonstrates the fact that if the surgeon drops his hand toward the plantar aspect of the foot, he will cut in an upward fashion. By doing this, as the osteotomy is rotated, the metatarsal head will rise slightly, alleviating plantar pressure.)

The medial eminence is resected, and the metatarsophalangeal joint is realigned as previously described.

Internal fixation is usually removed under local anesthesia 6 to 8 weeks following surgery.

Often, the minifragment screw used for internal fixation is removed if symptoms occur.

A midshaft diaphyseal osteotomy may be used for a bunionette deformity associated with either lateral metatarsal deviation or bowing or in the case of an increased 4–5 intermetatarsal angle. Metatarsophalangeal joint realignment combined with lateral eminence resection allows correction of the deviated fifth toe at the same time that the metatarsal abnormality is corrected.

Proximal Metatarsal Osteotomy

For correcting an increased 4–5 intermetatarsal angle, a proximal fifth metatarsal osteotomy has been advocated.[12, 15, 20] The rationale for this procedure is that it corrects the increased intermetatarsal angle at the site of the deformity. Controversy, however, surrounds osteotomy in the proximal region.

LeLievre[29] used a transverse osteotomy in the region of the styloid process. Diebold and Bejjani[12] did observe that "the risk of disruption of the transverse metatarsal joint is not negligible" with a very proximal fifth metatarsal osteotomy (Fig. 7–10A and B). In a large series of 72 patients (116 cases), Bishop[3] performed an opening wedge osteotomy of the proximal fifth metatarsal to diminish the 4–5 intermetatarsal angle. Esterholm and associates[14] performed a similar procedure in four cases. No long-term results were reported regarding the postoperative 4–5 intermetatarsal angle, frequency of delayed union (Fig. 7–10C to E) or nonunion, or development of transfer keratotic lesions in either of these series. Regnauld[34] used a closing wedge osteotomy

and stabilized it with a distal circlage wire between the fourth and fifth metatarsal bones. No results with this technique were reported.

In the only series which published significant follow-up with a proximal fifth metatarsal osteotomy, Diebold and Bejjani[12] performed a horizontal chevron osteotomy approximately 1 cm distal to the base of the fifth metatarsal. Immobilization was achieved using cross Steinmann pin fixation between the fourth and fifth metatarsals for 4 to 6 weeks. In 12 patients, excellent results were reported by 90 percent.

While Kaplan and colleagues[20] stated that

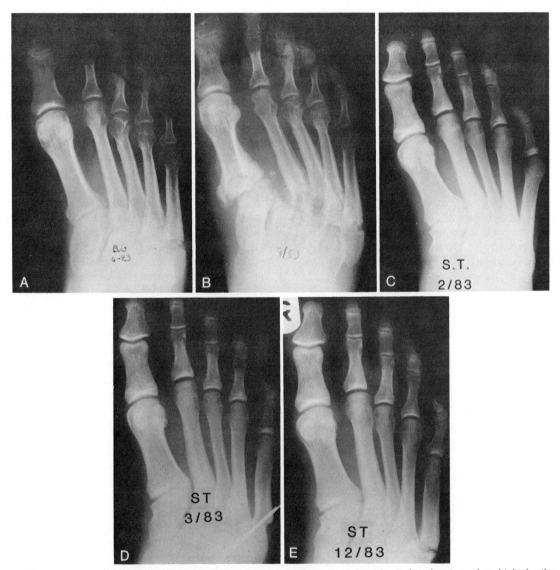

FIGURE 7–10. (A), Delayed union of the fifth metatarsal basilar osteotomy. (B), Delayed union of multiple basilar osteotomies. (C), Bunionette prior to basilar osteotomy. (D), Fixation of the basilar procedure. (E), Persistent delayed union of an osteotomy. (A and B from Mann RA, Coughlin MJ: The Video Textbook of Foot and Ankle Surgery. Medical Video Productions, St. Louis, 1991; C to E from Mann RA, Coughlin MJ: Surgery of the Foot and Ankle, 6th Ed. St. Louis, Mosby–Year Book, 1993, p 462.)

both proximal and distal osteotomies heal well because of the abundant vascular supply, Gerbert and associates[16] appreciated that the anastomosing arterial branches of the fourth intermetatarsal space are vulnerable to injury with a proximal fifth metatarsal osteotomy. This fact has been appreciated when delayed healing of fractures in the proximal 2 cm of the fifth metatarsal have occurred.* Diebold and Bejjani[12] reported that there was indeed poor healing potential of fractures in this region. Carp[5] hypothesized that the reason for delayed healing was the poor vascular supply in this region. Estersohn and colleagues[14] and Carp[5] noted the importance of the metaphyseal branch to the proximal fifth metatarsal bone, which enters on the medial aspect. Estersohn and associates[14] advised that this important vascular supply should be protected at the time of surgery.

Shereff and coworkers[36] reported on the intraosseous and extraosseous supply of the fifth metatarsal bone. The intraosseous supply eminates from a periosteal plexus, metaphyseal epiphyseal vessels as well as the nutrient artery. The extraosseous supply originates from the dorsal metatarsal artery as well as several branches of the lateral plantar artery. Shereff and associates[36] suggested that a fracture or osteotomy in the proximal 2 cm may injure both the intraosseous and extraosseous vascular supply, and may lead to delayed healing capacity.

Therefore, although a proximal fifth metatarsal osteotomy may correct the angulation at the site of maximum deformity, the potential for metatarsal-tarsal instability, delayed union, or nonunion (Fig. 7–10E) makes this area a somewhat less desirable alternative for surgical correction.

DISCUSSION

Many different procedures have been recommended for the treatment of the bunionette or tailor's bunion deformity. Excision of the lateral condyle; resection of the fifth metatarsal head; ray resection with or without fifth toe amputation; and distal, diaphyseal and proximal fifth metatarsal osteotomy have all been used to correct deformity. Unfortunately, the lack of long-term follow-up with most of these

procedures and the anecdotal reports on other techniques raise the question as to which of these procedures have long-term efficacy. The wide range of anatomic variation presenting with bunionette deformities complicates the choice of surgical correction. An enlarged fifth metatarsal head (with or without a pronation) may be treated with either a distal metatarsal osteotomy or with a lateral condylectomy and metatarsophalangeal joint realignment. When a plantar or plantar lateral keratotic lesion is present (without a significant increase in the 4–5 intermetatarsal angle) a distal oblique osteotomy as described by Kitaoka and Leventen[24] is preferable to the chevron procedure. A biplane diaphyseal fifth metatarsal osteotomy may also be used in this situation. When a pure lateral keratotic lesion is present, a chevron osteotomy is a relatively straightforward procedure that has inherent stability and may be used for this deformity. Kirschner wire fixation does help to ensure the stability of the osteotomy site. When an increased 4–5 intermetatarsal angle is associated with a bunionette deformity, or when the less common laterally deviated fifth metatarsal shaft is present, a diaphyseal metatarsal osteotomy with a lateral condylectomy and distal soft tissue realignment is an excellent means with which to correct this deformity.

The circulatory pattern described in the proximal fifth metatarsal[36] makes the possibility of vascular disruption a worrisome complication. Because of this possibility, a diaphyseal or distal metatarsal osteotomy offers a less risky location for metatarsal osteotomy.

Whether or not internal fixation is necessary for a fifth metatarsal osteotomy is still controversial. Malunion, nonunion, delayed union, and development of intractable plantar keratotic lesions in which floating osteotomies have been carried out indicate the necessity for fixation when there is instability at the osteotomy site. As Coughlin[7] stated, "the principles of osteotomy with internal fixation applied elsewhere in the musculoskeletal system apply equally as well to the foot."

Radiographic abnormalities associated with a bunionette deformity must be evaluated in analyzing the location of the deformity. The physical examination helps to ascertain the location of keratotic lesions, and when it is combined with the radiographic evaluation, it helps to define the appropriate means of treatment.

---

*See references 1, 5, 8, 10, 21, 27, 30, 40, and 44.

Conservative management of the symptomatic bunionette deformity includes the use of roomy footwear, padding, and trimming of keratotic lesions. Although conservative methods are effective in a large number of patients, chronic bursal thickening and the development of symptomatic keratoses may require operative treatment in certain patients.

Surgical versatility in the treatment of the symptomatic bunionette deformity is most important. Tailoring the surgical repair to the underlying pathology helps to determine whether a condylectomy, a distal soft tissue repair, a distal metatarsal osteotomy, or a diaphyseal osteotomy offers the best solution for the painful bunionette deformity.

References

1. Acker JH, Drez D: Nonoperative treatment of stress fractures of the proximal shaft of the fifth metatarsal (Jones fracture). Foot Ankle 7(3):152, 1986.
2. Amberry TR: *In* Weinstein F (Ed): Principles and Practice of Podiatry. Philadelphia, Lea & Febiger, 1968, pp 167–169.
3. Bishop J, Kahn A, Turba JE: Surgical correction of the splayfoot: The Giannestras procedure. Clin Orthop 146:234, 1980.
4. Brown JE: Functional and cosmetic correction of metatarsus latus (splay foot). Clin Orthop 14(166):166, 1959.
5. Carp L: Fracture of the fifth metatarsal bone. Ann Surg 86:308, 1927.
6. Coughlin MJ: Correction of the bunionette with fifth metatarsal osteotomy. Proceedings of the American Orthopaedic Foot and Ankle Society. Orthop Trans 12(1):30, 1987.
7. Coughlin, MJ: Bunionettes: Etiology and treatment. Instruct Course Lect 39:37–48, 1990.
8. Dameron TB: Fractures and anatomical variations of the proximal portion of the fifth metatarsal. J Bone Joint Surg 57A(6):788, 1975.
9. Davies H: Metatarsus quintus valgus. Br Med J 664, 1949.
10. DeLee JC, Evans JP, Julian J: Stress fracture of the fifth metatarsal. Am J Sports Med 11(5):349, 1983.
11. Dickson FD, Diveley RL: *In* Functional Disorders of the Foot, 3rd Ed. Philadelphia, JB Lippincott, 1953, p 230.
12. Diebold PF, Bejjani FJ: Basal osteotomy of the fifth metatarsal with intermetatarsal pinning: A new approach to Tailor's bunion. Foot Ankle 8(1):40, 1987.
13. DuVries H: *In* DuVries H (Ed) Surgery of the Foot, 2nd Ed. St. Louis, CV Mosby, 1965, pp 456–462.
14. Estersohn H, Scherer P, Bogdan R: A preliminary report on opening wedge osteotomy of the fifth metatarsal. Arch Podiatr Med Foot Surg 1(4):317, 1974.
15. Fallat LM, Buckholz J: An analysis of the Tailor's bunion by radiographic and anatomical display. J Am Podiatr Assoc 70(12):597, 1980.
16. Gerbert J, Sgarlato TE, Subotnik SI: Preliminary study of a closing wedge osteotomy of the fifth metatarsal for correction of a Tailor's bunion deformity. J Am Podiatr Assoc 62(6):212, 1972.
17. Giannestras NJ: Other problems of the foot. *In* Giannestras, NJ (Ed): Foot Disorders: Medical and Surgical Management. Philadelphia, Lea & Febiger, 1973.
18. Haber JH, Kraft J: Crescentic osteotomy for fifth metatarsal head lesions. J Foot Surg 19:66, 1980.
19. Hohmann F: *In* Bergman JG (Ed): Fuss und Bein. Berlin, 1951.
20. Kaplan EG, Kaplan G, Jacobs AM: Management of fifth metatarsal head lesion by biplane osteotomy. J Foot Surg 15(1):1, 1976.
21. Kavanaugh JH, Brower TD, Mann RV: The Jones fracture revisited. J Bone Joint Surg 60A(6):776, 1978.
22. Keating SE, DeVincentis A, Goller WL: Oblique fifth metatarsal osteotomy: A followup study. J Foot Surg 21(2):104, 1982.
23. Kelikian H: Deformities of the lesser toe. *In* Kelikian H (Ed): Hallux Valgus, Allied Deformities of the Forefoot and Metatarsalgia. Philadelphia, WB Saunders, 1965.
24. Kitaoka HB, Leventen E: Medial displacement metatarsal osteotomy for treatment of the painful bunionette. Clin Orthop 243:172, 1988.
25. Kitaoka HB, Nestor BJ, Bergmann AD: Radiologic anatomy of the painful bunionette. Presented at the Fourth Annual Summer Meeting of the American Orthopaedic Foot and Ankle Society, Minneapolis, Minnesota, 1988.
26. Leach RE, Igou R: Metatarsal osteotomy for bunionette deformity. Clin Orthop 100:171, 1974.
27. Lehman RC, Torg JS, Pavlov H, DeLee JC: Fractures of the base of the fifth metatarsal distal to the tuberosity: A review. Foot Ankle 7(4):245, 1987.
28. LeLievre J: Exostosis of the head of the fifth metatarsal bone, Tailor's bunion. LeConcours Med 78:4815, 1956.
29. LeLievre J: *In* Patholgie du Pied, 5th Ed. Paris, Masson et Cie, 1971.
30. Lichtblau S: Painful nonunion of a fracture of the fifth metatarsal. Clin Orthop 59:171, 1968.
31. Mann RA: Keratotic disorders of the plantar skin. *In* Mann RA (Ed): Surgery of the Foot, 5th Ed. St. Louis, CV Mosby, 1986.
32. McGlamry ED: Metatarsal shortening: Osteoplasty of head and osteotomy of shaft. J Am Podiatr Assoc 59:394, 1969.
33. McKeever DC: Excision of the fifth metatarsal head. Clin Orthop 13:321, 1959.
34. Regnauld B: *In* Technique Chirurgicales Du Pied. Paris, Masson et Cie, 1974.
35. Schoenhaus H, Rotman S, Meshon A: A review of normal metatarsal angles. J Am Podiatr Assoc 63(3):88, 1973.
36. Shereff MJ, Yang QM, Krummer FJ, Frey C: The vascular anatomy of the 5th metatarsal. Proceedings of the American Orthopaedic Foot and Ankle Society. Orthop Trans 12(1):30, 1988.
37. Sponsel KH: Bunionette correction by metatarsal osteotomy. Orthop Clin North Am 7(4):808, 1976.
38. Stewart M: Miscellaneous affections of the foot. *In* Edmonson S, Crenshaw AJ: Campbell's Operative Orthopaedics, 6th Ed. St. Louis, CV Mosby, 1980.

39. Throckmorton JK, Bradlee N: Transverse V sliding osteotomy: A new surgical procedure for the correction of Tailor's bunion deformity. J Foot Surg 18(3):117, 1978.
40. Torg JS, Balduine F, Zelko R, et al: Fractures of the base of the fifth metatarsal distal to the tuberosity. J Bone Joint Surg 66A:209, 1984.
41. Voutey H: Manueal De Chirurgie Orthopaedique et de Reeducational du Pied. Paris, Masson et Cie, 1978.
42. Weisberg MH: Resection of the fifth metatarsal head in lateral segment problems. J Am Podiatr Assoc 57:374, 1967.
43. Yancy HA: Congenital lateral bowing of the fifth metatarsal. Clin Orthop 62:203, 1969.
44. Zelko RR, Torg JS, Rachun A: Proximal diaphyseal fractures of the fifth metatarsal—treatment of the fracture and their complications in athletes. Am J Sports Med 7(2):95, 1979.

8
Intractable Plantar Keratoses

SALLY A. RUDICEL

An intractable plantar keratosis (IPK) is a callus that forms on the sole of the foot and does not resolve. It is a reactive proliferation of the epidermis caused by pressure of the metatarsal head on the plantar pad of the foot, and the condition is painful. The lesion has a hard keratotic core that invaginates the plantar skin. When the lesion is shaved, the margins are ill defined, but there is a hard keratotic core that is avascular. Histologically, there is fibrous tissue and necrosis with thickening and cornification. The increased height of the lesion increases the pressure, and thus, the pain worsens as the callus proliferates.

A callus must not be confused with a plantar wart. The plantar wart is usually *not* under a metatarsal head but is located elsewhere on a non–weight-bearing area of the foot. A plantar wart is also quite vascular when it is shaved, and it has discrete margins. Small, punctate areas seen in the center of the wart represent the end arteries. A wart is painful even with side-to-side pressure, whereas a callus is usually tender to direct pressure only.

The IPK is caused by abnormal pressure, either from poor shoewear, an abnormality in gait, poor mechanics of the foot, or a bony prominence. There are localized and diffuse IPKs.[7] The diffuse type has diffuse margins and is usually caused by shearing forces (Fig. 8–1). It is most commonly associated with rheumatoid arthritis and psoriatic arthritis, the cavus foot or a foot with claw toes, and atrophy of the fat pad. It is caused by an abnormality of gait or incompetency of the first ray, giving abnormal pressure to the lesser metatarsal heads. Patients with a hallux valgus deformity may develop a diffuse callus under the second

metatarsal head because of poor weight bearing under the first metatarsal head. The more localized type of IPK is usually associated with poor shoewear in which the foot is in a pointed-toed shoe or a short shoe in which the metatarsal heads are forced into the plantar fat pad as the toes are buckled under. This is true particularly in a high-heeled shoe, in which the metatarsophalangeal joints are dorsiflexed. Altered mechanics of the foot, such as a mal-aligned metatarsal fracture that is plantar-flexed, may also be the source of a keratosis.

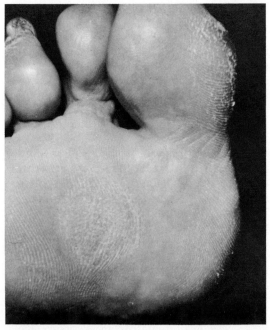

FIGURE 8–1. A discrete callus under the second metatarsal head.

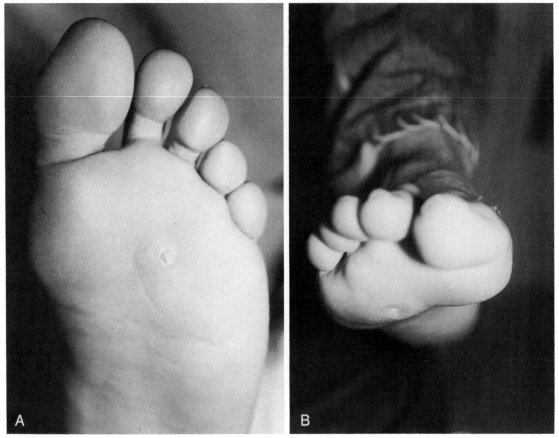

FIGURE 8–2. *(A)*, A localized callus under the third metatarsal head. *(B)*, Forefoot varus showing the pressure under the third metatarsal head leading to a callus.

Figure 8–2 *A* shows a localized IPK under the third metatarsal head, and Figure 8–2*B* shows a forefoot varus that may lead to pressure under the third metatarsal head. The discrete or localized keratosis has a deep core, with its apex centered over the bony prominence, and it can be quite hard.

Some authors have also attributed the formation of a callus under the second metatarsal to a long second metatarsal (Fig. 8–3).[12] However, a study by Dreeben and associates in 1989 did not confirm an increased incidence of metatarsalgia in feet with a longer second metatarsal. They did find, however, that feet with primary metatarsalgia did have an abnormal relationship of metatarsal head height and an elevation of plantar pressures. The quality of the plantar soft tissues and fat pad were believed to be as important as absolute thickness.[3] The symptomatic plantar tissues have also been implicated by some authors to be abnormal in patients with an IPK. Bonavilla showed an inflammatory-like reaction of the plantar tissues in biopsies of 10 patients with metatarsalgia.[1] Thus, there is some speculation that the keratosis is formed by a disease of the underlying fat pad in some cases rather than by a mechanical problem.

TREATMENT

Conservative Treatment

The initial treatment for the intractable plantar keratosis is conservative. The callus should be shaved, and pads and appropriate shoes should be used to cushion the area and to alleviate stress. A broad-toed, soft-soled, flat shoe with a metatarsal support proximal to the lesion should be used. This increases the distance between the bottom of the foot and the

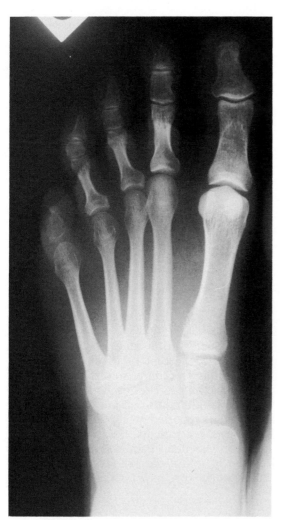

FIGURE 8–3. A long second metatarsal.

need to be changed with a metatarsal osteotomy to change the position of the bone.

TYPES OF LESIONS

Lesion Under Fibular Condyle

Frequently, well-localized lesions are caused by a prominent metatarsal condyle (Fig. 8–4). The fibular condyle is the usual offender. Conservative measures often fail to relieve the pain. The best surgical procedure for this problem is a DuVries arthroplasty, as described in 1953 by DuVries[4] and again in 1973 by Mann and DuVries.[9]

Technique

The operation consists of an arthroplasty of the metatarsophalangeal joint carried out through a dorsal hockey stick incision. The incision starts in the web space, is centered over the joint, and extends proximally. The extensor tendons are preserved and retracted. The joint capsule is entered longitudinally, and the collateral ligaments are divided. The metatarsal head is delivered out of the wound, and 2 to 3 mm of the articular surface of the metatarsal head is removed with an osteotome

ground, and places the stress proximal to the painful metatarsal head and callus instead of under it. The callus may need to be trimmed periodically. This makes the keratotic core much more superficial and less painful. Trimming may need to be done weekly at first and then every 6 to 8 weeks. If these measures do not provide satisfactory relief, surgery may be indicated.

Surgical Treatment

The method of treatment depends on the type of lesion and the source of the problem. The offending bony prominence may simply be removed, or the mechanics of the foot may

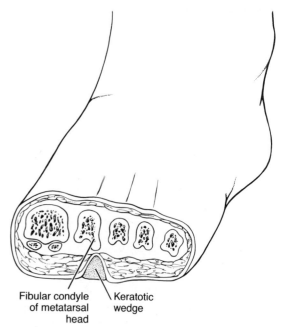

Fibular condyle of metatarsal head   Keratotic wedge

FIGURE 8–4. A prominent fibular condyle leading to a callus.

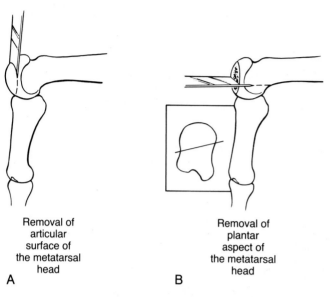

Removal of
articular
surface of
the metatarsal
head

A

Removal of
plantar
aspect of
the metatarsal
head

B

FIGURE 8–5. *(A)*, Excision of a portion of the metatarsal head in the DuVries arthroplasty. *(B)*, Excision of the plantar portion of the metatarsal head in the DuVries arthroplasty.

(Fig. 8–5*A*). The plantar condyle is then removed with an osteotome, removing more on the fibular than tibial side of the metatarsal head (Fig. 8–5*B*). The remaining edges of the metatarsal head are smoothed with a rasp or rongeur. Care should be taken not to fracture the metatarsal head. The capsule is repaired, the extensor tendon is allowed to fall back into place, and the skin is closed. A compressive dressing is applied, and the patient may ambulate in a wooden shoe. The foot is kept in a firm dressing for 4 to 6 weeks, and the patient may return to regular shoes as tolerated thereafter.

Most patients in the study of DuVries and Mann lost 25 percent of their joint motion following this procedure, so it is important to prescribe active exercises of the metatarsophalangeal joint after dressings are stopped. Mann and DuVries reported on 142 such operations. In all but seven patients, the callus was eliminated or lessened. Pain was eliminated or lessened in 138 of the 142 lesions.[9] The procedure works very well for this specific prob-

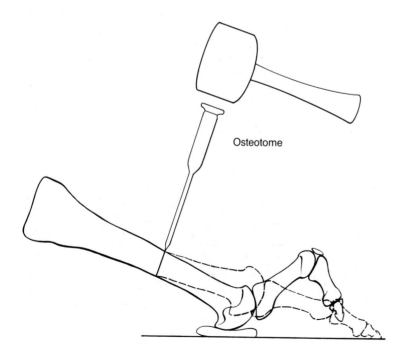

Osteotome

FIGURE 8–6. The midshaft greenstick osteotomy as described by Meisenbach.

lem when the condition is not responsive to conservative care.

Diffuse Lesion Under Metatarsal Head

A diffuse lesion under the metatarsal head is not caused by a prominent plantar condyle but rather by pressure from the entire metatarsal head. This may be caused by a congenital problem, by a metatarsal bone that is too long, or by a metatarsal bone that is in excessive plantar flexion, perhaps from an old fracture. Resection of the entire head of a metatarsal bone or overcorrection by an osteotomy may cause transfer metatarsalgia to an adjacent metatarsal head and the development of an IPK.

Again, conservative measures should be attempted. Proper shoes and metatarsal pads, as well as trimming the lesion, all may help. If these measures are insufficient, surgery may be indicated.

The metatarsal bone needs to be either shortened or placed in greater dorsiflexion, or both. Various type of osteotomies may be used to accomplish this.

One of the earliest types of osteotomies described was a greenstick osteotomy proposed by Meisenbach in 1916[11] and redescribed by Thomas in 1969.[13] It is a dorsal closing wedge osteotomy (Fig. 8–6). An osteotome is used to make an incision perpendicular to the shaft of the metatarsal, 3 cm from the metatarsophalangeal joint. The cut is made down to the plantar cortex. Digital pressure on the plantar surface of the metatarsal head then completes the fracture and allows the distal fragment to angulate dorsally. There is no fixation of the bone with this procedure, and the amount of correction is not precise. However, it has been described to work well by some authors.[13]

Other authors have described osteotomies at the neck of the metatarsal bone. Borggreve recommended excision of a dorsally based triangle in 1949.[2] Wolf described a distal greenstick dorsal wedge osteotomy in 1973.[14] He believed no fixation was necessary and that weight bearing would place the metatarsal head in the correct position. Helal described an oblique osteotomy in the distal half of the metatarsal shaft, in which he did not use fixation. He could shorten or angle the metatarsal bone, or both.[6]

Basal osteotomies of the metatarsal bone have been used as well. Mau recommended removal of a trapezoidal portion of the metatarsal bone, which would both shorten and dorsally angulate the metatarsal bone.[10] Giannestras described a step-cut osteotomy at the base of the metatarsal bone in 1954.[5] This procedure is technically difficult, and the fixation is tenuous. Mann has used a proximal dorsal wedge osteotomy with fixation by a screw or a tension band if plantar flexion of the metatarsal bone is the main problem (Fig. 8–7). However, if the metatarsal bone is too

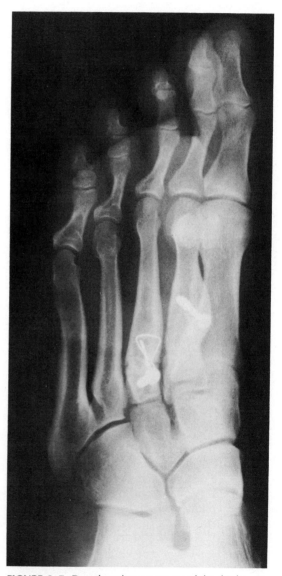

FIGURE 8–7. Dorsal wedge osteotomy of the third metatarsal showing tension band fixation.

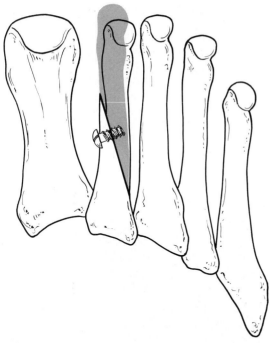

FIGURE 8–8. A long oblique sagittal osteotomy of the second metatarsal with screw fixation.

long, a long oblique sagittal osteotomy of the metatarsal bone may be performed, allowing the distal fragment to slide proximally 2 to 3 mm. The osteotomy is then fixed with a screw or wire (Fig. 8–8).[8] Fixation is believed to be important to hold the metatarsal in the appropriate position, since the main complication of the previously described procedures is transfer metatarsalgia because of inadequate correction. The larger bony surfaces with this osteotomy allow a greater surface area to promote healing.

Technique

A longitudinal incision is made over the shaft of the metatarsal. The extensor tendon is identified and retracted. The metatarsal shaft is cleared of the surrounding soft tissue and protected. A microsagittal saw is used to make a long, oblique osteotomy in the sagittal plane of the shaft. The distal fragment is displaced slightly proximally and fixed with a screw or wire. The skin is closed routinely, and the patient is allowed to ambulate in a compressive dressing and a wooden shoe for 4 to 6 weeks.

If the osteotomy is healed, activities may then begin as tolerated.

Lesion Under the First Metatarsal Head

Rarely, a patient may develop a diffuse IPK under the first metatarsal rather than the well-localized callus under the tibial sesamoid bone. This condition is usually due to a plantarflexed first metatarsal. If conservative measures fail, these patients may require a dorsal closing wedge osteotomy.

Technique

A small longitudinal incision is made over the base of the first metatarsal bone. The extensor tendon is identified and retracted. The bone is cleared of the surrounding soft tissue and protected. A microsagittal saw or sharp osteotome is used to make a dorsal closing wedge osteotomy approximately 1 cm from the proximal end of the metatarsal bone. Only 1 or 2 mm of bone needs to be resected at the base of the osteotomy. The osteotomy is then closed by dorsiflexing the distal metatarsal bone, and it is held by a pin or screw.

The major complication that can occur with all operative procedures in the correction of IPKs is the development of a transfer lesion. This occurs with excessive elevation of the corrected metatarsal bone. The author, therefore, prefers fixation of all osteotomies to place them in the desired position.

References

1. Bonavilla J: Histopathology of the heloma durum: Some significant features and their implications. Am Podiatry Assoc 58:423–427, 1968.
2. Borggreve J: Zur operativen Behandlung des kontrakten Spregfusses. Z Orthop 78:581–582, 1949.
3. Dreeben SM, et al: Metatarsal osteotomy for primary metatarsalgia: Radiographic and pedobarographic study. Foot Ankle 9(5):214–218, 1989.
4. DuVries HL: New approach to the treatment of intractable verruca plantaris. J Am Med Assoc 152(13):1202–1203, 1953.
5. Giannestras NJ: Shortening of the metatarsal shaft for the correction of plantar keratosis. Clin Orthop 225–231, 1954.
6. Helal B: Metatarsal osteotomy for metatarsalgia. J Bone Joint Surg 57:187–192, 1975.
7. Mann RA: Intractable plantar keratosis. Instr Course Lect 33:287–301, 1984.
8. Mann RA, personal communication, 1990.

9. Mann RA, DuVries HL: Intractable plantar keratosis. Orthop Clin North Am 4(1):67–73, 1973.
10. Mau C: Eine Operation des kontrakten Spreizfusses. Zentralbl Chir 67:667–670, 1940.
11. Meisenbach RO: Painful anterior arch of the foot: An operation for its relief by means of raising the arch. Am J Orthop Surg 14:206–211, 1916.
12. Morton DJ: Hypermobility of the first metatarsal bone: The interlinking factor between metatarsalgia and longitudinal arch strains. J Bone Joint Surg 10:187–196, 1928.
13. Thomas WH: Metatarsal osteotomy. Surg Clin North Am 49(4):879–882, 1969.
14. Wolf MD: Metatarsal osteotomy for the relief of painful metatarsal callosities. J Bone Joint Surg 55A(8):1760–1762, 1973.

9

Anatomy and Pathophysiology of the Lesser Toes

MARK S. MIZEL

An understanding of the anatomy of the lesser toes is necessary to appreciate their physiology and pathophysiology. A central dorsal structure is formed by the extensor digitorum longus tendon, which travels along the central aspect of the proximal phalanx (Fig. 9–1). This proceeds distally, and the tendon forms three slips. The central slip inserts into the proximal aspect of the middle phalanx, and the other two re-form into one tendon that inserts on the distal phalanx. On the plantar surface, the flexor digitorum longus tendon

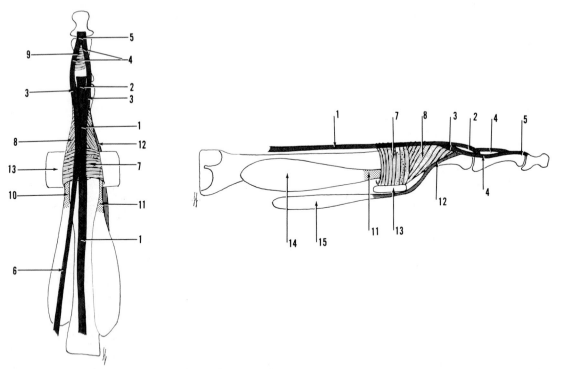

FIGURE 9–1. Extensor complex of a lesser toe. 1, Extensor digitorum longus tendon; 2, middle slip of the extensor tendon trifurcation; 3, 3', lateral slips of the extensor tendon trifurcation; 4, lateral tendons of the extensor tendon trifurcation; 5, terminal extensor tendon; 6, extensor digitorum brevis tendon; 7, transverse lamina of the extensor aponeurosis or extensor sling; 8, oblique component of the extensor aponeurosis forming the extensor hood or wing; 9, triangular ligament; 10, 11, interossei tendons; 12, lumbrical tendon; 13, deep transverse metatarsal ligament; 14, interosseous muscle; 15, lumbrical muscle. (From Sarrafian SK: Anatomy of the Foot and Ankle. Philadelphia, JB Lippincott, 1983, p 205.)

courses deep to the flexor digitorum brevis, which bifurcates and inserts at the middle aspect of the middle phalanx. The flexor digitorum longus tendon continues distally and inserts into the base of the distal phalanx. The extensor hood is connected by an extensor sling to the plantar plate under the metatarsophalangeal joint. The interossei tendons insert into the extensor hood,[11, 12] passing plantar to the axis of motion of the metatarsophalangeal joint and dorsal to the axis of the proximal and distal interphalangeal joints (Fig. 9–2). This gives the interossei the ability to flex the metatarsophalangeal joint while extending the proximal and distal interphalangeal joints, in a fashion analogous to the interossei of the hand. The lumbrical tendon passes deep to the transverse intermetatarsal ligament and then

inserts into the tibial side extensor hood, acting as an extensor of the proximal and distal interphalangeal joints. The antagonist groups for the metatarsophalangeal joint are the intrinsics (flexion) and the extensor digitorum longus tendon (extension); for the interphalangeal joints, they are the intrinsics (extension) and the flexor digitorum longus and brevis tendons (flexion) (Fig. 9–3). Given the weak action of the intrinsics for flexion of the metatarsophalangeal joint and extension at the proximal interphalangeal and distal interphalangeal joints, it becomes apparent why deformities of the digit are of hyperextension of the metatarsophalangeal joint, of hyperflexion of the proximal interphalangeal and distal interphalangeal joints, or both. The strongest structure preventing hyperextension of the metatar-

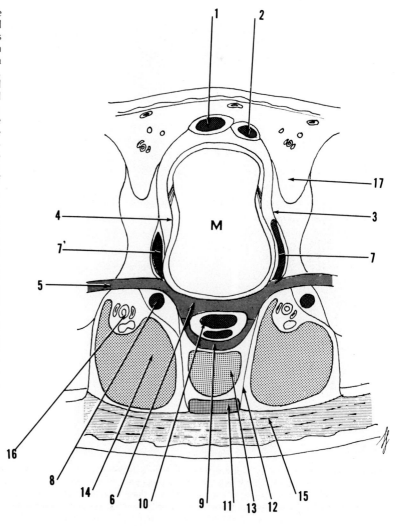

FIGURE 9–2. Cross section of the ball of the foot. M, metatarsal head; 1, extensor digitorum longus tendon; 2, extensor digitorum brevis tendon; 3, transverse lamina of the extensor aponeurosis; 4, capsule of the metatarsophalangeal joint; 5, deep transverse metatarsal ligament; 6, plantar plate; 7, 7', interossei muscles located in the narrow cleft formed by the capsule and transverse lamina (7) or incorporated in the split of the transverse lamina (7'); 8, lumbrical tendon in its own tunnel on the tibial side of the joint; 9, long flexor tunnel; 10, long flexor tendons; 11, longitudinal band of the plantar aponeurosis; 12, vertical thin fibrous band of the plantar aponeurosis forming a preflexor tendon space lodging a preflexor adipose cushion (13); 14, fat body on the plantar aspect of 5 covering the neurovascular bundle (16); 15, transverse component of the plantar aponeurois; 17, triangular adipofascial complex filling the intermetatarsal capitular space and carrying superficial nerves and vessels. (From Sarrafian SK: Anatomy of the Foot and Ankle. Philadelphia, JB Lippincott, 1983, p 243.)

Muscle antagonists

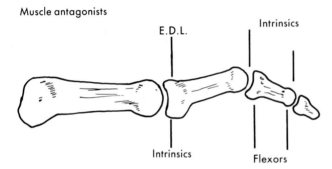

FIGURE 9–3. Relationship of intrinsic and extrinsic muscles about the lesser toe. E.D.L., extensor digitorum longus. (Reproduced by permission from Coughlin MJ, Mann RA: Lesser toe deformities. *In* Mann RA [Ed]: Surgery of the Foot, 5th Ed. St. Louis, 1986, The CV Mosby Co, p 140.)

sophalangeal joint is the plantar capsule and aponeurosis, which together form the plantar plate (Fig. 9–4).[6] This structure provides resistance to hyperextension and, along with the intrinsics, helps to bring the proximal phalanx to a neutral position. During a normal gait cycle, the motion of the toe at the metatarso-

phalangeal joint is passive extension. The plantar plate provides static forces to help return the toe to neutral, along with dynamic forces from the intrinsic flexors.

When the proximal phalanx is hyperextended, the extensor digitorum longus tendon is unable to extend the interphalangeal joints

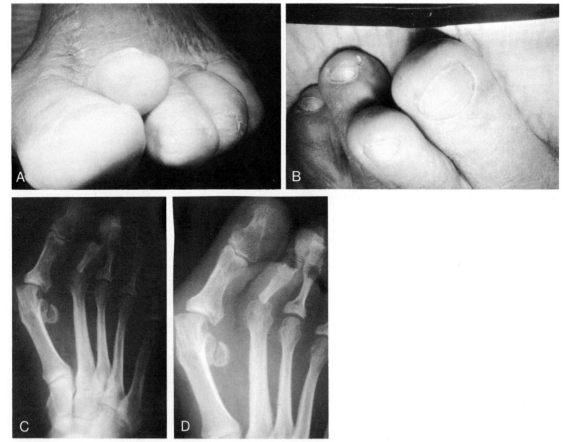

FIGURE 9–4. The importance of the plantar plate is demonstrated by this patient in whom a Keller-type procedure was performed on the second toe rendering the pad incompetent. As pictured here, the results demonstrate the dorsal migration of the second toe, with a subsequent increased valgus deformity of the great toe. This procedure is not recommended. *(A),* Elevated second toe at metatarsophalangeal joint. *(B),* Great toe underlaps and further displaces the second toe. *(C and D),* Resection of the proximal articulation and condylar flare of the proximal phalanx leads to further valgus of the great toe.

and the flexor digitorum longus tendon is unable to flex the metatarsophalangeal joint. Therefore, a foot placed in a shoe with a high heel with subsequent hyperextension of the metatarsophalangeal joint puts the toe in a position in which there is very little resistance to further extension of the metatarsophalangeal joint or flexion of the interphalangeal joints, which can easily explain the incidence of hammer toe deformities in women who wear stylish shoes.

HAMMER TOE DEFORMITIES

A hammer toe is usually a fixed flexion contracture at the proximal interphalangeal joint. A hammer toe causes pain when the dorsal aspect of the proximal interphalangeal joint rubs against the toe box. Conservative measures include the use of both a protective pad over the dorsal aspect of the distal interphalangeal joint and extra-depth shoes with a deeper toe box (Fig. 9–5).

The DuVries arthroplasty is a satisfactory surgical solution to this problem.[6] After resection of the distal condyle of the proximal phalanx, a fibrous joint forms, allowing a small amount of motion at the joint. Other procedures can also produce a satisfactory result.[5, 10]

The procedure is performed by removing an ellipse of skin over the dorsal aspect of the proximal interphalangeal joint, excising this callused skin, the extensor tendon, and the joint capsule (Fig. 9–6A to D). Following exposure of the joint, the collateral ligaments are cut, the distal condyle of the proximal phalanx is delivered into the wound, and the condyle of the proximal phalanx is then resected using a bone cutter (Fig. 9–6E). At this point, care should be taken to remove the entire condyle and to cut it at a plane perpendicular to the shaft of the proximal phalanx to avoid any prominent edges, which might cause irritation (Fig. 9–6F). The smallest amount possible of the shaft of the proximal phalanx should be removed to avoid a floppy distal toe. When the bone is cut, care should be taken to visualize the tips of the bone cutter to minimize the chance of injury to the neurovascular structures. Some surgeons carry out a tenotomy of the flexor digitorum brevis tendon at this point in the procedure. Other surgeons divide the flexor digitorum longus tendon. These tenotomies are accomplished as described in the next section (dorsally, through the resection site).

At this point, fixation of the toe and closure of the wound can be accomplished in either of two ways. With the first method, a smooth Kirschner wire can be brought distally from the joint out through the end of the toe; next, with the toe held in a satisfactorily corrected position, the pin can be brought in a retrograde fashion back into the proximal phalanx. The pin can be cut where it exits the toe and then bent. The extensor tendon can be repaired and the skin can be closed in separate layers. With the second method, the skin can be closed with a mattress suture. The deep portion of the suture picks up the skin and extensor tendon, and the superficial suture at the edge of the wound contains only skin.

An alternate method of closure and fixation does not use a Kirschner wire; instead, the skin is closed with mattress sutures, as previously described. Telfa bolsters are placed under each suture, allowing more leverage on the toe and holding it in satisfactory alignment (Fig. 9–6G).

If Telfa bolsters are used, they should be removed in approximately 7 to 10 days to avoid skin injury. The toe is then supported with tape for approximately 6 weeks, which helps to prevent recurrence (Fig. 9–6H). If a Kirschner wire is used, it can be removed in 3 weeks, and the toe can then be taped for 3 to 4 weeks. Swelling of the toe often persists for up to 6 months (Fig. 9–6I).

Dynamic Hammer Toe

A dynamic hammer toe is one in which the hammer toe deformity appears to be caused by a contracture of the flexor digitorum longus tendon. This deformity is not present with the ankle in an equinus position but is prominent with the foot and ankle in a neutral or dorsiflexed position. The deformity itself can also be resolved with passive plantar flexion of the toe at the metatarsophalangeal joint or passive elevation of the metatarsal head (Fig. 9–7).[3, 6] It is important to differentiate this from the fixed hammer toe deformity because the treatment is different (Fig. 9–8A to C). Two surgical procedures can produce satisfactory results. One method entails a resection of the distal condyle of the proximal phalanx as in a standard fixed hammer toe deformity, coupled

Text continued on page 84

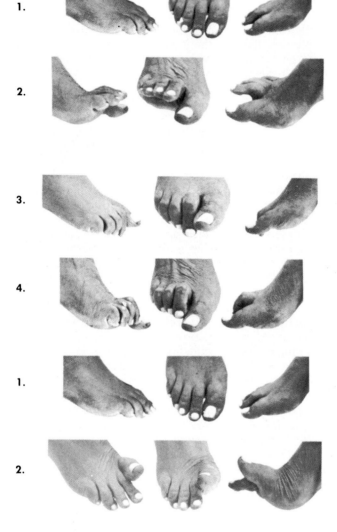

A

B

FIGURE 9–5. (A), Action of the muscles in clawtoe deformity (fresh cadaver foot). 1, At rest. 2, Tension on the extensor digitorum longus alone. Note the extension of the metatarsophalangeal joints and the minimal extension of the interphalangeal joints. 3, Tension on the flexor digitorum longus alone. Note that maximal flexion occurs in the interphalangeal joints. 4, Tension simultaneously on the extensor digitorum longus and the flexor digitorum longus. Note the resulting deformities in all but the great toe. (B), Action of the muscles in clawtoe deformity (cadaver foot). 1, At rest. 2, Tension on the extensor hallucis longus alone. Note the extension of the metatarsophalangeal and the interphalangeal joints. 3, Tension on the flexor hallucis longus alone. Note the maximal flexion in the interphalangeal joint. 4, Simultaneous tension on the extensor hallucis longus and the flexor hallucis longus, with resulting hammer toe deformity. (Reproduced by permission from Coughlin MJ, Mann RA: Lesser toe deformities. *In* Mann RA [Ed]: Surgery of the Foot, 5th Ed. St. Louis, 1986, The CV Mosby Co, p 136.)

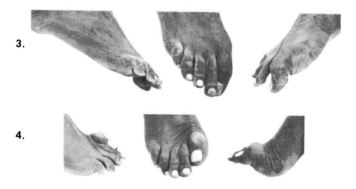

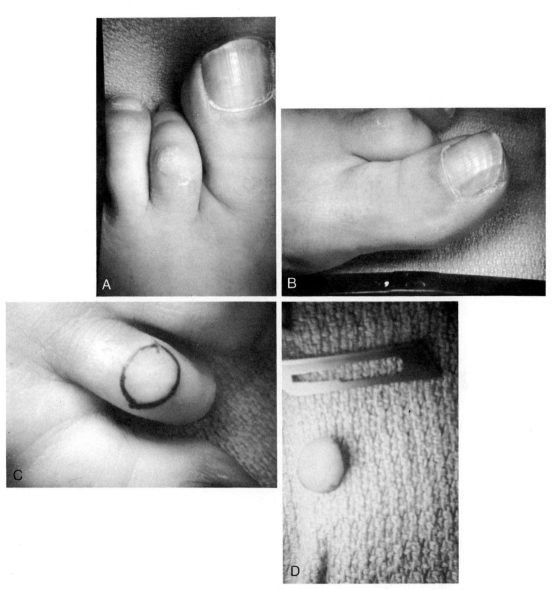

FIGURE 9–6. *(A* and *B),* Preoperative pictures of a patient with a fixed second hammer toe deformity. *(C),* The ellipse of skin that will be excised over the dorsal aspect of the proximal interphalangeal joint. *(D),* The ellipse of skin that has been excised.

Illustration continued on following page

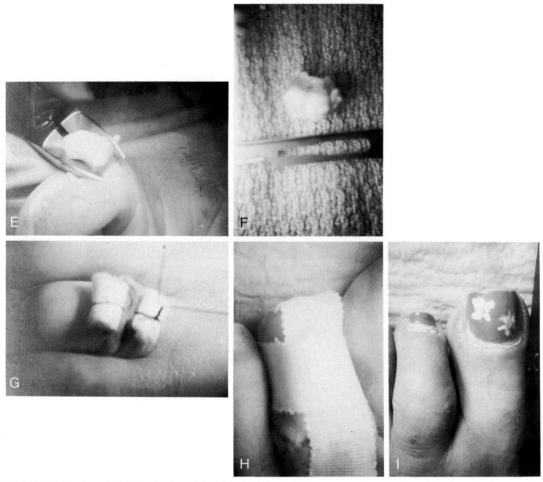

FIGURE 9–6 *Continued (E),* The distal condyle of the proximal phalanx as it is about to be removed with a bone cutter. Note that the tips extend beyond the bone. They can be visualized, to decrease the chance of inadvertent injury to the neurovascular bundle. *(F),* The excised condyle of bone. *(G),* Wound closure with bolsters of Telfa under each loop of the mattress suture to protect the skin, as well as to provide greater leverage. *(H),* Wrapping of the toe with tape after the removal of the suture and bolster approximately 10 days after the procedure. *(I),* The toe postoperatively. (From Mizel MS: Correction of hammertoe and mallet toe deformities. Operative Tech Orthop 2:189, 1992.)

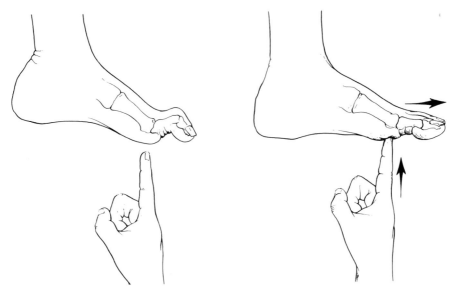

FIGURE 9–7. The push-up test. When the toes are easily flexible, pushing up on the metatarsal heads resolves the hammer toe deformity. (From Johnson KA: Surgery of the Foot and Ankle. New York, Raven Press, 1989, p 110.)

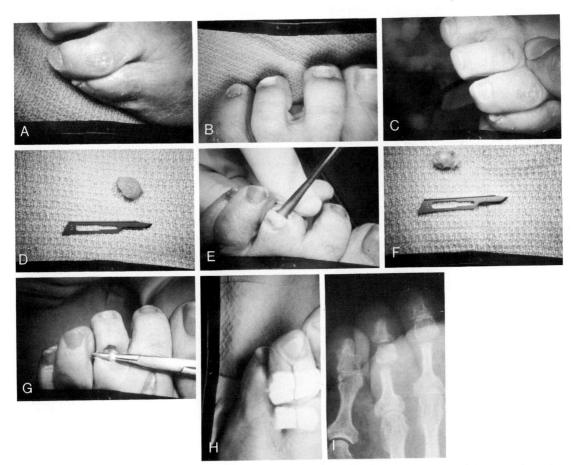

FIGURE 9–8. (A and B), Dynamic hammer toes of the third and fourth toes. (C), Resolution of the deformity with passive neutralization of the metatarsophalangeal joint. (D), The ellipse of skin that has been removed from the dorsal aspect of the interphalangeal joint. (E), Soft tissues elevated off the distal condyle. (F), The distal condyle that has been removed with a bone cutter. (G), A long flexor tendon that has been dissected free and elevated with a hemostat prior to its release. (H), The toe following closure with Telfa bolsters. (I), Postoperative x-ray study of the third and fourth toes.

with a tenotomy of the flexor digitorum longus tendon. The other method was described by Girdlestone and involves the transfer of the flexor digitorum longus tendon to the dorsum of the proximal phalanx to act as an extensor.[1, 8, 12, 13] Decompression of the toe by waist resection of the proximal phalanx has been described, but this author has had no personal experience with it.[7] Conservative treatment for this problem is aimed at relieving the symptoms with extra-depth shoes to allow for the increased toe height.

Surgical Treatment

Condylectomy and Flexor Tenotomy

An elliptical incision is made over the dorsal aspect of the proximal interphalangeal joint, and the extensor tendon is released along with the collateral ligaments at the proximal interphalangeal joint (Fig. 9–8D). With the soft tissue retracted, a bone cutter is used to resect the distal condyle (Fig. 9–8E), taking care to remove the entire condyle and a minimal amount of the shaft while avoiding injury to the neurovascular bundle. After removal of the condyle (Fig. 9–8F), the distal toe is held, a small amount of traction is applied, and a No. 11 blade is used in a longitudinal fashion to cut through the volar plate, staying in the center of the plate so as to minimize the possibility of injury to the neurovascular bundles. Following this, a small curved hemostat is used to dissect the flexor digitorum longus tendon free and to elevate it into the wound (Fig. 9–8G). Hyperflexion of the distal interphalangeal joint confirms that it is the flexor digitorum longus tendon. This tendon is then sharply cut. Following this, the toe is immobilized in a satisfactory position using either a smooth Kirschner wire or a 3–0 silk suture and a horizontal mattress stitch with Telfa bolsters (Fig. 9–8H), as in a standard hammer toe procedure. The remainder of the postoperative management remains the same as that used for repair of a static hammer toe (Fig. 9–8I).

Flexor Tendon Transfer (Girdlestone Procedure)

A Z-shaped incision is made from the flexor crease at the base of the toe, extending to the distal pulp. The long flexor tendon can then be identified, released distally, and carefully split along the longitudinal raphe with a No. 11 blade to create two tails (Fig. 9–9).

At this point, a longitudinal incision is made over the dorsal aspect of the metatarsophalangeal joint and the proximal aspect of the proximal phalanx. A hemostat is placed from the dorsal incision along the extensor hood to the middle of the plantar incision, taking care to avoid the neurovascular bundle. One of the tails of the flexor tendon is then brought up by the hemostat to the dorsal side of the toe. This is repeated so that both tails are situated on the dorsal aspect of the proximal phalanx, one medially and one laterally. If there is any element of a hyperextension deformity at the metatarsophalangeal joint, an extensor tenotomy can be performed at the level of the metatarsophalangeal joint, with release of the entire dorsal capsule. With the toe held in a slightly overcorrected position of metatarsophalangeal flexion and proximal interphalangeal extension, and the foot and ankle at neutral flexion and extension, both tails are sutured into place on the extensor hood, using a 3–0 suture. All wounds are then closed with interrupted sutures, with absorbable suture material used to close the plantar incisions. A compression dressing is applied, and the patient is allowed to ambulate in a postoperative wooden shoe for 3 weeks.

MALLET TOE DEFORMITIES

Mallet toe deformities are usually fixed and are symptomatic because of the constant striking of the distal tip of the toe on the ground. This results in a painful callus at the tip of the toe. Successful conservative treatment can be accomplished by placing a piece of felt or a padding device under the toe to elevate the tip off the ground. Correction of the mallet toe deformity requires release of the flexor digitorum longus tendon[3, 6] and usually removal of the distal condyles of the middle phalanx as well.

Surgical Treatment

An elliptical incision is made over the distal interphalangeal joint, and a small ellipse of skin is removed. The extensor tendon and collateral ligaments are released, with care taken to avoid injury to the neurovascular structures. The distal condyles of the middle phalanx are then resected using a bone cutter or a small power saw. Following this, a longitudinal incision is made in the midline of the plantar plate of the joint, and the flexor digitorum tendon is identified, elevated using a small hemostat, and then cut. The toe can then be held in a satisfactory position with a smooth 0.062- or 0.045-inch Kirschner wire, and the reapproximated wound can be closed with simple skin sutures after repair of the extensor mechanism. Alternatively, the wound can be closed with a mattress suture of 3–0 silk, taking care to pick up the skin and extensor tendons with the far throw and to pick up the skin only with the superficial stitch at the wound edge. Telfa bolsters are inserted, as for hammer toe repair, both to gain leverage and to prevent excess pressure on the skin. The smooth pin should remain in place for approximately 3 to 4 weeks, and following this, the toe should be held taped in position for approximately 3 weeks. If the mattress suture and the bolster are used, the sutures should be removed in approximately 7 to 10 days. The toe should be held taped in one position for 6 more weeks after surgery to allow satisfactory healing and fibrous tissue formation, no matter which closure is performed. The Kirschner wire can be removed after 3 weeks.

HARD CORNS

Hard corns are the result of the little toe's being pressed against the side of the toe box, with subsequent thickening of the skin at the site of increased pressure.[2, 3] Generally, hard corns occur at the level of the condyle of the proximal phalanx on the fifth toe. This condition is differentiated from the soft corns, which are found between toes, where moisture is present, and which subsequently form a soft skin callosity. Hard corns can be treated nonsurgically with protective pads that have a hole cut over the thickened skin or with the use of footwear that has a larger toe box.

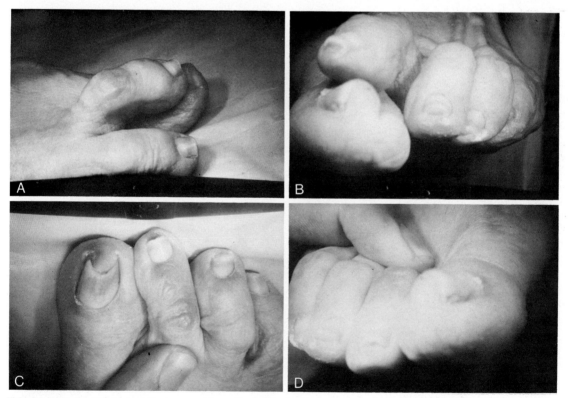

FIGURE 9–9. The Girdlestone-Taylor procedure. *(A and B),* The second hammer toe, which is associated with a hallux valgus deformity. *(C and D),* Correction of the hammer toe deformity with slight finger pressure.

Illustration continued on following page

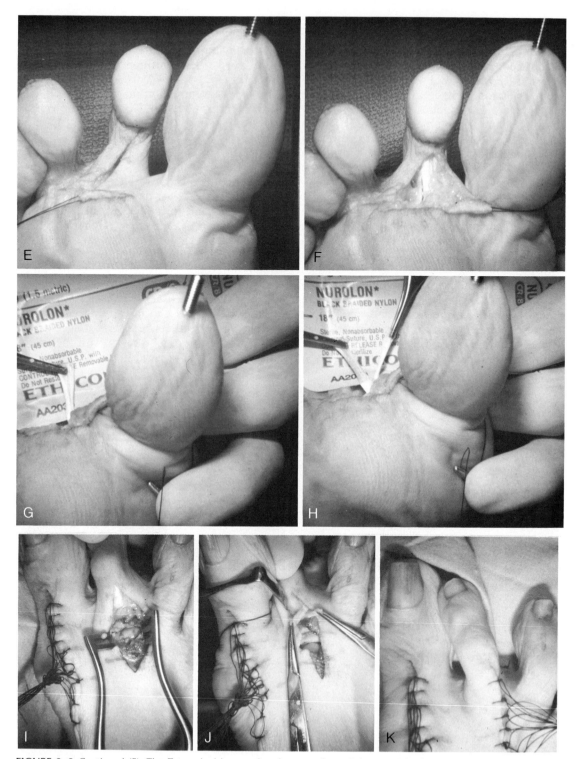

FIGURE 9–9 *Continued (E),* The Z-type incision on the plantar surface of the second toe after correction of the hallux valgus deformity. *(F),* The flexor tendons are exposed after longitudinal division of the sheath. *(G),* The flexor tendon has been released distally. *(H),* The long flexor tendon has been split along its raphe. *(I),* A dorsal incision over the second toe with release of the extensor tendon and dorsal capsule. *(J),* The flexor tendon tails have been brought up around each side of the proximal phalanx inside the neurovascular bundles. *(K),* Correction of the deformity.

Surgical Treatment

A longitudinal incision is made on the dorsum of the fifth toe, and a sharp dissection is carried down to the distal condyle of the proximal phalanx. Collateral ligaments are released along with the extensor tendon, and a condylectomy is then performed with a bone cutter or power saw. Following this, the skin incision is closed with interrupted sutures. The toe is protected for a period of 3 weeks postoperatively with a wooden shoe, with full weight bearing permitted immediately after surgery. It is important to remove the entire condyle and not to leave a small pointed spicule, which could be painful. The toe should be taped to provide support for 6 weeks (Fig. 9–10).

I always remove the entire condyle and rarely remove only a prominent corner. Removal of the entire condyle allows uniform stresses to the entire width of the shaft, preventing the distal aspect of the toe from falling into a varus or valgus position. In the little toe, stabilization with a pin or bolsters has not been necessary. With the use of a longitudinal incision, as was described, the toe remains stable. I have performed this procedure in this fashion (which I learned from R. A. Mann) for 10 years with no difficulty.

SOFT CORNS

A soft corn is a thickening of the skin between two toes that results from their pressing together.[2, 3, 6] These corns are referred to

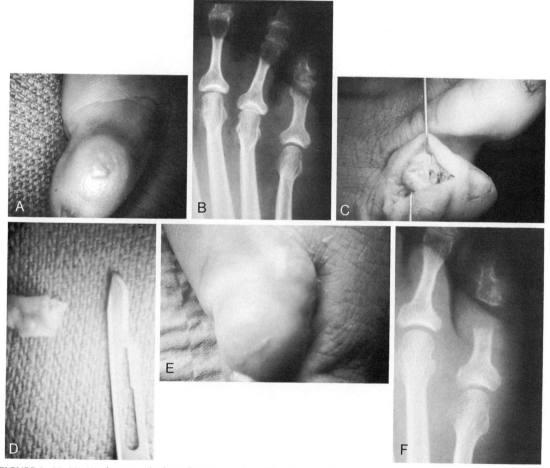

FIGURE 9–10. *(A)*, Hard corn at the lateral superior edge of the fifth toe. *(B)*, Preoperative x-ray study. *(C)*, The longitudinal incision has been made, and the distal condyle of the proximal phalanx has been identified. *(D)*, The distal condyle has been excised. *(E)*, The same toe 3 months postoperatively, with the hard corn now resolved. *(F)*, A postoperative x-ray study. Note that the entire condyle has been excised and no bony spicules are present.

as soft corns because of the moisture present between the toes, which maintains the thickened skin in a moist, soft form. Nonsurgical treatment consists of placement of a soft material, such as lamb's wool, between the toes to prevent the irritation.

Surgical Treatment

The surgical treatment of a soft corn consists of removing the bony prominence that is causing the irritation. This condition is often satisfactorily treated with removal of the condyle involved. Surgically, removal is done in a fash-

ion similar to a fixed hammer toe condylectomy. If there is any question about the location of the bony prominences involved, a lead marker can be placed over the soft corn and an x-ray study can be taken to better identify the offending bony prominences (Fig. 9–11).

(*Editor's note*: An alternative technique removes the intervening skin between bony prominences, and a partial syndactylization is performed between the adjacent toes. The syndactyly technique, described in Chapter 14, has particular validity in this situation. The resection arthroplasty described here by Mizel has particular merit in recurrent problems.)

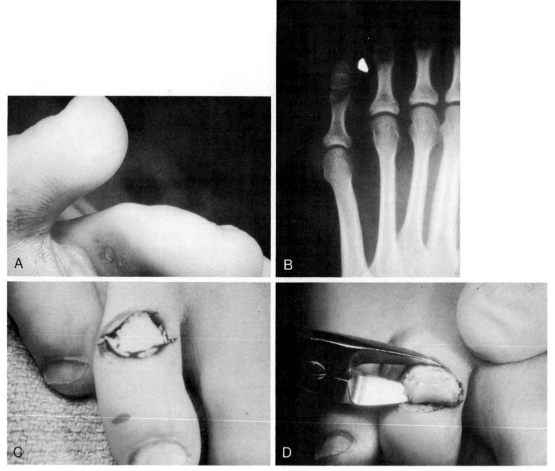

FIGURE 9–11. *(A)*, Preoperative picture of the soft corn on the lateral aspect of the fourth toe. *(B)*, Preoperative x-ray study with a lead marker placed over the lesion shows it to be at the level of the distal condyle of the proximal phalanx of the fourth toe. *(C)*, The ellipse of skin has been excised from the fourth toe. *(D)*, The bone cutter is positioned to excise the distal condyle of the proximal phalanx.

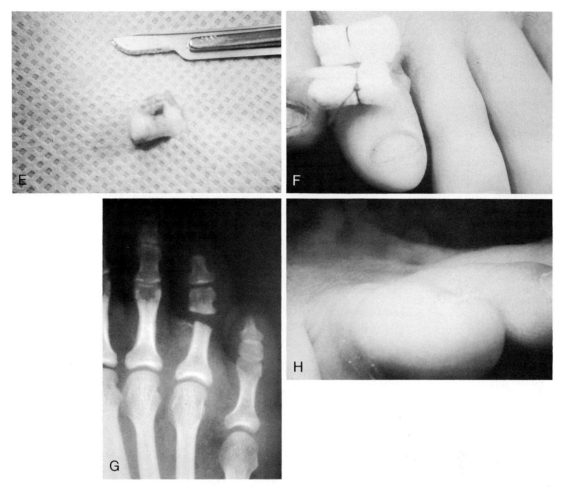

FIGURE 9–11 *Continued (E)*, The bony condyle has been removed. *(F)*, The toe with postoperative closure with Telfa bolsters. *(G)*, The postoperative x-ray study, in which the distal condyle has been removed. *(H)*, The toe with the soft corn resolved.

COCK-UP DEFORMITY OF THE FIFTH TOE

Some patients develop a significant cock-up deformity of the fifth toe, in which the proximal phalanx of the fifth toe is almost at a right angle to the metatarsal shaft. Treatment is basically aimed at realignment of both the metatarsophalangeal joint and the proximal interphalangeal joint. The Ruiz-Mora procedure has been very satisfactory in resolving this problem.[4]

Surgical Treatment

Ruiz-Mora Procedure

An elliptical incision is made on the plantar surface of the proximal phalanx of the fifth toe, with the long axis along the longitudinal axis of the toe, deviated slightly medially at the proximal aspect of the toe. The ellipse of skin is removed, and the proximal phalanx is then excised through this incision. Technically, disarticulation at the level of the proximal interphalangeal joint, with dissection carried out proximally, appears to be the easiest way to perform this procedure. The incision is then closed transversely to the long axis of the incision, bringing the toe into a mildly medially deviated plantar direction. The toe is then kept in a bulky dressing for approximately 1 1/2 weeks, after which it is held in position with tape for another 4 weeks. A wooden shoe is used for ambulation after surgery, and the patient continues to use it for approximately 6 weeks.

An alternate procedure has been described that includes reduction of the metatarsophalangeal joint (with lengthening of the soft tissues); reduction of the proximal interphalangeal joint, which is either passively reducible or requires the resection of the distal aspect of the proximal phalanx; and stabilization of the toe with a pin for 4 to 6 weeks. Flexor tendon transfer or syndactylization is occasionally necessary. The dorsal skin is usually contracted, and a 60-degree Z-plasty or use of a V-Y advancement flap is often necessary, along with tenotomy of the long extensor and dorsal capsulotomy.

References

1. Forrester-Brown MF: Tendon transplantation for the clawing of the great toe. J Bone Joint Surg 20:57, 1938.
2. Higgs SL: Hammer-toe. Postgrad Med J 6:130, 1931.
3. Jahss MH (Ed): Disorders of the Foot. Philadelphia, WB Saunders, 1982, pp 622–658.
4. Janecki CJ, Wilde AH: Results of phalangectomy of the fifth toe for hammer toe. J Bone Joint Surg 58:1005, 1976.
5. Johnson KA: Surgery of the Foot and Ankle. New York, Raven Press, 1989, pp 101–150.
6. Lambrinudi C: An operation for claw toes. Proc R Soc Med 21:239, 1927.
7. Lapidus PW: Operation for correction of hammer toe. J Bone Joint Surg 21:977, 1939.
8. Mann RA (Ed): Surgery of the Foot, 5th Ed. St. Louis, CV Mosby, 1986, pp 132–157.
9. McConnell BE: Correction of hammer toe deformity: A 10 year review of subperiosteal waist resection of proximal phalanx. Orthop Rev 8:65, 1970.
10. Parrish TF: Dynamic correction of claw toes. Orthop Clin North Am 4:97, 1973.
11. Sarrafian SK: Anatomy of the Foot and Ankle. Philadelphia, JB Lippincott, 1983.
12. Serrafian SK, Topouzian LK: Anatomy and physiology of the extensor apparatus of the toes. J Bone Joint Surg 51A:669, 1969.
13. Taylor RG: The treatment of claw toes by multiple transfers of flexor into extensor tendons. J Bone Joint Surg 33B:539, 1951.

10 *Disorders of the Toenails*

MICHAEL J. SHEREFF

$\mathbf{D}$isorders of the toenails are among the most common problems for which patients seek medical attention from the foot and ankle surgeon. These seemingly innocuous abnormalities may cause significant pain and deformity and may even interfere with the patient's ability to ambulate. Disorders of the nail that are commonly seen include those of congenital, traumatic, infectious, inflammatory, acquired, and neoplastic etiologies. The purpose of this chapter is to review the more common nail pathologies, with special emphasis on their treatment.

FUNCTIONAL ANATOMY OF THE TOENAIL

Anatomically, the nail consists of dorsal, intermediate, and ventral layers (Fig. 10–1A).[4, 8, 11] The dorsal nail plate is formed from the upper nail matrix. The intermediate nail plate is formed from the lower nail matrix, and the ventral plate is derived from the nail bed. The nail is covered proximally, medially, and laterally by the skin fold known as the eponychium, or nail wall (Fig. 10–1B). The slit, which is the site where the nail wall joins the nail bed, is known as the nail groove. It is generally believed that the longitudinal growth of the nail occurs primarily from the nail matrix.

INGROWN TOENAIL

Without a doubt, the most common abnormality of the nail seen in an orthopaedic practice is the ingrown toenail, also known as unguis incarnatus (Fig. 10–2).[1, 2, 4–6, 10] In the ingrown toenail, the nail margin grows into the soft lateral nail groove and surrounding skin of the nail wall. A small puncture wound is formed, and normal fungal and bacterial

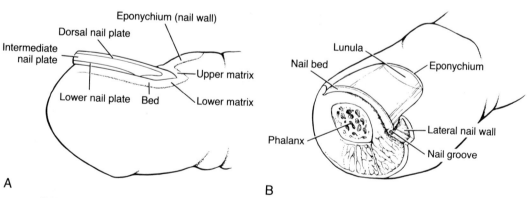

FIGURE 10–1. (A), Anatomic components of the toenail. (B), Cross-sectional anatomy of the nail.

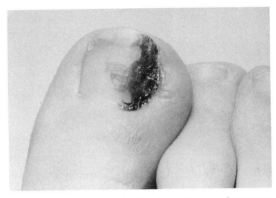

FIGURE 10–2. Photograph of patient with typical ingrown toenail (unguis incarnatus). Note the localized erythema, swelling, and hypertrophy of the nail fold.

flora present on the skin and nail surface invade the wound. This leads to a local inflammatory process that eventually may result in a paronychial infection.

Etiology

Several factors have been implicated in the etiology of the ingrown toenail. Tight, compressing shoes may force the soft nail wall into the nail margin. Tight socks are also thought to lead to local mechanical pressure. If the nail is cut too short, then on growing outward the corners may penetrate the skin. It is generally advised to cut the nail edge transversely at its distal margin. The incurvated nail (see Fig. 10–7), which is a congenital deformity in which the nail margin curves into the sides of the distal phalanx and takes on a horseshoe-shaped appearance when the toe is viewed axially, has been implicated in about 25 percent of cases of ingrown toenail. As one might imagine, this deformed nail has a greater tendency to project into the surrounding nail wall and eponychium.

Clinical Manifestations

The most common site of the ingrown nail is thought to be the lateral edge of the hallux nail. It should be noted, however, that any side of any nail may be involved. Patients complain of local pain as the most frequent symptom. Physical examination reveals localized tenderness, erythema, and swelling. Hypertrophy and granulation of the nail fold is quite common. Suppuration and purulent ex-

udate is seen in cases of paronychial infection. With severe chronic infection, destruction of bone and bulbous enlargement of the toe may be seen.

Laboratory Findings

Further diagnostic work-up may be appropriate if other concomitant lesions are suspected. An underlying bony prominence may often lead to mechanical impingement against the nail or nail bed. Anteroposterior and lateral x-ray studies may be helpful in revealing underlying pathology. If purulent exudate is present, obtaining a culture and sensitivity laboratory examination may help allow for selection of appropriate antibiotics.

Treatment

Nonoperative Treatment

Various conservative modalities of treatment may be helpful in caring for patients with this disorder. Soaking the involved toe three times each day in antiseptic solution may be beneficial. Of great importance is nail packing or nail training, which allows free drainage of what is in reality a localized abscess (Fig. 10–3). A wisp of cotton is inserted first under the nail at its distal corner and then is subsequently laid between the nail margin and skin fold. The initial packing should be performed by the physician. A digital block of local anesthetic may be required in advanced lesions. Afterward, the patient performs nail training after each antiseptic soak. If a small spike of nail is seen to be penetrating the skin, then this may be excised using either the anvil nail splitter or a pair of small iris scissors. If gross purulence is noted, then the patient is given oral antibiotics. A broad-spectrum antibiotic is begun, and once the culture and sensitivity are returned, the antibiotic may be changed. Appropriate footwear includes shoes with low heels and a high, wide toe box, which avoids placing mechanical pressure in the area of involvement. An open-toed sandal or shoe may be helpful.

Operative Treatment

In some cases, surgical treatment is necessary, particularly in those patients who present with a chronic, recurrent ingrown nail that has

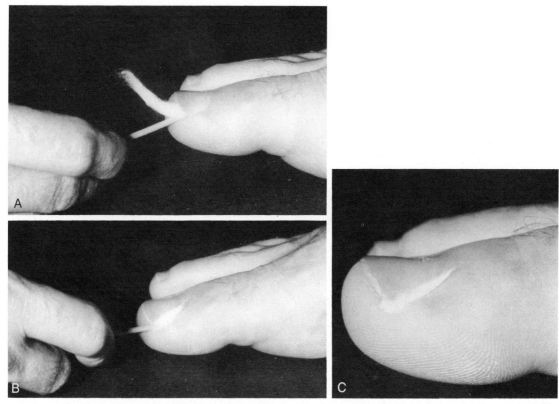

FIGURE 10–3. The technique of nail packing. *(A)*, A wisp of cotton is inserted under the nail at its distal corner. *(B)*, The cotton is subsequently laid between the nail margin and skin fold. *(C)*, Nail packing allows decompression of the mechanical impingement of the nail wall by the margin of the toenail.

proved to be recalcitrant to conservative measures. In these situations, the procedures found to be most effective include three classes of operative intervention. In the first type of procedure, a wedge resection of the nail margin, nail bed, nail matrix, and nail groove is performed (Fig. 10–4).[7, 14] This is commonly referred to as a Heifitz procedure. The Winograd procedure is very similar to the Heifitz procedure in many respects.

FIGURE 10–4. Intraoperative photograph showing wedge resection of the nail margin, bed, matrix, and groove.

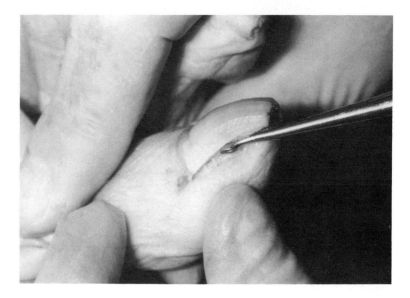

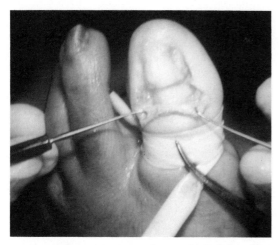

FIGURE 10–5. Intraoperative photograph depicting ablation of the entire nail and nail matrix.

The second type of nail procedure, called the Zadik procedure, includes ablation of the entire nail and nail matrix (Fig. 10–5).[15] This is particularly effective in those cases in which a severely incurvated nail is present.[4]

Finally, if recurrence of the lesion occurs after either of these two operations, then consideration can be given to the performance of a terminal Syme amputation, also known as a Thompson-Terwilliger procedure, in which the entire nail matrix and distal portion of the distal phalanx is removed (Fig. 10–6).[9, 13]

These three procedures are useful not only in unguis incarnatus but may be effective in many other nail disorders, as will be described later in this chapter.

OTHER NAIL DISORDERS

Congenital Nail Disorders

One of the most common congenital abnormalities seen is the previously mentioned incurvated nail (Fig. 10–7). This is a deformity in which the nail margin curves into the sides of the distal phalanx. This disorder may lead to chronic, recurrent ingrown nails and may prove to be quite painful in some patients. When this is the case, any of the three surgical procedures described for the ingrown toenail can be used to ablate the deformed nail.

Traumatic Disorders

Traumatic injuries to the toenail are common. These include subungual hematoma, which commonly occurs in the great toe and is often associated with athletic endeavors in which sudden deceleration occurs. The foot is propelled forward in the shoe and the toe jams against the toe box, leading to subungual hemorrhage. This is often associated with a stubbing injury to the hallux. If the toe is painful, then drainage of the subungual accumulation of blood is helpful. This can be accomplished by use of a flame-sterilized needle. Appropri-

FIGURE 10–6. Intraoperative photograph showing the terminal Syme amputation.

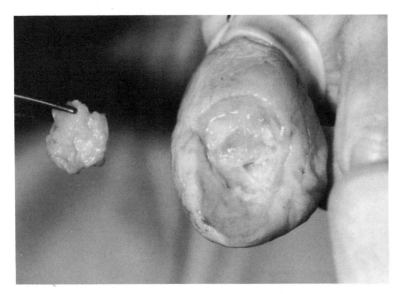

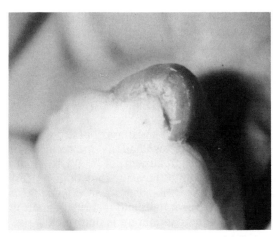

FIGURE 10–7. The incurvated nail is a congenital deformity in which the nail margin curves into the sides of the distal phalanx.

ate shoewear with a high, wide toe box may alleviate the symptoms.

Infectious Disorders

Onychomycosis is a fungal infection of the nail. Unfortunately, this condition often becomes a chronic relapsing problem and therapy is only of temporary value. The involved nail becomes brittle and thickens. Local pain and tenderness may occur. Treatment for this dis-

order is difficult. The use of topical antifungal ointments has proved to be of minimal value. The use of oral griseofulvin requires approximately 2 years of therapy in order to obtain a favorable response. Perhaps the most efficacious means of treatment includes periodic trimming of the thickened nail and appropriate shoewear. If conservative measures fail, consideration could be given for ablation of the nail.

Inflammatory Disorders

Psoriasis of the toenail may be associated with this cutaneous disorder. Pitting, yellowing, and shedding of the nail may occur. Medical therapy with appropriate rheumatologic and dermatologic medications may be helpful in some cases.

Acquired Disorders

Acquired disorders of the nail include onychogryphosis, also known as ram's horn nail (Fig. 10–8). This disorder most often involves the hallux but may also affect the lesser toes. The nails become thickened, darkened, and curved, and the condition may lead to localized pain and tenderness in some individuals. Conservative treatment includes nail trimming and

FIGURE 10–8. Onychogryphosis is an acquired disorder in which the nail becomes thickened, darkened, and curved.

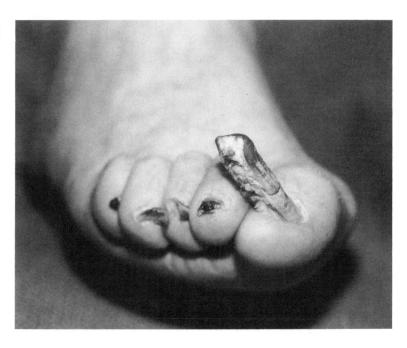

wearing wide toe box shoes. In recalcitrant, symptomatic cases, excision of the entire nail and nail matrix is often curative.

Another acquired disorder involves paraungual corns, which represent localized hyperkeratotic lesions in areas of excessive, mechanical pressure of the foot against the toe box of the shoe. These corns are commonly associated with underlapping fifth toes. Trimming of the paraungual corn and wearing appropriate shoewear may be helpful in some cases. Unfortunately, many patients require appropriate surgical intervention oriented toward the underlying pathology. The surgical procedure most often used in these cases is a terminal Syme-type amputation.

Neoplastic Lesions

Neoplastic lesions can occur. Most commonly seen is subungual exostosis, which is actually a proliferating fibrous cartilaginous cap that merges into mature trabecular bone at its base (Fig. 10–9). These lesions are uniformly benign and most commonly occur in the region of the hallux nail. The treatment of choice is local excision. The surgeon should attempt to preserve as much of the nail bed and matrix as possible. Unfortunately, recurrence is not uncommon and has been reported to occur in approximately 11 percent of patients.

SURGICAL TECHNIQUES

As becomes obvious from the preceding discussion, the same three surgical techniques are most often used for operative treatment of all nail disorders.[3, 8, 11, 12] In this section, these techniques are reviewed.

Wedge Resection of the Nail Margin, Matrix, and Groove (Fig. 10–10)

This procedure is most appropriate in cases of the chronic ingrown nail that are recalcitrant to conservative treatment.[3, 7, 8, 11, 14] It should be postponed until the acute infectious process has subsided. It is also most effective for recurrent ingrown nails and incurvated nails in which only the nail margin is deformed.

Operative Technique

The eponychium is incised for a distance of 5 mm from the point where the proposed nail excision meets the eponychium and then extending proximally, obliquely, and medialward (Fig. 10–10A). The root of the nail is exposed by elevating eponychial flaps. The nail is elevated with a small hemostat or elevator. The nail is incised longitudinally from its distal end to its root, and the fragment is removed (Fig. 10–10B). The nail bed and matrix are incised along the nail incision down to bone. The skin margin is incised to remove an elliptical wedge of tissue. The wedge is then removed en bloc. The matrix and bed are curetted to ensure complete removal of germinal material (Fig. 10–10C). One simple 4–0 nylon suture is applied at the corner of the incision to reapproximate the eponychial flap (Fig. 10–10E). The cavity thus formed is packed with Xeroform gauze. A sterile compression dressing is applied.

Postoperative Treatment

The compression dressing and Xeroform gauze are removed 24 to 36 hours after the operation. A small dressing may then be applied. If inflammation occurs, dilute betadine soaks are instituted three times a day for 20 minutes. The patient wears an open-toed wooden-soled shoe until the wound is healed.

Technical Pitfalls

Failure to remove the root of the nail or inadequate removal of germinal cells of the nail matrix may lead to a recurrence with

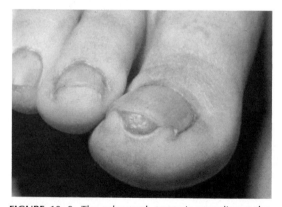

FIGURE 10–9. The subungual exostosis may disrupt the nail bed and result in deformity of the toenail.

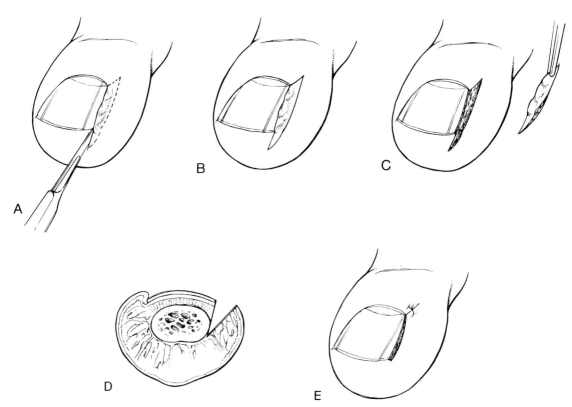

FIGURE 10–10. Surgical technique for wedge resection of the nail margin, matrix, and groove (see text).

regrowth of a portion of the nail. Failure to postpone surgery until the acute paronychial process has subsided may lead to chronic infection and delayed wound healing.

Potential Complications

Delayed wound healing and postoperative inflammation is a possible problem associated with this surgery. Recurrence of a nail horn, also known as an onychoma, has been described. Narrowing of the nail will occur and may lead to an unsightly appearance. The patient should be cautioned regarding this possibility during the preoperative discussion.

Ablation of the Nail and Nail Matrix
(Fig. 10–11)

This operation is most effective for patients with recurrent ingrown nail after the failure of less radical procedures. It is also effective in the alleviation of severe incurvation, onychomycosis, and onychogryphosis.[3, 8, 11, 15]

Operative Technique

An oblique incision 5 mm long is made in each corner of the nail from the base of the nail and extending through the eponychium proximally (Fig. 10–11 *A*). Eponychial flaps are elevated with a dental elevator and retracted proximally. The nail is elevated from the underlying nail matrix and bed with an elevator or with a hemostat. The nail is grasped with a Kocher clamp and is then avulsed. The nail matrix is incised transversely just proximal to the eponychium down to the periosteum of the underlying distal phalanx. The matrix is incised transversely just distal to the lunula. These transverse incisions are connected with a medial and lateral longitudinal incision to remove a rectangular segment including the entire matrix (Fig. 10–11*B*). All germinal material is removed with a scalpel and a curette. The undersurface of the eponychium is then excised by sharp dissection in order to remove the upper root matrix (Fig. 10–11*C*). One simple 4–0 nylon suture is inserted in each corner to reapproximate the eponychium (Fig.

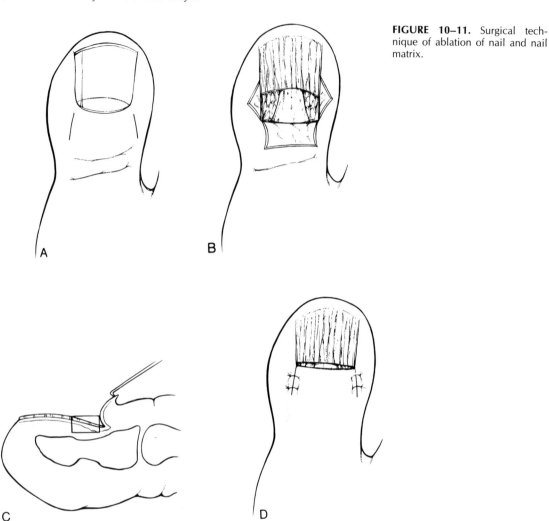

FIGURE 10–11. Surgical technique of ablation of nail and nail matrix.

A

B

C

D

10–11*D*). The defect thus formed is packed with Xeroform gauze. A compression dressing is applied.

Postoperative Treatment

The compression dressing and gauze is removed 24 to 36 hours after the operation, and a new dressing is applied. Some patients will have some local inflammation at the operative site. If this is the case, antiseptic soaks three times a day for 20 minutes will help alleviate this problem. Open-toed wooden-soled shoes are required until wound healing is complete.

Technical Pitfalls

Inadequate removal of nail matrix or failure to remove the root may lead to regrowth of a portion of the nail.

Potential Complications

Delayed wound healing with postoperative inflammation may be apparent. Regrowth of a portion of the nail (nail horn) may require further treatment.

Terminal Syme's Procedure (Fig. 10–12)

This procedure is particularly effective for a recurrent ingrown nail after prior attempts at surgical ablation have failed. It is also quite efficacious for paraungual lesions of the lesser toes (especially the fifth toe) and may be applicable to some subungual tumors. This operation is essentially a radical excision of the nail and nail bed combined with an amputation of the tuft of the distal phalanx.[3, 8, 9, 11, 13]

FIGURE 10–12. Surgical technique of the terminal Syme amputation.

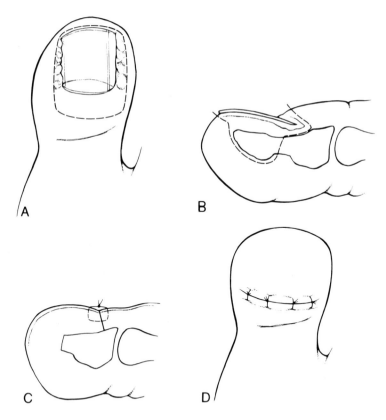

Operative Technique

An incision is made 5 mm proximal to the base of the nail and encircling the entire nail and nail bed (Fig. 10–12 *A*). The nail is completely excised by removing the nail, nail bed, and all soft tissues down to the distal phalanx (Fig. 10–12*B*). The plantar fat pad is separated from the tuft of the distal phalanx subperiosteally. The distal portion of the distal phalanx is excised with a saw or bone biter. The end of the phalanx is smoothed with a rasp. The plantar flap is brought over the stump of the phalanx and sutured to the dorsal skin with interrupted sutures of nonabsorbable material (Fig. 10–12*C* and *D*). A compression dressing is applied.

Postoperative Treatment

The compression dressing is removed after 24 hours. The patient wears an open-toed shoe until the sutures are removed.

Technical Pitfalls

Inadequate removal of bone may lead to areas of prominence, leading to mechanical impingement against the toe box of the shoe.

Inadequate tailoring of the plantar flap may lead to an unsightly bulbous stump.

Complications

Formation of an epithelioid inclusion cyst at the distal stump of the toe may cause tenderness. This lesion often requires surgical removal.

References

1. Bartlett R: A conservative operation for the cure of so-called ingrown toenail. JAMA 108:1257, 1937.
2. Bose B: A technique for excision of nail fold for ingrowing toenail. Surg Gynecol Obstet 132:511, 1971.
3. Brahms MA: Management of skin and nail problems. *In* Evarts CM (Ed): Surgery of the Musculoskeletal System. New York, Churchill Livingstone, 1983, p 239.
4. Dixon GL Jr: Treatment of ingrown toenail. Foot Ankle 3:254, 1983.
5. DuVries HL: Ingrown toenail: A review of the literature and personal observation. Chiropody Rec 27:155–166, 1944.
6. Fowler AW: Excision of the germinal matrix: A unified treatment for embedded toenail and onychogryphosis. Brit J Surg 45:382, 1958.
7. Heifetz CJ: Ingrown toenail: A clinical study. Am J Surg 37:298–315, 1937.
8. Johnson KA: Surgery of the Foot and Ankle. New York, Raven Press, 1989, pp 83–100.

9. Lapidus PW: Complete and permanent removal of toe nail in onychogryposis and subungual osteoma. Am J Surg 19:92, 1933.

10. Murray WR: Onychocryptosis: Principles of non-operative and operative care. Clin Orthop 142:96, 1979.

11. Richardson EG: The foot in adolescents and adults. *In* Crenshaw AH (Ed): Campbell's Operative Orthopaedics. St. Louis, CV Mosby, 1987, pp 829–988.

12. Seibert JS, Mann RA: Dermatology and disorders of the toenails. *In* Mann RA (Ed): Surgery of the Foot. St. Louis, CV Mosby, 1986, pp 394–420.

13. Thompson TC, Terwilliger C: The terminal Syme operation for ingrown toenail. Surg Clin North Am 31:575–584, 1951.

14. Winograd AM: A modification in the technique of operation for ingrown toe-nail. JAMA 92:229, 1929.

15. Zadik FR: Obliteration of the nailbed of the great toe without shortening of the terminal phalanx. J Bone Joint Surg 32B:66, 1950.

11

Morton's Neuroma— Interdigital Neuroma

J. CHRISTOPHER REYNOLDS

An interdigital neuroma (Morton's neuroma) is an entity in which the plantar interdigital nerves become entrapped, irritated, and compressed as they pass into the toes from the bottom of the foot. This condition classically is exhibited as a burning pain on the bottom of the foot in the area under the second, third, or fourth metatarsophalangeal joints. The pain may radiate to the toes, and symptoms are commonly increased by activity and decreased by rest.

In 1845, Durlacher first described this symptom complex in King George IV.[8] In 1875, Morton described an "affection" with pain in the area of the fourth metatarsophalangeal joint. Morton's cases described pain in and around the base of the proximal phalangeal fourth toe or fourth metatarsal head. Several surgical procedures were carried out and described by him as removing the head of the fourth metatarsal with relief of the pain. He reported that in one case "the nervous structures were all healthy as proved by microscopic examination." Morton believed the cause of the condition problem was in the relationship and mobility of the fourth and fifth metatarsal heads.[28] He did not describe what is currently believed to be the pathologic process; but, nevertheless, his name has been associated with this syndrome subsequently. Jones and Tubby, in 1898, suggested resection of a metatarsal head as the operation "par excellence" for this condition.[21]

Hoadley subsequently described the condition. He reported that surgical removal of the nerve cured the condition.[18] Betts, in 1940,

proposed the idea that a neuroma or irritated nerve was the cause of the condition and recommended surgical excision of the interdigital nerve, observing that the nerve was "thicker than the other digital nerves" because it received branches from the medial and lateral plantar nerves. Betts believed that this particular nerve (in the third interspace) was involved because of the tethering of these nerves by the flexor brevus muscle, which stretched the nerve underneath the deep transverse metatarsal ligament with dorsiflexion of the toes.[3] McElvenny, in 1943,[25] and Bickel and Dockerty,[4] in 1947, also attributed this phenomenon to degenerative and proliferative changes in the interdigital nerve.

Nissen, in 1948, postulated a more vascular degeneration basis for these symptoms, attributing the symptoms to ischemia of the nerve.[30] Mulder, in 1951, described a diagnostic test with a palpable click elicited by lateral pressure on the metatarsal heads, which he believed represented the "tumor escaping into the sole of the foot." He also described a thickened bursa secondarily between these metatarsal heads.[29] Nissen and Shephard also considered that a thickened bursa contributed to symptoms in some patients.[31, 36]

Reed and Bliss, in 1973, described the pathologic changes of the nerve itself and demonstrated fibrosis and fibrinoid degeneration and fibroelastic changes in the soft tissue around the neurovascular bundle.[34]

Ha'Eri and coworkers concluded that "repeated trauma in the connective tissue elements, including nerves and arteries in the interdigital clefts, led to a reactive overgrowth of connective tissue that disrupted the nerves and the arteries."[16]

Using the electron microscope, Lassman noted (1) sclerosis and edema of the endoneurium, (2) thickening and hyalinization of the basement membranes caused by multiple layers of basement membrane, (3) thickening of the perineurium, (4) deposition of an amorphous eosinophilic material built up by filaments of tubular structures, and (5) demyelinization and degeneration of the nerve fibers without signs of wallerian degeneration and local initial hyperplasia of the unmyelinated nerves followed by degeneration. He concluded that these findings were consistent with an entrapment neuropathy, although his findings were not typical of what others had described for compression neuropathies. He did not concur with the opinion of some authors who suggested that ischemia was the cause. In the absence of orthopedic abnormalities of the foot involved, he suggested that in addition to the chronic trauma, some metabolic or hormonal fractures were involved in the development of this condition.[23] Graham and Gauthier also suggest that the condition is an entrapment disorder.[12, 13] The pathologic description of any specimen removed at surgery generally reflects some report "typical of Morton's neuroma," "perineural fibrosis," or some similar finding. Johnson notes that pathologists almost always make a pathologic diagnosis of "neuroma."[20] He notes that, unfortunately, the pathologic diagnosis provided at surgery has not been reliable in predicting the failure or success of various operations on these conditions.[20]

Tate and Rusin theorized that in individuals with increased forefoot varus that "tissue under the fourth metatarsal head and between the third and fourth metatarsals would receive frictional forces for a longer duration of time during the gate cycle. Therefore, the communication between the medial and lateral plantar nerves would be subjected to abnormal shearing stress, which we theorize as the biomechanical etiology of the so-called Morton's neuroma."[37]

Mulder stated that abnormal mobility of the metatarsals results in a widening of the bursa between the heads, creating a space "into which the plantar tissue, including the plantar nerves and vessels, may enter, to be pinched by subsequent movements of the metatarsal

heads."[29] Gilmour, who studied the transmetatarsophalangeal bursa, notes that it was always thickened and that the bursal changes were primary and caused secondary compression on the neurovascular bundle.[10, 11]

In any event, most authors conclude that the problem represents some type of chronic entrapment neuropathy, with the common findings as described by Lassmann and with the changes primarily being degenerative in nature. In the absence of other consistent causative factors, which occur more frequently in women wearing high heels, most authors attribute the development of this condition to repetitive trauma.[7]

ANATOMY

The posterior tibial nerve passing below the medial malleolus divides into the medial and lateral plantar nerves, which subsequently divide into the interdigital nerves that course along the plantar aspect of the foot, with branches passing underneath the deep transverse metatarsal ligament and supplying sensation to the interspace and respective interdigital areas. These nerves supply most of the three of the four sides of the individual toe as well as the plantar aspect of the foot below the toes. The nerve leading to the third interspace receives contributions from the medial and lateral plantar nerves (see Fig. 11–10).

The third and fourth interspace has been described over the years as being the most common area for this condition[12, 20, 39]; but, in the author's experience, the incidence of neuroma has been almost identical in the second and third interspace. Other authors have also noted interdigital neuromas in the second as well as third interspace.[7, 17, 23, 24, 38] This casts doubts on Bett's theory of the tethering of the nerve to the third interspace.

PATIENTS' COMPLAINTS AND PHYSICAL FINDINGS

Patients commonly complain of plantar tenderness, pain radiating into the toes, burning pain, pain increased by walking, and relief by removing the shoe as well as relief by rest. The less common complaints include aching or sharp pain, pain up the leg or foot, numbness into the toes or foot, a cramping sensation, a popping or snapping sensation, or a lumpy feeling. The patient may present with a wide variety of symptoms, with the duration varying from a few months to many years. In most cases, the onset of symptoms is gradual.[26] The most common preoperative physical findings include subjective tenderness on the plantar aspect of the foot under the second or third interspace. Subjective numbness and pain radiating into the toe (50 percent) with plantar pressure is less common. Occasionally, a clicking sound can be palpated in the interspace, which is associated with pain and is called Mulder's click.[9, 29] If present, this is almost pathognomic of this condition. This click, however, is not the usual case in the author's experience because it is infrequently palpated. Squeezing the adjacent metatarsal heads together also frequently causes subjective discomfort. Dorsal palpation is usually painless. The patients usually have a normal gait, and there is no consistent type of foot or arch configuration in these patients.[24] In some patients, a synovial cyst may be present, usually in the second interspace. In these patients, one sees a spreading of the second and third toes and a thickened, doughy mass can be palpated in the interspace.

Occasionally, the patient has tenderness in the interspace between the first and second toes or the fourth and fifth toes. It has been reported that nerves have been removed in these areas, but finding a truly inflamed nerve or neuroma in these interspaces is rare.

The differential diagnosis includes metatarsophalangeal capsulitis or synovitis, intermetatarsal bursitis, arthritis, stress fracture of a metatarsal, plantar wart, and intractable plantar keratosis.

Plain x-ray evaluation is rarely beneficial, but it is performed to rule out some pathology that may be a factor prior to surgery. (The metatarsal heads may appear to be closer together than normally seen, suggesting a bony impingement.) Recently, Redd and associates have reported the use of ultrasonography that reviewed 134 intermetatarsal masses in 100 patients.[33] Forty-five percent of these patients underwent surgery, and the pathology confirmed the diagnosis. A nerve diameter of approximately 5 mm seemed to be the size that determined the need for surgery. The author had little experience with this approach, but it seems to be a relatively inexpensive adjunct for use in lesions that are difficult to

diagnose. The reliability of this approach inevitably depends on the interest and experience of the involved radiologist. Ultrasonography is considered less costly than the use of magnetic resonance imaging, which may also be used. Klenerman, Oh, and others have reported the use of nerve conduction studies for the diagnosis of Morton's neuroma but this method has been of little clinical value to the average practitioner at this point.[15, 22, 32]

THREE OPTIONS OF TREATMENT

Nonoperative Treatment

The majority of patients with this condition respond to conservative treatment. In the office, initial treatment is directed toward the use of a felt metatarsal pad (Hapad) or equivalent pad to be placed in the patient's shoe, with the pad placed just behind the area of maximum tenderness. The pads come in a variety of sizes, and often the patient must try several kinds of pads that can be placed in the shoe by the patient or by a pedorthotist. The author provides the patient with a pad and explains to him or her to place the pad in the shoe with a piece of cellophane tape in approximately the correct area and to move it back and forth until the point of maximum comfort is found, taking care to avoid placing the pad too far forward or too far back. It is necessary to give some guidance to the patient as to approximately the correct location to place the pad in the shoe. The author emphasizes to the patient that the pad will fail unless it is properly in place. This is usually behind the second and third or third and fourth metatarsal heads, or both. On occasion, when the area of maximum tenderness is poorly localized, a metatarsal support behind all the metatarsal heads has been used. In the author's experience, approximately two-thirds of patients respond with pads, although approximately 20 percent of this group wear the pads on an indefinite basis for continued relief.[35]

Nevertheless, most people are satisfactorily relieved and essentially cured by the use of the metatarsal pads. Proper shoewear for the pad is important, including shoes with a low heel, rounded toe, and a sufficiently sturdy sole to prevent forces of impact from the bottom of the foot to pass up to the sole distal to the pad. Anti-inflammatory medication can be used, but in the author's experience, it has rarely been beneficial.

In the last several years, the author has been injecting the interspace in patients who are unable to tolerate the pads or who find the pads provide little relief. Of note, a significant number of patients find that the presence of a pad, although theoretically placed to relieve symptoms, is so uncomfortable that it cannot be tolerated. In these patients, the author injects the appropriate interspace with a solution containing about 0.5 mL of bupivacaine and 0.5 mL of lidocaine with about 1 mL of a long-acting corticosteroid. The author injects the interspace from the top of the foot down in between the metatarsal heads to the bottom of the foot so that one actually feels the needle passing through the deep transverse metatarsal ligament with sort of a click as the needle almost penetrates the bottom of the skin. The patient sometimes notes that this approach reproduces their symptoms. At this point, the corticosteroid is injected. This method is both diagnostic and therapeutic, and most people achieve at least short-term relief. Greenfield and coworkers noted a high success rate with injection in persons who had trauma as the precipitating event. They noted that, with injection, 65 percent of the patients had no pain at the follow-up evaluation 2 years after the series of injections.[14]

The author has found the method to be beneficial in about 10 percent of patients, yielding, along with the use of pads, about a 75 percent success rate with nonoperative treatment. In an attempt to differentiate an intermetatarsal bursitis (which is infrequently diagnosed), the medication can be injected above the ligament. Freeman also notes some limited value for diagnostic injections.[9] Johnson has noted that injection of the interspace is not totally helpful in establishing a diagnosis because a normal nerve may be found at surgery when an injection has temporarily relieved the patient's symptoms. He attributes this, at least in part, to a placebo effect for the injection alone.[20] In Mann's series, use of injections was found to be of little help in establishing a diagnosis of neuroma.[24] If the patient achieves good results for several months after the injection, the author uses another injection, no more than three times over a 12-month period. If the patient fails to get any significant relief after the first injection, this technique is abandoned.

The author has found physical therapy, including the use of ultrasound or phonophoresis, is of minimal benefit. The majority of people with suspected interdigital neuroma do respond to the use of metatarsal pads, which is by far the most effective modality, plus the occasional use of corticosteroids, if properly injected. In the past, Morris suggested that surgery was the only approach that could benefit the patient,[27] but we have not found that to be the case and early surgery should be avoided. One must be diligent in trying to localize the area of maximum discomfort. Once conservative treatment has been exhausted, the physician should operate only on those patients who have symptoms or incapacitation by the neuroma sufficient to warrant surgery. Merkel and Johnson noted a higher success rate of conservative treatment in patients with symptoms of shorter duration, and they proposed, unless symptoms were totally disabling, at least a 2- to 3-month trial of conservative treatment before surgery.[26] One must be extremely cautious in approaching those patients whose symptoms are vague and changeable and in whom there are symptoms of neuromas in several locations.[26] Surgery should never be the first and only treatment modality.

Every attempt must be made to try to localize the most symptomatic interspace and to avoid exploring two interspaces if possible. Johnson reports that poor results from bilateral neuroma removal can be expected. He also reports a high incidence of good results with removal of neuroma from the third interspace alone.[20] In Mann's series, the results of removing neuromas from the second or third interspace were approximately equal.[24]

Operative Treatment

Surgical removal of an interdigital neuroma is carried out once the patient has failed a trial of conservative treatment, and when the physician believes he or she has localized the findings to one particular area, namely the interspace between the second and third or third and fourth metatarsal heads. Rarely, it is difficult or impossible to distinguish clearly which interspace is involved. The use of ultrasound may be helpful in these instances, as described earlier.

The surgical procedure is usually carried out

in the hospital or day surgery center under general or ankle block anesthesia. Under general anesthesia, a pneumatic calf or thigh tourniquet can be used. With the ankle block and the Esmarch wrapped around the ankle, the procedure has been found to be quite satisfactory and is well tolerated by most patients. The author has an anesthesiologist on standby and uses midazolam HCl (Versed, Roche) or a similar medication intravenously during the preoperative period and operative period. This anesthetic has made this type of procedure much more acceptable to the patients. Some surgeons have reported performing the operation without a tourniquet, but the author has personally found that using this technique makes it difficult to view the anatomy because it is such a small space and the tissue is rapidly discolored by even a small amount of bleeding.

A 3-cm incision is made over the dorsum of the foot over the involved interspace (Fig. 11–1). All bleeders are clamped and cauterized as visualized. Dissection is carried initially through the tissue longitudinally to try to protect the major blood vessels, and the superficial

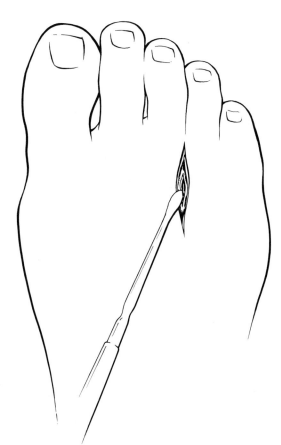

FIGURE 11–2. Dissection of the third interspace with Freer elevator.

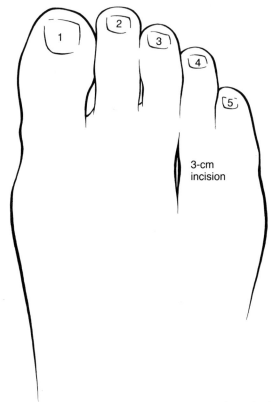

FIGURE 11–1. Incision through dorsal approach to third interspace.

3-cm incision

nerves are retracted to each side. Using the Freer elevator, a plane can be developed between the metatarsal heads (Fig. 11–2). The author then inserts an Army-Navy retractor in a longitudinal fashion, with the blade parallel to the metatarsals, down between the metatarsal heads. With a simple twist of the retractor, the metatarsals are spread allowing further dissection (Figs. 11–3 and 11–4) and insertion of either a Johnson neuroma retractor or, as the author prefers, a lamina spreader (Fig. 11–5). The Army-Navy retractor is then withdrawn.*

Occasionally, the use of the Johnson neuroma retractor (Fig. 11–6) prior to insertion of the Army-Navy retractor is helpful in establishing the interspace. Once the lamina spreader is in place, the soft tissue is disssected down and the deep transverse metatarsal ligament is visualized with blunt dissection. It is

---

*I attribute this technical innovation to Dr. John Gould, this book's editor.

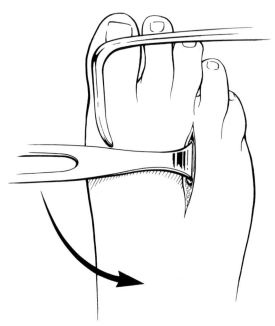

FIGURE 11–3. Army-Navy retractor inserted with blade parallel to metatarsal shafts.

recommended that loupe magnification be routinely used during these procedures.

The transverse metatarsal ligament is then carefully divided with a No. 15 blade, allowing further retraction of the metatarsals with the lamina spreader. Occasionally during this time, the patient (under block), will experience some discomfort as the metatarsals are spread. Injection of 2 percent plain lidocaine into the space or adjacent to the nerve will relieve this discomfort.

Once the transverse ligament is divided and the nerve is located as far proximally as possible, an attempt is made to identify the neuroma. It is much simpler to find the nerve proximally than try to find the nerve distally and carry it proximally. The interdigital neuroma is frequently found underneath the deep transverse metatarsal ligament or slightly distal to it, and sometimes a very tortuous nerve can be found distal to the ligament. Occasionally, the nerve is flattened or inflamed and no "true neuroma" is identified (Fig. 11–7).

If one is reasonably sure of the diagnosis at this point, the nerve should be gently retracted as far distally as possible and then resected, including any contributing branches that arise from under the adjacent metatarsal. The end of the resected nerve should lie well proximal to the deep transverse metatarsal ligament that

was divided because the ligament will invariably reconstitute in time. For this reason, it is not recommended to routinely release only the ligament, as has been described by Gauthier as his preferred method of surgical treatment.[12]

If a normal-appearing nerve is found in the interspace, one is faced with the dilemma of whether to remove it or not. It is this author's opinion that in these cases the nerve should be left alone after the ligament is carefully transected. With care and efficiency in the preoperative evaluation, this situation fortunately is infrequent. In cases in which one is unsure as to what may be found, the patient should be told preoperatively that the nerve may be left if there is reasonable doubt as to the diagnosis.

As noted previously, even when the nerve removed appears relatively normal, the condition will invariably be reported as "consistent

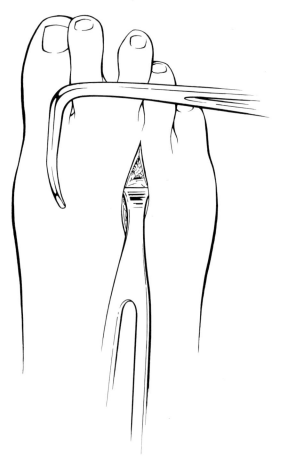

FIGURE 11–4. Twisted Army-Navy retractor spreading the adjacent metatarsals.

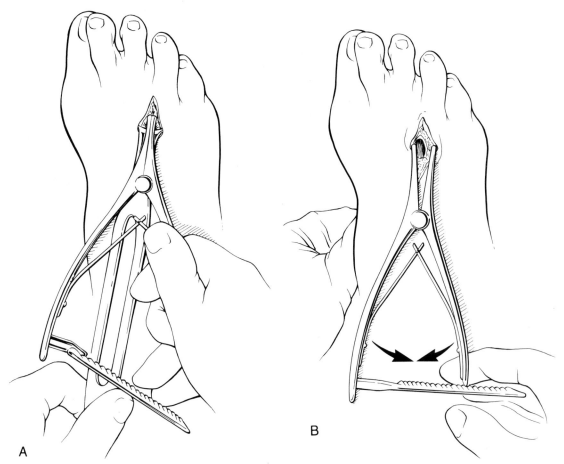

FIGURE 11–5. (*A* and *B*), Lamina spreader replaces the Army-Navy retractor, allowing interspace to be visualized.

with Morton's neuroma" on pathologic diagnosis.

In several instances, the author has found that when the nerve was left, where the deep

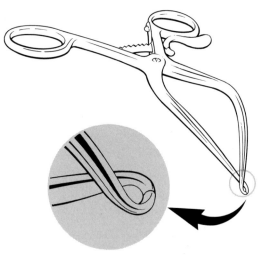

FIGURE 11–6. The Johnson neuroma retractor.

transverse metatarsal ligament was divided, and the nerve was carefully protected, that symptoms persisted that responded to later removal of the nerve. Nonetheless, unless the patient is properly informed, a normal-appearing nerve should not be removed. After all bleeders are clamped and cauterized, an attempt is made not to remove any more deep fat as far as is possible. With this technique, one is usually able to resect 2 to 3 cm of nerve proximal to the ligament (Fig. 11–8). If there is some question as to whether or not bleeding is present, it is best at this point to deflate the tourniquet and to control bleeding prior to skin closure.

The skin is usually closed with a dissolvable 4–0 suture or interrupted cotton sutures, and Steri-Strips are applied. If the surgery is performed under general anesthesia, the area is infiltrated with 0.5 percent bupivacaine local anesthetic prior to deflating the tourniquet. A circumferential bandage is applied as the tourniquet or Esmarch is removed. The author

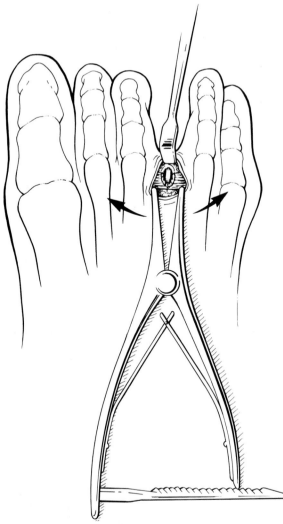

FIGURE 11–7. Exposed interspace with nerve pulled up distally from under ligaments.

prefers unfluffed fluffs with a 3-inch Kling gauze over the foot followed by a 1-inch adhesive tape and a snug bandage.

If symptoms are localized to one interspace alone, the author would explore this interspace and remove the pathologic nerve. In the case in which one is uncertain as to whether or not the neuroma is localized in one or more interspaces, the author believes that both interspaces should be explored. If the skin is flexible, a single incision can be made over the third metatarsal head. This method does require some retraction of the skin, and the author personally has found this incision produces complications and presents some prob-

lems with healing. An incision can be made over each interspace with as wide a skin bridge as possible. Exploration of both interspaces can be done with the deep transverse metatarsal ligament divided and the nerves inspected. The most abnormal nerve would then be resected by the author, and the other nerve would be carefully decompressed. Johnson has reported that he would explore the third interspace first if he were uncertain as to the interspace, noting that the pathology is most frequently found here and there are better results on removal.[20]

Postoperatively, the foot is bandaged by wrapping it with a 2-inch Kling roll and 1/2-inch tape changed weekly for a period of 3 weeks. The patient begins normal weight-bearing activities rapidly, and crutches are rarely necessary. A wooden surgical shoe is used during the 3-week postoperative period, and the patient progresses to normal activities as tolerated.

Postoperatively, as with all routine foot procedures, the patient is initially advised to rest, to keep the foot elevated above the heart as much as possible, to avoid getting the foot wet, and to avoid excess perspiration. The author continues to use prophylactic antibiotics (1 g intravenous cefazolin) prior to tourniquet inflation at the time of surgery.

In the United States, it is common for the initial removal of the neuroma to be from the dorsal aspect, but in the United Kingdom, the plantar approach is not infrequently used for the removal of a neuroma. The surgical scar from the plantar incision usually heals well with no problem. Burns and Stewart used a transverse plastic incision in the non–weight-bearing part of the foot, suggesting the approach had the "advantages of both the dorsal and plantar longitudinal incisions without their disadvantages."[6]

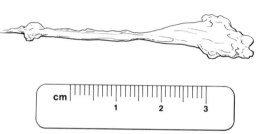

FIGURE 11–8. Neuroma adequately resected proximally.

Removal of Neuroma with Synovial Cyst

Occasionally, a patient will be found with tenderness in the interspaces suggesting an interdigital neuroma that is associated with a thick, doughy-feeling mass, accompanied by spreading between the toes, most commonly noted between the second and third toes. In this case, a synovial cyst has been described.[24] At surgery, a thick, poorly defined mass, which sometimes contains fluid, can be found in the interspace, rising up underneath the deep transmetatarsal ligament. Occasionally, the cyst could be found arising from the second metatarsophalangeal joint, which usually contains fluid. The cyst can be difficult to excise because it is poorly differentiated from the adjacent fat, and care should be taken in removing the cyst not to remove the excess fat from the interspace. Pathologic changes in the synovial cyst reveal fat with thin-walled fibrous tissue (Fig. 11–9).[24] In cases in which the toes have been deviated, I have performed a medial capsular release on the second metatarsophalangeal joint and a lateral capsular release on the third metatarsophalangeal joint. The toes are splinted together postoperatively, although frequently the toes will continue to deviate post-operatively even if they have been splinted. The patient should be advised of this possibility before the operation. Otherwise, the postoperative care for the patient with the synovial cyst is the same as for those without the cyst. Synovial cysts have not been frequently associated with any specific inflammatory condition, such as rheumatoid arthritis. Vainio, however, reported the incidence of Morton's neuroma as being one in 520 rheumatoid patients.[38]

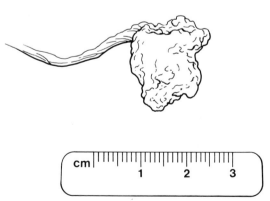

FIGURE 11–9. Synovial cyst encircling interdigital nerve.

The author's preferred approach has been described primarily in the section above. Specifically the author tries to define carefully one interspace involved and approach the foot from the dorsum with as little soft tissue dissection as possible, divide the deep transverse metatarsal ligament, remove the nerve as far proximally as possible, close the wound with a subcuticular suture, and splint the foot for 3 weeks. In cases in which more than one interspace is explored, the most pathologic-appearing nerve is removed and the deep transmetatarsal ligament divided on the other nerve.

Postoperative Results

Unfortunately, the results of neuroma removal are not completely satisfying. When the surgeon blithely assures the patient that the operation will be a complete success, he is doing himself and the patient a disservice by such a statement. In the past, some authors have noted that surgery resulted in a perfect cure.[3, 18] Mann reported in his series of neuroma removals that 71 percent were asymptomatic postoperatively, 9 percent significantly improved, 6 percent marginally improved, and 14 percent were surgical failures. These results were from a combined group of neuromas removed from the second and third interspaces, with the results being about the same for each interspace considered separately.[24] In the failure group, no reason was found why this group failed to do as well based on clinical examination or x-ray examination. This group did have a somewhat longer history of preoperative symptoms. Generally, all patients continue to improve for 3 to 4 months following surgery, with maximum improvement at about that point.

Johnson reported a preponderance of third interspace explorations (81 percent). He noted a rate of "patient satisfaction" of 90 percent when the third interspace was the only one involved. If both the second and third interspaces were explored, the satisfaction rate fell to 59 percent. A satisfaction rate of approximately 60 percent was noted in the patients with neuromas in the second interspace. Neuromas in the first or fourth interspaces were rare. His overall rate of dissatisfaction was 19 percent.[20] Bradley and Miller noted that 13 percent of patients had unsatisfactory results and 21.3 percent had some pain remaining.[5]

THE RECURRENT NEUROMA

A small but significant number of patients have significant discomfort after the initial procedure or present to the physician having had a neuroma removed at some time in the past noting a short period of limited relief after that surgery; this was followed by a persistence of disabling symptoms. These patients usually have some subjective numbness on the bottom of the foot under the appropriate interspace and have a scar on the dorsum of the foot over the interspace. Tenderness will be noted in the interspace with no mass palpated, and usually a positive Tinel sign can be elicited by tapping the plantar aspect of the foot about the level of the metatarsal heads. This area can be correlated to represent the area of the end of the involved nerve at the time of surgical exploration.

It is believed that the cause of discomfort in these instances are many: inadequate resection of the nerve, failure to remove the nerve at all in the initial procedure, new growth of the nerve, or scarring of the nerve to an adjacent metatarsal head.[24] In the failure group in which the discomfort was more subjective without a positive Tinel test, it is believed that some of the discomfort may represent a "phantom limb"–type of phenomenon rather than reentrapment or adherence of the nerve to the metatarsal or nerve regrowth. A positive Tinel sign confirms the diagnosis of recurrent neuroma. Johnson suggested that some functional component was not fully recognized prior to the initial surgery, and that this factor contributed to the failure.

In preoperative selection, one must be extremely conscientious in trying to assess whether or not a significant functional component exists in these patients prior to surgery. At the initial surgery, the surgeon actually produces a true "bulb neuroma," which forms as the nerve is cut. This may or may not be sensitive later.

Johnson, in discussing his removal of "secondary neuromas" using a plantar approach to the third interspace, noted that 50 percent of patients had complete satisfaction, 19.4 percent were satisfied with minimal reservations, and 8.3 percent were satisfied with reservations. He noted an overall dissatisfaction rate of 22.2 percent. He noted that in 65 percent of the cases, at reoperation, the original neuroma had not been removed. Johnson states that, rather than the "bulb neuroma" causing the "secondary neuroma" and persistent symptoms, that in most cases the initial nerve lesion had not been excised.[19, 20]

The author concurs with Johnson and his conclusion, especially when the patient presents with a small scar that is distally located. At reoperation in these patients, one will frequently find the nerve present in its entirety or resected only distal to the deep transverse metatarsal ligament under which is found the unresected neuroma.

In Mann's series, nine of eleven patients who were reoperated on through a dorsal approach (81 percent) noted good to excellent results after the second procedure. In some of these cases, the nerve was found tightly attached under a metatarsal bone and could be located in the proximal aspect of the wound with some difficulty.[24] In their series of 39 patients with a repeat operation (via a plantar approach), Becker and Baxter noted significant improvement in more than 80 percent of these patients.[2] These overall results from a second operation do not differ significantly from the results with the primary procedure. Findings such as partial regrowth of the nerve or the residual nerve being found scarred to an adjacent metatarsal head can be found in patients who have been operated on by an experienced foot surgeon using proper care and technique. Amis and colleagues studied cadaveric specimens, dividing the specimens into zones, and noted the presence of small plantar nerves off the common digital nerves being plantar digital nerve bundles that tethered the nerve and prevented the resected nerve from retraction proximally, resulting in the nerve from which the neuroma was resected to remain in the weight-bearing area of the foot (Figs. 11–10 and 11–11). They recommended a high proximal resection, at least 3 cm proximal to the proximal edge of the intermetatarsal ligament.[1]

If surgery is needed, there are proponents to using a dorsal approach (proposed by Mann) or using a plantar approach (proposed by Johnson and Baxter). Mann's surgeries were carried out through an extended dorsal approach. The nerve end could be resected well proximally to the deep transverse metatarsal ligament from a dorsal approach. Baxter recommends a transverse plantar incision, which allows better flexibility and side-to-side exploration if one is unsure as to where the neuroma lies

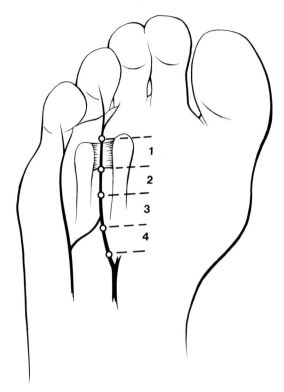

FIGURE 11–10. Plantar nerves.

(Figs. 11–12 and 11–13). This limits exploration distally, however.[2] Johnson reports a plantar longitudinal incision, starting over the underlying nerve and extending proximal to distal to ensure complete nerve or neuroma resection

(Figs. 11–14 and 11–15).[20] The plantar incisions are well tolerated, with good healing and minimal scar formation noted.

In either instance, the nerve lies superficial to the ligament between the metatarsal heads when approached from the plantar direction and lies adjacent to the lumbrical muscle and between the flexor tendons, which pass along the plantar surface of the metatarsals (Figs. 11–16 and 11–17).

Occasionally, some difficulty is encountered in localizing the nerve, which can be found often underneath one of the metatarsal heads. Every effort should be made preoperatively toward trying to pinpoint exactly where the most tender area is adjacent to the metatarsal area and where the positive Tinel sign is noted.

The nerve is identified and again resected as far proximally as possible and the wound closed in the same fashion with interrupted sutures if the incision is on a plantar surface. If a plantar incision is used, the patient is kept in a non–weight-bearing position or minimal weight-bearing position for about 2 weeks until the sutures are removed and immobilization is carried out for 1 or 2 more weeks.

In two instances, the author has removed a nerve a third time, and in both cases, a plantar approach was used. In both cases, the nerve, which had been previously resected by the author, was found to be partially regrown. In both these cases, these patients received satisfactory relief after the third excision.

FIGURE 11–11. Plantar-directed nerve bundles tethering digital and interdigital nerves.

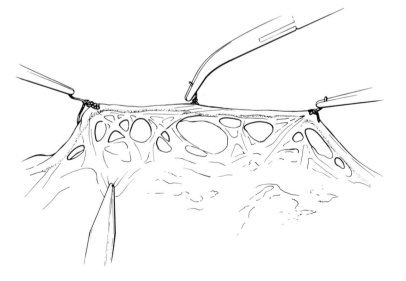

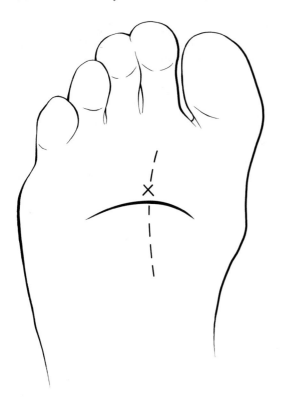

FIGURE 11–12. Transverse plantar incision with **x** marking location of a positive Tinel test.

REHABILITATION

The patient requires very little rehabilitation postoperatively. The patient is immobilized for about 3 weeks and progresses rapidly to nor-

mal ambulation. Physical therapy is seldom indicated. Occasionally, during the postoperative period, if the patient appears to be progressing poorly, an injection of corticosteroids in the area has been of relative benefit.

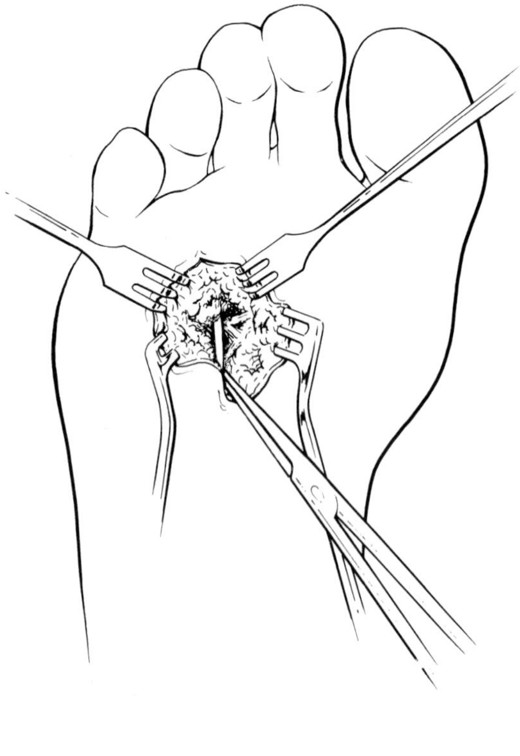

FIGURE 11–13. Nerve identified via transverse plantar approach.

FIGURE 11–14. Longitudinal plantar incision with x marking location of positive Tinel's test.

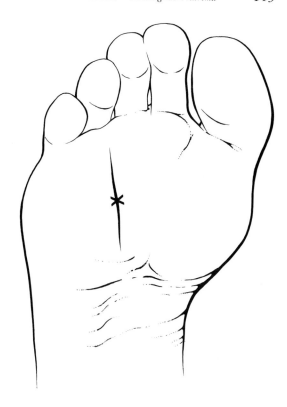

If the patient complains of pain on the plantar aspect of the foot, it needs to be emphasized to the patient that although the incision was from the top, the dissection was carried down to the bottom of the foot, and that this pain is to be expected. Occasionally, a patient notes no difference in sensation after surgery as compared with prior to surgery and

FIGURE 11–15. Hemostat on nerve located via longitudinal plantar incision.

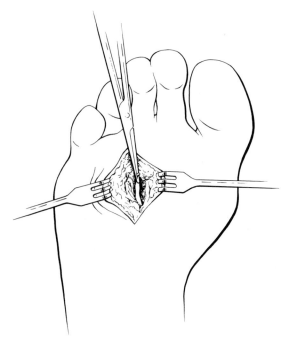

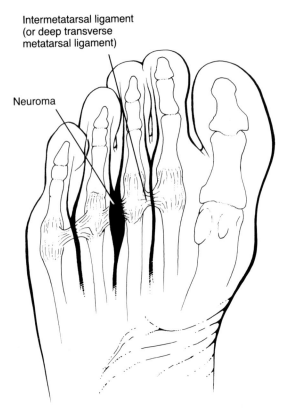

Intermetatarsal ligament
(or deep transverse
metatarsal ligament)

Neuroma

FIGURE 11–16. Nerve passing over deep metatarsal ligament as seen from the plantar aspect.

FIGURE 11–17. Transverse section through metatarsal heads demonstrating bones, ligament, tendon, and nerve.

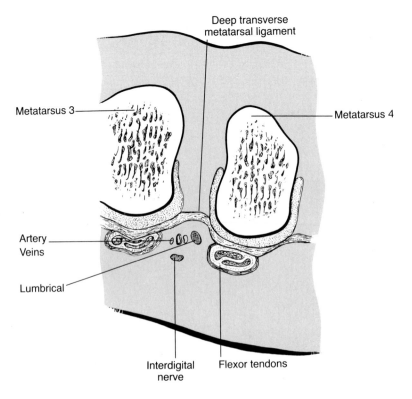

Deep transverse
metatarsal ligament

Metatarsus 3

Metatarsus 4

Artery
Veins

Lumbrical

Interdigital
nerve

Flexor tendons

questions whether the nerve was removed or not. In these instances, it is believed that sensory component of the nerve had gradually deteriorated over a period of time prior to removal so that when it was removed, no loss of sensation was noted. The patient's apprehension may be relieved by showing him or her the pathology report stating that the nerve has been removed.

COMPLICATIONS AND PITFALLS

As in all foot surgery, one of the complications of neuroma removal is of wound infection, with about 1 percent infection rate of all clean wounds reported. No increased incidence has been noted in these patients. This factor should be discussed with the patient preoperatively.

In most patients, the author routinely administers a cefazolin intravenously prior to application of the tourniquet. Wound dehiscence is uncommon, but complications usually result from hematoma formation in the wound. For this reason, attempts are made to control bleeding in the wound, and if there is any question about this, the tourniquet is deflated or removed. It is emphasized to the patient that numbness usually occurs in the interspace and on the plantar aspect of the foot, emphasizing that the operation is a *nerve removal*.

Postoperatively, as with all foot surgery, the patient may have some thickening in the area of the wound that may last several months and may be painful to the patient. Some of this pain can be avoided by having the patient elevate the foot as much as possible for a few days after surgery. There may be some limitation of motion in the adjacent metatarsophalangeal joints, particularly in cases in which a capsulotomy was carried out on adjacent metatarsophalangeal joints to correct diverting toes. Early range-of-motion exercises should be instituted for the adjacent metartarsophalangeal joints in an attempt to prevent residual stiffness with an incision on the plantar aspect of the foot. An occasional hypertrophic scar is present but is unusual, as noted earlier.

Johnson uses a cast postoperatively with a plantar incision in an attempt to minimize scar formation. The author uses a bulky dressing postoperatively and non–weight bearing with crutches for 2 to 3 weeks with a plantar incision.[20]

The most significant complication is failure to remove the nerve during the time of surgery. The nerve should be identified proximally and the deep transverse metatarsal ligament followed distally until its bifurcation is reached so as to avoid removing one of the adjacent lumbrical muscles that is mistaken for a nerve. The risk of this error happening can be diminished by using loupe magnification. Approaching the neuroma more distally, just at the beginning of the web space, and trying to identify the branches distally and following them proximally, is in the author's experience much more difficult and may result in insufficient removal of the nerve.

It should be emphasized to the patient that with excision of the interdigital neuroma, about 80 percent of patients are completely satisfied with the procedure and others may fail to demonstrate any significant improvement. Two-thirds of the patients in Mann's series noted subjective numbness in the plantar distribution of the resected nerve at the 2-year follow-up evaluation. In addition, 75 percent of the patients in this series noted persistent limitation in the type of shoes that could be worn postoperatively.[24]

In the management of interdigital neuromas, several options of treatment exist. First, are the options of conservative treatment, metatarsal pads, corticosteroid injections, and change of footwear. If conservative treatment fails and if signs and symptoms of neuroma are consistently incapacitating, then surgery is the next option. Surgery, as the primary basis, can be performed from a dorsal approach or a plantar approach. The nerve must be adequately visualized and resected well proximal to the deep transverse metatarsal ligament.

When primary surgery fails, one may use conservative treatment or surgery again, with a dorsal or plantar incision. With the plantar incision, one can use either a transverse or a longitudinal incision. A knowledge of plantar anatomy is essential to facilitate a relatively gentle localization of the nerve or neuroma when using a plantar approach.

References

1. Amis JA, Siverhus SW, Liwnicz BH: An anatomic basis for recurrence following Morton's neuroma ex-

cision. Presented at American Orthopaedic Foot and Ankle Society Meeting. Sun Valley, Idaho, 1989.

2. Beskin JL, Baxta DE: Recurrent pain following interdigital neurectomy. Foot Ankle 9:34–39, 1988.

3. Betts LD: Morton's metatarsalgia: Neuritis of the fourth digital nerve. Med J Aust I:514–515, 1940.

4. Bickel WH, Dockerty MB: Plantar neuromas, Morton's toe. Surg Gynecol Obstet 84:111–116, 1947.

5. Bradley N, Miller WA, Guans JP: Plantar neuroma: Analysis of results following surgical excision in 145 patients. South Med J 69:853–854, 1976.

6. Burns AE, Stewart WP: Morton's neuroma: Preliminary reports on neurectomy via transverse plantar excision. J Am Podiatry Assoc 72:135–141, 1982.

7. Dewberry JW, Christian JD, Beeton NL: Morton's neuroma. J Med Assoc Ga 62:144–146, 1973.

8. Durlacher L: Treatise on Corns, Bunions, the Diseases of Nails and the General Management of the Feet. London, Simkin, Marshall, 1845, p 52.

9. Freeman C: Morton's metatarsalgia. J Bone Joint Surg 67B:670, 1985.

10. Gilmour WN: Morton's Metatarsalgia. J Bone Joint Surg 55B:221, 1973.

11. Gilmour WN, Ecker JO, Harvey J: Morton's metatarsalgia J Bone Joint Surg 68B:333, 1986.

12. Gauthier G: Thomas Morton's disease: A nerve entrapment syndrome. Clin Orthop 142:90–92, 1979.

13. Graham CE, Graham DM: Morton's neuroma: A microscopic evaluation. Foot Ankle 5(2):150–153, 1984.

14. Greenfield J, Rea J, Ilfield FW: Morton's interdigital neuroma: Indications for treatment and local injections vs. surgery. Clin Orthop I85:142–144, 1984.

15. Guiloff RJ, Scadding JW, Klenerman L: Morton's metatarsalgia: Clinical, electrophysiological and histological observations. J Bone Joint Surg 66B:586–591, 1984.

16. Ha'Eri GB, Fornesier VL, Schatzer J: Morton's neuroma—pathogenesis and ultrastructure Clin Orthop 141:256–259, 1979.

17. Hauser ED: Interdigital neuroma of the foot. Surg Gynecol Obstet 133:265–267, 1971.

18. Hoadley AE: Six cases of metatarsalgia. Chicago Med Rec 5:32–37, 1893.

19. Johnson JE, Johnson KH, Unmi KK: Persistent pain after excision of an interdigital neuroma. J Bone Joint Surg 70A:651–657, 1988.

20. Johnson KA: Interdigital neuroma. *In* Surgery of the Foot and Ankle. New York, Raven Press, 1989, pp 69–82.

21. Jones R, Tubby AH: Metatarsalgia or Morton's disease. Ann Surg 28:297–328, 1898.

22. Klenerman GE, MacClellan RJ, Guiloff RJ, Scaddins JW: Morton's metatarsalgia: A retrospective and prospective study. J Bone Joint Surg 65B:220, 1983.

23. Lassman G: Morton's toe. Clin Orthop 142:73–84, 1979.

24. Mann RA, Reynolds JC: Interdigital neuroma—a critical clinical analysis. Foot Ankle 3(4):238–243, 1983.

25. McElvenny R: The etiology and surgical treatment of intractable pain about the fourth metatarsophalangeal joint (Morton's toe). J Bone Joint Surg 25:679, 1943.

26. Merkel KD, Johnson KE: Interdigital neuroma. *In* Gould JS (Ed): The Foot Book. Baltimore, Williams & Wilkins, 1986, pp 268–279.

27. Morris MH: Morton's metatarsalgia. Clin Orthop 127:203–207, 1977.

28. Morton TG: A peculiar and painful affliction of the fourth metatarso-phalangeal articulation. Am J Med Sci 71:37–45, 1876.

29. Mulder JD: The causative mechanism in Morton's metatarsalgia. J Bone Joint Surg 33B:74–95, 1951.

30. Nissen KI: Plantar digital neuritis. J Bone Joint Surg 30B:84–94, 1948.

31. Nissen KI: The etiology of Morton's metatarsalgia. J Bone Joint Surg 33B:293, 1951.

32. Oh SJ, Kim HS, Ahmad BK: Electrophysiological diagnosis of interdigital neuropathy of the foot. Muscle Nerve 7:218–225, 1984.

33. Redd RA, Peters UJ, Emery SE, et al: Morton's neuroma: Sonographic evaluation. Radiology 121:415–417, 1989.

34. Reed RJ, Bliss BO: Morton's neuroma, regressive and productive elastofibrosis. Arch Pathol 95:123–129, 1973.

35. Reynolds JC: Morton's neuroma. Presented at American Orthopaedic Foot and Ankle Society Meeting. Vail, Colorado, 1986.

36. Shephard E: Intermetatarsophalangeal bursitis—the causation of Morton's metatarsalgia. J Bone Joint Surg 57B:115, 1975.

37. Tate RO, Rusin JJ: Morton's neuroma, its ultrastructural anatomy and biomechanical etiology. J Am Podiatry Assoc 68:797–807, 1978.

38. Vainio K: Morton's metatarsalgia. Clin Orthop 142:85–89, 1979.

39. Winkler H, Feltner JB, Kimmelstiel P: Morton's metatarsalgia. J Bone Joint Surg 30A:496–500, 1948.

12

Implant Arthroplasty of the Foot

JUDITH W. SMITH
JOHN S. GOULD

SILICONE IMPLANTS

Implants of the foot have evolved from experience with implants of the hand. As early as 1965, articles began appearing in the engineering literature about the use of silicone material in biologic situations.[3] In 1966, Swanson published his first article on the use of silicone implants in the hand, and in 1968 first performed flexible implant resection arthroplasty of the great toe metatarsophalangeal joint for patients with rheumatoid arthritis, hallux valgus, and hallux rigidus.[33] Originally a single-stem silicone implant was used to replace the proximal third of the proximal phalanx (Fig. 12–1A to C).[33,35] In 1974, a high-performance silicone elastomer was developed that allowed construction of a flexible double-stem hinge implant (Fig. 12–2A to C).[33] In the metatarsophalangeal (MTP) joint, the hinge is placed to allow maximum extension, in an orientation opposite to that of metacarpal joint implants, which allow maximum flexion.

Grommets were first used in 1976 to reduce the fracture rate at the hinge site by preventing impingement of sharp bone edges (Fig. 12–3).[34]

Silicone implants have been used in the foot primarily for great toe MTP joint replacement.* Some surgeons have used silicone replacements for lesser toe MTP joints,[25] for proximal interphalangeal (IP) joints for hammer toe correction, and as toe caps for the lesser metatarsals following metatarsal head resection.[39] Silicone has also been used for arthroereisis, as a sinus tarsi plug to splint the hindfoot in neutral position during the healing phase after soft tissue reconstruction for planovalgus feet.[5] The silicone is subsequently removed. It has also been advocated as an injectable substance for conditions such as metatarsalgia to supplement the fat pad on the plantar aspect of the foot, but this use has not

*See references 7–9, 12, 13, 15, 17, 20, 21, 24–26, 29–31, 33, 35, 38.

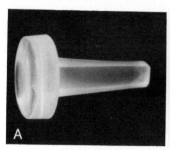 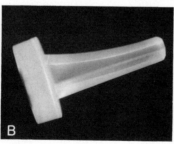 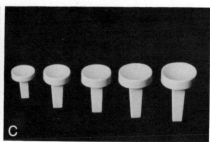

FIGURE 12–1. Single-stem silicone implants and sizers (Swanson, Dow Corning).

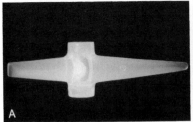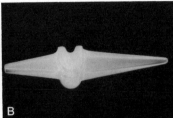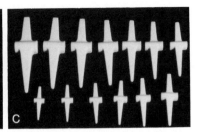

FIGURE 12–2. *(A to C),* Double-stem silicone implants and sizers (Swanson, Dow Corning).

been approved by the US Food and Drug Administration.[1]

Great toe MTP flexible implant arthroplasty was initially met with great enthusiasm.[8, 17, 35, 38] In 1981, Cracchiolo reported on 159 feet with double-stem silicone implants performed at two medical centers and followed for 18 months to 6 years, stating that all patients had pain relief and most had complete resolution of pain with improved function.[8] The majority of the patients had rheumatoid arthritis. However, more recent studies have reported less favorable results with silicone arthroplasty,[15, 19, 26, 27] and alternative methods for correcting MTP disorders have been advocated by several authors.[2, 6, 27, 36] Problems have developed for two major reasons: biomechanically, the function of the joints of the foot in weight bearing makes them less amenable to any type of arthroplasty in comparison to the joints of the hand, and silicone has been implicated in the development of silicone synovitis.[19, 27]

Single-stem implants, which articulate with

bone or cartilage, are subject to shear forces that cause an erasure effect, and the production of particulate matter results in silicone synovitis. We cannot advocate these devices because of their attendant complications. Problems with sinus formation and drainage when liquid injectable silicone has been used elsewhere in the body raise concerns about applications in the foot for metatarsalgia or fat pad loss. Cracchiolo has used double-stem flexible hinge prostheses for the minor MTP joints in rheumatoid patients with mixed results.[25] Silicone synovitis with use of the double-stem prosthesis in the great toe MTP joint has been infrequent except after the prosthesis has fractured. Although the incidence of fracture of the great toe prosthesis is unknown, studies of flexible hinges in the hand have reported fracture rates as high as 25 percent by 6 years.[11]

The more significant problem with the use of the prosthesis at the great toe MTP is the lack of normal toe-off due to instability of the joint and loss of the effective plantar fascia windlass mechanism. Even with the modification suggested by N. Gould (personal communication), in which the hinge is reversed to allow greater plantar flexion (hinge opens downward), normal toe-off strength is not restored. In our own series of 25 nonrheumatoid patients, a transfer lesion to the second metatarsal head occurred routinely despite maximal preservation of the plantar aspect of the metatarsal head (Figs. 12–4 and 12–5). As a result, we are reluctant to advise the use of the prosthesis in patients with hallux rigidus and generalized osteoarthritis. Weltmer and Cracchiolo, however, reported an 80-percent patient satisfaction rate in a series of 37 patients with 41 double-stem implants.[37]

We have continued to use the prosthesis in patients with collagen disorders, including psoriatic and rheumatoid arthritis. In particular, we consider the use of prosthetic replacement

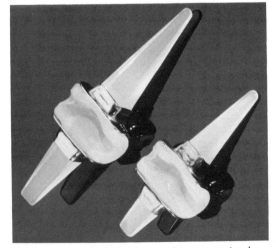

FIGURE 12–3. Silicone implants with grommets in place. Sizers are placed behind each implant.

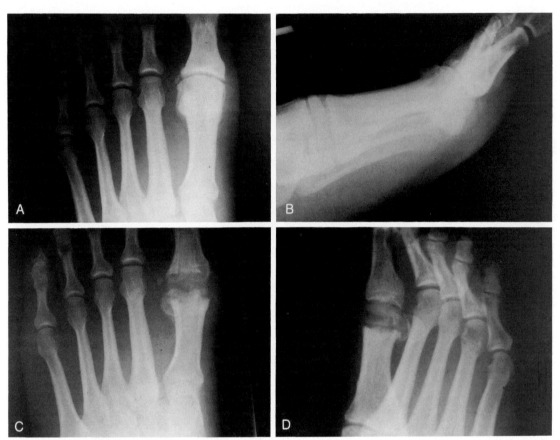

FIGURE 12–4. Radiographs of a 52-year-old male television announcer with hallux rigidus. The great toe metatarsophalangeal joint was replaced with a double-stem silicone prosthesis. Pain was relieved, but a transfer lesion to the second metatarsal developed within years.

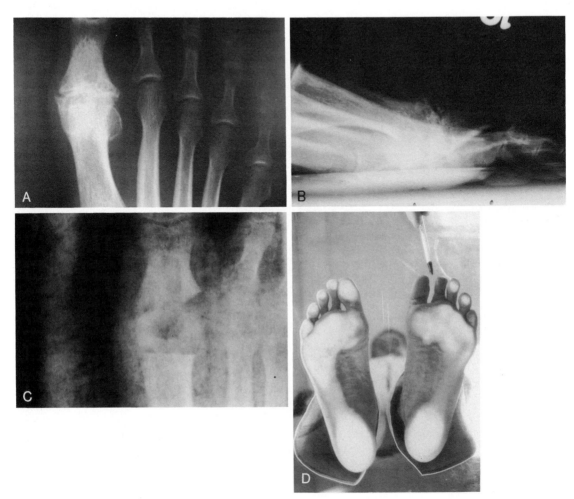

FIGURE 12–5. *(A to C)*, X-ray films of a 59-year-old male tennis player with advanced osteoarthritis of the hallux metatarsophalangeal joint and prosthetic replacement. *(D)*, Foot mirror view showing lack of great toe contact postoperatively. The second metatarsal head was also surgically elevated for the transfer lesion; the second toe also does not make contact. (The x-ray films and foot mirror view are of the same patient; the negative for *D* was reversed.)

in women wishing to wear heels of various heights and in patients with involvement of the adjacent first cuneiform–first metatarsal and IP joints. These patients have reasonable results in our experience, due to their typically more flatfooted gait and lower demand on the foot. We have also used the prosthesis in hallux rigidus and generalized arthritis in a first-stage resection arthroplasty. After a good pseudocapsule is formed (approximately 1 year), the prosthesis can be removed to leave a more stable "second-stage" arthroplasty.

SURFACE REPLACEMENT ARTHROPLASTY

Surface replacement arthroplasty and hemiarthroplasty in the foot continue to be attempted at the great toe MTP joint. Swanson developed an uncemented proximal phalangeal stemmed titanium implant (Figs. 12–6 and 12–7). Cemented total joint replacement prostheses have been developed by Johnson at the Mayo Clinic[15, 16] and by Sculco at The Hospital for Special Surgery (see Fig. 12–3).[22] Occasionally, attempts at resurfacing of other joints, such as the talonavicular joint, have been reported, but these are of historical interest only.[10]

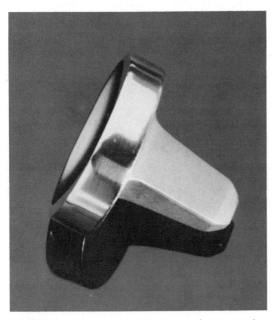

FIGURE 12–6. The Swanson titanium single-stem implant (Dow Corning).

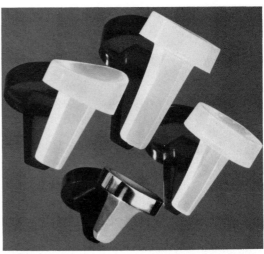

FIGURE 12–7. Single-stem implant models, including the titanium implant and a silicone angled-surface variety.

In general, these joint replacements have been unsuccessful. Johnson reported that implantation of his unconstrained resurfacing prosthesis in 25 patients gave results that were no better than those with resection arthroplasty, and he has discontinued its use.[15] Merkle and Sculco also reported poor results with the semiconstrained prosthesis in 15 feet and consider this implant experimental.[22]

TREATMENT OPTIONS

Surgical Alternatives

Almost any condition that causes disruption of first MTP joint function would theoretically be an indication for joint replacement, with the exception of prior joint sepsis, inadequate soft tissue coverage, or lack of active motors. Relative contraindications include significant peripheral vascular disease, chronic foot causalgia, multiple previous foot surgeries, previous failed implants, and significant loss of bone stock. Systemic diseases such as collagen vascular disorders and gout, osteoarthritis, and trauma can all lead to degenerative changes in the first MTP joint. Replacement arthroplasty might also be considered for pain following cheilectomy for hallux rigidus or intra-articular pathology related to a bunion problem. Unfortunately, currently available prostheses have been successful only in the low-demand patient, as noted earlier.

In considering joint replacement surgery, the surgeon must take into account the patient's age and general health, level of activity, weight, and occupation. Gender is also an important consideration. Women who wish to wear different height heels may prefer a mobile joint to a fused one, allowing them greater choice in shoewear. A careful history must be obtained, documenting all previous surgeries and determining any history of infection. The examination should focus on the neurovascular condition of the foot, previous surgical approaches and skin condition, deformity of the joint, range of motion of the MTP joint and whether or not motion is painful, and the condition of the surrounding joints in the foot. The patient should also be examined for other conditions that could affect outcome, such as generalized ligamentous laxity, pes planus, and severe hindfoot valgus.[28]

The major surgical alternatives to joint replacement are MTP joint arthrodesis or resection arthroplasty.[2, 6, 36] Arthrodesis of any joint is based upon the ability to maximize the bone contact area, stabilize and compress the bone, maintain the vascularity of the bone and soft tissues including the skin, and obtain an acceptable position for fusion. It may well be the best alternative in a young, active patient with isolated disease at the MTP joint. A successful arthrodesis provides a long-term solution without the risk of multiple additional surgeries requiring increasingly complex reconstructions. Cosmetically, it provides acceptable length and alignment and functionally provides good support for toe-off. As with any arthrodesis, the patient who has very little motion preoperatively is less likely to complain of loss of mobility following surgery. It is the patient with good range of motion preoperatively who often complains of stiffness postoperatively, even though the pain has been relieved.

Keller resection arthroplasty is a good alternative for the minimally ambulatory elderly patient. Problems with resection arthroplasty include loss of power, shortening, deformity, and development of a transfer lesion. Nevertheless, it can provide a simple solution in a specific population with limited goals.

Conservative Alternatives

Nonoperative options for great toe MTP arthritis and deformity are available. A stiff-soled shoe with a rocker bottom can provide relief by limiting motion at the joint during ambulation. The rocker should be placed behind the metatarsal heads, as opposed to the rocker used following ankle or hindfoot fusion, which is placed at about the level of the base of the fifth metatarsal. For deformity at the MTP joint, an extra depth shoe with a wide toe box and soft upper often provides a viable alternative. Many patients who are poor surgical candidates can be managed conservatively with good results.

TECHNIQUE OF SILICONE REPLACEMENT ARTHROPLASTY

Authors' Preferred Surgical Approach

For the first MTP prosthesis to have any chance of success, the hindfoot must be neutral and stable or reconstructed initially or simultaneously if collapsed into severe valgus.[28] In addition, the first ray must be aligned and the metatarsal and the first cuneiform–first metatarsal joint must be stable.[19, 24] If the joint is hypermobile, it should be fused; if the first metatarsal is in varus, an aligning basilar osteotomy must be done. The function of the IP joint and the alignment of the great toe distal to the MTP joint are also evaluated and are corrected if necessary.

Prophylactic intravenous antibiotics are used during the perioperative period. Meticulous attention is paid to the soft tissue technique intraoperatively. The MTP joint is approached through a dorsomedial incision, and the medial branch of the superficial peroneal nerve is identified and preserved (Figs. 12–8 and 12–9). The joint capsule is entered longitudinally, medial to the extensor hallucis longus. Preservation of the collateral ligaments is desirable but frequently not possible. In some patients, the collaterals are so attenuated that they provide little or no stability. The trial prostheses are used to determine the amount of bone that must be removed to create a space for the prosthesis. In most cases, a minimal amount of bone resection is performed (Fig. 12–10). Typically, the resection of the metatarsal head is performed distal to the collateral ligament origin, which will leave some of the plantar surface on the metatarsal head. An attempt is made to preserve the base

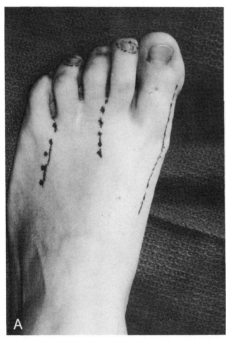

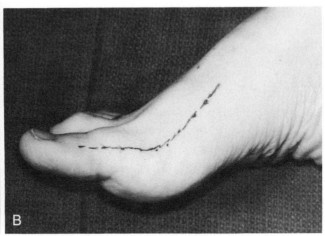

FIGURE 12–8. Anteroposterior *(A)* and lateral *(B)* views of the markings for the hallux metatarsophalangeal joint prosthetic arthroplasty incision. Resection arthroplasty incisions are marked for the lesser toes.

of the proximal phalanx with the attachments of the flexor brevis and plantar fascia. The metatarsal head is excised with a narrow microsagittal saw blade from dorsal to plantar perpendicular to the long axis of the metatarsal shaft. The proximal phalanx residual cartilage or irregularity is planed off by the saw to present a contiguous parallel surface (Fig. 12–11*A* and *B*).

The width of the prosthesis is chosen to match the width of the residual head without overlapping (Fig. 12–12). The opening into the medullary canal in the metatarsal is made with a sizing broach or a straight hemostat. With a Swanson blunt-ended burr, a truncated pyramid-shaped hole is created to match the shape of the prosthetic long (proximal) stem (Figs. 12–13 and 12–14).

On the proximal phalanx, a drill hole is made just dorsal to the center of the articular surface. Using a Swanson burr, an appropriately sized distal hole, also in the shape of a truncated pyramid, is made to match the shorter distal stem (Fig. 12–15). If the distal stem is longer than the medullary canal of the proximal phalanx, it may be shortened (Fig. 12–16). The trial prosthesis is usually fitted with the open side of the hinge facing dorsally,

although N. Gould (personal communication) reversed the alignment in his series (Fig. 12–17).

The determining factor in choosing an appropriately sized prosthesis is the metatarsal fit. The trial prosthesis is used for sizing first in the metatarsal medullary canal; once the correct size is determined, reaming of the proximal phalangeal canal is carried out. Following reaming, the trial prosthesis is inserted into the medullary canal of the metatarsal; the proximal phalanx is flexed, and the distal stem inserted into its medullary canal. Range of motion and stability are then tested. While some degree of pistoning of the prosthesis is acceptable and is actually the mode of function, buckling of the prosthesis must not occur when the joint is in extension, and impingement of the proximal phalanx and metatarsal inferior surfaces should not occur in flexion. If this does happen, an additional wafer of bone must be removed from the metatarsal to allow more space for the prosthesis (Figs. 12–18 and 12–19).

To prevent dust particle accumulation on the silicone prosthesis, the package should be opened just prior to insertion and the device put into a basin filled with saline solution.

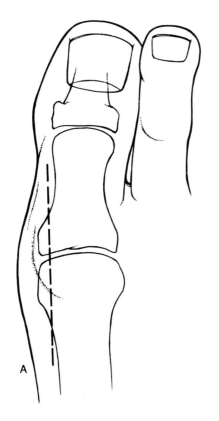

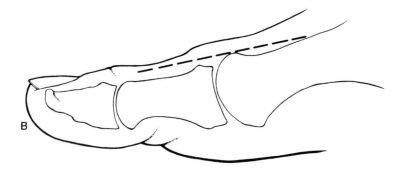

FIGURE 12–9. Anteroposterior *(A)* and lateral *(B)* views of the dorso-medial incision at the level of the great toe metatarsophalangeal joint.

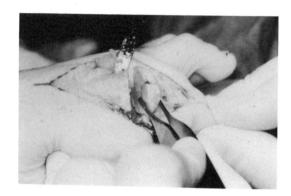

FIGURE 12–10. Bone resection is minimal but enough for adequate placement and motion of the "hinge" portion.

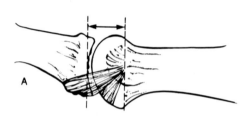

A

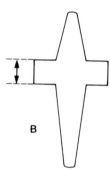

B

FIGURE 12–11. Level of joint resection. The metatarsal is cut perpendicular to the long axis of the shaft. The amount of bone removed *(A)* equals the width of the prosthetic hinge from stem to stem *(B)*. The cut in the metatarsal is made at the collateral ligament origin.

FIGURE 12–12. The width of the prosthetic center portion (hinge) should equal the width of the residual metatarsal stump surface.

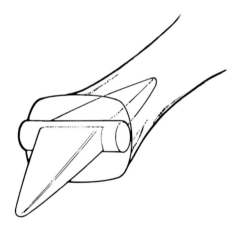

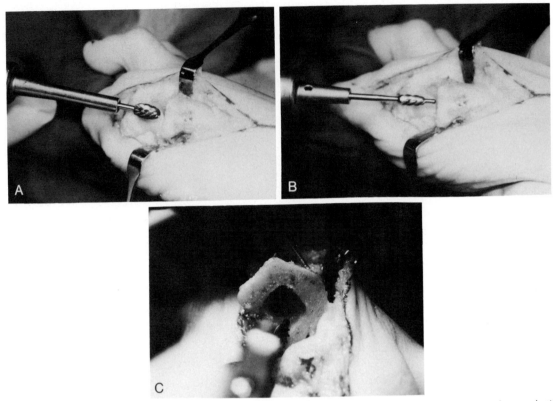

FIGURE 12–13. The Swanson blunt-tipped burr is used to ream and shape the metatarsal shaft to receive the prosthetic stem. The opening is rectangular. A pear-shaped burr *(A)* may be needed to initiate the reaming process.

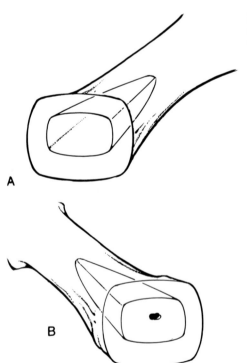

FIGURE 12–14. Burring of the medullary canals. *(A),* The metatarsal stump. The canal is burred in the shape of the prosthetic stem, a truncated pyramid or tapered parallelepiped. *(B),* The proximal phalanx. Reaming is centered just dorsal to the center of the articular surface to align with the center of the medullary canal.

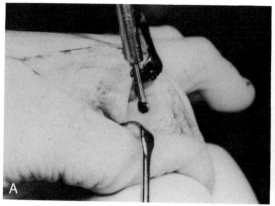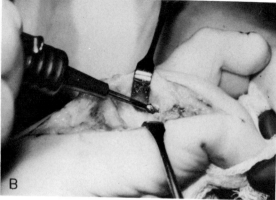

FIGURE 12–15. (*A* and *B*), Burring of the proximal phalanx.

Some surgeons prefer to add antibiotic solution to the saline as well. Thereafter, the prosthesis is handled only by smooth forceps to prevent tearing. (The prosthesis may be handled by the surgeon using a moist glove during positioning.) The surgeon then proceeds to insert the prosthesis and close the soft tissues (Fig. 12–20). The capsule is snugly closed with absorbable suture, and the skin with whatever technique the surgeon prefers. We use running subcuticular 4–0 polypropylene or interrupted locking horizontal mattress sutures of 5–0 nylon.

We carry out this procedure under tourniquet control. While the tourniquet may be released prior to capsular closure, we prefer to apply the dressing and then release the tourniquet. A subcutaneous silicone suction drain is utilized and brought out distally through a separate stab incision. A bulky, soft compressive dressing with a posterior plaster splint with a toe extension is applied with the ankle in neutral position. The drain is removed in 48 hours. The bulky dressing is changed at 3 to 4 days and the patient placed in a postoperative shoe. If an osteotomy has been performed concomitantly with the prosthetic arthroplasty, a short-leg walking cast is used preferentially at this point.

Rehabilitation

In the postoperative period, dressings are carefully applied so as to preserve alignment during capsular healing. Active and active assisted range-of-motion exercises are begun by the foot therapist at 2 weeks, with suture removal at 2 to 3 weeks, depending on the condition of the wound and the patient's estimated healing capacity.

FIGURE 12–16. Shortening of the distal stem on the prosthesis.

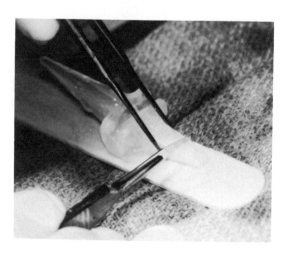

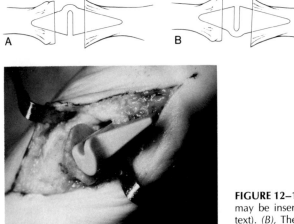

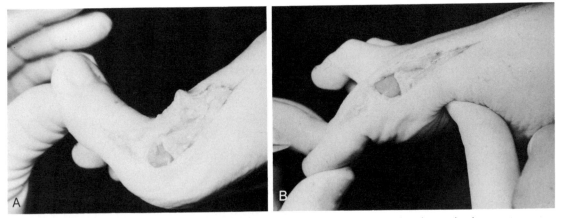

FIGURE 12–17. Orientation of the prosthetic hinges. *(A)*, The prosthesis may be inserted with the hinge opening plantarward (N. Gould; see text). *(B)*, The usual orientation places the hinge opening dorsalward. *(C)*, Trial sizing of the metatarsal side with the hinge opening dorsalward.

FIGURE 12–18. *(A* and *B)*, Testing of the prosthetic fit for buckling, excessive pistoning, or impingement.

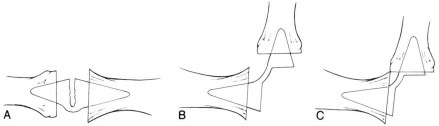

FIGURE 12–19. Checking the prosthetic fit. *(A)*, The prosthesis is checked in full extension to make certain there is no buckling of the hinge. *(B and C)*, The prosthesis is checked in dorsiflexion to look for excessive pistoning *(B)* and instability or impingement *(C)* of the metatarsal and phalangeal surfaces.

Dynamic splint devices have been fabricated to assist in toe dorsiflexion and plantar flexion. The patient is also encouraged to carry out proximal blocking of motion by manually holding the metatarsal shaft with one hand while attempting to flex and extend the MTP joint. It is also helpful to block IP motion with a static splint, thereby isolating motion to the MTP joint. When an osteotomy has been performed, motion is intitiated in the cast, with full mobilization after 4 weeks.

Complications and Salvage

Early complications include wound problems, infection,[27] inadequate range of motion, and recurrence of deformity. Late problems include infection, implant failure, silicone synovitis, and bone resorption, as well as deformity and development of a transer lesion. Salvage consists of removal of the prosthesis, resulting in a "second-stage" resection arthroplasty, prosthetic exchange, or arthrodesis with intercalary bone graft. If a resection arthroplasty is performed, the fibrous pseudocapsule that has formed around the prosthesis provides more stability than in a primary resection. If a patient has been pleased with an implant and has no significant silicone synovitis, exchange is an acceptable alternative. Arthrodesis, although perhaps more technically difficult, preserves both length and function of the great toe.

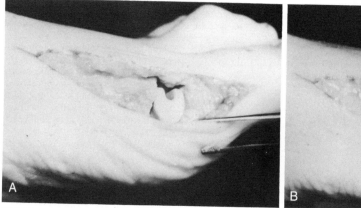
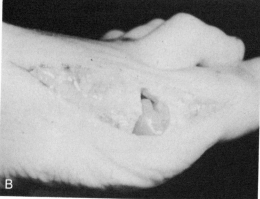

FIGURE 12–20. Final positioning of the prosthesis. *(A)*, The solid trial prosthesis is used to check the final fit. *(B)*, The clear implant is then inserted.

References

1. Balkin SW, Kaplin L: Pressure-related disorders of the foot treated by silicone fluid injection (scientific exhibit). American Academy of Orthopaedic Surgeons. Las Vegas, Nevada, February, 1989.
2. Barton NJ: Arthroplasty of the forefoot in rheumatoid arthritis. J Bone Joint Surg 55B:126–133, 1973.
3. Braley S: The silicones as tools in biological engineering. Med Electron Biol Engin 3:127–136, 1965.
4. Bonney G, Macnab T: Hallux valgus and hallux rigidus: A critical survey of operative results. J Bone Joint Surg 34B:366–385, 1952.
5. Clark WL, Hansen ST: The role of muscle balancing procedures in the planovalgus foot. Sixth Annual Summer Meeting, American Orthopaedic Foot and Ankle Society. Banff, Canada, June, 1990.
6. Coughlin MJ: Arthrodesis of the first metatarsophalangeal joint. Orthop Rev 19:177–186, 1990.
7. Cracchiolo A: Results of implant arthroplasty in the arthritic forefoot. Orthop Trans 4:150, 1980.
8. Cracchiolo A: Double stem silicone implant arthroplasty, hallux MTP joint. The foot—an advanced course in reconstructive and traumatic surgery. American Academy of Orthopaedic Surgeons. Tucson, Arizona, January, 1991.
9. Cracchiolo A, Swanson A, Swanson GD: The arthritic great toe metatarsophalangeal joint: A review of flexible silicone implant arthroplasty from two medical centers. Clin Orthop 157:64–69, 1981.
10. Daniels AU, Samuelson KM, Rusin KA: Talonavicular joint surface anatomy and prototype resurfacing prostheses. Foot Ankle 2:5–14, 1981.
11. Goldner JL, Gould JS, Urbaniak JR, et al: Metacarpophalangeal joint arthroplasties using silicone-Dacron prostheses (Niebauer type): Six and a half years' experience. J Hand Surg 2:200–211, 1977.
12. Gould N: Hallux rigidus: Cheilectomy or implant? Foot Ankle 1:315–320, 1981.
13. Jahss MH: Disorders of the Foot. Philadelphia, WB Saunders, 1982, pp 573–578.
14. Johnson KA: Total joint arthroplasty: The foot. Mayo Clin Proc 54:576–578, 1979.
15. Johnson KA: Surgery of the Foot and Ankle. New York, Raven Press, 1989, pp 29–34, 60–68.
16. Johnson KA, Buck PG: Total replacement arthroplasty of the first metatarsophalangeal joint. Foot Ankle 1:307–314, 1981.
17. Kampner SL: Total joint replacement in bunion surgery. Orthopaedics 1:275–284, 1978.
18. Kitaoka HB, Cahalan TD, Bleimeyer RR, et al: Revision of failed first metatarsophalangeal joint implant arthroplasty. Fifth Annual Summer Meeting, American Orthopaedic Foot and Ankle Society. Sun Valley, ID, August, 1989.
19. Lemon RA, Engber VD, McBeath AA: A complication of Silastic hemiarthroplasty in bunion surgery. Foot Ankle 4:262–265, 1983.
20. Lian GJ, Cracchiolo A: Double-stem silicone implant arthroplasty of the hallux metatarsophalangeal joint in the rheumatoid patient. Twentieth Annual Meeting, American Orthopaedic Foot and Ankle Society. New Orleans, February, 1990.
21. McAuliffe TB, Helal B: Replacement of the first metatarsophalangeal joint with a silicone elastomer ball-shaped spacer. Foot Ankle 10:257–262, 1990.
22. Merkle PF, Sculco TP: Prosthetic replacement of the first metatarsophalangeal joint. Foot Ankle 9:267–271, 1989.
23. Morton DJ: Hypermobility of the first metatarsal bone: The interlinking factor between metatarsalgia and longitudinal arch strains. J Bone Joint Surg 10:187–197, 1928.
24. Myers SR, Herndon JH: Silastic implant arthroplasty with proximal metatarsal osteotomy for painful hallux valgus. Foot Ankle 10:219–223, 1990.
25. Pfeiffer WH, Cracchiolo A, Dorey F: Double stem silicone implant arthroplasty of the hallux and lateral toe metatarsophalangeal joints in patients with rheumatoid arthritis. Sixth Annual Summer Meeting, American Orthopaedic Foot and Ankle Society. Banff, Canada, June, 1990.
26. Sethu A, O'Netto DC, Ramakrishan B, et al: Swanson's Silastic implants in the great toes. J Bone Joint Surg 62B:83–85, 1980.
27. Shereff MJ, Jahss MH: Complications of Silastic implant arthroplasty in the hallux. Foot Ankle 1:95–101, 1980.
28. Stockley I, Betts RP, Getty CJM, et al: The importance of the valgus hindfoot in forefoot surgery in rheumatoid arthritis. Fifth Annual Summer Meeting, American Orthopaedic Foot and Ankle Society. Sun Valley, ID, August, 1989.
29. Swanson AB: Implant arthroplasty for the great toe. Clin Orthop 85:75–81, 1972.
30. Swanson AB: Reconstructive surgery in the arthritic hand and foot. Clin Symp CIBA 31:1–32, 1979.
31. Swanson AB: Implant arthroplasty in disabilities of the great toe. AAOS Instruct Course Lect 21:227–235, 1972.
32. Swanson AB, Herndon JH: Flexible (silicone) implant arthroplasty of the metacarpophalangeal joint of the thumb. J Bone Joint Surg 59A:362–368, 1977.
33. Swanson AB, Lumsden RM, Braunohler WB, et al: Arthroplasty of the great toe with a silicone implant. In Bateman JE, Trott AW (Eds): The Foot and Ankle. New York, BC Decker, 1980, pp 137–142.
34. Swanson AB, Swanson GD: Treatment considerations and resource materials for flexible (silicone) implant arthroplasty. Grand Rapids, MI, Michigan State University Orthopaedic Research Department, 1987.
35. Swanson AB, Swanson GD, Mayhew DE, et al: Flexible hinge results in implant arthroplasty of the great toe. Rheumatology 11:136–152, 1987.
36. Watson MS: A long-term follow-up of forefoot arthroplasty. J Bone Joint Surg 56B:527–533, 1974.
37. Weltmer JB, Cracchiolo A: Double-stem silicone implant arthroplasty of the hallux metatarsophalangeal joint in the non-rheumatoid patient—a long term review. Fifth Annual Summer Meeting, American Orthopaedic Foot and Ankle Society. Sun Valley, ID, August, 1989.
38. Wenger RJ, Whalley RC: Total replacement of the first metatarsophalangeal joint. J Bone Joint Surg 60B:88–92, 1978.
39. Zang K: A conversation with Kerry Zang, DPM: Treatment of the arthritic foot with a new implant. San Diego, Educational Services Department, Sutter Biomedical.

13

Salvage of Failed Silicone Implants

JOHN S. GOULD

Although any procedure in foot surgery may have complications, the distinguishing feature of the problem in prosthetic arthroplasty is the presence of a sizeable foreign body, whose integrity is critical to the ultimate outcome. Because the frequent use of the great toe prostheses dates back to the early 1970s, we now have 20 years perspective with which to evaluate the problems of the device. Consequently, a chapter was devoted to these problems and their salvage. Complications may arise during and within the first few weeks of surgery, within the first few months, and unfortunately, several years after the procedure.

EARLY COMPLICATIONS

Nerve and vascular damage may compromise surgery in the great toe metatarsophalangeal joint area and is probably more common than has been reported by statistics owing to the rich neurovascular supply of the area. The extensiveness of the vascular supply, however, prevents this condition from being a significant clinical problem, whereas the many nerves passing through this area increases the risk of damage.

Vascular Damage

The risk of damage to the blood supply to the metatarsal head and proximal phalanx, which is of concern in various bunion proce-

dures, is not a problem here, because the head fragment is excised and the proximal phalanx merely is opened through its articular surface. The blood supply, passing distally, includes the two plantar digitals and the first dorsal metatarsal, which extends into the first web, anastomosing through a communicating artery to the plantar digitals, and then continuing as a dorsal artery.[4] Even with plantar digital vessel damage, the dorsal system is usually adequate to support the toe. Nevertheless, if the author were aware of damage to a proximal plantar digital, at the time of surgery, the author would release the tourniquet and evaluate the rapidity of refill and the color of the toe in order to decide whether or not to repair the damage at that time. Although initial spasm in the vessels may prolong the refill, the author would anticipate refill within a minute or two. If it is slow, the toe is pale (and later blue tinged), and a plantar digital artery or both are compromised, the author would do an immediate vascular repair. At this level, the digital vessel has an internal diameter greater than 1.0 mm and is relatively easily repaired with current microvascular technique. The operating surgeon or a colleague who specializes in microsurgery can repair the vessel, and the arthroplasty still can be completed.

If a single plantar digital vessel is intact, the blood supply to the toe should be essentially normal according to pulse volume recordings.

All patients with potential vascular compromise due to diabetes, arteriosclerotic peripheral vascular disease, and collagen disorders

131

warrant preoperative Doppler studies and toe pressure/ischemic index evaluations. All other patients should be evaluated by palpation of dorsalis pedis and posterior tibial pulses, the presence of hair growth on the foot and toes, and the appearance of the skin. Thin, hairless, violaceous skin indicates the possibility of an underlying vascular problem. When a patient with increased risk factors has superimposed vascular damage, the indication for immediate surgical repair is obviously heightened.

Nerve Damage

Nerves at risk during an arthroplasty of the first metatarsophalangeal joint include both hallucal digitals, including the common digital nerve to the great toe and the second toe; the deep peroneal nerve in the first web; and the superficial peroneal nerve branches to the first web and the medial side of the great toe.[3] Particular care to preserve the peroneal nerve branches should be made when performing the dorsomedial incision. Dissection in the first web can damage the superficial and deep peroneal nerve branches superficially and the fibular hallucal nerve under the intermetatarsal ligament. Although nerve injury may be a generic problem in foot surgery, the patient presenting with pain following what appears to be a successful procedure clinically and radiographically should be carefully evaluated for nerve injury.

The author's personal preference for treatment of these injured nerves includes the following: When an acute laceration occurs, it is immediately repaired. When a nerve is in continuity but is painful, the author tries a conservative regimen of manual desensitization, oral anti-inflammatory agents and drugs to improve peripheral circulation (e.g., calcium channel blockers), and transcutaneous nerve stimulation (TNS). Percutaneous steroids (iontophoresis) may also be used. When this approach fails, autogenous vein wrapping and, occasionally, implanted neurostimulators may be considered.[6] When a neuroma of the superficial or deep peroneal nerves is found and direct repair cannot be done, proximal resection is the initial surgery. Hallucal digital nerves are repaired with the use of nerve grafting, if necessary. Recalcitrant pain and recurrent neuromas have been treated with wandering nerve grafts or vein conduits, lead-

ing the nerve end into the distal leg and placing the end deep in a large muscle with relatively small excursion (e.g., the soleus or the arterior tibial muscle).

SKIN PROBLEMS

Although wound edge necrosis may be treated by dressings, débridements, and healing by secondary intention in many cases, a significant slough, exposing the subcutaneous tissues, should be rapidly débrided with the application of saline wet-to-dry dressings, followed by povidone-iodine (Betadine) dressings to stimulate granulation. If granulation forms in a few days, split-thickness skin grafting should be performed to cover the wound.

Unfortunately, there are several major problems with this method. If the prosthesis is exposed under the slough, granulation will, of course, not form over the device, rendering grafting impossible. If infection ensues under the slough, the tissue overlying the prosthesis will erode, exposing the device and infecting the deep tissues. A local transpositional flap may cover the critical area, but the length-to-width ratio of the flap must be 1:1 to avoid necrosis, and the skin in this area is not very mobile. Transposition of the abductor hallucis can be considered, but its arc of rotation on a short pedicle is minimal; the distal component is mostly tendon, and the muscle portion usually cannot be moved distally enough, even though the origin can be released and the muscle mobilized on its pedicle.

As a consequence of these factors, in order to save the prosthesis and the risk of deep infection when a skin slough occurs, rapid débridement followed by a free vascularized muscle flap is used. Typically, a small gracilis muscle flap is considered.[2, 5]

BONE, JOINT, AND PROSTHESIS PROBLEMS

In the past, angulation at the metatarsophalangeal joint was a common problem related to the use of prosthetic arthroplasty associated with bunion surgery.[10] This problem occurred because the surgeon failed to align the first metatarsal. Also, the problem occurred whether the single-stemmed or double-stemmed prosthesis was used. Prophylactically, if one considers prosthetic arthroplasty in the treatment of generalized arthritis associated with a bunion, a first metatarsal osteotomy at the base to align the first and second metatarsals, and soft tissue rebalancing at the joint (distal modified McBride) should accompany the arthroplasty. When the angulation occurs postoperatively due to a failure to carry out realignment, the arthroplasty must be performed again, the deformed or potentially damaged prosthesis must be exchanged, and the proper realigning procedure must be carried out.

Dislocation of the prosthesis may occur early because of failure of alignment or because an improperly sized prosthesis was used. Usually, the problem results from a small prosthesis with excessive pistoning, which can be rectified by exchange with a larger prosthesis. Too large a prosthesis may also dislocate and may be exchanged. If available, a tie-in silicone-Dacron great toe prosthesis may be more stable. At the time of revision surgery, the recommendations given for proper sizing and fit of the prosthesis in the proceeding chapter should be followed. If a stable construct cannot be achieved with these measures, the arthroplasty should be abandoned in favor of a pure resection arthroplasty, which is stabilized temporarily with Kirschner wires (0.062 inch), or a formal arthrodesis should be done. Use of temporary Kirschner wires through the prosthetic joint is not advised owing to the potentially increased risk of breakage or silicone synovitis. Cast stabilization cannot be considered reliable to protect an unstable prosthesis.

Sterile inflammation,[11, 12, 13] or persistent drainage from the operative site with negative cultures, may result because of failure to obtain proper cultures (e.g., anaerobes) but it also may occur because of contamination of the prosthesis by foreign particles, such as lint. When silicone protheses were first used, this was not an uncommon problem until it was known that silicone attracts such particles from the air. When the sterile package containing the prosthesis is opened, the device is placed under saline and not touched with dry gloves, or sponges or placed on towels prior to insertion. This is done to minimize lint build-up. In the event that sterile inflammation occurs, exchange of the prosthesis with an adequate washout should be sufficient. We have not encountered these problems since the early 1970s.

Infection of the implant, on the other hand, is a more significant but not insurmountable problem with silicone prostheses. It has been recommended that when inflammation occurs in the operative wound and a positive culture is obtained from the drainage, immobilization with casting and antibiotics may preserve a good outcome and save the prosthesis. When the infection is superficial, this method may be used. The author has used this approach when dealing with similar implants in the hand. Once the infection extends deeply, as evidenced by continuous pain on rest as well as pain with passive motion of the prosthetic joint, supportive radiologic evidence of bone erosions, and a positive culture, removal of the prosthesis and débridement of apparent infected tissue, including the pseudocapsule, is indicated. The administration of supportive intravenous antibiotics is also indicated. The author takes this rigorous approach, supporting the resection site with a Kirschner wire, if necessary but not routinely, and with the application of a walking cast. At the author's institution, with the support of the Infectious Disease Service intravenous antibiotics are administered via a Hickman catheter for at least 6 to 8 weeks, or until all signs of clinical infection are eradicated. The author has been consistently successful with this approach, although an exchange of the prosthesis has not been carried out, which would be theoretically possible once the infection has been eradicated. We leave a resection arthroplasty unless it proves to be painful. This condition is noted when the joint is moved passively, but pain at rest has been fully relieved. When pain does occur, we proceed to a formal arthrodesis (Fig. 13–1).

LATE COMPLICATIONS

Within months of the prosthetic arthroplasty, transfer lesions with callus formation and pain under the second metatarsal head, and even a stress fracture in the second or third metatarsal shaft have been encountered. To deal with this problem, total contact inserts for the patient's shoes are used initially, with placement of a metatarsal pad behind the second metatarsal head (and the third) and with relief under the prominent second metatarsal. A pedorthist may fill the relieved area with a shear-relieving material, such as a viscoelastic polymer. The callus is also pared or

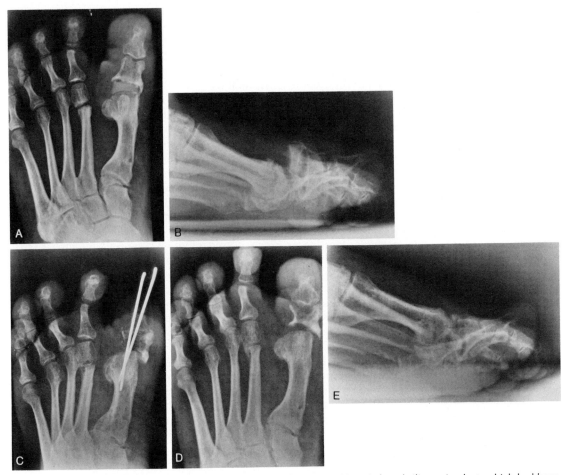

FIGURE 13–1. *(A)*, Anteroposterior radiograph of a 52-year-old woman with an infected silicone implant, which had been placed 15 months previously. The patient had been treated with oral antibiotics and was in severe pain. She also had a nonunion of a second metatarsal neck osteotomy, which had been performed concomitantly with the original procedure. *(B)*, Lateral projection reveals the dorsal dislocation of the single-stemmed implant and the erosion of the distal end of the implant into the interphalangeal joint. *(C)*, The patient underwent débridement of the silicone implant and other infected material, including a soft tissue absess in the first web space. The proximal phalanx was brought back into alignment and pinned in the desired position. The patient remained on intravenous antibiotics for 1 month, followed by oral antibiotics for a second month. The organism cultured was *Staphylococcus aureus.* *(D)*, The pins were removed at the 2-month postoperative interval. The second metatarsal fracture healed while in the wooden-soled shoe. *(E)*, The lateral view shows that the hallux is now reduced on the metatarsal head. (Courtesy of Francesca M. Thompson, M.D.)

shaved. An alternative method is to elevate the metatarsal head with an osteotomy either at the neck or base of the metatarsal bone. Unfortunately, the transfer lesion may continue to move laterally, requiring further management across the foot. As an alternative, many surgeons proceed to remove the prosthesis and carry out an arthrodesis of the metatarsophalangeal joint when the transfer lesion cannot be managed without surgery (Fig. 13–2).

In addition, pain may occur early after the surgery if a patient has arthritic changes not only of the metatarsophalangeal joint surfaces proper but also between the sesamoids and the inferior articular surface of the metatarsal head. When this occurs, we recommend performing metatarsophalangeal arthrodesis with or without sesamoid excision. The sesamoid resection is probably not necessary on a routine basis. Sesamoidectomy without removal of the prosthesis would be expected to cause muscle imbalance with a cockup or angular toe deformity.

Problems that occur later begin with prosthetic subsidence. This seems to occur in time

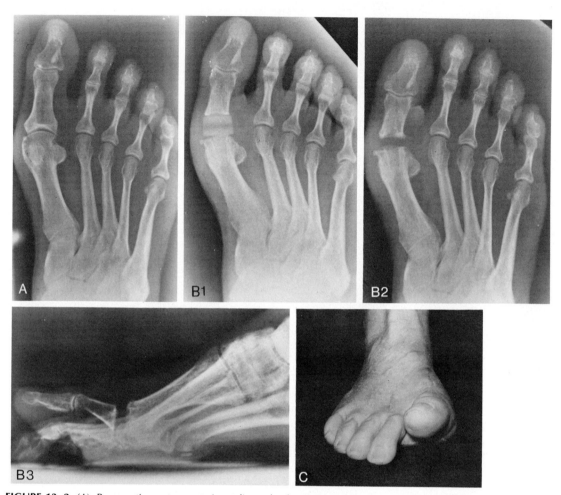

FIGURE 13–2. *(A)*, Preoperative anteroposterior radiograph of a 55-year-old woman who had been informed elsewhere that she had degenerative joint disease and who underwent prosthetic arthroplasty of the hallux metatarsophalangeal joint. *(B)*, Anteroposterior radiograph with the prosthesis in place. The patient had pain and loss of function with this double-stemmed prosthesis and a transfer lesion under the second and third metatarsal heads. An excisional arthroplasty was carried out by another surgeon. Anteroposterior and lateral views are shown. *(C)*, Clinically, the patient had a cock-up deformity of the nonfunctional hallux, with a fixed dorsiflexion position of 52 degrees. On the anteroposterior view, the alignment of the toe was reasonably satisfactory.

Illustration continued on following page

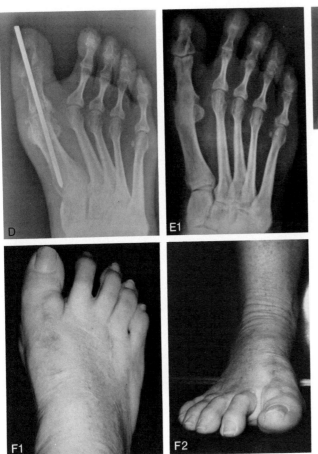

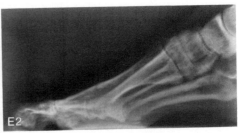

FIGURE 13-2 *Continued (D),* Two years after the implant surgery, the patient underwent an arthrodesis in which an iliac crest bone graft and threaded Steinmann pin fixation were used. Fixation was continued for 4 months while the patient ambulated in a wooden-soled postoperative shoe. *(E),* Anteroposterior and lateral views taken 2 years and 3 months after the arthrodesis. *(F),* Alignment of the toe on both anteroposterior and coronal views demonstrates good alignment of the toe. The dorsiflexion angle is 16 degrees, and the lateral metatarsalgia has been resolved. (Courtesy of Francesca M. Thompson, M.D.)

with most silicone prostheses, but it is not an immediate clinical problem. When bone impingement finally occurs, one needs to consider further surgical intervention.

Further problems with the prosthesis include breakage, prosthetic wear, and silicone synovitis.[11, 12, 13] Thorough studies on prosthetic breakage rates for metatarsophalangeal joint prostheses are not available, but extrapolation from experience with prostheses in the hand[1] suggests that one might anticipate breakage within only a few years of insertion, with an increasing frequency over time. Prosthetic exchange can be considered, as long as silicone synovitis is not a factor in the individual case.

Prosthetic wear occurs from both bending and shear forces. Although these prostheses may tolerate bending forces very well in vitro, such stress lead to tears and tear propagation in vivo. Avoiding the use of sharp metal instruments during insertion is recommended. Tears are then believed to occur from the bone edges on the metatarsal and proximal phalanx

stumps because prostheses were found to break at either side of the hinge. A change was subsequently made in the physical properties of the silicone to create cross linkages in the bonding and, therefore, to stop tear propagation. Later, grommets were added to further protect the silicone. Nevertheless, breakage still seems to occur,[7] although it is, perhaps, delayed.

Wear is readily seen on the single-stemmed prostheses (Fig. 13-3), where the prosthetic surface articulates with bone, cartilage, or another prosthesis (Fig. 13-4). Shear forces, however, with the single-stemmed prosthesis, edges of the double-stemmed prosthesis, and the broken double-stemmed prosthesis, particularly with the harder silicones, has an erasure effect with small particle formation. These particles cause synovitis with bone erosions and cyst formation in the involved and adjacent bones (Fig. 13-5).[9] Silicone has also been detected in regional lymph nodes. When this diagnosis is made, removal of the prosthesis, excision of the involved synovium, curettage of the cysts, bone grafting, and arthrodesis of the joint is the treatment of choice.

SALVAGE PROCEDURES

General salvage techniques for the above-mentioned complications already have been described. Two techniques, secondary excisional arthroplasty and arthrodesis, demand further comment.

Kitaoka and associates have reported that excisional arthroplasty after a failed prosthesis has been successful.[8] The author has had a similar experience. In the series conducted by the author and by Kitaoka and associates the techniques are similar. The original incision is opened, and the pseudocapsule also opened longitudinally. A small curved elevator is placed around the hinge, and the prosthesis gently prized out of the joint. If the prosthesis is broken and the stems remain in the medul-

lary canals, they may be grasped with a Brown-Adson forceps, a fine-pointed rongeur, or with the aid of a curette. The author curettes the pseudocapsule in the medullary canals as well, and may use a Swanson blunt-ended burr on a power tool, if necessary. Often, capsule removal is easily started with a curette and then grasped with a rongeur, removing the entire intramedullary capsule in one maneuver. The capsule between the bone ends is preserved, closed, and purse-stringed, if possible (dorsal to plantar, or medial to lateral) to create, in effect, an interpositional tissue (Fig. 13–6).

When an arthrodesis is performed, the main problem is loss of bone stock and, hence, length of the toe. To compensate, an interpositional bone graft from the iliac crest is used. After filling the depths of the medullary canals or cysts with cancellous bone, the author fashions a football-shaped graft from the rim of the iliac crest, which may be tricortical, and place either end within the well-reamed med-

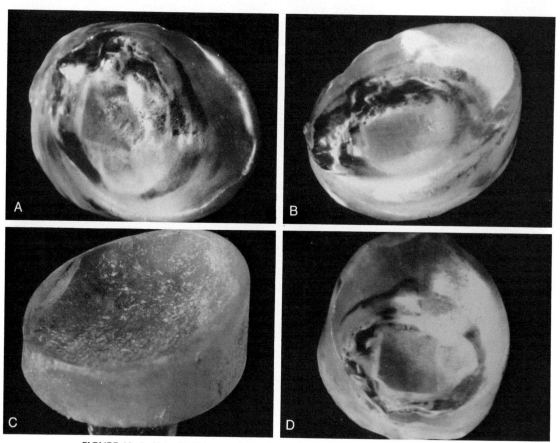

FIGURE 13–3. *(A to D)*, Wear on the surfaces of single-stemmed prostheses.

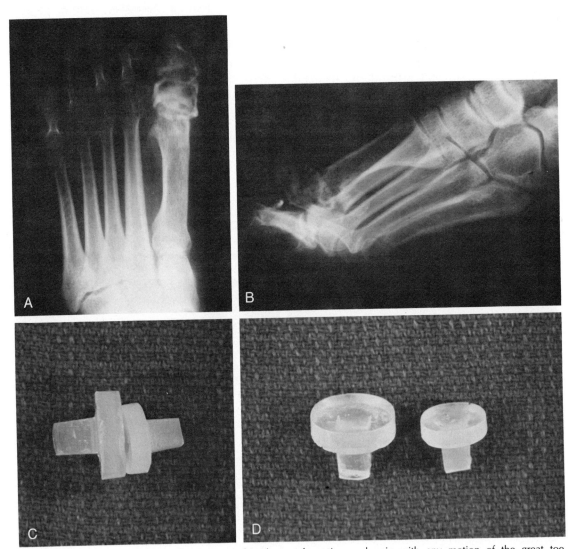

FIGURE 13–4. *(A to D)*, This patient presented with cyst formation and pain with any motion of the great toe metatarsophalangeal joint. At surgery, it was apparent that two single-stemmed prostheses had been used, with one each placed in the metatarsal and proximal phalanx. Erosion had occurred on the prostheses, and significant synovitis was present. After removal of the devices, leaving the patient with an excisional arthroplasty, the pain was relieved successfully.

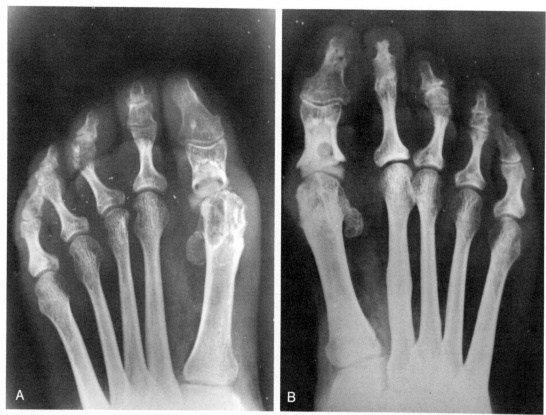

FIGURE 13–5. *(A and B)*, Fifty-year-old man, 3 years after the placement of silicone implants associated with hallux valgus procedures. Significant cyst formation is noted. The patient's feet were salvaged with an iliac crest bone graft and arthrodeses.

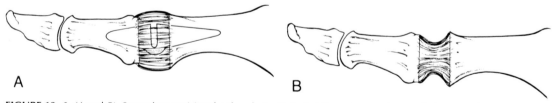

FIGURE 13–6. *(A and B)*, Secondary excisional arthroplasty. Note that the outer pseudocapsule is retained and imbricated.

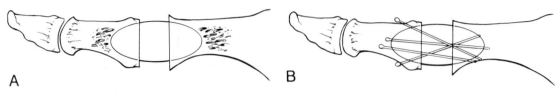

FIGURE 13–7. Arthrodesis following prosthetic failure. *(A),* A football-shaped iliac crest tricortical graft is used. Trimming of the bone is carried out with a bone saw. *(B),* Fixation may be carried out with any number of devices, including threaded Kirschner wires, Steinmann pins, or plate and screws.

ullary canals of the metatarsal and proximal phalanx. This construct may then be fixed with the hardware of choice. The author uses multiple-buried threaded 0.062-inch Kirschner wires, drilled from the proximal phalanx cortex medially, across the graft, and across the metatarsal cortex (Fig. 13–7). Various plates and screws are good alternatives.

In summary, although silicone implants for the hallux have numerous shortcomings and complications, currently they represent the only implants available that have been used with success, and they are retrievable, as noted above. Silicone-Dacron implants are considerably more difficult to excise, and use of cemented or porous coated implants would provide more formidable challenges if we can extrapolate our experiences in the hand and elsewhere in the body.

References

1. Goldner JL, Gould JS, Urbaniak JR, McCollum DE: Metacarpophalangeal joint arthroplasties using silicone-Dacron prostheses (Niebauer type): Six and a half years experience. J Hand Surg 2:200–211, 1977.
2. Gould JS: Reconstruction of soft tissue injuries of the foot and ankle with microsurgical techniques. Orthopedics 10:151–157, 1987.
3. Gould JS: Ancillary studies—Neurologic. *In* Gould JS (Ed): The Foot Book. Baltimore, Williams & Wilkins, 1988, pp 8–14.
4. Gould JS: Ancillary studies—Vascular: Doppler, pulse volume recordings, thermograms. *In* Gould JS (Ed): The Foot Book. Baltimore, Williams and Wilkins, 1988, pp 15–22.
5. Gould JS: Management of soft tissue loss on the plantar aspect of the foot. Instr Course Lect 39:121–126, 1990.
6. Gould JS: Treatment of the painful injured nerve in continuity. *In* Gelberman RH (Ed): Operative Nerve Repair and Reconstruction. Philadelphia, JB Lippincott, 1991, pp 1541–1550.
7. Herndon JH: Personal communication, 1991.
8. Kitaoka HB, Cahalan TD, Bleimeyer RR, et al: Revision of the failed first metatarsophalangeal joint implant arthroplasty. Fifth Annual Summer Meeting, American Orthopaedic Foot and Ankle Society. Sun Valley, Idaho, August 1989.
9. Lemon RA, Engber VD, McBeath AA: A complication of Silastic hemiarthroplasty in bunion surgery. Foot Ankle 4:262–265, 1983.
10. Sethu A, O'Netto DC, Ramakrishan B, et al: Swanson's Silastic implants in the great toes. J Bone Joint Surg 62B:83–85, 1980.
11. Shereff MJ, Jahss MH: Complications of Silastic implant arthroplasty in the hallux. Foot Ankle 1:95–101, 1980.
12. Swanson AB: Complications of silicone elastomer prostheses. JAMA 238:939, 1977.
13. Swanson AB, Lumsden RM II, Swanson GD: Silicone implant arthroplasty of the great toe. Clin Orthop 142:30–43, 1979.

14 Rheumatoid Arthritis of the Forefoot

ANDREA CRACCHIOLO III

PATHOLOGY

Rheumatoid arthritis (RA) is a systemic disease that frequently involves the foot. The etiology is still unknown; however, susceptibility to most rheumatic diseases is strongly influenced by human leukocyte antigens (HLA). With the advent of HLA typing, our understanding of the pathology of immune diseases has improved considerably, as exemplified by the recognition of the close association between HLA-B27 and susceptibility to ankylosing spondylitis. More than 90 percent of white ankylosing spondylitic patients studied carried the B27 antigen, in contrast to only 8 to 9 percent of normal white controls. More recent population studies in several different ethnic groups have confirmed the strong association between rheumatoid arthritis and HLA-DR4, with an incidence of 70 to 75 percent. A small but significant number of racial groups have shown an association with DR1 antigen.[29] Although these studies may be helpful in the diagnosis of a specific type of arthritis, the role of these human leukocyte antigens in producing or mediating the disease is still unclear.

The clinical diagnosis of rheumatoid arthritis can be difficult, particularly early in the disease. Recently, the American College of Rheumatology proposed revised criteria for the classification of rheumatoid arthritis that demonstrated a 91- to 94-percent sensitivity and an 89-percent specificity for RA when compared with non-RA rheumatic disease control subjects.[1] Occasionally, rheumatoid arthritis presents in the forefoot. Metatarsalgia is by far the earliest symptom, although rarely the hindfoot or the ankle is the initial focus of the disease. An inflammation of the synovium, of unknown etiology, is the primary pathologic mechanism in rheumatoid arthritis, and since there are many synovial joints within the foot, active rheumatoid disease can produce widespread foot pain. The rheumatoid synovial membrane proliferates, becomes thickened and inflamed, and is infiltrated with mononuclear cells. Joint swelling can probably be best appreciated in the forefoot in the metatarsophalangeal (MTP) joints. Swelling can also be seen surrounding the tendon sheaths across the dorsum of the ankle, along the posterior tibialis tendon, and occasionally in the peroneal tendons. Swelling of the hindfoot is most obvious over the talonavicular joint medially and over the sinus tarsi laterally. Ankle synovitis is best seen anteriorly.

The classic findings of rheumatoid arthritis in the forefoot include hallux valgus with obvious intra-articular involvement of the MTP joints. As the toes drift laterally with dorsal subluxation or dislocation, the metatarsal heads are directed more plantarward, the toes show a hammer toe or a clawtoe deformity, and the protective plantar fat pad is drawn further forward from its normal location underneath the metatarsal heads. Large bursae with overlying calluses are frequently seen under the plantar aspect of the forefoot, most prominently under the second and third metatarsal heads and, at times, under the hallux.

Synovitis of the MTP joints usually occurs early in the disease. In a population of RA patients studied in a medical rheumatology clinic, Spiegel and Spiegel[33] found synovitis in 65 percent of patients with a disease duration of 1 to 3 years, while only 18 percent of patients having disease for more than 10 years showed any synovitis. There appeared to be equal involvement of all the MTP joints. Dorsal corns, usually occurring over the proximal interphalangeal (PIP) joint, are also common in the subluxated or dislocated toes. A mallet toe deformity can affect the second and third toes. Nail deformities are a result of both the disease and the abnormal position of the toes. Web space pathology usually includes the presence of an intermetatarsal bursa. Neuroma-like symptoms can be an early sign of forefoot involvement due to pressure on the digital nerve from an enlarged intermetatarsal bursa.[2] In 1975, Shepard[32] reported 24 patients with metatarsal bursitis with nerve compression, and RA was the diagnosis in seven, with eight more being diagnosed with RA from 4 months to 4 years later. Recently, Dedrick[16] reported three women with spreading of the second and third toes, two of whom had pain. At operation, an interdigital rheumatoid nodule was found; further work-up indicated a diagnosis of RA, and two were seropositive. Synovitis within the tarsal tunnel can lead to neurapraxia of the posterior tibial nerve, although this is an unusual finding. Other forefoot deformities, such as hallux varus with varus drift of the second and third toes, can occur but these are more unusual. Occasionally, the second toe is in varus lying over or under an abnormal hallux valgus.

Hindfoot and ankle pathology is more subtle, can progress rapidly, and frequently affects the forefoot. The hindfoot and forefoot are joined together through many structures, including the plantar fascia and the short toe flexors. Normally the hindfoot is aligned in about 7 degrees of valgus during weight bearing. The weight-bearing line of the body normally falls to the medial side of the axis of the subtalar joint. When moving through a gait cycle, going from heel to strike to toe-off, the leg will externally rotate and the hindfoot and heel, supported in part by a normal posterior tibial tendon, will invert so that the heel can rise off the ground. Several factors can upset hindfoot stability in the rheumatoid patient. First, there is frequently synovitis of the hindfoot joints. Second, loss of articular cartilage and erosion of the talonavicular and subtalar joints give a persistent valgus of the hindfoot.

The talonavicular joint becomes unstable, with the head of the talus drifting medially and plantarward.[18] The calcaneus can also butt against the distal fibula so that the patient complains of pain at the lateral malleolus.[10] Third, the posterior tibial tendon may be ruptured,[17] and even if it is not, the altered hindfoot mechanics do not allow it to function effectively as the medial stabilizer of the hindfoot. This increases the valgus of the hindfoot and produces pronation of the midfoot and forefoot. Spiegel and Spiegel[33] found that only 8 percent of patients with disease of less than 5 years' duration had moderate to severe hindfoot deformities. However, 25 percent of patients suffering from disease for more than 5 years had abnormal hindfoot valgus on weight bearing. Other abnormalities of the ankle or the knee, usually valgus deformities, can contribute to the malalignment of the foot.

Ankle disease has far fewer symptoms, and when rheumatoid patients complain of ankle pain, the majority are actually experiencing hindfoot pain. Ankle synovitis may be well tolerated but can result in a narrowing of the ankle joint with gradual loss of motion. However, ankle instability can also occur from erosions of the dome of the talus and ligament instability, so that a valgus deformity may result from pathology within the tibiotalar joint rather than the hindfoot. It is essential to distinguish between hindfoot and ankle pathology. Either one or all three of the hindfoot joints may require surgical arthrodesis to correct the deformity and relieve pain. Less frequently, the ankle joint destruction is advanced and will require surgical arthrodesis. Fortunately, with fusion of the ankle in the proper position[26] and use of newer methods of internal fixation,[31] ankle arthrodesis can be a most satisfactory procedure.

Seronegative spondyloarthropathies that can affect the foot include ankylosing spondylitis, Reiter's syndrome, and psoriatic arthritis.[5, 11]

RADIOGRAPHIC EVALUATION

The most common radiographic abnormalities seen in rheumatoid arthritis are classic joint erosions, and the most frequently involved joints are the metatarsophalangeal (MTP) joints, the metatarsocuneiform joints, and the talonavicular joint. The MTP joints are usually subluxated or dislocated, and extensive periarticular osteoporosis may be seen.[22] Osteoporosis of the MTP joints is often the earliest sign of the disease. Although all of these joints are usually involved, the earliest changes may be seen in the first, fourth, and fifth joints.[21] Erosions of the metatarsal heads occur at the margins of the articular cartilage and the synovial reflections and are caused by the inflammatory pannus tissue. They are detected along the medial side of the heads except for the fourth metatarsal head, where they initially occur on the lateral side. A standard set of radiographs should be obtained when evaluating any rheumatoid patient with significant involvement of the foot (Fig. 14–1A to D). These should include a weight-bearing view of the foot in the anteroposterior and lateral positions. A weight-bearing anteroposterior view of the ankles is mandatory. Some measurements of pronation and hindfoot valgus can be made on the lateral weight-bearing radiograph by measuring the lateral talometatarsal angle. Comparison radiographs are always helpful, and significant changes may be seen within 3 to 6 months.

DIAGNOSTIC MANEUVERS

Although patients may be referred from other specialists, such as rheumatologists, patients with foot pain often self-refer directly to an orthopaedic surgeon. It may be inappropriate for an orthopedist to launch into a complete rheumatologic evaluation; however, the diagnosis should always be considered in the differential diagnosis of foot pain, especially when evidence of a specific mechanical problem is lacking. Rheumatoid arthritis is most commonly a disease of younger women. Bilateral symmetrical pain is another clue to an arthritic disease. In men, heel pain, especially when bilateral, suggests a diagnosis of ankylosing spondylitis or one of the other rheumatic diseases such as Reiter's syndrome. Should there be clinical evidence of a systemic arthritic disease, the physical examination should be expanded. One should evaluate other joints, particularly the hands, sacroiliac joints, and the spine, and appropriate radiographs may be indicated. Basic laboratory studies include sedimentation rate, rheumatoid factor, antinuclear antibody, and perhaps serum uric acid levels. Radionuclide bone scans can identify multiple areas of synovitis.

However, the best method of diagnosing a systemic inflammatory disease is still a thorough and specific history and physical examination.

One should evaluate the entire foot and ankle in patients with rheumatoid arthritis who present with symptoms predominantly involving the forefoot. These patients have a systemic disease that has produced these deformities; therefore, it is important to assess any and all factors that affect the patient's forefoot pathology.

At times it is impossible clinically or radiographically to determine the origin of hindfoot and ankle pain when both areas may be involved. Differential injections of a local anesthetic with a small amount of corticosteroid can help in establishing the area of involvement. When both the hindfoot and ankle are involved, it is usually best to inject the ankle through an anteromedial approach to avoid any infiltration of the local anesthetic laterally into the subtalar joint. The subtalar joint is injected downward and medially through the sinus tarsi, keeping well away from the lateral recess of the ankle synovium. Usually if the correct area is injected, the patient will have significant relief of symptoms. However, in 15 to 20 percent, there is a communication between the ankle and hindfoot joints, and pain relief from an injection in one area may be misleading.

NONOPERATIVE TREATMENT

Conservative care should be given to the rheumatoid foot either prior to or following an operative procedure. Skin and nail care is frequently needed, and this includes trimming of the nails and paring down of painful hard calluses. It is frequently difficult for rheumatoid patients to cut their own toenails due to upper extremity involvement. Aspiration and injection of any swollen joint or an intermetatarsal bursa using small amounts of corticosteroids and a local anesthetic give temporary relief of pain.

The most important aspect of nonoperative care is proper shoewear.[9] Usually a shoe must be specially selected or modified to fit the patient's deformity. Shoes do not correct deformities; rather, they accomodate the deformities and thus reduce pain. Since the forefoot is the most common area of symptoms and pathology, shoes with a wider and deeper toe box should be worn. Such shoes are commercially available and do not need to be custom manufactured.

It is important to remember that any modification on the inside of the shoe can affect the fit. Thus if an orthotic device or any other material is added to the inside of the shoe, the patient may need a shoe at least one size larger. The most common such modification is an anterior support, otherwise known as a metatarsal pad. This support should be fitted so that the apex of the pad is just proximal to the area of maximum tenderness or callus formation, usually between the second and third metatarsal heads. A longitudinal arch support is also helpful as it gives more plantar surface contact to better distribute skin pressure. Some rheumatoid patients have very thin atrophic skin and an atrophic plantar fat pad that is usually out of position due to the pathology, and they may find a Plastizote (polyethylene foam) liner quite helpful. Excavations under painful areas of the insole can also reduce tenderness and callus formation. The excavation can be filled with some type of shear-reducing material such as Spenco or Sorbothane. Mild pronation and valgus deformities can be controlled to some degree by stiffening the counters of the shoe, usually by laminating them with fiberglass. A wider heel or an outflare heel can reinforce the hindfoot and better stabilize that area.

Occasionally, if there is significant ankle involvement as well as hindfoot involvement, an ankle-foot orthosis (AFO) can temporarily stabilize the foot. Whenever there is significant ankle stiffness or following ankle arthrodesis, a solid-ankle, cushioned-heel shoe with a rocker-bottom sole is very helpful for improved ambulation.[13] These modifications should also be incorporated in the shoe of a patient requiring an AFO. Since rheumatoid patients frequently have upper extremity pathology, Velcro straps are preferable to laces.

SURGICAL CORRECTION OF RHEUMATOID DEFORMITIES

Preoperative Considerations

The patient should be fully informed about the planned operative procedure and any potential systemic and local complications. It is important to assess the patient and the foot more specifically with regard to certain preoperative factors. Any areas of *sepsis,* such as an infected toenail, must be cleared. *Skin lesions,* such as distal leg ulcers or poor skin over various prominences such as corns or calluses, must be treated and healed preoperatively if possible. The foot can be kept in a sandal or some other very wide shoe until these areas heal or the toebox of the shoe can be cut out over painful draining dorsal skin areas.

The *peripheral circulation* must be assessed. The circulation is usually adequate in rheumatoid patients, but one should palpate for pulses. If there is a history of vasculitis or ulcers on the lower legs, then it may be necessary to obtain Doppler flow studies. One can also review the radiographs to see whether there are significant calcifications in the vessels. The occasional rheumatoid patient with coexistent peripheral vascular disease or diabetes should have Doppler flow studies and possibly a vascular surgical consultation preoperatively. Usually a tourniquet is used in performing these various operative procedures so it is essential that adequate peripheral circulation be present. Because of frequent problems with skin about the ankle, it may be best to place the tourniquet high on the thigh where there is much more muscle and subcutaneous tissues. If a minor operation is being considered, a tourniquet can be used at the ankle if the skin is in good condition. However, in major forefoot reconstructive procedures where there are severe deformities, the ankle tourniquet is too constrictive. It tends to bind down the tendons and does not allow free movement of the toes, making the correction of deformities much more difficult.

Medications must be adjusted. Certainly anyone who is currently taking corticosteroids or who has been on a daily dose of corticosteroids for several months within 18 months of the operation needs an increased amount on the day of surgery. Various dosage scales exist, but frequently 75 to 100 mg of an injectable corticosteroid (usually Solu-Cortef) is administered about 1 hour before the operation. A similar dose is given approximately every 8 hours for the first 24 hours and then a smaller dose, usually 50 to 75 mg every 8 hours, is given for the next 1 or 2 days. Patients should then resume their usual daily dose of oral corticosteroids. These patients are at risk for impaired wound healing and sepsis and have a higher incidence of delayed union or nonunion following osteotomy or arthrodesis.

Patients taking methotrexate should discontinue their weekly dose 1 week before the planned operation and for 2 weeks following the operation, as this medication causes delayed wound healing. It may not be the drug that causes the problem as much as the specific type of rheumatoid disease that requires methotrexate. In any case, it is probably safer to temporarily discontinue it.

Other *areas of rheumatoid involvement* should be considered. For example, cervical spinal radiographs should be obtained to be certain that there is no instability at C1–C2 and in the subaxial areas of the cervical spine. Consideration of other joints is likewise important. Many of these patients will have undergone hip or knee replacements and they should receive appropriate antibiotic coverage for the first 48 hours. Patients who do not have other implants and are not receiving an implant in the foot do not require routine antibiotic prophylaxis.

It is sometimes helpful to have the patient consult a *physical therapist* to determine what type of assistance will be necessary for walking postoperatively. Patients with deformed upper extremities may not be able to use the traditional crutches or walkers and need a special upper extremity support. At times, an occupational therapy evaluation is useful to determine what postoperative aids will assist the patient in the convalescent period.

Timing of Operations

While the forefoot is usually the most involved site, some patients may require surgical correction in other areas. In a patient with painful forefoot and hindfoot deformities, it may be best to correct the hindfoot first. Forefoot deformities may recur in patients with significant pronation and valgus deformity of the foot. At times, it may be necessary to perform a more minor procedure to allow for skin healing and to eliminate sepsis. Examples are treatment of an infected toenail or excision of a proximal interphalangeal (PIP) joint to eliminate an ulcerated dorsal corn.

It is usually unwise to perform extensive bilateral forefoot surgery. Even with an advanced deformity, the patient can better rely on the unoperated foot to ambulate. Thus by placing less stress on the operated foot, wound healing is improved. Operations on the ipsilateral forefoot and hindfoot should also be avoided as this may produce extensive swelling leading to problems with wound healing. The safest course is to proceed with a properly planned forefoot reconstruction unilaterally and to operate on the opposite side 4 to 6 weeks later after wound healing is complete.

Forefoot Procedures

Incisions

Dorsal incisions provide excellent exposure of the MTP joints (Fig. 14–1). Longitudinal incisions usually heal well and are more helpful in reconstructive procedures of the forefoot. Three incisions are usually required: a dorsal medial incision to expose the hallux MTP joint, an incision over the second web space, and a third incision over the fourth web space (Fig. 14–2). The latter two incisions allow access to the second, third, fourth, and fifth MTP joints. When forefoot pathology is severe, especially when there is advanced angular deviation of the toes, exposure is facilitated by operating on the four lateral MTP joints before operating on the hallux. It is frequently difficult to gain full correction of the hallux MTP joint first when there is severe deformity of the second through fifth joints. A dorsal transverse approach gives wide exposure of all the MTP joints and can be used if these joints are going to be completely excised. However, skin closure and wound healing are more difficult with this incision. The plantar approach to the MTP joints also gives good exposure and is the easiest approach to the dislocated metatarsal heads (Fig. 14–3). Large calluses on the plantar surface are frequently caused by bursae that overlie the dislocated metatarsal head, and these should be excised. Occasionally rheumatoid nodules are also present. The transverse incision is placed at the level of the metatarsal necks, to the heel side of the dislocated MTP heads. If the tissues are handled carefully and if gentle skin traction is utilized, this is a perfectly safe incision that heals well. Abnormal PIP joints are usually approached through dorsal transverse or longitudinal incisions. A web space incision is also most helpful and is described later.

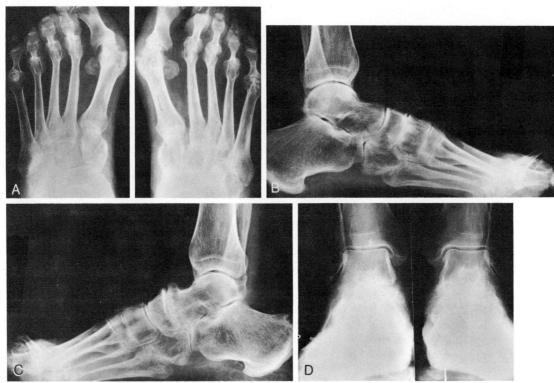

FIGURE 14–1. (A), Weight-bearing radiographs of the foot and ankle are essential in evaluating a patient with rheumatoid arthritis. Since these patients may have deformities in any of the areas and since all three anatomic areas are interrelated, it is best not to depend solely on the history and physical examination but to obtain these views. The anteroposterior radiograph gives excellent information about the forefoot and midfoot. (B and C), Lateral weight-bearing radiographs give some indication as to the status of the ankle joint as well as the subtalar joint and transverse tarsal joints. The lateral radiograph does not give significant information about the forefoot. However, it is very important to measure the lateral talo–first metatarsal angle. A line drawn through the axis of the talus should follow the intramedullary shaft of the first metatarsal in a foot unless there is significant pronation or cavus deformity. Pronation is common in patients with rheumatoid arthritis. (D), The anteroposterior weight-bearing view of the ankle demonstrates the status of the ankle joint. If there is valgus deformity of the hindfoot, it is very difficult to determine from clinical examination alone whether the valgus deformity is in the hindfoot area or may be due, in part or entirely, to a valgus deformity of the ankle joint.

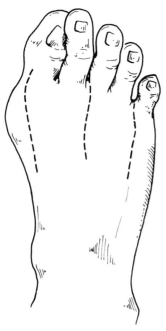

Dorsal
Longitudinal
Incisions

FIGURE 14–2. Three dorsal longitudinal incisions are used to expose the metatarsophalangeal joints. In a severe deformity, the second and fourth web space incisions are usually made first. The incision should retain as much subcutaneous tissue and fat as possible. The metatarsophalangeal joint is approached only when the extensor tendons are visualized. The incision over the hallux can be made somewhat more medially to avoid the dorsal cutaneous nerve to the hallux, or can be made directly over the dorsum of the hallux just medial to the extensor hallucis longus. (From Gould JS [Ed]: The Foot Book. Baltimore, Williams & Wilkins, 1988, p 246. © 1988, The Williams & Wilkins Company, Baltimore.)

146

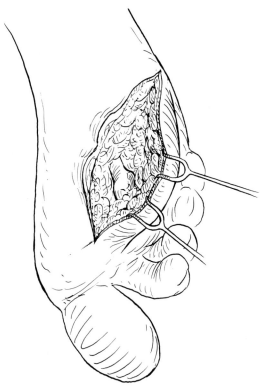

FIGURE 14–3. A plantar approach can be used with care to expose the lateral four metatarsal heads. This incision is placed on the heel side of the fat pad and *not* at the base of the toes. It is very easy to do this with the patient in the prone position, but this should only be done when there is no surgery planned for the hallux or when the hallux metatarsal head is to be excised. Otherwise, this incision can also be easily performed with the patient supine; the operating table is tilted head down (Trendelenberg's position), and the foot may be elevated by placing a soft roll under the ankle. (From Gould JS [Ed]: The Foot Book. Baltimore, Williams & Wilkins, 1988, p 249. © 1988, The Williams & Wilkins Company, Baltimore.)

Midfoot joints are also generally approached through dorsal incisions. However, little midfoot pathology is seen in the rheumatoid patient. Occasionally, it is necessary to expose the metatarsocuneiform joint, as this may require an arthrodesis.

Patient Positioning

The patient should be positioned so that both the lateral and the medial sides of the foot are easily accessible. Because of the normal external rotation of the hip in a supine patient, it is necessary to place a support or towel roll under the ipsilateral buttock to internally rotate the hip and keep the foot in a neutral position.

Soft Tissue Procedures

Early in the disease, patients may exhibit specific localized symptoms rather than generalized metatarsalgia, including bunion-like symptoms or interdigital neuroma pain, which may emanate from the second or third web space. Patients with known rheumatoid arthritis who have hallux valgus and painful bunions must be carefully assessed before any reconstructive procedure. The reason for this is obvious: if the systemic disease progresses, the joint may become destroyed, requiring yet another operation. One or two isolated swollen MTP joints, resistant to conservative care, might be considered for synovectomy. This operation may only give temporary relief but is a reasonable approach, particularly if the symptoms are unremitting and do not respond to medications, aspiration, injection, or shoe modification. Web space pain may be an early sign of rheumatoid disease.[2] An inflamed intermetatarsal bursa can cause a Morton's metatarsalgia either from pressure on the digital nerve or from the painful bursa itself. Excision of the bursa can have diagnostic as well as treatment implications, as pathologic evaluation may suggest the diagnosis of RA.

Excisional Arthroplasties

Historically, the destroyed MTP joint has been excised in patients with rheumatoid arthritis. This operation has been performed for many years, and almost all conceivable varieties of excisional arthroplasty have been described. Clayton[6] popularized excision of both the metatarsal head and the base of the proximal phalanx. The sesamoids were excised only if they were fused to the bottom of the metatarsal head or grossly deformed. After extensive clinical experience, Clayton observed that even if one or two joints were relatively spared by the disease, they should also be excised, so that in general all MTP joints should be included in the forefoot operation. He also emphasized that if the patient is followed long enough, the postoperative foot will gradually deteriorate. Rheumatoid disease is progressive in most patients and if deformities increase in the remaining joints of the foot, particularly the hindfoot joints, then forefoot deformities may recur. This is a particular problem if a patient has a coexisting planovalgus deformity of the foot or develops such a deformity following forefoot surgery. Excision of the MTP joints gives a somewhat unpredictable result as it is not possible to determine the final position of any of the toes. Also, when the base of the proximal phalanx is resected, the majority of toe function is lost. Thus one should avoid the indiscriminate resection of the bone as the sole method of correcting the forefoot deformity: it is as important to realign the soft tissue structures as it is to resect the bone.

Operative Results

McGarvey and Johnson[30] reviewed 20 different series involving more than 1730 RA forefoot reconstructions done between 1959 and the present. Overall, they estimate an average success rate of approximately 85 percent (range, 55 to 100 percent). Most of these studies report "success" using the patients' subjective response to their operation. Thus it is difficult to know which procedure is the best. In fact, when Barton[3] reviewed three different types of excisional arthroplasty in 65 feet, he was unable to find major differences in the clinical results. Hasselo and coworkers[23] also followed up 26 patients (45 feet) from 4 months to 15 years and were able to conclude only that forefoot surgery in RA was beneficial but that the benefit may not be long lasting. A more detailed clinical analysis was performed by McGarvey and Johnson,[30] who for an average of 4.9 years followed up 29 patients (49 feet) who had undergone a Keller arthroplasty along with excision of the lateral four metatarsophalangeal joints. Only 16 patients (33 percent) were fully satisfied, although 82 percent were willing to undergo the procedure again. Twenty-one patients (43 percent) had some reservations regarding the final result. The major complaint was hallux valgus and pain (53 percent). Perhaps this could be minimized by either performing an arthrodesis of the hallux MTP joint or inserting a double-stem silicone implant.

Betts and associates[4] and Stockley and colleagues[34] used foot pressure studies to assess the results of forefoot surgery in RA. Stockley studied 35 RA patients (60 feet) prospectively with a 36.5-month mean follow-up using a clinical and dynamic pedobarographic evaluation both pre- and postoperatively. All patients had resection of the metatarsal heads, and although all had preoperative pain, only 70 percent had abnormal plantar pressures. At follow-up, 91 percent were satisfied as to function and mobility but only 70 percent were completely pain free. Of the 18 feet with some postoperative pain, 13 had abnormal plantar pressures. The most common area of pain was under the stump of the first metatarsal. The operation used by Stockley and coworkers, which resects the first metatarsal head, resulted in a 73-percent incidence of hallux valgus. Thus it appears that both the Keller operation,[30] which resects the base of the proximal phalanx, and excision of the first metatarsal head will result in residual hallux valgus. Also of interest is Stockley's finding that maximum postoperative pressure was found under the first metatarsal in 67 percent. Moreover, these pressures were increased three-fold as compared with preoperative pressures. Again, this seems to indicate the need for a more definitive reconstruction of the hallux MTP joint.

Surgical Correction of the Lateral Four Metatarsophalangeal Joints

Currently there are at least three basic surgical techniques for correcting the rheumatoid deformities in the lateral four metatarsophalangeal joints, all of which include excision of bone, usually the metatarsal head. The metatarsal head is most frequently resected because it is usually grossly destroyed and pushed plantarward by the dorsally dislocated toes. One must then decide whether to resect the base of the proximal phalanx. This is usually not necessary, and excision of the proximal one third usually results in complete loss of control of the toe. If not surgically syndactylized, the toe may become floppy. Thus excising the entire base of the proximal phalanx should be done only for severe deformity, for revision surgical procedures, and when syndactylization can also be performed.

Usually it is best to perform RA forefoot surgery under tourniquet control. Obviously this is not essential, but the continued bleeding from this very vascular area adds to the length and difficulty of the procedure. A thigh-high tourniquet is preferred because there are usually gross deformities of the toes, and a tourniquet applied above the ankle tends to bind the tendons, interfering with the soft tissue correction of the toe deformities. Also, these operations require about 90 minutes to perform and there is little subcutaneous tissue in the distal leg, so the nerves may be more vulnerable to the tourniquet pressure. Vasculitis and peripheral vascular disease are contraindications to tourniquet use.

Plantar Plate Arthroplasty

This procedure developed by Clayton,[7] appears to be a distinct improvement in the technique of excisional arthroplasty. Through two longitudinal dorsal incisions made as previously described, the lateral four MTP joints are approached in sequence.[12] If the joints are severely dislocated, it is best to perform both incisions and to release the extensor tendons dorsally to all four joints before attempting to expose the metatarsal heads. One must use caution and treat the tissues gently, especially when there is severe deformity. All viable subcutaneous fat should be preserved so that a single layer of skin and subcutaneous tissue is created; this aids in wound closure and wound healing. The short extensors to the toe are lateral to the long extensors and should be released since the toe is usually deviated laterally. The long extensors can be lengthened using a Z cut technique or divided by a long oblique incision. The dorsal capsule of the dislocated MTP joint is incised transversely.

After both collateral ligaments are released from the head, it should be possible to deliver the head into the wound. However, in severe deformities this may be difficult, especially for the second and third metatarsal heads, and it may be necessary to make both skin incisions and release the tendons, capsule, and ligaments to all four lateral MTP joints before gaining enough exposure to excise the metatarsal heads. One should not spend an undue amount of time or inflict more soft tissue trauma simply to gain an optimal exposure to proceed with excision of the head. In such patients, it is better to excise all or part of the head in situ and then adjust the length of the metatarsals when exposure is facilitated after the heads are removed. It is important to excise the metatarsal head in an oblique direction, removing more bone from the plantar aspect of the distal metatarsal (Fig. 14–4) as plantar bone regrowth can occur and cause a painful callus. Sufficient bone should be excised and soft tissue released to allow for approximately a 1.5- to 2.0-cm space to exist between the resected end of the metatarsal and the proximal phalanx. This can be checked by inspection or by placing the tip of the index finger within the resected area within minimum traction on the toe. Also, one should check for any residual spike of bone at the plantar side of the osteotomy area, which should be removed. Generally the second and third metatarsals are of equal length following excision of the head. Because it is by far the shortest metatarsal, the fifth never ends up being too long. Therefore, it is important to carefully check the length of the fourth metatarsal to be certain it is significantly shorter than the second and third metatarsals.

A small amount of the base of the proximal

FIGURE 14–4. It is best to resect the lateral metatarsal heads using an oblique osteotomy. A power oscillating saw can be used, and care should be taken to avoid leaving any bony spike on the plantar surface of the resected metatarsal.

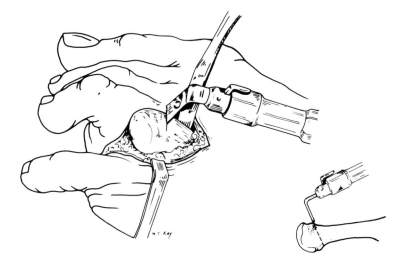

phalanx can also be resected, especially if the deformity is severe. This frees the plantar (volar) plate, and it can be placed over the resected end of the metatarsal and transfixed with a 0.062-inch Kirschner wire passed retrograde through the toe and then across the plate and into the metatarsal shaft (Fig. 14–5). Exposing the plantar plate is important as this structure helps centralize the flexor tendons under the involved ray. Maintaining this position while healing occurs improves the soft tissue realignment of the toes and the forefoot. This procedure also allows the surgeon to inspect the flexor tendon, which is easily seen after the plantar plate has been released. One can then determine that the tendon is intact (which is usually the case) and that there is no significant synovitis. It is possible to do a limited tenosynovectomy even through this incision.

At times, it is neither necessary nor advisable to resect the base of the proximal phalanx, particularly if the deformity is not severe. The plate can be dissected away from the base of the proximal phalanx without injuring the underlying flexor tendon and be utilized in the plantar plate arthroplasty. The use of a No. 11 scalpel blade facilitates this dissection. It is best not to advance the Kirschner wire across the base of the metatarsal as this "skewers" the toe, leaving it immobile and perhaps jeopardizing its vascular supply. It is better to extend the wire into the intramedullary canal of the metatarsal only about 2 to 3 cm so that it stabilizes the alignment but does not cause any undue tension on the toe. The end of the Kirschner wire should be cut and immediately covered with a rubber or metal cap so that the operating team is not injured by the protruding pin. Depending on the type of rheumatoid arthritis, the wires should stay in place for 3 to 6 weeks. In patients with "stiff" rheumatoid disease the wires can be removed at about 3 weeks; those with "loose" disease should have the wires in place for about 5 to 6 weeks. The wires are removed easily in the clinic with only a mild discomfort. The use of a 0.062-inch Kirschner wire is preferred because it is large enough to minimize any significant movement of the skin about the wire. This prevents secondary skin necrosis or sepsis about the pin site and allows the pins to remain in place for several weeks if necessary as they are well tolerated.

If there is some subcutaneous tissue, a few 4–0 absorbable sutures are placed and the skin

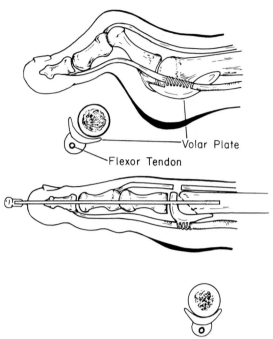

FIGURE 14–5. The results of excisional arthroplasty of the lateral metatarsals may improve if one can balance the extensor and flexor tendons and soft tissues. In rheumatoid arthritis, the toes usually have a marked lateral drift. Both the flexor and the extensor tendons are displaced laterally. Once the metatarsal head has been resected, it is usually easy to find the plantar plate, if it exists. Should the dorsal dislocation of the second and third toes be severe, then the plate is frequently eroded or completely destroyed. If the plate is present, it can be carefully resected from the base of the proximal phalanx using a No. 11 scalpel blade. Alternatively, a small amount of the base of the proximal phalanx can be resected with a power oscillating saw. Just underneath the plate is the flexor hallucis longus, which can be inspected and is usually intact, although there may be surrounding tenosynovitis. Placing the plate between the resected bone ends and securing it with a short 0.062-inch Kirschner wire centralizes the flexor tendon, and this is probably more important than the interposition of the plate. It is important not to pass the Kirschner wire more than about 2 cm into the metatarsal canal. Placing the wire across the base of the metatarsal tends to "skewer" the toe and may interfere with its blood supply. A Kirschner wire simply aids in holding the already corrected position of the toe because it is difficult to do this with any type of external dressing. If the wire is placed before the toe deformity is completely corrected, the deformity will recur when the wire is removed. The end of the wire should be covered with a protective device so that the patient and members of the operating room team are not injured by the sharp edge. (From Gould JS [Ed]: The Foot Book. Baltimore, Williams & Wilkins, 1988, p 251. © 1988, The Williams & Wilkins Company, Baltimore.)

is closed with a 4–0 nonabsorbable suture. Prior to dressing the wounds, a flat silicone drain about 3 inches long is inserted as a wick drain (Fig. 14–6). A sterile compression dress-

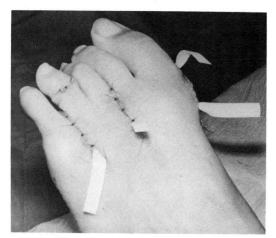

FIGURE 14–6. It is best to use interrupted sutures to close the wounds of a patient with rheumatoid arthritis. Following placement of these sutures, a very thin, flat silicone drain, approximately 3 to 4 cm long, is carefully placed into the base of the incision. This wick drain is satisfactory to remove the excess blood that forms in the wound when the tourniquet is released. It is better to evacuate excessive blood from this area via the drain and a compressive dressing than to allow excessive swelling of the forefoot postoperatively.

ing is placed and then the thigh-high tourniquet is deflated. The combination of good wound closure, the drain, and the dressing allows minimal wound hematoma. It is impossible to achieve hemostasis before closure so deflating the tourniquet early is not helpful and in fact adds to swelling in the operative site. Moreover, the ends of the metatarsal heads have been resected and bone bleeding from the intramedullary canals can be treated only with compression. The skin of RA patients is fragile and delayed healing is common.

Excisional Arthroplasty

This procedure can also be performed through a web space incision as described by Daly and Johnson.[15] The incision is centered on the lateral side of the second toe and the medial side of the third toe and then is extended proximally in the second web space (Fig. 14–7A). A marking pen is used to outline the incision on the lateral side of the second toe, which should be placed just above the flexion creases to avoid injury to the neurovascular bundle. The second and third toes are then pressed together, outlining the position of the incision on the third toe. The incision is

carried into the web space for a few centimeters at the apex of these two lines. This incision was originally used in excising the base of the proximal phalanx of the second and third toes, but this approach also allows excision of the head of the metatarsal as well as the base of the proximal phalanx. If there is a severe deformity, the incision can be carried more proximal in the web space. By extending the incision distally, it is also possible to remove the head of the proximal phalanx if necessary. The procedure is also performed on toes four and five. The adjacent plantar edges of the incision are sutured together with interrupted 4–0 plain catgut (Fig. 14–7B). Then the dorsal side of the incision is closed, creating a syndactylization between the adjacent two toes (Fig. 14–7C). Another type of syndactylization is described by Kelikian[25] in which a wedge of skin is removed from between the toes, resulting in good skin healing but a poor cosmetic appearance. Kirschner wires are not used. Syndactylization is particularly useful in patients with a "loose" type of rheumatoid arthritis, in patients with poor dorsal skin, and in some patients who require revision forefoot surgery. Its only disadvantage is that one may not be able to realign the flexor tendon under the affected ray.

Plantar Approach

Kates described a procedure in which the dislocated MTP joints are approached plantarly with only the metatarsal heads being resected.[24] It is important to remember that the plantar incision should not be made at the base of the toes but rather proximally to the metatarsal heads. The incision is a gentle curve with the convex side pointing distally (see Fig. 14–3). It is much easier to perform this operation with the patient prone, but it is not necessary, and good access can be achieved with the patient supine and the operating table appropriately positioned. Following excision of the metatarsal heads, it is also possible to release the extensor tendons under direct vision. Excision of some of the redundant skin (as much as 2 cm from the proximal [calcaneal] side of the incision) may also be helpful and may keep the fat pad more accurately repositioned. The incision has a slight advantage in that the operative scar does not show. It is especially useful when the dorsal skin is poor

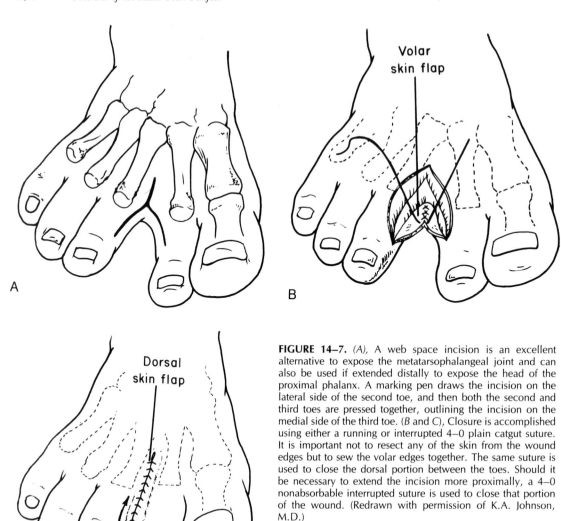

FIGURE 14–7. (A), A web space incision is an excellent alternative to expose the metatarsophalangeal joint and can also be used if extended distally to expose the head of the proximal phalanx. A marking pen draws the incision on the lateral side of the second toe, and then both the second and third toes are pressed together, outlining the incision on the medial side of the third toe. (B and C), Closure is accomplished using either a running or interrupted 4–0 plain catgut suture. It is important not to resect any of the skin from the wound edges but to sew the volar edges together. The same suture is used to close the dorsal portion between the toes. Should it be necessary to extend the incision more proximally, a 4–0 nonabsorbable interrupted suture is used to close that portion of the wound. (Redrawn with permission of K.A. Johnson, M.D.)

or when the patient has inappropriately placed dorsal scars from previous operations. In 1959, Fowler[19] combined both the dorsal and the plantar approaches to the rheumatoid forefoot. He did most of his bony surgery through a dorsal incision and then used the plantar incision to excise an ellipse of skin and draw the toes into more plantar flexion.

SURGICAL CORRECTION OF HALLUX PATHOLOGY

Occasionally (perhaps rarely), the hallux metatarsophalangeal joint may be spared of significant disease, and it should not be operated upon if there is no synovitis or malalignment. However, if there is significant synovitis, an arthrotomy should be performed through a longitudinal incision and a synovectomy done. If there is a significant hallux valgus deformity with a good joint space, this must be corrected to accomodate the more normal realignment of the lateral four toes. Correction of the lateral drift of the toes (especially toes two and three) may cause impingement on the hallux, in which case a distal metatarsal (chevron) osteotomy, sometimes accompanied by a phalangeal (Akin) osteotomy to properly realign the hallux, should be done. However, in most cases there is significant destruction of the joint and frequently there is significant lateral drift. Two options for treating this joint surgically are arthrodesis and double-stem silicone implant arthroplasty.

Arthrodesis

Many techniques are used to surgically arthrodese the MTP joint. It may be best to use two flat surfaces so that there is some intrinsic stability to the arthrodesis site.[27] However, all types of peg or ball and socket bony preparations can be utilized. The lateral rays will be shorter after all or part of the MTP joint has been excised; therefore, it is important to resect sufficient amounts of the metatarsal head and the base of the proximal phalanx so that the first ray will not be overly long. The final position of the hallux is also important. Although 15 to 20 degrees of valgus may be the optimum position for the hallux, there may be further lateral drift of the lateral toes with time, so one may wish to select a bit more valgus (20 to 25 degrees). About 15 degrees of dorsiflexion as measured from the floor or about 30 degrees as measured from the first metatarsal is adequate. There should be no pronation of the toe and the toenail should point directly dorsally. The hallux should not protrude more than 1 cm beyond the second toe at the end of the procedure.

Internal fixation is accomplished using a variety of techniques. Multiple 0.062-inch Kirschner wires, either threaded or plain, have been used, and 3.5-mm cortical screws placed as lag screws can be employed if the quality of bone is good and if the medial flare of the proximal phalanx can be salvaged (Fig. 14–8A to E). Two screws are essential. Usually the joint is held in the correct fusion position with a 0.062-inch Kirschner wire passed from the dorsal surface of the phalanx across the metatarsal head plantarward. Then the first screw is placed from the medial side of the base of the proximal phalanx across the joint in a proximal lateral direction. The Kirschner wire is then removed and the second screw is placed in its path (Fig. 14–8B and C). Recently, Mann[28] and Coughlin[8] reported on the use of a five- or six-hole 1/4 tubular plate fixed with 3.5-mm cortical screws dorsally to hold the bony surfaces together until arthrodesis occurs. The plate must be bent to allow the proper

angle of dorsiflexion. This method may be useful if significant amounts of bone graft are required for the arthrodesis. Unfortunately, the dorsal position of the plate allows it to act only as a neutralizing force so that internal fixation may be suboptimal. Such patients may require more rigid external support in the form of a short leg cast. All three of these methods (wires, screws, and plates) share the advantage of not crossing the interphalangeal joint. Mann and Thompson[27] utilized two heavy (9/64-inch [3.6 mm] and 1/8-inch [3.2 mm]), double-ended, threaded Steinmann pins to fix the arthrodesis site. These have the disadvantage of crossing the interphalangeal joint but do not necessarily cause further damage to the joint. The average time to radiographic fusion in their study was 97 days (range, 62 to 150 days) (Fig. 14–9A and B). None of the patients had bilateral procedures performed simultaneously, and the interval between operations in bilateral cases was 5 months.

Implant Arthroplasty of the Hallux Metatarsophalangeal Joint

Implant arthroplasty of the hallux MTP joint is possible using an implant manufactured of a high-performance silicone elastomer.[13, 35] This operation is indicated when the aim is to restore more normal forefoot alignment and maintain some hallux function. An ideal candidate for this procedure is a rheumatoid patient with a subluxated or dislocated MTP joint with adequate bone stock and overlying skin and without evidence of sepsis or vascular insufficiency. Implants should always be used as an alternative in a patient who otherwise would have an excision of the joint or an arthrodesis. They can also be most helpful for salvage in patients with an unsatisfactory result following excision of the hallux MTP joint.

Several features of this operation are noteworthy.[12] Intravenous prophylactic antibiotics should be given preoperatively and continued per os for 2 to 3 days postoperatively. The operative procedure emphasizes soft tissue balancing with release of contracted tissues, usually on the lateral side of the joint, repositioning of the sesamoids whenever possible, and careful closure of the capsule on the medial side both to the distal phalanx when it has been detached and always to the medial distal metatarsal. Capsular closure is best done by

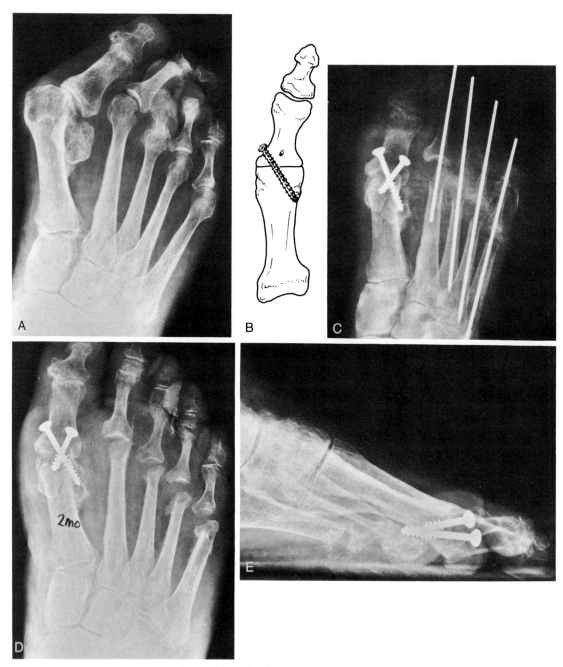

FIGURE 14–8 *See legend on opposite page*

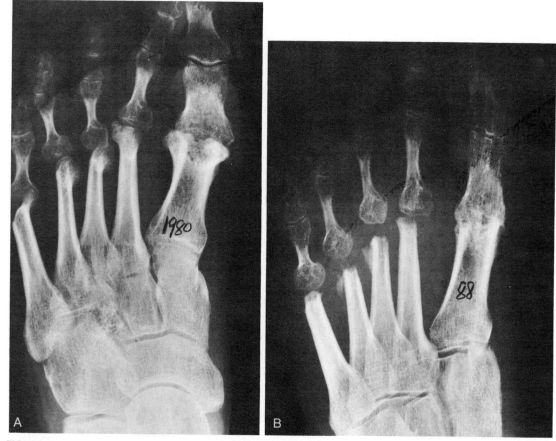

FIGURE 14–9. (A), Anteroposterior radiograph of the left foot of a 58-year-old woman with rheumatoid arthritis who had undergone previous excisional arthroplasty 8 years earlier. The lateral four toes are still satisfactorily aligned, but the patient is complaining of pain across the metatarsophalangeal joint area and more severe pain over the hallux. (B), A radiograph performed 6 years following arthrodesis of what remained of the hallux metatarsophalangeal joint and removal of a small amount of bone from each of the lateral four metatarsals. Due to poor bone quality, arthrodesis required the use of two large threaded Steinmann pins across the entire toe. The pin tracks can be seen. There is some increase in the arthritic deformity of the interphalangeal joint, but the patient had no pain and was satisfied.

FIGURE 14–8. (A), Anteroposterior weight-bearing radiograph of a patient with advanced rheumatoid deformities of the right forefoot.

(B), This technique of arthrodesis creates two planar surfaces at the base of the proximal phalanx and the metatarsal head. These surfaces are then held together by a 0.062-inch Kirschner wire placed from the dorsum of the proximal phalanx into the metatarsal head. The Kirschner wire holds the toe in the optimum position selected for arthrodesis. A screw is then placed from the medial side of the proximal phalanx across the arthrodesis site and into the metatarsal head in a medial lateral direction, engaging the opposite cortex of the metatarsal shaft. The Kirschner wire is then removed, and one can carefully test the stability of the arthrodesis using only one screw. Should this screw provide only minimum fixation, usually seen when the bone is quite osteoporotic, then it should be removed and an alternative method of internal fixation should be selected. However, if the screw and arthrodesis site are stable, then the second screw can be passed using the hole made by the Kirschner wire.

(C), The hallux arthrodesis has been secured using two screws. The Kirschner wires have been placed across the lateral four metatarsophalangeal joints. This postoperative radiograph shows optimal placement of the wire across the second ray, but the wires across the third, fourth, and fifth rays are too long. It is easy to measure the length of the wire, which needs to be carefully withdrawn to adjust a more optimum length. The excess wire should be cut and the protective cap reapplied.

(D and E), Anteroposterior and lateral radiographs obtained 2 months following this patient's forefoot reconstruction. There is satisfactory evidence of early fusion across the hallux metatarsophalangeal joint, and the lateral toes are well aligned. At this point, it is probably safe to allow the patient out of a wooden-soled shoe and into an athletic shoe of some type. Usually, due to the swelling, the patient needs shoes approximately one to one and one-half times the usual size. Later, the patient should fit into the same shoe size as before the operation; however, if severe deformities were corrected, the patient may need a shoe a half-size smaller.

suturing the capsule directly to the bone through small 1.5-mm drill holes. There is no need to excise extra bone in order to place a large implant (Fig. 14–10*A*). Usually a size 0, 1, or 2 double-stem implant will be satisfactory. Preparation of the intermedullary canals must be meticulous. I prefer to use a hand broach initially to compact the cancellous bone and then finish with a pilot burr if necessary. All rough bone edges must be eliminated and reduction with a trial implant must show optimal correction of the hallux deformity (Fig. 14–10*B*). Currently, we are utilizing titanium grommets but experience with over 7 years of follow-up indicates that given proper patient selection, fracture of these implants occurs very rarely as does silicone synovitis, particularly in rheumatoid patients (Fig. 14–10*C*). Wound closure is important and a flat silicone drain is recommended (see Fig. 14–6).

Postoperative care is one of the most important features of the operation, with dressing changes being done by the surgeon. All corrections must be obtained at the time the operation is complete, and the corrected position is simply held by the dressings. Weekly dressing changes may be needed for at least 6 weeks to hold the hallux in the corrected position. At 2 to 3 weeks, joint motion can be started, but this may vary depending on the condition of the wound and the patient.

REOPERATIONS OF THE FOREFOOT

Reoperations on the foot of an RA patient may be necessary if deformities have not been adequately corrected or recur. Several factors should be considered when a second or even a third operation is being contemplated. At times the forefoot deformity is secondary to changes occurring either in the hindfoot or the ankle and so the entire foot must be reassessed, both clinically and radiographically. The same general goals apply to revision surgeries as to primary procedures: pain relief and more comfortable shoewear. There may be an increased incidence of delayed wound healing, and the toes themselves may be at greater risk for vascular injury and even necrosis if there have been previous extensive surgical procedures. Obviously a reoperation will mean that the patient has had the disease for a longer time and is older and may be taking more potent medications. There may be specific causes for the recurrent forefoot deformities. The first operation may not have com-

FIGURE 14–10. *(A)*, Correction of the hallux deformity using a double-stemmed silicone implant is a procedure that relies mostly on soft tissue corrections and release rather than bony resection. The head of the metatarsal should be excised using a power oscillating saw. Only sufficient amounts of head need to be excised to accept the hinged portion of the implant. There should be enough of the metatarsal head remaining, especially on the plantar surface, to articulate with the sesamoid bones. Only the base of the proximal phalanx is resected, and this should be as thin as possible. If the attachments of the short toe flexors are divided, they should be resutured into the remainder of the base of the proximal phalanx. It is not necessary to use the largest possible implant, and in fact, this should be avoided since the lateral four rays will be somewhat shortened by removal of at least the head of the metatarsal. Therefore, a size 0, 1, or possibly in a large person, a No. 2 double-stemmed implant, is sufficient for this procedure.

(B), It is essential to be certain that the hallux ray has been completely corrected prior to placing the silicone implant. Thus, after soft tissue release and bony resection, a trial implant of the appropriate size should be placed across the joint. The surgeon must be satisfied that a realignment of the hallux ray has been established. If there is severe deformity of the forefoot, this part of the procedure should follow whatever has been done to correct the lateral four toes, including placement of Kirschner wires. If the forefoot deformity is not severe, then it is possible to start with the hallux ray. The trial implant should be left in place and then the lateral four joints operated on. When the latter steps have been completed, then one can return to the hallux ray, remove the trial implant, place the actual double-stemmed implant, and then close the medial capsule of the hallux. Following this, all skin incisions are sutured.

(C), Anteroposterior radiograph of a 42-year-old woman with rheumatoid arthritis 2 years following forefoot arthroplasty. Titanium grommets have been placed about the stems of a No. 1 implant. One can see a small amount of bone production at the lateral side of the base of the proximal phalanx. The implant appears to be completely secure within the intramedullary canals. This patient had such severe metatarsus primus varus that it was necessary to perform a closing wedge osteotomy at the base of the proximal phalanx. Since the bone was osteoporotic, power-driven titanium staples were adequate for fixation. It is not usually necessary to perform an osteotomy at the base of the first metatarsal. However, it is necessary to completely correct the deformity of the hallux ray just as one would do in any type of reconstructive hallux valgus deformity. If the bone quality is sufficient, a screw is preferable to secure any osteotomy at the base of the hallux metatarsal. The lateral four metatarsophalangeal joints were reconstructed using the plantar plate arthroplasty, and their alignment has been well maintained.

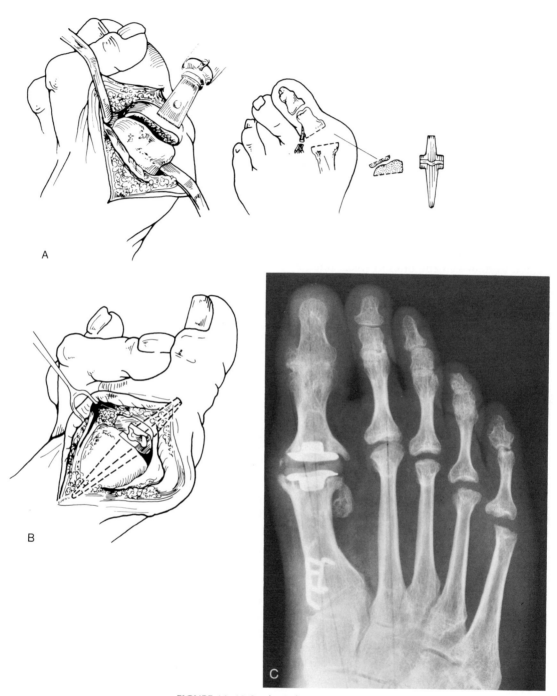

FIGURE 14–10 *See legend on opposite page*

pletely corrected the forefoot deformities. If an excisional arthroplasty was performed, insufficient bone may have been removed or regrowth of bone at the resected plantar end of the metatarsal may have occurred. Perhaps only one or two metatarsals were operated on at the first procedure and now the patient requires reconstruction of the entire forefoot. It is not possible to correct recurrent lateral drift of all four toes by operating on only one or two. If this is the case, it will usually be necessary to revise the excisional arthroplasty of the joints that were previously excised so that all the toes can be realigned. Syndactylization may be useful in such cases. Hammer toes that were not previously corrected or have developed since previous operations usually need surgical correction as well. At times, the hallux interphalangeal joint becomes arthritic or malaligned, usually in valgus. This may be treated by débridement and soft tissue release, holding the corrected position with a Kirschner wire for several weeks. However, if the joint is painful and destroyed, then arthrodesis should be performed. If the hallux metatarsophalangeal joint has already been fused, it may be difficult to obtain a good result with fusion of both joints of the hallux.

Failure of operations to the hallux metatarsophalangeal joint have several causes. A previous Keller or Mayo excision of the joint may have led to an unstable and frequently malaligned toe. If sufficient bone exists, a double-stem silicone implant might be considered if the soft tissues are viable. Otherwise, an arthrodesis with or without a bone graft should be considered. Internal fixation may be a technical problem if there is insufficient bone. It is usually difficult to use screws, particularly if a significant portion of the base of the proximal phalanx has been removed. Other options include multiple Kirschner wire fixation, large threaded Steinmann pins, or if there is enough bone on the proximal phalanx to accept at least two screws, stabilization with a 1/3 tubular plate. Usually it is not necessary to lengthen the hallux ray, particularly if the lateral metatarsal heads or joints have been excised. However, a bone graft may be required to gain a solid arthrodesis.

A second reason for failed hallux surgery is failure of arthrodesis. The nonunion may be painful or the hallux malaligned. It is important to determine the causative factors, which may include medications, poor bone quality,

and poor surgical technique. A second complication of arthrodesis is a malalignment of the fusion angle and this usually occurs when a toe is fused with insufficient dorsiflexion. A dorsal wedge osteotomy can be performed, which requires some type of internal fixation. The arthrodesis may have left the hallux ray overly long. This is corrected by resecting sufficient bone from the fusion site, thus shortening the ray and refusing the hallux.

The third type of problem is a failed double-stem implant. Patients with rheumatoid arthritis usually do not show evidence of silicone synovitis, as they are usually not active enough to fragment the implant. However, implants can fail if they have been placed incorrectly, if there is recurrent lateral drift of the hallux, or if the implant becomes infected. In revising a failed implant, one has three choices. If the alignment of the toe is basically satisfactory, one can simply remove the implant through a limited dorsal incision and leave all of the surrounding collagen tissue intact. However, if the implant has become septic, all infected soft tissue must be thoroughly débrided, even if the alignment is satisfactory. The toe should be stabilized with soft dressings and the infection treated. The amount of time intravenous antibiotics are given depends on the circumstances of the individual infection. For example, an acute infection that seems to involve only the soft tissues may require only 7 to 10 days of intravenous antibiotics, followed by oral antibiotics until the wound is healed, usually within 2 to 3 weeks. Osteomyelitis is rare, so prolonged intravenous antibiotics are usually unnecessary. If the patient has further difficulties with the hallux, then an arthrodesis can be considered, but this is probably best done at a later date after the infection has been eradicated. If the implant has fractured and the joint becomes painful, it can be replaced with a new implant. This should be done only if the patient has had a good long-term result with the implant. If a crack is seen on radiography but the patient is asymptomatic and there is no evidence of silicone synovitis, the implant should not be removed. However, if the silicone implant has failed, it can be removed and an arthrodesis attempted. This is a bit more difficult because the intramedullary bone is gone, making the arthrodesis technically more demanding. We prefer to use a block of bone from the iliac crest shaped to fit in both intramedullary canals. Alternatively, both canals can be packed with cancellous bone. Internal fixation usually consists of either a 1/3 tubular plate placed dorsally as a neutralizing plate or multiple 0.062-inch Kirschner wires.

Forefoot reconstructive operations can provide the rheumatoid patient with relief of pain and improved ambulation and shoewear. Proper patient selection and preparation are important. However, it must always be kept in mind that rheumatoid patients have a chronic disease and that deformities may be progressive, making proper patient assessment and follow-up essential.

References

1. Arnett FC, Edworthy SM, Block DA, et al: The American Rheumatism Association 1987 revised criteria for the classification of rheumatoid arthritis. Arthritis Rheum 31:315–324, 1988.
2. Auerbach MS, Shephard E, Vernon-Roberts B: Morton's metatarsalgia due to intermetatarso-phalangeal bursitis as an early manifestation of rheumatoid arthritis. Clin Orthop 167:214, 1982.
3. Barton NJ: Arthroplasty of the forefoot in rheumatoid arthritis. J Bone Joint Surg 55B:126–133, 1973.
4. Betts RP, Stockley I, Getty CJM, et al: Foot pressure studies in the assessment of forefoot arthroplasty in the rheumatoid foot. Foot Ankle 8:315–326, 1988.
5. Bluestone R: Collagen diseases affecting the foot. Foot Ankle 2:311–317, 1982.
6. Clayton ML: Evolution of surgery of the forefoot in rheumatoid arthritis. J Bone Joint Surg 64B:640, 1982.
7. Clayton ML: Personal communication.
8. Coughlin MJ: First metatarsophalangeal joint arthrodesis using cup shaped power reamers and small fragment plate fixation. Presented at 20th Annual Meeting, American Foot and Ankle Society, New Orleans, LA, February 20, 1990.
9. Cracchiolo A: The use of shoes to treat foot disorders. Orthop Rev 8:73–83, 1979.
10. Cracchiolo A: Pearson S, Kitaoka H, Grace D: Hindfoot arthrodesis in adults utilizing a dowel graft technique. Clin Orthop 257:193–203, 1990.
11. Cracchiolo A: Arthritic diseases of the foot and ankle. Foot Ankle 2:309–341, 3:2–44, 1982.
12. Cracchiolo A: Rheumatoid arthritis of the foot and ankle. *In* Gould J (Ed): The Foot Book. Baltimore, Williams & Wilkins, 1988, pp 239–267.
13. Cracchiolo A, Swanson A, Swanson GD: The arthritic great toe metatarsophalangeal joint: A review of flexible silicone implant arthroplasty from two medical centers. Clin Orthop 157:64–69, 1981.
14. Cracchiolo A: Surgery for rheumatoid disease. Instruct Course Lect 33:386–404, 1984.
15. Daly PJ, Johnson KA: Treatment of painful subluxation and dislocation at the second and third metatarsophalangeal joints by proximal phalanx excision and subtalar webbing. Clin Orthop, in press.
16. Dedrick DK, McCune WS, Smith WS: Rheumatoid arthritis presenting as spreading of the toes. J Bone Joint Surg 72A:463–464, 1990.
17. Downey DT, Simkin PA, Marc LA, et al: Tibialis posterior tendon rupture: A cause of rheumatoid flat feet. Arthritis Rheum 31:441–446, 1988.
18. Elbaor JE, Thomas WK, Weinfeld MS, et al: Talonavicular arthrodesis for rheumatoid arthritis of the hindfoot. Orthop Clin North Am 7:827–836, 1976.
19. Fowler AW: The method of forefoot reconstruction. J Bone Joint Surg 41B:507–513, 1959.
20. Gainor BJ, Epstein RG, Henstorf JE, et al: Metatarsal head resection for rheumatoid deformities of the forefoot. Clin Orthop 230:207–213, 1988.
21. Gold RH, Bassett LW: Radiologic evaluation of the arthritic foot. Foot Ankle 2:332–341, 1982.
22. Guerra J, Resnick D: Arthritides affecting the foot: Radiographic-pathologic correlation. Foot Ankle 2:325–331, 1982.
23. Hasselo LG, Wilkens RF, Toomey HE, et al: Forefoot surgery in rheumatoid arthritis: Subjective assessment of outcomes. Foot Ankle 8:148–151, 1987.
24. Kates A, Kessel L, Kay A: Arthroplasty of the forefoot. J Bone Joint Surg 49B:552–557, 1967.
25. Kelikian H: Hallux Valgus, Allied Deformities of the Forefoot, and Metatarsalgia. Philadelphia, WB Saunders, 1965.
26. King HA, Watkins TB, Samuelson KM: Analysis of foot position in ankle arthrodesis and its influence in gait. Foot Ankle 1:44–49, 1980.
27. Mann RA, Thompson FM: Arthrodesis of the first metatarsophalangeal joint for hallux valgus in rheumatoid arthritis. J Bone Joint Surg 66A:687–692, 1984.
28. Mann RA: Hallux rigidus. Instruct Course Lect 39:15–21, 1990.
29. McDermott M, McDevitt HO: Immunogenetics of rheumatic diseases. Bull Rheum Dis 38:1–10, 1988.
30. McGarvey SR, Johnson KA: Keller arthroplasty in combination with resection arthroplasty of the lesser metatarsophalangeal joints in rheumatoid arthritis. Foot Ankle 9:75–80, 1988.
31. Morgan CD, Henke JA, Bailey RW, et al: Long term results of tibiotalar arthrodesis. J Bone Joint Surg 67A:546–550, 1985.
32. Shepard E: Intermetatarsophalangeal bursitis in the causation of Morton's metatarsalgia. *In* Proceedings of the British Orthopaedic Association. J Bone Joint Surg 57B:115–116, 1975.
33. Spiegel TM, Spiegel JS: Rheumatoid arthritis in the foot and ankle—diagnosis, pathology, and treatment. Foot Ankle 2:318–324, 1982.
34. Stockley I, Betts RP, Eng C, et al: A prospective study of forefoot arthroplasty. Clin Orthop 248:213–218, 1989.
35. Swanson AB, Swanson GD, et al: Flexible (silicone) implant arthroplasty in the small joints of the extremities: Concepts, physical and biological considerations, experimental and clinical results. *In* Rubin LR (Ed): Biomaterials and Reconstructive Surgery. St. Louis, CV Mosby, 1983, pp 595–623.

Editor
ROBERT S. ADELAAR

15 Degenerative Problems of the Midtarsal Joints

SAUL G. TREVINO
NORMAN LICHT

Degenerative processes of the midtarsal joints are common. The factors that influence their course are not well described in the medical literature. The midtarsal region is a broad anatomic area between the Lisfranc articulations and the transverse tarsal joints, which includes the talonavicular and the calcaneocuboid joints.

The specific stresses in these areas are complex.[3, 8–10] One can classify midfoot degenerative conditions into four broad categories (Table 15–1). The first category is aging in the midtarsal joints or premature aging that is due to abnormal biomechanical overloads. The sec-

ond category is degeneration of the posterior tibial tendon, which influences and accelerates early arthritic changes. Patients are frequently predisposed to this condition by the "innocuous" flatfoot. Post-traumatic arthritis, the third category, is most commonly caused by injuries to the Lisfranc joints. The fourth category is neuropathic arthritis, of which diabetes is the prototype. Clues to the degenerative processes can be gathered by observing the pattern of breakdown in cases of progressive flatfoot and neuropathic collapse of the midfoot.

ANATOMIC FEATURES

The midtarsal region consists of the three cuneiforms and the cuboid and navicular bones. Distally, except for the navicular, these bones articulate with the five metatarsals. Proximally, the unit articulates with the talus and calcaneus. The cuneiforms, along with the cuboid, form a transverse arcade or arch, which functions as a roof for the plantar neurovascular and tendinous structures.

Within this unit of bones, there is a great deal of stability lent by the intertarsal ligaments. In regard to stability, the most significant ligaments bridge between the first ray and the middle cuneiform. The first ray can be defined as the first metatarsal and the medial cuneiform. The three sets of interosseous ligaments correspond to the first, second, and third cuneiform–metatarsal spaces. The first cuneiform–metatarsal space is occupied by the

---

TABLE 15–1. CLASSIFICATION OF MIDFOOT DEGENERATIVE CONDITIONS

Degenerative
  Early
    Hypermobility stress syndromes
    Dorsal spurs
  Late
    Diastasis of the first metatarsal–cuneiform joint
    Isolated tarsometatarsal arthritis
    Panmidtarsal arthritis

Posterior tibial insufficiency syndrome

Post-traumatic arthritis
  Lisfranc's region
  Midtarsal region
  Transverse tarsal region

Neuropathic arthritis

163

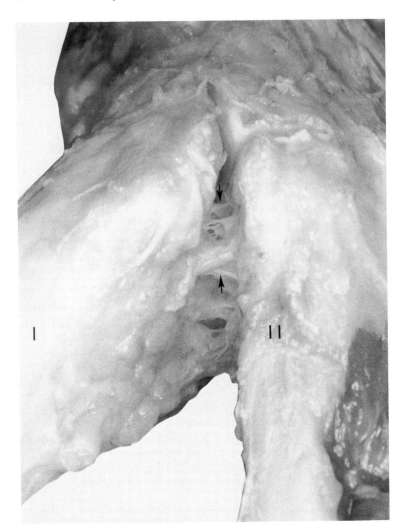

FIGURE 15–1. Frontal view of the Lisfranc and the accessory ligament. The foot is viewed from distal to proximal; the Lisfranc ligament *(bracketed by arrows)* is dorsal to the accessory ligament. This figure demonstrates the size and location of these ligaments between the first and second metatarsals.

FIGURE 15–2. Lateral aspect of the first metatarsal and medial cuneiform bone. The origins of the Lisfranc ligament *(A)*, first intercuneiform ligament *(B)*, and accessory ligament *(C)* are not shown. The insertion of the peroneus longus tendon *(D)* expands the first metatarsal–first cuneiform joint. The articulating facets of the first cuneiform bone are dorsal to the origins of these ligaments. The facets are small, and the majority of the lateral aspect of the first cuneiform bone is nonarticular. Fixation is placed through this nonarticular area.

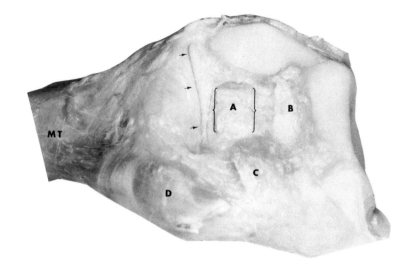

medial interosseous ligament, or the Lisfranc ligament (Fig. 15–1). It arises from the lateral plantar surface of the first cuneiform and inserts onto the lower half of the medial plantar surface of the second metatarsal. Two other ligaments contribute to the stability of the first ray: the accessory medial interosseous ligament and the plantar intercuneiform ligament (Fig. 15–2). The Lisfranc ligament is the strongest of the three. In contrast, the lateral rays are stabilized by the recessed position of the second metatarsal with the three cuneiforms and by multiple intermetatarsal ligaments.[12] Thus, the ligaments of the first ray are far more vulnerable to repeated stresses of ordinary ambulation than are those of the lateral tarsometatarsal joints.

FUNCTIONAL ANALYSIS OF MIDTARSAL JOINTS

From gait analysis, the critical function of the foot is to convert from a flexible phase at heel strike to a rigid lever arm at toe-off. At toe-off, the foot develops a supinated posture, locking the transverse tarsal joint, which accomplishes the conversion from a flexible to a rigid structure.

Two basic degenerative patterns are observed. One is the simple aging of multiple related joints, with gradual evidence of breakdown in the midtarsal joints. The most common location of degenerative overload is the first metatarsal–cuneiform joint, caused by compressive loads about twice as great as those on the lateral tarsometatarsal joints.[9] Repetitive stress causes the gradual evolution of degenerative joint disease. A common manifestation of this process is the dorsal spur.

The second pattern is accelerated by altered gait biomechanics: that is, when the foot fails to convert from the flexible to the fixed or rigid position at toe-off. A patient at risk is simply one who does not reconstitute the longitudinal arch at toe-off. Clinically, this is seen most commonly in patients with hypermobility, in those with the incompetent posterior tibialis tendon syndrome, or, most dramatically, in those with an acute neuropathic joint. This repetitive overload initially presents as midtarsal pain. With time, these subacute overloads result in ligamentous laxity at the medial intercuneiform joint or the first metatarsal–cuneiform joint.

TABLE 15–2. STAGES OF PROGRESSIVE MIDFOOT BREAKDOWN
1. Increased stress of the Lisfranc ligament with gradual laxity
2. Diastasis of the intercuneiform region
3. Progressive dorsal excursion of the first ray–medial cuneiform segment
4. Fixed deformities of forefoot varus and collapse of the longitudinal arch at the navicular-cuneiform joint

The progression of this laxity can be divided into four stages (Table 15–2). Hypermobility of the first ray represents the first stage of the second pattern. Although this condition can be hereditary, other factors may accelerate it (e.g., inflammatory arthritis, trauma, or a neuropathic process).

The second stage of midfoot breakdown is diastasis. With stress, a gradual stretching of the primary stabilizers of the first ray occurs, with the radiographic presentation of increased space between the base of the first ray and the base of the second metatarsal. An associated radiographic change is rounding off of the flat first metatarsal–cuneiform joint. This observation can be explained by the pronation movement that occurs through the first metatarsal–cuneiform region. There is not only dorsal displacement of the first ray but also eversion along the longitudinal axis of the first metatarsal. The rotation of the first ray results in a rounded appearance of the base of the first metatarsal. Anatomically, this can be demonstrated by division of the Lisfranc ligament and the associated plantar intercuneiform ligament (Fig. 15–3).

The third stage is an exaggeration of the hypermobility but without contracture. With time, this hypermobility leads to a dorsiflexed first ray and an abducted forefoot. Proximally, the first ray displacement occurs at the navicular-cuneiform joint with the associated breakdown of the longitudinal arch. Lateral rays are subluxed at the transverse tarsal joints, with subluxation at the calcaneocuboid joint. Lateral radiographs demonstrate the loss of the normal cascade of the metatarsals (Fig. 15–4). There is a relative elevation of the fifth metatarsal relative to the cuboid. On radiographs, flattening of the longitudinal arch is noted, as

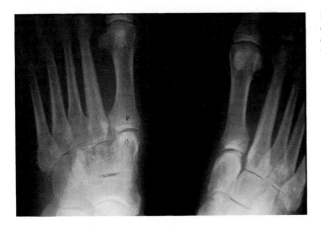

FIGURE 15–3. Diastasis (widening) between the base of the first and second metatarsals. Note the rounding off of the articular surface of the first metatarsal due to the pronation of the first ray.

is shifting of the relationship of the medial cuneiform to the base of the fifth metatarsal. The fifth metatarsal is now either at the same level as or plantar to the shaft.[4]

The fourth and final stage is a rigid flatfoot with contractures of forefoot abduction and varus. The contractures can be demonstrated by placing the hindfoot in the neutral position, which reveals the fixed varus position of the forefoot (Fig. 15–5). With progression of the arthritis, a plantar prominence occurs that is painful to direct stress. These findings will be compounded by any breakdown that may also be occurring in the hindfoot. The combination of hindfoot and forefoot decompensation leads to a rocker-bottom foot.

Neuropathic joints exhibit a similar sequence but can result in a more severe pattern of breakdown, resulting not only in deformities but also in multiple fractures.[2] The process can abruptly accelerate from a "foot at risk" into complete collapse in less than a week (Fig. 15–6).

Understanding these patterns and stages, one may approach midfoot arthritis with a logical strategy. The classification helps to place the individual in a temporal spectrum of disease. The urgency and aggressiveness of treatment depend on the presence of neuropathic or posterior tibial insufficiency. Surgery is reserved for those with persistent pain or structural problems not amenable to conservative treatment.

DIAGNOSIS AND WORK-UP

History

In an adult, the first symptom is aching over the midtarsal region. Pain can be present in the absence of a spur. The presentation of the symptoms is usually of an arthritic nature. Pain is usually present in the morning and improves initially with activity but is usually worse at the end of the day. Pain is aggravated by

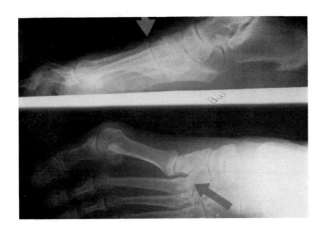

FIGURE 15–4. *(Top),* Loss of the normal cascade pattern between the first and fifth metatarsals *(arrow).* There is a dorsal shift on the base of the fifth metatarsal relative to the medial cuneiform. *(Bottom),* Destructive changes at the base of the second metatarsotarsal joint as well as widening between the medial cuneiform and the base of the second metatarsal.

walking up stairs or by any forceful plantar-flexed movement. It is important to have the patient point out the precise location of the pain, because not all prominences are symptomatic. A possible association with pain is the complaint of swelling and local heat. These symptoms are usually minor; however, in a neuropathic process, they may indicate the onset of severe breakdown of the forefoot, with swelling and heat over the affected area being disproportionate relative to the patient's pain.

One commonly sees dorsal spurs in adults with midfoot arthritis. The most common locations are over the first or second metatarsal–cuneiform regions. The patient will complain of pain with shoes that is due to increased pressure on the dorsum of the foot. Associated with the prominence is occasional numbness in the distribution of the deep peroneal nerve.[13] When the condition is in an advanced stage, patients will complain of a plantar prominence under the first metatarsal, which represents the overgrowth of the arthritic joint. Secondary skin changes are frequently present, with callosities and associated inflammatory bursas. In an insensitive foot, these prominences frequently lead to skin breakdown and infection.

In contrast, dorsal spurs can occur in young individuals without arthritis. This finding is similar to dorsal bossing in the hand and does not represent a degenerative process. This condition usually presents as a problem with shoe fit. Other conditions that should be considered are prior tarsometatarsal injuries and inflammatory diseases. Prior injuries fre-

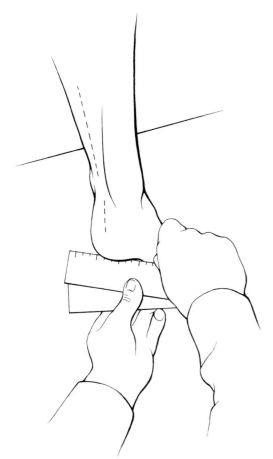

FIGURE 15–5. A fixed forefoot varus deformity is demonstrated by holding the hindfoot in neutral and dorsiflexing the foot by pressure on the distal fifth metatarsal without inverting or everting the heel. The angles obtained by the goniometer represent the degrees of forefoot varus. Dotted lines represent the longitudinal axis of the lower leg relative to the heel axis.

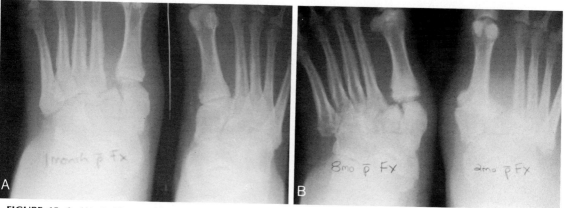

FIGURE 15–6. (A), A 45-year-old patient with diabetic neuropathy is treated for a neuropathic Lisfranc joint. (B), Six months into the treatment, the patient presents with an acute fracture-dislocation of the opposite foot.

quently result in diffuse bony prominences in this area, as well as an abducted forefoot.

Physical Examination

A comprehensive biomechanical examination of the foot is essential. Fixed rotational deformities often go unrecognized if they are not specifically searched for. Before surgery is considered, determine the mobility and the alignment between the hindfoot and forefoot. Place the hindfoot in the neutral position by moving the forefoot until the talonavicular joint is felt to be aligned medially. While the hindfoot is kept in neutral, determine the degree of forefoot abduction or adduction and inversion or eversion by passively moving the forefoot. Total mobility should be assessed (see Fig. 15–5). A fusion that does not address and correct rotational deformity will lead to a predictable poor result. Beware of combined forefoot and hindfoot deformities, which require intense evaluation in regard to alignment. Individuals with adjacent loose joints will be better able to compensate for any stiffening procedure.

Determine which joints are symptomatic. The precise location may be difficult to determine because of patients' inability to localize their pain and because of the close proximity of the joints. Aids in preoperative evaluation include selective stress testing of different joints and injection of anesthetic into individual joints.

Radiology

Radiographic work-up should include weight-bearing anteroposterior and lateral views of the feet. Oblique views especially help in locating the specific site of any degenerative process. By thorough examination of the radiographs, causes of dorsiflexion of the first ray can be identified. A predisposition to increased stress in the midfoot is caused by a dorsiflexed first ray, which can be secondary to metatarsus primus varus, first ray elevation due to technically flawed metatarsal osteotomies for splayfoot, or subluxation of the first metatarsal–cuneiform joint (Fig. 15–7). The last is not an uncommon finding in the elderly, but weight-bearing radiographs are needed for diagnosis. Common degenerative patterns occur in the distal midtarsal articulations. The most common are first metatarsal to medial cuneiform, second metatarsal to middle cuneiform, and third metatarsal to lateral cuneiform. Anteroposterior and lateral tomograms aid in assessing the degree of the arthritic process (Fig. 15–8). In difficult cases, bone scans help to localize more active areas or occult disease.

Computed tomography can assist in evaluating the more proximal hindfoot joints, which may be jeopardized by an arthrodesis. This can assist in preoperative planning and in predicting outcome. A mixed result may develop from an arthrodesis because of increased stress placed on already compromised adjacent joints.

TREATMENT

To treat the patient effectively, one should diagnose the cause of the arthritis, the stage of the arthritis, and the precise location of symptoms. Patients with post-traumatic or degenerative arthritis frequently respond well to conservative modalities. Posterior tibial insuf-

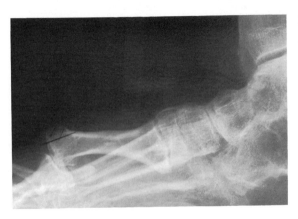

FIGURE 15–7. Severe arthritis of the first metatarsal–cuneiform and calcaneocuboid joint with marked dorsiflexion.

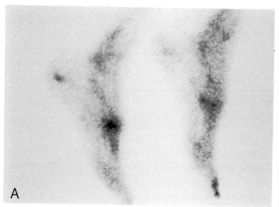 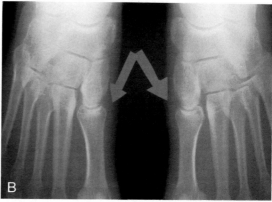

FIGURE 15–8. (A), A positive bone scan localizing the degenerative process in a patient who presented with midfoot pain. (B), The arrow represents the level at which slight diastasis between the first and second metatarsals occurs in this patient.

ficiency syndrome presents frequently with both hindfoot and forefoot deformities; thus, it is a difficult management problem. Neuropathic joints have the greatest risk from surgery because the outcome is unpredictable owing to the progressive nature of the disease. Although the initial surgery may be technically successful, the long-term prognosis is guarded because of overload to adjacent joints, ulceration related to decreased flexibility, and patients' loss of sensation.

In the majority of cases, conservative modalities should be the initial form of treatment. Patients who do not respond, however, will need surgical treatment.

Nonoperative Treatment

The basis of nonoperative treatment is to decrease stress to the midfoot and to accommodate any bony prominence with appropriate footwear.

The goal of shoe modifications is to decrease the stress at toe-off. With the use of a full-length flexible steel shank, this can be accomplished. Further, stress reduction can be accomplished with rockering of the sole. Thus, the ideal shoe prescription should include any or all of the following features: accommodative insole, flexible steel shank, and rocker sole with shock-absorbing crepe. Medial forefoot buildup (posting) of the orthosis can compensate for varying degrees of first ray elevation. The insole should be constructed to accommodate deformities and be of a soft enough material to cushion any bony prominence. The tongue of the shoe may be padded with appropriate material, if needed, to relieve bony

prominences as well as local nerve irritation. In diabetic patients who are not operative candidates, total contact casting should be used to treat any acute problems. Later, they should be prescribed an ankle-foot orthosis to contain the arthropathy, along with the comprehensive shoe prescription. For obese patients, a patellar tendon–bearing ankle-foot orthosis should be a consideration.

Anti-inflammatory drugs can also be prescribed. Local steroid injections may be useful as a temporizing treatment. These measures should be used before operative therapy is considered.

Surgical Procedures

Surgical procedures of the midfoot can be divided into three categories: exostectomies, arthroplasties, and arthrodeses. In general, the majority of the procedures performed are arthrodeses. In a few selected incidences, arthroplasties can be considered.

Exostectomies

The usual indication for surgical excision of dorsal spurs is the presence of a painful prominence with the failure of nonoperative treatment with modified shoes. Most dorsal spurs are restricted to the first and second metatarsal–cuneiform joints. The main technical problems are inadequate débridement, inadequate postoperative immobilization, iatrogenic neuromas, and residual arthritis. Some instability results from this intervention; thus, adequate immobilization is needed. A generous amount of bone should be resected because of frequent postoperative overgrowth.

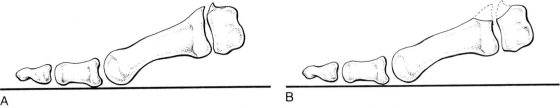

FIGURE 15–9. *(A and B),* Moderate resection for dorsal spurs.

Technique

Use the anteromedial approach to the midfoot. Curve the incision away from the apex to avoid pressure-sensitive scars with shoewear. Identify any branches of the superficial peroneal nerve, as well as the deep peroneal nerve. The circumference of the spur should be outlined by sharp dissection. Use a small curved osteotome to remove the prominence and create a gentle concavity (Fig. 15–9). A small amount of bone wax is used to minimize postoperative bleeding.

A variation of this approach is used when plantar or medial spurs are present. These are commonly at the base of the first metatarsal–cuneiform joint or the fifth metatarsal–cuboid joint. The incision should ideally avoid any weight-bearing area. Again, generous amounts of bone should be removed in the routine fashion.

Rehabilitation

Plan for 6 weeks of immobilization. In younger individuals, use a removable cast brace or a stiff postoperative shoe. In contrast, older individuals will probably have less morbidity with a short-leg walking cast to stabilize their degenerative joint disease. Minimize postoperative swelling with elastic wraps, contrast baths, and elevation. Later, consider using accommodative insoles to minimize further midfoot stress.

Arthroplasty

There is limited use of formal arthroplasty in the midfoot, with two exceptions: isolated traumatic arthritis of the calcaneocuboid joint or of the talonavicular joint. Isolated fusion is possible; however, to maintain subtalar motion, a limited resection arthroplasty of the talonavicular joint can be performed. A cheilectomy of the talonavicular joint can be performed that is quite similar to that performed for hallux rigidus. However, the arthroplasty and rehabilitation of the calcaneocuboid joint are more complex. Surgery is indicated for limited traumatic arthritis of this joint. The ideal candidate has less than 50% involvement of the joint and has no abduction deformity of the forefoot (Fig. 15–10). By resection of this joint, shortening of the lateral column of the foot will occur and will predispose to more abduction.

Technique

Use the extended Ollier incision to expose the calcaneocuboid joint. Care is taken to

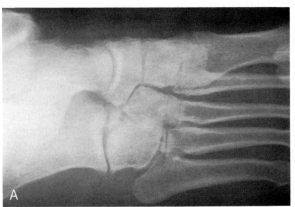
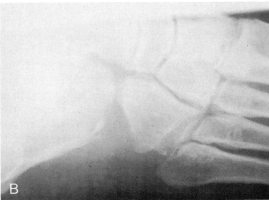

FIGURE 15–10. *(A),* The arthritic process in the calcaneocuboid joint. *(B),* One year after resection of the calcaneocuboid joint.

preserve the extensor digitorum brevis muscle by sharp subperiosteal dissection over the joint. Incise the capsule in the direction of the joint. The cuboid is saddle shaped, with the bifurcate ligament originating from the medial aspect. Be sure to free the joint well to allow complete access. A resection is carried out on both sides of the joint so that the degenerative cartilage is removed. If less than one-fourth of the joint is involved, that portion can be excised. A thin layer of bone wax is then applied to the raw surfaces to inhibit bony overgrowth. With the resection arthroplasty technique, the digitorum brevis muscle is used as an interpositional material. Divide the undersurface of the muscle sharply to leave the dorsal aspect for closure. The proximal ends of the muscle are sutured with a 2–0 absorbable suture. They are brought under the talonavicular joint to the medial side of the foot with Keith's needles. The sutures are tied through a small stab wound so that external buttons are not necessary. After closure, the foot is kept in a plantarflexed and inverted position and is immobilized in a short-leg splint.

Rehabilitation

The goal of this procedure is to maximize motion. Postoperatively, the foot is placed in a splint for 7 to 10 days. Once the initial pain has subsided, the patient is instructed on exercises for range of motion, elevation, and tissue massage. Weight bearing is not started until 4 to 6 weeks postoperatively. A comprehensive physical therapy program is started at the end of the sixth week to encourage subtalar motion and to decrease the equinus deformity that may be present. There are no late follow-up clinical series for this procedure. If symptoms persist postoperatively, the salvage procedure is a limited outside fusion of the calcaneocuboid joint.

Midfoot Fusions

General Considerations

Fusion of the midtarsal region can be approached by three methods: the dowel technique, the inlay bone graft technique, and the resurfacing technique. In cases in which primarily two joints without significant deformities are involved, either the dowel technique or the resurfacing procedure is of value. Inlay grafts are suggested in areas in which extensive

dissection is needed. The advantages and disadvantages of these techniques are discussed in the following sections.

Dowel Technique

After adequate exposure, use a bone biopsy set or trephine to core out the affected joints. Establish the proper location (if in doubt, use intraoperative radiographs with pin localization) and then place the sleeve of the trephine in the proper plane and angle. Use the cutting trephine in as many areas as needed, each time checking the graft to ensure that the chosen articulated surfaces have been removed. A trephine of around 7.5 mm in diameter is of adequate size. In a similar fashion, the bone graft is obtained from the anterior iliac crest. With surgical experience, the graft may be taken with one or multiple stab incisions. The thickest portion of the anterior iliac crest is approximately 1 inch proximal to the superior iliac spine. Direct the trephine toward the midline and slightly inferior to the crest. Soft tissue should be removed from the plug before it is inserted into the recipient area. Postoperative stabilization of the midfoot is performed with pins or screws as needed.

The advantages of the dowel technique are limited dissection, less postoperative pain, and reduced operative time. Johnson and Johnson were able to obtain excellent or good results in nine of 13 patients.[5]

The disadvantages are the need for special biopsy equipment, the potential for poor fit of the graft with delayed union, and the danger of intra-abdominal injury from biopsy equipment. The dowel technique is not feasible when a significant reduction of the displaced joints is needed because of the instability of the mobilized joints.[11]

Inlay Technique

The use of a trough to span more diffuse patterns can be a helpful technique. A trough allows for extensive débridement of the multiple affected joints and is a solution to the limited exposure of tight joints. Using either a power sagittal saw or osteotome, the surgeon develops a trough over the required areas. Smaller joints can be fused by the resurfacing arthrodesis technique to complement the inlay grafts in the larger joints. Split bicortical grafts are used. This places cancellous bone adjacent to the fusion site, and the cortical portion provides inherent stability. This technique is useful in cases of diffuse involvement of the intertarsal midfoot region.[6] The precise carpentry, extensive exposure, need for large bone grafts, and difficulty in correcting deformities limit this technique.

Resurfacing Technique

The resurfacing technique employs the removal of all involved articulating surfaces down to bleeding subchondral bone, as well as any scar or fibrous debris. Potential gaps are minimized by being filled with cancellous grafts. Use a sequential approach to gain access to all affected joints. Divide the capsule and ligaments in line with the joints to allow dorsal exposure. Remove the remaining joint surfaces with curettes and thin osteotomes. Use a small lamina spreader to access the joint, then drill multiple holes to weaken the surface. Beware of angulation of the drill bit deep in the bony tissues, which could result in breakage. Further denude the joint with a burr or cross-hatching cuts with an osteotome. The ultimate goal is to create a broad surface of bleeding subchondral bone with minimal bone resection. The alignment can be changed by the placement of a graft or by direct manipulation of the loosened joints. In difficult cases, an external fixator can be used to regain alignment. Accomplish fixation with cortical screws using a lag technique; 3.5- or 4-mm screws are preferable. Partially threaded cancellous screws are more susceptible to breakage and are difficult to remove at a later date. An alternate fixation is accomplished with large Steinmann pins.

Authors' Preferred Treatment

From past experience with triple arthrodesis and Lapidus' bunionectomies, we became disenchanted with any method that required shortening of the foot or difficult biplane cuts. The resurfacing technique gives the most flexibility with the least morbidity. Using an extensile approach to the anteromedial aspect of the midfoot has been helpful for orientation, avoidance of skin necrosis, and prevention of neuromas (Fig. 15–11).

The patient is positioned so that the ipsilateral hip is elevated to facilitate the obtaining of bone graft, as well as to place the foot in a neutral and plantigrade position. Because of the close proximity of the intertarsal and metatarsal joints, the plantigrade position facilitates the establishment of proper screw placement by fluoroscopic control.

After proper positioning, the leg is exsanguinated with an Esmarch bandage. A curvilinear incision is started over the midportion of the navicular and extended over the medial aspect of the third metatarsal base and to the distal one-third of the first metatarsal (see Fig. 15–11A). This provides an extensile approach to the middle two-thirds of the midtarsal area. The path of the incision avoids the apex of the foot, thus minimizing sensitive scars. It also avoids multiple small incisions, which lead to inadequate exposure and skin necrosis.

With the use of 2.5-power magnification and the extensile incision, the multiple fine extensions of the medial branch of the superficial peroneal nerve can be easily identified. Divide the fascia lateral to the extensor hallucis longus tendon and retract the tendon medially. The dorsalis pedis artery and deep peroneal nerve are located just inferior to the musculotendinous junction of the extensor hallucis longus tendon. By subperiosteal dissection, the neurovascular structures can be mobilized laterally (see Fig. 15–11B). Be careful of the first proximal perforating artery. Capsulotomies are then made to expose the bases of the first and second metatarsals, as well as the interval between the medial and lateral cuneiforms. If necessary, the exposure can be extended to include joints up to the talus.

The lateral portions of the second and third metatarsals are approached via a deep fascial incision lateral to the dorsalis pedis artery (see Fig. 15–11C). Again, a subperiosteal dissection is carried out to expose the affected joints. For lateral exposure, a straight longitudinal incision is made between the fourth and fifth metatarsals.

After a meticulous débridement of cartilage, scar tissue, and bone, bleeding subchondral bone is seen. Excessive bone removal should be avoided. A common mistake is to débride only the superior surface of the first metatarsal–cuneiform joint. A small lamina spreader is useful to see the inferior surface and to allow adequate débridement. This instrument can be used for the exposure of the intercuneiform region as well.

The most common patterns of midfoot breakdown and possible surgical constructs are summarized in Table 15–3. The first pattern is incompetence or arthritis of the first metatarsal–cuneiform joint. After thorough prepara-

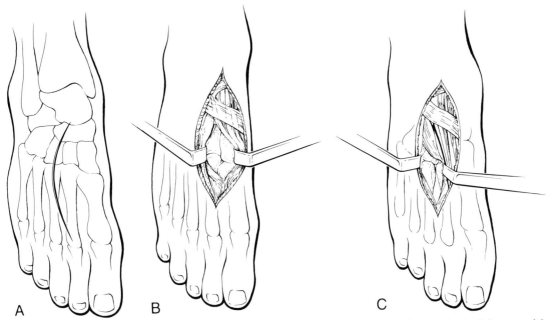

FIGURE 15–11. *(A),* A curvilinear incision is made from the lateral one-third of the navicular over the medial aspect of the base of the third metatarsal to the neck of the second metatarsal. The superficial branches of the medial branch of the superficial peroneal nerve are encountered in this region. From this exposure, the bases of the first, second, and third metatarsals, as well as the intercuneiform articulations, can be débrided and internally fixed. *(B),* The medial aspect of the midfoot can be approached by retracting the superficial branches of the superficial peroneal nerve and dividing the fascia overlying the extensor hallucis longus tendon. First, identify and divide transversely the capsule of the first metatarsal–cuneiform joint as well as the medial and middle cuneiforms. Then, by subperiosteal dissection, the base of the second metatarsal can be exposed. *(C),* Frequently the lateral exposure is needed to expose the bases of the second and third metatarsals. The neurovascular bundle is not mobilized, but the interval between the extensor hallucis brevis and the extensor digitorum longus is used to expose these bones. Fixation of the bases with lag techniques is then quite easy.

tion of the joint, a 3.5-mm lagged cortical screw is placed across the first metatarsal–cuneiform joint. A stabilization screw is placed across the bases of the first and second metatarsals. Special points are to align the first ray in a neutral position in the lateral plane and to avoid dorsiflexion. In all these procedures, a small rectangular inlay graft can be used to enhance the fusion.

The second pattern is overload of the second metatarsal–cuneiform joint, which is usually associated with a short or hypermobile first ray. Both problems are addressed by an arthrodesis of the respective joints using a similar lag technique. Again, use a stabilization screw for the first metatarsal. Also, place the first ray in a neutral position or, if necessary, in a plantarflexed position so as to unweigh the second metatarsal. An opening wedge iliac graft can be useful.

The diastasis pattern requires a reduction between the first and second metatarsals. After preparing the medial two metatarsal-cuneiform joints, use a reduction clamp to compress the gap. The incompetent Lisfranc ligament is reconstructed by placing a lag screw between the first cuneiform and the base of the second metatarsal (Fig. 15–12). The previously described technique is used for the first metatarsal–cuneiform joint.

The fourth common pattern of the global type involves the bases of all the metatarsals, or at least the lateral four.[1, 11] All the involved joints need to be prepared and mobilized. If mobilization is difficult, a small distractor can be placed in the calcaneus and fifth metatarsal to aid in reduction. Fixation at the individual bases is performed for the medial three metatarsals. Temporary fixation is adequate for the lateral two rays. Sangeorzan and colleagues, in their limited series on salvage of Lisfranc's injuries, did not find an improvement in patients who had fusion of the lateral two joints.[11]

Although bone grafting is optional for these procedures, we use iliac crest grafts on the majority of our patients. By using a window technique in the ilium and curetting only cancellous bone graft, morbidity has been quite

TABLE 15–3. **SURGICAL OPTIONS FOR SPECIFIC TYPES OF MIDFOOT BREAKDOWN**

DEGENERATIVE PATTERNS

I. Arthritic or decompensated first metatarsal–medial cuneiform joint

SURGICAL OPTIONS

Fusion of the first metatarsal–cuneiform joint with two-screw fixation and an iliac crest bone graft

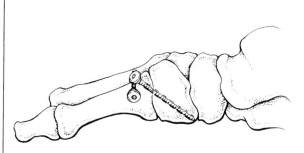

Type I

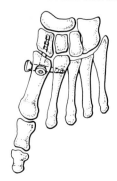

II. Overload, degenerative joint disease, or both of the second metatarsal with an incompetent first ray; short or hypermobile first ray

Fusion of the first and second metatarsal–cuneiform joints with the optional use of a stabilization screw for the first metatarsophalangeal joint and an iliac crest bone graft

III. Diastasis

Reduction of the Lisfranc ligament region with a lag screw between the first cuneiform and the base of the second metatarsal and an iliac crest bone graft

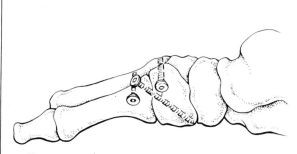

Types II and III

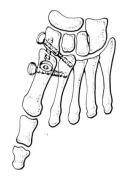

IV. Global involvement

   a. Trauma

   b. Charcot's foot
   c. Rheumatoid arthritis

Reduction of subluxation with an optional small distractor
   a. Screws at the bases of the first, second, and third metararsal–cuneiform joints
   b. Optional pin fixation for the fourth and fifth rays
   c. Iliac crest bone grafting

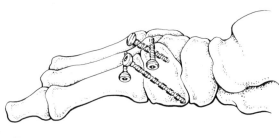

Type IV

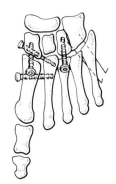

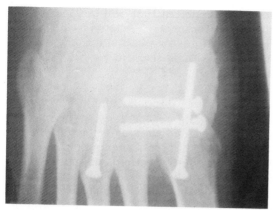

FIGURE 15–12. Postoperative film demonstrating reduction of the diastasis between the second metatarsal and the medial cuneiform. This fixation was also used for arthrodesis of the intercuneiform region as well as the bases of the second and third metatarsals. (See Fig. 15–4 [bottom] for a preoperative view of the diastasis.)

minimal. Without the use of bone graft, mobilization techniques can be slow and there is a higher risk of delayed union.

We use 3.5-mm cortical screws and an AO lag technique. With a decompensated diastasis pattern, we suggest a fully threaded cancellous screw lagged from the medial border of the medial cuneiform to the base of the second metatarsal. This fixation stabilizes the medial first ray to the lateral metatarsals, a function similar to that of the Lisfranc ligament. In addition, stability is established across the area of the individual tarsometatarsal joints by placing individual screws from the bases of the individual metatarsals into the adjacent cuneiform or cuboid. In these cases, partially threaded cancellous screws are used to avoid contact with adjacent navicular articulation. In summary, this method allows both inherent medial and lateral stability, as well as tarsometatarsal control.

Rehabilitation

In both proximal and distal midfoot arthrodeses, immobilization is modified depending on the degree of stability achieved at the time of surgery. In general, there is a period of 4 to 6 weeks of non–weight bearing in a short-leg cast, followed by 6 weeks of immobilization in a walking cast. Radiographs are taken at 6 and 12 weeks to assess the extent of healing. If, at 12 weeks, the patient appears clinically healed, a removable short-leg brace is used for prolonged weight bearing in conjunction with a custom-molded insert and a

flexible steel-shank shoe for less strenuous activities. Brace use is gradually discontinued as swelling and pain subside. Residual postoperative swelling lasts from 3 to 6 months, depending on multiple factors. Swelling may be improved by the use of contrast baths, elevation, and compression socks. Arthralgia in adjacent joints may develop, owing to changes in mechanical loading. Patients should be advised of this condition and informed that an adaptive period related to it may be necessary.

Complications and Pitfalls

Incisional Hazards

Operative neuromas about the dorsum of the foot are especially common.[13] Operative neuromas about the dorsum of the foot are especially common, and for this reason Kenzora has named this the N-zone.[7] Neuromas have been associated with pain syndromes as well as with sympathetic dystrophy. They are frequently symptomatic on the dorsum of the foot because they are compressed by normal shoewear over bony prominences. Most incisions advocated in the past have been multiple short longitudinal incisions that limit the visualization of the tiny nerves that give rise to neuromas. The best treatment is prevention with the use of surgical loupes and a thorough knowledge of the local anatomy. Therefore, before surgery, perform a thorough examination for visible and palpable nerves in the operative field. One can usually examine and locate the following nerves: the superficial peroneal nerve, the deep peroneal nerve, the communicating sural nerve, and the saphenous nerve. The lateral branch of the superficial peroneal nerve is frequently visible, but for others, running an instrument such as a hemostat over the nerve may be required to locate them. Most iatrogenic injuries occur in the area in which the superficial peroneal nerve runs over the deep peroneal nerve. The details of the surgical approach have been listed in the previous section.

Options for salvage are neurolysis of adherent nerves; resection of neuroma with neurorrhaphy; or resection of the proximal portion of the nerve and burying it in muscle, fat, or bone. At times, it is advisable to ligate the stump above the ankle to avoid stretching the nerve on plantar flexion of the ankle or to avoid local pressure from shoewear.

Infection

Infections can be minimized by the use of prophylactic antibiotics, surgical drains, and sterile surgical technique. Postoperative wound infections are uncommon in this location but should be treated by standard protocols.

Failed Fusions

Although failed fusions occur, not all are symptomatic; attention should be directed only to the symptomatic ones. The talonavicular joint is the most common site of failure. Nonunions can be minimized through the use of adequate exposures, stable fixation, and appropriate postoperative immobilization. In a symptomatic failed arthrodesis, further surgery can be fruitful. Previous hardware should be removed. Broken hardware can remain if it does not obstruct the reduction or interfere with new fixation. Although autogenous iliac bone graft is used in resurfacing procedures, local bone graft is usually sufficient in reperformed fusions. In our experience, slotted inlay grafts are successful.[5] A rectangular slot is made across the joint. Via the slot, a majority of the nonunited surface can be débrided further until bleeding cancellous bone is observed. Bone graft can be taken from adjacent bone or, if necessary, from appropriate distant sites. The fusion site is internally fixed through new portals to allow for better purchase.

Breakdown in Adjacent Joints

Even when surgery has been successful, future stress on adjacent joints may predispose a patient to painful symptoms or breakdown. Most patients have an adaptive period of 6 to 12 months after surgery before they return to optimum condition. During this period, shoe adaptations are used to balance the stress on the foot. A well-molded insole in a shoe with a flexible steel shank is advisable. After this adaptive period, further corrections may not be necessary.

Patients with a history of spinal disorders, neuropathy, or signs of high tolerance to pain can demonstrate dramatic breakdown in adjacent structures after surgery. In patients with potential neuropathy, prolonged immobilization is necessary for fusion. Total contact casting is frequently used, which predisposes to disuse osteoporosis and potential stress fractures. After completion of plaster immobilization, we recommend bracing with an ankle-foot orthosis and a shoe with a flexible steel shank and rocker sole. After clinical healing, the goal is to allow patients to function with an insole in a rigid-sole shoe.

Malalignment

As previously discussed, the most common late finding with degeneration of the midfoot is that of longitudinal arch collapse, forefoot varus, and abduction of the forefoot. Conservative treatment can include an insole with a longitudinal arch along with forefoot posting. In patients who are not candidates for surgery, advanced deformities can be treated with an ankle-foot orthosis or a double upright brace and medial T-strap.

Salvage surgery can consist of an isolated navicular-cuneiform fusion for the loss of the arch. The abduction can be relieved with a closing medial osteotomy of the cuneiform or navicular area. If the hindfoot is in severe valgus, a triple arthrodesis or subtalar fusion may allow correction of a portion of the longitudinal sag and abducted deformity. The hindfoot must be rotated internally to compensate for abduction deformity before fusion. If this is extensive, a more radical transtarsal wedge can be performed.

References

1. Arntz CT, Hansen ST: Dislocations and fracture dislocations of the tarsometatarsal joints. Orthop Clin North Am 18:105, 1987.
2. Cohn BT, Brahms MA: Diabetic arthropathy of the first metatarsal cuneiform joint. Orthop Rev 16:38, 1987.
3. Donatelli R: The Biomechanics of the Foot and Ankle. Philadelphia, FA Davis Company, 1990.
4. Faciszewski T, Burks T, Manaster BJ: Subtle injuries of the Lisfranc joint. J Bone Joint Surg 72A:1519, 1990.
5. Johnson JE, Johnson KA: Dowel arthrodesis for degenerative arthritis of the tarsometatarsal (Lisfranc) joints. Foot Ankle 5:243, 1986.
6. Johnson K: Surgery of the Foot and Ankle. New York, Raven Press, 1989.
7. Kenzora JE: Sensory nerve neuromas—Leading to failed foot surgery. Foot Ankle 7(2):110–117, 1986.
8. Manter JT: Movements of the subtalar and transverse tarsal joints. Anat Rec 80:396, 1947.
9. Manter JT: Distribution of compression forces in the joints of the human foot. Anat Rec 96:313, 1946.
10. Oatis CA: Biomechanics of the foot and ankle under static conditions. Phys Ther 68:1815, 1988.
11. Sangeorzan BJ, Veith RG, Hansen ST: Salvage of Lisfranc's tarsometatarsal joint by arthrodesis. Foot Ankle 4:193, 1990.
12. Sarrafian SK: Anatomy of the Foot and Ankle. Philadelphia, JB Lippincott, 1983.
13. Schon L, Baxter D: Neuropathies of the foot and ankle. Clin Sports Med 9:489, 1989.

16 *Charcot-Marie-Tooth Disease*

ROGER A. MANN

This chapter does not present a complete discussion of Charcot-Marie-Tooth disease (CMT) but discusses the surgical treatment of the problems encountered in the mature foot. The spectrum of bony deformities that occurs in CMT tends to follow a pattern: this includes a varus deformity of the calcaneus, adduction of the forefoot, and plantar flexion of the first metatarsal.

This pattern of deformity is due to the fact that the most common muscle weakness in CMT is that of the peroneus brevis and the tibialis anterior. This weakness leaves the tibialis posterior and peroneus longus relatively unopposed, which I believe accounts for the varus deformity of the calcaneus and adduction of the forefoot from the former and the plantar flexion of the first metatarsal from the latter. Because of the muscle imbalance and the adduction and varus configuration of the foot, the plantar aponeurosis often becomes severely contracted.

The toe deformity that is observed is usually a clawtoe deformity of various degree that can be either flexible or fixed. This deformity is due to an imbalance between the intrinsic and extrinsic muscles. A cock-up deformity of the first metatarsophalangeal joint may also be present because of the use of the extensor hallucis longus as an accessory dorsiflexor of the ankle joint.

Planning surgery about the foot in patients with CMT begins with a detailed physical examination. Only in this way can an accurate treatment plan be formulated. In general, if the foot can be realigned by carrying out osteotomies and tendon transfers rather than an arthrodesis, the patient will have a supple foot, which is usually more functional than a rigid one. Obviously, if the deformity is too severe, a stabilization procedure is indicated.

PHYSICAL EXAMINATION

In the physical examination, the physician first has the patient stand and carefully observes the foot, noting the position of the calcaneus (degree of varus) and that of the forefoot (degree of adduction). The patient then walks, and careful note is made of foot placement and of whether a cock-up deformity occurs at the first metatarsophalangeal joint, which would indicate weakness of the tibialis anterior muscle.

Physical examination of the ankle joint must determine whether there is adequate dorsiflexion and what the strength of the dorsiflexors is. When checking for dorsiflexion of the ankle joint, the physician needs to be careful that the degree of dorsiflexion is in relation to the calcaneus and not to the forefoot, which is often in an equinus position. Next, the motion of the subtalar joint is determined. The degrees of inversion and eversion are noted, as is the motor function present. The main invertor of the subtalar joint is the tibialis posterior, and the main evertor is the peroneus brevis. The physician must also note through what arc the rotation of the subtalar joint is occurring: that is, can the subtalar joint be brought into valgus, or is all the motion carried out with the subtalar joint in a varus position? This is important because if the subtalar joint cannot be brought into valgus and no motor function exists to hold it in valgus, probably an osteotomy alone will not be adequate to correct the problem.

The transverse tarsal joint, which is the talonavicular and calcaneocuboid, is evaluated next. The degrees of adduction and abduction are determined. Again, it is important to see, by holding the foot in an adducted position, whether the foot can be brought into some semblance of normal alignment or if a fixed bony deformity is present. The metatarsophalangeal joint motion is determined, as is the muscle strength, with particular attention paid to whether a cock-up deformity of the first metatarsophalangeal joint is present. The other metatarsophalangeal joints are observed to see whether there is any fixed dorsiflexion contracture or whether the deformity is only a dynamic one that can be passively corrected. The interphalangeal joints of the lesser toes are checked for evidence of a dynamic versus a fixed deformity.

The posture of the forefoot is carefully observed in relation to the hindfoot. To carry this out, the calcaneus is placed in line with the tibia and the forefoot is observed in relation to the calcaneus. The forefoot is almost invariably in valgus, with the first and sometimes the second and third metatarsals in a plantarflexed position. The plantar aponeurosis is palpated, and it is usually noted to be contracted, almost holding the forefoot in a plantarflexed and somewhat adducted position. It is this forefoot posture (adduction and plantar flexion of the first ray), along with the varus configuration of the calcaneus and the weak peroneus brevis, that creates an unstable ankle with a tendency to invert with weight bearing.

The basic goal in the treatment of the foot with CMT is to create a stable plantigrade foot. If the flexibility of the foot can be maintained, the patient will have the most functional foot; however, this may not be achievable and an arthrodesis may be necessary.

In creating a plantigrade foot, the physician should start with the calcaneus and work forward.

CREATION OF A PLANTIGRADE FOOT

Calcaneus

As a general rule, the calcaneus is not in an equinus position but is almost invariably in a varus position. If a calcaneal osteotomy (Dwyer's procedure) can be performed that can place the alignment of the heel into valgus, it is preferable to a subtalar arthrodesis. If a mild equinus contracture is present, then along with the correction of the varus deformity of the calcaneus the osteotomy can be permitted to slide proximally to correct the equinus. However, if a significant contracture of the Achilles tendon is present, a tendo Achillis lengthening should be carried out after the calcaneal osteotomy is made. As a general rule, the peroneus longus muscle has adequate strength but the peroneus brevis muscle is quite weak. To increase the eversion strength and the stability of the subtalar joint, the peroneus longus is detached as it starts to pass under the cuboid and is then woven through the peroneus brevis, placing the peroneus brevis under the maximum amount of tension possible. This helps to reinforce the eversion stability of the subtalar joint.

Surgical Technique for Calcaneal Osteotomy (Dwyer's Procedure)[1]
(Fig. 16–1)

1. After adequate anesthetic has been administered, a tourniquet is used about the thigh. A bolster is used under the involved side to tilt the patient, making exposure of the lateral side of the heel easier.

2. An incision starting about 1 cm posterior to the fibula is carried obliquely toward the area of the plantar aspect of the calcaneocuboid articulation. The incision is deepened through subcutaneous tissue and fat, and the sural nerve is identified and carefully protected.

3. The peroneal tendons within their sheaths are reflected proximally off the calcaneus. In this way, the calcaneus is exposed from behind the fibular malleolus to the level of the calcaneocuboid joint.

4. With a wide-blade saw, an oblique osteotomy is produced that begins proximally about 1 cm posterior to the subtalar joint and ends about 1 cm proximal to the calcaneocuboid joint on the plantar aspect of the foot. This cut is then deepened, staying as perpendicular to the long axis of the leg as possible until the cortex on the medial side is encountered.

5. A wedge of calcaneus measuring from 5 to 10 mm, depending on the severity of the deformity, is removed by making a second cut

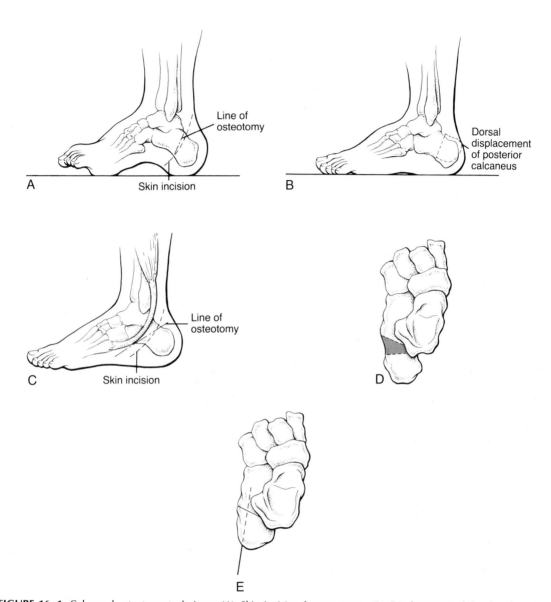

FIGURE 16–1. Calcaneal osteotomy technique. *(A)*, Skin incision for pes cavus. *(B)*, Displacement of the dorsal wedge. *(C)*, Skin incision for heel varus. *(D)*, Wedge removal. *(E)*, Pin fixation.

parallel to the first but somewhat more plantar to it and angulated toward the apex of the first cut. The bone is removed, and the osteotomy site is manipulated and closed lateralward.

6. At this point, the alignment of the calcaneus in relation to the long axis of the tibia must be carefully assessed. It is imperative that the calcaneus be brought into valgus; if it is not, more bone must be removed from the calcaneus.

7. The osteotomy site can be stabilized with a Steinmann pin, which is brought up through the heel and into the calcaneus, but caution must be exercised so that the posterior facet of the subtalar joint is not violated by the pin. Another option is to use multiple staples to hold the osteotomy in a closed position.

8. The subcutaneous tissue and skin are closed in a routine manner.

Surgical Technique for Calcaneal Osteotomy (Samilson's Procedure)[2]

1. The lateral aspect of the calcaneus is approached as outlined in steps 1 to 3 of Dwyer's procedure.

2. The osteotomy is somewhat more vertically oriented because the posterior fragment needs to be displaced superiorly. The initial cut begins about 5 mm posterior to the subtalar joint and is angulated anteriorly about 40 degrees. This cut exits through the plantar aspect of the calcaneus about 3 cm proximal to the calcaneocuboid joint.

3. If a varus deformity is also present, which is usually the case, a lateral closing wedge is removed from the posterior fragment. The wedge is 4 to 8 mm in width.

4. After the osteotomy site is manipulated, it is displaced superiorly about 1 cm. The displacement is made easier if the foot is brought into plantar flexion, the posterior fragment is displaced superiorly, and the foot is brought back up into dorsiflexion.

5. Fixation is achieved by a Steinmann pin brought up from the tip of the heel across the osteotomy site.

Surgical Technique for Transfer of the Peroneus Longus into the Peroneus Brevis

1. Through the same incision with which the calcaneus has been exposed, the peroneus lon-

gus tendon sheath is opened and the tendon is exposed to the point where it passes beneath the cuboid.

2. At the site where the peroneus longus starts to pass beneath the cuboid, it is sutured to the periosteum and the tendon is sectioned.

3. Two sutures are woven through the proximal end of the peroneus longus tendon. The peroneus brevis tendon sheath is opened starting at the tip of the fibula distal to its insertion into the base of the fifth metatarsal.

4. With a Pulvertaft type of weave, the peroneus longus is brought through the peroneus brevis tendon and is pulled as distally as possible as the subtalar joint is brought into maximum eversion. It is important that as this is done, the peroneus brevis is put under some tension proximally so that it is not pulled distally with the peroneus longus tendon; otherwise, the effective pull of the peroneus longus will be diminished.

5. The peroneus longus is secured into the brevis by multiple cross sutures. The subcutaneous tissue and skin are closed in a routine manner.

Plantar Aponeurosis

The plantar aponeurosis is almost always severely contracted in patients with advanced CMT. Whether this is a primary or a secondary change is not known. However, the plantar aponeurosis should be released off of its origin on the calcaneus and medially along the abductor hallucis fascia to release the forefoot contracture.

Surgical Technique for Release of the Plantar Aponeurosis

1. A longitudinal medial plantar skin incision is made starting proximally almost in line with the tip of the tibial malleolus and carried distally along the plantar aponeurosis.

2. This incision is deepened to the plantar aponeurosis, and with a small elevator, the origin of the plantar fascia is carefully exposed plantarward and along its medialward extension, which surrounds the abductor hallucis muscle.

3. Under direct vision, the plantar fascia is cut as an assistant applies dorsiflexion pressure to the metatarsal heads. This step must be performed very cautiously in order to avoid

damage to any of the nervous structures in the area. As complete a fascial release as possible is carried out on the plantar aspect, as well as along the heavy fascia that invests the abductor hallucis muscle. When this has been achieved, there usually is about 2 cm of separation of the fascia. This allows the forefoot to move into a more plantigrade position.

4. The subcutaneous tissue and skin are closed in a routine manner.

Forefoot Valgus

The remaining deformity after the hindfoot has been corrected is forefoot valgus. Forefoot valgus is brought about by the plantar flexion of the first, sometimes the second, and occasionally the third metatarsal. Following os calcis osteotomy and plantar fasciotomy, as the foot is brought into neutral position towards dorsiflexion, the calcaneus is in a slight degree of valgus. Because the plantar fascia has been released, the foot can be brought out of some of its adducted position. However, there still is plantar flexion of the first, the second, and sometimes the third metatarsal, and this must be dealt with to create a plantigrade foot that will not have a tendency to invert the subtalar joint when weight is borne by the forefoot.

Surgical Technique for Metatarsal Osteotomy (Dorsal Closing Wedge)

1. A longitudinal dorsal incision is centered over the base of the first metatarsal and carried down through subcutaneous tissue and fat. The extensor hallucis longus tendon is identified and moved medially or laterally, as is convenient.

2. The first metatarsal–cuneiform articulation is identified, and the surgeon moves distally to this approximately 1 cm. The periosteum around the metatarsal is stripped medially and laterally.

3. The osteotomy at the base of the first metatarsal is carried out with a small sagittal saw. The first cut is made parallel to the first metatarsal–cuneiform articulation, leaving a hinge of bone on the plantar aspect of the first metatarsal.

4. An appropriate wedge of bone is removed, which is anywhere from 3 to 10 mm,

preferably leaving the base of the metatarsal intact.

5. The osteotomy site is manipulated and brought up into dorsiflexion, leaving the plantar periosteum intact. The relationship of the first metatarsal to the fourth and fifth metatarsals is then carefully determined. The goal is the creation of a neutral forefoot, or possibly one in which there is a slight degree of forefoot varus.

6. If insufficient bone has been removed the first time, more bone is taken from the distal cut in order to bring the first metatarsal up into proper alignment. Once this has been achieved, fixation can be carried out in one of several ways.

7. Fixation can be achieved by placing a staple or by using an oblique screw. However, I prefer the technique of placing one screw vertically into the proximal fragment, placing a loop of 22-gauge wire through the dorsal third of the metatarsal, closing the osteotomy site, and tightening the wire for firm fixation.

8. If necessary, the second and possibly the third metatarsals are osteotomized in a similar way. As the surgeon proceeds laterally across the foot, the size of the wedge diminishes.

9. All the wounds are closed, and the foot is carefully inspected. At this point, the patient should have a plantigrade foot, with the hindfoot in valgus and the forefoot in neutral position. One metatarsal head should not protrude more plantarward than another, and if it does, it should be osteotomized and brought up into line with the first and second metatarsal heads.

Correction of Cock-Up Deformity of the First Metatarsophalangeal Joint

If there is weakness of the tibialis anterior, so that the extensor hallucis longus helps to dorsiflex the ankle joint, a first toe Jones procedure is indicated to improve dorsiflexion strength at the ankle. In this procedure, an arthrodesis of the interphalangeal joint of the great toe is performed, and the extensor hallucis longus tendon is transposed proximally through the neck of the first metatarsal. As a general rule, the first toe Jones procedure can be carried out at the same time as the first metatarsal osteotomy, but if hindfoot surgery is also carried out, I prefer to delay the forefoot surgery for 1 month.

Surgical Technique for a First Toe Jones Procedure[3]

1. A longitudinal dorsal incision is made over the distal one-third of the first metatarsal, exposing the extensor hallucis longus tendon. The tendon is then carefully denuded of its soft tissue as far distally as possible.

2. An elliptical dorsal incision is made over the interphalangeal joint of the great toe, releasing the extensor hallucis longus tendon. Working distally and proximally, the surgeon frees the extensor hallucis longus tendon and brings it back into the proximal wound.

3. The first metatarsal is exposed approximately 1 cm proximal to the articular surface. If an extension contracture of the metatarsophalangeal joint is present, it is released at this time with a medial and lateral dorsal capsulotomy.

4. After the distal portion of the metatarsal has been exposed, a hole of an adequate size to accommodate the extensor hallucis longus tendon is produced.

5. A suture is passed through the tip of the extensor hallucis longus tendon and through the drill hole made in the distal portion of the metatarsal. The tendon is not secured until the interphalangeal joint arthrodesis has been carried out.

6. The interphalangeal joint is prepared for fusion by excision of the articular surfaces with a small sagittal saw. This cut is made so as to produce a slight degree of plantar flexion (about 5 degrees) and 2 to 3 degrees of valgus.

7. A 2.5-mm drill bit is selected, and a hole is drilled from the proximal portion of the distal phalanx through the tip of the toe. Where the drill bit comes through the skin, a transverse cut of adequate size is made in the skin, and a 3.5-mm tap is used to tap the hole in the distal phalanx.

8. A 4.0-mm cancellous screw of adequate length, usually 30 to 35 mm, is placed into the hole in the tip of the toe, and when the screw head is just visible, the screw is advanced another 2 mm. The interphalangeal joint is brought together firmly, and the screw is screwed into the proximal phalanx. If the bone is quite hard, a drill hole can be made in the proximal phalanx, but usually this is not necessary.

9. If adequate fixation has been achieved, no further fixation is indicated. However, if any wobble is present at the osteotomy site,

an oblique 0.045-inch Kirschner wire is passed across the intended arthrodesis site.

10. Once the arthrodesis site has been fixed, the extensor hallucis longus tendon is tightened through the metatarsal while the foot is brought up into as much dorsiflexion as possible. The extensor hallucis longus tendon is sutured back onto itself.

11. The wounds are closed in a routine fashion, and a short-leg cast is applied, with the foot held in neutral position and with weight bearing as tolerated for approximately 5 weeks.

Correction of Clawtoes

The clawtoe deformity in CMT can be either a fixed or a flexible deformity. If a fixed deformity is present, release of the extensor tendons and a dorsal capsulotomy must be carried out. If the deformity is only dynamic and the metatarsophalangeal joints can be brought into a normal degree of plantar flexion, the tendons and capsule do not need to be released. The same applies for the interphalangeal joints: namely, if a fixed contracture is present, a DuVries type of condylectomy or an interphalangeal joint fusion is carried out. If, however, a dynamic deformity is present, then a flexor tendon transfer (Girdlestone's procedure[4, 5]) is all that is indicated.

Surgical Technique for the Girdlestone Procedure and Release of the Dorsal Capsules

1. The initial skin incision is made over the dorsal aspect of each toe, starting at the middle of the middle phalanx and carried proximally along the extensor tendon to the metatarsophalangeal joint.

2. The long and short extensor tendons, along with the dorsal, medial, and lateral capsule, are cut. The metatarsophalangeal joint is brought down into approximately 20 degrees of plantar flexion to be sure that an adequate release has been achieved.

3. Through a small transverse incision on the plantar aspect of the foot at the level of the proximal flexion crease, the flexor tendon sheath is exposed.

4. The flexor tendon sheath is opened with a No. 11 blade, and three tendon strands are noted.

5. The middle of the three tendons—namely, the flexor digitorum longus tendon—is pulled into the wound and is released distally from its insertion into the base of the distal phalanx through a small stab wound.

6. The flexor digitorum longus tendon is pulled into the wound. A raphe runs through the middle of the tendon; this is split and two tails are created.

7. At the distal portion of the dorsal wound, the proximal interphalangeal joint is opened and the distal portion of the proximal phalanx is exposed. With a bone cutter, the condyles are generously removed. This permits the fixed hammer toe deformity to be corrected. If the toe cannot be brought into correct alignment, more bone should be removed from the phalanx to decompress the joint. The proximal interphalangeal joint is fixed with a 0.045-inch Kirschner for 4 weeks. If only a dynamic deformity exists, it is not necessary to excise the distal portion of the proximal phalanx.

8. With the use of a Kelly clamp, a tunnel is created on either side of the extensor hood mechanism and presents through the wound on the plantar aspect of the foot.

9. A small mosquito clamp is placed into this wound from dorsal to plantar in order to bring up a tail of the flexor tendon on either side of the extensor hood. As the flexor tendon is brought up, the metatarsophalangeal joint is placed into approximately 15 degrees of plantar flexion while the ankle joint is in equinus. This places maximum tension on the flexor digitorum longus tendon, and it is sutured into the dorsal hood.

10. This procedure is carried out for all of the lesser toes to correct the clawing.

11. The skin is closed in a routine manner. If this procedure is carried out with a first toe Jones procedure, the patient is casted, but if this is carried out as an isolated procedure on the lesser toes, only a wooden shoe is necessary for approximately 3 weeks.

12. It is important for the patient to appreciate that after this procedure, although the toes are usually well aligned, they do not have good selective control to flex the interphalangeal joints.

References

1. Dwyer FC: Osteotomy of the calcaneus for pes cavus. J Bone Joint Surg 41B:80, 1959.
2. Samilson RL: Crescentic osteotomy of the os calcis for calcaneo-cavus feet. *In* Bateman JE (Ed): Foot Science. Philadelphia, WB Saunders, 1976, p 18.
3. Jones R: An operation for paralytic calcaneocavus. Am J Orthop Surg 5:371, 1908.
4. Girdlestone GR: Physiotherapy for hand and foot. J Chartered Soc Physiother 32:167, 1947.
5. Taylor RG: The treatment of claw toes by multiple transfers of flexor into extensor tendons. J Bone Joint Surg 33B:539, 1951.

17 Nerve Compression Syndromes of the Foot and Ankle

GEORGE B. HOLMES, JR.

Nerve compression syndromes involve the mechanical impingement of one or more of the peripheral nerves about the foot and ankle. The compression may be an acute or a chronic process to a sensory, motor, or mixed nerve. The simplest and most common nerve entrapments of the foot are superficial neuromas, which result from acute or repetitive trauma. Interdigital neuromas are associated with compression or injury of the common digital nerve. Compression of the posterior tibial nerve results in the tarsal tunnel syndrome. The discussion that follows focuses on the anatomy, pathophysiology, diagnosis, and treatment of these three nerve compression syndromes.

SUPERFICIAL NEUROMA

Because of the paucity of subcutaneous fat and soft tissues on the dorsum of the foot, the superficial nerves in this area are particularly prone to injury (Fig. 17–1). Most prone to injury are the superficial branches of the intermediate dorsal and medial dorsal cutaneous branches of the superficial peroneal nerve, the lateral dorsal cutaneous nerve, and the branches of the sural nerve. The causes of entrapment include (1) chronically tight shoewear, (2) acute blunt trauma or laceration, and (3) scarring or entrapment from an adjacent injury or previous surgery. Measures to prevent injury to these structures include the use of appropriate shoewear and the use of longitudinal incisions rather than transverse ones.

Patients with a neuroma present with a chief complaint of pain associated with tingling, burning, or numbness. The differential diagnosis includes ganglion cyst, stress fracture, and tendinitis. Tight straps across the dorsum of the foot may accentuate the symptoms experienced by the patient. A thorough history taking along with an appreciation of the surface anatomy of the foot usually allows the examiner to localize the specific area of involvement. The subsequent physical examination must include visual inspection, testing of active and passive range of motion, and a thorough neurovascular examination. Direct observation may indicate a previous scar or injury at the site of involvement. Palpation is another important element in the diagnosis of neuroma. Direct tapping over the area of the neuroma should elicit a well-circumscribed area of pain. There may be distal or proximal radiation of pain consistent with the anatomic course of the involved nerve. Patients may also indicate an area of partial or complete loss of sensation distal to the neuroma site.

When the diagnosis of a neuroma has been confirmed, the initial approach to this problem is conservative. If the history suggests that tight shoewear initiated the neuroma, shoe modification is one early step in the management of this condition. This step should be augmented with a program of desensitization using a shower or gentle daily massage. In my experience, less than half of patients will have complete satisfaction with this form of treatment.

With persistent symptoms, a local injection of a few milliliters of lidocaine (Xylocaine) or

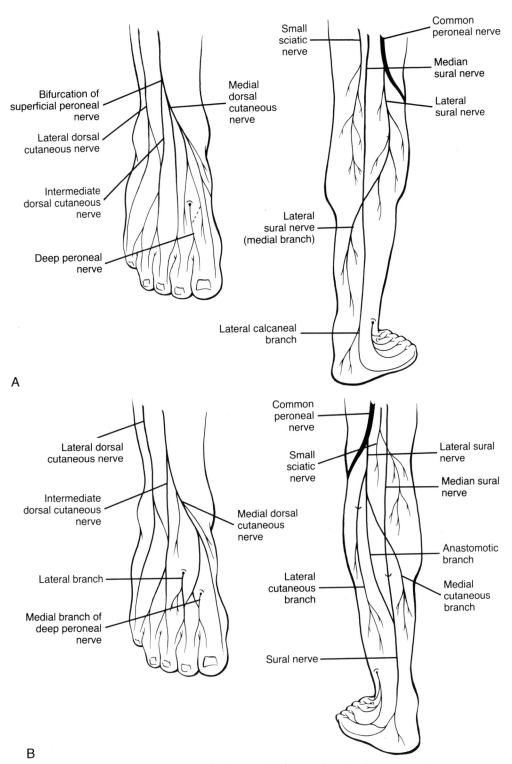

FIGURE 17–1. (*A* and *B*), Superficial nerves of the leg, foot, and ankle.

bupivacaine (Marcaine) subcutaneously proximal to the lesion may be useful in confirming the diagnosis. Within a few minutes, there should be complete resolution of pain distal to the location of the injection. The addition of a subcutaneous corticosteroid may also be attempted before operative intervention is undertaken.

Surgical intervention may be necessary if conservative measures fail to diminish the patient's symptoms significantly. Surgery can be performed on an outpatient basis with local, regional, or general anesthesia. It is preferable to use an incision in line with the anatomic course of the nerve. This allows adequate extension proximal and distal to the neuroma and does not risk injury to adjacent nerves. Normal nerve tissue must be identified proximal to the neuroma. This should then be used as a guide to the area of the neuroma. Transection of the neuroma should occur proximally through normal nerve tissue and distal to the bulbous enlargement of the nerve. The proximal stump is then placed in an area that is deep and protected from repetitive trauma. This can be accomplished by various means, such as placement under fascia or muscle. Some surgeons recommend burying the nerve within an adjacent bone. The important goal is to place the stump deep and preferably in an area not subjected to excessive motion or trauma. Small dissolvable sutures affix the nerve to these deeper structures. In addition, the care used in the planning and execution of the surgery should be maintained during the closure. Care should be taken not to entrap any superficial nerves with the suture during the closure.

Postoperatively, the foot is placed in a light compressive dressing. Patients are given a postoperative wooden shoe and are allowed to ambulate as tolerated. Elevation and rest are strongly recommended for the first 24 to 48 hours after surgery. Sutures are generally removed 5 to 7 days after surgery. A compressive dressing is worn by the patient for 1 to 2 weeks. A sandal or a wide shoe is then worn until the postoperative swelling has resolved completely.

The presentation of a patient with multiple neuromas is not entirely uncommon. This problem demands a greater emphasis on conservative management. It is very difficult to achieve satisfactory surgical results in a foot or ankle with several painful neuromas. If conservative measures prove unsuccessful, it is important to identify at least one or two areas on which to concentrate surgical attempts.

Patients can also present with recurrent pain after previous surgical excision of a neuroma. The same diagnostic approach used for a new neuroma is used for evaluating a recurrent neuroma. Once the diagnosis of a recurrent neuroma is made, the usual conservative modalities should not be bypassed before surgery is considered.

Perhaps the most difficult management problem is the patient with a neuroma and associated reflex sympathetic dystrophy. A detailed discussion of reflex sympathetic dystrophy is beyond the scope of this section. However, painful foci such as neuromas have been postulated to be initiators of reflex sympathetic dystrophy.[3] Nonoperative management is the basis of treatment for patients with combined neuroma and reflex sympathetic dystrophy. Conservative modalities for neuromas are augmented with a regimen of physical therapy (range-of-motion, desensitization, and mobilization techniques), mild analgesics, anti-inflammatory agents, nerve blocks, epidural blocks, and psychological counseling. If surgery is attempted, it should be performed in a quiescent phase of the disease and should be augmented with nerve blocks and judicious physical therapy postoperatively.

INTERDIGITAL NEUROMA

Interdigital neuroma, or Morton's neuroma, is the syndrome of pain associated with injury or compression of the interdigital nerves. The exact etiology of interdigital neuroma is unknown; however, anatomic, extrinsic, and traumatic factors have been identified as probable causes of this syndrome.[7]

The interdigital nerves are the continuation of the medial and lateral plantar branches of the posterior tibial nerve. The first, second, and third common digital nerves branch from the medial plantar nerve. The common digital nerve to the fourth interspace and the proper digital nerve of the small toe originate from the lateral plantar nerve. A communicating branch between the third and fourth common digital nerves imposes a tethering effect on the nerve to the third interspace. Consequently, this site is a frequent location of the formation of an interdigital neuroma. Other factors implicated include differential metatarsal mobility, trauma to the plantar aspect of the forefoot, and extrinsic pressure on the metatarsal heads from tight shoes and high-heeled shoes. These factors, singularly or in combination, lead to edema, thickening, and nerve degeneration in and about the interdigital nerves.

The symptoms of interdigital neuroma occur most frequently in women. Mann and Reynolds have observed a female-to-male ratio of about 12:1, with an average age of 55 years for both men and women.[9] Classically, interdigital neuroma occurs unilaterally in the third interspace. Some 15 percent of patients may present with bilateral neuromas.[9] Most authors emphasize that the occurrence of more than one neuroma in the same foot is quite rare.[1, 9] Interdigital neuromas also occur with the same relative frequency in the second and third interspaces. The pain is most frequently described as burning and is localized to the plantar aspect of the forefoot between the metatarsal heads. There may also be proximal radiation of pain and distal numbness of the adjacent toes. Patients generally report the exacerbation of pain while wearing certain shoes, such as narrow-toe shoes or, for women, high-heeled shoes. Many patients indicate that their pain decreases over the weekend or during vacation, when they tend to wear more comfortable shoes.

Direct palpation of the plantar aspect of the suspected interspace will produce sharp pain localized to that specific interspace. Associated tingling of the toes adjacent to the interspace may also occur. With two hands, medial-lateral pressure to the foot and dorsal-plantar pressure are simultaneously applied to each interspace of the forefoot in turn. This can be very helpful in isolating the pain to a specific intermetatarsal space. If several interspaces are painful, alternative diagnoses must strongly be considered. In all cases of suspected interdigital neuroma, the possibility of (1) tarsal tunnel syndrome; (2) atrophy of the plantar fat pad; (3) synovitis, subluxation, or dislocation of the metatarsophalangeal joint; (4) intractable plantar keratoses; and (5) lumbar disk disease must be kept in mind.

Sometimes the injection of an anesthetic agent into the interspace of a suspected neuroma is helpful in confirming the diagnosis. An injection of lidocaine, bupivacaine, or mepivacaine temporarily eliminates the pain localized to a specific interspace. The addition

of an injection of a corticosteroid has been effective for more long-term relief of pain, as long as it is not injected into the fat pad.

With the diagnosis of an interdigital neuroma firmly supported by the history and physical examination, the initial treatment plan is conservative. The patient is encouraged to wear a broad shoe with a soft sole. Women should wear flat shoes or low-heeled shoes in lieu of high-heeled shoes. These modifications allow the metatarsals to spread and thus decrease the pressures on the interdigital nerves. This treatment plan can be augmented with the use of a soft metatarsal pad just proximal to the metatarsal heads.

Only about 30 percent of patients demonstrate a long-term satisfactory response to conservative measures. The remainder usually require surgical excision of the neuroma, and approximately 80 percent of this group have a successful result. The neuroma may be approached from the dorsal or the plantar aspect of the foot. Proponents of the dorsal approach indicate the advantages of an adequate exposure without the risk of a painful plantar incision.[4, 5, 8] The advocates of a plantar incision cite the better visualization of the neuroma, the absence of painful plantar scars, and the localization of the incision in the non–weight-bearing area of the interspace.[2, 10] My preference for both primary and recurrent interdigital neuromas is the dorsal approach as described by Mann.[8]

The procedure is carried out using a tourniquet under regional block or general anesthesia. The incision extends from the web space proximally for about 1 inch (Fig. 17–2). The two metatarsal heads on either side of the nerve are spread with a Weitlaner retractor. The transverse metatarsal ligament, which is under tension, is transected, allowing visualization of the common digital nerve. After blunt dissection, the nerve is pulled distally and is then transected as far proximally as possible. The terminal branches of the nerve are then cut, after which the proximal stump of the nerve is positioned more proximally by dorsiflexing the ankle. The closure is confined to the skin. The foot is then maintained in a compression dressing for 2 to 3 weeks. About 80 percent of patients will be asymptomatic or have a significant improvement after surgery.

A recurrent interdigital neuroma should be evaluated and treated as if it were a new neuroma. A dorsal incision is preferred if an

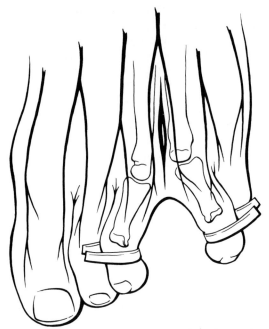

FIGURE 17–2. Dorsal interdigital approach for the excision of Morton's neuroma.

inadequate proximal resection was performed with the initial surgery. A plantar approach is usually preferred if the original dorsal procedure had an adequate proximal margin.

TARSAL TUNNEL SYNDROME

Tarsal tunnel syndrome (TTS) is the resultant neuropathy from extrinsic or intrinsic pressure on the posterior tibial nerve or on one of its branches as it courses beneath the flexor retinaculum. The posterior tibial nerve passes from the soleus muscle to the calcaneal canal. In the upper portion of the leg, it lies within the deep posterior compartment, between the posterior tibial muscle and the flexor digitorum longus muscle. Distally, the posterior tibial nerve is located between the flexor digitorum longus and the flexor hallucis longus muscles.

The posterior tibial nerve courses behind the medial malleolus (Fig. 17–3). The division into the various branches usually occurs proximal to the medial malleolus. Its branches include (1) the cutaneous branches, (2) the articular branches, (3) the vascular branches, (4) the calcaneal branch, and (5) the medial and lateral plantar branches.

The calcaneal branch originates from the posterior tibial nerve in the distal third of the leg; infrequently, however, it can branch from the medial plantar nerve. It supplies sensation to the medial and posterior aspects of the heel.

The medial plantar branch is the anterior terminal division of the posterior tibial nerve. Distal to the medial malleolus, it passes along the superior border of the abductor hallucis and the flexor sheath of the flexor hallucis longus. It supplies sensory branches to the medial sole of the foot and motor branches to the abductor hallucis and flexor digitorum brevis. It provides branches to the talonavicular and calcaneonavicular joints. Distally, the medial three common digital nerves of the foot and the medial plantar cutaneous nerve of the

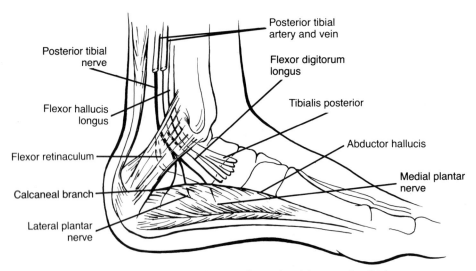

FIGURE 17–3. Anatomy of the tarsal tunnel and the posterior tibial nerve.

great toe also originate from the medial plantar nerve.

The lateral plantar nerve is smaller than the medial plantar nerve. As it passes distal to the medial malleolus, the lateral plantar nerve goes through the substance of the abductor hallucis muscle and then further divides into several more branches. These include (1) the motor branches to the abductor digiti quinti and the quadratus plantae; (2) the lateral plantar cutaneous nerve to the fifth toe; (3) the fourth common digital nerve; (4) the motor branches to the lumbricals and to the second, third, and fourth interossei; and (5) the branches to the transverse head of the adductor hallucis and muscles of the first interosseous space.

The roof of the tarsal tunnel is formed by the flexor retinaculum. The proximal and inferior borders of the tarsal tunnel are formed by the corresponding inferior and superior aspects of the flexor retinaculum. The bony floor consists of the inferomedial aspect of the tibia, the medial wall of the talus, and the superior aspect of the calcaneus. This bony canal is often referred to as the tibiotalocalcaneal tunnel, or Richet's tunnel.

This wealth of anatomy can be simplified: the posterior tibial nerve supplies sensation to the heel, the plantar aspect of the foot, and the toes. It also supplies motor branches to the intrinsic muscles of the foot. Any combination of these functions may be compromised by a compression neuropathy of the posterior tibial nerve or one of its branches.

About half of the patients who present with TTS relate a history of a previous sprain, ankle fracture, crush injury, flatfoot, or fracture-dislocation about the foot and ankle. Compression of the nerve can be caused by engorgement of the venous plexus, increased pronation, ganglion formation, or impingement from an exostosis or fracture fragment. An equal number of patients have no historical clues as to the cause of the nerve compression. For many patients, no specific cause is found even after decompression of the nerve.

The chief complaint is a diffuse burning or tingling pain that is localized to the plantar aspect of the foot. Occasionally, the pain may be isolated to the distribution of only one of the branches of the posterior tibial nerve. This discomfort may be worse at night and may radiate proximally. Physical examination can elicit Tinel's sign over the tarsal tunnel behind the medial malleolus at the abductor hallucis longus origin.

Plain radiographs are mandatory in the work-up of a patient with suspected TTS. Computed tomography and magnetic resonance imaging have allowed more effective visualization of the bone and soft tissue structures about the tarsal tunnel but are certainly not part of the standard evaluation. The presence of a ganglion, lipoma, or exostosis can be indicated by these more sensitive studies.

Electrodiagnostic studies can be helpful in confirming the diagnosis of TTS. The examiner must determine three parameters: (1) the conduction velocity of the posterior tibial nerve, (2) the terminal latency of the medial plantar nerve to the abductor hallucis, and (3) the terminal latency of the lateral plantar nerve to the abductor digiti quinti. The diagnosis of TTS is supported by a terminal latency of the medial plantar nerve to the abductor hallucis of greater than 6.2 msec. The terminal latency of the lateral plantar nerve to the abductor digiti quinti must be greater than 7 msec. Finally, the difference in the terminal latency of the medial and lateral plantar nerves should be greater than 1 msec.

Three criteria must be met to confirm the diagnosis of TTS.[6] The patient must have a history of pain that is congruent with the anatomy of the posterior tibial nerve. The physical examination must verify the presence of Tinel's sign over the posterior tibial nerve or one of its branches. Finally, electrodiagnostic findings must be positive. If these criteria are not met, surgery should not be performed. (*Editor's note*: Although I strongly agree with the first two criteria, the requirement for positive electrodiagnostic studies is more controversial. Unpublished data from our center suggest that abnormal pressure threshold findings (Semmes-Weinstein monofilaments) have a very high correlation with relief obtained from tarsal tunnel release, more so than the presence of normal or abnormal electromyographic or NCS findings. Nevertheless, the author's careful, conservative approach and cautions should be given serious consideration, at least until statistically significant data suggest otherwise.) This will keep the patient's foot ache from becoming a greater headache for the physician. If any uncertainty exists about the diagnosis of TTS, lumbar disk disease, interdigital neuroma, diffuse peripheral neuropathy, and a variant of heel pain syndrome should be considered in the differential diagnosis. Physicians should be particularly guarded in the diagnosis of TTS in patients who present with bilateral symptoms.

The initial treatment is conservative. It consists of a reduction in the activity contributing to the problem and the use of anti-inflammatory medication. Anatomic problems such as excessive hindfoot valgus or varus, which can contribute to compression of the posterior tibial nerve, may be helped by the use of orthotics. A trial period of casting or splinting may be helpful. The use of local injections of corticosteroids is not recommended in the treatment of TTS, but local blocks are helpful in diagnosing the condition. Conservative modalities are employed for at least 6 to 8 weeks. This allows adequate time to observe the response to these measures and to obtain all necessary electrodiagnostic studies. Further, this period affords the patient time to gain a full appreciation of the complex nature of this syndrome. If these conservative measures fail to significantly reduce the patient's discomfort, surgical exploration and decompression should be considered. If no specific cause of the compression neuropathy is found, no more than 75 percent of patients can be expected to have satisfactory relief of pain with surgery.[7] A less favorable outcome should be anticipated if the patient has had long-standing symptoms.

There are four key points in the surgical technique for exploration and decompression of the tarsal tunnel. First, the most common mistake is making an incision of inadequate length. The incision must extend from just proximal to the posterior aspect of the medial malleolus to a point just proximal and slightly inferior to the navicular (Fig. 17–4). This is necessary to visualize the normal proximal portion of the posterior tibial nerve and the distal lateral and medial plantar branches. The procedure demands adequate visualization of the normal proximal portion of the posterior tibial nerve using loupe magnification. An adequate incision also allows an accurate assessment of the patency of distal soft tissue canals through which the main branches travel. It is also important to preserve the delicate multiple calcaneal branches of the posterior tibial nerve to the heel. Therefore, particular care must be taken during the proximal dissection. Finally, there must be a complete release of the flexor retinaculum and the fascial slings of the abductor hallucis muscle. At the time of closure,

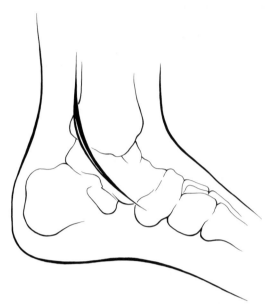

FIGURE 17–4. Incision for release of the tarsal tunnel.

the retinaculum must not be repaired because this would potentially form a constriction on the nerve.

Second, this procedure is best carried out under tourniquet control. My preference is to have the patient in the supine position, but the prone position is also acceptable. Minimal manipulation of the nerve and its branches should be adhered to throughout the procedure. The skin should be handled with all possible care in order to prevent wound problems in the area of the incision. Because of the increased potential for wound problems, I do not instill steroids into the wound before closure. Postoperatively, patients are placed in a short-leg Robert Jones dressing for 7 to 10 days. This is then changed to a removable walking brace or short-leg walking cast for an additional 1 to 2 weeks.

Third, patients experience a gradual decrease in pain over the course of several months after decompression. The length of time required for improvement is in part determined by the duration of symptoms prior to surgery. The longer the duration of symptoms was, the slower and less complete is the expected recovery. There may actually be a period of paradoxic increase in pain, which is related to the healing process. In some cases, a slowly advancing Tinel sign can be elicited along the posterior tibial nerve or its branches during this regenerative process. The swift recovery seen after decompression for carpal tunnel syndrome is generally not witnessed after decompression for TTS. Vigorous physical therapy after decompression of the posterior tibial nerve is not generally helpful. Patience, supervised active range-of-motion exercises, the application of mild heat, the use of nonsteroidal anti-inflammatory agents, and the use of nonrestrictive shoewear seem to be the most important elements in patient recovery.

Fourth, one postoperative complication of tarsal tunnel decompression is numbness of the heel secondary to injury of the calcaneal branches. This complication may be avoided by employing a meticulous dissection and adequate visualization at the time of surgery. The most common problem involves inadequate exposure and inadequate decompression. Another potential problem is slow or inadequate wound healing. Again, close attention should be paid to the careful handling of soft tissues and the avoidance of thin skin flaps. The potential for persistent pain, numbness, and burning after release of the tarsal tunnel should be thoroughly discussed with the patient. Recurrent or unresolved symptoms do not generally respond well to reoperation.

Caution, re-examination, and electromyographic studies should be employed before re-exploration of a previous tarsal tunnel release is embarked on.

References

1. Bordelon RL: Surgical and Conservative Foot Care. Thorofare, NJ, Slack, 1988, p 119.
2. Kargas DE: Plantar excision of primary interdigital neuromas. Foot Ankle 9:120, 1988.
3. Lankford LL, Thompson JE: Reflex sympathetic dystrophy, upper and lower extremity: Diagnosis and management. *In* Instructional Course Lectures, American Academy of Orthopaedic Surgeons, Vol 26. St. Louis, CV Mosby, 1977.
4. McElvenny RT: The etiology and surgical treatment of intractable pain about the fourth metatarsophalangeal joint (Morton's toe). J Bone Joint Surg 25:675, 1943.
5. McKeever DC: Surgical approach for neuroma of plantar digital nerve (Morton's metatarsalgia). J Bone Joint Surg 34A:490, 1952.
6. Mann RA: The tarsal tunnel syndrome. Orthop Clin North Am 5:109, 1974.
7. Mann RA: Surgery of the Foot, 5th Ed. St. Louis, CV Mosby, 1986, p 200.
8. Mann RA: Surgery of the Foot, 5th Ed. St. Louis, CV Mosby, 1986, p 203.
9. Mann RA, Reynolds JD: Interdigital neuroma. A critical clinical analysis. Foot Ankle 3:238, 1983.
10. Nissen KL: Plantar digital neuritis. J Bone Joint Surg 30B:84, 1948.

18 *Heel Pain Syndrome and Entrapment Neuropathies About the Foot and Ankle*

LEW C. SCHON
DONALD E. BAXTER

HEEL PAIN SYNDROME

Some of the confusion in diagnosing and treating heel pain stems from the complexity of the local anatomy. The causes of heel pain include seronegative arthritides, heel spur fracture, calcaneal stress fracture, plantar fasciitis, bursitis, complete or partial plantar fascia rupture, lumbosacral radiculopathy, and entrapment of the nerve to the abductor digiti quinti muscle. Often, several conditions coexist, which may further confuse the clinician.

Anatomy. The posterior tibial nerve ramifies into three branches: the calcaneal nerves, the lateral plantar nerve, and the medial plantar nerve (Fig. 18–1). Most commonly, the calcaneal nerve or nerves penetrate the laciniate ligament or pass below it and provide sensation to the skin of the posterior and posteromedial aspect of the heel. The posterior tibial nerve subsequently divides into the lateral plantar nerve and the medial plantar nerve in the retromalleolar region. These nerves are separated by a fibrous septum, which originates from the calcaneus and inserts onto the deep fascia of the abductor hallucis muscle. Just after it branches off from the posterior tibial nerve, the lateral plantar nerve has its first branch. This first branch courses between the deep fascia of the abductor hallucis muscle and the medial fascia of the quadratus plantae muscle (Fig. 18–2). After it passes the quadratus plantae, it changes direction and courses

laterally in a horizontal plane, first between the quadratus plantae and the flexor digitorum brevis and then between the flexor digitorum brevis and the os calcis.[54]

This first branch of the lateral plantar nerve has three major divisions (Fig. 18–3). Proximally, the nerve divides and provides sensation to the periosteum of the medial process of the calcaneal tuberosity. As the first branch passes dorsally to the flexor digitorum brevis, a branch of it innervates this muscle. Distally, the terminal branch is a mixed (sensorimotor) nerve that innervates the abductor digiti quinti muscle. The branch that provides sensation to the periosteum of the calcaneal tuberosity often innervates the long plantar ligament and occasionally innervates the quadratus plantae muscle.[4, 5, 24, 54]

The plantar fascia originates from the medial tubercle on the posterior tuberosity of the os calcis. It is plantar to the heel spur that is found by radiographic studies in both symptomatic and asymptomatic patients. The heel spur actually lies within the substance of the origin of the flexor digitorum brevis. The plantar fascia is quite thick and in its proximal aspect may measure 2 to 4 mm. It fuses posteromedially to the investing fascia of the abductor hallucis muscle.

Etiology. Heel pain syndrome may involve pathology of any of the anatomic structures in this region. The coexistence of several processes often cannot be excluded, even by an astute examiner. Chronic inflammation of the

192

FIGURE 18–1. The posterior tibial nerve divides into the calcaneal, lateral plantar, and medial plantar nerves.

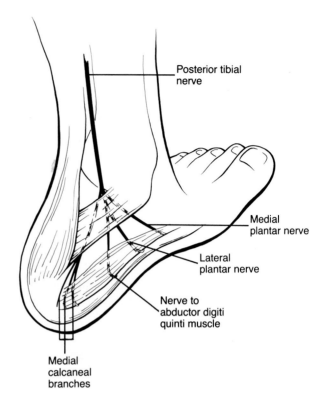

Posterior tibial nerve

Medial plantar nerve

Lateral plantar nerve

Nerve to abductor digiti quinti muscle

Medial calcaneal branches

fat pad of the heel may follow an acute traumatic event, such as a fall from a height with impaction of the heel, or may evolve from repetitive microinjury. In a shearing injury, the fat pad may actually separate from the calcaneus, with disruption of the complex fibrous septa and their compartments. Fat pad atrophy or insufficiency of the fat pad may be due to chronic diseases, hereditary predisposition, or the aging process.[28, 43]

Plantar fasciitis results from repetitive microtrauma to the plantar fascia at its origin on the medial calcaneal tuberosity. The plantar fascia is a stress-relieving structure that spans the bones and joints of the foot. With each step, forces are transmitted by the plantar

FIGURE 18–2. The first branch of the lateral plantar nerve courses between the abductor hallucis and the quadratus plantae and then runs laterally between the latter muscle and the flexor digitorum brevis.

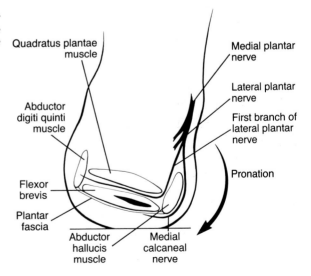

Quadratus plantae muscle

Medial plantar nerve

Lateral plantar nerve

First branch of lateral plantar nerve

Abductor digiti quinti muscle

Pronation

Flexor brevis

Plantar fascia

Abductor hallucis muscle

Medial calcaneal nerve

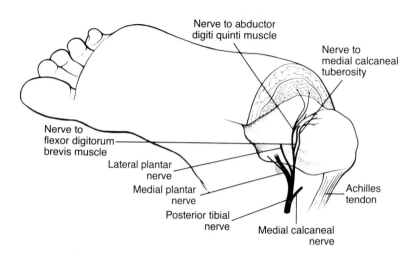

FIGURE 18–3. The first branch of the lateral plantar nerve divides into three major branches.

fascia, redistributing loads throughout the foot. Concentrated stress transfer occurs at the fascia-bone junction, making this region vulnerable to fatigue failure and microtears. Conceptually, the plantar fascia is like a rope attached to a plaster wall. With each pull on the rope, stresses are absorbed by the wall and rope at their junction. Eventually, fatiguing will occur, with cracking of the plaster or fraying of the rope at this interface. (This process is similar to that which occurs in lateral epicondylitis, or "tennis elbow.") Fortunately, unlike the conceptual model, the body has the capability to heal itself with either new bone or fibrous tissue. During this healing phase, repetitive insults lead to more inflammation and swelling. This accounts for the chronic nature of the condition. At times the entire plantar fascia can be involved, with progression from the heel into the midfoot region.

Acute ruptures of the plantar fascia may occur during rigorous athletic activity, but these injuries are rare.[35] Seronegative arthropathies may cause peritendinous or perifascial inflammatory conditions.[15, 17-19] These enthesopathies may involve the fat pad, the fascia of the surrounding muscles, the plantar fascia, or the periosteum. Periostitis of the medial calcaneal tuberosity, often demonstrated by a technetium scan, may be seen in seronegative arthropathy or degenerative insertional plantar fasciitis.[58, 71]

Heel pain may also be caused by either acute or stress fractures of the medial calcaneal tuberosity, the body of the calcaneus, or the heel spur.[1, 22, 51] Osteoporosis due to aging, metabolic disease, nutritional deficiencies, or endocrine imbalance predispose patients to these bone injuries.

The entrapment of the first branch of the lateral plantar nerve between the deep fascia of the abductor hallucis muscle and the medial caudal margin of the quadratus plantae muscle is also a cause of the heel pain syndrome.* This is an under-recognized condition that occurs concomitantly with other pathologic processes. Additionally, a "double-crush" syndrome, in which a more proximal nerve compression increases the susceptibility of the nerve to a more distal entrapment, may be noted in patients with this condition.[33, 49, 56, 58a, 69] Inflammatory processes and local edema may affect the nerve as it courses over the plantar side of the long plantar ligament or in the osteomuscular tunnel between the flexor digitorum brevis and the calcaneus. Heel pain may be partially or completely due to lumbosacral radiculopathy, sciatica, posterior tibial nerve compression by a popliteal cyst, or tarsal tunnel syndrome.

Other causes of heel pain include bursitis, phlebitis of the calcaneal venous plexus, bone and soft tissue tumors, infections, and foreign bodies.

History. Heel pain may be described as dull, aching, or sharp. It may have a neuritic component with radiation up the medial aspect of the leg or into the lateral aspect of the heel. The pain is typically exacerbated with walking, running, or prolonged standing, and it usually responds to rest and elevation of the feet. A neurologic cause may be suspected if the pain

---

*See references 4–6, 8, 25, 29, 38, 47, 52–54, and 67.

persists despite non–weight bearing and rest. A patient with inflammation around the plantar fascia from degenerative disease, seronegative enthesopathy, or venous stasis may have increased pain in the morning, which gradually wanes during the first few hours of activity. A history of back problems, radiculopathy, tarsal tunnel syndrome, diabetes, thyroid disease, and alcohol consumption should be noted.

Physical Examination. The key to successful diagnosis of the painful heel syndrome is a thorough knowledge of the regional anatomy. Patients with fat pad atrophy will have pain with palpation of their sparse subcutaneous tissues. Point tenderness may also be noted over the medial calcaneal tuberosity or more posteriorly in the center of the heel, although often more diffuse pain is found in this condition. Insertional plantar fasciitis causes maximal discomfort with palpation over the medial calcaneal tuberosity and the proximal 1 to 2 cm of the plantar fascia. Although dorsiflexing the toes may increase the pain in plantar fasciitis,[10, 26] it also increases the pain with flexor digitorum longus or flexor hallucis longus tendinitis. A stress fracture of the body of the calcaneus causes tenderness along the medial wall of the calcaneus, the lateral wall, or both.

Proximal and distal nerve entrapments should be excluded by palpation along the course of the tibial nerve and its branches. A neurologic examination including testing of motor nerves, sensory nerves, reflexes, and vibratory perception should be performed. The pathognomonic finding in patients with entrapment of the first branch of the lateral plantar nerve is point tenderness to palpation where the nerve courses deep to the abductor hallucis and over the quadratus plantae in the proximal medial aspect of the heel. This point is located at the junction of the plantar and medial skin approximately 5 cm anterior to the posterior border of the heel (Fig. 18–4). The neuritic symptomatology of burning, shooting, stabbing, tingling, electric, or sharp pain should be reproduced. At times, there is radiation of the pain proximally and distally with this maneuver. The tenderness is usually quite exquisite and causes a marked withdrawal response.

Diagnostic Tests. If properly placed, a local injection of 1-percent lidocaine with or without corticosteroid may relieve symptoms of plantar fasciitis or nerve entrapment. The needle

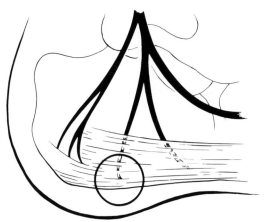

FIGURE 18–4. The point of maximum tenderness when the first branch is involved in the heel pain syndrome.

should be introduced medially along the junction of the medial and plantar skin approximately 4 to 5 cm anterior to the posterior aspect of the heel. It is directed laterally toward the medial process of the calcaneal tuberosity. In this manner, the periosteum, the first branch of the lateral plantar nerve, and the perifascial tissue can be infiltrated.

Radiographs of the heel should include a lateral and a posterior tangential view. Some authors have recommended oblique views to examine the anatomy more closely when a stress fracture is suspected. Bone scans findings are often positive with degenerative insertional plantar fasciitis, enthesopathies, or stress fractures of the calcaneus. Electrodiagnostic studies may also be helpful in further distinguishing between more proximal nerve compression syndromes and neuropathies.[58a]

Conservative Treatment. Conservative treatment should consist of a shock-absorbent heel cup or pad (Viscoheel, Hapad, or Tuli's), soft-soled shoes, contrast baths, deep massage, and anti-inflammatory agents. Patients with hypermobility and excessive pronation may benefit from a medial longitudinal arch support or a UCBL (University of California Biomechanics Laboratory) orthosis. In some cases, an orthosis designed with a heel well to relieve local pressures may be useful. In addition, 3/16-inch tapered heel elevations with or without medial heel wedges may be of benefit. As previously mentioned, an injection of local anesthesia with steroid may provide some relief.

Gastrocnemius stretching exercises should

be instituted three times a day for at least 4 weeks (stretching is especially important if there is a tight heel cord). Athletes, especially runners, are advised to decrease the duration of their workout for several weeks and then to increase their distances gradually. Cross-training varies stresses while permitting progressively strenuous activities. Changing running shoes and running surfaces should also reduce the symptoms. A minimum of 6 to 12 months of conservative treatment must be tried before surgery is considered. If the previously mentioned modalities are given a fair trial, the vast majority of patients will not require operative intervention.*

Surgical Treatment. Different surgical approaches addressing the painful heel syndrome have been proposed. There are advocates of medial, lateral, or plantar incisions with minimal, moderate, or extensile exposure. Some surgeons resect, some release, and some avoid the plantar fascia. Many resect the spur, whereas some do not. Some osteotomize the calcaneus, while others drill it. Various authors recommend releasing or resecting the calcaneal nerve or the first branch of the lateral plantar nerve.

Perhaps the most popular technique was described by DuVries[12] and by Steindler and Smith.[64] They advocated resecting the heel spur through a medial longitudinal incision parallel to the plantar fascia. In general, variable results have been reported with this tech-

---

*See references 1, 6–8, 10, 13–15, 29, 34, 41, 55, 61, and 62.

nique. The patients commonly experienced medial heel numbness postoperatively.[41, 62, 64]

Bateman recommended approaching the heel spur from the lateral side, thus avoiding the calcaneal nerves.[3] He resected the spur using a reciprocating saw, smoothed the region with a burr, and packed the area with surgical gauze to prevent spur recurrence.

Kenzora advocates a direct plantar approach via a midline longitudinal incision through the weight-bearing portion of the heel. He incises the plantar fascia longitudinally and reflects it off the medial tubercle. He resects the heel spur and then releases the first branch of the lateral plantar nerve. No attempt is made to repair the incised plantar fascia. He reported good or excellent results in six patients after a short follow-up.[29]

Authors' Preferred Surgical Approach. The patient is placed on the operating room table in the supine position. Ankle block anesthesia is most frequently used. Depending on the surgeon's discretion, a tourniquet may or may not be used. An oblique 4-cm incision is made over the medial aspect of the heel (Fig. 18–5). Blunt and sharp dissection is carried out down through the subcutaneous tissue, avoiding the occasional branches of the medial calcaneal nerve. The superficial fascia of the abductor hallucis muscle is divided, and the muscle is retracted superiorly. The medial edge of the plantar fascia is identified using a small periosteal elevator. A 3 × 5-mm rectangle of the plantar fascia is removed medially to facilitate exposure of the plantar spur and the first branch of the lateral plantar nerve (Fig. 18–

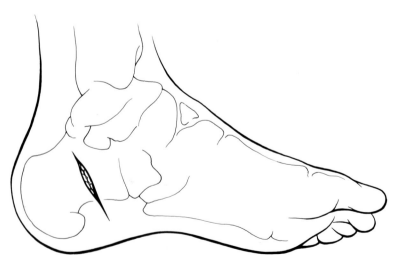

FIGURE 18–5. The medial incision.

FIGURE 18–6. Excision of a portion of the plantar fascia and deep fascia of the abductor hallucis.

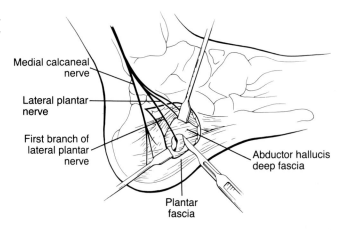

Medial calcaneal nerve

Lateral plantar nerve

First branch of lateral plantar nerve

Abductor hallucis deep fascia

Plantar fascia

6). The deep fascia of the abductor hallucis muscle is then incised where the first branch of the lateral plantar nerve courses over the quadratus plantae muscle (Fig. 18–7). When a heel spur is present, a Freer elevator is passed both plantar and dorsal to the spur. Because the spur commonly lies within the substance of the flexor digitorum brevis, a portion of this muscle is swept from the spur. Next, with an osteotome and a rongeur, the spur is removed. Throughout the procedure, careful dissection must be used to avoid cutting the vein or artery that may accompany the nerve. A small hemostat is used to palpate along the course of the nerve to ensure that it is free from any impingement proximally and distally. If the medial caudal border of the quadratus plantae is unyielding and prominent, this muscle is

released. Finally, the wound is closed with 4–0 interrupted horizontal mattress sutures. No deep sutures are used. A bulky compression dressing is applied.

Patients are allowed to begin weight bearing in a postoperative shoe as tolerated. Once the sutures are removed, patients may begin biking and swimming. At 4 weeks, patients start low-impact aerobic exercises as tolerated. Usually, by 5 to 8 weeks, athletes may begin running. In general, it takes patients 3 months to be able to resume full sports activities without symptomatology.

Complications and Pitfalls. Although Baxter and coworkers reported good or excellent results in the overwhelming majority of patients, certain pitfalls may occur.[4–6] Prolonged recovery periods may be seen in patients in

FIGURE 18–7. Release of the deep fascia of the abductor hallucis.

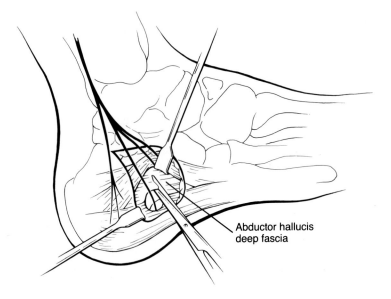

Abductor hallucis deep fascia

whom the venous plexus is disrupted. Therefore, it is imperative that the surgeon use gentle blunt dissection and at least 2.5-power magnification. Resection of more than one-third of the plantar fascia may also prolong the recovery time. All efforts should be made to avoid cutting the calcaneal branches of the posterior tibial nerve or the first branch of the lateral plantar nerve itself because this may lead to painful neuromas. Additionally, some patients develop a reflex sympathetic dysfunction or dystrophy after release of the nerve, even with the most gentle surgical technique. This is typically associated with a poorer prognosis.

On a long-term basis, some patients (usually long-distance runners) who have had partial or complete resection of the plantar fascia can develop a strain of the lateral aspect of the arch. This condition is caused by excessive resultant stress on the remaining plantar fascia or on midtarsal or hindfoot bones or joints. Although no permanent deleterious consequences have been noted, this lateral arch sprain may take several months to resolve. Often a well-molded, high-density Plastizote medial longitudinal arch support is necessary. In some cases, a short-leg cast may be applied for 2 to 6 weeks to successfully eliminate this pain.

SUPERFICIAL PERONEAL NERVE ENTRAPMENT

Although entrapment of the superficial peroneal nerve commonly occurs after trauma or surgical procedures, a less well known nerve entrapment exists where the nerve pierces the deep fascia of the lateral or occasionally the anterior compartment.

Anatomy. The common peroneal nerve branches into the superficial peroneal nerve, which courses through the anterolateral compartment of the leg. After innervating the peroneus brevis and longus, it travels between the anterior intermuscular septum and the fascia of the lateral compartment. The nerve usually pierces the deep fascia approximately 10.5 to 12.5 cm above the tip of the lateral malleolus. Subsequently, it divides into the intermediate dorsocutaneous nerve and the medial dorsocutaneous nerve at approximately 6.4 cm above the lateral malleolus. The division of the superficial peroneal nerve occasionally occurs more proximally, and the nerve

may pierce the fascia at different locations. In this case, the medial dorsocutaneous nerve pierces the fascia at approximately 13 cm proximal to the tip of the fibula, and the intermediate dorsocutaneous nerve pierces the fascia at 5 cm proximal to this site. The intermediate branch provides sensation to the dorsolateral aspect of the ankle and to portions of the third, fourth, and fifth toes. The medial dorsocutaneous nerve provides sensation over the dorsomedial aspect of the ankle and the medial aspect of the hallux, as well as over the second and third toes.[57]

Etiology. According to clinical and anatomic studies, the superficial peroneal nerve becomes entrapped at its point of exit from the deep fascia. In most cases, the fascial edge impinges on the nerve. Fascial defects often lead to muscle herniation, which may further compromise the nerve. Styf observed that the nerve coursed within a low-compliance fibrotic tunnel between the fascia of the lateral compartment in the anterior muscular septum in nearly half of his patients.[66] He postulated that this predisposed them to the syndrome. Chronic lateral ankle instability is another etiologic factor, because it causes recurrent stretching of the nerve (Fig. 18–8). The nerve may also be stretched when the fascia shifts after an anterior compartment fasciotomy.

History. Patients with superficial peroneal nerve entrapment may complain of other foot and ankle problems that misdirect the clinician's attention away from this smoldering neuropathy. Frequently, patients recall several years of pain over the lateral ankle and the dorsum of the foot. Only one-third, however, have numbness or paresthesias along the distribution of the nerve. In some cases, patients only note vague pain at the junction of the middle and distal third of the leg, which may or may not be associated with local swelling. Physical activity ranging from walking, jogging, running, or squatting may exacerbate the condition. Nocturnal pain is atypical. Although rest and avoidance of the offending activity often relieve the symptoms, leg crossing with the lateral aspect of the affected leg pressed against the contralateral knee induces symptoms. When the activities are resumed, symptoms recur. A quarter of the patients have a history of previous ankle sprain or trauma.* It is important to distinguish between an entrapment neuropathy and a direct nerve injury.

---

*See references 2, 30, 37, 39, 59, 63, and 66.

FIGURE 18–8. Superficial peroneal nerve entrapment is associated with a history of ankle sprain.

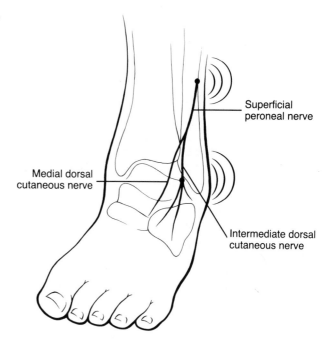

Superficial peroneal nerve

Medial dorsal cutaneous nerve

Intermediate dorsal cutaneous nerve

Physical Examination. As with all nerve entrapment syndromes, examination should take into consideration the entire course of the nerve. This includes examination of the lower back, the sciatic notch, and the common peroneal nerve where it courses around the neck of the fibula. Typically, point tenderness is found approximately 10.5 to 12.5 cm above the distal fibula. Roughly 60 percent of patients will also have a palpable fascial defect with or without a muscle bulge in this location (Fig. 18–9). Palpation or percussion may cause radiation of the pain proximally and distally with or without paresthesias and numbness. Exacerbations of the symptoms may be noted when the patient actively dorsiflexes and everts the foot against resistance while the nerve is percussed or palpated. The symptoms may also be elicited with passive plantar flexion and inversion of the foot with and without percussion along the course of the nerve. Decreased sensation with light touch and pinprick is not common.

Diagnostic Tests. Most cases are confirmed without the need for electrodiagnostic testing. In Styf's series, conduction velocities were often diminished in symptomatic legs.[66] Compartment pressures before and after exercise may be recorded in cases of suspected lateral compartment syndrome. A local injection of anesthetic in the region of compression is useful in establishing the diagnosis.

Differential Diagnosis. The differential diagnosis of entrapment of the superficial peroneal nerve includes lateral compartment syndrome, varicose veins, stress fracture of the fibula or tibia, peroneal muscle sprain, herniated disk, bony entrapment of the superficial peroneal nerve following fracture, and ischemic pain secondary to atheromatous disease.* A soft tissue tumor may also compress the nerve or one of its branches (Fig. 18–10). Neuropathy of the common peroneal nerve has been well described and may occur in athletes after injuries to the lateral collateral and anterior cruciate ligaments.[23, 45, 60, 68, 70] It also may occur following direct trauma to the nerve in its vulnerable position superficial to the fibula.

Conservative Treatment. Any underlying associated injury should be treated symptomatically, and this treatment may result in resolution of the syndrome. Avoidance of the offending activity is important. Injections of steroid and local anesthetic are effective approximately 25 percent of the time. Most cases resolve or become less symptomatic with alteration of activity or adequate rest.

Surgical Treatment. Some controversy surrounds the ideal method of treatment. Styf treated his patients with complete fasciotomy

---

*See references 2, 16, 30, 37, 39, 40, 44, 63, 65, and 66.

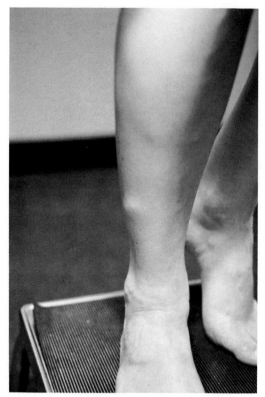

FIGURE 18–9. A 29-year-old female runner with muscle herniation and superficial peroneal nerve entrapment.

Koons[2] all reported that limited fasciotomy gave excellent results in their six patients. The latter agrees with our experience.

Authors' Preferred Surgical Approach. Prior to the operation, the physician must note the exact distance from the tip of the distal fibula to the area of compression. The patient is positioned in the supine position, and a 4- to 8-cm incision is made over the point of maximal tenderness (Fig. 18–11). Blunt and sharp dissection is carried out down to the fascia, and the nerve is identified as it pierces through the fascia. The fascia is released both proximally and distally until the nerve is able to move back and forth freely. The skin is then closed with a nylon suture, and a light compression dressing is applied. Postoperatively, the patient is encouraged to walk as tolerated. Range-of-motion exercises of the foot and ankle are encouraged. The patient can usually progress rapidly to high-impact activities. However, prolonged intense activity may be limited for several months.

Complications and Pitfalls. Perhaps the most difficult part of this operation is determining the extent of release. A complete fasciotomy as advocated by Styf and others may leave the patient with some peroneal muscle weakness.[66] However, unless the patient is an athlete, it is unlikely to be a significant problem. If too limited a fasciotomy is performed, the nerve may become compressed by a new fascial edge proximally. One final pitfall is failure to recognize a more distal piercing of the fascia by the intermediate dorsocutaneous nerve. Thus, it is imperative preoperatively to note the exact point of nerve entrapment.

of the lateral compartment and reported that only nine of the 19 patients were completely satisfied, although 13 of the 19 had increased physical ability and decreased pain.[66] Mackey and colleagues reported excellent results in six patients treated with neurolysis.[40] Kernohan and colleagues,[30] Lowdon,[37] and Banerjee and

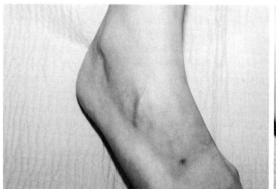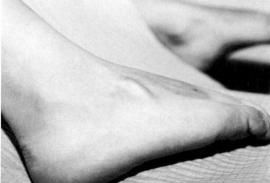

FIGURE 18–10. A 26-year-old female tennis player with compression of the intermediate dorsocutaneous nerve secondary to a subcutaneous mass.

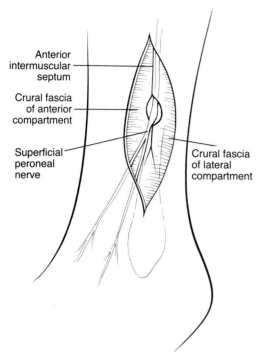

FIGURE 18–11. Superficial peroneal nerve penetrating the fascia of the lateral compartment.

In cases of superficial peroneal nerve entrapment that occur following direct or indirect nerve trauma (i.e., crush or stretch injuries), especially in association with a neurologic deficit, a postoperative neuritis may ensue. Occasionally, a reinnervation causalgia or frank reflex sympathetic dystrophy may develop. These patients often require aggressive medical management consisting of tricyclic antidepressants, alpha-adrenergic blockers, analgesics, or a combination of these agents, in conjunction with local nerve blocks, sympathetic nerve blocks, and physical therapy. Recovery may take several months to years.

DEEP PERONEAL NERVE ENTRAPMENT

The deep peroneal nerve entrapment syndrome has been commonly labeled the *anterior tarsal tunnel syndrome.* Although this name is "catchy," it does not specify the particular point of nerve compression. Several sites of entrapment may exist and must be identified.

Anatomy. The deep peroneal nerve lies between the extensor hallucis longus and the tibialis anticus in the middle third of the leg.

At approximately 3 to 5 cm above the ankle joint, it travels between the extensor digitorum longus and the extensor hallucis longus. Approximately 1 cm above the ankle joint, the motor division to the extensor digitorum brevis branches off the nerve. The medial division continues along the dorsalis pedis artery, running superficial to the talonavicular joint. While running between the extensor hallucis brevis and the tendon of the extensor hallucis longus, it courses over the middle cuneiform and the bases of the first and second metatarsals. Thereafter, it courses along the lateral border of the first metatarsal, passing deep to the extensor hallucis brevis. Once it pierces the dorsal aponeurosis of the foot, it supplies sensation to the web space and the adjacent borders of the first and second toes (Fig. 18–12).[57]

Etiology. Entrapment of the deep peroneal nerve may occur in several areas. Most commonly, the nerve is compressed underneath the oblique inferior medial band of the inferior extensor retinaculum. Prominent ridges of the talonavicular joint often contribute to compression in this location (Fig. 18–13). A more

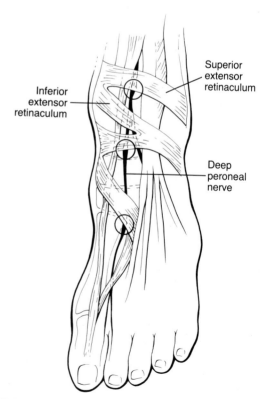

FIGURE 18–12. The deep peroneal nerve may be entrapped in several locations along its course.

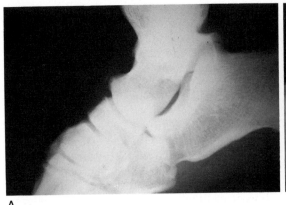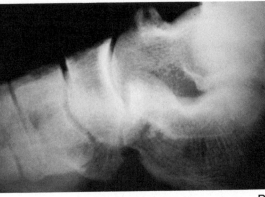

A   B

FIGURE 18–13. (*A*), A 19-year-old college sprinter with entrapment of the deep peroneal nerve secondary to a talonavicular osteophyte and capsular calcification. (*B*), A 35-year-old runner with deep peroneal nerve entrapment secondary to a talar osteophyte.

proximal entrapment may occur under the superior edge of the inferior retinaculum where the extensor hallucis longus crosses over the nerve.[9, 31, 42] Distally, the nerve may be entrapped under the oblique tendon of the extensor hallucis brevis.[31] Hypertrophic ridges of the first or second metatarsal–cuneiform joints or an os intermetatarseum may also be responsible for compression syndromes.[47] Recurrent episodes of ankle sprain with the foot in supination and plantar flexion stretch the nerve over the talonavicular joint.[9] Repetitive blows to the dorsum of the foot or tight-fitting shoes or boots may cause nerve entrapment as well.[20, 32, 36, 42] External compression may also occur in joggers who wear keys under the tongue of their running shoes or from sit-up bars.[59] Excessive stretch on the nerve may also result from osteophytes of the distal tibia, talus, navicular, cuneiforms, or metatarsal bases. Although we have seen cases of stretch neurapraxia that began following arthroscopy, direct nerve trauma is a more frequent cause in these situations.

History. Entrapment of the deep peroneal nerve often causes pain on the dorsal aspect of the foot. Occasionally, there is radiation to the first web space. Often pain will be noted when the patient is wearing certain types of shoes or boots. The pain usually resolves with rest and removal of any constricting apparatus. A history of injury or ankle sprain is often elicited. It is imperative to determine whether the symptoms began following a crush or a more violent neurologic insult because these conditions carry a more guarded prognosis than the entrapment syndromes.

Physical Examination. After palpation prox-

imally along the course of the nerve, beginning at the common peroneal nerve, the specific site of entrapment distally must be identified. The pain may be exacerbated with extremes of foot and ankle positioning. Occasionally, diminished sensation is found in the first web space. When the entrapment occurs above the ankle joint, the extensor digitorum brevis may be weak or atrophied. Vague tenderness in the anterior compartment with or without swelling should alert the clinician to the possibility of exertional compartment syndrome or, infrequently, to causalgia.

Diagnostic Tests. Injection of a local anesthetic in the area of entrapment may be useful. Electromyography and nerve conduction velocity testing can distinguish between compressions proximal or distal to the ankle. Radiographs of the ankle and hindfoot are imperative because accessory bones, osteophytes, or other bony abnormalities may be present.

Differential Diagnosis. The most critical aspect of evaluating deep peroneal nerve compression is excluding compression of the common peroneal nerve. The latter entity has been well described in the literature. Compression of the common peroneal nerve has been associated with venous pathology, knee operations, ankle sprains, direct trauma, ganglions, Baker's cysts, cross-legged sitting, and instability of the proximal tibiofibular joint.[23, 31, 45, 60, 68, 70] Subtalar pathology may produce a poorly characterized pain that may mimic a deep peroneal nerve entrapment. In this case, injection of local anesthetic into the subtalar joint is helpful.[31]

Conservative Treatment. The condition usually responds to rest and the elimination of external factors that precipitate the syndrome. Padding may be applied along the course of the nerve to alleviate compression from shoes or straps. Injection of a local anesthetic combined with a steroid may be successful. When an external factor is not responsible and the patient does not respond to conservative modalities, surgery is often warranted.

Surgical Treatment. The patient is placed in the supine position on the operating room table. An ankle block or general or regional anesthesia is used, and a dorsal incision is made over the point of entrapment. Over the ankle joint, a gentle S-incision is used. If two areas of entrapment are expected, two incisions are used: one at the ankle and the other over the midfoot. It is important when approaching the nerve not to confuse the dorsomedial cutaneous branch of the superficial peroneal nerve with the deep peroneal nerve. The inferior extensor retinaculum is incised, and bony prominences are resected. Occasionally, the extensor hallucis brevis tendon requires excision. Postoperatively, the patient is placed in a light compression dressing and is allowed to begin partial weight bearing after 1 week. After 2 weeks, the patient may begin swimming and water workouts. Low-impact exercises may be resumed by 4 weeks, with gradual return to full activity by 8 weeks.

Complications and Pitfalls. Cases involving crush injuries or direct neurologic trauma may in certain individuals result in postoperative causalgia or reflex sympathetic dystrophy. Bowstringing of the extensor tendons may result from overly aggressive retinacular release. Neuritis or painful neuroma can follow inadvertent injury of the dorsomedial cutaneous nerve.

SURAL NERVE ENTRAPMENT

Most typically, sural nerve entrapment occurs following a specific trauma or surgical procedure. A discrete but uncommon entity of sural nerve entrapment over the posterolateral border of the Achilles tendon has also been identified.[27, 59]

Anatomy. The medial sural nerve branches off the tibial nerve in the popliteal fascia. It penetrates the deep aponeurosis of the gastrocnemius in the midportion of the leg. In 40 to 80 percent of the population, the medial

sural nerve is joined by an anastomotic branch of the lateral sural nerve, which originates from the common peroneal nerve. In the lower third of the leg, the sural nerve runs along the border of the Achilles tendon, and at various points it crosses over the posterolateral edge of the tendon. It begins to ramify above the ankle joint, supplying sensation to the lateral heel and occasionally anastomosing with the intermediate dorsocutaneous nerve. Typically, the nerve courses inferior to the peroneal sheaths in a subcutaneous manner. It branches distally, providing sensation to the lateral aspect of the foot and occasionally to the fourth and fifth toes.[57]

Etiology. The sural nerve is particularly vulnerable to entrapment following fractures of the calcaneus or fifth metatarsal.[21, 50, 59] Nerve entrapment may result from recurrent ankle sprains with secondary fibrosis around the nerve.[11, 50] Ganglions originating from the calcaneocuboid joint or the peroneal sheaths have been reported.[50] Compression by myositis ossificans circumscripta at the musculotendinous junction of the Achilles tendon has been reported.[27] Similarly, Achilles tendinitis with nerve entrapment over the posterolateral edge of the tendon must also be considered (Figs. 18–14 and 18–15).[59]

History. Characteristically, a history of bone or soft tissue injury is obtained. Shooting pains and paresthesias are quite common with sural nerve entrapment. Often shoes or straps may exacerbate the condition.

Physical Examination. Both the medial and lateral sural nerves should be examined from their proximal origins. A point of local tenderness with or without a positive Tinel sign is frequently noted. Decreased sensation and numbness can usually be detected.

Diagnostic Tests. Radiographs must be obtained to rule out fracture or bony residuals of trauma. Myositis ossificans at the posterior aspect of the Achilles tendon may also be found. The use of electrodiagnostic testing has not been reported with this entrapment syndrome. Injection of local anesthetic is valuable in identifying the point of entrapment.

Differential Diagnosis. The differential diagnosis includes more proximal nerve entrapments in the popliteal space. Rarely, a lateral plantar nerve entrapment may resemble entrapment of the sural nerve. Recognition of direct nerve injury or diffuse peripheral neuropathy is critical. Electrodiagnostic studies may be helpful in these situations.

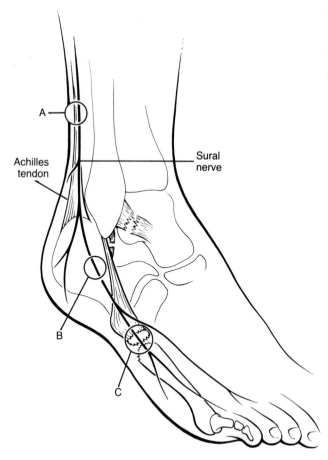

FIGURE 18–14. The sural nerve may be entrapped at several sites. A, entrapment from myositis ossificans circumscripta or the edge of the Achilles tendon; B, entrapment from chronic ankle instability or calcaneal fracture; C, entrapment from fifth metatarsal fracture.

Conservative Treatment. Conservative treatment consisting of rest, the application of ice, nonsteroidal anti-inflammatory drugs, transcutaneous electrical nerve stimulation, and local injection of steroid may be tried. When the entrapment is mechanical in etiology (i.e., a bony prominence compressing the nerve), release may be necessary.

Surgical Treatment. The patient is placed on the operative table in the supine position. A large bolster is placed under the ipsilateral buttock to rotate the foot internally. The incision should be made over the region of presumed entrapment. In the region of the ankle joint, beginning approximately 5 cm above the tip of the lateral malleolus, the first branches of the nerve may be encountered. All efforts should be made to preserve these branches. The lesser saphenous vein is often encountered superficial to the nerve. Once the area of aponeurotic, fibrotic, or bony impingement is relieved, the nerve sometimes may be transferred away from the area of pathology. The wound is then closed with nylon suture. A light compression dressing is applied. Occasionally, we use a short-leg cast for the first 2 weeks to prevent any inadvertent inversion injuries during the period of recovery.

If inadequate soft tissue protection is present at the site of entrapment, it may be prudent to excise the nerve and bury it in bone or more proximally in muscle. This is especially useful in locations that are subjected to compression from shoes.

Complications and Pitfalls. Postoperative neuritis, neuroma, causalgia, or reflex sympathetic dystrophy may occur.

SAPHENOUS NERVE ENTRAPMENT

The femoral nerve terminates in the saphenous nerve and runs alongside the superficial femoral artery in the lower third of the thigh.

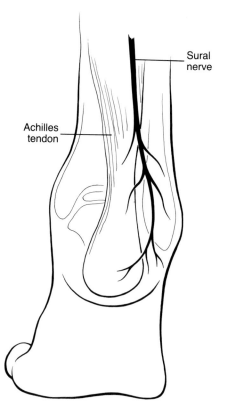

FIGURE 18–15. Entrapment of the sural nerve over the posterolateral edge of the Achilles tendon.

It enters Hunter's canal and pierces the subsartorial fascia approximately 10 cm proximal to the medial femoral condyle. Frequently, the nerve branches just before it courses through the fascia, dividing into an infrapatellar branch and a descending branch. The descending branch is subcutaneous and courses posterior to the medial border of the tibia in conjunction with the greater saphenous vein. At approximately 15 cm from the medial malleolus, it branches into two terminal divisions, one of which provides sensation at the medial aspect of the ankle and the other of which provides sensation to the medial side of the foot (Fig. 18–16).[31, 46, 57, 72]

Etiology. Saphenous nerve entrapment occurs where the nerve leaves Hunter's canal. Hyperextension of the knee and torsional forces may play a role in the development of this syndrome. In one series, 67 percent of these entrapments were associated with previous knee surgery.[72] Mozes and colleagues reported a high correlation with vascular dis-

ease.[46] Kopell and Thompson found that genu varum, internal tibial torsion, and obesity are etiologic factors.[31] Saphenous vein stripping or harvesting of a vein graft may directly injure the nerve but rarely causes entrapment neuropathy. In one series, neurologic symptoms occurred in 12.5 percent of patients after stripping of the vein.[48]

History. Patients complain of medial knee, leg, or foot pain. It is exacerbated by prolonged walking, standing, and quadriceps exercises. The pain is often burning in character and may occur at night. Symptoms of intermittent claudication with fatigue and heaviness of the leg may also be present.[46] A history of knee injury is common.

Kopell and Thompson reported on a group of patients who presented with symptoms of both saphenous nerve entrapment and interdigital neuroma.[31] They postulated that patients' avoidance of knee extension resulted in a flexed posture that effectively shortened the limb. This necessitated walking with the foot plantarflexed. The subsequent development of the interdigital neuroma was due to the hyperextension of the metatarsophalangeal joints.

Physical Examination. Point tenderness over Hunter's canal approximately 10 cm above the medial femoral condyle is characteristic. Patients may or may not have sensory changes. Hyperextension of the thigh may cause the pain to radiate down the leg.

Diagnostic Tests. Anesthetic block at the area of entrapment is often diagnostic. Electrodiagnostic testing has not been reported in this syndrome.

Differential Diagnosis. The differential diagnosis of saphenous nerve entrapment should include chronic venous insufficiency, phlebitis, proximal nerve root compression, arterial diseases, and arthrosis of the hip or knee.[46] Many cases are misdiagnosed as patellofemoral disorder or chondromalacia patellae.

Conservative Treatment. Mozes and colleagues reported that 12 of 32 patients responded to local anesthetic and corticosteroid injections.[46] Worth and colleagues[72] and Kopell and Thompson[31] were unable to successfully treat this condition with injections.

Surgical Treatment. The patient should be placed in the supine position. Under general endotracheal anesthesia or spinal anesthesia, a 10-cm incision is made along the anterior border of the sartorius muscle in the lower

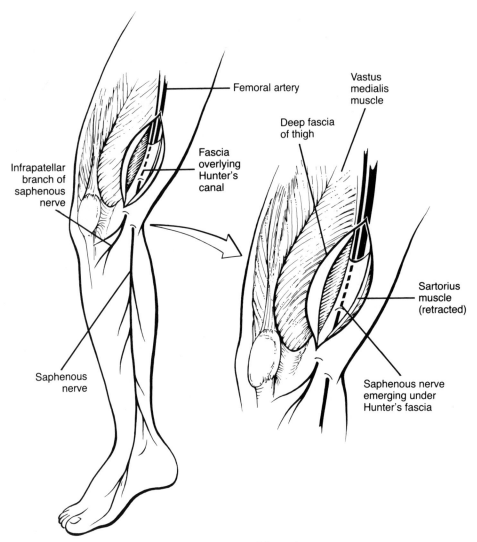

FIGURE 18–16. The course of the saphenous nerve.

third of the thigh. The fibrous roof of Hunter's canal is released, freeing up the perforating nerves.[31, 46] If preoperative symptoms are primarily in the inferior medial aspect of the knee, a neurectomy may be advisable. Worth and coworkers recommended resecting a segment, applying a ligature, and treating the proximal end of the nerve with alcohol.[72]

References

1. Amis J, Jennings L, Graham O, et al: Painful heel syndrome: Radiographic and treatment assessment. Foot Ankle 9:91, 1988.
2. Banerjee T, Koons DD: Superficial peroneal nerve entrapment: Report of two cases. J Neurosurg 55:991, 1981.
3. Bateman JE: The adult heel. *In* Jahss MH (Ed): Disorders of the Foot and Ankle, Vol 2, 2nd Ed. Philadelphia, WB Saunders, 1992, p 1372.
4. Baxter DE, Pfeffer GB: Treatment of chronic heel pain by surgical release of the first branch of the lateral plantar nerve. Submitted for publication.
5. Baxter DE, Pfeffer GB, Thigpen M: Chronic heel pain treatment rationale. Orthop Clin North Am 20:563, 1989.
6. Baxter DE, Thigpen CM: Heel pain: Operative results. Foot Ankle 5:16, 1984.
7. Blockley MJ: Painful heel, controlled trail of value of hydrocortisone. Br Med J 1:1277, 1956.
8. Bordelon RL: Subcalcaneal pain: A method of evaluation and plan for treatment. Clin Orthop 177:49, 1983.
9. Borges LF, Halle HM, Selkoe DJ, Welch K: The anterior tarsal tunnel syndrome: Report of two cases. J Neurosurg 54:89, 1981.
10. Campbell JW, Inman VT: Treatment of plantar fas-

ciitis and calcaneal spurs with the UCBL shoe insert. Clin Orthop 103:57, 1974.

11. Colbert DS, Cunningham F, Mackey D: Sural nerve entrapment: Case report. J Ir Med Assoc 68:544, 1975.
12. DuVries HL: Heel spurs (calcaneal spurs). Arch Surg 74:536, 1957.
13. Eggers GWN: Shoe pad for treatment of common painful conditions of the foot. J Bone Joint Surg 39A:219, 1957.
14. Freidberg JA: The diagnosis and treatment of common painful conditions of the foot. Instr Course Lect 14:238, 1957.
15. Furey JG: Plantar fasciitis. J Bone Joint Surg 57A:672, 1975.
16. Garfin S, Mubarak SJ, Owen CA: Exertional anterolateral compartment syndrome: Case report with fascial defect, muscle herniation, and superficial peroneal nerve entrapment. J Bone Joint Surg 59A:404, 1977.
17. Gerster JC: Plantar fasciitis and Achilles' tendinitis among 150 cases of seronegative spondarthritis. Rheum Rehabil 19:218, 1980.
18. Gerster JC, Vischer T, Bennani A, Fallet G: The painful heel. Ann Rheum Dis 36:343, 1977.
19. Gerster JC, Piccinin P: Enthesopathy of the heel in juvenile onset seronegative B-27 positive spondyloarthropathy. J Rheumatol 12:310, 1985.
20. Gessini L, Jandolo B, Peitrangel A: The anterior tarsal tunnel syndrome: Report of four cases. J Bone Joint Surg 66A:786, 1984.
21. Gould N, Trevino S: Sural nerve entrapment by avulsion fracture at the base of the fifth metatarsal bone. Foot Ankle 2:153, 1981.
22. Graham CE: Painful heel syndrome: Rationale of diagnosis and treatment. Foot Ankle 3:261, 1983.
23. Haimovici H: Peroneal sensory neuropathy entrapment syndrome. Arch Surg 105:586, 1972.
24. Heimkes B, Posel P, Stotz S, Wolf K: The proximal and distal tarsal tunnel syndromes: An anatomic study. Int Orthop 11:193, 1987.
25. Henricson AS, Westlin NE: Chronic calcaneal pain in athletes: Entrapment of the calcaneal nerve? Am J Sports Med 12:152, 1984.
26. Hicks JH: The plantar aponeurosis and the arch. J Anat 88:25, 1954.
27. Husson JL, Blouet JM, Masse A: Le syndrome du de file de 1 aponevrose superficielle posterieure surale. Int Orthop 11:245, 1987.
28. Jorgensen U: Achillodynia and loss of heel pad shock absorbency. Am J Sports Med 13:128, 1985.
29. Kenzora JE: The painful heel syndrome: An entrapment neuropathy. Bull Hosp Jt Dis Orthop Inst 47:178, 1987.
30. Kernohan J, Levack B, Wilson JN: Entrapment of the superficial peroneal nerve: Three case reports. J Bone Joint Surg 67B:60, 1985.
31. Kopell HP, Thompson WAL: Peripheral Entrapment Neuropathies. Malabar, FL, RE Krieger Publishing Company, 1976.
32. Krause KH, Witt T, Ross A: The anterior tarsal tunnel syndrome. J Neurol 217:67, 1977.
33. Kupersmith MJ, Lieberman AN, Sphielholz N: Neuropathy with susceptibility to compression aggravated by herniated disc. Arch Neurol 36:645, 1979.
34. Lapidus PW, Guidotti FP: Painful heel: Report of three hundred twenty-three patients with three

hundred sixty-four painful heels. Clin Orthop 39:178, 1965.
35. Leach R, Jones R, Silva T: Rupture of the plantar fascia in athletes. J Bone Joint Surg 60A:537, 1978.
36. Lindenbaum BL: Ski boot compression syndrome. Clin Orthop 140:19, 1979.
37. Lowdon IMR: Superficial peroneal nerve entrapment: A case report. J Bone Joint Surg 67B:58, 1985.
38. Lutter LD: Surgical decisions in athletes' subcalcaneal pain. Am J Sports Med 14:481, 1986.
39. McAuliffe TB, Fiddian NJ, Browett JP: Entrapment neuropathy of the superficial peroneal nerve: A bilateral case. J Bone Joint Surg 67B:62, 1985.
40. Mackey D, Colbert DS, Chater EH: Musculocutaneous nerve entrapment. Ir J Med Sci 146:100, 1977.
41. Mann RA, Baxter DE, Lutter LL: Running symposium. Foot Ankle 1:191, 1981.
42. Marinacci AA: Neurological syndrome of the tarsal tunnels. Bull LA Neurol Soc 33:98, 1968.
43. Miller WE: The heel pad. Am J Sports Med 10:19, 1982.
44. Mino DE, Hughes EC: Bony entrapment of the superficial peroneal nerve. Clin Orthop 185:203, 1984.
45. Moller BN, Kadin S: Entrapment of the common peroneal nerve. Am J Sports Med 15:90, 1987.
46. Mozes M, Oukmine G, Nathan H: Saphenous nerve entrapment simulating vascular disorder. Surgery 77:299, 1975.
47. Murphy PC, Baxter DE: Nerve entrapment of the foot and ankle in runners. Clin Sports Med 4:753, 1987.
48. Negus D: Should the incontinent saphenous veins be stripped down to the ankle? Phlebologie 40:753, 1987.
49. Nemoto K, Matsumoto N, Tazaki K, et al: An experimental study on the "double crush" hypothesis. J Hand Surg 12A:552, 1987.
50. Pringle RM, Protheroe K, Mukherjee SK: Entrapment neuropathy of the sural nerve. J Bone Joint Surg 56B: 465, 1974.
51. Protzman RR, Griffs CG: Stress fracture in men and women undergoing military training. J Bone Joint Surg 59A:825, 1977.
52. Przyluki H, Jones CL: Entrapment neuropathy of muscle branch of the lateral plantar nerve. J Am Podiatr Med Assoc 71:119, 1981.
53. Roegholt MN: Een nervus calcaneus inferior als overbrenger, Van de pijn bij calcaneodynie of calcaneuss poor en de daaruit volgend therapie. Ned Tijdschr Geneeskd 84:1898, 1940.
54. Rondhuis JJ, Huson A: The first branch of the lateral plantar nerve and heel pain. Acta Morphol Neerl Scand 24:269, 1986.
55. Rubin G, Witten M: Plantar calcaneal spurs. Am J Orthop 5:38, 1963.
56. Saal JA, Dillingham MF, Gamburd RS, Fanton GS: The pseudoradicular syndrome: Lower extremity peripheral nerve entrapment masquerading as lumbar radiculopathy. Spine 13:926, 1988.
57. Sarrafian SK: Anatomy of the Foot and Ankle. Philadelphia, JB Lippincott, 1983.
58. Sewell JR, Black CM, Chapman AH, et al: Quantitative scintigraphy in diagnosis and management of plantar fasciitis (calcaneal periostitis): Concise communication. J Nucl Med 21:633, 1980.
58a. Schon LC, Glennon TC, Baxter DE: Heel pain syndrome: Electrodiagnostic support for nerve entrapment. Foot Ankle, in press.

59. Schon LC, Baxter DE: Neuropathies of the foot and ankle in athletes. Clin Sports Med 9:489, 1990.
60. Sidey JD: Weak ankles: A study of common peroneal entrapment neuropathy. Br Med J 3:623, 1969.
61. Snook GA, Chrisman DO: The management of sub-calcaneal pain. Clin Orthop 82:163, 1972.
62. Spiegl PV, Johnson KA: Heel pain syndrome: Which treatment to choose? J Musculoskeletal Med 1:66, 1984.
63. Sridhara CR, Izzo KL: Terminal sensory branches of the superficial peroneal nerve: An entrapment syndrome. Arch Phys Med Rehabil 66:789, 1985.
64. Steindler A, Smith AR: Spurs of the os calcis. Surg Gynecol Obstet 66:663, 1938.
65. Styf J: Diagnosis of exercise-induced pain in the anterior aspect of the lower leg. Am J Sports Med 16:165, 1988.
66. Styf J: Entrapment of the superficial peroneal nerve: Diagnosis and results of decompression. J Bone Joint Surg 71B:131, 1989.
67. Tanz SS: Heel pain. Clin Orthop 288:169, 1963.
68. Turco VJ, Spinella AJ: Anterolateral dislocation of the head of the fibula in sports. Am J Sports Med 13:209, 1985.
69. Upton RM, McComas AJ: The double crush syndrome in nerve entrapment syndromes. Lancet 2:359, 1973.
70. Vastamaki M: Decompression for peroneal nerve entrapment. Acta Orthop Scand 57:551, 1986.
71. William PL, Smibert JG, Cox R, et al: Imaging study of the painful heel syndrome. Foot Ankle 7:345, 1987.
72. Worth RM, Kettelkamp DB, Defalque RJ, et al: Saphenous nerve entrapment: A cause of knee pain. Am J Sports Med 12:80, 1984.

19

Surgical Treatment and Reconstruction of the Diabetic Foot

JAMES W. BRODSKY

Four basic underlying conditions in the diabetic foot lead to clinical problems requiring surgical reconstruction. Basic comprehension of these conditions is essential to proper surgical care. These conditions are neuropathy, ischemia, infection, and deformity.

The first of these conditions, neuropathy, is the most important underlying cause of diabetic foot problems. Sensory neuropathy is the most significant because the insensitivity allows occult injury, often of devastating proportions, to occur without the patient's knowledge. However, autonomic and motor neuropathies also contribute to the pathophysiology of diabetic foot lesions. Autonomic neuropathy leads to dryness and loss of skin flexibility. Cracking and fissuring lead to loss of the normal protective barrier of the skin, and these openings are portals for infection in the diabetic foot. Motor neuropathy, usually expressed as clawing of the toes, is the presumed result of dysfunction of the intrinsic muscles of the foot. The hyperextended metatarsophalangeal joint of clawed toes increases the downward pressure against the metatarsal head, thus exacerbating the classic neurotrophic ulceration in the forefoot of the diabetic patient.

Second, ischemia plays a major role in the creation of diabetic foot lesions. The presence of a painful lesion or condition of the foot in a patient with significant insensitivity, especially one who has already developed neuropathic ulceration, is a sign of ischemia. Ischemia generally causes gangrenous changes and pain but is *not* the primary cause of ulcerations.

It is a widely held misconception that diabetic ulcers occur primarily because of circulatory impairment.

Diabetic ulcers are primarily due to the combination of insensitivity and the presence of unrelieved pressure. This pressure may take the form of a bony prominence from within against the skin and soft tissues or may be an external pressure, such as the pressure of a shoe against the fifth toe, or on the medial or lateral border of the foot. Nonhealing lesions must be evaluated for the adequacy of vascularity, and guidelines have been established with regard to the minimal perfusion that is likely to allow a diabetic lesion to heal.[14, 16]

Orthopaedic operative treatment of the diabetic foot frequently requires concomitant vascular reconstruction to allow an ulcer to heal, to resolve an infection, or to permit foot salvage (i.e., a successful amputation at a more distal level).

Third, diabetics are recognized as having an unusual persistence of foot infections. To some extent, this is synonymous with the issue of neuropathy and unrecognized injury. Basic science studies do indicate alterations in immune system function relative to infection in diabetics, and clinical experiences demonstrate that infection can be precipitous and even catastrophic. Prompt care of infection requires not only appropriate surgical intervention but also attention to the use of appropriate antibiotic regimens.

Fourth, underlying deformities in the forefoot, midfoot, or hindfoot are the second most important source of neurotrophic ulceration.

209

It is the combination of insensitivity and intrinsic pressure caused by bony deformity that invariably leads to neuropathic ulcerations. The ulcers of insensitivity do not occur without a combination of altered sensation and pressure. Although most pressure arises from underlying bony prominences, it may also take the form of shear stress on the skin, for example blisters or abrasions. Much of the surgery for the diabetic foot consists of correcting deformity or relieving bony prominences that contribute to the pressure of ulceration. This concept, although a simple one, is central to understanding reconstructive procedures in the diabetic foot.

The clinical problems in the diabetic foot reviewed in this chapter are infection (including abscess and osteomyelitis), neuropathic ulceration, gangrene, and Charcot's joints. For each of these, a brief discussion of general principles is followed by specific problem-solving approaches to the individual lesions.

PREOPERATIVE CARE

Treatment of the diabetic foot is truly an interdisciplinary undertaking, and the "team" approach of many medical subspecialists and disciplines, including nurses, physical and occupational therapists, orthotists, prosthetists, social workers, and others, has been documented as effective by multiple authors. Patients require management of their diabetes (glucose control and general medical care) by a primary care physician or endocrinologist. Vascular evaluation is essential in any presurgical diabetic patient, and it begins with Doppler arterial screening. If Doppler ultrasonography indicates ankle-to-arm pressure ratios below 0.45, or if the pulse-volume recordings fail to indicate pulsatile flow and artificially elevated pressures are recorded (e.g., ankle-to-arm ratios of greater than 1.0), a vascular surgery consultation is recommended. Most often, the vascular surgeons follow noninvasive studies such as the Doppler with arteriography for a definitive evaluation of the arterial patency of the lower extremity. In cases in which inadequate vascularity is present, vascular reconstruction is usually considered *before* orthopaedic surgery on the foot, except in the most emergent of cases.

Vascular reconstruction alternatives include in situ and reversed saphenous vein graft bypass. The distal arterial insufficiency in diabetics differs from that in nondiabetics in the common pattern of diffuse narrowing of all three vessels distal to the trifurcation of the popliteal artery. Distal bypass procedures to the ankle level are commonly required. In centers with expertise in interventional radiology, balloon angioplasty can be effective in selected cases for relieving isolated stenotic lesions of the distal leg.

Appropriate culture for aerobic and anaerobic organisms and use of the proper antimicrobial regimen are essential to healing diabetic foot infections, as are proper surgery, revascularization, and glucose management. The typical diabetic foot infection is polymicrobial and often includes gram-positive cocci, gram-negative (enteric) rods, and anaerobic organisms. Therefore, broad-spectrum antibiotics or combination-drug regimens are required to cover these diverse organisms. Some of the new antibiotics, such as the third-generation cephalosporins, or others such as ampicillin-sulbactam or imipenem are applicable because of their broad coverage.

Regardless of which drug regimen is selected empirically at the onset of treatment, the choice of antibiotics should be modified according to the specific organisms cultured before the initial antibiotics are given. Consultation with an infectious disease specialist is often appropriate.

In the not-uncommon situation in which the patient has been pretreated with a low dose of oral antibiotics as an outpatient, obtaining accurate culture findings can be difficult, if not impossible. The pretreatment antibiotics may be sufficient to prevent positive culture findings but inadequate to eradicate the infection. In these situations, biopsy of the bone through an incision separate from the site of drainage may be required to obtain the best cultures of bone and to determine histologically whether evidence of osteomyelitis is present. The presence of inflammatory cells within the marrow indicates infection within the bone and can directly affect the decision on the required length of treatment with intravenous antibiotics.

INFECTION

Diagnosis

Diagnostic imaging is necessary less often to determine the presence of infection than to establish its extent. Bone scans can be helpful in cases of osteomyelitis but are limited by their lack of specificity. Charcot's neuroarthropathy can produce positive ^{99}Tc bone scan findings of an intensity equal to that of osteomyelitis. Soft tissue lesions adjacent to periosteum but not invading it can likewise produce false-positive scan findings. The use of "triple-phase" scans indicates the presence of soft tissue inflammation and increased local vascularity, but these scans do not distinguish between osseous infection and noninfected inflammation such as a Charcot joint and are therefore generally unhelpful.

Gallium scan findings can likewise be positive in the inflammatory or later stages of Charcot's arthropathy. An indium scan is more specific for infection because it is based on "labeled" white blood cells.[17]

The use of magnetic resonance imaging represents the greatest advancement in the diagnosis of diabetic foot infection, and the parameters for its use are still evolving. One of its greatest uses is determining the marrow changes in early osteomyelitis, before changes are seen on plain radiographs. The marrow changes of osteomyelitis are visible on magnetic resonance images not only sooner than on radiographs but also earlier than on bone scans. These changes, which are basically those of marrow edema (i.e., normal marrow fat is replaced by water, which has a different density and signal intensity), are not specific for osteomyelitis. For example, they can be produced by trauma as well. They are represented by the loss of the normal bright signal of marrow fat on the T_1-weighted images and by the increased brightness on the heavily weighted T_2 images.

Magnetic resonance imaging is particularly useful in delineating the extent of abscess formation, especially in the deep plantar space. This representation of soft tissue makes magnetic resonance imaging more applicable in preoperative surgical planning than is computed tomography, although the latter also has a place.

Abscess

Abscess formation in the diabetic foot does not always present as the classic loculated region of free-flowing pus. Sometimes the purulence is thin, watery, and scant material, diffusely spread within an area of tissue necrosis in which there is no loculated fluid.

Surgical Approaches for Abscess Drainage

Web Space

When the abscess occurs in the web space (most often, it occurs in the first web space between the great and second toes), the surgeon should determine where the abscess is pointing (i.e., dorsal versus plantar). At times the abscess points toward the web space itself, and the incision should begin at the base of the web. Incision of the web is seldom adequate in itself, and the incision must be carried from the web either dorsally, plantarward, or both to expose the entire web and the intrinsic muscles within it. This is basically a websplitting incision that can extend 270 degrees from the dorsum of the foot to the plantar surface of the foot and still result in a viable foot (Fig. 19–1). (This is the same type of incision used with excision of a single ray.) If the abscess is adequately drained and if the necrotic tissue is properly resected, this type of abscess can sometimes heal even without the loss of a digit. However, if the capsule or tissues of a metatarsophalangeal joint desiccate after being exposed, the ray will probably need to be excised.

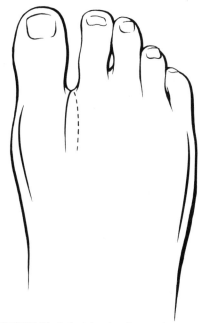

FIGURE 19–1. Incision for abscess drainage.

Plantar Abscess

Plantar abscesses can be drained either through plantar incisions or through incisions along the medial or lateral border of the foot. Although an incision on the plantar surface can heal and re-epithelialization can produce excellent weight-bearing skin, it is still preferable to keep the incision off the weight-bearing surface if possible. In this case, incisions on the medial or lateral border of the foot are preferable if the abscess extends to the foot border.

Longitudinal incisions on the plantar surface are generally preferable to curvilinear ones. The surgeon should make certain that the incision is adequate for full visualization to allow débridement of all necrotic tissue. The wound will heal more rapidly with a longer incision that allows resection of all necrotic plantar fascia than, for example, with a shorter but inadequate incision meant to "spare" the patient a more extensive procedure.

Osteomyelitis

Forefoot

The vast majority of osteomyelitis evaluated in the foot occurs in the forefoot region. Specific surgical interventions are discussed and illustrated in the following sections.

First Metatarsophalangeal Joint

Osteomyelitis within the sesamoids of the great toe is not uncommon, and involvement of the medial sesamoid occurs more commonly than that of the lateral sesamoid. It is often necessary to obtain special sesamoid radiographic views to determine if erosion of the plantar cortex of the sesamoid bone is present. Occasionally, bone scanning is helpful, although fracture and severe sesamoiditis can also produce positive scan findings.

In a case of incipient sesamoid infection, partial resection of the bone can be accomplished. This resection is similar to that which would be performed for chronic ulceration in the absence of osteomyelitis (see the later section on ulceration). In this situation, resection of the plantar half of the bone with a small oscillating saw has the advantage of not requiring tendon repairs; thus, it has a low

likelihood of producing postoperative varus or valgus deformity of the hallux. Partial excision of the lateral sesamoid is seldom necessary because of its diminished weight bearing and small size compared with the medial sesamoid.

Partial Sesamoid Excision. Partial excision of the medial sesamoid is relatively simple and is performed through an incision on the medial border of the foot. Careful scissor dissection is required to identify the sensory nerves of the great toe, primarily the proper plantar digital nerve.

Dissection is performed through the fibers of the abductor hallucis and periosteum, which are peeled down plantarward, rather than by entering the metatarsal-sesamoid joint. The plantar half of the bone is then resected with a saw and smoothed with a rasp (Fig. 19–2).

Complete Sesamoid Excision. When osteomyelitis is established and the entire sesamoid must be resected, it is important to make the incision through the metatarsal-sesamoid joint and to dissect out and excise the sesamoid very carefully, preserving the fibers of the flexor hallucis brevis that surround it.[1] The flexor hallucis brevis mechanism must then be reconstructed with multiple absorbable sutures to retard the occurrence of postoperative valgus deformity (in the case of a medial sesamoid excision). Because of the associated insensitivity, diabetics have an increased risk of such deformity after sesamoid excision.

Proximal Metatarsal Osteotomy. For larger or recalcitrant ulcerations in the first metatarsophalangeal joint region, partial or total sesamoidectomy may be insufficient to relieve the pressure and should be accompanied by or replaced by a dorsiflexion osteotomy of the first metatarsal.[5] This osteotomy is generally performed at the base of the metatarsal as a dorsally based closing wedge osteotomy. Internal fixation with screws is advised.

Metatarsal Head Resection. Osteomyelitis occurring within the metatarsal heads is a difficult problem. The often quoted caveat against metatarsal head resection is only partially true. On one hand, it can lead to transfer lesions and subsequent ulceration at adjacent metatarsal heads. However, in severely recalcitrant ulcerations, resection of part or all of the single metatarsal head is usually preferable to a metatarsal osteotomy. The osteotomy can proceed to a nonunion because of the underlying neuropathy and can subsequently lead to

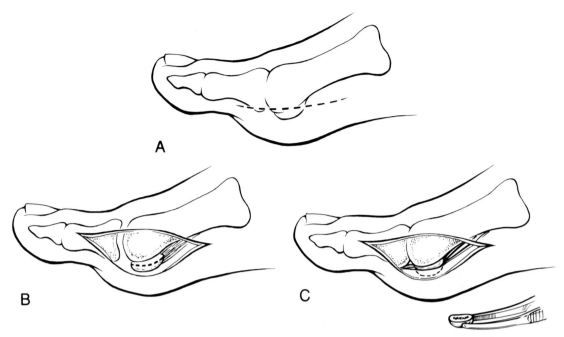

FIGURE 19–2. Medial sesamoid excision (partial). *(A)*, Medial incision, plantar to the midaxis of the first metatarsophalangeal joint. *(B)*, Exposure of the medial sesamoid. *(C)*, Resection of the plantar half of the medial sesamoid.

more widespread Charcot's changes in the foot. Many patients with solitary metatarsal head resections function well with a custom-molded insole in an extra-depth shoe postoperatively.

A modification of the DuVries condylectomy[9] is a reasonable intermediate solution that can precede resection of the entire metatarsal head and offers a diminished risk of transfer ulceration at adjacent metatarsals. However, this can be used primarily for recalcitrant ulcerations and not in situations of osteomyelitis. Once the transfer lesion has occurred beneath the metatarsal head adjacent to one previously resected, the surgeon can consider resection of yet another metatarsal head or a condylectomy. However, once transfer ulcerations have occurred on two occasions, the patient should have a transmetatarsal amputation or a modified Hoffmann procedure for resection of all the lesser metatarsal heads.[7]

The metatarsal heads should be resected using a dorsal incision that is subsequently loosely closed. The plantar ulcer is left open and is débrided in an elliptical fashion to enhance drainage. Resection should be done with a saw because it produces less splintering of cortical bone than does an osteotome. The distal end is beveled such that the cut is made

from distally on the dorsal surface in a proximal and plantar direction (Fig. 19–3). All adjacent nonviable and avascular tissue, including tendon and plantar plates, should be débrided as necessary when infection is present.

Pitfalls. In all cases, it is preferable to resect the metatarsal, even if it is very far proximal, rather than to disarticulate it at its base in the midfoot. The latter leads to instability and potential Charcot's midfoot breakdown.

Toes

Single-toe amputation is a successful procedure for isolated osteomyelitis within the digit,

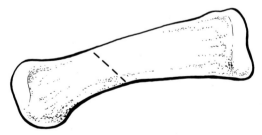

FIGURE 19–3. Angle of bone resection in a modified Hoffmann or single-metatarsal resection.

especially if it occurs at the proximal interphalangeal joint, for example in a patient with pre-existing clawtoe who has experienced dorsal shoe pressure.

However, for osteomyelitis at the tip of the toe, partial toe amputation is advisable. This simple procedure preserves the base of the proximal phalanx and at least some of the proximal phalangeal shaft. The remnant of the toe serves as a "spacer" to deter drift of the adjacent toes into the space created by digit amputation and enhances weight bearing on the corresponding metatarsal head by preserving the plantar fascia at its attachment on the base of the proximal phalanx.

Osteomyelitis of the great toe is more problematic. Every effort should be made to preserve the base of the proximal phalanx in order to spare the attachment of the plantar fascia and enhance the remaining function of the sesamoids and their soft tissue sling. Weight bearing is improved and the risk of secondary transfer metatarsalgia is diminished by preserving the base of the toe and its plantar fascia attachment. Cosmetically, of course, 1 cm of proximal phalanx will appear to be "total" toe amputation to the patient, because in every digit the base of the proximal phalanx lies proximal to the base of the toe web. The

key to toe amputation is to preserve more soft tissue than bone and to close the wound primarily whenever possible (Fig. 19–4).

Midfoot

Osteomyelitis of the midfoot usually occurs secondary to ulceration. This ulceration is usually due to bony prominences caused by midfoot collapse in Charcot's foot (see the later section on Charcot's arthropathy).

Hindfoot

Osteomyelitis of the hindfoot is an especially challenging and difficult problem. When osteomyelitis occurs over the navicular tuberosity or the base of the fifth metatarsal and is due to shoe or cast pressure, the bony prominence can be resected and the posterior tibialis tendon or peroneus brevis tendon, respectively, can be repaired. When osteomyelitis occurs at the base of the fifth metatarsal, if the peroneus brevis is not reattached, it can be sutured to the peroneus longus. Reattachment can usually be avoided if the tendon is split longitudinally.

However, when osteomyelitis occurs within the calcaneus itself, it is a vexing problem because of the paucity of well-vascularized soft tissue coverage and because the fat pad is relatively avascular tissue, even in the best situation. A total contact cast is less effective in the hindfoot than in the forefoot because hindfoot ulcers are more often due to shoe pressure than to the pressure of weight bearing against the plantar surface of the foot. Disease in the posterior tibial artery and its branches prevents healing, and this area of the vascular supply needs to be evaluated.

Salvaging the foot with osteomyelitis of the calcaneus is often impossible or heroic. Free tissue transfer can be required if the ulcer is directly over the posterior tuberosity of bone. Significant danger exists for recurring breakdown because the "free" flap and its overlying skin graft are also insensitive. The use of a postoperative polypropylene ankle-foot orthosis can diminish this effect to some extent.

When the Achilles tendon is exposed and a free flap cannot be formed rapidly, the tendon desiccates and requires débridement. Achilles tendon resection does not necessarily make the foot useless, and below-knee amputation can be avoided if the patient is treated with a polypropylene ankle-foot orthosis.

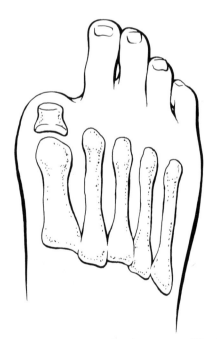

FIGURE 19–4. Toe amputation for osteomyelitis of the great toe.

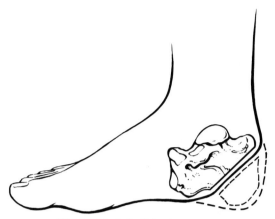

FIGURE 19–5. Partial calcanectomy.

Partial calcanectomy of the posterior tubercle is a viable option in diabetics (Fig. 19–5). Vascularity of the tissue, especially the branches to the heel pad that arise from the posterior tibial vessel just above the level of the foot, is a key consideration. Partial calcanectomy can allow primary closure without free tissue transfer by diminishing the amount of the bony prominence that must be covered by the available soft tissue.[3]

Most patients require permanent use of an ankle-foot orthosis after partial calcanectomy, although this is not always the case. Some patients can achieve partial function of the residual Achilles tendon after calcanectomy if the procedure has been performed for osteomyelitis in the absence of a necrotic tendon. The posterior tubercle is best approached through an Achilles tendon–splitting incision. The Achilles tendon is left within the two full-thickness soft tissue flaps that are made from skin to periosteum, and the bone is shelled out and cut with a saw or osteotome. Dissection should be subperiosteal but must not "dig in" to the bone, which would leave bone fragments behind.

Principles of Surgery for the Diabetic Foot with Regard to Osteomyelitis and Ulceration

Microbiology

Cultures of the sinus tract have been well documented to be unreliable in representing the microorganisms of a deep wound.[12] There-fore, it is important to obtain culture samples from deep sites at the time of surgery, sampling both bone and soft tissue and submitting all samples for culture of both aerobic and anaerobic organisms. Proper technique is critical in obtaining satisfactory anaerobic cultures, which are necessary for the selection of proper antibiotic regimens.

Many diabetics have surgery after partial or incomplete treatment with oral antibiotics. This use of antibiotics is often sufficient to suppress culture growth but not sufficient to cure the underlying infection (as noted in the previous section). It is especially advisable in these cases but generally advisable in all cases in which bone is removed from the diabetic foot that samples of the bone closest to the ulcer be submitted for culture and that the remaining specimens be submitted for analysis of permanent pathologic sections. A request should be made to examine the bone for histologic evidence of marrow inflammation to document the presence or absence of osteomyelitis.

Drainage

Diabetic surgical wounds in cases of osteomyelitis, abscess, or chronic grade II or greater ulceration require adequate drainage. One alternative is suction drainage. However, a short course of wound irrigation is clinically efficacious, although there are no controlled studies of its use.[8] The irrigation system can be left in place as long as 48 hours, but 12 to 24 hours is usually sufficient. A No. 8 pediatric feeding tube is placed through a tiny stab incision proximal to the wound. It is then attached to sterile intravenous line extension tubing and from there to a liter of normal saline or Ringer's lactate solution. This irrigation is performed without antibiotics because of the risk of absorption of medications through the wound. In the case of previous use of aminoglycoside antibiotics, there was some risk of adverse effects in diabetic patients with pre-existing renal impairment.

Irrigation is generally performed at 30 to 60 mL/hr, which is moderated according to the size of the wound. A large, bulky, soft bandage is applied around the foot and ankle to absorb the draining fluid that effluxes between the loosely placed sutures. The irrigation system is removed at the first bandage change.

SURGICAL TREATMENT OF RECURRENT AND RECALCITRANT ULCERATION

Surgical treatment is seldom the primary therapeutic choice for noninfected ulcers but is reserved for the difficult ulcers that fail to respond to nonsurgical pressure-relieving measures. The principle of surgical treatment is the resection of bony projections or the diminution of bony prominences producing the pressure that, in combination with insensitivity, is always present in diabetic ulcers. Surgical relief of pressure is indicated by the failure of nonsurgical methods such as shoe modification, the use of a prefabricated walking brace, or the application of a total contact cast.

The following principles apply to surgery that is intended to relieve pressure in recurrent or chronic persistent ulceration. A separate incision is usually made either on the border of the foot or dorsally. The bony prominence should not be excised through the ulcer itself. It is preferable to avoid plantar incisions if possible. The ulcer should generally be left open and débrided at the time of the surgery in order to enhance drainage due to gravity. The surgical incision can often be loosely closed, depending on the degree of soft tissue infection. If any doubt remains, the incision should be left open and the patient should be returned to the operating room in several days for repeated irrigation, débridement, and delayed closure. It is imperative to remember to collect samples for both aerobic and anaerobic cultures from both the soft tissue and bone. Once the acute surgical wounds have healed, the residual ulcer can be treated with external pressure relief, as was done preoperatively with either shoe modifications or total contact casts.

Midfoot plantar ulcerations are almost invariably caused by Charcot's joints until proven otherwise, because the longitudinal arch does not normally exhibit bony prominence to the degree that would produce ulceration.

Toe Ulcers

Chronic ulceration of the toes should initially be treated conservatively, as is the case with most other diabetic foot problems, but when bone has been exposed or osteomyelitis occurs, partial amputation is indicated.

Chronic ulcerations on the great toe most commonly occur at the medial plantar side of the interphalangeal joint. This ulceration is caused by the width of the phalanges at the joint, and the pressure under this area is accentuated by pronation of the foot and toe.

Partial phalangectomies of a portion of both the proximal and distal phalanges at the joint (resection arthroplasty), with reduction of their medial prominence, usually causes the ulcer to resolve. The latter reduction is generally performed in a sagittal plane with the saw blade angled plantarward and laterally in order to remove more bone in the area of increased pressure (Fig. 19–6). If this treatment fails, dorsiflexion osteotomy at the base of the proximal phalanx is the second alternative.

First Metatarsophalangeal Joint Ulcers

Plantar ulcers beneath the first metatarsophalangeal joint are particularly problematic. These ulcers are usually caused by pressure beneath the medial sesamoid and should be

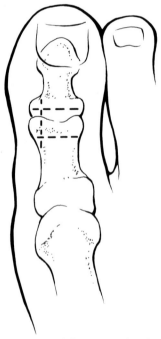

FIGURE 19–6. Lines of bone resection in surgery for recalcitrant ulceration of the hallux interphalangeal joint.

treated with the same technique outlined previously in the section on osteomyelitis, which starts with partial or complete sesamoid excision. This excision can be followed or accompanied by dorsiflexion osteotomy of the first metatarsal.

Middle Metatarsal Ulcers

Recalcitrant ulcers occurring beneath the lesser metatarsal heads that are resistant to conservative measures and in which there has been exposed tendon or bone are treated initially with débridement. A procedure for relief of pressure must then be selected: this procedure is usually condylectomy,[9] osteotomy, or metatarsal head resection. If the bone is not infected, it is preferable not to excise the metatarsal head because of the transfer pressure to adjacent metatarsals discussed previously. Condylectomy is preferred over osteotomy because it does not require bone healing the way osteotomy does.

If osteotomy is elected, it should be because metatarsal head resection cannot or should not be done. In general, a patient with excision of a single metatarsal head in a neuropathic foot can function very well with properly molded shoe insoles postoperatively. Patients with multiple-metatarsal resections, however, do not do well unless they have had a pan–metatarsal head resection (i.e., a modified Hoffmann procedure).[7]

When an osteotomy is performed, internal fixation is necessary. Nonunion can progress to a more widespread Charcot change. It is therefore important to evaluate the level of the patient's neuropathy before osteotomy is considered. If the patient has very dense neuropathy, an osteotomy is less desirable. The patient must always be warned about the risk of transfer metatarsal pressure and subsequent secondary ulceration. In this clinical situation, no technique of osteotomy has proved to be superior.

When severe metatarsal pressure produces ulceration and surgical intervention is required, it is important to correct concurrent toe deformity. Metatarsal head resection itself can also produce increased toe elevation.

A clawtoe contributes to plantar ulceration through depression of the metatarsal head by the hyperextended base of the proximal phalanx. Surgical correction includes proximal interphalangeal joint arthroplasty, extensive metatarsophalangeal capsulotomy (including the medial, lateral, and dorsal sides), and extensor tendon lengthening. If the deformity is extremely severe or the correction cannot be maintained, a flexor-to-extensor tendon transfer may be required.

In surgery for ulceration of the lesser metatarsals, a dorsal incision should be used. If all of the metatarsal heads will be excised, one incision for two metatarsals can be used in the second and fourth interspaces (Fig. 19–7). Subcutaneous sutures should not be placed; instead, closure should be with nonabsorbable skin sutures, although often these should include the subcutaneous tissue.

The Hoffmann procedure is equally applicable for chronic ulcerations and for chronic recurrent osteomyelitis. These conditions represent different stages in the continuum of chronic ulceration. Patients undergoing metatarsal head resection should be warned that the foot will be shorter and the toes will be floppy and less controlled. Surgical technique

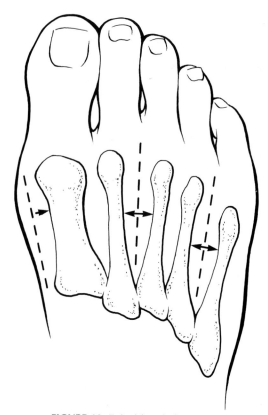

FIGURE 19–7. Incisions in interspaces.

includes the use of an oscillating saw. The cuts should be angled from dorsal and distal to plantar and proximal, as noted previously, and each metatarsal should be cut at least 2 to 3 mm shorter than the one medial to it. More than a 3-mm difference should be made between the fourth and fifth metatarsals because the latter is more mobile and more likely to produce recurrent ulceration. Unless the wound is grossly infected, it should be closed primarily but somewhat loosely, with or without drains. When infection is present, the wound can be left open. Sutures should generally be left in place for an absolute minimum of 2 weeks and often for 3 to 6 weeks.

Fifth Metatarsal Ulcers

The fifth metatarsal is particularly susceptible to ulceration in any condition in which the hindfoot is in the varus position. This is true not only at the metatarsal head but especially at the fifth metatarsal base. When an ulceration exists in the fifth metatarsal head, a condylectomy is more easily performed here because a lateral approach can be used. Condylectomy is performed through a horizontal incision along the lateral border of the foot (Fig. 19–8).

Severe ulcers of the base of the fifth metatarsal often cannot be corrected by local bone resection alone and require correction of hindfoot varus with calcaneal osteotomy or triple arthrodesis. This is primarily a problem in Charcot's foot, although it is not a common occurrence. Partial excision of the base of the

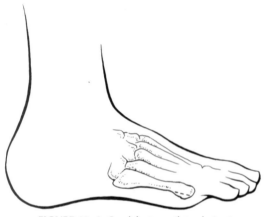

FIGURE 19–8. Condylectomy (lateral view).

fifth metatarsal with repair of the peroneus brevis is still the preferred initial surgical intervention.

Hindfoot and Ankle Ulcers

Hindfoot ulcers should be suspected of being potentially more likely to have a vascular component because they are the exception to the rule that ulcerations occur primarily over bony prominences. Ulcers over the heel pad are more often ischemic, and a vascular evaluation and early vascular consultation are necessary. These ulcers are less amenable to treatment with total contact casting than are forefoot and midfoot ulcers.

Once satisfactory vascularity has been documented or has been established by vascular reconstruction, small gangrenous areas in the heel pad can be excised and the incision can be closed with primary or delayed primary closure. However, the relative avascularity of the tissue leads to a higher number of failures.

Varus and valgus angulation, especially the former, can expose the malleoli to excessive pressure, which can lead to ulceration as well, especially in a Charcot hindfoot in which the lateral malleolus has produced an ulceration. There are two potential ways to correct this, and often both are required. The first method is partial resection of the lateral portion of the lateral malleolus. The disadvantage of this procedure is weakening of the malleolus, which could lead to neuropathic fracture. More often, it is necessary to correct the varus position with an osteotomy of the calcaneus or an arthrodesis of the hindfoot or ankle. Both of these are high-risk procedures that can lead to further neuropathic change and nonunion.

AMPUTATION

The principles of amputation of the diabetic foot are straightforward. First, it is imperative to save a maximum of skin and soft tissue. When a toe or forefoot is being amputated, the incision should be made right at the line of demarcation between viable and nonviable tissue. Even in the case of gangrene, it is best to save the maximum amount of even potentially viable skin. More can always be resected later. The difference of 1 cm of soft tissue may mean the difference in an entire amputation level if the soft tissue cannot be closed over what is already maximally resected bone. Second, closure of the wound is the key to a successful outcome. It is always preferable to achieve primary or delayed primary closure of the wound. Delayed primary closure can be performed between 3 and 14 days after the initial débridement or amputation of the gangrenous part. In general, it is best to try to achieve closure within 7 to 10 days because contraction of the flaps can lead to bulky, less mobile soft tissue with which to cover the remaining or exposed bone. The surgeon is advised to be creative with the flaps: in other words, to use whatever soft tissue is available, even if it means making unorthodox medial or lateral flaps rather than standard dorsal and plantar flaps. Saving additional soft tissue often means the difference between achieving closure with local tissue and having to use a flap or skin graft, both of which have higher morbidity and a greater complication rate. It is especially worthwhile to maximize available plantar skin for closure of the wound after partial foot amputation because this specialized dermis tolerates weight bearing and generally holds up better with the trauma inflicted on the insensitive foot.

A balance is always required between the amount of soft tissue preserved and the amount of bone resected over which the soft tissue must achieve closure. Many situations arise in partial amputation of the diabetic foot in which it is necessary to remove additional viable bone in order to create sufficient soft tissue for coverage of the area. In some cases, this means sacrificing a portion of a ray that is not actually infected or gangrenous itself. When saving a technically viable ray requires leaving the wound open for many months because insufficient soft tissue is available to close the wound, the result is "more foot," but the foot is not available for the patient to actually use. In other words, the morbidity may not be worth salvage of the additional ray. Again, the goal is to achieve primary or delayed primary closure for rapid rehabilitation of the extremity as well as of the patient.

If the wound is left completely open to granulate, it may take between 2 and 6 months to close. This can ultimately produce an unstable scar and much unnecessary debility while the patient spends the many months inactive or non–weight bearing waiting for the wound to fill in slowly.

Most amputations are performed for infection, but occasionally a foot amputation or partial foot amputation is performed in the presence of deformity itself. The latter is especially true in cases of severe Charcot's joint.

Toe Amputation

In a toe or partial toe amputation, the toe is filleted. The incision can be a fish-mouth–type or a racket-type incision. In order to close the wound primarily, a significant amount of skin must be present distal to the level of bone resection. For example, some of the skin overlying at least one-third to one-half of the proximal phalanx of the lesser toe must be viable to achieve closure of a metatarsophalangeal joint disarticulation.

Partial amputation of the toe, when possible, is a reasonable and viable alternative, as noted previously in the section on osteomyelitis. The stump of the amputated toe, which prevents or retards drift of the adjacent two toes toward one another, is important because such subsequent deformity can often lead to pressure ulceration and amputation of the adjacent digits in a "domino" fashion. If the entire toe is amputated, it is often advisable for the patient to use a foam spacer between the toes postoperatively to prevent such a drift.

Ray Amputation

Ray amputations are one of the most important areas in which closure is allowed by adequate resection of bone. Resection of a metatarsal head has often been described as being strictly contraindicated. This is not necessarily the case in the diabetic foot, and if the metatarsal head is extensively involved with osteomyelitis, it should be resected along with the distal one-half to two-thirds of the metatarsal. It is important in this situation, in particular, to save the base of the metatarsal. Resection of the entire metatarsal bone including disarticulation at the base produces significant tarsometatarsal instability that frequently leads to Charcot's breakdown of the midfoot and the many problems that this produces.

Saving the metatarsal head whenever possible has the benefit of preventing the maldistribution of pressure beneath the reduced number of metatarsal heads that remain. Such a transfer lesion can occur and can lead to ulceration, osteomyelitis, and infection of the adjacent residual metatarsal heads. Once two or more metatarsal heads have been resected, it is necessary to consider a transmetatarsal amputation.

Technique

The incision should be made dorsally directly over the ray. The surgeon cuts down to the bone sharply and performs a subperiosteal dissection, elevating full-thickness flaps when possible. Dissection is limited out into the subcutaneous plane. The ray is resected with a micro–oscillating saw, with irrigation as necessary to prevent burning of the residual bone. The bone should be beveled as described earlier so that the remaining edge does not have a sharp plantar corner (see Fig. 19–3).

Partial Foot Amputation

Partial foot amputation generally signifies the resection of multiple rays from either the medial or the lateral portion of the foot. A lateral partial foot amputation is generally more functional than a medial partial foot amputation. More of the latter amputations eventually require conversion to transmetatarsal or more proximal amputations. Regardless of which side of the forefoot is resected, once these patients have healed postoperatively, they require special inserts and shoe modifications. Resection of a single ray is not as significant on the lateral half of the forefoot as on the medial portion, but single-ray resection can still lead to major complications when it is the first ray that has been resected.

This is the most critical situation for saving the maximum amount of skin and soft tissue. The creation of irregular flaps to save plantar skin is most important in this type of amputation. This is a successful procedure in many cases because it allows the patient to use a nearly normal shoe with the insert. These patients do not require a high-top shoe to hold onto the foot, as is often the case in transmetatarsal amputation, in which the shortened foot is not long enough for a low-quarter lace-up shoe. In general, partial foot amputations like the transmetatarsal amputation have the advantage of saving dorsiflexion function through the anterior tibialis tendon. It is best

to save the insertion of the peroneus brevis as well, if possible, in order to balance the foot and prevent a varus deformity.

Transmetatarsal Amputation

Transmetatarsal amputations are indicated in cases of wider involvement with gangrene or infection across the forefoot, failed medial or lateral partial forefoot amputation, or multiple metatarsal head resection with residual infection. A high-top conversion of the shoe in order to hold the throat of the shoe onto the shortened foot is usually necessary, as is a shoe insert with a built-in toe filler.

Technique

Transmetatarsal amputation should be done with a saw. This procedure is similar to the modified Hoffmann procedure but more proximal. If necessary, one metatarsal base can be resected, especially if it is on the lateral side, but whenever possible the bases should be preserved. It is especially important to preserve the base of the first metatarsal because it affects the insertion of the anterior tibialis tendon. If the first metatarsal base is resected, the tendon may still have adequate attachment to the cuneiform. If the tendon does not have adequate attachment, it should be resutured into bone to preserve its function.

A long plantar flap is generally preferable for transmetatarsal amputations, but the inability to produce such a flap is not a strict contraindication to this amputation (Fig. 19–9). A tendo Achillis lengthening should be considered at the time of transmetatarsal amputation as needed. Careful attention is required to evaluate the foot for an equinus contracture. The tight Achilles tendon is more difficult to appreciate once the forefoot has been removed. However, such residual equinus contracture is the most common cause of failure of a transmetatarsal amputation. If the patient has recurring ulcerations on the plantar distal edge of the transmetatarsal amputation stump, a fixed or functional equinus contracture of the Achilles tendon should be sought as the source. The Achilles tendon lengthening can be performed either as an open or as a percutaneous-type procedure. Complete section of the tendo Achillis is not advised in this situation.

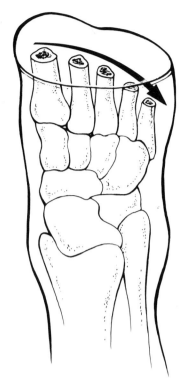

FIGURE 19–9. Transmetatarsal amputation.

Chopart's Amputation

Chopart's amputation[6] (disarticulation to the calcanocuboid and talonavicular joints) should include the creation of a plantar flap, and if the plantar skin is severely compromised in the hindfoot, this amputation is probably not viable. This amputation has the advantage of producing less shortening than the Syme procedure because the entire heel is retained. Many complications have been reported with this amputation in the past, primarily related to the equinus contracture from the loss of the anterior tibialis and peroneal tendons to balance the force of the triceps surae. Achilles tendon lengthening or section is required in all Chopart's amputations in diabetics. Many patients with Chopart's amputation still require a prosthesis, just as a Syme amputee would, but a few can function with only a modified shoe. The determining factor is the amount of sensitivity and concentration of pressure on the residual foot. Because the foot is so short, and the weight-bearing area is therefore small, breakdown is a significant danger.

Syme's Amputation

The technique of Syme's amputation has been very well described by Wagner.[13] Syme's amputees often do better with an insensitive foot than do patients with normal sensation, probably because symptomatic neuroma formation is distinctly unusual in diabetics.

The two-stage Syme amputation as described by Wagner is necessary only if infection is present in the very proximal portion of the foot at the time of amputation. For example, if the amputation is being performed for dry gangrene, it is advisable to proceed with a one-stage procedure in which the malleoli are trimmed at the time of primary closure. Previous authors have emphasized resection of too much of the flare of the distal tibial metaphysis. The metaphyseal flare of the distal tibia contributes to prosthetic fit, and I generally advise not resecting any of the medial or lateral portions of the distal tibial metaphyseal flare (Fig. 19–10). Syme's amputations are the most technically demanding of all foot amputations but are very rewarding. They have great advantages of enhanced function when compared with below-knee amputations. Less effort and less oxygen consumption are required, as has been documented in the studies by Waters and colleagues.[15] Rehabilitation is also significantly easier for Syme's amputees. Their mechanical advantage is greater in that the residual limb is longer. Their residual limb also has the advantage of being at least partially weight bearing on its end portion, relieving some of the pressure that is borne entirely through the proximal tibial metaphysis in a below-knee amputation. The end weight-bearing stump also has the benefit of retaining skin, which is normally weight-bearing skin and has less tendency for ulceration and breakdown than does the distal skin in a below-knee amputation.

Postoperatively, the amputation stump should be protected in a rigid dressing such as a bivalved cast or splint for approximately 6 weeks.

SURGICAL PROBLEMS OF CHARCOT'S FOOT

The vast majority of Charcot's feet in diabetics are best managed by nonsurgical means.[2] Immobilization is the initial treatment advised in almost all cases. Surgical interven-

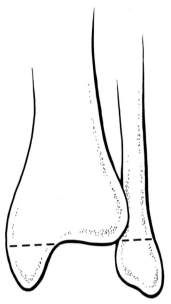

FIGURE 19–10. Lines of resection of the distal tibia and fibula for a Syme amputation.

tion is limited to specific problems. It is not the usual goal of surgical treatment of the Charcot foot to produce anatomic restoration of the fractured or dislocated joints. Such an attempt has a high failure rate and subjects the patient to unnecessary risks. Accepting some deformity and allowing conservative treatment to heal the Charcot foot usually results in a viable limb that continues to function. Overly aggressive surgical intervention in the Charcot foot, especially in inexperienced hands, has a very high complication rate and, ultimately, a very high amputation rate.

There are two basic indications for surgical intervention in Charcot's foot. The first is for treatment of the recurrent or recalcitrant plantar ulceration produced by the increased pressure (usually in the midfoot region) on the plantar surface. The pressure is caused by the architectural disruption and collapse of the tarsal bones. An example of this is the classic rocker-bottom foot. The second indication is the failure of other conservative management for the plantar ulceration, including weight-bearing modification and total contact casting, among others (i.e., the same treatment protocol as for treatment of forefoot plantar ulceration). If the patient has not had an adequate trial of conservative therapy, surgical intervention should usually be delayed. Plantar

exostectomy of the bony prominence is advised for severe and recurring ulcerations.

Plantar Exostectomy

The incisions should be made along the medial or lateral border of the foot. A full-thickness flap should be created from skin down to bone, and a subperiosteal dissection of the entire flap should then be performed. Very careful attention should be paid to hemostasis because these feet tend to be hypervascular and bleed a great deal in the postoperative period.

The clinical decision must be made about how much bone to resect. Insufficient resection of bone allows recurrence of the ulceration, whereas excessive resection can lead to instability and further collapse. The bone should be resected with large osteotomes or a small oscillating saw. The wound should always be drained, and closure should generally be performed loosely to allow drainage to occur. Delayed healing of part or the entire length of the wound is common, but the vast majority of these wounds, if adequately treated in the postoperative period, go on to close and heal.

Postoperative cast treatment is most helpful and is advised in most cases, not only for protection of the soft tissue wound but also for protection against secondary destabilization of the midfoot after bone resection. Such immobilization in the cast is usually required for a minimum of 2 months but often for as long as 6 or 8 months.

Plantar ulcerations can recur if the midfoot continues to shift downward in the postoperative period. Plantar incisions over the ulceration are possible but generally less desirable because healing will occur if an adequate amount of bone is resected. Ulcer excision itself is usually not necessary, although if the wound is grossly purulent, it should be débrided. If the ulceration is acutely infected, it is important to débride and treat the ulceration and to deal with the acute infection before the exostectomy is performed.

Arthrodesis of Charcot's Foot

Arthrodesis of Charcot's foot is required infrequently, if not rarely, and it is to be considered a salvage procedure only.[18] If the deformity is so great that it will lead to deep ulceration, osteomyelitis, and amputation and if only arthrodesis will realign and salvage the foot, arthrodesis is indicated. This operation is most often considered for Charcot's joints in the hindfoot or ankle because midfoot Charcot's joints tend to stabilize more readily with adequate immobilization. The primary indications are instability and severe deformity, but instability is not a common long-term problem in the midfoot region.[2]

Midfoot fusion is indicated if gross disruption of the midfoot architecture produces deformity and a bony prominence that threatens severe skin breakdown not amenable to exostectomy. In such cases, the midfoot and metatarsal bases are generally displaced in a lateral direction, exposing the skin to pressure over the isolated or dislocated medial cuneiform bone. Despite a flattened foot or even a rocker-bottom deformity, most midfoot Charcot's joints heal with spontaneous osseous consolidation without surgical intervention.[2]

When performing arthrodesis of a Charcot foot, the surgeon must keep in mind that complications are generally significant and that failures tend to result in amputation. Gentle technique is advised, especially in handling the skin.

Internal fixation is required in arthrodesis of a Charcot joint, but this does not preclude the use of external immobilization with a cast as well. Rigid fixation is preferable, especially with screws. Many Charcot's joints have softened bone as a result of localized resorption related to the hypervascularity. A significant failure rate has been reported even in the best of series.[10]

A high proportion of fusions of Charcot's ankles and hindfeet fail to attain bony arthrodesis and result in fibrous ankylosis. Despite this, if the ankylosis is relatively stable, the patient can have a successful result.

The nature of this salvage procedure is such that it should not be attempted unless failure to operate would subject the patient to such severe pressure, deformity, or ulceration that osteomyelitis would occur and amputation would be required otherwise. The reason for this is that the failed arthrodesis in a Charcot foot is often treatable only by amputation. This general approach to the indications is necessary to achieve a reasonable risk-to-benefit ratio for this difficult procedure. The underlying neuropathy that produced the Charcot

breakdown in the first place is still present and can lead, of course, to similar breakdown of the arthrodesis.

The timing of arthrodesis for Charcot's foot can be critical. It is best performed early, in the first few weeks of an Eichenholtz[4] stage I disintegration (acute inflammation), or later, late in an Eichenholtz stage II disintegration, when bony coalescence has occurred. Between these two points, the hypervascularity of the Charcot joint leads to osteopenia, which makes this an exceptionally difficult procedure and one in which rigid fixation is most difficult to attain. Anecdotally, these feet are noted to bleed heavily at the time of the procedure; these reports of bleeding are related to the observation by many authors of hypervascularity in the Charcot joint. This relatively good vascularity has been documented.[2]

Lastly, both doctor and patient must be prepared for very slow healing of this arthrodesis. The patient should be warned that immobilization in a cast followed by use of a total contact ankle-foot orthosis will be necessary for a minimum of 1 year. Many patients, especially those whose arthrodeses result in fibrous ankylosis, require permanent bracing with an anterior and posterior shell polypropylene ankle-foot orthosis (total contact ankle-foot orthosis). Nonetheless, the procedure may be worthwhile in cases in which deformity is so severe that even the fabrication of a brace is untenable preoperatively. Bone grafting is generally recommended in these arthrodeses whenever possible.

POSTOPERATIVE CARE

Once the appropriate surgical intervention has been undertaken and the patient obtains a satisfactory result, which is generally defined as healing of the foot, appropriate follow-up care is essential. Without appropriate outpatient management postoperatively, incomplete healing or recurrence is the rule rather than the exception.

Appropriate shoe modification and manufacture of shoe insoles are required to protect the foot and to make the result of the surgery lasting. To ignore these conservative measures is to condemn the patient to an even higher rate of recurring problems and procedures than is already the case given the chronic nature of the underlying disease.

CONCLUSIONS

The problems of the diabetic foot are many and varied, and surgical intervention should always be undertaken with a measure of caution. Surgery in a diabetic foot is not completely contraindicated, as was preached in the past, but it must be practiced with circumspection and care and with strict indications for its use. The team approach includes adequate treatment of infection, adequate control of hyperglycemia and other diabetic complications such as nephropathy, and adequate revascularization. All are essential parts of successful orthopaedic surgery for the diabetic foot. There is no clinical problem in orthopaedics that is more interdisciplinary than surgery for the diabetic foot. Therefore, it requires more than the ordinary amount of skill on the part of the orthopaedic surgeon to manage these problems. Despite this, the orthopaedic surgeon is uniquely qualified to deal with the diabetic foot because of the osseous procedures required and because of the subsequent need for rehabilitation and for shoe and prosthetic management.

References

1. Brodsky JW: Sesamoid excision for painful nonunion. Twenty-first Annual Winter Meeting, American Orthopedic Foot and Ankle Society. Anaheim, CA, March 1991.
2. Brodsky JW, Kwong PK, Wagner FW, Chambers RB: The diabetic foot. *In* Mann RA, Coughlin MJ (Eds): Surgery of the Foot and Ankle. St. Louis, CV Mosby, 1992.
3. Crandall RC, Wagner FW: Partial and total calcanectomy. J Bone Joint Surg 63A:152–155, 1981.
4. Eichenholtz SN: Charcot joints. Springfield, IL, Charles C Thomas, 1966.
5. Hammerschlag W: Dorsiflexion osteotomy of the first metatarsal for diabetic ulcers. Nineteenth Annual Meeting, American Orthopedic Foot and Ankle Society. Las Vegas, NV, February 1989.
6. Jacobs RL: The diabetic foot. *In* Jahss MH (Ed): Disorders of the Foot and Ankle. Philadelphia, WB Saunders, 1991.
7. Jacobs RL: Hoffmann procedure in the diabetic. Foot Ankle 3:142, 1982.
8. Kritter AE: A technique for salvage of the infected diabetic gangrenous foot. Orthop Clin North Am 4:21, 1973.
9. Mann RA: Keratotic disorders of the plantar skin. *In* Mann RA (Ed): Surgery of the Foot, 5th Ed. St. Louis, CV Mosby, 1986, pp 191–192.
10. Meyerson M, Quill G: Arthrodesis of the Charcot foot and ankle. Fifth Annual Summer Meeting, American Orthopedic Foot and Ankle Society. Sun Valley, ID, August 1989.
11. Sapico FL, Canawati HN, Witte JL, et al: Quantitative aerobic and anaerobic bacteriology in infected diabetic feet. J Clin Microbiol 12:413–420, 1980.
12. Sharp CS, Bessmen AN, Wagner FW Jr, et al: Microbiology of superficial and deep tissues in infected diabetic gangrene. Surg Gynecol Obstet 149:217–219, 1979.
13. Wagner FW Jr: The diabetic foot and amputations of the foot. *In* Mann RA (Ed): Surgery of the Foot, 5th Ed. St. Louis, CV Mosby, 1986, pp 421–455.
14. Wagner FW Jr: The dysvascular foot: A system for diagnosis and treatment. Foot Ankle 2:64–122, 1981.
15. Waters RL, Perry J, Antonelli E, Hislop H: Energy cost of walking of amputees: The influence of level of amputations. J Bone Joint Surg 58A:42–46, 1976.
16. Brodsky JW: Outpatient diagnosis and care of the diabetic foot. Instruct Course Lect 42, 1993.
17. Gould JS, Erickson SJ, Collier BD, Bernstein BM: Surgical management of ulcers, soft tissue, infections and osteomyelitis in the diabetic foot. Instruct Course Lect 42, 1993.
18. Harrelson JM: The diabetic foot: Charcot arthropathy. Instruct Course Lect 42, 1993.

20 Hemiplegic Disorders of the Foot

LANDRUS L. PFEFFINGER

SPASTIC HEMIPLEGIA

General Considerations

The term *spastic hemiplegia* is used for the neural deficit that may occur in patients who have cerebral palsy or who have had a traumatic injury to the brain or a cerebrovascular accident. *Cerebral palsy* is generally taken to mean a nonprogressive disorder that begins either in utero or within the first 2 years of life with a selective loss of muscle control. Many of the characteristics seen in patients who have cerebral palsy are similar to those in patients who have suffered head trauma or a cerebrovascular accident. The primary difference in treating the patient with adult-onset spastic hemiplegia versus the patient with cerebral palsy is skeletal immaturity. In the patient with cerebral palsy, the potential for bony deformities to occur is significant, whereas in the patient with adult-onset spastic hemiplegia, in whom the skeleton is mature, this potential is essentially nonexistent. Therefore, stabilization procedures such as fusions are required. They are often performed in combination with corrective procedures for alignment, such as wedge osteotomies. A separate discussion of spastic hemiplegia in patients with skeletal immaturity follows the section on adult-onset spastic hemiplegia.

Adult-Onset Spastic Hemiplegia

For the purposes of discussion, I have selected as an example the elderly patient who has suffered a cerebrovascular accident. A cerebrovascular accident may be due to either a cerebral thrombus with infarction, an embolus with infarction, an intracerebral hemorrhage, a subarachnoid hemorrhage from an aneurysm, or an arteriovenous malformation. It is important to determine the underlying cause of the cerebrovascular accident, not only for treatment but also for preventing recurrence. It is of little value to the patient to correct any deformities if the risk of recurrence with further deficits is significant. Cerebrovascular disease is often associated with either systemic or local disease such as diabetes mellitus, hypertension, coronary artery disease with mild myocardial infarction, and valvular heart disease with arrhythmias. Any of these conditions can carry negative prognostic weight and must therefore be addressed in the overall care of the patient. The highest mortality occurs within the first 3 weeks after a stroke, and during this period the first 24 hours is the most predictive in terms of survival. Of the patients who survive the first 3 weeks, the median survival is between 3 and 4 years. For patients older than 70 years of age, mortality increases significantly in all phases (i.e., acute, intermediate, and late) after a stroke. Of the various forms of cerebrovascular accident, cerebral thrombosis has the best prognosis for survival. Computed tomography and magnetic resonance imaging have considerably improved the ability to distinguish hemorrhage from infarction.

Of patients who survive their cerebrovascular accidents long term, approximately 84 percent can be expected to go on to live in their

225

own homes. The level of function within this environment depends on patients' mobility, ability for self-care, and communication. In terms of mobility, patients who develop extensor spasticity in the lower extremities are more likely to ambulate at an early stage. The few patients with persistent flaccidity are more dependent on orthotics and functional electric stimulation technology. Patients who demonstrate early spontaneous neurologic recovery (i.e., within the first 4 to 6 weeks) seem to fare better in the long term than those who do not. In all cases, however, most authors agree that no spontaneous neurologic recovery can be expected beyond 6 months after a stroke. No evidence shows that comprehensive rehabilitation increases neurologic recovery, but strong evidence suggests that functional recovery is significantly improved through a rehabilitation program, which can include surgical intervention for deformities about the foot and ankle.

Preoperative Assessment of Stroke Patients

Obviously, not every patient who has had a stroke is a candidate for corrective surgery for spastic deformities about the foot and ankle. There are certain minimum requirements for independent ambulation. Among these are the *cognitive skills*: that is, patients' ability to learn and to perform safely within their environment. Without this ability, certain patients will require continued custodial care for their own safety, even though they may be able to ambulate. Patients must also have the *energy capacity* to meet the specific physiologic demands created during walking. For example, patients who suffer severe chronic obstructive pulmonary disease may demonstrate severe limitations secondary to poor oxygenation and would also be poor surgical candidates. Other patients with moderate to severe coronary artery disease, congestive heart failure, or both would also find independent ambulation difficult. Patients must also demonstrate *motor control* that is adequate to meet the postural demands of walking. Neck strength must be at least fair; trunk strength may be poor; and the uninvolved upper extremity must have good strength if it is used for support. The uninvolved lower extremity should have good to

normal strength, and the nonpostural muscles must have fair to good strength.

In terms of *balance,* either two-limb momentary standing balance without hand support or single-limb standing balance with hand support must be demonstrated.

In terms of *sensation,* proprioception deficit can be compensated for by visual keys or an orthosis, such as an ankle-foot orthosis. In terms of perceptual integration, patients need to be aware of all body parts, particularly the lower extremities, and of body position in space.

In addition to these minimal requirements for independent ambulation, the risk of anesthesia must also be weighed as part of the overall preoperative analysis of the patient. Patients who are receiving adequate treatment for any underlying medical problem, even though they have suffered a cerebrovascular accident, can be safely anesthetized after an initial period of 6 to 9 months from the time of their stroke.

After the surgeon has established that the patient has attained the minimal requirements for independent ambulation and that anesthesia poses no significant risk for the patient, further evaluation is still needed. For most orthopaedic surgeons, this evaluation includes critical clinical observation of the patient during ambulation to determine which muscles are contributing to the deformity observed. In more sophisticated settings, a more precise delineation of the offending muscles can be obtained by percutaneous or in some cases surface electrodes placed for dynamic electromyographic analysis. In studies performed by Perry and colleagues at Rancho Los Amigos Hospital, in which the authors evaluated patients with dynamic electromyography after stroke, the following general conclusions were based on the 40 patients examined.[1] First, premature firing of the triceps surae due to the release of primitive locomotor control mechanisms and a hyperactive stretch response during limb loading were the most important causes of equinus. Second, prolonged firing of the tibialis anterior during stance and inactivity of the peroneus brevis were the principal factors responsible for the varus component of the equinus varus deformity. Premature or continuous activity of the flexor hallucis longus and the flexor digitorum longus was also noted in a significant number of patients. This activity can contribute to the equinus deformity of the ankle as well as to toe curling. Posterior tibialis muscle activity was noted to occur prematurely in stance; therefore, the investigators did not consider it to play a significant role in the production of stance varus. In addition, the posterior tibialis was not considered a good candidate for transfer to the anterior aspect of the foot because only four of 28 patients studied with equinus or equinus varus deformity had significant posterior tibialis activity during swing phase. On the other hand, the flexor hallucis longus showed significant swing-phase activity in 20 of these patients and was therefore considered a more likely candidate for transfer.

Surgical Correction of Foot and Ankle Deformities

Toe Curling

Toe curling is a common problem after cerebrovascular accidents. It differs from toe clawing in that the toe extensors are usually inactive. Surgical correction for this problem is indicated when toe curling causes pain. If only one or two toes are involved, an open tenotomy is performed at the base of each toe. If all the toes are involved, the flexor hallucis longus and flexor digitorum longus are sectioned distal to the quadratus plantae muscle in the sole of the foot. For this, an incision is made on the medial border of the foot along the anterior margin of the abductor hallucis (Fig. 20–1). The abductor hallucis is then reflected plantarward, and the tendons are localized between the first and third subfascial layers of the plantar aspect of the foot. The

same incision can also be used to detach the lateral portion of the anterior tibial tendon when the split anterior tibial tendon transfer procedure is simultaneously performed for correction of varus deformity. An intrinsic plus deformity—that is, flexion of the metatarsophalangeal joints and extension of the interphalangeal joints—may occur subsequent to sectioning the long flexors of the toes, but this rarely causes discomfort.

Equinus Deformity

Spastic plantar flexion of the ankle results in weight bearing on the forefoot without heel contact, backward extension of the tibia, and hyperextension of the knee. This deformity commonly responds to the use of a rigid ankle-foot orthosis that restricts plantar flexion. The heel height may be increased to compensate for mild equinus deformity; however, more than 2 cm of heel elevation results in difficulty in walking for the hemiplegic patient.

Surgical correction of equinus is indicated when an ankle-foot orthosis is not able to control plantar flexion. The patient's heel should be firmly in contact with the sole of the shoe, and the patient should not walk with a hyperextension thrust of the knee. While the patient stands in one position, pistoning out of the counter of the shoe is usually not noted; however, it can be observed as the patient starts to walk and spasticity increases. To observe this, a mark is placed on the patient's sock at the top of the counter of the shoe while the heel is firmly in contact with the sole of the shoe. The patient is then observed during walking, and the mark is noted to rise above the level of the counter of the shoe, demonstrating the pistoning (Fig. 20–2).

FIGURE 20–1. Release of the flexor hallucis longus and the flexor digitorum longus through a medial incision. Either one or both may be used to transfer anteriorly. The same incision is used in the split anterior tibial tendon procedure. (From Waters RL, Perry J, Garland D: Surgical correction of gait abnormalities following strokes. Clin Orthop 131:57, 1978.)

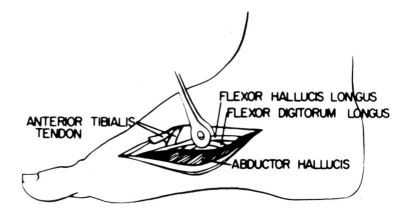

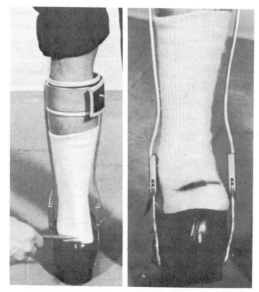

FIGURE 20–2. Pistoning noted during walking by marking a sock as indicated. (From Waters RL, Perry J, Garland D: Surgical correction of gait abnormalities following strokes. Clin Orthop 131:57, 1978.)

The potential benefits of surgical correction can be demonstrated by a posterior tibial nerve block performed at the level of the popliteal fossa. Assuming there is no contracture of the triceps surae, pistoning will no longer be observed after a block has been obtained.

Lengthening of the Achilles tendon may be either an open or a percutaneous procedure. The percutaneous method as described by Hoke is simple and decreases surgery time and morbidity by decreasing dissection when compared with the open procedure (Fig. 20–3).[2] At surgery, the knee is fully extended and the ankle is dorsiflexed to place tension on the Achilles tendon, drawing it posteriorly away from the neurovascular bundle medially. After the tenotomy has been performed, the ankle is dorsiflexed to a neutral position but not beyond this point. At the end of the procedure, a short-leg walking cast is applied with the ankle at approximately 5 degrees of plantar flexion to prevent further stretch of the Achilles tendon during walking. Excessive lengthening of the Achilles tendon results in plantar flexion weakness, loss of control of the tibia, and instability of the ankle. The cast is worn approximately 6 weeks, and then the ankle is protected in an ankle-foot orthosis for an additional 6 weeks.

Release of the long toe flexors is usually performed at the time of the Achilles tendon lengthening, even if toe flexion is not painful. This is done for a number of reasons: (1) these flexors can be spastic and cause curling of the toes; (2) with correction of the equinus deformity, relative shortening of the long toe flexors occurs, and with it toe curling; and (3) the toe flexors can be transferred to the anterior aspect of the foot to assist in dorsiflexion of the ankle, particularly if they are active during swing phase.

Most patients require an ankle-foot orthosis after Achilles tendon lengthening, either because the patient has weak dorsiflexion of the foot and thus requires an ankle-foot orthosis to prevent footdrop or because it is often difficult to lengthen the Achilles tendon just the right amount. This may result in plantar flexion weakness or mild persistent equinus. Additionally, in patients who lack good proprioception, an ankle-foot orthosis provides necessary sensory input to the patient.

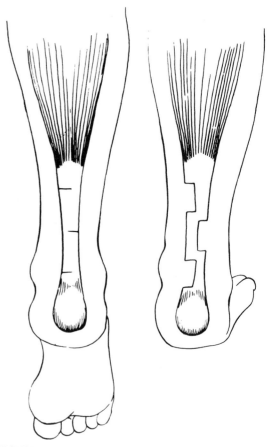

FIGURE 20–3. Hoke's technique for Achilles tendon lengthening. (From Waters RL, Perry J, Garland D: Surgical correction of gait abnormalities following strokes. Clin Orthop 131:58, 1978.)

Plantar Flexion Weakness

It is important to differentiate patients with plantar flexion weakness from those with equinus deformity of the ankle because both groups demonstrate hyperextension of the knee. Patients with plantar flexion weakness bear weight primarily on the heel rather than on the forefoot, in contrast to patients with equinus. Knee hyperextension due to plantar flexion weakness is corrected by an orthosis that restricts excessive plantar flexion, whereas knee hyperextension caused by equinus deformity is corrected by Achilles tendon lengthening.

Inadequate Dorsiflexion

Inadequate dorsiflexion or footdrop during swing phase is due to inactivity or paresis of the anterior tibial muscle, and it can occasionally occur in patients without equinus deformity. Gait analysis generally fails to demonstrate any muscle that is suitable for transfer to assist in dorsiflexion during the swing phase. In general, this deformity is corrected by an ankle-foot orthosis, although stimulation of the peroneal nerve using floor contacts in the sole of the shoe has been tried. However, I have occasionally transferred long toe flexor tendons through the interosseous membrane to the anterior aspect of the foot and sutured them into the second and third cuneiforms, which creates a tenodesis effect that is usually sufficient to clear the foot during swing phase.

Varus Deformity

Varus deformity results in the patient's walking along the lateral aspect of the foot. If this deformity is not corrected by a well-fitted orthosis, it will require surgical correction. The five muscle groups that contribute to a varus deformity because they lie medial to the subtalar joint axis are the soleus, the flexor hallucis longus, the flexor digitorum longus, the posterior tibial, and the anterior tibial muscles. When the soleus contributes to the varus deformity, equinus is also present; therefore, Achilles tendon lengthening will diminish its deforming forces. Sectioning of the long toe flexors similarly diminishes their contribution to the varus deformity.

Lengthening of the tibialis posterior tendon is generally not indicated in patients who have had strokes because, unlike patients with cerebral palsy, they do not usually have a fixed varus deformity of the hindfoot. If the posterior tibial tendon is released or lengthened in association with a split anterior tibial tendon procedure (SPLATT), calcaneovalgus deformity may occur in conjunction with excessive eversion of the forepart of the forefoot. This results in collapse of the longitudinal arch and pain along the medial border of the foot—in short, the opposite of the deformity for which correction was attempted.

The SPLATT procedure is performed in the following manner (Fig. 20–4). Through an incision along the medial border of the foot, just dorsal to the anterior margin of the abductor hallucis longus, dissection is carried down through the subcutaneous tissue, and hemostasis is maintained with electrocautery. The lateral two-thirds of the tendon is freed from its insertion, and a Bunnell-type suture is placed around the free end. The next incision is placed over the musculotendinous junction of the tibialis anterior muscle, which is generally approximately one handbreadth above the level of the ankle joint. The pretibial muscle fascia is divided. A long hemostat or similar instrument is passed over the tendon from proximal to distal. The tendon suture is then delivered to the proximal incision. Through the application of traction to the suture, the musculotendinous junction is split in a longitudinal manner.

The third incision is then placed over the area of the third cuneiform and the cuboid bones. A 1/4-inch drill bit is used to place a hole between the cuboid and the cuneiform. This hole can be further enlarged using curettes. The lateral portion of the tibial tendon is then passed distally in a subcutaneous manner, pulled through the cuboid, pulled medially through the cuneiform, and sutured onto itself. (*Editor's note:* A wire loop suture passer is useful to grasp the tendon suture and pass it and the tendon through the bone. Tension on the transfer is determined by placing the ankle and midfoot in neutral position and temporarily suturing the tendon at 50 percent of its elastic excursion. The tension on this limb of the tendon should be compared with that of the medial limb in the proximal wound. It should be slightly tighter.) A short-leg walking cast is applied. After 6 weeks, the cast is removed and the tendon is further protected for an additional 4 1/2 months with an ankle-foot orthosis that prevents plantar flexion during walking and with a posterior splint at night during rest.

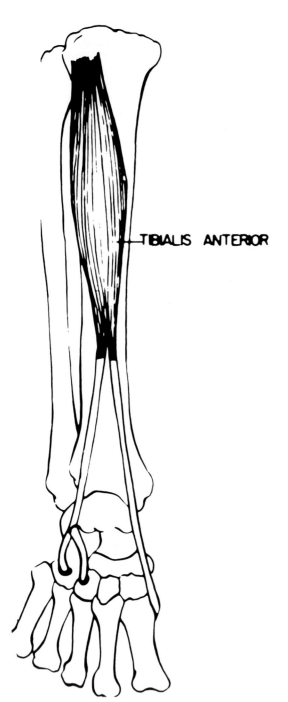

deformity, a combined Achilles tendon lengthening, SPLATT procedure, and toe flexor release are performed simultaneously.[2] Transfer of the long toe flexor is also indicated, particularly if flexion of the toes is noted during swing phase, because this transfer may assist in dorsiflexion (Fig. 20–5). Patients are protected in an ankle-foot orthosis for 4 1/2 months after 6 weeks of cast immobilization. There may be a tendency for footdrop to recur secondary to plantar flexion thrust of the ankle at heel strike or an imbalance between the anterior and posterior muscle groups. No attempt should be made to correct any resultant plantar flexion deformity with another Achilles tendon lengthening if the equinus deformity is mild. Doing so can create plantar flexion weakness and instability of the ankle. Transfer of the flexor hallucis longus or flexor digitorum longus through the interosseous membrane

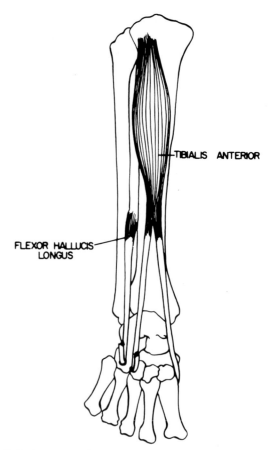

FIGURE 20–4. Split anterior tibial tendon transfer. (From Waters RL, Perry J, Garland D: Surgical correction of gait abnormalities following strokes. Clin Orthop 131:59, 1978.)

Equinovarus Deformity

The equinovarus deformity associated with toe curling is the most common that occurs in the patient who has had a stroke. For this

FIGURE 20–5. Split anterior tibial tendon transfer combined with transfer of the flexor hallucis longus. (From Waters RL, Perry J, Garland D: Surgical correction of gait abnormalities following strokes. Clin Orthop 131:60, 1978.)

may assist in dorsiflexion. When these muscles are active during swing phase, they can help prevent recurrence of the equinus deformity. If both the flexor hallucis longus and the flexor digitorum longus are active, only the former is transferred. They are transferred through the interosseous membrane and through the same holes used to pass the lateral portion of the anterior tibial tendon in the SPLATT procedure.

Discussion

As was indicated previously, careful preoperative assessment of the hemiplegic patient is required to determine not only which patients can tolerate anesthesia but also which can benefit from the surgical procedure. A careful analysis of gait abnormalities must be made to determine the correct surgical procedure to perform. It is important not only for the patient but also for those who care for the patient to realize the goals of surgery and the limitations of any surgical procedure. Improvement of gait is to be anticipated, but normal gait is *not*. Some patients can walk without a brace after surgical correction, whereas others, although their deformity has been corrected, still require a brace because they lack proprioception and have knee instability. Pinzur and colleagues studied 54 adult patients with acquired spastic equinus and equinus deformities about the foot and ankle that were treated with Achilles tendon lengthening, lateral transfer of the anterior tibial tendon (similar to the SPLATT procedure), and appropriate muscle releases.[3] All their patients had preoperative dynamic electromyographic and electrogoniometric studies to assist in planning of the surgical procedures and to provide a baseline assessment of the dynamic deformities. In all patients, the operation was performed at least 1 year after the onset of hemiplegia. The investigators demonstrated that in an average follow-up of 30 months, the equinus deformity was corrected in all patients and 59 percent of them were brace-free.

More important, these studies suggested that the spastic equinus deformity was a major dynamic derangement of the gait of adults with acquired hemiplegia and that correction of this deformity, although it did not fully correct any related deformities of the hip and knee, improved gait sufficiently so that few patients required any further surgery. Pinzur and colleagues recommended that only the equinus deformity about the ankle be corrected as an initial procedure for this type of patient. They believe that the results were predictable in terms of improving patients' gaits and thus reduced patients' energy demands for gait. I concur with their finding, and after correcting the deformity about the foot and ankle, I have not had to correct any proximal deformities of either the hip or the knee.

CEREBRAL PALSY

As noted previously, cerebral palsy is generally defined as a nonprogressive disorder that begins either in utero or within the first 2 years of life with a selective loss of muscle control.[4] Basically five types can be distinguished clinically: (1) spastic paralysis, (2) athetosis, (3) ataxia, (4) tremor, and (5) rigidity. The incidence of each is as follows: spastic paralysis, 50 percent; athetosis, 25 percent; ataxia, 7 percent; tremor, 1 percent; and rigidity, 7 percent. In the remaining 10 percent of cases, more than one type is present.

Cerebral palsy may have its origin in either the perinatal, prenatal, or postnatal period. Approximately 37 percent of cases can be attributed to either trauma at birth or anoxia. Prematurity, in which the infant is susceptible to intracranial hemorrhage, accounts for approximately 32 percent of cases. Congenital defects are responsible for approximately 11 percent of cases, and postnatal causes such as encephalitis account for 7 percent. Unfortunately, the illegal use of drugs has also contributed to the high incidence of cerebral palsy in infants whose mothers used drugs during pregnancy.

In cerebral palsy, surgery is indicated most often in the patient with spastic paralysis. The objective of surgery is to correct physical deformities that can interfere with the patient's overall rehabilitation or basic nursing care. Surgery should be considered part of the overall management of these patients, as are physical, speech, and occupational therapy and appropriate bracing.

As with the adult patient with spastic hemiplegia, careful clinical assessment of the patient is needed to determine the underlying causes of deformity and to select patients who will benefit most from surgical intervention.

Children who have overwhelming disabilities, severe medical problems, uncontrollable or frequent convulsive disorders, and a poor social environment and who lack motivation should not be considered serious candidates for surgery. Mental deficiency alone should not make surgical intervention inadvisable.

Unnecessary delays in performing surgery may only prolong nonproductive and expensive physical therapy modalities. The goals of surgery should be realistic, and the benefits of surgery must, as in all cases, be weighed against the potential risks to the patient.

In the patient with cerebral palsy, surgery is useful to correct deformities, whether they are static or dynamic: dynamic to balance muscle power, and static to stabilize uncontrollable joints. Static or fixed deformities are corrected primarily by tendon lengthening, capsulotomy, fasciotomy, and osteotomy of the tarsal bones for varus or valgus deformity. Dynamic deformities are partially corrected by tenotomies or musculotendinous lengthening procedures. Most tendon transfers to balance the muscle power about a joint work more in theory than in practice and in my opinion serve more as a tenodesis. Function training after out-of-phase transfers may be difficult enough in patients with full mental capacities, let alone in a child with diminished mental capacity.

Neurectomy of some of the motor branches of nerves to a particular muscle is based on the idea that this procedure will result in diminished strength of the muscle and in equal strength of its antagonist muscle. Again, this idea is rarely realized in practice. I have no experience with this type of treatment and do not believe it should be considered in the overall armamentarium of surgical procedures. In my opinion, the results are too unpredictable because it is nearly impossible to measure the power of the muscles the surgeon is trying to balance.

Unstable joints are not easily corrected by muscle balancing procedures because the muscles may eventually stretch and a deformity may recur. In cerebral palsy, triple arthrodesis is useful in stabilizing the unbalanced foot, and the Grice extra-articular arthrodesis of the subtalar joint is valuable in correcting an equinovalgus deformity. Soft tissue procedures may be combined with bone procedures such as fusions and wedge osteotomies; however, if there is any concern about the condition of the skin in doing so, staging of these procedures is strongly recommended.

With regard to the foot and ankle, the following deformities may occur in the patient with cerebral palsy: (1) equinus, (2) valgus, (3) varus, and (4) clawing of the toes.

Surgical Correction of Equinus Deformity

Surgical correction of equinus deformity is indicated when conservative care has failed or when the deformity is of such magnitude and severity that conservative treatment would be inappropriate. Because this deformity will recur until growth is complete, surgery should be postponed until that time, if possible. However, if the offending muscles are contributing to the development of a bony deformity, early surgery should be performed. Early surgical intervention should also be considered if the chances for increased mobilization of the patient are good or if ease of nursing care for the severely involved patient can be enhanced. Basically, three types of operations are used in correcting an equinus deformity. The first is neurectomy of one or more branches of the tibial nerve to either the gastrocnemius or the soleus. As indicated earlier, I have no experience with this procedure, and I believe its results are too unpredictable. The second procedure is release of the triceps surae by distal transplantation of the heads of origin of the gastrocnemius (as included in the Silfverskiöld procedure[5]), lengthening of the tendon of the gastrocnemius alone (the Vulpius or Strayer procedures[5]), or lengthening of the tendo calcaneus. Third, advancement of the insertion of the tendo calcaneus to decrease its moment arm and thus its power for plantar flexion has been described. I have had no experience with this procedure either. By far the most common procedure is Achilles tendon lengthening for correction of the equinus deformity. This procedure was described in an earlier section. Either the percutaneous Hoke technique or an open tenotomy with Z-lengthening of the tendon can be used.

The Silfverskiöld test was an important advancement in the analysis and treatment of spastic equinus contracture. In the awake child, it is not easy to differentiate gastrocnemius spasticity from contracture. Under anesthesia, however, the spastic reflex is eliminated; thus, the determination is easily made. Silfverskiöld determined that there were two types of deformities: in one, the equinus cannot be corrected when the knee is fully extended but can be passively corrected when the knee is flexed to 90 degrees; in the second deformity, no change in the position of the knee results in the correction of the deformity.[5] In the first type, the deformity is caused chiefly by contracture of the gastrocnemius muscle, and the procedure of choice is release and transplantation of the heads of the gastrocnemius muscle distal to the knee joint. The Strayer and Vulpius procedures are the preferred alternatives.[5]

In the Strayer procedure, a posterior longitudinal incision of approximately 10 to 15 cm is made over the midcalf (Fig. 20–6). The medial sural cutaneous nerve is identified and retracted. The fascia is split to expose the gastrocnemius muscle, and the gastrocnemius muscle is separated from the underlying soleus by blunt dissection proximal to where the tendons of the gastrocnemius and the soleus

join. The gastrocnemius tendon is then severed, the foot is dorsiflexed to a neutral position, and a gap of approximately 2 to 2.5 cm appears between the ends of the tendons. The gastrocnemius is further freed from the underlying soleus to allow it to retract proximally. The proximal portion of the gastrocnemius aponeurotic tendon is then sutured to the underlying soleus with nonabsorbable suture, and the wound is closed with interrupted sutures. A long-leg cast is applied from the groin to the toes, with the knee in extension and the ankle in neutral position. The cast is maintained for approximately 4 to 6 weeks, after which night splints are used until skeletal maturity.

The Vulpius procedure is essentially the same as the Strayer procedure; however, the aponeurotic tendon of the gastrocnemius is incised in an inverted V-shaped incision (Fig. 20–7). Placing the ankle in neutral position

FIGURE 20–6. Lengthening of the gastrocnemius by Strayer's technique. (From Strayer LM Jr: J Bone Joint Surg 32A:671, 1950.)

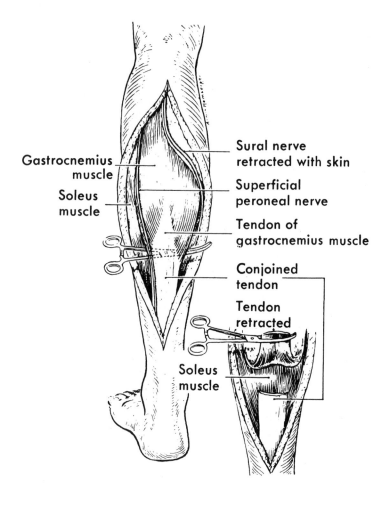

Gastrocnemius muscle

Soleus muscle

Sural nerve retracted with skin

Superficial peroneal nerve

Tendon of gastrocnemius muscle

Conjoined tendon

Tendon retracted

Soleus muscle

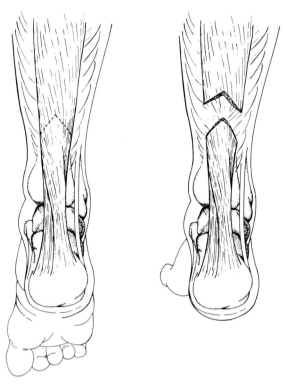

FIGURE 20–7. Lengthening of the gastrocnemius by Vulpius' technique. (Reproduced by permission from Sage FP: *Cerebral plasy. In* Crenshaw AH [Ed]: *Campbell's Operative Orthopaedics*, 7th Ed. St. Louis, 1987, The CV Mosby Co, p 2862; courtesy of Drs. E.L. Compere and W.T. Schnute.)

with the knee extended separates the segments of the tendons. If the aponeurosis of the soleus muscle is also tight, it too is divided, but the muscle itself is not disturbed. Again, a long-leg cast is applied for approximately 4 to 6 weeks, and subsequent night splinting is used until skeletal maturity is reached.

For the equinus deformity caused by contracture of both the gastrocnemius and the soleus, lengthening the Achilles tendon is appropriate. The tendon should be lengthened only to such a degree that allows the foot to come to a neutral position. A short-leg cast is then applied for 6 weeks, after which posterior splinting at night is indicated until skeletal maturity to help prevent recurrence of the deformity.

Correction of Varus or Valgus Deformity

Varus deformity of the foot in cerebral palsy may be caused by overpull of the tibialis pos-terior or any other muscle lying medial to the subtalar joint axis associated with either actual or relative weakness of any muscle lying lateral to the subtalar axis (i.e., an evertor muscle). Conversely, valgus deformity may be caused by overpull of the peroneal muscles or other evertor muscles associated with either relative or actual weakness of an invertor muscle. The triceps surae is the primary deforming factor in a valgus deformity. Ankle dorsiflexion is blocked, and dorsiflexion consequently occurs through the midpart of the foot. To accomplish this, the calcaneus must roll into a valgus position to allow the head of the talus to rotate medially and unlock the transverse tarsal joints to make the foot more supple. As the talus drops into a more medial and vertical position, the forepart of the foot comes into a more valgus position. This can be easily demonstrated on a standing radiograph of the foot: on a lateral view, the talus will be vertical in its orientation, and on an anteroposterior view, the head of the talus will show marked medial rotation. Thus, release of the contracted triceps surae, by any of the appropriate methods described previously, is the first step in correcting a valgus deformity of the foot.

An opening wedge osteotomy can also be performed as a modification of the Dwyer osteotomy. It can be performed by interposing either autologous or homologous bone graft. Varus deformity can be corrected by closing wedge osteotomy and stapling. Another technique is a through-and-through osteotomy in an oblique cephalad to caudad plane posterior to the subtalar joint in which the posterior fragment to which the Achilles tendon is attached is displayed medially. This, of course, would be for a valgus type of deformity, to place the triceps surae insertion medial to the subtalar joint axis.

The Grice subtalar extra-articular arthrodesis is considered the procedure of choice for stabilizing a planovalgus foot in patients with cerebral palsy, particularly those between 4 and 9 years of age. This procedure has been described in many texts and is not included in this chapter. There are a number of pitfalls to this procedure. First, the procedure should be preceded or accompanied by operations that correct deformities caused by soft tissue contracture, such as release of the triceps surae, as well as by operations that balance muscle power. Second, the dislocation or subluxation of the talar head off the sustentaculum tali should be reduced before the grafts are inserted. Autogenous graft is preferred over homogenous graft from a bone bank. The grafts should lie at a right angle to the motion of the subtalar joint axis as seen on a lateral radiograph of the foot and parallel to the weight-bearing axis of the leg, ankle, and foot. The extremity must be immobilized until bony fusion is solid. This usually requires 8 weeks in a long-leg cast followed by 4 weeks in a short-leg walking cast.

When the spastic tibialis posterior muscle is the principal cause of varus and internal rotation deformity of the foot, rerouting its tendon anteriorly through the interosseous membrane to the peroneal brevis tendon is, in my opinion, the procedure of choice (Fig. 20–8). It not only establishes a tenodesis but also eliminates the dynamic deforming force. Clinically, when the posterior tibial tendon is the primary de-

forming force, it is noted to be prominent subcutaneously through its distal course. In addition, the forepart of the foot is noted to be in adduction, varus deformity of the heel is present, and the metatarsals are in plantar flexion. This contrasts with the situation in which the tibialis anterior muscle creates the varus deformity, in which in addition to the varus deformity of the heel and adduction of the forepart of the foot, there is prominence of the tibialis anterior tendon and subcutaneous tissue, the forepart of the foot is supinated more, and the metatarsals are in less plantar flexion. If the tibialis anterior is the offending force, a SPLATT transfer is performed, with the lateral half of the tendon inserting into the peroneus brevis or into a drill hole into the cuboid and third cuneiform (as described earlier).

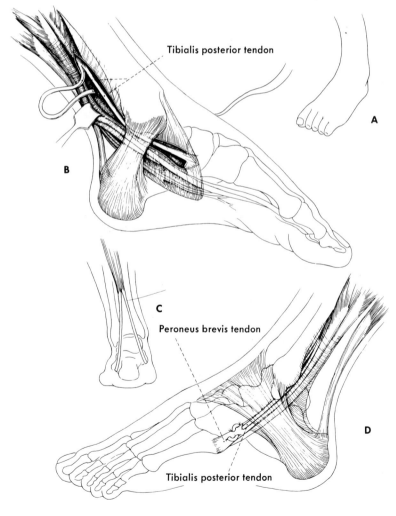

FIGURE 20–8. Kaufer's split transfer of the tibialis posterior tendon for varus deformity. *(A)*, Varus deformity. *(B)*, Medial view, harvesting one-half of the posterior tibial tendon. *(C)*, Posterior view. *(D)*, Attachment of the split portion to the peroneus brevis insertion. (Reproduced by permission from Sage FP: Cerebral plasy. *In* Crenshaw AH [Ed]: Campbell's Operative Orthopaedics, 7th Ed. St. Louis, 1987, The CV Mosby Co, p 2868; courtesy of Dr. H. Kaufer.)

In both cases, the strength, as well as it can be determined, should be rated at least good in motor power, and the tension of the transfer portion should be such that it brings the foot into a neutral position at the ankle and thus avoids a calcaneus deformity of the foot. In addition, excessive tension of the transfer portion may create a valgus deformity of the foot.

Correction of Toe Clawing

Some authors advocate neurectomy of the lateral plantar nerve, plantar capsulotomy of the first metatarsophalangeal joint, and division of the heads at the insertion of the flexor hallucis brevis. I have no experience with this procedure and prefer open tenotomy. This procedure has been described in the previous sections.

PARALYTIC FOOTDROP

Paralytic footdrop, or talipes equinus, is caused by a muscle imbalance between the muscles lying anterior and those lying posterior to the axis of the ankle joint. This condition can be secondary to poliomyelitis; to an injury to the muscles of the anterior compartment of the leg, such as occurs in the anterior compartment syndrome; or to a specific injury to the peroneal nerves to the muscles of the anterior compartment, such as occurs with gunshot wounds or fractures about the head and neck of the fibula. If the footdrop is a chronic condition that has essentially been left untreated, contracture of the posterior capsule of the ankle can also occur and may require surgical release. If the deformity occurs prior to skeletal maturity, such as in a child stricken with polio, bony deformities such as equinus calcaneus can also occur. Imbalance between the muscles medial and lateral to the subtalar joint axis can result in either equinovarus or equinovalgus deformity; however, these deformities are not considered in this section.

Nonsurgical treatment of this condition involves the use of a well-fitted ankle-foot orthosis made of lightweight polypropylene material that helps to support the foot in a neutral position. If stretching of the Achilles tendon and muscle complex is required, a spring-loaded double-upright metal brace can be used. If nonsurgical forms of treatment fail, Achilles tendon lengthening with or without

posterior capsular release is indicated. This would bring the foot into a neutral position, which could then be maintained by a polypropylene ankle-foot orthosis.

In lieu of using a polypropylene brace, a stabilization procedure can be performed to prevent recurrence of the equinus deformity. This could be either a posterior bone block, a Lambrinudi procedure, a pantalar arthrodesis, or an arthrodesis of the ankle joint. The first two operations make the use of an ankle-foot orthosis unnecessary by eliminating plantar flexion of the ankle while retaining dorsiflexion. The posterior bone block and Lambrinudi's procedure are the two procedures most often used for talipes equinus deformity and are described in the following sections.

Posterior Bone Block Procedure

The posterior bone block procedure as devised by Campbell is the use of a bone block located along the posterior aspect of the talus and the superior aspect of the calcaneus, which acts much like a doorstop in preventing plantar flexion of the ankle (Fig. 20–9).[5] This procedure should be combined with appropriate tendon transfers to assist in active dorsiflexion whenever possible. It will correct a deformity produced by the effects of gravity or a minor muscle imbalance, but it cannot be expected to maintain correction against a severe muscle imbalance. It is usually combined with triple arthrodesis to help stabilize medial and lateral instability. The following complications have been noted with the posterior bone block procedure: (1) degenerative arthritis, which occurred in the ankle joint in approximately 44 percent of the cases studied long term and is considered secondary either to instability about the foot or to the development of avascular necrosis of the talus; (2) recurrence of the deformity secondary to muscle imbalance, as mentioned earlier; (3) fibrous or bony ankylosis of the ankle joint secondary to the posterior bone block; and (4) flattening of the talus, which occurred in approximately 25 percent of cases and was secondary to avascular necrosis.

Technique

An incision of approximately 10 cm is made along the medial border of the Achilles tendon. If this tendon is contracted, a Z-length-

FIGURE 20–9. Posterior bone block procedure. *(a),* Skin incision. *(A),* Completed operation. *(B),* Bone graft across the posterior tibia, ankle, and subtalar joint. *(C),* Reflecting graft from the calcaneus. (Reproduced by permission from Ingram AJ: Paralytic disorders. *In* Crenshaw AH [Ed]: Campbell's Operative Orthopaedics, 7th Ed. St. Louis, 1987, The CV Mosby Co, p 2953.)

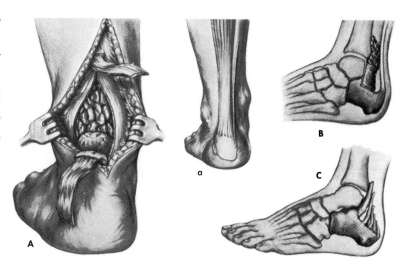

ening is performed. Otherwise, it is retracted laterally. Subsequently, using a periosteal elevator, the posterior surfaces of the tibia, ankle joint, and subtalar joint and the cephalad surface of the calcaneus are exposed. The foot is dorsiflexed and the posterior surface of the talus is exposed. The exposed portion of the talus and that of the subtalar joint are resected, and the cephalad portion of the calcaneus is excavated as illustrated (see Fig. 20–9). The posterior surface of the tibia should not be denuded; otherwise, the bone block may fuse to it and create a fusion of the ankle joint. When a triple arthrodesis has been performed in conjunction with this procedure, the bony fragments removed for the triple arthrodesis are used for the posterior bone block. Additional cancellous bone may be obtained from the anterior ilium.

The wound is subsequently closed in layers, and the Achilles tendon is repaired if it has been lengthened. The extremity is then immobilized in a long-leg cast with the ankle in neutral position or in slight dorsiflexion, and the foot is properly aligned with the knee. Approximately 2 weeks after surgery, the patient is prepared for general anesthesia. The alignment is again adjusted if necessary, and radiographs are obtained. A cast boot is then applied, and the patient is allowed on crutches. Subsequently, a walking cast is applied and is worn until consolidation is complete, which is usually in approximately 3 months. The bone block should then be protected by an ankle-foot orthosis that prevents footdrop but allows dorsiflexion. This orthosis is worn for approximately 6 months.

Lambrinudi's Procedure

In the Lambrinudi procedure, the plantar and distal aspect of the talus is excised in a wedge-like manner so that the talus remains in equinus at the ankle joint, leaving the rest of the foot in the desired degree of plantar flexion (Fig. 20–10). This procedure has many of the same complications that occur in the posterior bone block procedure: (1) recurrence of deformity, which is caused by pseudarthrosis at the talonavicular joint or by stretching of the anterior ligaments of the ankle; (2) residual deformity, which may be caused by inappropriate or inadequate tendon transfers; (3) tarsal arthritis; (4) pseudarthrosis, which has been noted in the talonavicular as well as in the calcaneocuboid joint; and (5) arthritis of the ankle joint, which may be secondary to the development of avascular necrosis. As with the posterior bone block procedure, appropriate transfers should be performed when possible to diminish any significant muscle imbalance.

Technique

The Lambrinudi operation must be preceded by appropriate radiographs and tracings. A lateral view is obtained with the foot and ankle in extreme plantar flexion. The film is traced, the tracings are then cut into three pieces along the outlines of the subtalar and midtarsal joints. From these tracings, the exact amount of bone to be removed from the talus can be determined preoperatively. The talus is cut along its plantar and distal aspect in such a

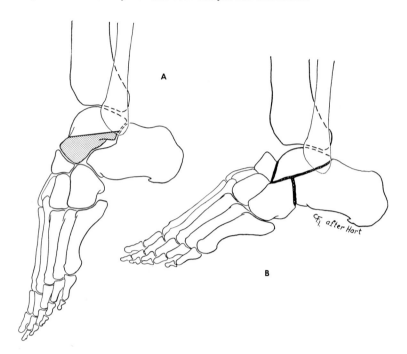

FIGURE 20–10. Lambrinudi's procedure for dropfoot. The shaded area is resected (A), and the remaining talus is wedged into the inferior aspect of the navicular (B). (From Hart VL: J Bone Joint Surg 22:937, 1940.)

manner that when the talonavicular and calcaneocuboid joints are fitted to it, the foot will be in slight equinus with relationship to the leg. Five to 10 degrees of plantar flexion is desirable.

Through a long, lateral, curved incision, the peroneal tendons are sectioned in a Z-like manner, and the talonavicular and calcaneocuboid joints are exposed by dissecting under the extensor brevis and lifting it and the fat of the sinus tarsi as a large flap based distally. All lateral interosseous and fibular collateral ligaments are divided to allow the medial dislocation of the subtalar joint. With a small oscillating saw, the predetermined wedge of bone is removed from the distal parts of the neck and body of the talus. The cartilage and bone from the superior aspect of the calcaneus are removed to form a plane parallel to the longitudinal axis of the foot. Subsequent osteotomies of the inferior part of the talonavicular and calcaneocuboid joints are performed to correct any lateral deformity. The distal part of the talus is then wedged into the remaining portion of the navicular, and the calcaneal and talar surfaces are approximated. Care should be taken to make certain that the talus is wedged firmly into the navicular and is also medial to allow correct alignment of the foot. Lateral radiographs are obtained, and if satisfactory position of the talus is demon-strated, the peroneal tendons are sutured and the wound is closed in layers.

Postoperative treatment in terms of cast immobilization is the same as that for a posterior bone block procedure.

Split Transfer of the Tibialis Posterior Tendon

Technique

The incision starts at the level of the navicular tuberosity and follows the course of the posterior tibial tendon inferiorly and posteriorly to the medial malleolus and then to the midline of the Achilles tendon. Next, the tibialis posterior tendon and the neurovascular bundle are exposed. The posterior tibial tendon sheath is excised except for a small 1-cm band at the level of the medial malleolus. This helps prevent subluxation of the posterior tibial tendon anteriorly. The posterior tibial tendon is then split into dorsal and plantar halves. The tendon is split into halves from the level of the navicular tuberosity to the musculotendinous junction and then beyond the level of the tuberosity to the plantar aspect of the foot. The part that extends to the plantar aspect of the foot is the longest portion of the split tendon, and it is withdrawn at the proximal aspect of the wound. If necessary, the Achilles tendon is then lengthened at this time through the same extended incision. The toe flexor tendons and neurovascular bundle are retracted posteriorly to allow the split portion of the tibial tendon to be brought directly against the posterior aspect of the distal tibia. Next, the peroneal tendon sheath is exposed from the tip of the lateral malleolus to the insertion of the peroneus brevis. The split portion of the posterior tibial tendon is then brought into the peroneal tendon sheath posterior to the lateral malleolus, and the segment of the split posterior tibial tendon is sutured to the insertion of the peroneus brevis with the foot in the corrected position. That is, the forefoot is abducted and pronated and in tension so that the foot dangles in a neutral position. The wound is closed in layers, and a long-leg plaster cast is applied with the foot in the corrected position. The long-leg cast is removed at 8 weeks, and a short-leg walking cast is then applied for another 8 weeks. After this, all external support is discontinued (see Fig. 20–8).

Acknowledgment

My thanks to Mrs. Terri Mesplé for her assistance and patience in preparing this manuscript.

References

1. Perry J, Waters RL, Perrin T: Electromyographic analysis of equinovarus following stroke. Clin Orthop 131:47, 1978.
2. Waters RL, Perry J, Garland D: Surgical correction of gait abnormalities following strokes. Clin Orthop 131:54–63, 1978.
3. Pinzur MS, Sherman R, DiMonte-Levine P, et al: Adult-onset hemiplegia: changes in gait after muscle-balancing procedures to correct the equinus deformity. J Bone Joint Surg 68A:1249–1257, 1986.
4. Winters TF, Gage JR, Hicks RH: Gait patterns in spastic hemiplegia in children and young adults. J Bone Joint Surg 69A:437–441, 1987.
5. Ingram AJ: Miscellaneous affections of the nervous system. *In* Edmonson AS, Crenshaw AH (Eds): Campbell's Operative Orthopaedics, Vol 2, 6th Ed. St. Louis, CV Mosby, 1980, pp 1579–1588.

21 *Foot Tumors*

KENNETH A. JAFFE

FRAZIER K. JONES

Although bone and soft tissue tumors about the foot and ankle are rare, a working knowledge of these tumors and masses is of great practical importance to the surgeon. The key to successful management of any tumor or reactive process is a thorough understanding of its biologic behavior and natural history. This knowledge is based on accurate physical, diagnostic, radiographic, and histologic evaluation. The method of treatment depends on the neoplastic nature of the lesion as well as on its actual anatomic location and involvement with local structures. The treatment of these tumors also requires both a consideration of their possible life-threatening nature and an understanding of the principles of foot surgery.

GENERAL WORK-UP FOR BONE TUMORS AND SOFT TISSUE TUMORS OF THE FOOT

To fully evaluate patients with lesions of the foot and ankle, the surgeon must undertake a systematic approach to avoid any pitfalls. Lesions of the foot can be quite misleading; many nontumorous conditions can present like tumors and can appear to be quite aggressive. For these reasons, the work-up is divided into four categories: (1) complete history and physical examination, (2) radiographic staging, (3) diagnosis, and (4) treatment.

The radiographic staging is designed to provide information on the diagnosis and the anatomic extent of the lesion. A definitive diagnosis almost always requires a biopsy. Only after these first two phases are complete

can a rational treatment plan be established and carried out. In formulating the treatment plan, the surgeon must consider the histologic type of tumor, the local extent, and the possibility of recurrent disease.[19] Clinical factors such as patient age, size, occupation, lifestyle, and expectations also play key roles in determining what treatment options are available.

Staging Techniques

As stated previously, the purpose of radiographic staging of tumors is two-fold. The first reason is to obtain information concerning the probable diagnosis, and the second is to define the anatomic extent of the lesion.[19] The extent of the necessary work-up depends on the expected diagnosis.

Plain Radiography

The first study obtained in most instances is a plain radiograph. Plain radiographs provide the most general diagnostic information. This information, in combination with the clinical presentation, gives some indication as to whether the tumor is malignant or benign and determines the extent and type of the subsequent staging studies.[19] Plain radiographs demonstrate which bone is involved, which region of this bone is involved, the extent and type of destruction, and the amount of reactive bone formed. Radiographs may also give some clue as to the type of matrix being formed by the lesion. The pattern of bone destruction and the reaction to that destruction have been well described and can be used to place the lesion in one of a few major categories.[30] These categories are based on the biologic aggressiveness of the lesion and are used to direct the remainder of the diagnostic work-up.

Radioisotope Scanning

Skeletal scintigraphy is most commonly performed using [99mTc]-labeled phosphonates. [99mTc] is incorporated into sites of tumor, bone repair, and reactive bone. Increased isotope uptake also occurs in areas of increased vascularity seen in the flow phase of the three-phase bone scan. The two major functions of this study are to provide an estimation of the local intramedullary extent of the tumor and to screen for other areas of skeletal involvement. To accomplish these goals, it is necessary to obtain anterior and posterior views of the entire skeleton, with toned-down views and two planes of the involved bone, and of any other areas of increased uptake. The extent and intensity of increased uptake may give information about the biologic aggressiveness of the tumor.[18]

Computed Tomography

Computed tomography (CT) has aided greatly in the evaluation of foot tumors. CT enables the diagnostician to view a lesion and the surrounding anatomic structures in an axial plane. New programs can also offer three-dimensional reconstruction, as well as the ability to view structures from different angles, to remove certain structures (disarticulate joints), or to eliminate the soft tissue. CT is the best study for evaluating cortical penetration and osseous detail. It is also valuable in the assessment of matrix calcification or ossification.[53] Adding contrast aids in the identification of vascular structures, as well as in the enhancement of well-vascularized lesions.

Magnetic Resonance Imaging

Magnetic resonance imaging (MRI) studies include axial images with T_1 and T_2 weighting, as well as longitudinal images in either the sagittal or coronal plane. MRI is the most accurate method of evaluating both the intramedullary extent of a bone tumor and its soft tissue components and relationship to neurovascular structures.

The role of MRI in the work-up of musculoskeletal tumors of the foot is becoming better

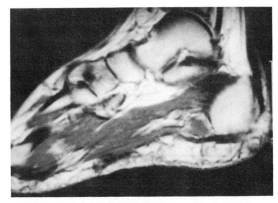

FIGURE 21–1. Magnetic resonance image of the foot.

defined. Although many possible pulse sequences can be used for tumor imaging, the most popular has been spin-echo imaging. This sequence is technically easy to implement and provides information about hydrogen density, T_1, and T_2 weighted images. Another advantage of using MRI is that by varying pulse repetition time (TR) and echo time (TE), the radiologist can drastically change the contrast level between different tissues. This process can be very helpful in trying to distinguish tumor from surrounding normal tissue (Fig. 21–1).[53]

In some instances, MRI is able to determine tumor histology[27, 40] or to determine if tumors are fluid filled. Lipomas have T_1, T_2, and hydrogen density values that are virtually identical to those of normal subcutaneous fat. However, when spin-echo imaging is used, lipomas reveal a characteristically high intensity that remains high at most spin-echo pulse sequences. Fluid content may be suspected in a lesion with a very long T_1 or T_2 time. Such lesions therefore appear relatively low in intensity on a T_1-weighted sequence and become substantially brighter on a more T_2-weighted sequence (Fig. 21–2).

The use of intravenous paramagnetic contrast agents in musculoskeletal imaging also helps to improve the contrast between tumor and normal tissue.

Staging Musculoskeletal Tumors

Benign Lesions

Stage 1: Benign–Latent. Stage 1 lesions have a benign histologic pattern, are always intracapsular, and do not metastasize.[11] Radio-

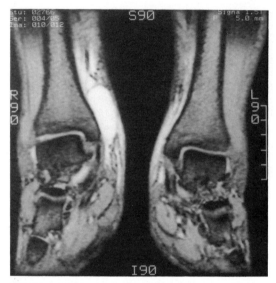

FIGURE 21–2. Synovial cyst (right ankle) mimicking soft tissue tumor on magnetic resonance imaging.

graphically, bony lesions are rimmed by mature reactive bone and either remain static in size or heal spontaneously. They are usually relatively inactive on isotope scanning. The CT scan shows a mature cortical rim. Clinically, patients are often asymptomatic and discover their lesions incidentally. The lesions seldom cause pathologic fractures, but if they do, these fractures are often obliterated by the callus.

Stage 2: Benign–Active. Stage 2 lesions have benign cytologic characteristics, remain intracapsular, and do not metastasize. Radiographically, they are rimmed by reactive bone, but they often slowly expand. Although they remain intracompartmental, they are less contained by contact inhibition and may deform or distort the barriers to extension. They may show active isotope uptake and have a moderate neovascular reaction on angiography. CT scanning usually shows a very thin but intact immature border of reactive bone. These lesions often cause symptoms and actively enlarge. They may be associated with a pathologic fracture and seldom heal spontaneously.

Stage 3: Benign–Aggressive. Stage 3 lesions have predominantly benign cytologic features, although an occasional mitotic figure may be seen. The lesions often are extracapsular and occasionally cross compartmental barriers. Radiographic features are correspondingly aggressive—poor containment by reactive bone;

increased isotope uptake, which is occult beyond the radiographic limits; and a brisk neovascular reaction on angiography. The overall impression is of a quasi- or pseudomalignant process, and distinguishing such a lesion from a low-grade sarcoma may be difficult.

Malignant Lesions

Staging of malignant tumors is dependent on the histologic grade, the presence or absence of metastasis, and whether the tumor is intracompartmental (A) or extracompartmental (B) in location.[10, 12]

Low-Grade Sarcoma (Stage I). Low-grade lesions (stage I) have invasive capability but a low risk of distant metastasis. They often present as a slow-growing, painless mass. These lesions stimulate generous amounts of reactive bone and fibrous tissue to form a pseudocapsule. Low-grade lesions progress relentlessly given enough time, but they seldom cross articular cartilage, joint capsules, tendon sheaths, nerve sheaths, or major vascular structures. Soft tissue lesions are soft, nontender, fixed, and superficial. Bony lesions have a reactive rim of bone, Codman's triangles, and endosteal scalloping. Radioisotope scans show uptake slightly beyond the radiographic limits of the lesion. Angiography shows little neovascularity. Histologic features include an even cell-to-matrix ratio, mature matrices, malignant cytology, various amounts of hemorrhage and necrosis, and pseudocapsule interruption. These lesions rarely have skip lesions, lymph node metastasis, or extracompartmental spread. Pulmonary metastasis is a late sequela.

High-Grade Sarcoma (Stage II). High-grade sarcomas (stage II) are destructive lesions that are uninhibited by natural barriers. They rapidly escape their compartment of origin and invade almost any nearby structure. Soft tissue lesions are large, hard, deep, and tender, and they stimulate a surrounding inflammatory reaction. Bony lesions show rapid destruction of nearby structures. Isotope scans show uptake far beyond that suggested on other studies and can suggest skip lesions. Angiograms show prominent neovasculature. Histologic features show a high cell-to-matrix ratio, immature matrices, malignant cytology, little encapsulation, and skip lesions; these lesions have significant risks of lymphatic or hematogenous metastasis (Table 21–1).

From Enneking WF, Spanier SS, Goodman MA: A system for the surgical staging of musculoskeletal sarcoma. Clin Orthop 153:106–120, 1980.

TABLE 21–1. STAGES OF MUSCULOSKELETAL TUMORS

BENIGN
1. Latent
2. Active
3. Aggressive

MALIGNANT
I. Low grade without metastasis
   A. Intracompartmental
   B. Extracompartmental
II. High grade without metastasis
   A. Intracompartmental
   B. Extracompartmental
III. Low and high grade with metastasis
   A. Intracompartmental
   B. Extracompartmental

Biopsy

The biopsy is an important step in the management of bone or soft tissue tumors. A principle that permeates orthopaedic oncology is the need for a multidisciplinary approach to the diagnosis and management of neoplasms.[46] The accurate staging of the local lesion should be completed before biopsy. Changes induced by the biopsy may alter the lesion enough to make it difficult to determine the extent of disease after biopsy, or they may introduce confusing artifacts on the special studies. The biopsy procedure must be planned as carefully as the definitive procedure. Details of the biopsy procedure should be the responsibility of the person who will ultimately treat the patient. Several methods of biopsy are used, with the choice of method depending on the presumptive clinical diagnosis.

Needle biopsy is the simplest method for obtaining tissue. The limitation of this method is the small size of the tissue sample, which may make diagnosis difficult. This technique is gaining in popularity as more cytologists and pathologists have developed experience in interpreting needle biopsy findings. The path of the needle must be placed in such a way that the needle track can be subsequently excised at the time of the definitive resection. The most common indication for needle biopsy is a deep-seated bone or soft tissue lesion in which the presumptive diagnosis is malignant disease. It can also be used to rule out recurrent disease. Open biopsy is used more commonly in diagnosing lesions that appear benign. These are best approached with incisions that match the anatomic creases and avoid the weight-bearing surfaces.[11] Benign lesions are best managed by marginal excision for both biopsy and treatment because of the ease with which these lesions may be transplanted inadvertently or extended by incisional biopsy and because of the difficulty that such implants cause in subsequent management. Conversely, the surgeon should approach open biopsy of malignant lesions through longitudinal incisions, bearing in mind the approaches to be used in subsequent wide or radical local procedures.

In the distal tibial epiphysis and talus, particular care must be taken to avoid contaminating the anterior and posteromedial neurovascular bundles while obtaining tissue for biopsy. The biopsy should be carried out in a fashion that permits adequate exposure for subsequent wide excision without inadvertent contamination of these vital structures. Medial lesions are best approached by a longitudinal anteromedial incision on the medial side of the tibialis anterior in the sulcus between the muscle and the anterior margin of the medial malleolus (Fig. 21–3). Lateral lesions call for the use of a longitudinal incision through the sulcus between the lateral malleolus and the lateral margin of the common extensor tendon (Fig. 21–4). Posterior lesions in the body of the talus are best approached through a posterolateral incision just lateral to the edge of the Achilles tendon (Fig. 21–5). Lesions in the os calcis are best approached by either a medial or a lateral incision that parallels the border of the transition from weight-bearing to non–weight-bearing skin of the heel (Fig. 21–6). Direct incision to bone through skin and fat with minimal retraction of the subcutaneous flap inhibits potential extension, whereas incisions that parallel the course of the tendons in their sheaths encourage extension. Surgeons making incisions for biopsies of lesions within a particular ray should keep in mind the possibility of ray resection and should make incisions in such a way that allows subsequent re-excision without prejudice to the necessary flaps for reconstruction.

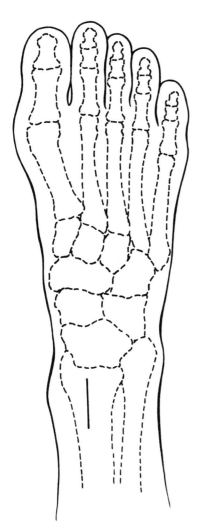

FIGURE 21–3. Medial distal tibia. Longitudinal anteromedial incision on the medial side of the tibialis anterior.

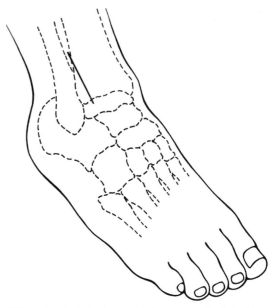

FIGURE 21–4. Lateral distal tibia. Longitudinal incision through the sulcus between the lateral malleolus and the lateral margin of the common extensor tendon.

Surgical Considerations

The foot and ankle are in many ways analogous to the wrist and the hand.[11] The ankle has many complex extensions that make extraarticular en bloc removal by a local procedure quite difficult. Like the distal radius and ulna, the distal tibia and fibula are tightly bound together, in this case by the tibiofibular ligament, which is an extension of the intraosseous membrane. The articular cartilage at the ends of the malleoli is a good barrier, but the relatively thin cortices about the epiphyseal regions are perforated by multiple large vascular channels that make extension into the periarticular soft tissues quite easy. Each of

the bones of the hindfoot and tarsal region forms separate compartments and is bounded with articular cartilage, which is quite impenetrable. However, these bones include multiple vascular perforations, and extensions into the surrounding soft tissues occur readily. The

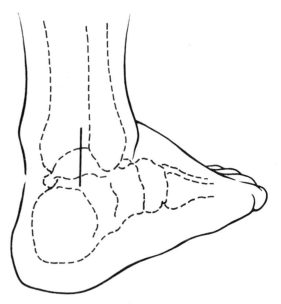

FIGURE 21–5. Posterior talus. Posterolateral approach just lateral to the edge of the Achilles tendon.

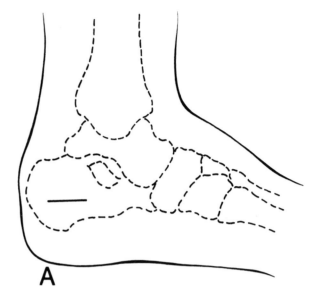

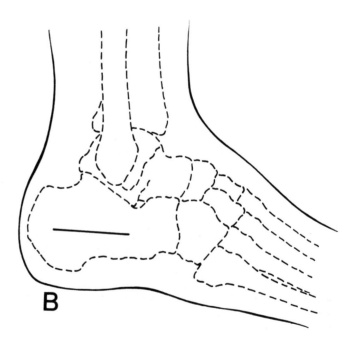

FIGURE 21–6. Os calcis. Lesions are best approached by either a medial *(A)* or a lateral *(B)* incision that parallels the border of the transition from weight-bearing to non–weight-bearing skin of the heel.

rays of the foot form individual compartments that contain the metatarsal shaft, the phalanges, the interphalangeal joints, and the surrounding soft tissues. The fascial planes between the rays that lead to the periarticular soft tissues of the midfoot have no barriers to proximal or distal extension and are extracompartmental, as are all the periarticular soft tissues about the midfoot and ankle joint.

Surgical Resection

Intralesional is the term used for an operation in which the tumor is removed from within the pseudocapsule.[10, 12] This type of resection leaves macroscopic tumor within the patient and is not appropriate for any sarcoma that is to be treated with surgery. An incisional biopsy is an intralesional operation, as are all curettages.

Marginal is the term used for an operation in which the removal of the tumor is through its pseudocapsule. This is a shell-out. Sarcomas infiltrate their pseudocapsules, and a resection through the pseudocapsule leaves microscopic tumor in the patient. A marginal resection is not adequate surgery for a sarcoma unless an excellent adjuvant is used to manage the microscopic disease.

Wide is the term used for an operation in which the tumor is removed along with a surrounding cuff of normal, uninvolved tissue. This procedure is often called an en bloc resection, and it is adequate for all sarcomas except those with skip lesions. A wide margin is the most common margin used in the surgical management of sarcomas and is successful in controlling the primary tumor in at least 95 percent of even the highest-grade tumors.

Radical is the term used for an operation in which the entire compartment or compartments involved with the tumor are removed. Usually this removal is accomplished with an amputation, but occasionally a soft tissue tumor can be resected with a radical margin without the necessity for amputation. A radical margin has the lowest possible risk of a local recurrence and is recommended for recurrent tumor or for patients who want the safest surgical resection (Table 21–2).

Surgical Procedures

Curettage is the treatment of choice for stage 1 and stage 2 benign lesions about the foot and ankle. Occasionally, the lesion involves the subchondral cortices of the bone, and overtreatment by marginal excision, with intra-articular dissection and sacrifice of portions of the articular cartilage of the foot, may be indicated. The disability from excision and joint fusion is minimal compared with the potential degree of disability that would result from undertreatment and subsequent recurrence. Bone grafting is recommended for large defects and for support of the subchondral bone. In stage 2 lesions, in which the possibility of local recurrence is increased, an augmented curettage could be performed using phenol, liquid nitrogen, or methyl methacrylate. Reconstruction following loss of an articular surface is best accomplished by an arthrodesis.

Stage 3 and 1-A lesions should be managed definitively by wide excision. The procedure often entails segmental removal of a significant portion of the bone and soft tissue. Depending on the area involved, the following is a guide for surgical exposure and reconstruction.

TABLE 21–2. SURGICAL MARGINS*

TYPE	PLANE OF DISSECTION	RESULT
Intralesional	Piecemeal debulking or curettage	Leaves macroscopic disease
Marginal	Shell-out en bloc through pseudocapsule or reactive zone	May leave either satellite or skip lesions
Wide	Intracompartmental en bloc with cuff of normal tissue	May leave skip lesions
Radical	Extracompartmental en bloc, entire compartment	No residual

*The plane of dissection used to achieve a particular margin is shown, as is the result of that margin in terms of residual lesion remaining in the wound.

From Enneking WF, Spanier SS, Goodman MA: A system for the surgical staging of musculoskeletal sarcoma. Clin Orthop 153:106–120, 1980.

Bone Tumors

Distal Tibia. Wide excision of the distal tibial metaphysis and epiphysis often entails loss of the articulating surface of the tibial component of the ankle joint. Satisfactory exposure may be obtained by parallel medial and lateral incisions rather than by straight anterior or transverse incisions that expose the neurovascular bundles to contamination. The reconstruction options after wide excision of the distal tibia include fusion of the ankle in a functional position using autogenous intercalary cortical or corticocancellous grafts from the fibula or iliac crest. This fills the defect between the dome of the talus and the osteotomy of the tibia. Alternatives include the use of an osteoarticular allograft in which the joint surface could be reconstructed and would allow almost-normal motion. Should degenerative changes occur at a later date, an arthrodesis could then easily be performed (Fig. 21–7).

Distal Fibula. If a stage 2 sarcoma involves just the distal fibula, a wide resection could be satisfactorily obtained by excision of the fibula along with the surrounding muscles. If necessary, reconstruction of the distal third could be achieved by a primary ankle arthrodesis. The resulting valgus instability could be controlled with a short-leg orthosis or, alternatively, with a primary ankle arthrodesis.

Talus. Reconstruction after excision of a significant portion of or all of the talus for aggressive low-grade lesions may be satisfactorily accomplished by a pantalar arthrodesis. The articular cartilages at the distal tibia and subtalar joint are removed, and the os calcis is internally fixed at the tibia. The cartilage of the tarsal navicular is removed so that it and the anterior tibia can be fused. Both malleoli are excised and used as graft to fill the gaps between the tarsal navicular and the tibia. If the more distal head and neck of the talus can be preserved, the articular surface of the tibia is brought into apposition with the superior articulating facets of the os calcis, and the cancellous surface of the transected neck to the talus is fixed to a matching bed on the anterior margin of the tibia to achieve a Blair-like arthrodesis.

Foot. Wide excision of lesions in the os calcis often means disarticulation of the os calcis. To achieve wide margins in aggressive

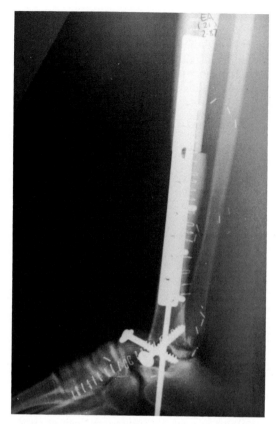

FIGURE 21–7. Resected distal tibia and talus reconstructed with allograft pantalar arthrodesis.

lesions of single tarsal bones, a complete resection is indicated. This area can be satisfactorily reconstructed by corticocancellous autografts with the appropriate intertarsal arthrodesis. Satisfactory wide margins can be obtained for lesions within the shafts of the metatarsals by segmental excision, and reconstruction can be accomplished with intercalary autogenous cortical grafts. Fixation with longitudinal transfixion wires regularly achieves union, although a high likelihood of fatigue fracture exists because of the high stress concentration in this area.

High-grade lesions in the os calcis and talus are best managed by below-knee amputations in order to achieve adequate margins. Lesions distal to the talonavicular or calcaneocuboid joints can be managed with a Syme-type ankle disarticulation. Stage 2 lesions within a ray can be managed by radical resection of that compartment if they are distal to the metatarsophalangeal joint. In the more proximal portion of the ray, resections often require removal of the ray on either side of the affected ray. This procedure usually produces a significant functional deficit, and a Syme-type amputation is therefore indicated.

Soft Tissue and Tumor-Like Lesions

Stage 1 and 2 benign soft tissue lesions require a marginal excision. The excision should be done under tourniquet control in order to give a bloodless field. A frozen section should be taken and examined to ensure that no evidence of malignancy exists. Primary soft tissue closures can usually be achieved without difficulty.

Stage 3 and I soft tissue lesions require a wide excision. Frequently, these lesions extend into the underlying bone and en bloc resection may lead to a significant amount of disability. Skin coverage is often a problem because local flaps are seldom available. For these reasons, a partial amputation may best serve the patient.

Stage 2 soft tissue lesions in the foot require amputation to achieve a radical margin. Lesions in the toe distal to the metatarsophalangeal joint require ray resection; lesions in the midfoot require a Syme amputation; and lesions in the hindfoot and the periarticular soft tissues of the ankle require below-knee amputations above the musculotendinous junction.

Limb-sparing surgery for stage 2 soft tissue sarcomas of the foot is a feasible but still inconsistently achievable goal. Several anatomic factors particular to the foot militate against obtaining the high success rates of combined-modality treatment reported for extremity sarcomas in general.[35] These treatment techniques require administration of a high dose of radiation or a combination of radiation and regional infusion of chemotherapeutic agents. Such radiation doses are poorly tolerated by the tissues of the foot, in contrast to the more proximal tissues of the arm and leg. The numerous tissue compartments of the foot are prone to the development of acute edema. Fibrosis and obliteration of lymphatic vessels also predispose the patient to stiffness, with resulting loss of function. Nonhealing ulcers and persistent pain may result in the need for amputation despite successful control of the

sarcoma. For these reasons, adjuvant treatment coupled with more conservative surgery is indicated less often in the foot than elsewhere for comparable lesions.

SOFT TISSUE AND TUMOR-LIKE LESIONS

Tumor-Like Lesions

Ganglia

A ganglion is a tumor-like collection of viscous fluid encapsulated by a fibrous sheath. It is most often found on the dorsum of the wrist but can occasionally be found on the dorsum of the foot or at the ankle level, and it is one of the most commonly encountered tumor-like lesions.[26] These lesions often are associated with tendon sheaths and may communicate with the nearest joint capsule. When found at the ankle level, the lesion often appears between the tibialis anterior and extensor digitorum longus tendons. As a whole, these lesions can account for as many as 30 percent of the soft tissue tumors of the foot. The lesions occur in patients who are between 20 and 60 years of age, with the average age being about 40 years. This is slightly older than the 25-year average for the dorsal wrist ganglion. Women are more commonly affected than men.

Ganglia range in size from 1 to 3 cm. Symptoms include pain, discomfort, and cosmetic worries. An occasional patient may have joint instability or paresthesia (from cutaneous nerve compression). Physical examination findings show a soft, movable, cystic-feeling mass. The mass tends to become more tense with age and can obstruct the smooth gliding of nearby tendons if it is allowed to reach a significant size. Radiographs usually show nothing but a small soft tissue mass, but they may show extension into adjacent bone.[20, 50] The etiology of this lesion has never been elucidated. Theories have included repetitive trauma, connective tissue defects, joint capsule herniation, and articular tissue irritation.[48] Regardless of the initiating factor, the ganglion appears to go through a staged development.[13] The first phase is dominated by the liquefaction of swollen fibroblasts, producing excessive interstitial fluid. The next phase begins to show peripheral collagen organization and coalescence of liquefied material. The final phase is characterized by a proliferation of the fibro-blastic rim or capsule. The ganglionic fluid is a viscous, honey-colored fluid rich in hyaluronic acid and mucopolysaccharides.

Treatment varies widely. The most common method is marginal excision of the lesion (Fig. 21–8). However, this can yield recurrence rates of up to 20 to 30 percent and leaves a scar that can be cosmetically unacceptable. For these reasons, other clinicians have searched for alternative methods. In the early stages, if the capsule has not excessively matured, the ganglion can be ruptured by manipulation, and the fluid can be massaged into nearby tissue. The fluid will gradually be resorbed. If the ganglion reappears, this process can be repeated until the capsule matures. Aspiration of the ganglion with subsequent injection of steroids and local anesthetics can provide a safe and simple alternative to operative therapy. Others have tried subcutaneous dissection of the ganglion with a stab incision and rupture of the structure with a tenotome. This procedure can be performed under local anesthesia,

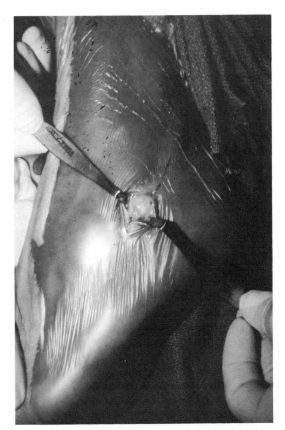

FIGURE 21–8. Ganglion cyst along the peroneal tendon.

but extreme caution must be used if the ganglion lies near a major neurovascular structure. Bony lesions can be treated by curettage or marginal excision with bone grafting.[42]

Giant Cell Tumor of Tendon Sheath

Giant cell tumor of tendon sheath is a benign lesion originally described by Chassaignac as a "cancer of tendon sheaths."[7] This tumor can occur at any age but most commonly affects people in their third or fourth decade of life. There is a slight female predominance. Giant cell tumor of tendon sheath is the second most common neoplasm found in the hand, but it can also be found in the foot.

The cell of origin is thought to be the synovial cell; therefore, the lesion naturally occurs around joints or along tendon sheaths. These tumors tend to occupy the dorsal aspect of the foot, especially around the ankle. These tumors are small and slow growing, and they can often remain the same size for years. Their exact etiology is unknown, but previous trauma may be associated with their occurrence. The typical presentation is a slow-growing, painless nodule that is soft but remains fixed to deep tissue. These tumors range from 0.5 to 4.0 cm in diameter, with lesions of the foot typically being larger than those found in the hand. The nodules remain immobile with tendinous or ligamentous manipulation. They are solid and therefore not compressible or translucent.

Gross pathologic findings show a small lobulated mass with an irregular surface. These masses typically have a mottled pink-gray appearance with some intermittent yellow and brown staining.[25] Microscopically, they are moderately cellular, with sheets or whorls of rounded or ovoid synovial cells. These cells lie on a background of hypocellular fibrillar matrix. Multinucleated giant cells are scattered in a random fashion, and areas of large foam-filled macrophages or histiocytes are present. Mitoses are rare (usually fewer than three per high-power field).

Giant cell tumor of tendon sheath has the capacity to recur locally in 10 to 20 percent of patients.[13] The recurrences have been shown to take place more commonly from lesions that are hypercellular or have increased mitoses. Local excision with a small cuff of tissue is the treatment of choice.

Pigmented Villonodular Synovitis

Pigmented villonodular synovitis (synovial xanthoma or villous synovitis) is a benign tumor-like lesion involving the synovial tissues of joints, tendon sheaths, and bursae. This lesion is characterized by villous overgrowth and pigmentation of the synovial membrane. Pigmented villonodular synovitis usually occurs in the knee but can involve any region of the foot and is especially common in the ankle.

The exact pathogenesis of pigmented villonodular synovitis is not known. Theories have ranged from neoplastic disorders to localized disturbances of lipid metabolism, post-traumatic reactions, or inflammation.[14] The most widely accepted view is that inflammation somehow plays a role, but the triggering mechanism has not been determined. Regardless of whether the patient has a localized or diffuse form, the pathology is the same. The joint fluid is usually xanthochromic or chocolate colored. The involved synovium is the consistency of rubber and is covered by a mixture of gray-yellow villi. Histologically, pigmented villonodular synovitis is characterized by a one- to three-layer pigmented synovial lining. The pigmentation, hemosiderin, is contained in the round synovial fibroblasts or type B lining cells. This soft tissue lesion can violate bone via a pressure-like phenomenon to cause localized osteoporosis, cystic degeneration, or pathologic fracture. Conventional radiography shows this bony violation in addition to a generalized soft tissue enlargement.

Symptoms depend on the form of pigmented villonodular synovitis found. Localized pigmented villonodular synovitis causes mild to moderate intermittent pain and swelling. Occasionally, a mass or nodule may be felt. The diffuse form is characterized by a generalized soft tissue swelling, which causes progressive pain but with surprisingly little discomfort compared with the degree of swelling (Fig. 21–9). The form of disease present also determines the best treatment. The localized form is best controlled by complete extracapsular or wide excision of the soft tissue component with curettage and bone grafting of the intraosseous component. The diffuse form may require a more extensive excision.

Benign Soft Tissue Tumors

Plantar Fibromatosis

Plantar fibromatosis (Dupuytren's disease) is a disease of the plantar fascia. It is a relatively rare, benign, often bilateral multinodular lesion occurring in the plantar fascia, usually in the non–weight-bearing area of the medial longitudinal arch. It is characterized by invasion of the plantar fascia by an overgrowth of fibroblasts that appear to infiltrate and produce nodular thickening. These benign lesions begin as small, painless masses, but after a variable time, they may progress to several centimeters in diameter and constitute a space-occupying lesion.[37] The mass may be locally aggressive, may extend into the overlying fat or fibrous tissue, and may adhere to the overlying skin and deep muscles, but it does not invade adjacent nerves or blood vessels. The incidence of plantar fibromatosis as a unique disease entity or as part of a syndrome is unknown. Plantar fibromatosis has been reported to appear at an earlier age than Dupuytren's disease of the hands.[1] The peak occurrence is in patients between 50 and 60

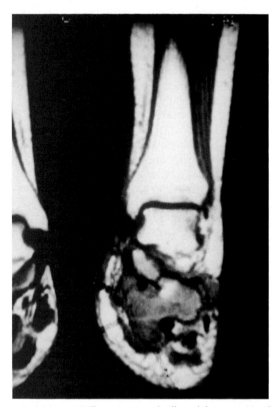

FIGURE 21–9. Diffuse pigmented villonodular synovitis of the foot.

years of age, with a slight male predominance. There is a possible familial precedence for this condition. Plantar fibromatosis has an association with epilepsy, alcoholism, and diabetes. Multiple hypotheses about the etiology of this lesion have been advocated, but they are controversial. The proposed causes include trauma, neuropathy, biochemical and metabolic disturbances, endocrinopathy, faulty development, local infections, genetic factors, chronic intoxication, senility, and occupational factors.

The natural history of the disease can be classified into three phases: (1) the proliferation phase, with increased fibroblastic activity and cellular proliferation, as well as perivascular round cell infiltration; (2) the active (involutional) phase, in which the nodules are formed; and (3) the residual phase, in which the fibroblastic activity is reduced and maturation of the collagen and tissue contracture take place.

Because plantar fibromatosis is a benign lesion, it has not been found to metastasize. Pathologists may easily confuse a recurrent plantar mass that is unencapsulated, has mitotic figures, and has an aggressive appearance with a malignant mass.[2] Differential diagnoses include fibroma, fibrosarcoma, and neurofibroma.

The treatment of plantar fibromatosis is symptomatic and may vary. If the lesion becomes symptomatic, special orthotic footwear may be indicated.[8] If the nodules are large and painful enough to be disabling, wide surgical excision is indicated. Surgical excision should take several considerations into account. A lazy-S incision is the incision of choice (Fig. 21–10).[6] It begins about 2 cm posterior to the head of the first metatarsal. It proceeds posteriorly in a lazy-S curve that traverses the medial half of the plantar surface and avoids any potential weight-bearing area that underlies a bony prominence. The exposure need not extend distal to the heads of the metatarsals because few fascial bands proceed to the toes.

This approach affords the benefits of good exposure and minimum compromise of skin circulation, and it allows the healing contracture to be multidirectional. A medial approach from the side of the foot should be avoided because this compromises the collateral venous network between the dorsal and plantar sur-

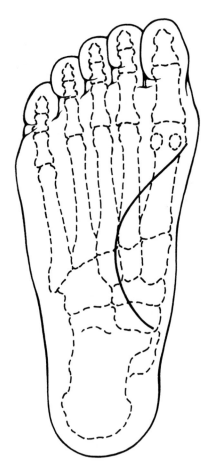

FIGURE 21–10. A lazy-S incision for resection of plantar fibromatosis.

faces. Once identified, the nodular boundary should be distinguished from the adjacent normal plantar aponeurosis. Because recurrence of the mass has been suggested to be caused by inadequate excision, dissection of the nodule involving the plantar aponeurosis should be carried out en bloc as a wide excision.[16] The surgeon should be cognizant of the location of the flexor hallucis longus tendon and the medial plantar nerve. The closure and dressing should eliminate dead space to avoid possible hematoma. Tension sutures and a compression dressing help to avoid edema. Immobilization with a posterior splint is encouraged until the sutures are removed. The patient should remain non–weight bearing for an appropriate period. Despite meticulous surgical dissection, patients may experience benign recurrences in the future.

Neurofibroma

Neurofibroma is the most common neurogenic tumor of the foot. The tumor can be solitary or multicentric. Neurofibroma is located in the central portion of the peripheral nerve, and its removal requires interference with nerve function. In neurofibromatosis, many peripheral nerves are involved. Associated with this dysplastic condition, severe deformity of the subadjacent bones of the foot is often seen, as are extensive soft tissue hypertrophy and localized gigantism.

Lipoma

Lipomas are the most common benign soft tissue tumors involving the foot and ankle. They consist entirely of mature fat cells and most often become apparent in the fifth and sixth decades of life. Location and size of the tumor determine the type of symptoms. Subcutaneous masses are usually quite mobile, and dimpling of the skin occurs on movement. Pain is rare, but it may occur secondary to compression of peripheral nerves. Deep-seated lipomas may restrict movement and give a sense of fullness.

Radiographs are quite helpful in the diagnosis of lipomas. The mass presents as a globular radiolucent area that may have areas of calcification. MRI and CT scans can clearly delineate the mass, and the lesion has the same tissue density as the surrounding subcutaneous fat (Fig. 21–11).

Subcutaneous lipomas are soft, well circumscribed, and thinly encapsulated. At the time of surgery, it may be difficult to delineate the lipomas from the surrounding subcutaneous tissue. The treatment can consist of observation if the mass is not painful or causing any functional deficit. Surgical treatment consists of marginal resection; the lipoma recurrence rate after resection is less than 5 percent. Malignant changes are exceedingly rare.

Malignant Soft Tissue Tumors

Malignant soft tissue tumors of the foot are rare. Because of the infrequency of these lesions, awareness of their existence is quite important to the physician specializing in the care of the foot. The biologic behavior of these sarcomas conforms to that of soft tissue sar-

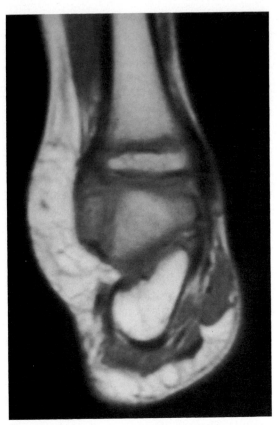

FIGURE 21–11. Magnetic resonance image of a lipoma in a young child. The lesion has the same signal intensity as the subcutaneous fat, which makes it quite difficult to delineate the margins of the lesion.

comas in general. The pathologic grade of malignancy and the size of the tumor constitute two of the most important prognostic determinants. A number of options are available for the treatment of sarcomas of the foot: (1) limited wide excision; (2) partial amputation; (3) high amputation; and (4) wide excision with adjuvant irradiation, regional chemotherapy, or both. In deliberating on the type of treatment, the clinician should consider the prognostic factors for each tumor, the applicability of the treatment method to the pathologic and anatomic situation, the expected functional result, and the potential risk of local treatment failure and tumor recurrence.[35]

Malignant Fibrous Histiocytoma

Malignant fibrous histiocytoma is a diverse sarcoma that can occur in soft tissue or bone. This tumor is the most common soft tissue sarcoma of later adult life, usually occurring in the sixth to seventh decade.[13] Malignant fibrous histiocytoma of bone has an even age distribution. Males are affected slightly more often, and whites are more commonly affected than blacks or Asians. The soft tissue variety is found throughout the lower extremities, upper extremities, and retroperitoneal area. Bony lesions most commonly affect the femur, tibia, pelvis, and humerus. The foot is not commonly affected by either variety. Soft tissue tumors have been known to occur in areas that have had previous radiation exposure, and bony lesions have arisen in pre-existing Paget's disease and bony infarcts.

The usual symptom of bone and soft tissue malignant fibrous histiocytoma is a slow-growing, painless mass of several months' duration that may cause a pathologic fracture. The radiographic features of malignant fibrous histiocytoma show obvious malignant destruction when this tumor occurs in bone. These tumors often resemble metastatic carcinoma, malignant lymphoma, or osteosarcoma. Malignant fibrous histiocytoma of the soft tissues of the foot generally shows only soft tissue swelling with an increase in radiopacity. Bone scans show intense uptake in the region of the tumor.

Gross pathologic findings show a fibrous tumor that is usually gray-brown or yellow (from lipid content). Necrotic zones are usually present. When involving bone, the lesion widely destroys cortical and cancellous bone and causes periosteal reaction. Soft tissue lesions can show heterotopic bone formation. Microscopically, the tumor can be divided into five subgroups: storiform-pleomorphic, myxoid, giant cell, inflammatory, and angiomatoid. However, a basic pattern is repeated. Multinucleated giant cells have a histiocytic appearance, with grooving of nuclei, large nucleoli, and a prominent foamy cytoplasmic mass. These cells are located on a background of storiform fibrosis. Chronic inflammation can be present, with lymphocytes occurring in small clusters. Most of these tumors are highly malignant, with many mitotic figures and high nuclear anisocytosis.

Because of the malignant nature of this lesion, aggressive therapy is indicated. Wide resection is the least conservative method that should be attempted, and radical procedures are often considered.[52] If resection is not possible without causing severe disability, amputation with prosthetic replacement is a consid-

eration. Adjuvant chemotherapy may yield better results.[43]

Synovial Cell Sarcoma

Synovial cell sarcoma is a soft tissue lesion occurring primarily in the periarticular areas. The lesion usually lies close to a tendon sheath, bursa, or joint capsule. It is the most common soft tissue sarcoma of the foot[22] and constitutes approximately 10 percent of soft tissue sarcomas. The foot is the second most common site of involvement after the knee. This is a disease of adolescents and young adults, primarily between the ages of 15 and 40. Males are affected slightly more often than females.

Patients most often present with a slow-growing, painful mass. Many patients have symptoms for 2 to 4 years before seeking attention. Sometimes patients may complain only of pain or tenderness without a mass being present. There is no definite etiology, but some patients have a history of antecedent trauma. Physical examination findings are significant for a soft, tender mass. The mechanism for this tenderness is not known, and an inflammatory process has never been proven to exist. Radiographic findings may be of benefit in diagnosing this lesion. On plain film, these lesions typically appear as round or oval lobulated soft tissue masses in proximity to a joint. The underlying bone is involved in only 20 percent of cases. Occasionally, spotty focal calcification is noted at the periphery of the soft tissue lesion. Angiography shows prominent neovasculature, and bone scans show increased uptake.

Gross pathologic findings depend on tumor growth rate and location. Slow-growing tumors are often enveloped by pseudocapsules that are adherent to nearby structures such as tendon or joint capsule. They are usually gray-white and 3 to 5 cm in diameter. Less differentiated lesions have less encapsulation and may outgrow the blood supply to yield cystic or hemorrhagic necrosis. Microscopically, the tumor is composed of two lines of cells. Epithelial cells resembling carcinoma and spindle cells resembling fibrosarcoma are present. The varying ratios of such cells indicate four types of synovial cell sarcoma: biphasic, monophasic fibrous, monophasic epithelial, and poorly differentiated forms.

The overall survival rate is 35 to 50 percent over 5 years. The prognosis is more dependent on tumor size than on tumor site or type or on the treatment modality employed. If the tumor is smaller than 5 cm, the 5-year survival rate is 75 percent, but it drops to 25 percent if the tumor is larger than 5 cm. The most widely used therapy is wide or radical excision, but in the foot, amputation is often required to gain local control because of possible proximal spread along tendon sheaths.[35] Local recurrence is the predominant concern, but metastasis can occur to lung, lymph nodes, and bone marrow. Because of the risk of local recurrence, some clinicians advocate adjuvant radiotherapy, but extreme care would need to be taken in the foot area. Trials of chemotherapy to prevent or suppress micrometastasis have been instituted, but the results are not yet known.

BONE LESIONS

Benign Tumor-Like Lesions

Giant Cell Reparative Process

Giant cell reparative granuloma is a benign non-neoplastic process linked to intraosseous hemorrhage that is found in the mandible or maxilla.[24] Similar lesions have been found in the short tubular bones of the hands and feet.[31] The presenting symptoms usually are pain and swelling for periods ranging from a few days to a few years.

Conventional radiography shows a soft tissue mass that may cause adjacent joint degeneration or cortical erosion, depending on the site of involvement. Bony changes, which can occur in 10 percent of cases, are more common with the foot nodules than with their counterparts in the hand. The mass erodes and sometimes blows out the cortex but is always well contained by the periosteum.[39] Although seldom necessary, CT or MRI may further delineate which structures are involved.

Microscopically, the lesional tissues consist of well-differentiated connective tissue and giant cells. Areas of hemorrhage are an almost constant finding, and scattered histiocytes, many of which contain phagocytosed pigment, are common. Giant cells are usually located around areas of hemorrhage. Bony trabeculae giving the appearance of metaplastic bone formation may also be present.

The differential diagnosis includes giant cell tumor, chondroblastoma, aneurysmal bone cyst, and the brown tumor of hyperparathyroidism. These lesions possess a capacity to recur locally. Intralesional excision with or without bone grafting is the usual treatment of choice, and the area of resection can always be extended if local recurrence becomes a problem.

Aneurysmal Bone Cyst

Aneurysmal bone cyst is a benign lesion characterized by cyst-like walls of predominantly fibrous tissue filled with free-flowing blood. In its early to middle phases of development, it is easily mistaken both radiographically and pathologically for a malignant tumor because of its great rate of growth, tremendous destruction of bone, and marked cellular exuberance. Almost all cases of aneurysmal bone cyst are associated with a precursor lesion such as fibrous dysplasia, giant cell tumor, chondroblastoma, or osteoblastoma. The most common clinical features are pain, swelling, or both. The lesions usually involve the tarsal or metatarsal bones of the foot. Radiographically, the lesion may be located in almost any site or portion of the bone (Fig. 21–12). It may also begin within the medullary canal, the periosteum, or the cortex. If it begins within the medullary canal, the lesion can be centrally or eccentrically placed. It can be associated with massive destruction of the bone or may be well circumscribed. Large lesions are more suggestive of malignant tumors. The treatment of aneurysmal bone cyst is usually curettage, but local recurrence is reported in approximately 20 percent of cases.[4] Total resection is the treatment of choice in certain metatarsal lesions in which the functional deficit is mini-

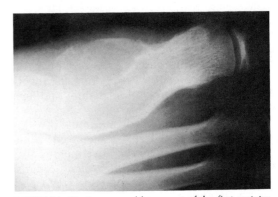

FIGURE 21–12. Aneurysmal bone cyst of the first metatarsal.

mal and the complications of local recurrence would be severe.

Unicameral Bone Cyst

Unicameral bone cysts are benign, solitary, fluid-filled lesions that usually involve the long bones of the body but have a predilection for the os calcis.[47] The cysts are filled with a clear yellow or serosanguineous fluid. The membrane of the cyst is lined with flat to slightly plump layers of cells. Patients usually present with pain due to incipient or actual pathologic fracture. Radiographically, pure lysis with or without loculation is seen, as are sharp borders. The cortical edges generally are smoothly curved to modestly scalloped. Many cases have a radiographic pathognomonic sign, a sliver of cortical bone in the bottom of the lytic lesion (fallen fragment sign). MRI reveals an intramedullary unilocular white shadow, brighter than subcutaneous fat, a finding that is consistent with a fluid-filled cyst.

The unicameral bone cyst is completely benign but is prone to local recurrences or fractures. Treatment in the past has been curettage and bone grafting. Injection of a corticosteroid into the cavity has resulted in resorption of the cyst, with healing and complete bone repair (Fig. 21-13).[41, 42]

Giant Cell Tumor

Giant cell tumor is a benign bone tumor that is most often found in the epiphyseal region of long bones. Such lesions constitute approximately 5 to 8 percent of primary bone tumors. The bones of the foot may be primary sites of involvement.[3] Seventy percent of pa-

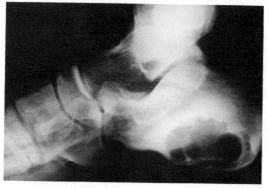

FIGURE 21-13. Lateral radiograph of a unicameral bone cyst of the os calcis.

tients are 20 to 40 years of age. Rarely is this tumor seen in patients with open growth plates. The presenting symptom of patients with giant cell tumors involving the bones of the foot is pain from the weakened bone. Patients also report local swelling, tenderness, and limitation of movement. Radiographs show "geographic destruction." The lesions may be concentrically located; however, most are eccentric, with cortical erosion and enlargement of bone contours, and they can abut the border of the articular cartilage. Bone scans often show increased uptake at the site of involvement. CT and MRI are also useful in determining the extent of the lesion.

Histologically, osteoclast-like giant cells are quite prominent. These giant cells can be quite large and are filled with many nuclei, which tend to collect near the cell center. Also present are spindle stromal cell elements containing a single nucleus similar to those within the giant cells. Mitotic activity may be present, and most cases show five to 10 mitoses per 10 high-power fields. Greater numbers or atypical mitoses are strongly suggestive of a sarcoma admixed with benign giant cells.

The locally aggressive nature of these tumors and their tendency to occur in juxta-articular locations cause difficulty in the management of giant cell tumors.[15] The challenge in treating this tumor is to rid the patient of the neoplasm while leaving a functioning joint. A curettage-intralesional resection results in a local recurrence rate that is prohibitively high—50 percent.[9] Marginal or wide resection controls the tumor but may be overly destructive in some cases. To determine the proper treatment, the surgeon must consider three factors: (1) whether the bone involved is expendable, (2) whether complete destruction of the involved bone has occurred, and (3) what is the host-tumor interaction. Occasionally, a tumor enlists enough of a host bone response that local containment seems to be taking place. At the other end of the spectrum is the tumor that has rapid local extension with no containment whatsoever. It is logical that treatment would be more aggressive in the latter case than in the former. A successful adjuvant method is the use of liquid nitrogen or phenol for more thorough local removal.[32, 33] The major complication noted is fracture through necrotic bone. This may be reduced by cortical strut grafting and autografting (Fig. 21-14). Another method is the use of methyl methacry-

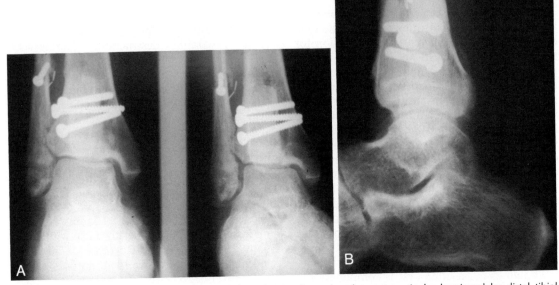

FIGURE 21–14. Anteroposterior mortise *(A)* and lateral *(B)* radiographs of an osteoarticular hemicondylar distal tibial allograft used for reconstruction after resection of a giant cell tumor.

late.[38] It has been postulated that the additional heat from the curing of the acrylic might add some additional tumor control. The juxtaposition to articular cartilage and the mechanical demands for weight bearing may make this material biomechanically less desirable than bone graft in the foot. If marginal resection is required, reconstruction by arthrodesis is warranted. When located in the hindfoot, giant cell tumors may require amputation for control.

Chondroblastoma

Chondroblastoma is a fairly uncommon benign cartilaginous tumor. It has a predilection for the epiphyseal region of long bones but can also affect the foot, especially the calcaneus.[28] The presenting symptoms are usually related to impairment of joint function. Patients present with impaired range of motion, joint pain and tenderness, synovial effusion, and limping. Radiographically, there is an eccentric lucency in the epiphysis, with a thin sclerotic margin. Histologically, the cells are polygonal, round, or oval. They have slightly indented nuclei, even chromatin, inconspicuous nucleoli, granular cytoplasm, and a distinct

cytoplasmic border. Various numbers of mitotic figures, multinucleated giant cells, fine trabeculae of calcification, and small foci of cartilaginous tissue also are found. The treatment of chondroblastoma usually consists of marginal resection. Depending on the site and size of the lesion, bone grafting may be indicated. There is a 20 percent incidence of local recurrence with this form of treatment, and if the tumor does recur, wide resection is indicated.

Osteoid Osteoma

Osteoid osteoma was first described in 1935, and it has become a well-recognized pathologic entity. The foot is a relatively common site for presentation, and a review of the literature indicates that all of the bones in this region may be affected, although the talus seems to be a site of predilection.[5] The lesion is primarily one of adolescents and young adults, and males seem to be affected twice as often as females.

The presenting symptom is predominantly pain at night, for which aspirin provides significant relief.[21] The pain may be exacerbated by weight bearing and walking. On physical examination, an area of local tenderness is usually identified. Muscle atrophy of the lower extremity is seen, as is decreased range of motion of the joint adjacent to the involved bone.

Osteoid osteoma is generally classified according to anatomic location—cortical, cancellous, or subperiosteal. Cortical lesions are the most common, and the subperiosteal region is the least common location. However, cancellous and subperiosteal localizations are known to be more frequent than cortical involvement in the small bones of the hands and feet. The radiographic characteristics of subperiosteal and cancellous osteoid osteomas differ from those of the more common cortical lesions. The cortical lesions consist of a radiolucent nidus less than 2 cm in diameter, and they frequently contain a region of demineralization centrally. Around the nidus, the cortex may be sclerotic. This sclerosis may be so extensive that special radiologic techniques such as tomography are required to visualize the nidus (Fig. 21–15).

Cancellous as well as subperiosteal lesions may be difficult to diagnose and thus difficult to treat appropriately. In subperiosteal lesions, a sclerotic response is usually absent for unknown reasons. There may be no cortical response, and often only a small, irregular lytic erosion is evident. Cancellous lesions are even more difficult to delineate on plain radiographs.

When the clinical symptoms suggest an osteoid osteoma, other diagnostic modalities are recommended. Because these lesions are quite vascular, a three-phase radionuclide scan shows quite increased uptake. Further localization can be accomplished by either polytomography or CT.

Articular subperiosteal osteoid osteomas may be especially difficult to diagnose because they frequently produce clinical symptoms and signs and radiographic features of an acute monoarticular arthritis. Joint pain relieved by aspirin is also a characteristic of early degenerative arthritis, which is diagnosed much more frequently than osteoid osteoma, and is therefore not pathognomonic for any diagnosis. Other differentials in diagnosis have included Brodie's bone abscess, enostosis (bone island), osteonecrosis, and stress fracture.

Although controversy still exists about the pathogenesis and natural history of the lesion,

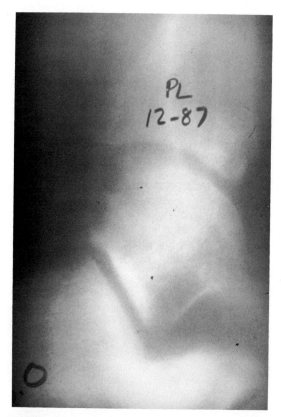

FIGURE 21–15. Lateral tomogram of subperiosteal osteoid osteoma of the os calcis.

complete surgical excision of the lesion is the treatment of choice.[44] If the lesion is incompletely removed, recurrence is a distinct possibility. The symptoms will be minimally changed in the postoperative period or will recur within a few months. Accurate preoperative localization is important for surgical planning. An incision is made in the area that would give the best exposure to allow for adequate resection and reconstruction. Some studies report the use of intraoperative technetium bone scanning with a sterile detection probe to localize the lesion in bone and to ensure that the excised specimen has the same increased activity. When the lesion is subperiosteal in location, a peg- or dowel-shaped autogenous bone graft can be obtained from the iliac crest. Postoperatively, patients are placed in a short-leg cast and are allowed partial weight bearing. When complete surgical removal is accomplished, patients have significant relief of pain.

Enchondroma

Enchondromas are common benign bone tumors that most often occur in the phalangeal bones of the foot. They are composed of benign hyaline cartilage. Multiple enchondromatosis (Ollier's disease) may be found in other bones of the foot as well, and malignant transformation of these lesions to chondrosarcomas may occur. Patients with enchondromas are usually asymptomatic, unless a pathologic fracture occurs through the lesion. The typical radiographic appearance is a geographic punched-out lesion with a sharp, reactive edge and spiculed calcification (Fig. 21–16). The treatment is intralesional resection and bone grafting.

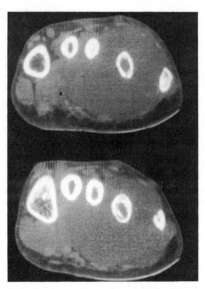

FIGURE 21–17. Computed tomographic scan illustrating the dramatic soft tissue mass surrounding Ewing's sarcoma involving the fourth metatarsal. (From Leeson MC, Smith MJ: Ewing's sarcoma of the foot. Foot Ankle 10:150, 1989. © American Orthopaedic Foot and Ankle Society 1989.)

Malignant Bone Tumors

Ewing's Sarcoma

Ewing's sarcoma is an aggressive primary malignant tumor of bone that generally affects children and young adults. It has historically been associated with a dismal prognosis because of a fulminant course of local recurrence and early metastasis to bone, lung, and abdominal viscera. Although it is one of the most common primary malignant tumors arising in the bones of the foot, involvement of the foot is unusual, with fewer than 40 cases reported in the literature (Fig. 21–17). Distal extremity lesions have been associated with both decreased rates of local recurrence and an increased incidence of metastasis at the time of initial presentation.[23] Current treatment has focused on chemotherapy, radiation therapy, and surgery where indicated. This therapy aims to eliminate both the primary tumor and metastatic disease. Aggressive multiagent chemotherapy is used to control micrometastasis and to assist in achieving permanent local control.

Some controversy still exists concerning the role of surgery, radiation therapy, or both in the management of the primary site of Ewing's sarcoma.[29] Although successful in the treat-

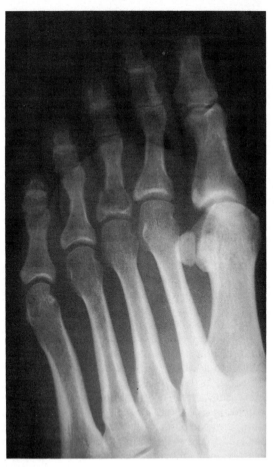

FIGURE 21–16. Pathologic fracture of the third proximal phalanx through an enchondroma. This is treated by intralesional curettage and bone grafting.

ment of local disease, radiation therapy is not without its own morbidity. In the skeletally immature population, whole bone irradiation may cause epiphyseal injury, which may lead to significant limb length discrepancy and angular deformities. An additional morbidity of radiation therapy is local recurrence in irradiated primary sites; this carries an almost uniformly fatal prognosis.

Current indications for surgery in patients with Ewing's sarcoma include relatively small tumors, tumors that are easily accessible surgically, and tumors in expendable anatomic sites. Ewing's sarcoma of the foot meets all of these criteria. A distal extremity tumor or a foot tumor lends itself to amputation because of tumor size and surgical accessibility and because of the excellent functional results in young patients with below-knee amputation.

In a large series, patients who underwent complete surgical excision of the primary tumor had a better survival rate (75 percent at 5 years) than those who did not undergo resection (34 percent at 5 years).[45] When the benefits of amputation and its morbidity are considered, in addition to the hazards of irradiating these young patients, below-knee amputation is an excellent alternative in the treatment of patients with Ewing's sarcoma of the foot.

Chondrosarcoma

Chondrosarcoma is the third most common primary malignant tumor of bone but is rarely located in the foot.[36] All reported cases of pedal chondrosarcoma are distributed equally between the short tubular bones and the tarsus. Chondrosarcoma may arise from a preexisting enchondroma. The existence of multiple enchondromatosis—Ollier's disease and Maffucci's syndrome—undoubtedly enhances the probability of malignant changes. Males are usually more frequently affected by pedal chondrosarcoma than are females.

The majority of patients with chondrosarcoma of the foot complain of progressive swelling and pain—symptoms identical to those of chondrosarcoma elsewhere in the body. A history of trauma is sometimes noted, but it is likely that the injury called attention to a previously existing neoplasm.

Radiographs usually show a centrally placed, expanding lesion that is predominantly lytic (Fig. 21–18). The area of bone destruction is apt to contain small scattered foci of calcifica-

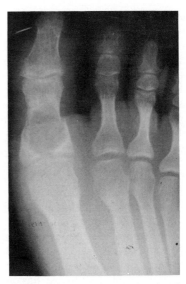

FIGURE 21–18. Pathologic fracture of a chondrosarcoma involving the proximal phalanx of the great toe.

tion or ossification. In some cases, the cortex is slightly thickened, whereas in others, the cortices are attenuated and perforated. Extension of the tumor into the adjacent soft tissue is commonly observed. The subchondral bone may be destroyed, and the adjacent bone on the other side of the joint may be involved. Typically, subperiosteal new bone formation is absent. The differential diagnosis includes enchondroma, osteogenic sarcoma, and tuberculosis. The findings of enchondroma significantly resemble those of chondrosarcoma. However, an enchondroma does not perforate the cortex to form a soft tissue neoplastic mass, nor does an enchondroma destroy the subchondral plate to invade the adjacent bone on the other side of the joint. Ordinarily, the enchondroma is sharply delineated by a thin margin of cortical bone. Serial radiographs may show considerable enlargement of the chondrosarcoma. Osteogenic sarcoma in the short tubular bones also shows cortical perforation in the soft tissue mass. However, this tumor often shows sclerosis of the affected bone, a finding not commonly observed in chondrosarcoma. In addition, subperiosteal new bone formation perpendicular to the shaft will probably occur. Spotty calcification within the osseous lesion and cortical thickening are usually absent in osteogenic sarcoma. Tuberculosis also may imitate chondrosarcoma, with bone destruction and a soft tissue mass of several months' duration. However, patients with tuberculous involvement of the phalanx or metacarpals are likely to show significant subperiosteal new bone formation, and a sinus tract may be present. Cortical thickening and spotty calcification of the osseous lesion are usually absent.

Histologically, chondrosarcomas are poorly differentiated. The cells show variation in size and shape, with bizarre nuclei and multinucleated malignant chondrocytes.

The treatment of chondrosarcoma is surgical. When a phalanx is involved, disarticulation at the joint proximal to the lesion is the proper therapy. When a metatarsal is involved, resection of the ray including an adequate margin of normal bone is indicated. For a tarsal lesion, it may be necessary to perform a below-knee amputation, although the possibility of carrying out a local en bloc resection could be considered. Curettage has no place in the treatment of chondrosarcoma. Because chondrosarcoma is resistant to radiation therapy, this form of treatment should be used only when the patient refuses surgical intervention. The survival rate of patients with chondrosarcoma is quite variable because pulmonary metastasis does occur. It is important to note that chondrosarcoma frequently has a very slow evolution, even with inadequate treatment.

Osteogenic Sarcoma

Osteogenic sarcoma is an extremely rare tumor in the foot and ankle.[51] Because of its tremendous range of characteristics, osteosarcoma can be misinterpreted as many other benign and malignant entities, most of which require radically different therapeutic approaches. Osteosarcoma is by definition a mesenchymally derived malignant tumor that produces osteoid, bone, or both.[34] Other elements, such as malignant cartilage or malignant fibrous tissue, may or may not be produced. Implicit in this definition is the fact that tumor cells produce the osseous matrices and that the osseous matrices must be neither reactive nor metaplastic. Osteogenic sarcoma most commonly occurs in the first and second decades of life. The predominant symptom is pain, which at first may be slight and intermittent. Pain probably results from weakening of the bone with the development of stress fractures. With time, extraosseous extension may occur, which may cause swelling and nerve compression. Patients may have elevated serum alkaline phosphatase values at the time

of presentation. Radiographs show a sclerotic, expansile, destructive bone lesion. Cartilage tends to resist penetration by this neoplasm. Another radiographic finding is periosteal reaction.

Once the clinical suspicion of osteosarcoma is entertained, a staging work-up is of vital importance. The local extent of the tumor can be delineated further by CT, as well as by MRI. ^{99m}Tc scans show markedly increased uptake at the site of tumor and may be helpful as a whole body screening method for metastasis. CT scans are also used to evaluate patients for the presence of lung metastasis.

The treatment of choice is to remove the tumor with wide margins. Because these tumors often present in advanced stages with extraosseous tumor extension, ablative surgery—below-knee amputation—is most often the surgical treatment of choice for pedal lesions.[5] Local control is achieved by surgery, and adjuvant chemotherapy is given to control microscopic systemic disease. Several different protocols for chemotherapy currently yield 5-year survival rates as high as 75 percent.[49]

Lymphoma of Bone

Primary lymphocytic lymphoma of bone is a rare tumor that can be found in the foot or ankle region. This entity was once labeled primary "reticulum cell" sarcoma.[34] This tumor can affect persons in all age groups, but it is rarely noted in patients 10 years of age or younger. Pain, swelling, or both with increased warmth are the usual complaints. Constitutionally, these patients appear to be in good health in comparison with those with secondary malignant lymphomas. Radiographically, these lesions appear as ill-defined mixed lytic-blastic lesions. Also associated with the tumor is a large soft tissue mass. In some cases, extensive permeative destruction is evident, mimicking a sarcomatous lesion. This lymphoma can be mistaken for Ewing's sarcoma, both clinically and pathologically. Histologically, sheets of cells with quite round, hyperchromatic, lymphoid-appearing nuclei are seen. The differential diagnosis includes osteomyelitis, neuroblastoma, Ewing's sarcoma, and multiple myeloma. Special stains as well as immunologic marker studies may be required to differentiate the tumor. The treatment for lesions in the foot and ankle favors primary ablative surgical procedures because irradiation may result in local necrosis that is disabling or may fail to halt the growth of the primary tumor. Chemotherapy provides subjective and objective relief for many patients with disseminated lymphoma.

Metastatic Tumors of the Foot

Metastatic tumor of the foot and ankle is rare. Although metastatic tumor of the skeleton occurs in at least 20 to 30 percent of patients with malignancy, only a small fraction of these patients will have acrometastasis: that is, metastasis to the hands or feet. Foot or ankle pain may be the presenting symptom of an occult malignancy.[17] If metastatic disease is not kept in the differential diagnosis of foot pain, diagnosis and treatment may be delayed. Osteomyelitis, gout, rheumatoid arthritis, Reiter's syndrome, Paget's disease, and ligamentous sprains are diagnostic considerations in these patients. Making the correct diagnosis is often quite difficult. Plain radiography, bone scanning, and conventional or computed tomography may aid in the diagnostic process.

The survival rate after diagnosis of acrometastasis is quite variable. Because of the variation in survival rates, individualization of treatment is required to maintain mobility, relieve pain, and avoid unnecessary hospitalization and surgical morbidity. Radiation therapy can provide significant relief of symptoms in some patients with isolated painful intraosseous metastasis.[18] Cast immobilization or bracing may be useful in conjunction with radiation therapy to decrease stress across the weakened, diseased bone. Many patients fail to achieve satisfactory pain control with nonsurgical treatment, or they have local extension of the disease; these patients may require amputation if sufficient longevity is anticipated. For patients with phalangeal metastasis, digital or ray resection is effective treatment of the local disease, allowing the rapid resumption of ambulation without pain. Consideration should be given to early surgical ablation of these lesions to provide rapid relief of pain, to eliminate open draining of the wound, and to improve function.

References

1. Allen RA, Woolner LB, Ghormley RK: Soft-tissue tumors of the sole. J Bone Joint Surg 37A:14–26, 1955.
2. Aviles E, Arlen M, Miller T: Plantar fibromatosis. Surgery 69:117–120, 1971.
3. Burns TP, Weiss M, Snyder M, Hopson CN: Giant cell tumor of the metatarsal. Foot Ankle 8:223–226, 1988.
4. Campanacci M, Capanna R, Picci P: Unicameral and aneurysmal bone cysts. Clin Orthop 204:25–36, 1986.
5. Capanna R, Van Horn JR, Ayala A, et al: Osteoid osteoma and osteoblastoma of the talus. Skeletal Radiol 15:360–364, 1986.
6. Cavolo DJ, Sherwood GF: Dupuytren's disease of the plantar fascia. J Foot Surg 21:12–15, 1982.
7. Chassaignac CME: Cancer de la gaine des tendons. Gaz Hop Civ Milit 47:185–186, 1952.
8. Curtin JW: Fibromatosis of the plantar fascia. J Bone Joint Surg 47A:1605–1608, 1965.
9. Dunham WK, Calhoun JC: The surgical treatment of giant cell tumor of bone. Alabama J Med Sci 22:258–265, 1985.
10. Enneking WF: Musculoskeletal Tumor Surgery. New York, Churchill Livingstone, 1983.
11. Enneking WF: System of staging musculoskeletal neoplasms. Clin Orthop 204:9–24, 1986.
12. Enneking WF, Spanier SS, Goodman MA: System for the surgical staging of musculoskeletal sarcoma. Clin Orthop 153:106–120, 1980.
13. Enzinger FM, Weiss SW: Soft Tissue Tumors, 2nd Ed. St. Louis, CV Mosby, 1985.
14. Flandry F, Hughston JC: Pigmented villonodular synovitis. J Bone Joint Surg 69A:942–949, 1987.
15. Goldenberg RR, Campbell CJ, Portis RB: Giant cell tumor of bone: An analysis of 218 cases. J Bone Joint Surg 52A:619–664, 1970.
16. Haedicke GJ, Sturim HS: Plantar fibromatosis. Plast Reconstr Surg 83:296–299, 1989.
17. Hattrup SJ, Amadio PC, Sim FH, Lombardi RM: Metastatic tumors of the foot and ankle. Foot Ankle 8:243–247, 1988.
18. Healey JH, Turnbull ADM, Miedema B, Lane JM: Acrometastases. J Bone Joint Surg 68A:743–746, 1986.
19. Heare TC, Enneking WF, Heare MH: Staging techniques and biopsy of bone tumors. Orthop Clin North Am 20:273, 1989.
20. Kambolis C, Bullough PG, Jaffe HL: Ganglionic cystic defects of bone. J Bone Joint Surg 55A:496–505, 1973.
21. Kenzora JE, Abrams RC: Problems encountered in the diagnosis and treatment of osteoid osteoma of the talus. Foot Ankle 2:172–178, 1981.
22. Kirby EJ, Shereff MJ, Lewis MM: Soft-tissue tumors and tumor-like lesions of the foot. J Bone Joint Surg 71A:621–626, 1989.
23. Kliman M, Harwood AR, Jenkin RD, et al: Radical radiotherapy as primary treatment for Ewing's sarcoma distal to the elbow and knee. Clin Orthop 165:233–238, 1982.
24. Jaffe HL: Giant cell reparative granuloma, traumatic bone cyst and fibrous (fibro-osseous) dysplasia of the jaw bones. Oral Surg 6:159–175, 1953.
25. Jones FE, Soule EH, Coventry MB: Fibrous histiocytoma of synovium (giant cell tumor of tendon sheath, pigmented nodular synovitis). J Bone Joint Surg 51A:76–86, 1969.
26. Kliman ME, Freiberg A: Ganglia of the foot and ankle. Foot Ankle 3:45–46, 1982.
27. Kransdorf MJ, Jelinek JS, Moser RP, et al: Soft tissue masses: Diagnosis using MR imaging. AJR Am J Roentgenol 153:541, 1989.

28. Kricun ME, Kricun R, Haskin ME: Chondroblastoma of the calcaneus: Radiographic features with emphasis on location. AJR Am J Roentgenol 128:613–616, 1977.
29. Leeson MC, Smith MJ: Ewing's sarcoma of the foot. Foot Ankle 10:147–151, 1989.
30. Lodwick GS, Wilson AJ, Farrell C, et al: Determining growth rates of focal lesions of bone from radiographs. Radiology 134:577, 1980.
31. Lorenzo JC, Dorfman HD: Giant cell reparative granuloma of short tubular bones of the hands and feet. Am J Surg Pathol 4:551–563, 1980.
32. Malawer MM, Vance R: Giant cell tumor and aneurysmal bone cyst of the talus: Clinicopathological review and two case reports. Foot Ankle 1:235–244, 1981.
33. Marcove RC, Weiss ID, Vaghairvalla MR, et al: Cryosurgery in the treatment of giant cell tumors of bone: Report of 52 consecutive cases. Cancer 41:957–969, 1978.
34. Mirra JM: Bone tumors. Clinical, radiologic, and pathologic correlations. Philadelphia, Lea & Febiger, 1989.
35. Owens JC, Shiu MH, Smith R, Hajdu SI: Soft tissue sarcomas of the hand and foot. Cancer 55:2010–2018, 1985.
36. Pachter MR, Alpert M: Chondrosarcoma of the foot skeleton. J Bone Joint Surg 46A:601–607, 1964.
37. Pedersen HE, Day AJ: Dupuytren's disease of the foot. JAMA 154:33–35, 1954.
38. Person BM, Wouters H: Curettage and acrylic cementation in surgery of giant cell tumors of bone. Clin Orthop 120:125–143, 1976.
39. Picci P, Baldini N, Sudanese A, et al: Giant cell reparative granuloma and other giant cell lesions of the bones of the hands and feet. Skeletal Radiol 15:415–421, 1986.
40. Richardson ML, Kiloyne RF, Gillespy T, et al: Magnetic resonance imaging of musculoskeletal neoplasms. Radiol Clin North Am 24:259–267, 1986.
41. Scaglietti O, Marchetti PG, Bartolozzi P: The effects of methylprednisolone acetate in the treatment of bone cysts: Results of three years follow-up. J Bone Joint Surg 61B:200–204, 1979.
42. Schajowicz F, Sainz MC, Slullitel JA: Juxta-articular bone cysts (intra-osseous ganglia). J Bone Joint Surg 61B:107–116, 1979.
43. Seale KS, Lange TA, Monson D, Hackbarth DA: Soft tissue tumors of the foot and ankle. Foot Ankle 9:19–27, 1988.
44. Shereff MJ, Cullivan WT, Johnson KA: Osteoid-osteoma of the foot. J Bone Joint Surg 65A:638–641, 1983.
45. Shirley SK, Askin FB, Gilula LA, et al: Ewing's sarcoma in bones of the hands and feet. J Clin Oncol 3:686–697, 1985.
46. Simon MA: Biopsy of musculoskeletal tumors. J Bone Joint Surg 64A:1253–1257, 1982.
47. Smith RW, Smith CF: Solitary unicameral bone cyst of the calcaneus. J Bone Joint Surg 56A:45–56, 1974.
48. Soren A: Pathogenesis and treatment of ganglia. Clin Orthop 48:173–179, 1966.
49. Unni KK: Bone Tumors. New York, Churchill Livingstone, 1988.
50. Willems D, Mulier JC, Martens M, Verhelst M: Ganglion cysts of bone. Acta Orthop Scand 44:655–662, 1973.
51. Wu KK: Osteogenic sarcoma of the foot. J Foot Surg 26:269–271, 1987.
52. Wu KK: Malignant fibrous histiocytoma of the foot. J Foot Surg 29:298–303, 1990.
53. Zimmer WD, Berquist TH, McLeod RA, et al: Bone tumors: Magnetic resonance imaging versus computed tomography. Radiology 155:709, 1985.

22

Management of Foot Infections

JEFFREY E. JOHNSON
REGINALD L. HALL

Bacterial infections are one of the most common presenting problems in patients with foot complaints. As in infections in the hand, the initial presenting symptoms are often subtle and easily overlooked. The key to proper treatment is the accurate initial characterization of the infectious process as involving either the superficial or the deep structures of the foot. This chapter provides a framework for evaluating foot infections and discusses their surgical management.

Most foot infections occur because bacteria gain access to the superficial or deep structures through an opening in the skin caused by a puncture wound, blister, laceration, ulcer, ingrown toenail, or surgical procedure. Hematogenous infection about the foot and ankle is rare but may occur in a child or immunocompromised host. Foot infections in diabetics, however, are most often associated with a break in the skin through a vascular or neurotrophic ulcer or skin fissure.

CLASSIFICATION

Infections of the foot can be classified as affecting either the superficial or the deep structures. Superficial structures include the epidermis, dermis, subcutaneous adipose tissue, and adventitial bursae, which are superficial to the deep investing fascia about the bone and muscle compartments of the foot. The deep structures include the tendons, bones, and muscles, which are deep to the investing fascia. Superficial infections often respond to local wound care and antibiotics.

Deep foot infections more often require surgical intervention and a more prolonged course of antibiotics and can lead to permanent sequelae.

EVALUATION

Clinical symptoms of a foot infection include pain at rest as well as with activity that is often throbbing. When pain is out of proportion to the extent of surgery during the early postoperative period (especially 5 to 14 days postoperatively) infection should be considered. Swelling and erythema are usually present and purulent drainage may be evident. There is usually tenderness over the affected area and with motion of the nearby joints.

The physical examination can be misleading, especially following trauma or in the face of an acute neuropathic arthropathy (Charcot's foot) when there is pre-existing swelling, erythema, and often pain. Lymphangitic streaks over the dorsum of the foot and increased warmth of the overlying skin are helpful signs that can be present with either superficial or deep infection. Fever is an unreliable sign and often is not present unless there is a significant bacteremia.

Laboratory Evaluations

A white blood cell count with differential and an erythrocyte sedimentation rate should be obtained when the diagnosis of infection is in question. Even with a deep infection, the

263

white blood cell count differential and erythrocyte sedimentation rate may be normal; however, an elevated white blood cell count, an increase in the percent of polymorphonuclear lymphocytes, or an elevated erythrocyte sedimentation rate may indicate a deep infection. These can also be elevated with severe trauma.

Radiographic Evaluation

Anteroposterior (AP), lateral, and oblique x-ray studies of the foot should be obtained in all cases of suspected deep foot infection. With toe involvement, coned down or magnified views of the involved digits can also be obtained in AP, lateral, and oblique projections, holding the adjacent toes out of the plane of the x-ray to prevent their superimposition.

The radiographs should be scrutinized for evidence of soft tissue swelling, foreign bodies, subcutaneous gas, and irregularity or displacement of the deep fat planes. Imaging of these soft tissue changes is more easily accomplished with low kilovolt soft tissue radiography or xerography than with routine radiographs.[6, 8, 12, 33] Radiographic changes within the bone consistent with osteomyelitis are usually not evident for 10 to 14 days or until 35 to 50 percent of the bone has been destroyed.[18, 20, 52] Bone and periosteal abnormalities vary with age, the type of bone involved, and the causative organism.[1]

Acute hematogenous osteomyelitis produces swelling of the deep soft tissues adjacent to the involved bone within 2 to 3 days, causing irregularity or displacement of the deep fat planes.[1] As the soft tissue involvement progresses, the deep tissue infection spreads superficially. This is in contrast to cellulitis, in which the superficial tissue is involved initially with progression to the deep tissues, periosteum, cortex, and finally medullary bone. With hematogenous osteomyelitis the reverse of this pattern is seen, with initial soft tissue swelling, followed by medullary involvement before involvement of the cortex or periosteum.[1] The periosteal changes may be extensive, forming a dense involucrum (sclerotic sheath usually around sequestra) that surrounds the shaft of tubular bones. Radiographs may demonstrate adjacent abcesses in the soft tissues, and areas of necrotic or dead bone (sequestra) may also

be evident that often appear more dense than the surrounding cortical regions. Sequestra are usually not evident for at least 3 weeks and size variation may make them difficult to identify using conventional radiographs.[1] Tomography can be useful in identification of subtle sequestra.

Trispiral tomography or computed tomography (CT) can be helpful in identifying, localizing, or determining the extent of infectious bone lesions in the foot, especially in the midfoot and hindfoot. The CT scan should be made in 2-mm slices in two planes. In the midfoot, the preferred scanning planes are axial cuts in the plane of the metatarsal shafts and coronal cuts perpendicular to the plane of the metatarsal shafts. For the hindfoot, axial cuts parallel to the plantar surface of the foot and coronal cuts as close to perpendicular to the axial cut as possible provide the best visualization.

Nuclear Imaging

Technetium-99m pyrophosphate or methylene diphosphonate scans can detect and localize bone and joint infections in the foot as well as other parts of the skeleton. Areas of osteomyelitis almost always show increased uptake on bone scintigraphy; however, early images may demonstrate a photopenic area surrounding the joint space when there is a joint space infection. As the infection progresses, the uptake in the joint increases.[1] A three-phase technetium bone scan using both early "blood pool" images and delayed images will enhance the specificity of isotope imaging.[1] Osteomyelitis appears as a focal area of increased uptake in bone on both early and late images. Patients with cellulitius have diffuse increased uptake in soft tissue areas on both early and delayed studies without definite focal bone uptake.[1]

Further isotope studies are useful in patients with suspected infection when technetium-99m scans are normal or equivocal or when there is an associated fracture, recent surgery, or other reason for uptake on the bone scan. Gallium-67– and indium-111–labeled leukocyte scans are particularly useful in these situations.

Diagnostic problems are encountered in diabetic patients with suspected osteomyelitis because of the difficulty in differentiating neuropathic osteoarthropathy from sites of infection. However, bone scintigraphy is still useful in diabetic patients with suspected osteomyelitis.[38, 39, 45, 60] Seldin and colleagues[60] demonstrated increased blood flow during the arterial phase of the technetium scan flow study in diabetics with osteomyelitis, whereas neuropathic joints with soft tissue pathology showed increased venous flow.

Indium scans may demonstrate uptake in diabetic osteoarthropathy without infection. Indium-111–labeled leukocytes are more useful in excluding infection than in diagnosing it in the face of diabetic neuropathic osteoarthropathy.[38] Schauwecker[58] and Patel and colleagues[47] showed that the ability to determine that the infection is in bone rather than adjacent soft tissue was greater with simultaneous technetium bone scan and indium-111 leukocyte studies. When indium-111 activity is present, the simultaneous studies can differentiate between bone and soft tissue involvement 89 percent of the time. Therefore, once the bone is violated by an insult that causes increased bone turnover, such as surgery, fracture, or neuropathic osteoarthropathy, the bone scan becomes less specific. Since indium-111 leukocytes are not usually incorporated into the areas of increased bone turnover, the combination of technetium and indium is more specific for infection in these complex cases.

Combined use of bone scans and gallium-67 studies is also worthwhile in patients with previous violation of the involved bone in the setting of suspected infection. Similar uptake patterns with both tracers with only mild to moderate gallium uptake indicate that no infection is present. If patterns of uptake are incongruent, there is a very high probability that the patient has osteomyelitis, a joint space infection, cellulitis, synovitis, or a combination thereof.[55] The specificity for osteomyelitis is much higher for the combination of indium and technetium than for that of gallium and technetium for the diabetic foot.[47]

The technetium-99m bone scan is an excellent screening test for osteomyelitis. In areas of violated bone or osteomyelitis superimposed on other conditions that affect tracer uptake (e.g., bone infarction, diabetic neuropathic osteoarthropathy) the addition of an indium-111 leukocyte scan will increase the diagnostic yield.[1, 47]

Magnetic Resonance Imaging and Computed Tomography

Magnetic resonance imaging (MRI) by virtue of its soft tissue contrast, multiple plane views, improved resolution with surface coils, and lack of beam hardening artifact from cortical bone is an excellent technique for evaluation of the foot and ankle. MRI can indicate infection earlier than routine radiographs and can more clearly demonstrate the extent of bone and soft tissue involvement.[1] It is especially useful in infections not associated with previous trauma or surgical intervention. Computed tomography (CT) is most useful in evaluating subtle cortical changes and in identifying sequestra. Like MRI, CT is sensitive and can detect subtle bone changes earlier than routine radiographs. Subtle soft tissue abnormalities and involvement of the tendon sheaths and deep muscle compartments of the foot can be easily seen with MRI. Sinograms may also be useful in chronic soft tissue fistula to identify the extent of bone or soft tissue involvement.[1]

Cultures

Aerobic and anaerobic cultures and gram staining should be obtained for material from draining, open wounds suspected of being infected or from the aspirate of a superficial or deep abscess. Wound swabbing is much less valuable in identifying pathogenic organisms than aspirations of abcesses or deep cultures from soft tissue or bone.

In the case of a significant infection, empiric therapy to cover the most likely organisms is instituted while awaiting culture results. Specific antibiotic therapy can then be given after identification of the organism and sensitivities.

MICROBIOLOGY OF FOOT INFECTIONS

The vast majority of diabetic foot infections are polymicrobial.[2, 3, 5, 6] While the predominate isolate varies from study to study, bacteroides and staphylococcal species are the most common pathogens, followed closely by the streptococcal species (particularly group D streptococci and enterococci).[2, 3, 5-7] The most commonly encountered gram-positive aerobe isolate is *Staphylococcus aureus* and the most common gram-negative species is *Pseudomonas aeruginosa*. Bacteroides species are the most common anaerobes isolated, followed closely by peptococci.[2, 3, 5–7]

The bacterial organism identified most frequently in debilitated patients (alcoholism, diabetes, hypogammaglobulinemia), with hematogenous osteomyelitis is *Staphylococcus aureus*, and the most common gram-negative bacteria are *Escherichia coli, Pseudomonas aeruginosa, Klebsiella spp*, and *Aerobacter spp*.[15, 65] Beta-hemolytic streptococcal infections are not uncommon in infants.

Puncture wounds of the foot are colonized with *Pseudomonas* in a high percentage of cases.[7, 32, 40, 44, 53] Fungal and mycobacterial infections should also be considered in debilitated individuals or in recent immigrants from third world countries.

SUPERFICIAL INFECTIONS

Superficial bacterial infections are common and often caused or aggravated by footwear. An overgrown or deformed toenail can cause irritation and blistering of the surrounding skin due to pressure against the toe by the shoe. Inadequate shoe fit or cushioning can lead to excessive metatarsal head weight-bearing pressure and subsequent ulcer formation in diabetics or other patients with insensitive feet. Not wearing shoes may be as harmful as wearing poorly fitting footwear since the foot is subject to puncture wounds and lacerations.

Paronychia

A paronychia is an infection of the soft tissue adjacent to the nail margins. It usually involves the medial or lateral margin of the nail but may extend proximally to involve the eponychium. If the proximal fold is involved, the infection is termed an eponychia. The causative organism is most often *Staphylococcus aureus*.[11, 17] Cellulitis with associated pain and swelling is the first clinical manifestation. In the early cellulitis stage, treatment with antibiotics, warm soaks, and a roomy shoe or open-toed sandal may lead to resolution without surgical intervention. The infection may progress to form a localized abcess, which is usually superficial.

Surgical Treatment

If the abscess is superficial it may be drained under local anesthesia, but often a digital or metacarpal block with a local anesthetic is helpful. A scalpel with a No. 11 blade can be placed flat against the nail and extended into the nail fold medially, laterally, and proximally to decompress the abscess (Fig. 22–1). This is followed by warm soaks two to three times daily and antibiotics if there is significant associated cellulitis.

In some cases, excision of the medial or lateral one-quarter to one-third of the nail may allow spontaneous decompression of the nail sulcus. This can be accomplished by elevation of the edge of the affected nail with a blunt elevator back to the proximal border of the nail. Scissors are then used to longitudinally incise the nail and remove the nail margin from the nail fold to decompress the abscess (Fig. 22–2).

If it appears that the abscess extends into the deep soft tissues of the toe or into the distal phalanx bone, débridement of the deep tissues must be performed with curettement of

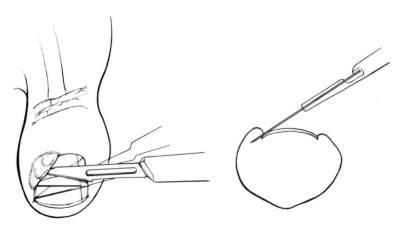

FIGURE 22–1. Drainage of paronychia by incision alone. Scalpel blade is kept tangential to nail plate, and incision is made in sulcus.

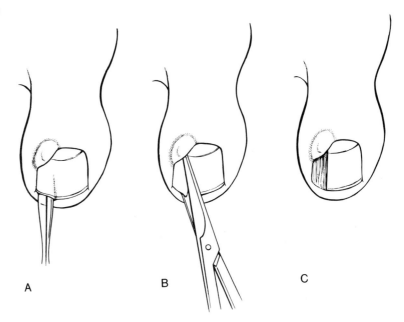

FIGURE 22–2. *(A)*, Elevation of lateral nail. *(B)*, Excision of lateral one-quarter to one-third of nail. *(C)*, Decompressed paronychia.

A B C

the involved bone. This requires removal of the margin of the nail to gain access to the nail fold. The wound is then packed open for 24 hours, a compression dressing is applied, and foot soaks are given two to three times daily with an antiseptic soap solution. Amputation of the distal phalanx may be required for osteomyelitis or inability to obtain soft tissue coverage.

Eponychia

If the infection should extend to involve the eponychium, several techniques may be used.

Marsupialization (Fig. 22–3). A crescent-shaped elliptical incision is made in the skin overlying the abscess and the ellipse is excised.[31] This keeps the skin edges open to allow drainage without the use of a wick and theoretically may yield a more cosmetic result since the nail itself is not disturbed.

Proximal Nail Excision Without Excision (Fig. 22–4). The proximal nail is often loose because of the accumulation of pus in the region of the lunula in the proximal nail fold. Therefore, the eponychial fold can be bluntly elevated and the proximal one-third of the nail cut transversely with the scissors and removed. A gauze wick can then be inserted under the eponychium into the abscess and soaks begun after the gauze is removed at 48 hours.

Proximal Nail Excision with Single or Double Incision (Fig. 22–5). A single dorsal longitudinal incision can be made from the midpoint of the paronychia to the edge of the proximal nail. The nail is elevated and the proximal one-third is excised. A wick is inserted into the abscess cavity after evacuation and at 48 hours warm antiseptic soaks are begun. The double incision technique uses two longitudinal incisions beginning at the margin of the nail fold and extending proximally for 5 to 7 mm. The entire eponychium is elevated as a proximally based flap, the exposed proximal one-third of the nail is excised and packed with a gauze wick, and soaks are begun at 48 hours.

Chronic Suppurative Paronychia

The chronic suppurative paronychia is treated as an acute paronychia except that a radiograph should be obtained to look for underlying osteomyelitis, a subungual exostosis, or a retained foreign body. One should also consider the existence of an overlooked or resistant bacterial infection, granulomatous disease, or neoplasm. Biopsy should be performed at the time of surgical treatment.

Often the paronychia or eponychia does not involve the nail matrix plantar to the nail surface. In this case adequate drainage can be obtained without excising the proximal nail.

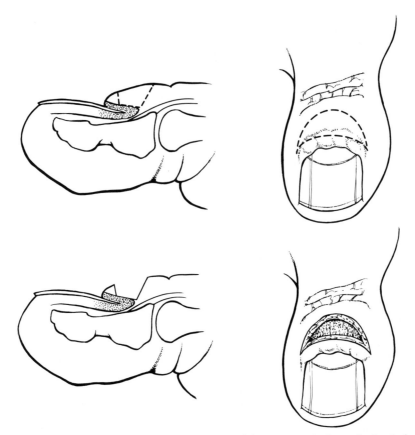

FIGURE 22–3. Method of eponychial marsupialization. (Adapted from Keyser J, Eaton R: Surgical cure of chronic paronychia by eponychial marsupialization. Plast Reconstr Surg 58:66, 1976.)

Authors' Preferred Method of Treatment

For eponychia and paronychia, with the toe anesthetized, a No. 11 blade is placed flat against the nail and slid under the proximal nail fold or the lateral nail margin into the abscess as shown in Figure 22–1. The abscess cavity is then milked of its contents and irrigated with a small syringe. A small gauze wick is placed into the abscess cavity and removed at 48 hours during the first foot soak. A 1-week course of oral antibiotics is usually sufficient in association with foot soaks in an antiseptic soap solution two to three times daily.

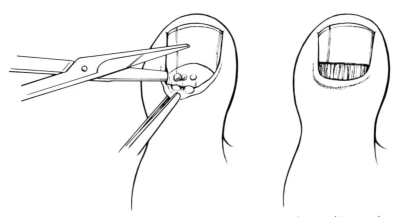

FIGURE 22–4. Method of proximal nail excision without incision. *(A)*, Retraction of eponychium, and excision of proximal nail. *(B)*, Appearance after excision of proximal nail.

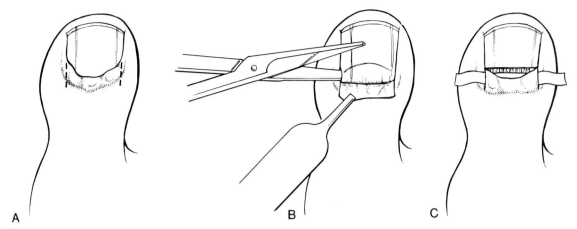

FIGURE 22–5. *(A),* Outline of incisions to expose base of nail. *(B),* Elevation of eponychial fold, and resection of proximal one-third of nail. *(C),* Gauze wick prevents premature closure of cavity.

If the sterile nail matrix is involved on the plantar side, the double incision technique (see Fig. 22–5) is used to raise the proximally based eponychial flap, and the proximal one-third of the nail is excised as described previously. Even if it is necessary to excise some of the nail to allow drainage of an abscess plantar to the nail surface, avulsion of the entire nail should be avoided, since any retained nail will help splint the soft tissues and the nail bed and completely avulsed nails may regrow with some deformity.

Felon

A felon is a closed space infection of the distal pulp of the terminal phalanx that occurs most commonly in the fingers but can occasionally affect a toe, primarily the great toe. It often follows an injury or puncture wound of the distal phalanx, but may be secondary to a neglected paronychia or subungual abscess. *Staphylococcus aureus* is the most common etiologic organism, but gram-negative bacilli are also implicated.[11, 49]

Diagnosis may be difficult because early objective signs are minimal despite the often significant pain. This in itself may be a clue to the diagnosis. The pain is often constant and severe and there may be swelling of the volar tip with marked tenderness to palpation. If the infection progresses to involve the bone, the pain may actually decrease as bone necrosis occurs. If there is no spontaneous or surgical decompression, the process may cause oblit-

eration of the digital vessels and a slough of the pulp of the digit may result.[45]

Treatment

Early in the infection or when the diagnosis is in doubt, rest and elevation of the extremity and administration of antistaphylococcal antibiotics are instituted. If there is no response within 24 to 48 hours incision and drainage should be undertaken. The surgical incision for drainage of the pulp space should allow adequate drainage with good functional and cosmetic result, should avoid the neurovascular bundle, and should be distal enough to avoid the flexor sheath and the distal interphalangeal joint.[45] The pulp consists of fat with interspersed trabeculations of fascial strands[17] and these should be divided to provide adequate decompression. Surgical drainage is usually performed under regional or general anesthesia. The abscess cavity is then loosely packed with gauze, which is removed at 24 to 48 hours when antiseptic soap soaks are begun for 5 minutes two to three times daily. Emperic therapy with a broad-spectrum antibiotic with good staphylococcal coverage is given pending culture and sensitivity results.

Lateral Incision (Fig. 22–6). A lateral incision is made just dorsal to the midlateral line beginning at the proximal extent of the nail and extending distally to the nail tip. The scalpel is inserted through the skin to bone and the incision is extended distally into the pulp space taking care to divide all the fascial septae.

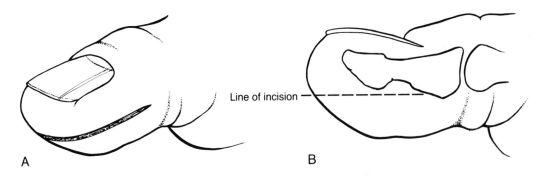

A   B

Line of incision -------

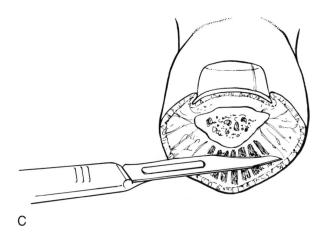

C

FIGURE 22–6. Lateral incision for drainage of felon. *(A),* Location of lateral incision. *(B),* Sagittal section showing purulence in pulp space between multiple septae. *(C),* Division of multiple septae to ensure adequate drainage.

Fishmouth Incision (Fig. 22–7*A*). The fishmouth incision is essentially the same as the hockey stick except that it is continued around the tip of the toe to the opposite side. A disadvantage of this incision is the potential for devascularizing the plantar pulp tip and for the development of an unsightly, tender scar with a bulbous mobile toe pad.

Hockey Stick Incision (Fig. 22–7*B*). The hockey stick incision is made above the midlateral line and 0.5 cm distal to the distal flexion crease of the toe. The incision is extended distally in a plane 1 mm plantar to the edge of the nail bed and around the tip of the toe (approximately 2 mm anterior to the nail) to the distal corner of the nail on the opposite side. The incision is carried through the skin to bone, then distally into the pulp to divide the fascial septae. Care is taken not to dissect too far into the plantar aspect of the toe pulp because adequate drainage will be impossible.[45]

Plantar Incision (Fig. 22–7*C* and *D*). This incision is most appropriate in the presence of a sinus or puncture wound on the plantar aspect of the toe. A transverse or longitudinal plantar incision is made over the central portion of the abscess, and the sinus or puncture tract can be ellipsed. This incision may have a greater tendency to remain open and allow drainage but placing a scar on the weight-bearing surface of the toe may be a disadvantage.

Through-and-Through Incision (Fig. 22–7*E*). The through-and-through incision is a combination of two lateral incisions that are connected through the volar pulp space, thereby decompressing the abscess. The incision is not carried around the tip of the toe as in the fishmouth incision. Gauze is inserted from one side to the other through the pulp space to keep it open.

Authors' Preferred Surgical Approach

For most cases of felon a hockey stick incision is made. Care is taken to avoid entering the germinal or sterile nail matrix dorsally or

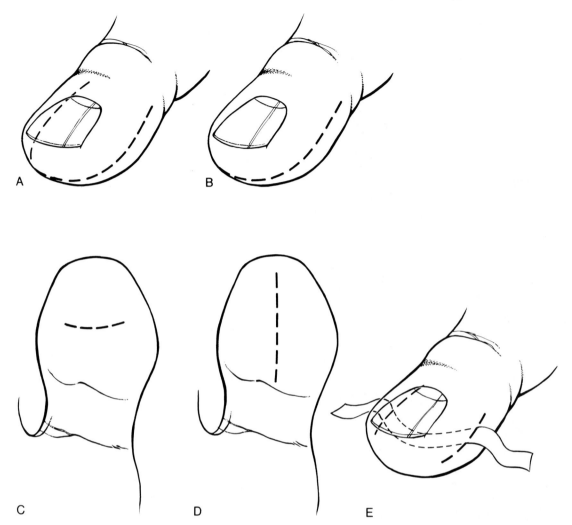

FIGURE 22–7. Other incisions for drainage of felon. *(A)*, Fishmouth incision. *(B)*, Hockey stick incision. *(C)*, Transverse plantar incision. *(D)*, Longitudinal plantar incision. *(E)*, Tibial and fibular lateral incisions and placement of wick.

the neurovascular bundle plantarward. If there is a plantar puncture wound or sinus, a plantar longitudinal incision is made. The wound is loosely packed open with gauze and at 24 to 48 hours warm soaks in a dilute antiseptic solution are begun. As infection clears, the wound will close secondarily. Closure with sutures is not necessary and will impede proper drainage of the wound.

DEEP INFECTIONS

Web Space Infection

Infections of the web space of the foot are often caused by a fissure, ulcer, or blister near the web space that becomes infected. Pain and swelling are localized to the web space and the adjacent toes may become splayed.[43, 57] The bacteria often gain access to the skin on the plantar aspect of the foot as a subepidermal collection of pus. Because of the insertion of the longitudinal fibers of the plantar aponeurosis into the plantar skin, a web space abscess cannot track superficially between the skin and plantar fascia, and as a result, the infection extends dorsally instead of peripherally.[9, 66]

Treatment

Incision plus drainage is the treatment of choice if there is evidence of abscess formation clinically or radiographically or if there is no improvement 24 to 48 hours after beginning antibiotics.

Plantar Incision (L-Shaped). A transverse incision is made over the base of the affected proximal phalanx just distal to the weight-bearing area (Fig. 22–8*A*) and a second longitudinal limb of incision is made at an angle of 60 to 90 degrees to the first. The longitudinal limb is extended between the metatarsal heads to the level of the metatarsal neck. Sharp dissection is carried down to the level of the transverse vesiculae of the plantar aponeu-

rosis. A dissecting clamp can then be positioned beneath the aponeurosis, which is divided longitudinally. Care is taken to protect the neurovascular bundle, which lies directly beneath the aponeurosis. Blunt dissection and spreading with the clamp are continued until the clamp can be felt to tent the skin on the dorsal surface of the web space. A dorsal incision can then be centered over the clamp if necessary.

The deep transverse metatarsal ligament may or may not have to be transected, depending on the extent of the infection. Copious

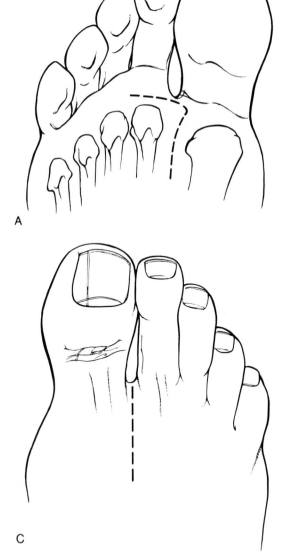

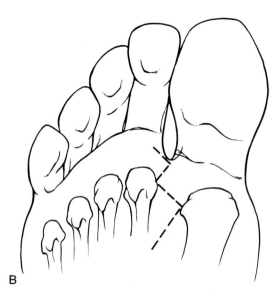

A

B

C

FIGURE 22–8. Incisions for drainage of web space infection. *(A)*, Plantar L-shaped incision. *(B)*, Brunner-type plantar incision. *(C)*, Dorsal incision to be used in conjunction with *A* and *B* to complete through-and-through drainage.

through-and-through irrigation is carried out and the wound is loosely packed with gauze. At 24 to 48 hours the gauze is removed and daily pack changes are begun.

Plantar Incision (Brunner Zig-Zag). An oblique incision is made beginning at the junction of the most proximal skin crease and the glabrous skin (Fig. 22–8*B*). The incision should extend obliquely across the base of the proximal phalanx to the edge of the metatarsal head and then obliquely through the interval between the metatarsal heads, taking care to keep the limbs of the incision at 60 to 90 degrees to one another in a zig-zag configuration. If more proximal dissection is necessary, a longitudinal extension can be made between the metatarsal heads. The deep dissection and postoperative care are the same as for the transverse incision.

Authors' Preferred Surgical Treatment

The Brunner zig-zag incision is made as described when an abscess of the web space is identified. Blunt dissection to the dorsal skin and a longitudinal dorsal incision are often made to allow through-and-through irrigation (Fig. 22–8*C*). The plantar incision can then be loosely approximated with nonabsorbable skin sutures at the corners of the zig-zags and the wound packed open with the gauze exiting dorsally. This allows a more rapid closure of the plantar wound but still permits adequate wound drainage. A first-generation cephalosporin, occasionally with an aminoglycoside and penicillin, is begun pending aerobic and anaerobic cultures. After 24 to 48 hours the foot is soaked in warm dilute povidone iodine solution or Hibiclens solution for 5 minutes three times daily. The gauze packing is removed at the first soak, and a dry gauze pack is applied between soaks. No weight bearing is permitted until the plantar wound begins to close, then a postoperative sandal is worn.

Puncture Wounds of the Foot

Puncture wounds of the foot are common and can lead to significant problems. Fitzgerald and Cowan found that 0.8 percent of emergency room visits by children over 9 years old were for puncture wounds of the foot, 98 percent of which were caused by stepping on a nail.[23] Patients with insensitive feet are also

at significant risk for puncture wounds. Puncture wounds are often undertreated, since many physicians do not associate them with significant sequelae. Fitzgerald, however, reported serious complications in 3.3 percent of patients, including 1.8 percent with osteomyelitis,[23] and Houston reported a late infection rate of 10 percent.[28] In those patients who developed osteomyelitis, *Pseudomonas* was the most common organism isolated, followed by *Staphylococcus* and *Escherichia coli*.[32, 40, 50, 53]

Initial evaluation consists of a detailed history to determine the type of shoe worn, the type of penetrating object, the estimated depth of penetration, the local environment in which the puncture occurred, and the presence of any associated disease such as diabetes mellitus, peripheral neuropathy, or peripheral vascular disease.

The wound often appears benign without evidence of infection. An x-ray study should be obtained to localize any foreign bodies and to rule out penetration to bone, which may require more aggressive treatment. Xeroradiography may be helpful in identifying radiolucent foreign bodies. Tetanus prophylaxis should be updated and the wound cleansed. This is often not sufficient treatment, however, and exploration of the wound with débridement is indicated when there has been deep penetration (deep to the plantar fascia), when bone or joint penetration is suspected, or when there is a possibility of retained foreign material (Fig. 22–9). Débridement may also be indicated for a superficial puncture if the wound was grossly contaminated. In these situations antibiotic coverage with a first-generation cephalosporin is added. Additional antibiotic coverage is needed for fecal contamination (anaerobes) or if the puncture occurred through a shoe (*Pseudomonas*).

In the acute injury, the puncture wound should be ellipsed to keep it from closing prematurely. If there has been gross contamination, a core of subcutaneous tissue including the puncture tract is excised and the wound is copiously irrigated then loosely packed with a wick of gauze to keep the tract open for drainage. At 24 to 48 hours the packing is removed and warm soaks in an antiseptic soap solution are begun for 5 minutes three to four times daily.

With an established infection, an incision is made directly over the puncture site and blunt dissection with a hemostat is carried out until the depth of penetration has been established. If there is evidence of bone or joint involvement

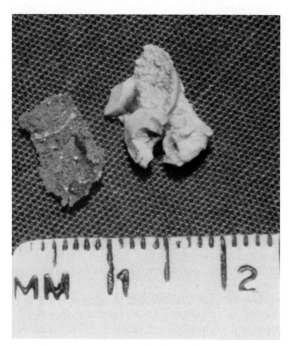

FIGURE 22–9. Pieces of sole material removed from the deep central compartment of the foot following a nail puncture wound through a tennis shoe.

(either by patient history or radiography), then the bone is curetted and the joint opened and thoroughly irrigated.

Authors' Preferred Surgical Treatment

With an acute puncture wound that is known to be superficial to the plantar fascia, tetanus prophylaxis is updated and the wound is cleansed and watched expectantly. If there is a question about the depth of penetration or proof of deep tissue penetration, the puncture wound is excised (Fig. 22–10) under local, regional, or general anesthesia and probed to its depth. The wound is copiously irrigated with at least 1 L of sterile normal saline solution through a 14- or 16-gauge plastic intravenous catheter attached to the tubing of an elevated IV bag. The wound is packed with a wick, which is removed at 24 to 48 hours, and soaked in a warm povidone iodine or Hibiclens solution for 5 minutes three to four times daily. For prophylaxis, an oral first-generation cephalosporin is given for 48 hours unless gross contamination is known to have occurred, in which case a 10-day course is given. If the puncture occurs through a shoe, antibiotic pro-

phylaxis with ciprofloxacin, which has *Pseudomonas* coverage, is used. If there is deep penetration with fecal contamination (e.g., from a barnyard), penicillin is added for anaerobic coverage. The patient is seen every 2 to 3 days for the next 10 days to ensure continued progress. If there has been gross contamination, admission for intravenous prophylactic antibiotic administration may be prudent.

Tenosynovitis

Isolated purulent tenosynovitis of the foot is rare and tends to occur in combination with a plantar abscess. In these cases the tenosynovitis probably begins first and then goes on to suppurate and decompress into the plantar spaces of the foot, producing a plantar abscess.

Tenosynovitis of the foot most often follows penetrating trauma, but also can arise as a proximal extension from an infected toe, most commonly in diabetes or peripheral vascular disease, or in other immunocompromised patients. An isolated purulent tenosynovitis in the foot presents with at least three of Kanavel's four cardinal signs of flexor tendon sheath infection: swelling of the involved digit(s), tenderness along the course of the tendon sheath, and pain with passive extension of the toes. In addition there may be pain with dorsiflexion, inversion, or eversion of the foot due to motion of the tendon units that cross the ankle. Examination should ensure that the pain is along the entire tendon sheath as opposed to being present in only one area, which might indicate a more localized infection not affecting the tendon sheath.[45]

Tendon Sheath Anatomy

The tendons of the foot and ankle lie within fibrous or fibro-osseous tunnels that are surrounded by synovial tendon sheaths to provide a smooth gliding surface and appropriate directional pull. The sheath consists of a visceral and a parietal layer that form a cavity closed at both ends. The anatomy of the tendon sheaths about the foot has been described by Jones[29] and is illustrated in Figures 22–11 and 22–12. Note that the long flexor tendon sheaths have a malleolar and a plantar component that are not continuous. The most

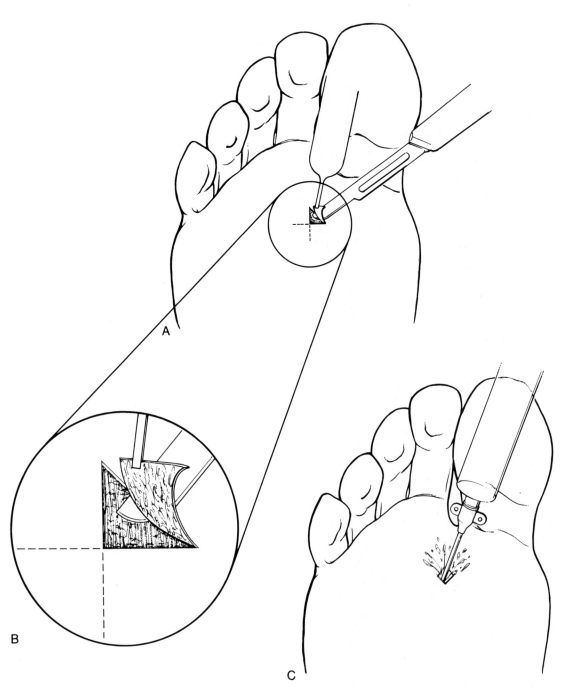

FIGURE 22–10. Technique for débridement and irrigation of puncture wound. *(A),* Cruciate incision is centered over puncture wound, and flaps created are excised. *(B),* Magnification view of *A*. *(C),* Irrigation of wound with a plastic intravenous catheter attached to bag of intravenous tubing.

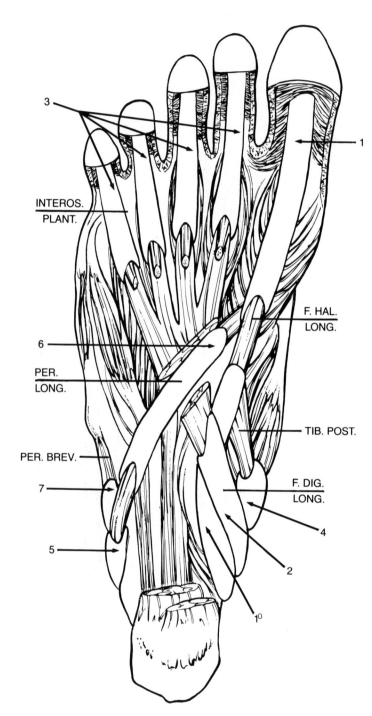

FIGURE 22–11. Tendon sheaths of the plantar aspect of the foot (1, distal tendon sheath of flexor hallucis longus; 1°, proximal tendon sheath of flexor hallucis longus; 2, proximal tendon sheath of flexor digitorum longus; 3, distal digital tendon sheath of flexor digitorum longus; 4, tendon sheath of tibialis posterior; 5, proximal tendon sheath of peroneus longus; 6, distal tendon sheath of peroneus longus; and 7, tendon sheath of peroneus brevis). (Modified from Jones FW: Structure and Function as Seen in the Foot. 2nd ed. London, Bailliere, Tindall, and Cox, 1949, pp 229–245.)

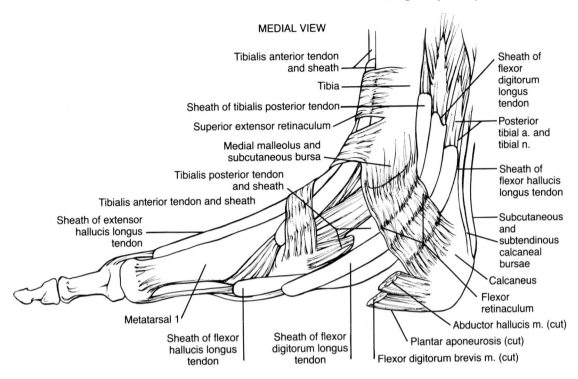

MEDIAL VIEW

Tibialis anterior tendon and sheath

Tibia

Sheath of tibialis posterior tendon

Superior extensor retinaculum

Medial malleolus and subcutaneous bursa

Tibialis posterior tendon and sheath

Tibialis anterior tendon and sheath

Sheath of extensor hallucis longus tendon

Metatarsal 1

Sheath of flexor hallucis longus tendon

Sheath of flexor digitorum longus tendon

Sheath of flexor digitorum longus tendon

Posterior tibial a. and tibial n.

Sheath of flexor hallucis longus tendon

Subcutaneous and subtendinous calcaneal bursae

Calcaneus

Flexor retinaculum

Abductor hallucis m. (cut)

Plantar aponeurosis (cut)

Flexor digitorum brevis m. (cut)

FIGURE 22–12. Tendon sheaths of the medial and plantar medial aspect of foot. (Redrawn from Hamilton WG: Surgical anatomy of the foot. CIBA Found Symp 37[3]:4, 1985. Copyright 1985 Ciba-Geigy Corporation. Reproduced with permission from the Clinical Symposia by Frank H. Netter, M.D. All rights reserved.)

distal extension of the sheaths is to the level of the distal interphalangeal (DIP) joint of the toes or the interphalangeal (IP) joint in the case of the hallux. The sheaths of the flexor hallicus longus (FHL) and the flexor digitorum longus (FDL) are in direct contact as the tendons cross beneath the foot at the master knot of Henry.[26] Proximal communications between the long toe flexors and the tibialis posterior tendon sheath have also been demonstrated.[26] Injection studies of the tendon sheaths show the weakest point to be the proximal portion of the sheath where it is unprotected by the outer fibrous sheath.[26] Based on these studies the pattern of spread of infection has been postulated for each tendon.

1. Flexor hallucis longus (FHL). An infection starting in the FHL sheath in the great toe remains localized within that sheath until pressure from the infection causes it to rupture, probably at the proximal end, and spread along the tendon toward the medial side of the ankle and the medial leg space or into the medial plantar spaces.[26] If the infection starts in the malleolar sheath of the FHL, proximal

spread into the sheath behind the malleolus will occur in addition to extension distally along the tendon into the great toe and possibly into the medial plantar spaces.

2. Flexor tendons of the lesser toes. Infections of the FDL and flexor digitorum brevis (FDB) tendons of the lesser toes usually rupture proximally with extension of the infection into the central plantar space. Should the infection start in the malleolar sheath of the FDL, proximal extension may occur into the other sheaths behind the malleolus, with potential distal extension to the junction of the long toe flexors and the FHL and into the central or medial plantar spaces.

3. Tibialis posterior tendon. Tenosynovitis of the tibialis posterior tendon may extend to the medial leg space as well as distally along the medial aspect of the foot.

4. Peroneus longus and brevis tendons. An infection in the malleolar portion of the peroneal tendon sheath can spread proximally into the lateral leg space and/or distally into the foot via rupture of the sheath or through a normal communication between it and the plantar sheath. Infections originating in the

plantar sheath of the peronei will initially remain localized in the sheath or the medial spaces of the foot with potential for spread along the tendons proximally.

5. Extensor tendons. Infections in the long toe extensors tend to remain localized within the sheaths and do not extend to form deep abscesses.

Treatment

Nevaiser outlined several tenets of treatment for early tenosynovitis of the hand that are also applicable to the foot.[45] If the patient is seen within the first 24 to 48 hours, nonoperative treatment is likely to be successful. The patient should be admitted to the hospital and the foot placed at rest with a compression dressing, posterior splint, and elevation and administration of intravenous broad-spectrum antibiotics. If the patient responds to treatment within 24 to 48 hours, oral antibiotics can be substituted and treatment continued on an outpatient basis with weight-bearing avoided until symptoms abate.

Surgical drainage should be performed if there is no definitive improvement 24 to 48 hours after the start of nonoperative treatment or if the duration of symptoms is unclear. Untreated purulent tenosynovitis can cause tendon ischemia and necrosis as well as an abscess in the deep plantar space. Considering the anatomy and pattern of extension along the tendon sheaths, surgical drainage should have two aims: (1) adequate drainage of the tendon sheath and (2) adequate drainage of any fascial spaces that may be secondarily affected. Unlike in the hand, where regaining or maintaining motion is of the utmost importance, the primary goal in the foot is eradication of the infection through surgical incisions that will result in a pain-free and plantigrade foot. Additional goals are prevention of (1) painful scars on the weight-bearing areas of the foot, (2) any equinus contracture at the ankle, and (3) claw or hammer toe deformities secondary to soft tissue contracture. In general, the tendon sheaths are best approached via incisions directly over them.

Surgical Techniques

Combination Linear and Brunner-type Incision

Special efforts should be made to identify the portion of the sheath that is most tender.

A plantar linear incision is outlined along the appropriate metatarsal, extending from the middle of the metatarsal distal to the level of the metatarsal neck. The distal portion of the incision should extend up to but not onto the weight-bearing area. The dissection is carried down to the plantar fascia. A small opening is made in the fascia and a curved hemostat inserted beneath the plantar fascia to dissect any soft tissue off of the dorsal surface of the aponeurosis. The fascia is incised in line with the incision. Blunt dissection is carried out until the flexor tendon sheath can be identified. The proximal extent of the fibrous sheath should be identifiable. The sheath is incised and if pus is seen, it may be opened for the length of the initial incision. A Brunner-type incision is made on the plantar aspect of the toe if the infection extends into the distal portion of the tendon sheath. After the skin incision, careful dissection is performed until the tendon sheath is identified to avoid damage to the neurovascular bundles. A longitudinal incision is made through the sheath over the middle and proximal phalanges. These should be separate incisions skipping the sheath overlying the PIP and DIP joints. A small plastic tube such as from a 21-gauge butterfly catheter can then be threaded proximally to distally to irrigate the tendon sheath until the effluent is clear. The wound is then closed loosely over a drain.

Curvilinear Plantar Incision

As described by Loeffler and Ballard,[35] the incision begins posterior to the medial malleolus, extending laterally and distally to the midline and then distally to end between the first and second metatarsals (Fig. 22–13). The entire incision or any part of it may be used depending on the clinical situation. For drainage of a flexor tenosynovitis, the incision may begin at the level of the metatarsal head between the first and second rays and extend proximally. At the level of the navicular, the incisions should begin to curve dorsally toward a point 1 cm posterior to the medial malleolus. If more proximal exposure is necessary, the incision can be extended proximally along the course of the neurovascular bundle. The incision should be made through the plantar skin down to the level of the plantar aponeurosis without undermining the skin flaps. The plantar aponeurosis should be excised in line with the skin incision, taking care to protect the

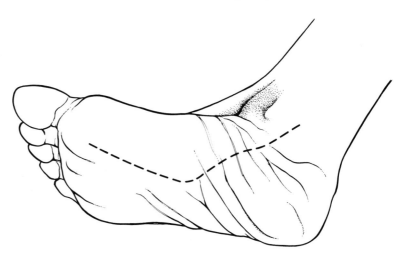

FIGURE 22–13. Skin incision for curvilinear plantar approach to the foot. (Modified from Loeffler RD, Ballard A: Plantar fascial spaces of the foot and a proposed surgical approach. Foot Ankle 1(1):13, 1980. © American Orthopaedic Foot and Ankle Society 1980.)

medial plantar nerve and artery, which lie directly beneath the plantar fascia in the fore-foot. The dissection is begun over the area that is most symptomatic and then extended proximally or distally as needed. This incision may also be extended distally onto the plantar aspect of the great toe through a zig-zag Brunner-type incision. The Brunner incision is begun just distal to the sesamoids and angled toward the proximal flexion crease of the great toe at a 45-degree angle. It can then be angled toward the fibular side of the great toe at the interphalangeal joint level. The flap is elevated to expose the FHL tendon to the interphalangeal joint level.

Proximal to the level of the navicular, the dissection is extended by carefully dividing the abductor hallucis muscle including the deep investing fascia. The tendon sheaths are then followed proximally, and if needed the flexor retinaculum just proximal to the medial malleolus is divided. The neurovascular bundle lies in the fat immediately beneath the retinaculum. A dissecting hemostat can be used to dissect posterior to the neurovascular bundle to identify the sheath of the flexor hallucis longus tendon. Dissection anterior to the neurovascular bundle reveals the sheath of the flexor digitorum longus and posterior tibial tendons.

Infections of the Fascial Spaces of the Sole of the Foot

Potential fascial spaces are present in the central, medial, and lateral compartments, as described by Grodinsky.[25] There are four fas-cial spaces in the central compartment and one fascial space in each of the medial and lateral compartments as shown in Figures 22–14 and 22–15. Grodinsky found that an injection into any one of the fascial spaces of the central compartment often revealed multiple communications among the four fascial spaces.[25] Infection in one space within the central compartment is likely to spread to another, and care must be taken to ensure that all the spaces in the middle compartment are explored. Infection may also spread from the central compartment to the dorsal subcutaneous regions.

Incisions for Draining Fascial Spaces

Central Compartment

Because of the potential for communication between fascial spaces of the central compartment, any technique for drainage must allow access to the entire compartment to ensure adequate drainage.

Medial Incision A medial incision can be used to gain access to the middle compartment as well as the medial compartment by the technique described by Myerson for an acute compartment syndrome fasciotomy (Fig. 22–16).[42] A curved linear incision is made starting at the level of the navicular–first cuneiform joint and extending distally along the inferior margin of the first metatarsal to the level of the metatarsal neck. Dissection is carried through the subcutaneous tissue, and the abductor hallucis muscle fascia can be split to decompress the medial compartment. Through dissection beneath the first metatarsal, the abductor hallucis and flexor hallucis brevis may be retracted plantarward and the medial inter-

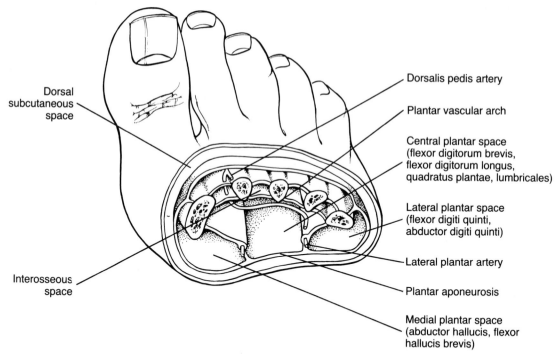

FIGURE 22–14. Plantar compartments of the distal foot.

muscular septum incised to gain access to the central compartment. Each of the fascial spaces of the central compartment can then be identified and opened by blunt dissection. Care

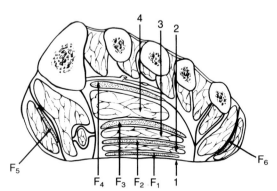

FIGURE 22–15. Fascial spaces of the sole of the foot. Central compartment: F_1, fascial space between central plantar aponeurosis (1) and flexor digitorum brevis (2); F_2, fascial space between flexor digitorum brevis (2) and quadratus plantae (3); F_3, fascial space between quadratus plantae (3) and oblique head of adductor hallucis (4); F_4, fascial space between adductor hallucis (4) and interosseous fascia. Medial compartment: F_5, fascial space located between investing fascia of abductor hallucis and deep surface of muscle. Lateral compartment: F_6, fascial space located between investing fascia of abductor digiti quinti and deep surface of muscle. (Modified from Grodinsky M: A study of the fascial spaces of the foot and their bearing on infections. Surg Gynecol Obstet 49:737, 1929. By permission of Surgery, Gynecology and Obstetrics.)

must be taken to divide all the septae of the first fascial space. Infections of the interosseous compartments and lateral compartment will not drain well through the medial incision and if involved should be approached directly.

Curvilinear Plantar Incision. The curvilinear plantar incision[35] is a gently curving incision that begins between the first and second metatarsals at the level of the metatarsophalangeal (MTP) joints and extends longitudinally down the sole of the foot, curving medially to just behind the medial malleolus as described previously (see Fig. 22–13). All of the fascial spaces of the central and medial compartments can be drained via this approach. This incision has the advantage of allowing direct visualization of the neurovascular structures as well as each division of the central compartment. A disadvantage is the plantar location, although it is located in an area of minimal weight bearing.

Medial Compartment

The potential fascial space of the medial compartment is located between the investing fascia of the abductor hallucis and the deep surface of the muscle. This space is decompressed directly through the medial incision (see Fig. 22–16).

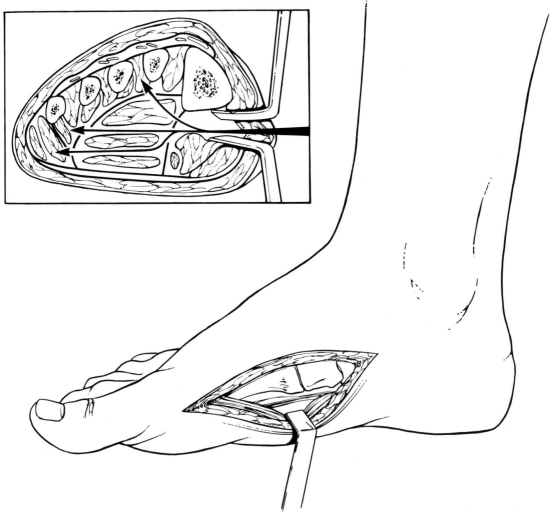

FIGURE 22–16. Medial approach for drainage of plantar spaces of the foot. (Modified from Myerson M: Experimental decompression of the fascial compartments of the foot. The basis for fasciotomy in acute compartment syndrome. Foot Ankle 8[6]:308–314, 1988. © American Orthopaedic Foot and Ankle Society 1988.)

Lateral Compartment

The fascial space of the lateral compartment is a potential space located between the deep surface of the abductor digiti quinti and the investing fascia. It extends from the os calcis to the level of the fifth metatarsal head. Drainage of this compartment can be done through a curved linear incision centered at the junction of the dorsal and plantar skin on the lateral side of the foot. The incision begins just proximal to the fifth metatarsal head and ends approximately 1 cm proximal to the insertion of the peroneus brevis into the base of the fifth metatarsal. Dissection is carried through the subcutaneous tissue to the deep fascia, taking care to avoid the terminal branches of the sural nerve. The fascia overlying the abductor digiti quinti can be identified and incised in line with the incision. Any necrotic tissue is débrided and the wound copiously irrigated and lightly packed open. The packing can be removed at 48 hours and dressing changes started. The wound may be allowed to heal by secondary intention or closed over a drain after a second débridement in 48 hours.

Heel Space

Infections in the heel space are most often secondary to the entrance of bacteria through cracks in overly callused skin[61] or puncture wounds. A true infection of the heel space involves the subcutaneous fat of the heel pad as opposed to an intradermal infection.

The primary symptoms are steadily increasing pain, associated swelling of the soft tissue covering the sides of the calcaneus, and overlying tenderness.[61]

Drainage of the heel space is accomplished through a longitudinal medial or lateral incision (Fig. 22–17). The incision is placed 5 mm below the junction of the plantar and dorsal skin to the deep fascia, which is incised in line with the skin incision. The fibrous septae are then divided to drain areas of loculated pus. The wound is copiously irrigated and loosely packed open with gauze. At 48 hours the pack is removed and dressing changes and local

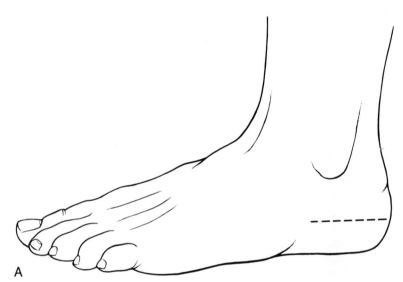

A

FIGURE 22–17. Lateral incision for heel pad abscess or calcaneal osteomyelitis.

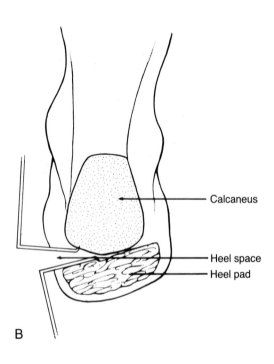

Calcaneus

Heel space
Heel pad

B

wound care begun. A posterior splint is used to hold the foot in the neutral position and the patient is kept non–weight-bearing until healing has occurred.

Dorsal Interosseous Compartments

Infections of the dorsal interosseous compartments are likely to remain localized and can easily be drained through a dorsal longitudinal incision. If there is involvement of the interosseous compartment secondary to extension from the middle compartment, through-and-through drainage is necessary. This can be accomplished by making an additional longitudinal incision centered over the area of the infection.

A longitudinal dorsal incision should be centered over the abscess (Fig. 22–18). Dissection is carried through the skin and subcutaneous tissue and then blunt dissection is used within the interosseous compartment. If extension from a deep layer is suspected, the blunt tip of a hemostat can penetrate through the inter-

osseous fascia into the middle compartment. Once the tip of the clamp is palpated plantarward, a curvilinear or Brunner-type incision can be made on the plantar surface centered over the clamp. The wound may then be irrigated through the dorsal and plantar wounds.

Authors' Preferred Surgical Treatment

A fascial space abscess of the medial or lateral compartment is approached directly through a longitudinal incision overlying the respective space. If the central compartment fascial spaces are involved but the infection seems localized to that area without dorsal extension, adequate decompression is obtained via the medial curvilinear incision (see Fig. 22–16). The medial incision may need to be extended proximally and distally to give adequate exposure. If, however, the foot is swollen both dorsally and plantarward and if there may be associated flexor tenosynovitis, a longitudinal plantar incision is made as in Figure

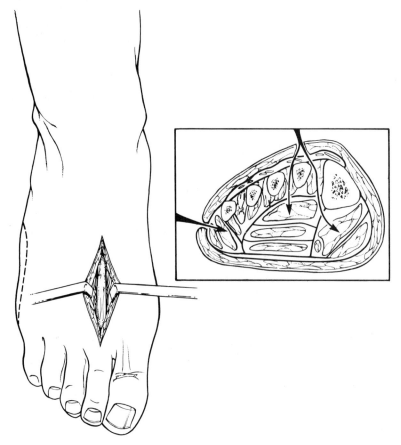

FIGURE 22–18. Incisions for drainage of plantar spaces through dorsal and lateral approaches.

22–13 and a dorsal longitudinal incision is added if needed (see Fig. 22–18).

Postoperative Care

After decompression, the fascial space is copiously irrigated with 3 L of sterile normal saline and loosely packed with iodoform gauze, and a compression splint is applied with the foot in the neutral position. After 48 hours the patient is returned to the operating room and the wound again irrigated and débrided as necessary and closed over a suction drain. The drain is removed in 1 to 2 days. The patient is kept non–weight bearing and intravenous antibiotics are continued until significant improvement in the wound is seen.

Septic Arthritis

Septic arthritis refers to a pyogenic infection involving a synovial joint. Septic arthritis of the joints in the foot is rare and tends to occur more frequently in children (4%).[24] Septic arthritis may occur as a result of hematogenous spread from a distant source; however, spread from an adjacent focus of infection or direct innoculation through a penetrating joint injury are more common etiologies.[13, 64] Local trauma, degenerative joint disease, and neuropathic and crystalline arthropathies are associated with increased incidence of pyogenic arthritis. *Staphylococcus aureus* and beta-hemolytic streptococci are the most common offending organisms.[2, 10, 19, 30, 37, 45] *Pseudomonas* and anaerobic organisms may also be present, especially in patients with diabetes mellitus.

Clinically, the most common finding is exquisite pain with motion. Joint effusion and erythema may or may not be present. Swelling and joint effusion are most often detected in the ankle as opposed to the smaller joints in the foot.

The earliest radiographic finding in septic arthritis is periarticular soft tissue swelling, followed by juxta-articular osteoporosis.[1] Occasionally, air is seen in the joint as a result of gas-forming bacteria (e.g., *Clostridia perfringens, Clostridia welchii, Escherichia coli,* anaerobic streptococci).[4, 58]

Definitive diagnosis of septic arthritis is made by aspiration and joint fluid analysis. The fluid should be examined for aerobic and anaerobic culture, sensitivities, gram stain, cell count, and crystal analysis. Fluid is often unobtainable from the small joints of the foot. In these instances, a saline lavage can be performed or nuclear medicine scans and radiographic correlations can be used to make a presumptive diagnosis.

Aspiration of the interphalangeal joints of the toe is performed through a dorsal approach after sterile preparation and draping with or without local anesthesia. In general, the largest bore needle possible is chosen. For the interphalangeal joints a 20-gauge needle can be used to approach the joint medial or lateral to the extensor tendon aiming toward the center of the digit. The metatarsophalangeal joints can be approached similarly with an 18- or 20-gauge needle. Treatment of septic arthritis of the joints of the foot with multiple joint aspirations, as has been advocated for other joints, is not recommended.

Surgical Drainage

Interphalangeal Joints

The interphalangeal joints are drained through a dorsal lateral incision centered over the joint. Dissection is carried through the subcutaneous tissue and the joint capsule is opened just lateral to the extensor tendon. Cultures are obtained. Any proliferative synovium found is excised and the joint copiously irrigated. The incision is left open to allow drainage and secondary closure.

Metatarsophalangeal Joints

When septic arthritis of the metatarsophalangeal (MTP) joints is secondary to puncture or contiguous spread from a plantar ulcer, drainage should include débridement of the puncture tract, sinus, or ulcer. A dorsal lateral incision 2 to 3 cm long is then made longitudinally over the affected MTP joint just lateral to the extensor tendon. Dissection is carried through the subcutaneous tissue, and the dorsal capsule is incised longitudinally. Cultures are obtained and any proliferative synovium is excised and the joint copiously irrigated. In the case of an associated plantar wound, through-and-through irrigation is done. The plantar wound is then closed, if possible, leaving a gauze packing or small Silastic drain to keep the dorsal wound open to allow drainage. The skin is loosely approximated on either side of the drain and a bulky dressing applied with the foot held in the neutral position. At 48 hours the drain is removed and dressing changes and antibiotics are continued until the wound is closed. The patient is allowed to ambulate in a postoperative shoe once the wound has shown signs of significant improvement.

Intertarsal Joints

Septic arthritis of the intertarsal joints is drained through a dorsal longitudinal incision approximately 2 to 3 cm in length centered over the involved joint. Dissection is carried through the skin, and care is taken to identify the dorsal cutaneous nerves. Dissection is carried through the subcutaneous tissue and deep fascia and the capsule is incised parallel to the joint. Cultures are obtained, and any proliferative synovium is excised and the joint copiously irrigated. A gauze wick is placed at the opening of the joint to hold the soft tissues open for 24 to 48 hours to allow joint drainage. Intravenous antibiotics are begun emperically pending culture results and a bulky compressive dressing with the foot in the neutral position is applied. The small gauze pack is removed at 48 hours and daily dressing changes performed until the wound closes secondarily. Weight bearing is limited until the wound has closed.

Osteomyelitis

In contrast to septic arthritis, osteomyelitis of the foot is not an uncommon problem. The most common pathogenic mechanisms are direct traumatic penetration of the bone or contiguous spread from an adjacent soft tissue infection.[40, 63, 64, 66] Osteomyelitis of the foot occurs more frequently in infants and children and there is a slight male predominance. The calcaneus is reportedly the most common site (6 to 8%), followed by the metatarsals, cuboid, talus, phalanges, and cuneiforms in order of decreasing frequency.[52, 61]

Diagnosis

Acute osteomyelitis can be suspected on the basis of clinical symptoms and physical examination, radiography, magnetic resonance imaging (MRI), and nuclear medicine scans.

However, the definitive diagnosis can be made only by a positive culture from the bone. A reasonable attempt should be made to determine the pathogenic organism prior to committing the patient to a long course of antibiotics. In acute osteomyelitis, the organism can be recovered through needle aspiration of the interosseous space, subperiosteal space, or surrounding soft tissue in the case of continuous spread from a soft tissue infection. Wound cultures of a draining sinus or ulcer can be helpful but are less accurate.

If there are not significant radiographic findings but there is uptake on bone scan, positive culture, or gram staining, antibiotic therapy is begun. Initial emperical therapy should cover the most common organisms and then should be tailored by the organism sensitivities.

Surgical Treatment

Indications for surgical débridement of an acute osteomyelitis are:

1. Clinical, radiographic, or MRI diagnosis of abscess formation.
2. Presence of acute osteomyelitis in a severely septic patient or compromised host.
3. Failure of the patient to improve despite appropriate parenteral antibiotics in 48 to 72 hours.

Phalanges

Osteomyelitis of the proximal, middle, or distal phalanges is usually treated by partial or complete amputation of the toe or a ray resection. When the infection is confined to the mid or distal phalanx, amputation through the proximal interphalangeal (PIP) joint is satisfactory.

Under adequate anesthesia, dorsal and plantar proximally based fishmouth-shaped flaps are made over the involved toe. The flap begins at the level of the head of the proximal phalanx and extends to the mid-middle phalanx. Dissection is carried through the subcutaneous tissue from skin directly to bone throughout the extent of the incision. The collateral ligaments surrounding the PIP joint are cut along with the flexor and extensor tendons, and the joint is disarticulated. Using a small rongeur the articular surface on the head of the proximal phalanx is removed and the end of the bone smoothed. The wound is copiously irrigated and the skin closed with nylon sutures. A bulky forefoot dressing is applied.

If infection involves the proximal phalanx, a disarticulation at the metatarsophalangeal level or a ray resection can be carried out. A ray resection gives a more cosmetic result and is especially indicated when the second toe is involved. When the second toe is amputated at the MTP joint level, the resulting gap between the first and third toes will allow a valgus deviation of the great toe causing an acquired hallux valgus deformity in some patients.

Disarticulation at the MTP joint level is performed through a racquet-shaped incision around the base of the toe. Sharp dissection is taken straight through the skin to the bone at that level. No undermining of the flaps is done. The base of the proximal phalanx is subperiosteally exposed and the collateral ligaments about the joint divided. The flexor and extensor tendons are pulled down and transected and allowed to retract proximally. The cartilage on the metatarsal head is removed and the end of the bone smoothed with a rongeur. The wound is copiously irrigated and the elliptical racquet-shaped incision is then closed longitudinally with nylon sutures. A small silicone drain can be placed in the wound. A forefoot compression dressing is applied; this is changed and the drain removed at 48 hours.

Metatarsal Ray Resection

A ray resection differs from disarticulation in that the proximal end of the racquet incision is carried dorsally along the line of the affected metatarsal. Dissection is carried through the subcutaneous tissue. The dorsal cutaneous nerves are identified, and the extensor tendon is divided in the proximal end of the wound at a level approximately 1 cm distal to the base of the metatarsal. Dissection is carried through the subcutaneous tissue to the bone and the metatarsal is subperiosteally exposed. Using a small oscillating saw the metatarsal is osteotomized at the metaphyseal-diaphyseal junction and the metatarsal is removed. The wound is copiously irrigated. The soft tissue envelope around the removed metatarsal is closed with interrupted absorbable sutures and the skin closed with interrupted nylon sutures over a small silicone drain. A compression foot dressing is applied with a splint to hold the ankle in the neutral position. The dressing is changed

and the drain removed at 48 hours. Once the wound has healed, a short leg walking cast is applied for 2 to 3 weeks until soft tissue healing is complete.

Metatarsal Osteomyelitis

If limited to the metatarsal head, osteomyelitis can be treated with a metatarsal head resection. If there is an associated plantar ulcer, excision of the metatarsal head is performed through a dorsal longitudinal incision and the plantar ulcer is elliptically excised and closed, leaving the dorsal wound open to close secondarily. If the metatarsal shaft is involved, a ray resection is performed as described in the preceding section.

To avoid complications, care must be taken to excise all the infected or devitalized tissues in the soft tissue envelope around the metatarsal. When performing a first or second ray amputation, the surgeon must be careful to avoid injury to the first dorsal metatarsal artery, which courses between the bases of the first and second metatarsals as a distal extension of the dorsalis pedis artery.

Authors' Preferred Surgical Approach

Metatarsal head resection is performed through a dorsal longitudinal incision approximately 3 cm in length overlying the affected MTP joint. Dissection is carried through the subcutaneous tissue, and the extensor tendon is identified and retracted. The head and neck region of the metatarsal head is exposed and the collateral ligaments are divided on each side of the MTP joint. With an oscillating saw, an oblique osteotomy is made through the distal metatarsal shaft in a dorsal-distal to plantar-proximal direction. The proximal end of the distal metatarsal fragment is then elevated dorsally by grasping the bone with a clamp, and the metatarsal head is sharply released of all soft tissue attachments.

If there is an associated plantar wound, the wound edges are débrided and any necrotic tissue at the base of the wound is excised. Copious irrigation of the wound is done with at least 2 L of normal saline solution. The plantar wound is closed with nonabsorbable sutures. The dorsal wound is packed open and a compression dressing is applied to hold the ankle and foot in the neutral position. The pack is removed at 48 hours and dressing changes are begun. The wound is then allowed to close by secondary intention.

If multiple metatarsals are involved, a transmetatarsal amputation may be necessary. However, even if one or two rays on the medial or lateral side of the foot can be saved, function is better and less shoewear modification is required than in a patient with a transmetatarsal amputation stump.

Involvement of one or both of the sesamoid bones beneath the first metatarsal head is treated with sesamoidectomy. Since the dorsal articular surface of the sesamoid articulates with the first metatarsal head, a concurrent intra-articular infection is possible, which may require more extensive débridement. The tibial sesamoid is excised through a plantar medial approach unless there is an overlying ulcer or sinus. The fibular sesamoid is excised through a curvilinear plantar approach or a dorsal web space approach between the first and second metatarsal heads. Care must be taken not to damage the plantar digital nerves during sesamoid excision.

Tarsal Osteomyelitis

Osteomyelitis of the tarsal bones localized to a single bone in the midfoot is treated by open débridement, curettage with removal of all infected bone, and then by loose closure of the wound over a suction drain to allow the wound to heal by secondary intention.

If more than one tarsal bone is affected or the talus is significantly involved, extensive débridement is carried out and the patient kept non–weight bearing. Once the infection has been eradicated, a delayed reconstructive procedure with an arthrodesis is indicated. If there is associated significant peripheral vascular disease, neuropathic arthropathy, or a large soft tissue defect, a below-knee amputation may be indicated.

Calcaneal Osteomyelitis

If limited to a small area within the bone such as the tuberosity section, osteomyelitis of the calcaneus can be approached through a medial, lateral, or combined medial-lateral incision.

Medial Approach

With the patient in the supine position, a linear incision is made paralleling the plantar

aspect of the heel at a level just above the junction of the plantar skin with the glabrous skin of the foot. The incision begins 2.5 cm anterior to the medial malleolus and extends posterior to the insertion of the Achilles tendon. The inferior border of the abductor hallucis muscle is identified and retracted dorsally, exposing the medial wall of the calcaneus. The dissection is continued distally dividing the plantar aponeurosis and the muscles attached to the calcaneus as needed. The cortex can be drilled or windowed with curettage of the involved region.

Lateral Approach

With the patient supine with a sandbag beneath the involved hip, a linear incision is made over the lateral aspect of the heel beginning 2.5 cm anterior to the medial malleolus and extending posteriorly to the insertion of the Achilles tendon. The posterior end of the incision can be curved proximally along the edge of the Achilles tendon making an L-shaped incision to gain more exposure to the tuberosity. Care should be taken to avoid damage to the sural nerve.

The U Approach

With the patient prone on the operating table a U-shaped incision is made over the heel with the medial and lateral arms of the U similar to those incisions previously described for the medial and lateral approach (Fig. 22–19). The U is placed approximately 0.5 to 1 cm above the most distal palpable portion of the calcaneus. It is extended medially or laterally as needed for adequate exposure. The skin flaps are undermined at the junction of the subcutaneous tissue and the periosteum. The periosteum is incised in line with the skin incision and the plantar soft tissues are stripped from the calcaneus. All infected bone and devitalized soft tissue are excised and the wound irrigated with 2 to 3 L of sterile saline. The wound is packed open and a compressive short leg splint is applied to hold the foot in the neutral position. At 48 hours the patient is returned to the operating room and a second débridement and irrigation is carried out and the wound closed over a suction drain. The drain is removed once drainage has ceased, usually by 48 hours, and dressing changes and continued splinting continued until the wound

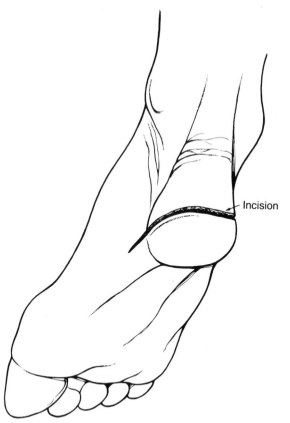

Incision

FIGURE 22–19. Surgical exposure of the calcaneus through a U-shaped or circumferential heel incision. (Modified from Bank SW, Laufman H: An Atlas of Surgical Exposures of the Extremities. Philadelphia, WB Saunders Company, 1953, p 379.)

closes. A short leg cast is applied until the patient is able to ambulate with full weight bearing. Skin flap necrosis of the heel pad is a potential complication of this incision.

Calcaneal osteomyelitis is often associated with a soft tissue wound or sinus, which must be completely excised at the time of débridement. If local soft tissue coverage cannot be accomplished, a free soft tissue transfer flap is indicated. If the patient has significant diabetes or peripheral vascular disease or is otherwise not a candidate for free tissue transfer, a Syme or below-knee amputation is indicated. If soft tissue coverage can be obtained, even if there has been an almost complete calcanectomy, adequate pedorthic management with a Plastizote-lined heel cup and a high-top extradepth shoe will usually allow functional ambulation. Aggressive pedorthic management with close follow-up is especially necessary

following free tissue transfer to the heel to prevent future skin breakdown over the insensate flap.

Postoperative Infections

Postoperative wound infections remain a major concern when considering surgical intervention. In 1983, Miller reported a gross infection rate of 2.2 percent (41 of 1841 clean operative foot and ankle cases). This study excluded cases in which there was a compound fracture, open wound, toenail procedure, or concurrent superficial infection.[41] No prophylactic antibiotics were administered. Thirty-seven of the postoperative infections healed without further surgery. Only one patient (0.05%) developed permanent sequelae as a result of the infection. This rate of infection compares favorably to that in other studies, even those in which prophylactic antibiotics were given.[43, 48]

Antibiotic prophylaxis to prevent postoperative wound infection has gained a place in the armamentarium of an increasing number of orthopaedic surgeons. Prophylactic antibiotics are probably advisable when performing foot and ankle surgery when there is the chance of local contamination (e.g., from toenails), when hardware is used, and when significant soft tissue dissection and exposure are performed, but more study is required to substantiate this recommendation.

Infections of Foot Implants

Wound infection following elective foot surgery in uncompromised patients is uncommon. When it does occur, it is usually treatable with antibiotics and local wound care. If infection occurs about a pin site, removal of the pin, local wound care, and antibiotics are usually adequate. If a postoperative infection involves the deep structures or an abscess develops, treatment is as previously described for deep infections of the foot.

Clostridial Infections

Although clostridial infections are rare, they are a strong diagnostic consideration whenever there is an injury resulting in devitalization of tissue and contamination by a foreign body, soil, or feces. The causative organism may be any one of six of the gram-positive rods that belong to the clostridial species, the most important of which is *Clostridia perfringens*. Found primarily in soil and in the feces of most animals, including humans,[21] these organisms are obligate anaerobes that cannot multiply in the relatively high oxidation-reduction potentials found in healthy tissues.

Clostridial infection requires contamination and an area of decreased oxidation-reduction potential, which can result from several factors. The foremost is circulatory failure due to direct trauma to vessels, pressure from tourniquets, casts, or dressings, or severe local edema. Other causative factors are foreign bodies, necrotic tissue or hemorrhage in the wound, and the other bacteria.[21]

Clostridial infections are classified into three types: clostridial contamination, clostridial cellulitus, and clostridial myonecrosis or gas gangrene. Clostridial contamination refers to when the organism is present in the wound but there is no evidence of clinical disease. Clostridial cellulitus is seen when there is infection with clinical evidence of disease but no evidence of dead muscle. The hallmark of Clostridial myonecrosis is the presence of dead muscle in addition to toxin production, which results in severe clinical disease.[16] In patients with clostridial myonecrosis, there is production of one of a variety of potent toxins that cause the local tissue damage and systemic toxicity.

The diagnosis is made primarily on clinical grounds and requires a high index of suspicion. Clostridial cellulitus usually involves the subcutaneous and fascial planes. There may be crepitus in the subcutaneous tissue, but muscle in general is not affected. Often the patient is only mildly toxic. This form of clostridial infection may be more common in the foot because there is less muscle than in the leg.[51]

The onset of clostridial myonecrosis is often heralded by marked local pain and edema via destruction of local tissues. The patient may have tachycardia with only a mild fever, and there is often rapid destruction of local tissue and subsequent profound toxemia.[21] Gram stain of the involved region may be helpful. In anaerobic cellulitis there is often an abundance of leukocytes, gram-positive rods, and some other associated bacterial flora. In clostridial myonecrosis there is usually an abundance of gram-positive rods and associated bacterial flora but few if any leukocytes.[21]

Prophylaxis and Treatment

As in many conditions, prevention is much easier than cure. It is critical to recognize wounds that have the potential for the development of clostridial infection. Any wound in which there has been marked tissue trauma with potential devitalization, (e.g., crush injury or an open fracture) should be closely monitored for development of gas gangrene. Surgical débridement without primary closure is vital in the treatment of these wounds and the prevention of gas gangrene. Once the patient presents with gas gangrene (clostridial myonecrosis), treatment is three-fold. Most important is aggressive débridement of all devitalized tissue combined with antibiotics (usually penicillin) and hyperbaric oxygen therapy. The use of antitoxin is still controversial, but it may prove an effective addition to débridement, antibiotics, and hyperbaric therapy.

Nonclostridial gas gangrene is more common than previously thought and is an important consideration in the differential diagnosis of clostridial gas gangrene. Nonclostridial gas gangrene has been reported in up to 17 percent of diabetic patients with vascular problems.[3] The clinical characteristics range from severe to benign toxicity. Because the causative organism is usually a gram-negative rod or enterococcus, the diagnosis of this syndrome and its differentiation from clostridial gas gangrene is important for appropriate treatment.

References

1. Berquist TH, Brown ML: Infection. *In* Berquist TH (Ed): Radiology of the Foot and Ankle. New York, Raven Press, 1989, pp 277–313.
2. Berney S, Goldstein M, Bishko F: Clinical and diagnostic features of tuberculous arthritis. Am J Med 53:36–42, 1972.
3. Bessman AN, Wagner W: Nonclostridial gas gangrene: Report of 48 cases and review of the literature. JAMA 233:958–963, 1975.
4. Blixnak J, Ramsey J: Emphysematous septic arthritis due to E. coli. J Bone Joint Surg 58A:138–139, 1976.
5. Bojsen Moller F, Flagstad KE: Plantar aponeurosis and internal architecture of the ball of the foot. J Anat 121:599–611, 1976.
6. Bonakdapour A, Gaine VD: Radiology of osteomyelitis. Orthop Clin North Am 14:21–37, 1983.
7. Brand RA, Black H: Pseudomonas osteomyelitis following puncture wounds in children. J Bone Joint Surg 56A:1637–1642, 1974.
8. Brown ML, Kamida C, Berquist TH, et al: An imaging approach to musculoskeletal infections. *In* Berquist TH (Ed): Imaging of Orthopaedic Trauma and

Surgery. Philadelphia, WB Saunders, 1986, pp 731–753.

9. Burkhalter W: Deep space infections. Hand Clin 5:553–559, 1989.

10. Butt WP: The radiology of infection. Clin Orthop 96:20–30, 1973.

11. Canales FL, Newmeyer WL, Kilgore ES: The treatment of felons and paronychias. Hand Clin 5:515–523, 1989.

12. Capitano MA, Kirkpatrick JA: Early roentgen observations in acute osteomyelitis. AJR 188:488–496, 1970.

13. Chused MJ, Jacobs WM, Sty JR: Pseudomonas arthritis following puncture wounds of the foot. J Pediatr 94:429–432, 1979.

14. Cierny G, Mader JT, Pennick JJ: A clinical staging system for adult osteomyelitis. Contemp Orthop, 10:17–37, 1985.

15. Clawson DK, Dunn W: Management of common bacterial infections of bone and joints. J Bone Joint Surg 49A:164–182, 1967.

16. Colwill MR, Mandsleu RH: The management of gas gangrene with hyperbaric oxygen therapy. J Bone Joint Surg 50B:732–742, 1968.

17. Crandon JH: Lesser infections of the hand. *In* Flynns J (Ed): Hand Surgery. Baltimore, Williams & Wilkins, 1966, pp 803–814.

18. Curtiss PH: Some uncommon forms of osteomyelitis. Clin Orthop 96:84–87, 1973.

19. Curtiss PH: The pathophysiology of joint infection. Clin Orthop 96:129–135, 1973.

20. Dalinka MK, Lally JF, Konwer G: The radiology of osseous and articular infection. CRC Radiol Nucl Med 7:1–64, 1975.

21. DeHaven KE, Evarts CM: The continuing problem of gas gangrene: A review and report of illustrative cases. J Trauma 11:983–991, 1971.

22. Fierer J, Daneel D, Davis C: The fetid foot: Lower extremity infections in patients with diabetes mellitus. Rev Infect Dis 1:210–217, 1979.

23. Fitzgerald RH, Cowan JDE: Puncture wounds of the foot, Orthop Clin North Am 6:965–972, 1975.

24. Gillespie R: Septic arthritis of childhood. Clin Orthop 96:152–159, 1973.

25. Grodinsky M: A study of the fascial spaces of the foot and their bearing on infections. Surg Gynecol Obstet 49:737–752, 1929.

26. Grodinsky M: A study of the tendon sheaths of the foot and their relation to infection. Surg Gynecol Obstet 51:460–468, 1930.

27. Grodinsky M: Foot infections of peridigital origin: Routes of spread and methods of treatment. Ann Surg 94:274–285, 1931.

28. Houston AN, Roy WA, Faust RA, et al: Tetanus prophylaxis in the treatment of puncture wounds of patients in the deep South. J Trauma 2:439–450, 1962.

29. Jones FW: Structure and Function as Seen in the Foot, 2nd Ed. London, Baillière, Tindall, and Cox, 1949, pp 229–245.

30. Kelly PJ: Bacterial arthritis in adults. Orthop Clin North Am 6:973–982, 1975.

31. Keyser J, Eaton RG: Surgical cure of chronic paronychia by eponychial marsupialization. Plast Reconstr Surg 58:66–70, 1976.

32. Lang AG, Peterson HA: Osteomyelitis following puncture wounds of the foot in children. J Trauma 16:993–999, 1976.

33. Lee, SM, Lee RGL, Wilinsky J, et al: Magnification radiography in osteomyelitis. Skel Radiol 15:625–627, 1986.

34. Livingston R, Jacobs R, Karmody A: Plantar abscesses in the diabetic patient. Foot Ankle 5:205–213, 1985.

35. Loeffler RD, Ballard A: Plantar fascial spaces of the foot and ankle: Proposed surgical approach. Foot Ankle 1:11–14, 1980.

36. Louie TJ, Bartlett JG, Tally FP, et al: Aerobic and anaerobic bacteria in diabetic foot ulcers. Ann Intern Med 85(4):461–463, 1976.

37. McClatcheg WM: Pseudopodia from Hemophilus influenzae in the adult. Arthritis Rheum 22:681–683, 1979.

38. Mauer AH, Millmond SH, Knight LC, et al: Infection in diabetic osteoarthropathy: Use of indium labeled leukocytes for diagnosis. Radiology 161:221–225, 1986.

39. Mendelson EB, Fisher MR, Deschler TW: Osteomyelitis in the diabetic foot: A difficult diagnostic challenge. Radiographics 3:248–261, 1983.

40. Miller EH, Semian DW: Gram-negative osteomyelitis following puncture wounds of the foot. J Bone Joint Surg 57A:535–537, 1975.

41. Miller WA: Postoperative wound infection in foot and ankle surgery. Foot Ankle 4:102–104, 1983.

42. Myerson M: Experimental decompression of the fascial compartments of the foot: The basis for fasciotomy in acute compartment syndromes. Foot Ankle 8:308–314, 1988.

43. Nelson CL: Prevention of sepsis. Clin Orthop 222:66–72, 1987.

44. Neviaser RJ: Infections. *In* Green DP (Ed): Operative Hand Surgery, Vol 2. New York, Churchill Livingstone, 1982, pp 771–791.

45. Park HM, Wheat J, Siddiiqui A: Scintigraphic evaluation of diabetic osteomyelitis. J Nucl Med 23:569–573, 1982.

46. Paterson DC: Acute suppurative arthritis in infancy and childhood. J Bone Joint Surg 52A:474–482, 1970.

47. Patel NC, Kennedy EJ, Johnson JE, et al: Diabetic pedal osteomyelitis: Diagnostic efficacy of In-111 WBC imaging. J Nucl Med 32:963, 1991.

48. Pavel A, Smith R, Ballard A, et al: Prophylactic antibiotics in clean orthopaedic surgery. J Bone Joint Surg 56A:777–782, 1974.

49. Perry A, Gottlieb L, Zachary L: Fingerstick felons. Ann Plast Surg 20:249–251, 1988.

50. Peterson HA, Tressler HA, Lange AG, et al: Puncture wounds of the foot. Minn Med 56:787–794, 1973.

51. Pollock SF: Infectious disorders of the foot. *In* Mann RA (Ed): Surgery of the Foot. St. Louis, CV Mosby, 1986, pp 387–389.

52. Resnick D, Niwayama G: Diagnosis of Bone and Joint Disorders, Vol. 4. Philadelphia, WB Saunders, 1988.

53. Riegler HF, Routson GW: Complications of deep puncture wounds of the foot. J Trauma 19:18–72, 1979.

54. Rubb JE: Primary acute hematogenous osteomyelitis of an isolated metatarsal in children. Acta Orthop Scand 55:334–338, 1984.

55. Rosenthall L, Lisbona R, Hernandez M: 99m Tc-PP and 67 Ga-citrate imaging following insertion of orthopaedic appliance. Radiology 133:717–721, 1979.

56. Sapico FL, Witte JL, Canawati HN, et al: The infected

foot of the diabetic patient: Quantitative microbiology and analysis of clinical features. Rev Infect Dis (Suppl) 6:171–176, 1984.

57. Sarrafian SK: Anatomy of the Foot and Ankle: Descriptive, Topographic, Functional. Philadelphia, JB Lippincott, 1983, pp 107–142.

58. Schauwecker DS: Osteomyelitis: Diagnosis with In-111 labeled leukocytes. Radiology 171:141–146, 1989.

59. Riff MJ: Clostridium perfringens septic arthritis. Clin Orthop 139:92–95, 1979.

60. Seldin DW, Heiken JP, Beldman F, et al: Effect of soft tissue pathology on detection of pedal osteomyelitis. J Nucl Med 26:988–993, 1985.

61. Selvapandian AJ: Infections of the foot. *In* Jahss MH (Ed): Disorders of the Foot, Vol 2. Philadelphia, WB Saunders, 1982, pp 1398–1420.

62. Sharp CS, Bessman AN, Wagner FW, et al: Microbiology of superficial and deep tissues in infected diabetic gangrene. Surg Gynecol Obstet 149:217–219, 1979.

63. Steinbeck HL: Infection in bone. Sem Roentgenol 1:337–369, 1966.

64. Swischuk LF, Jorgenson FJ, Jorgenson A, et al: Wooden splinter induced pseudotumors and osteomyelitis-like lesions of bone and soft tissues. AJR 122:176–179, 1974.

65. Waldvogel FA, Medoff G, Swartz MN: Osteomyelitis: A review of clinical features. Therapeutic considerations and unusual aspects. N Engl J Med 282:198–205, 1970.

66. Whitehouse WM, Smith WS: Osteomyelitis of the feet. Sem Roentgenol 5:867–877, 1970.

23 The Rheumatoid Hindfoot

JAMES A. NUNLEY
CLAUDE T. MOORMAN III

Involvement of the hindfoot with rheumatoid arthritis is a common and often disabling process.[5] More than 90 percent of rheumatoid patients experience foot pain at some point in the course of their disease.[33] Painful feet are the sole presenting symptom of rheumatoid arthritis in 28 percent of patients, whereas 8 percent have foot pain as their major disability.[25] The subtalar, talonavicular, and calcaneocuboid joints constitute the joints of the hindfoot; they are second only to the forefoot in the frequency and severity of involvement with rheumatoid disease.[29, 36] Two large series have shown that there is some disability relating to the hindfoot in 42 percent of rheumatoid patients; in 34 percent hindfoot symptoms were the predominant complaint, and in 16 per cent hindfoot pain was most responsible for difficulty with walking.[18, 19]

PATHOPHYSIOLOGY

The mechanism of destruction in rheumatoid arthritis is poorly understood. A synovitis that invades and erodes bone, ligament, capsule, and cartilage is the end result of this disease process.[26, 31, 32] Hindfoot disease appears to begin as a tenosynovitis of the tendons surrounding the ankle and hindfoot, most frequently the tibialis posterior and the peroneals. This tenosynovitis frequently interferes with the ability of the tibialis posterior to function as a static and dynamic stabilizer of the medial longitudinal arch of the foot. With prolonged tenosynovitis, this tendon may elongate and become weakened and dysfunctional, or it may

rupture, resulting in a planovalgus deformity of the hindfoot.[9] In addition to the tibialis posterior, other structures that stabilize the talocalcaneonavicular joints are the ligaments (deltoid and lateral ankle ligaments), other tendons (e.g., the flexor digitorum longus), and the bone architecture.[20]

A planovalgus deformity is the most common deformity seen in the rheumatoid hindfoot; it was noted in 87.4 percent of rheumatoid hindfeet followed up by Vahvanen, whereas varus deformity was much less common, being seen between 4 and 10 percent of the time.[35, 37] Valgus hindfoot deformity is significant in that it predisposes the patient to lateral calcaneofibular impingement, which can cause the lateral "ankle" pain common in later stages of rheumatoid hindfoot disease. Varus deformity is usually seen in patients who have been at bed rest for prolonged periods and who are inadequately splinted.

CLINICAL PRESENTATION

Symptoms and signs of rheumatoid hindfoot involvement are often variable and inconsistent. The clinical picture varies with the severity of the disease at presentation.[20] As the swelling in the tendon sheaths becomes severe, patients may complain of pain in the region of the tibialis posterior or laterally in the peroneals. Additionally, the Achilles tendon insertion, plantar fascia origin, and retrocalcaneal bursae are sites of early painful involvement.[31] These patients often have difficulty in localizing their symptoms and may present with the vague complaint of pain in the "ankle."[10] Later in the clinical course, the pain generally shifts from the medial to the lateral side of the ankle in response to impingement of the peroneal tendons between the lateral malleolus, the talus, and the calcaneus.

On physical examination, tenosynovitis with swelling and tenderness of the posterior tibial tendon and over the sinus tarsi is an early finding and may also be associated with tarsal tunnel syndrome.[15, 23, 31] Most patients have a painless range of motion through a functional arc in the talocrural joint. Later in the disease process, as the tenosynovitis becomes progressive, rupture of the tibialis posterior tendon has been reported, as has a deterioration of the ligamentous architecture of the hindfoot joints.[17] Patients with significant tenosynovitis

and those with rupture of the tibialis posterior tendon demonstrate weakness of inversion of the foot when the ankle is plantarflexed.[24] In the standing position, loss of the medial longitudinal arch and an increase in hindfoot valgus and pronation are observed (Fig. 23–1). Findings of the single-legged toe raise test may be positive: that is, as the patient attempts to stand on the toes of one foot, the heel will *not* invert. Another significant finding is peroneal spasm on rapid inversion of the hindfoot; this leads to a closer examination of the subtalar and transverse tarsal joints for evidence of joint involvement.[10]

Midtarsal and subtalar joint involvement is present in 68 percent of patients, and it often results in collapse of the medial longitudinal arch with weight bearing.[11, 25] This loss of the

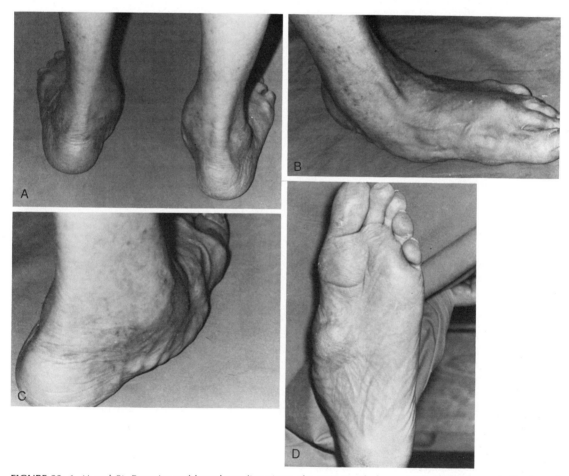

FIGURE 23–1. *(A and B)*, Posterior and lateral standing views of a patient with rheumatoid arthritis demonstrating loss of posterior tibial tendon function, collapse of the medial longitudinal arch, and increased hindfoot valgus on the left. *(C)*, Note the prominence of the head of the talus along the medial foot, which is associated with forefoot pronation. *(D)*, Callosity on the posterior medial aspect of the same foot.

medial arch results in abduction through the subtalar joint and pronation in the midtarsal region.[25] Moderate to severe deformity of the hindfoot is present in 8 percent of patients who have had the disease for less than 5 years, and significant hindfoot valgus is present in more than 25 percent of patients with a disease duration of longer than 5 years.[31]

Minaker and Little found flexible flatfoot in 52 percent of their rheumatoid patients and rigid flatfoot in 16 percent; gait abnormalities were present in 88 percent. These rheumatoid patients demonstrate a characteristic "shuffling" gait with absent heel strike while the knee and hip are maintained in slight flexion. Forefoot push-off is absent, and their stride is shortened by abbreviation of both the swing and stance phases.[25] Marshall and colleagues showed through gait analysis that alteration of the subtalar axis resulted in a loss of plantar flexion at heel strike and in a late heel rise.[22] In these patients, pain on hindfoot examination was present in 98.6 percent, swelling in the region of the subtalar joint was found in 98.3 percent, and limitation of subtalar range of motion was noted in 96.6 percent.[35] Spontaneous ankylosis of the subtalar joint occurred in only two of 484 adults (0.4 percent) in Vahvanen's series.[34]

RADIOGRAPHIC CHANGES

Radiographic changes mirror the clinical progression in the rheumatoid hindfoot. The disease process is for the most part symmetrical, and radiographs initially reveal soft tissue swelling and periarticular edema.[20] Loss of the normal retrocalcaneal triangle of radiolucent fat signifies retrocalcaneal bursitis due to inflammation of the Achilles tendon.[13] Reactive periosteal new bone formation may occur at capsular, tendinous, or plantar aponeurosis attachments. A progression to generalized osteoporosis, joint space narrowing, bony erosion, malalignment, and subluxation is often the natural history.[27] Hypertrophic spurring and subchondral sclerosis, which are present in 48 percent of these patients, occur with the onset of secondary osteoarthritis, usually late in the disease course.[13, 25]

Changes in the foot generally appear first in the forefoot, followed by the midtarsal, subtalar, and ankle joints in decreasing frequency.[20] The talonavicular joint is usually the first of the tarsal joints to be involved, and it often demonstrates the most severe narrowing.[13, 35] Osteoporosis is seen in the periarticular regions in 68 percent of patients, most commonly in the calcaneocuboid joint, where the changes are moderate or severe in 90.5 percent.[25, 35] With the progression of ligamentous laxity and increased hindfoot valgus, there is frequently evidence of calcaneofibular impingement, which is seen best on the standing anteroposterior radiograph of the ankle; hypertrophy, bending, and occasional fracture of the fibula have also been reported.[20, 21] Bony ankylosis is seen spontaneously in 25 percent of tarsal joints followed up for 19 years.[19]

Standard radiographs should include standing anteroposterior and lateral views of both the foot and ankle and the weight-bearing tibiocalcaneal Morrey view (Fig. 23–2).[4] This last radiograph is used to assess the important tibiocalcaneal alignment.[20] Computed tomography is useful for ruling out tarsal coalition and for depicting the bone and soft tissue anatomy in the coronal plane; computed tomography is also the best imaging method for obtaining quantitative information about bony relationships and for planning surgical correction of deformity.[30] Many parameters are helpful in the radiographic assessment of hindfoot deformity: they include the talocalcaneal angle, the talometatarsal-1 angle, the arch height-to-length ratio, and the calcaneal pitch angle.

TREATMENT

Treatment of the rheumatoid hindfoot requires a team approach, with input from primary care practitioners, rheumatologists, and orthotists, as well as orthopaedic surgeons.[3] Our approach typically begins with medical therapy including nonsteroidal anti-inflammatory drugs and other pharmacologic intervention under the care of the rheumatologist. If the initial therapy is ineffective, patients are considered for a graduated sequence of treatment progressing from injections to orthoses, synovectomy, selective joint fusion, and often finally to triple arthrodesis. Authors have reported success with talonavicular and subtalar resurfacing prostheses and supramalleolar osteotomy, although our experience with these techniques is limited.[8, 29]

In patients with increased hindfoot valgus secondary to tibialis posterior tenosynovitis or

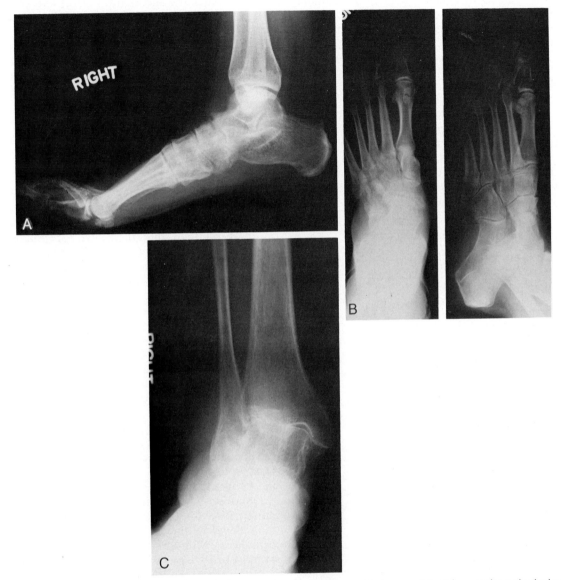

FIGURE 23–2. *(A)*, Standing lateral radiograph demonstrating severe rheumatoid changes at the talonavicular and subtalar joints. *(B)*, Standing anteroposterior and oblique radiographs demonstrating severe changes at the talonavicular joint. *(C)*, Standing anteroposterior radiograph of the ankle and hindfoot (Morrey's view) demonstrating severe ankle valgus.

dysfunction or in those with true joint involvement seen before their deformity has become *fixed*, a UCBL (University of California Biomechanics Laboratory) insert may be helpful in countering the tendency to valgus angulation.[7] Specially designed extra-depth shoes with molded Plastizote liners may minimize pressure points in deformed feet, and the molded arch supports can minimize symptoms of synovitis by relieving pressure on the posterior tibial tendon and the medial arch.

Surgical Technique

Surgical treatment ideally begins with synovectomy in the early stages of the disease process.[6] In patients in whom tibialis posterior tenosynovitis persists for longer than 6 months despite maximal medical treatment and footwear modification, we have had excellent results with simple synovial resection.

Tibialis Posterior Tenosynovectomy

1. The exposure for the tibialis posterior tenosynovectomy is best obtained using an incision in line with the course of the posterior tibial tendon and extending posterior to the medial malleolus, avoiding the greater saphenous vein (Fig. 23–3A).
2. The flexor retinaculum overlying the tendon above and below the medial malleolus is incised longitudinally to allow good exposure. The thickened retinaculum at the level of the medial malleolus is left intact to avoid dislocation of the tendon postoperatively (Fig. 23–3B).
3. The tendon and its synovium are now available for inspection, and synovectomy is performed carefully using scissors, cutting in line with the longitudinal axis of the tendon to avoid injury to the adjacent flexor digitorum longus tendon as well as to the neurovascular bundle (Fig. 23–3C).
4. The flexor retinaculum is repaired to prevent subluxation of the tendon, and a short-leg splint is applied.

Aftercare. If the tenosynovectomy was performed early and if the tendon has good sustenance and is functional, the splint is removed when the wound has healed and a molded arch support is provided. The patient is placed on a program of tibialis posterior strengthening exercises. If the tendon is severely diseased and a segment of it has been resected and repaired, a cast is worn for 6 weeks. (Tenosyn-

ovectomy would be performed only if the talonavicular and subtalar joints are normal; if they are abnormal, a fusion is performed.) In cases in which the tibialis posterior is clearly ruptured or the talonavicular joint alone is involved, selective fusion of the talonavicular joint is frequently successful.[28] Fogel and colleagues, in a retrospective review with an average follow-up of 9.5 years, demonstrated that talonavicular fusion is successful in providing satisfactory pain relief.[12] However, their patients did have difficulty with ambulation on uneven ground and demonstrated decreased subtalar motion at follow-up. When isolated talonavicular fusion is indicated, we use a technique similar to that described by Elbaor and colleagues.[10]

Talonavicular Fusion

1. A medial approach is developed through a 7-cm incision extending several centimeters more distal than that described for tibialis posterior synovectomy (see Fig. 23–3A).
2. The tibialis posterior tendon is protected, the tuberosity of the talus is removed, and the cancellous bone is saved for grafting.
3. The joint surfaces are cleared of articular surface and rasped to promote healing (Fig. 23–3D).
4. The bone graft, either local or autogenous, is packed into the defect, and fixation is maintained with a cannulated screw or a pneumatic staple (Fig. 23–3E).

Supramalleolar Osteotomy

Supramalleolar osteotomy as described by Heywood is an option for the realignment of the varus hindfoot.[16] Equinovarus position of the hindfoot with limited tarsal motion is the prerequisite for consideration of this procedure. Seven of nine of Heywood's patients had pain relief with this procedure, although an average of 10 degrees of ankle motion was lost postoperatively.

Triple Arthrodesis

The standard by which all surgical treatments of hindfoot deformity must be judged is the triple arthrodesis. Results with this procedure have been reliable, predictable, and beneficial, and they can be expected to last for upwards of 30 years.[14] Vahvanen reported on the largest series, 290 rheumatoid patients,

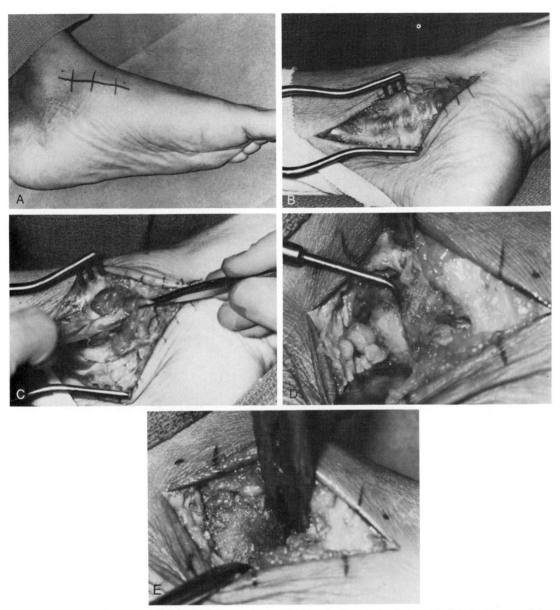

FIGURE 23–3. Technique for posterior tibial synovectomy and isolated talonavicular fusion. *(A)*, Skin incision parallel to the course of the posterior tibial tendon. *(B)*, Rheumatoid synovium bulging from the posterior tibial tendon sheath. *(C)*, Partial rupture of the posterior tibial tendon; rheumatoid synovium is in the forceps. *(D)*, Probe outlines the diseased talonavicular joint. *(E)*, Removal of any remaining cartilage to expose cancellous bone for isolated talonavicular fusion.

with good results found in 85 percent,[34] whereas Adam and Ranawat reported good results in 88 percent.[1] Our preferred technique combines both medial and lateral approaches to the hindfoot.

1. A medial incision is made along the axis of the tibialis posterior tendon, as described previously for synovectomy, to expose the talonavicular joint medially. This approach can be used to perform a synovectomy of the tibialis posterior tendon at the same time as a fusion if necessary (Fig. 23–4A).

2. The talonavicular joint is minimally resected back to cancellous bone surfaces. We have found no advantage to the use of dowel grafts or bone wedge resections and believe this practice is unnecessary, except in patients with severe cavus deformity (Fig. 23–4B).

3. A lateral incision is made longitudinally, starting above the sural nerve at the tip of the fibula and extending down over the sinus tarsi (Fig. 23–4C).

4. The sinus tarsi is cleared of the short toe extensors, and the beak of the calcaneus is osteotomized and saved for later bone graft (Fig. 23–4D).

5. Soft tissue is reflected anteriorly to expose the calcaneocuboid joint, and this joint is resected minimally, as was done with the talonavicular joint medially. The majority of patients with rheumatoid arthritis have normal bone structures of the talus, navicular, calcaneus, and cuboid; thus, even with *severe* deformity, wedge resections are *not* necessary to realign the foot. Realignment is done by soft tissue release alone. We believe that fixation should be rigid and durable. (*Editor's note:* I totally agree with the authors' contention that wedges are not needed for this triple arthrodesis. However, alignment of the subtalar and midtarsal joints is critical, as also stated. The pronated valgus foot has a closed sinus tarsi: that is, the anterior wall of the talar component of the posterior facet approximates the prom-

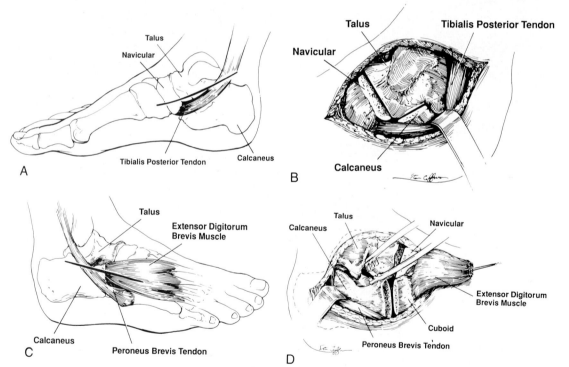

FIGURE 23–4. Triple arthrodesis. *(A)*, Medial incision made slightly superior to the posterior tibial tendon sheath. *(B)*, The posterior tibial tendon may be retracted inferiorly or may be transected to allow exposure of the talonavicular and portions of the subtalar joint. Joint surfaces are denuded of articular cartilage and prepared for subsequent internal fixation. *(C)*, Lateral skin incision made paralleling a line drawn from the tip of the lateral malleolus toward the fourth toe. *(D)*, The extensor digitorum brevis muscle has been detached and the contents of the sinus tarsi have been excised, allowing débridement of the calcaneocuboid joint and the lateral-most portion of the talonavicular joint. With a laminar spreader under the head of the talus and on top of the calcaneus, the posterior facet of the subtalar joint can more easily be visualized and débrided.

inence of the anterior process of the calcaneus. The posterior facet is reduced to a slight valgus to neutral position by rotating the calcaneus under the talus. The sinus tarsi or posterior facet is *not* wedged or "booked open" to achieve reduction. I carry out this operation with the patient supine, with a pad under the affected side hip, with the hip and knee flexed (for lateral exposure), and with a padded roll or "mailbox" to maintain knee flexion. To check talocalcaneal reduction, the knee is ex-

tended and the thigh flexed at the hip. The heel is then viewed from behind. I use a temporary Steinmann pin across the subtalar joint, inserted through the heel, before initiating permanent fixation. The authors' guide pin can serve the same purpose.

The problem to deal with at the midtarsal (talonavicular and calcaneocuboid) joint in the patient with prior deformity is rotation: that is, pronation or supination of the forefoot. In the chronic valgus hindfoot, the compensatory

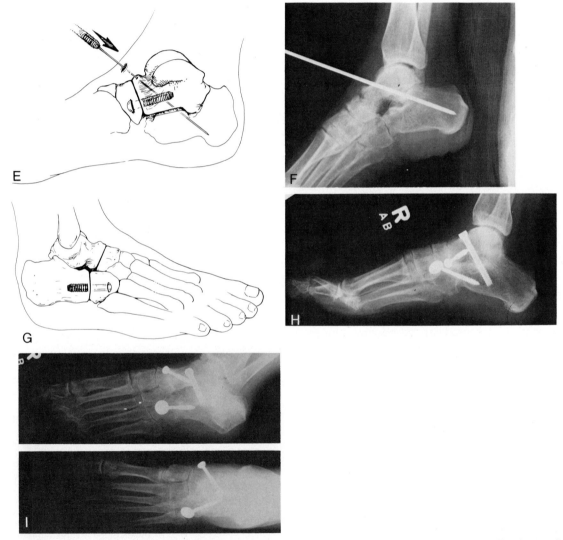

FIGURE 23–4 *Continued (E),* Rigid internal fixation of the subtalar joint is accomplished by making a small stab wound over the anterior aspect of the foot. A guide wire is inserted and checked radiographically to confirm that it crosses the subtalar joint. A cannulated screw is then placed to the proper depth over a cannulated guide pin. In a similar manner, a cannulated guide pin is inserted across the navicular into the body of the talus and is exchanged for a screw as well. *(F),* Guide wire inserted prior to insertion of the cannulated screw. *(G),* Through a separate stab incision at the base of the fourth metatarsal, a screw is placed across the calcaneocuboid joint. *(H and I),* Appearance of a solidly united triple arthrodesis showing the three screws that were used in the fusion.

position of the structures distal to the midtarsal joint is supination. This must be reduced and visualized by inspecting the plane of rotation of the toes and metatarsals relative to the hindfoot. Again, temporary pin fixation may be needed before final stabilization. My sequence of reduction is subtalar followed by midtarsal.)

6. The lateral capsule of the navicular is cleared of soft tissue, and a lamina spreader is inserted under the neck of the talus to expose the subtalar joint. We have found this step to be indispensable in exposing the posterior facet of the subtalar joint. The articular cartilage is next removed from the subtalar joint (see Fig. 23–4*D*).

7. A 6.5- or 7.0-mm cannulated screw is used for fixation across the talocalcaneal fusion. A small incision is made over the neck of the talus, and hemostats are used to dissect bluntly to bone. In this way, injury to the dorsalis pedis artery or the peroneal nerve can be avoided. With carefully placed retraction, a guide pin is inserted from the talus into the calcaneus (Fig. 23–4*E*). The position and depth of the guide pin are confirmed with a lateral radiograph (Fig. 23–4*F*). Next, a cannulated screw of appropriate length is inserted to compress the joints. All of the threads on the screw should be in the calcaneus to avoid distraction at the fusion site.

8. Fixation of the talonavicular and calcaneocuboid joints is accomplished with cannulated 6.5-mm screws in large adults or 4.0-mm screws in smaller patients. Pneumatic staples have also been used for the talonavicular and calcaneocuboid joints (Fig. 23–4*G* to *I*). Cancellous bone from the osteotomized beak of the calcaneus or autogenous iliac crest bone graft is packed into any remaining gaps.

Aftercare. Both wounds are drained, and a short-leg splint is applied. This splint is converted to a short-leg cast when the sutures are removed. Partial weight bearing is allowed for the first 6 weeks. At 6 weeks, the patient is fitted with a removable brace, and full weight bearing is allowed until healing is complete (generally 12 weeks after surgery).

Complications. Although the majority of patients have vast improvement with triple arthrodesis, there are several well-described complications.[2] The most common problems are secondary degeneration of the ankle joint, nonunion, and the failure to achieve a plantigrade foot. Wilson and colleagues have shown that 20 percent of patients followed up for 20 years postoperatively develop significant arthritis in the ankle joint.[38] In Vahvanen's series, just under 10 percent of his rheumatoid patients required subsequent ankle arthrodesis. Nonunion occurs in one of the three joints 9 percent of the time.[35] It is most common in the talonavicular joint. Patients are particularly dissatisfied when residual or iatrogenic deformity prevents achievement of a plantigrade foot. Avoidance of this complication requires careful attention at the time of surgery.

CONCLUSIONS

Rheumatoid involvement of the hindfoot is one of the most common and disabling manifestations of rheumatoid arthritis. Only recently have recognition of this condition and appropriate intervention been available to the average patient. A multidisciplinary approach involving early diagnosis by the primary care physician and medical management by medical practitioners is crucial. Refractory cases can be successfully managed with a graduated series of surgical procedures, ranging from simple tenosynovectomy to triple arthrodesis. Although not without complications, these procedures have been excellent in minimizing the suffering and increasing the quality of life for these patients.

References

1. Adam W, Ranawat C: Arthrodesis of the hindfoot in rheumatoid arthritis. Orthop Clin North Am 7:827, 1976.
2. Angus P, Cowell H: Triple arthrodesis: A critical long-term review. J Bone Joint Surg 68B:260, 1986.
3. Benson G, Johnson E Jr: Management of the foot in rheumatoid arthritis. Arthritis Rheum 5:19, 1962.
4. Buck P, Morrey B, Chao E: The optimum position for arthrodesis of the ankle: A gait study of the knee and ankle. J Bone Joint Surg 69A:1052, 1987.
5. Calabro J: A critical evaluation of the diagnostic features of the feet in rheumatoid arthritis. Arthritis Rheum 5:19, 1962.
6. Clayton M: Surgical treatment of the rheumatoid foot. *In* Giannestras N (Ed): Foot Disorders: Medical and Surgical Management. Philadelphia, Lea & Febiger, 1967, p 319.
7. Colson J, Berglund G: An effective orthotic design for controlling the unstable subtalar joint. Orthot Prosthet 33:1, 1979.

8. Daniels A, Samuelson K, Rusin K: Talonavicular joint surface anatomy and prototype resurfacing prostheses. Foot Ankle 2:5, 1981.
9. Downey D, Simkin P, Mack L, et al: Tibialis posterior tendon rupture: A cause of rheumatoid flat foot. Arthritis Rheum 31:441, 1988.
10. Elbaor J, Thomas W, Weinfeld M, et al: Talonavicular arthrodesis for rheumatoid arthritis of the rheumatoid hindfoot. Orthop Clin North Am 7:821, 1976.
11. Elftman H: The transverse tarsal joint and its control. Clin Orthop 16:41, 1960.
12. Fogel G, Katoh Y, Rand J, et al: Talonavicular arthrodesis for isolated arthrosis: 9.5-year results and gait analysis. Foot Ankle 3:105, 1982.
13. Gold R, Bassett L: Radiologic evaluation of the arthritis foot. Foot Ankle 2:332, 1982.
14. Goldner J: Advances in care of the foot: 1800–1987. Orthopedics 10:12, 1987.
15. Grabois M, Puentas J, Lidsky M: Tarsal tunnel syndrome in rheumatoid arthritis. Arch Phys Med Rehabil 62:401, 1981.
16. Heywood A: Supramalleolar osteotomy in the management of the rheumatoid hindfoot. Clin Orthop 177:76, 1983.
17. Kellgren J, Ball J: Tendon lesions in rheumatoid arthritis: Clinico-pathological study. Ann Rheum Dis 9:48, 1950.
18. King J, Burke D, Freeman M: The incidence of pain in the rheumatoid hindfoot and the significance of calcaneofibular impingement. Int Orthop 2:255, 1978.
19. Kirkup J: Ankle and tarsal joints in rheumatoid arthritis. Scand J Rheumatol 3:50, 1974.
20. Kitaoka H: Rheumatoid hindfoot. Orthop Clin North Am 20:4, 1989.
21. Lloyd D, Agarwal A: Tarsal tunnel syndrome, a presenting feature of rheumatoid arthritis. BMJ 3:32, 1970.
22. Marshall R, Myers D, Palmer D: Disturbance of gait due to rheumatoid disease. J Rheumatol 7:617, 1980.
23. McGuigan L, Burke D, Fleming A: Tarsal tunnel syndrome and peripheral neuropathy in rheumatoid disease. Ann Rheum Dis 42:128, 1983.
24. Milgrom C, Giladi M, Simkin A, et al: The normal range of subtalar inversion and eversion in young males as measured by three different techniques. Foot Ankle 6:143, 1985.
25. Minaker K, Little H: Painful feet in rheumatoid arthritis. Can Med Assoc J 109:724, 1973.
26. Rana N: Juvenile rheumatoid arthritis of the foot. Foot Ankle 3:2, 1982.
27. Resnick D: Roentgen features of the rheumatoid mid- and hindfoot. J Can Assoc Radiol 27:99, 1976.
28. Ruff M, Turner R: Selective hindfoot arthrodesis in rheumatoid arthritis. Orthopedics 7:49, 1984.
29. Samuelson K, Freeman M, Tuke M: Implant arthroplasty in the adult hindfoot. Clin Orthop 177:67, 1983.
30. Seltzer S, Weissman B, Braunstein E, et al: Computed tomography of the hindfoot with rheumatoid arthritis. Arthritis Rheum 28:1234, 1985.
31. Spiegel T, Spiegel J: Rheumatoid arthritis in the foot and ankle: Diagnosis, pathology, and treatment: The relationship between foot and ankle deformity and disease duration in 50 patients. Foot Ankle 2:318, 1982.
32. Thomas W: Surgery of the foot in rheumatod arthritis. Orthop Clin North Am 6:831, 1975.
33. Thould A, Simon G: Assessment of radiological changes in the hands and feet in rheumatoid arthritis: Their correlation with prognosis. Ann Rheum Dis 25:220, 1966.
34. Vahvanen V: Rheumatoid arthritis of the TC or pantalar joints in rheumatoid arthritis. Acta Orthop Scand 40:642, 1969.
35. Vahvanen V: Rheumatoid arthritis in the pantalar joints: A follow-up study of triple arthrodesis on 292 adult feet. Acta Orthop Scand Suppl 107:9, 1967.
36. Vainio K: Rheumatoid foot: Clinical study with pathological and roentgenographical comments. Ann Chir Gynaecol Suppl 45:1, 1956.
37. Vidigal E, Jacoby R, Dixon A, et al: The foot in chronic rheumatoid arthritis. Ann Rheum Dis 34:292, 1975.
38. Wilson F Jr, Fay G, Lamotte P, et al: Triple arthrodesis: A study of the factors affecting fusion after three hundred and one procedures. J Bone Joint Surg 47A:340–348.

24

Microsurgical Reconstruction of the Foot and Ankle

WILLIAM W. DZWIERZYNSKI
JOHN S. GOULD

Soft tissue reconstructions of the foot and ankle region have advanced rapidly. Today, the reconstructive surgeon can save many extremities that only recently would have been lost to amputation. The advent of free microvascular tissue transfer has led the surgical advances in lower extremity reconstruction.[1-3] Although microsurgical advances have had the greatest impact, most reconstructive surgery of the foot still involves local tissue transfer and grafting. The reconstructive microsurgeon must have a good understanding of both local tissue options and distant tissue transfer to reconstruct the foot successfully.

The foot and ankle area is unique and requires special attention in any type of reconstructive procedure. Reconstruction of the foot requires a balance of functional consideration and attention to durability. The stress that is placed on the foot during normal ambulation is great, and for a reconstruction to be successful, it must be durable.

In this chapter, five areas of the foot and ankle are discussed individually: the plantar foot, the heel, the dorsum, the anterior ankle, and the posterior ankle.[4] Each area of the foot has special requirements and special needs for reconstruction. The plantar foot needs durable coverage because it is the primary weight-bearing surface. The heel also requires durable coverage and thick tissue is needed to replace its specialized fat pad. Thin coverage is required for the malleoli area, and ultrathin coverage is needed over the Achilles tendon and the dorsum of the foot. The unique reconstructive needs of each of these special areas are discussed separately; however, many reconstructive options are similar for different areas of the foot.

TIMING OF RECONSTRUCTION

The importance of early wound coverage was first shown by Godina.[5] Wounds that were débrided on the day of injury and covered with a free tissue flap within 72 hours did better than those that had delayed closure. Wounds treated by early coverage were compared with groups in which free tissue transfer was performed later than 72 hours but before 6 weeks after injury, and with a group that had free tissue transfer later than 6 weeks after injury. The rate of free flap failure in the early-surgery group was less than 1 percent. In the intermediate and later groups the failure rate was 12 percent. Infection rates were 1.5 percent in the group treated early and 17.5 percent in the delayed-treatment groups.[5] When faced with a complex reconstruction, the surgeon need not delay reconstruction to determine tissue "viability." Clinicians since Godina, however, have shown that reconstruction may not need to take place immediately or within 72 hours, but it should definitely be performed within the first 2 weeks.

PLANTAR FOOT

Reconstruction of the plantar foot is a difficult surgical challenge. The plantar area is composed of highly sensitive and durable gla-brous skin, which is found only in this area and on the palm of the hand. To replace the skin of this area with "like skin," only the contralateral side is truly equivalent. Although some authors have described cross-foot flaps, today this is seldom an appropriate reconstructive option. The reconstructed tissue in this area must be able to tolerate the stress of ambulation and the shear force associated with normal footwear. The tissue, ideally, should have adequate sensibility because it is in such a high-shear area. Durability is important in the reconstructed tissue, particularly in the weight-bearing areas of the metatarsal heads.

When local tissue is available, it provides the best reconstructive options. Skin may be transposed from the non–weight-bearing arch to cover defects in weight-bearing surfaces. Hildalgo and Shaw extensively described the anatomy of the plantar foot and applications of skin flaps in this area.[6-8] Through careful design of the plantar flaps and careful execution of flap transfer, normal sensibility may be preserved. The medial plantar artery supplies blood to the skin over the non–weight-bearing sole of the foot, and a flap based on this artery is useful for coverage of the entire plantar surface of the heel.[9] The lateral plantar artery can also be used as the basis of a flap that includes both skin and fascia. A proximally based flap will cover calcaneal defects to the level of the Achilles tendon, and if the flap is based distally, although it is not a sensory flap, it can be used to cover metatarsal head defects.[10] Another flap based on the lateral calcaneal artery can be used to provide sensory skin coverage up to the heel.

The muscles of the foot, on the plantar surface, are grouped into four levels. The neurovascular structures run between the first and second levels. The first level of muscles is important to the reconstructive surgeon. Muscles in this level may be rotated or transposed to fill a defect without impairing foot function. Bostwick described the use of the flexor digitorum brevis flap for plantar reconstruction.[11] This flap can be mobilized as a musculocutaneous flap or as a muscle-only flap to cover a defect in the heel.[12] The flexor hallucis brevis flap, described by Ger, will cover the medial and anterior sole.[12] The abductor hallucis brevis, also initially described by Ger, will cover defects of the heel or of the medial malleolus. The abductor digiti minimi will

cover defects of the lateral malleolus and heel. All of these muscles can be harvested with minimal functional loss in the foot; however, the dissection involved in harvesting these local muscle flaps is tedious. The role of local muscle flaps in plantar reconstruction is questionable at best. Many authors have described their personal success with local foot flaps, but it is often difficult to duplicate these results. At times, these flaps can leave the patient with more donor site problems than the original defect.

Another option for reconstruction of the metatarsal head area is the fillet toe flap (Fig. 24–1).[13] This option necessitates loss of a toe, but this loss is of only minor cosmetic consequence. The greatest advantage of the fillet flap is that it provides tissue with similar skin quality and sensibility for reconstruction. To obtain the fillet flap, the toe is opened plantarly and the nail and bone are dissected out of the skin and subcutaneous tissue envelope. The toe is now free and can be rotated to close a defect on the sole. For more proximal defects on the plantar surface, the vascular pedicle can be dissected and the flap can be transferred as an island flap.[14]

Free tissue transfer to the plantar area can be by a cutaneous flap or by a muscle flap covered with a split-thickness skin graft. Muscle flaps tailor well over bony surfaces, develop a fibrous shear plane with the bone,[15] and adhere well to the bone, minimizing swivel. These flaps require split-thickness skin graft coverage; the graft usually hypertrophies and provides very acceptable coverage.[16] Sensibility is limited in the free muscle flaps, but they are well tolerated, particularly with well-molded and cushioning pedorthic devices.

Many surgeons prefer to use a cutaneous flap in plantar foot reconstruction because a skin graft is not required. Cutaneous flaps have the potential for reinnervation,[17] either by di-

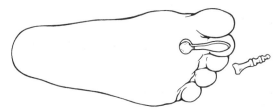

FIGURE 24–1. Fillet toe flap. The phalanges are removed through a plantar incision, preserving the neurovascular pedicle.

rect neurotization or by sensory ingrowth from the periphery.[18] Choices for cutaneous flaps in the reconstruction of a plantar defect include the scapular flap, the lateral arm flap, and the radial forearm flap.[19] The scapular flap provides thick skin coverage and allows spontaneous reinnervation. The lateral arm flap and the radial forearm flap are somewhat softer than the scapular flap and provide neurocutaneous innervation.[20] The radial forearm flap is discussed later in this chapter.

Scapular Flap

The scapular flap is a purely cutaneous flap that originates from the subscapular vessels. Because it is purely cutaneous, it is usually fairly thin and is well suited for foot reconstruction. The donor site defect is well concealed by clothing (unlike that of the radial forearm or lateral arm flap). Dissection of the flap is straightforward. The axillary-subscapular arterial pedicle should be well known to any reconstructive microsurgeon. If the flap taken

is based only on the circumflex scapular artery, the pedicle length is only 3 cm. However, this length can be increased by dissection to the axillary artery.[21]

Technique of Elevation

The patient is positioned in a prone or lateral decubitus position, whichever allows the donor and recipient site teams to work with greatest ease. The flap can be oriented either horizontally or vertically (the parascapular flap [22]), or these two areas can be combined for a larger flap. The horizontal flap is oriented midway between the scapular spine and the inferior scapular border (Fig. 24–2). The flap can extend from the deltoid region to the midline of the back and can be up to 12 cm in width and still allow primary closure of the defect. The vascular pedicle of the scapular flap arises out of the triangular space bordered by the teres minor muscle superiorly, the teres major muscle inferiorly, and the long head of the triceps laterally. After the flap is marked, the dissection is begun at its distal portion. The flap is

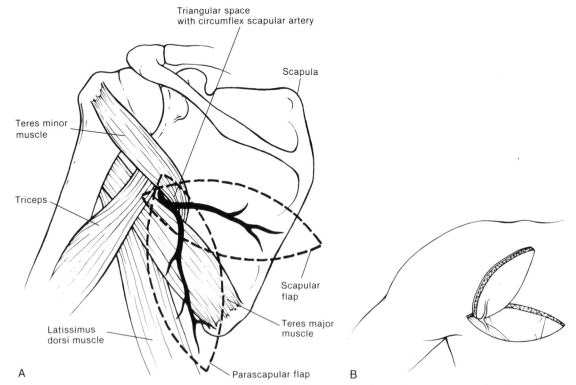

FIGURE 24–2. Scapular flap. *(A)*, Anatomy and surface landmarks of the scapular and parascapular fasciocutaneous flaps. *(B)*, The scapular fasciocutaneous flap is elevated from medial to lateral and is attached by the circumflex scapular pedicle.

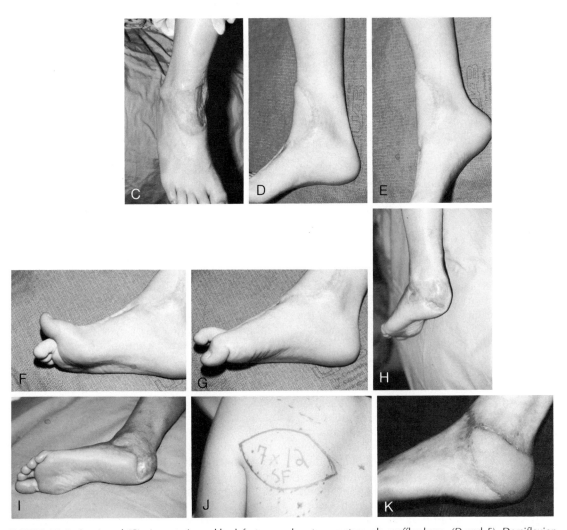

FIGURE 24–2 *Continued (C)*, An anterior ankle defect secondary to a motorcycle muffler burn. *(D and E)*, Dorsiflexion and plantar flexion are possible after replacement of the skin graft with a scapular flap and reconstruction of the anterior tibial tendon under the flap. *(F and G)*, Dorsiflexion and plantar flexion of the great toe after flap transfer and reconstruction of the extensor hallucis tendon under the flap. *(H and I)*, A defect of the heel previously covered with an unstable skin graft. *(J)*, Outline of the scapular flap. *(K)*, The inset and subsequently defatted scapular flap. *(C, D, F to I, and K from Gould JS: Reconstruction of soft tissue injuries of the foot and ankle with microsurgical techniques. Orthopedics 10:153–155, 1987. J from Gould JS: Management of soft tissue loss on the plantar aspect of the foot. Instruct Course Lect 39:123, 1990.)*

elevated in a plane superficial to the infraspinatus muscle. Dissection continues until the lateral border of the scapula is reached; at this point, the vascular pedicle must be identified. This is the most difficult portion of the dissection. The circumflex scapular artery must be identified as it emerges from the triangular space. Dissection proceeds around the pedicle medially and laterally in the triangular space to gain additional length on the vascular pedicle. If further length is desired, the pedicle may be extended up to the axillary artery.

Branches to the latissimus dorsi and serratus anterior muscles must be ligated to free the flap up to its axillary artery origin. If cutaneous innervation is required, the lateral branches of the dorsal cutaneous nerves must be protected as they enter the flap in its medial aspect. Multiple nerves innervate the flap, and multiple nerves must be anastomosed to ensure adequate innervation. The skin defect can be closed primarily after flap harvest. The patient must be warned that the scar usually hypertrophies and may require later revision.[23]

Lateral Arm Flap

The lateral arm flap is a thin fasciocutaneous flap based on vessels of the deep brachial artery.[24] Because of its relative ease of harvest and its location, which does not require complex patient positioning, this flap is one of the most popular fasciocutaneous flaps among microsurgeons. Drawbacks of this flap are that it may be bulky in some women and that the cosmetic defect is obvious on the upper arm and may be bothersome. The vascular pedicle is relatively small, usually averaging 1.5 mm in diameter.

Technique of Elevation

The patient is placed on the operating table in the supine position, with the arm extended. The flap is marked preoperatively: it is centered on the lateral intermuscular septum between the insertion of the deltoid muscle and the lateral epicondyle (Fig. 24–3). It is helpful to perform this dissection using a sterile tourniquet. The dissection is started on the posterior edge of the flap and proceeds to the deep fascia of the arm. The plane of the dissection is between the deep fascia and the underlying muscles. The pedicle arises in the intermuscular septum between the triceps and the brachialis muscles. Following the vascular pedicle proximally, the surgeon identifies the radial nerve; this must be visualized and protected during the dissection. To facilitate dissection of the flap, it is often helpful to place the patient's arm across the chest to avoid dissecting on the undersurface of the arm. The posterior cutaneous nerve of the forearm runs through the flap and must be taken with the flap, whether the flap is neurotized or not. An area of numbness will occur on the posterior forearm, and the patient must be warned of this preoperatively. The vascular pedicle must be traced back to its origin off the deep brachial vessels to gain sufficient pedicle length. If the planned flap is less than 6 cm in width, the skin defect may be closed primarily; otherwise, the donor site must be skin grafted.[25, 26]

HEEL

Heel defects may involve the weight-bearing heel or the non–weight-bearing posterior heel.[8] There is a significant difference in the management of these areas. As with coverage of the plantar surface of the foot, the reconstructed tissue of the weight-bearing heel must be durable. Many options have been described, from simple to quite complex.

If the patient is fortunate enough to have retained some soft tissue on the heel, use of a thick split-thickness or a full-thickness skin graft *may* provide a good reconstruction option for the weight-bearing heel. Placing a skin graft on a weight-bearing surface increases the risk of skin graft loss and the risk of hyperkeratosis over the graft.[27] However, some surgeons have reported very good success rates with skin grafts on weight-bearing surfaces.[28] The morbidity of a skin graft is small compared with that of other types of reconstruction in this area, and for the selected patient, skin grafting is a good option. Many times, the defect in the heel does not leave sufficient soft tissue coverage suitable for skin grafting, and more complicated methods of reconstruction must be sought. Local muscle flaps are available for heel reconstruction. However, caveats must be heeded to avoid complications: the defect must be relatively small, and excess tension must never be placed on local flaps in this area, or failure is likely to occur.

The abductor hallucis and the flexor digitorum brevis muscles are useful for reconstruction of small heel defects. (Fig. 24–4).[10] Although the dissection of these muscles is difficult, the surgery is still more limited than that of a free flap for coverage of a similar defect. These muscles are transferred without a cutaneous paddle (the attached overlying skin) and must be covered with a skin graft. The flexor digitorum brevis muscle is harvested through a midline plantar incision and is turned back onto itself at its calcaneal origin. Care must be taken in its dissection not to interfere with the sensory nerves in the sole of the foot. In a manner similar to that used with the flexor digitorum brevis muscle, the abductor hallucis muscle can be used to cover heel defects with very little donor site morbidity.[29] The abductor arises from the medial surface of the calcaneous and inserts into the medial surface of the proximal phalanx of the big toe. Harvest of this muscle is through an incision along the medial border of the sole. It must be remembered that for these muscles to remain viable, their delicate vascular pedicle must be preserved, although the origin and insertion of the muscle can be released. Only small defects

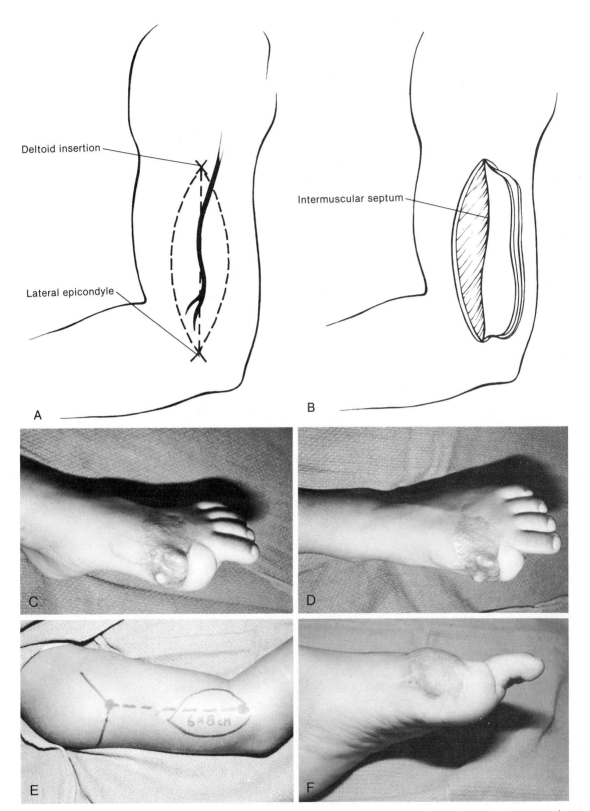

FIGURE 24–3. Lateral arm flap. *(A)*, The posterior descending branch of the deep brachial artery lies in the intermuscular septum. *(B)*, The lateral arm flap is elevated deep to the arm fascia laterally and medially down to the intermuscular septum. *(C and D)*, A defect on the dorsomedial first metatarsal with an unstable skin graft. *(E)*, Outline of a small lateral arm flap. *(F)*, The inset flap. (Photographs and case presentation courtesy of Douglas P. Hanel, M.D.)

307

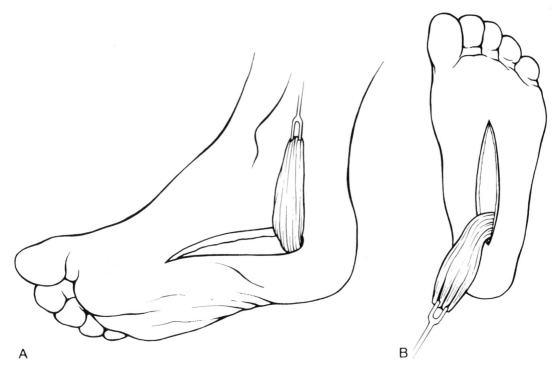

A   B

FIGURE 24–4. Abductor hallucis and flexor digitorum brevis muscle flaps. *(A)*, The abductor hallucis muscle is elevated from a medial foot incision to reach the medial malleolus. *(B)*, The flexor digitorum brevis is harvested through a midline plantar incision.

can be covered with these muscles. For larger defects of the heel, an instep flap may be used.

Instep Flap

Originally described by Shanahan and Gingrass,[9] the medial plantar or instep flap is a local flap that can provide innervated skin, fascia, and muscle coverage to the entire weight-bearing surface of the heel. The donor site of this flap is the non–weight-bearing arch of the foot. The instep flap is supplied with blood by the medial plantar artery, which is a terminal branch of the posterior tibial artery. In elderly or diabetic patients, the patency of this artery must be assessed with Doppler scanning.

Technique of Elevation

The design of the flap is first marked on the plantar surface of the foot (Fig. 24–5). Dissection of the flap is started distally at the level of the plantar arch. The incision is made down through the plantar fascia. At this level,

branches from the medial plantar artery to the digits are encountered. These digital branches are ligated and divided. Preoperative assessment of the dorsal circulation is essential to ensure that this maneuver does not compromise toe circulation. Nerve branches from the plantar cutaneous nerve are identified and carefully dissected from the medial plantar nerve. An interfascicular dissection is used to free the digital branches from the sensory branches to the flap. Small branches to the edge of the skin flap must be preserved to protect sensation in the flap. Branches to the muscle should also be protected. The artery and nerve branches are followed as they pass under the flexor digitorum brevis muscle. At this point, the muscle tendon is transected proximally to allow access to the neurovascular bundle. To achieve better rotation of the flap, the proximal attachments of the plantar fascia are divided, allowing the flap to rotate easily to the heel. The flexor digitorum brevis muscle can be taken with the flap if desired. The flap is inset with a two-layer suture closure, and the patient is confined to strict bed rest during the first 5 postoperative days.

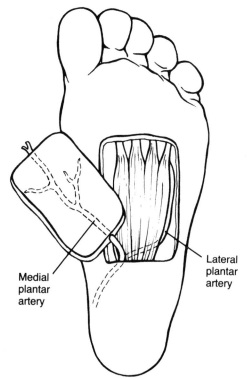

Medial
plantar
artery

Lateral
plantar
artery

FIGURE 24–5. Instep flap (medial plantar artery flap). Based on the medial plantar artery, the instep flap is raised on the plane superficial to the flexor digitorum brevis muscle.

Free Tissue Transfer

As with reconstruction of the plantar foot, free flap reconstruction in the heel can be performed either with cutaneous flaps or with muscle flaps. Cutaneous flaps have the advantage of providing neurotized skin coverage. No skin graft is needed, as it is with the use of a muscle flap. A disadvantage of cutaneous flaps is that they may be quite bulky, especially in an overweight person. Debulking of these flaps may be a postoperative problem. Like skin elsewhere on the body, a cutaneous flap may lose and gain subcutaneous fat as a person's overall weight changes. The flap options for cutaneous free flap reconstruction of the heel include the scapular flap and the lateral arm flap; these flaps were described in the previous section.

Muscle flaps offer the advantage of being easy to contour around the os calcis. They usually provide a quite durable reconstructed area in the heel. If a muscle flap is to be used, the two best choices are the latissimus dorsi muscle and the rectus abdominis muscle. Each of these muscles can be elevated as a free flap with relative ease; each has long vascular pedicles and minimum donor site morbidity. These muscles are of sufficient bulk to cover large soft tissue defects.

Rectus Abdominis Muscle Flap

The rectus abdominis muscle is one of the workhorse flaps of lower extremity reconstruction. In 1982, Bunkis and colleagues[30] and Cunningham and colleagues[31] first used the rectus abdominis muscle for microvascular free flap transfer. The rectus abdominis muscle is a large muscle that fills contour defects well and readily accepts a skin graft. Elevation of the flap is technically easy, and the vascular pedicle is large. The deep inferior epigastric artery has a diameter of 2 to 3 mm, and its accompanying vein has a diameter of 3 to 4 mm. The length of the pedicle is usually 10 cm, which means that this flap can be used in lower extremity reconstruction without the need for vein grafting. Although skin can be transferred with the muscle, the subcutaneous tissue in the lower abdomen is usually quite extensive, and the resultant flap will be too bulky. For heel reconstruction, the rectus abdominis flap is harvested without a skin paddle, and a skin graft is applied to the muscle.

Technique of Elevation

Before dissection of the rectus flap, a determination must be made as to which rectus muscle will be harvested. The vascular pedicle arises on the deep inferolateral surface of the muscle. The location of the defect and the available recipient vessels determines whether the right or the left rectus muscle should be used. The rectus abdominis muscle flap can be harvested through a paramedian incision or through a low transverse Pfannenstiel-type incision. The low transverse incision is usually reserved for women, in whom a cosmetic scar is more important. Dissection through the transverse incision is more difficult, and the full extent of the rectus muscle cannot always be harvested. The usual method of flap dissection is through a paramedian incision (Fig. 24–6). After the paramedian skin incision is made, the superior rectus fascia is opened longitudinally throughout the entire length of the rectus muscle. At the inferior portion of the fascia,

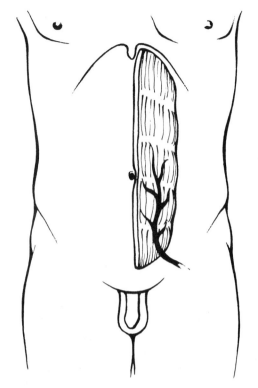

FIGURE 24–6. Rectus abdominis flap. The inferior epigastric artery is the dominant vessel supplying blood to the rectus abdominis muscle. The skin may be harvested with the muscle, but usually the muscle is taken alone.

the incision is gently curved laterally over the vascular pedicle. The muscle is dissected from the superior fascia medially and laterally. All perforating vessels are cauterized with a bipolar electrocautery unit. Dissection is continued around the posterior side of the muscle, freeing the muscle from the posterior rectus fascia. The vascular pedicle, the deep inferior epigastric vessels, can be identified at this point.[32, 33] The artery is easily palpated on the undersurface of the muscle. The vessels are followed to their origin at the inferolateral aspect of the muscle. Dissection of the pedicle under loupe magnification aids in dividing small arterial and venous branches from the main pedicle. The superior insertion of the rectus muscle is divided with the monopolar electrocautery unit, and the muscle is flipped over onto itself to facilitate exposure in the pedicle dissection. The vascular pedicle is traced to the femoral vessels, yielding a pedicle of 10 cm in length. After flap transfer, the superior rectus fascia is closed with a continuous-suture technique.

The subcutaneous tissue is drained with closed suction drains to prevent seroma formation. As the free flap harvest takes place, a second surgical team can be preparing the recipient site in the foot.

Latissimus Dorsi Flap

The latissimus dorsi muscle flap is a large reliable muscle flap. Described by Baudet and colleagues[34] and Ricbourg and colleagues,[35] the free latissimus flap is based on the thoracodorsal artery, a terminal branch of the axillary artery. The latissimus dorsi is a large flat muscle that acts primarily as an adductor and medial rotator of the arm. After the latissimus dorsi is harvested as a free flap, all of its major upper extremity functions are duplicated by other muscles in the area. The latissimus dorsi is a large muscle, so that contour defects can easily be filled, but the muscle itself is quite thin, so that it can provide thin, aesthetic coverage. A disadvantage to the use of this flap is its location on the back. The patient needs to be placed either in a prone position or in the lateral decubitus position, either of which may preclude an approach using two operating teams.

The vascular pedicle, the thoracodorsal artery, arises from the subscapular artery, which is a branch of the axillary artery. The latissimus dorsi flap is usually harvested by dissecting up to the origin of the subscapular artery from the axillary artery to obtain the greatest pedicle length. At its origin, the subscapular artery is at least 2 mm in diameter. The latissimus dorsi flap may be raised with or without the overlying skin, but for most reconstructions in the foot or ankle, only the muscle is used.

Technique of Elevation

Depending on the defect to be covered, the patient is placed on the operating table in either the prone or the lateral decubitus position. Adequate padding is important to protect the patient against pressure-related injuries. An inflatable bean bag and axillary rollers are used. The incision for harvesting the muscle extends from the axilla to the lower lateral back. The lateral border of the latissimus muscle can be palpated, and this serves as a guide for the incision. Skin flaps are elevated, leaving the filmy fascia on the surface of the muscle (Fig. 24–7). The dissection is continued from the lateral edge of the muscle to the muscle origin on the thoracic spine. The muscle is elevated from distal to proximal in the well-defined plane below the muscle. As the muscle is elevated, the thoracodorsal pedicle can be seen on the underside of the muscle. The pedicle is followed as it comes off the subscapular artery from the axillary artery. The circumflex scapular artery and branch to the serratus anterior artery are divided to allow greater pedicle length.[36] After dissection of the pedicle to the axillary artery, the muscle is transected at its humeral attachment.[37] To prevent postoperative scar formation in the axilla, one or two Z-plasties are performed when the axillary portion of the incision is closed.

For smaller defects that do not require the entire bulk of the latissimus muscle, a tailored latissimus dorsi muscle flap can be used.[38] As the latissimus is elevated and its vascular pedicle is identified, two main branches of the thoracodorsal artery can be seen. The muscle can be harvested on the lateral branch, leaving the medial portion of the muscle and its nerve supply intact. If a tailored latissimus free flap is used, it is important to identify the thora-

codorsal nerve and to protect it from operative injury. The nerve to the lateral muscle is divided, and an interfascicular dissection is performed to free the medial portion of the nerve. The lateral portion of the muscle is dissected intramuscularly from the remaining muscle. Careful dissection is required so as not to injure the arterial supply or the medial nerve. Finally, the muscle is freed before its tendinous insertion to allow continued function of the remaining muscle.

DORSUM OF THE FOOT

Although the dorsum of the foot is not subjected to the constant stress of weight bearing, as are the plantar surface of the foot and the heel, it must stand up to the stress of modern footwear. Special modifications, including soft leather (deerskin) uppers lined with polyethylene foam (Plastizote), help to decrease the potential for breakdown. Coverage of the dorsal foot must be thin so that a patient may continue to wear relatively normal shoes (Fig. 24–8). Coverage over the dorsum

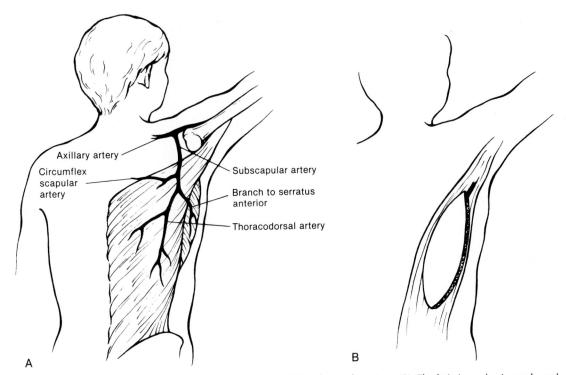

A

B

FIGURE 24–7. Latissimus dorsi flap. *(A)*, Vascular anatomy of the subscapular artery. *(B)*, The latissimus dorsi muscle and skin pedicle are elevated through a dorsolateral incision.

Illustration continued on following page

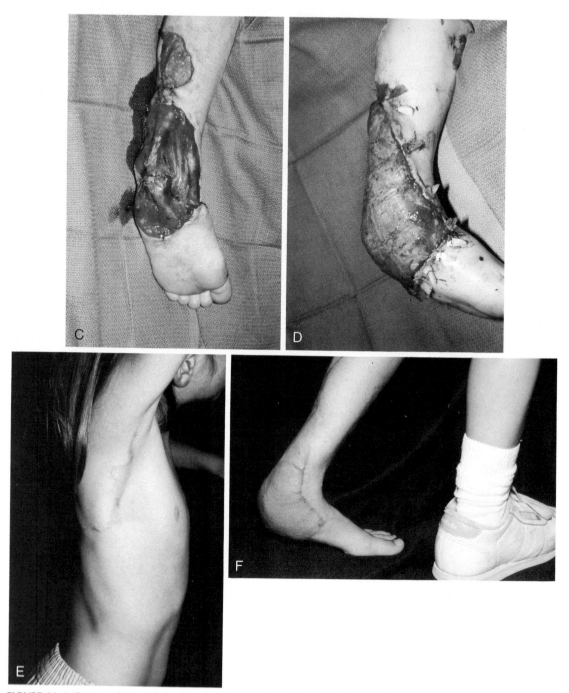

FIGURE 24–7 *Continued (C)*, A large defect of the posterior ankle and heel. *(D)*, A latissimus dorsi muscle flap covered with a meshed split-thickness skin graft. *(E)*, The donor site defect. *(F)*, The healed flap. (Photographs and case presentation courtesy of Douglas P. Hanel, M.D.)

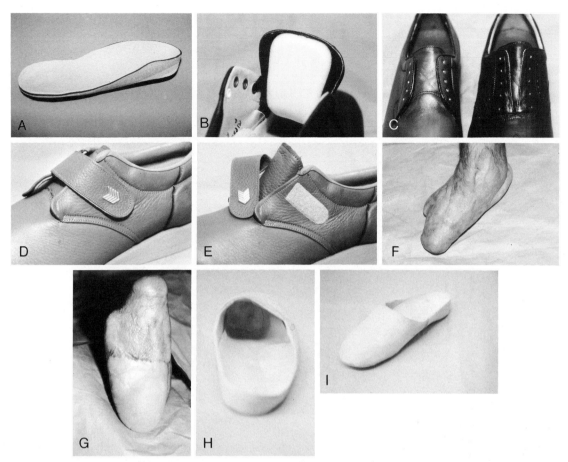

FIGURE 24–8. Shoe modifications to decrease the potential for soft tissue breakdown. *(A)*, A three-ply insert (soft polyethylene foam, micropore rubber, and dense Plastizote and cork) to evenly distribute weight bearing on the insensate plantar surface. *(B)*, A Plastizote-padded shoe tongue. *(C)*, A Blucher-cut design for lacing *(left)* allows more flexibility in lacing than the Bal design *(right)*. *(D and E)*, A Velcro fastener instead of lacing decreases the potential for abrasion over the dorsum of the foot. *(F and G)*, A foot with a split-thickness graft requires extraordinary pedorthic measures to prevent breakdown. *(H and I)*, A perfectly contoured Plastizote inner-shoe insert decreases shear and fills out the shoe in this partial foot amputation.

of the foot must also protect the underlying tendons of the dorsal foot.[4] Currently, the best option for reconstruction of the dorsal foot is skin grafting, if paratenon remains over the tendons. Skin grafts will not "take" over exposed tendon or bone, and alternative methods of reconstruction are required. No satisfactory local tissue flap exists for deeper wounds on the dorsum of the foot. If a wound cannot be covered by a skin graft, distant tissue transfer is usually required.

Free muscle flaps can be used to cover dorsal foot wounds, but this may not be the optimal reconstructive solution because muscle flaps, unless they are tailored, are far bulkier than the tissue of the normal dorsal foot (Fig. 24–9). Occasionally free muscle flaps are useful if

a large deep space is present (Fig. 24–10). Free fascial or fasciocutaneous flaps are excellent for many microsurgical reconstructions of the foot. Fascial flaps provide a very satisfactory reconstructive alternative. They provide thin, durable coverage and a surface for unaltered tendon gliding. The cutaneous flap options for free tissue transfer in the dorsal foot are the lateral arm and scapular flaps, which have already been discussed, and the radial forearm flap.

Radial Forearm Flap

The radial artery fascial and fasciocutaneous flaps provide thin, reliable donor tissue for

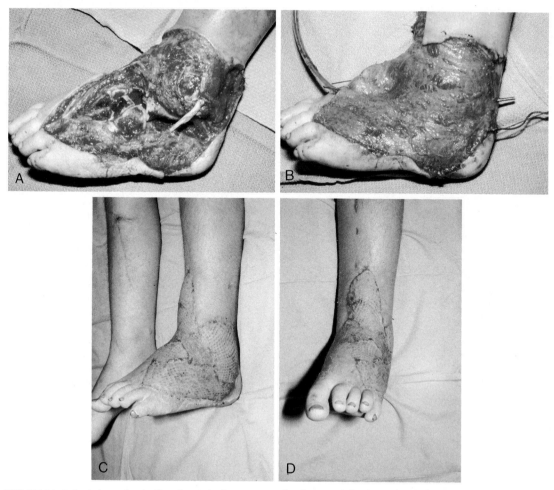

FIGURE 24–9. Latissimus dorsi tailored muscle flap to cover the dorsum of the foot. *(A)*, A dorsal foot and ankle defect. *(B)*, The defect is covered with a thinned latissimus dorsi muscle flap and subsequently covered with a meshed split-thickness skin graft. *(C and D)*, The healed flap. Note the thin and optimal contouring of this flap. (Courtesy of Douglas P. Hanel, M.D.)

microvascular transfer. The flap is based on the radial artery and its venae comitantes. The flap has a long pedicle and an arterial diameter of 2 to 3 mm.[39] A skin island of up to one-half the circumference of the wrist and almost the entire length of the forearm may be included with the flap. Only a very narrow skin island can be taken if primary closure of the donor site is planned. Usually the donor site must be skin grafted; this leaves a visible and often conspicuous donor site defect. The radial forearm flap may be taken as a purely fascial flap, which avoids skin grafting of the donor site. A neurosensory flap can be fashioned by including the lateral cutaneous nerve of the forearm or the anterior branch of the medial cutaneous

nerve of the forearm. Disadvantages of this flap include an unaesthetic donor site scar and the sacrifice of the radial artery, although this can be reconstructed with a long vein graft, which may or may not remain patent. It is imperative to perform an Allen test before flap transfer. The flap may be hair bearing in males, leading to unacceptable recipient site hair.

Technique of Elevation

The flap is based over the radial artery either proximally or distally on the forearm; distal flaps are thin, but proximally based flaps are usually unacceptably bulky. An Allen test is performed preoperatively to ensure a patent

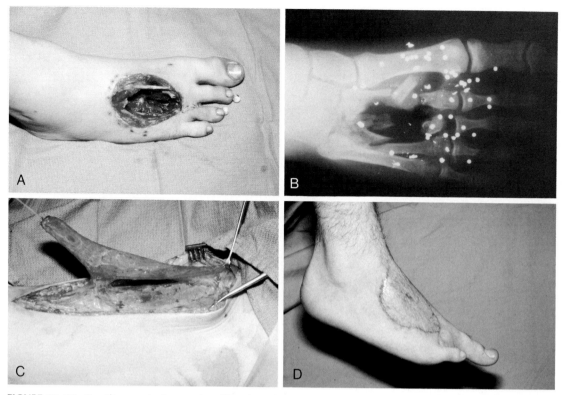

FIGURE 24–10. Gracilis muscle flap used to fill a through-and-through defect of the foot. *(A)*, A through-and-through shotgun defect of the forefoot. *(B)*, Radiograph of a skeletal defect. *(C)*, Elevation of the gracilis muscle flap. *(D)*, The completed reconstruction. (Courtesy of Douglas P. Hanel, M.D.)

ulnar artery and palmar arch. The planned skin resection and the superficial veins of the skin are marked before tourniquet inflation. Elevation of the flap is started down through the deep fascia of the wrist (Fig. 24–11). When the skin portion of the flap is being dissected, the superficial veins are not divided but are followed proximally in the forearm. They are more reliable than the venae comitantes and are not divided but are followed proximally in the forearm, and are used for venous anastomosis. If the flap is to be directly innervated, superficial nerves are also dissected with the flap. The flap is dissected deep to the forearm fascia, taking care not to strip peritenon off the superficial tendons in order to enhance the likelihood of satisfactory take of the donor site skin graft. The dissection continues until the radial artery is identified in the cleft between the flexor carpi radialis and the brachioradialis muscles. Small arterial and venous branches are ligated and divided from the vascular pedicle. The dissection is continued until adequate pedicle length is achieved.

The superficial radial nerve, which lies lateral to the radial artery in the proximal forearm, is left undisturbed. To ensure proper venous outflow, venous anastomosis is performed on a cutaneous vein and on the venae comitantes.[40] The donor site is covered with a nonmeshed skin graft over the peritenon of the flexor tendons. A protective splint must be used over the donor site. The fascial flap is dissected in the same manner as the fasciocutaneous flap, except that the skin is not harvested. The fascial flap is elevated both on its superficial and on its deep surfaces. Brachial fascia overlying the lateral arm can be taken without the skin in the manner described for that flap in the earlier section.

ANTERIOR ANKLE

Defects in the anterior ankle usually involve significant damage to tendons, nerves, and bones in this area. Defects in this area are

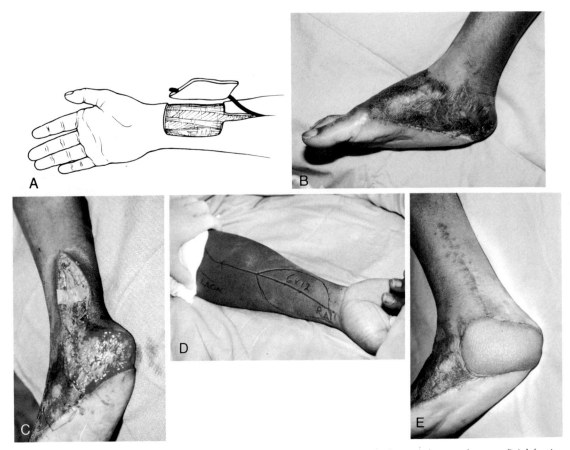

FIGURE 24–11. Radial artery forearm flap. *(A),* The radial artery forearm flap is elevated deep to the superficial fascia, leaving the peritenon of the flexor tendons intact. *(B),* A posteromedial defect of the heel covered with an unstable skin graft and with a painful neuroma of the medial calcaneal branch of the posterior tibial nerve. *(C),* Excision of the grafted area with exposure of the nerve and recipient vessels. *(D),* Outlining the radial forearm flap. *(E),* The healed neurovascular forearm flap. Direct neurotization was provided by suture of the medial calcaneal nerve to the lateral antebrachial cutaneous in the flap.

treated in a manner similar to defects in the dorsal foot. If significant soft tissue is present, a skin graft may be used to cover the defect. Thin coverage is needed in this area, but most important is the provision of a smooth gliding surface for tendon excursion.[41]

Local tissue options for anterior ankle reconstruction are limited to skin grafting and use of the dorsalis pedis flap. The skin, subcutaneous tissue, and superficial fascia of the dorsal foot may be rotated on the pedicle of the dorsalis pedis artery. Sensory innervation of this flap is by means of the superficial peroneal nerve. The dissection of the dorsalis pedis flap is very tedious, and the donor site defect may be as troublesome as the original defect. This flap should be used only by surgeons experienced in its dissection.

Free tissue transfer options for the anterior ankle include the scapular and lateral arm flaps and the tensor fascia lata flap (Fig. 24–12). These fasciocutaneous flaps may be somewhat bulky, but they allow good tendon gliding and a very satisfactory reconstruction.

POSTERIOR ANKLE

Defects of the posterior ankle require a flap that is able to cover the Achilles tendon and the nerves and tendons of the medial malleolus area. Small isolated lesions over the Achilles tendon area can be covered with local fasciocutaneous flaps from the calf or dorsum of the foot. These flaps are limited in size and rotation, and they are not acceptable for larger

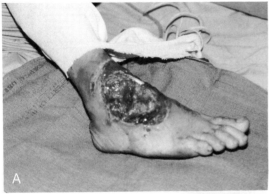
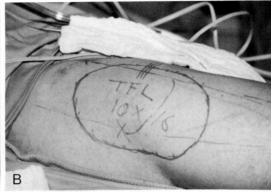
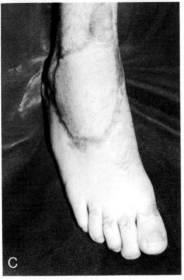

FIGURE 24–12. Tensor fascia lata flap. *(A)*, Anterior ankle defect secondary to a go-cart accident. *(B)*, Outlining the tensor fascia lata flap. *(C)*, The healed defatted flap. (From Gould JS: Reconstruction of soft tissue injuries of the foot and ankle with microsurgical techniques. Orthopedics 10:152, 1987.)

defects. The dorsalis pedis flap is useful for defects of both malleoli and the medial, lateral, and posterior aspects of the foot. This flap can also be used as a free flap (Fig. 24–13).[41]

The choice of coverage for the posterior ankle depends on the type of defect and on which structures require coverage. Soft tissue defects directly over the Achilles tendon require coverage that will allow smooth tendon gliding. Coverage of this area must be thin enough to be cosmetically acceptable and to allow normal, matched footwear to be worn. The scapular fasciocutaneous flap is an option for these defects. Defects with bony loss or large dead spaces are best treated with muscle flap transfer and split-thickness skin grafting. The gracilis, rectus, and latissimus dorsi muscle flaps are most commonly used (Fig. 24–14).

Gracilis Flap

The greatest advantage to the use of the gracilis muscle flap is the lack of a donor site defect. After the muscle is harvested, the functional loss is negligible and the cosmetic defect is minimal. The gracilis muscle may be harvested with a skin pedicle, but the distal skin circulation is precarious, and its use may also result in a bulky flap. The muscle-alone gracilis flap is of greatest use in lower extremity reconstruction. This muscle is especially useful to cover small defects (see Fig. 24–10).[42]

The gracilis flap is easy to elevate, and its pedicle is consistent in location, diameter, and length. The vascular pedicle of the gracilis muscle arises from the deep femoral artery. There are usually one or two minor pedicles

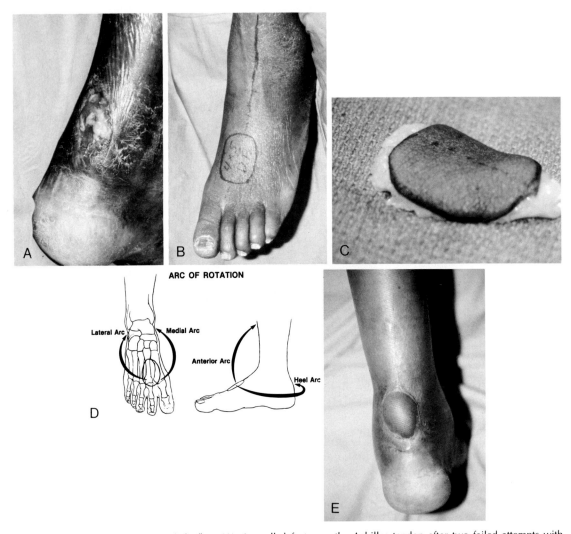

FIGURE 24–13. Dorsalis pedis pedicle flap. *(A)*, A small defect over the Achilles tendon after two failed attempts with split-thickness skin grafting. *(B)*, Outlining the small dorsalis pedis flap. *(C)*, The dissected flap. The pedicle is to the right. *(D)*, The arc of rotation of the flap. *(E)*, The healed defect. (From Gould JS: The dorsalis pedis island pedicle flap for small defects of the foot and ankle. Orthopedics 9:868–869, 1986.)

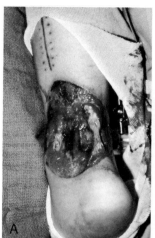 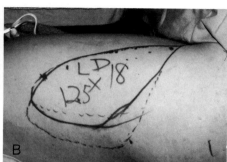 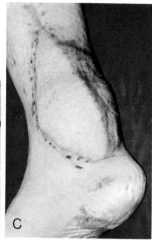

FIGURE 24–14. Use of the combined latissimus dorsi muscular and musculocutaneous flap for a posterior ankle defect. (A), A posteromedial defect requiring thick coverage medially behind the malleolus and thin coverage over the Achilles tendon. (B), Outlining the muscle and the myocutaneous latissimus dorsi flap. (C), The healed flap. (A and C from Gould JS: Reconstruction of soft tissue injuries of the foot and ankle with microsurgical techniques. Orthopedics 10:154, 1987.)

to the muscle; however, they are not required to support the muscle as a free flap.[43]

Technique of Elevation

The muscle is harvested with the patient in a supine, frog-legged position. The outline of the muscle can easily be identified when the leg is abducted (Fig. 24–15). Drawing a line between the pubic bone and the medial condyle of the femur locates the anterior border of the gracilis. The gracilis muscle is easily confused with the adductor magnus muscle, and the skin pedicle for the gracilis musculocutaneous flap may be erroneously located. The distal gracilis tendon should be identified through a distal incision on the medial leg to ensure proper muscle selection. The tendon of the gracilis muscle is long and thin distally. Identification of the muscle before flap dissection is especially important if a skin paddle is to be harvested with the muscle. The incision to harvest the muscle is made posterior to the line connecting the pubic tubercle to the medial condyle. Dissection is continued from medially and laterally around the gracilis muscle. The main vascular pedicle is located in the proximal one-third of the muscle lying between the adductor longus and adductor magnus muscles. Branches to the adductor longus muscle must be ligated and divided. The vascular

pedicle can be traced to its origin from the deep femoral artery. A pedicle length of 6 cm can be obtained, and a pedicle diameter of approximately 2 cm can be anticipated.

FREE TISSUE TRANSFER RECIPIENT SITE

In performing free tissue transfer in the lower extremity, great care must be taken in the recipient site dissection. The concept of "zone of injury" must always be observed. Bone and soft tissue injury may be limited to the foot, but the vascular injury may extent far more proximally.[44] In the trauma patient, the vasculature may be compromised by the tracking of hematoma or serous fluid along vascular planes. The recipient vessel must be dissected until normal-looking vessels are found.[45] To avoid the zone of injury, it is often necessary to use long vein grafts. It is often wise to obtain lower extremity angiograms prior to free tissue transfer. Angiography is useful in the smoker or the diabetic patient. Preoperative angiography may reveal proximal lesions, which must be dealt with before free tissue transfer in order to ensure optimal arterial inflow.[46] Angiography may also reveal unsuspected vascular occlusion in the trauma patient.

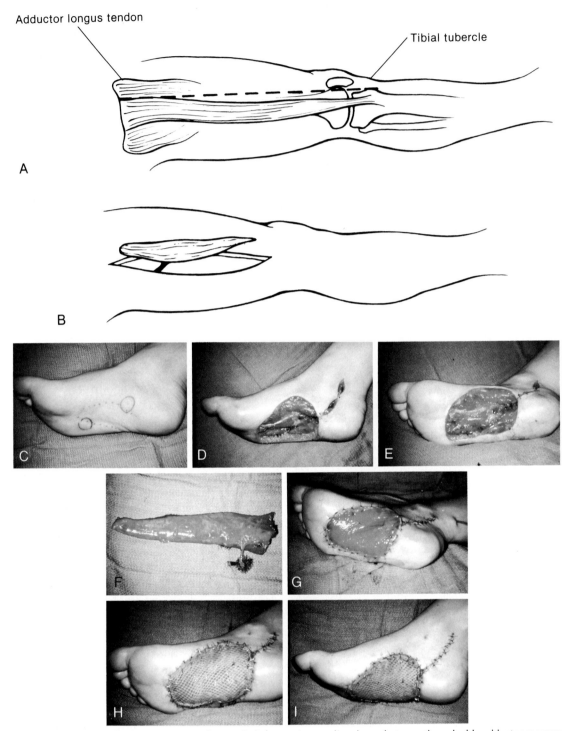

FIGURE 24–15. Gracilis flap. *(A),* The gracilis muscle lies posterior to a line drawn between the palpable adductor magnus tendon and the tibial tubercle when the leg is abducted. *(B),* The tendon of the gracilis muscle is located distally, and the muscle is dissected after identification of the vascular pedicle on the anterior surface of the muscle. *(C),* Recurrent plantar fibromatosis requiring an extensive en bloc resection. *(D and E),* The defect after resection. *(F),* The gracilis muscle free flap. *(G),* The defect filled with vascularized flap. *(H and I),* Meshed split-thickness skin coverage of the muscle. The foot is fully functional, with an excellent cosmetic result, no breakdown, and no detected tumor recurrence 1 year after the flap procedure.

POSTOPERATIVE CARE

In the postoperative period, the patient with a microsurgical or local flap reconstruction must be well hydrated to avoid vasoconstriction. Diuretic and vasoconstrictive medications should be avoided. The extremity must be elevated to improve venous outflow. For the first postoperative week, the patient is usually maintained at strict bed rest. Dependency of the extremity is undertaken very slowly during the next few weeks.

The care of the patient who has had foot reconstruction does not end with the surgery. Because of the special needs of the foot, ongoing care must be provided to assist with normal ambulation and to prevent late breakdown of the reconstructed tissue. Pedorthics plays a major role in the rehabilitation of the patient. Irregular surfaces and surfaces with diminished sensibility must be protected from injury. To protect troublesome areas, a mold of the foot is fabricated using a conforming wax, plaster, or foam material. From this mold, an impression of the foot can be made. Shoe inserts are then custom-made to cushion the foot and evenly distribute weight bearing when problem areas are seen on the impression. Gait analysis may sometimes be required to analyze the patient's needs for other orthotics or shoe modifications.[47]

SUMMARY

Soft tissue reconstruction of the foot and ankle is a complicated surgical endeavor. Each area of the foot must be considered separately in regard to reconstructive needs. Microsurgical techniques are now commonly used in the salvage of complicated foot and ankle reconstructions; however, a reconstructive hierarchy must be remembered. The foot should be reconstructed with the simplest surgical option that will ensure good function. This option often includes microsurgical free tissue transfer. The reconstructive microsurgeon must closely orchestrate the soft tissue reconstruction with the bony reconstruction and with postoperative pedorthics. Successful management of these complicated cases depends on careful planning, meticulous surgery, and good postoperative support.

References

1. Khouri RK, Shaw WW: Reconstruction of the lower extremity with microvascular free flaps: A 10 year experience with 304 consecutive cases. J Trauma 29:1086–94, 1989.
2. Sinha AK, Wood MB, Irons GB: Free tissue transfer for reconstruction of the weight bearing portion of the foot. Clin Orthop 242:269–71, 1989.
3. Woods MB, Irons GB, Cooney WP: Foot reconstruction by free flap transfer. Foot Ankle 4:2–7, 1983.
4. Gould JS: Reconstruction of soft tissue injuries of the foot and ankle with microsurgical techniques. Orthopedics 10:151–157, 1987.
5. Godina M: Early microsurgical reconstruction of complex trauma of the extremities. Plast Reconstr Surg 78:285–292, 1986.
6. Hidalgo DA, Shaw WW: Anatomic basis of plantar flap design. Plast Reconstr Surg 78:627–636, 1978.
7. Shaw WW, Hidalgo DA: Anatomic basis of plantar flap design: Clinical applications. Plast Reconstr Surg 78:637–49, 1978.
8. Hidalgo DA, Shaw WW: Reconstruction of foot injuries. Clin Plast Surg 13:663–680, 1986.
9. Shanahan RE, Gingrass RP: Medial plantar sensory flap for coverage of heel defects. Plast Reconstr Surg 64:295–298, 1979.
10. Ger R: The technique of muscle transposition and the operative treatment of traumatic and ulcerative lesions. J Trauma 2:502, 1971.
11. Bostwick J III: Reconstruction of the heel pad by muscle transposition and split skin graft. Surg Gynecol Obstet 143:973–974, 1976.
12. Ger R: The surgical management of ulcers of the heel. Surg Gynecol Obstet 140:909–911, 1975.
13. Emmett AJ: The fillet toe flap. Br J Plast Surg 29:19–21, 1976.
14. Synder GB, Edgerton MT: The principle of the island neurovascular flap in the management of ulcerated anaesthetic weight bearing areas of the lower extremity. Plast Reconstr Surg 36:518–528, 1965.
15. Stevenson TR, Mathes SJ: Management of foot injuries with free muscle flaps. Plast Reconstr Surg 78:665–669, 1986.
16. May JW Jr, Rohrich RJ: Foot reconstruction using free microvascular muscle flaps with skin grafts. Clin Plast Surg 13:681–689, 1986.
17. Chang KN, Buncke HJ: Sensory reinnervation in reconstruction of the foot. Foot Ankle 7:124–132, 1986.
18. Brown CJ, Mackinnon SE, Dellon AL, Bain JR: The sensory potential of free flap donor sites. Ann Plast Surg 23:135–140, 1989.
19. Hallock GG, Rice DC, Keblish PA, Arangio GA: Restoration of the foot using the radial forearm flap. Ann Plast Surg 20:14–25, 1988.
20. Wyble EJ, Yakuboff KP, Clark RG, Neale HW: Use of free fasciocutaneous and muscle flaps for reconstruction of the foot. Ann Plast Surg 24:101–108, 1990.
21. Gilbert A, Teot L: The free scapula flap. Plast Reconstr Surg 69:601–604, 1982.
22. Nassif TM, Vidal L, Bouet JL, Baudet J: The parascapular flap: A new cutaneous microsurgical free flap. Plast Reconstr Surg 69:591–600, 1982.

23. O'Brien B, Morrison W: Reconstructive Microsurgery. Edinburgh, Churchill Livingstone, 1987.
24. Cromack GC, Lamberty BG: Fasciocutaneous vessels in the upper arm; Application to the design of new fasciocutaneous flaps. Plast Reconstr Surg 74:244–249, 1984.
25. Matloub HS, Sanger JR, Godina, M: The lateral arm flap. *In* William HB: Transactions of the VIII International Congress of Plastic Surgery. Montreal, International Society of Plastic and Reconstructive Surgery, 1983, p 132.
26. Katsaros J, Schusterman M, Beppe M, et al: The lateral upper arm flap: Anatomy and clinical applications. Ann Plast Surg 12:489–500, 1984.
27. Sommerland BC, McGrouther DA: Resurfacing the sole: Long term followup and comparison of techniques. Br J Plast Surg 31:107, 1978.
28. Woltering EA, Thorpe WP, Reed JK Jr, Rosenberg SA: Split thickness skin grafting of the plantar surface of the foot after wide excision of neoplasms of the skin. Surg Gynecol Obstet 149:229–232, 1979.
29. McGraw JB, Arnold PG: McGraw & Arnolds Atlas of Muscle and Musculocutaneous Flaps. Norfolk, Hampton Press, 1986.
30. Bunkis J, Walton R, Mathes S: The versatile rectus abdominis flap. Fifty-first Annual Convention, American Society of Plastic and Reconstructive Surgery. Honolulu, HI, October 1982.
31. Cunningham B, Christiansen M, Diessel T, Shonsi A: The rectus abdominis muscle: A useful free flap donor site. Fifty-first Annual Convention, American Society of Plastic and Reconstructive Surgery. Honolulu, HI, October 1982.
32. Bunkis J, Walton R, Mathes S: The rectus abdominis free flap for lower extremity reconstruction. Ann Plast Surg 11:373–380, 1983.
33. Pennington DG, Lai MF, Pelly AD: The rectus abdominis myocutaneous free flap. Br J Plast Surg 33:277–282, 1980.
34. Baudet J, Guimberteau J, Nascimento E: Successful clinical transfer of two free thoracodorsal axillary flaps. Plast Reconstr Surg 58:680–688, 1976.
35. Ricbourg B, Lassau J, Violete A, Merland S: A propos del'artere mammaire ext. orgine, territorre et interet pour les transplants cutanes libris. Arch Anat Pathol 23:317–322, 1975.
36. Maxwell GP, Stueber K, Hoopes JE: A free latissimus dorsi myocutaneous flap: Case report. Plast Reconstr Surg 62:462–469, 1978.
37. Watson JS, Craig RD, Orton CI: The free latissimus dorsi myocutaneous flap. Plast Reconstr Surg 64:299–305, 1979.
38. Bartlet SP, May JW, Yaremchuk MJ: The dorsi myocutaneous muscle; A fresh cadaver study of the primary neurovascular pedicle. Plast Reconstr Surg 67:631–635, 1981.
39. Song R, Gao Y, Song Y, et al: The forearm flap. Clin Plast Surg 9:21–26, 1982.
40. Muhlbauer W, Heindl E, Stock W: The forearm flap. Plast Reconstr Surg 70:336–344, 1982.
41. Gould JS: The dorsalis pedis island pedicle flap for small defects of the foot and ankle. Orthopedics 9:867–871, 1986.
42. Mathes SJ, Alpert BS, Chang N: Use of muscle flap in chronic osteomyelitis; Experimental and clinical correlation. Plast Reconstr Surg 69:815–828, 1982.
43. Harii K, Ohmori K, Sekiquck J: The free gracilis musculocutaneous flap. Plast Reconstr Surg 57:294–303, 1976.
44. Acland RD: Refinements in lower extremity free flap. Clin Plast Surg 17:733–744, 1990.
45. Grotting JC: Prevention of complications and correction of postoperative problems in microsurgery of the lower extremity. Clin Plast Surg 18:485–489, 1991.
46. Koman LA, Pospisil RF, Nunley JA, Urbaniak JR: Value of contrast arteriography in composite tissue transfer. Clin Orthop 172:195–206, 1983.
47. May JW, Hall MJ, Simon SR: Free microvascular muscle flaps with skin graft reconstruction of extensive defects of the foot: A clinical and gait analysis study. Plast Reconstr Surg 75:627–641, 1985.

PART **III** *TRAUMA OF THE*

ADULT FOOT AND

ANKLE

Editor
LAMAR L. FLEMING

25 Fractures and Dislocations of the Ankle

MICHAEL E. MILLER

Fractures and dislocations of the ankle joint are common injuries that have been the subject of orthopaedic treatises for more than 200 years.[25, 44] During the last 50 years, much debate over the management of these injuries has centered around the issues of closed treatment versus surgical intervention. This debate has often been clouded by a lack of understanding of the biomechanics of the normal ankle joint and by an accompanying misunderstanding of the mechanics of injury. This chapter first reviews the mechanics and pathomechanics of ankle joint injury and then discusses classification systems useful in inferring a rationale for treatment. The clinical patterns of injury that require surgical management are covered in two sections: ankle mortise disruptions and fractures of the tibial plafond. Finally, open fracture-dislocations are discussed, along with a brief presentation of progress in allograft reconstruction of the distal tibia.

ANKLE JOINT BIOMECHANICS

Inman's classic work on the anatomy and mechanics of the ankle joint represents our best understanding of this complex structure.[20] This book, which has unfortunately been out of print for several years, rigorously investigates the relationship of the talus to the tibia and fibula and clearly explains how and why ankle joint motion occurs. The talar surface constitutes a *frustum* (Fig. 25–1), a section of a cone, that is broader anteriorly than posteriorly. The base of the cone is lateral, and the narrow end of the cone is medial. The trochlea,

the superior articular surface of the talus, tends to cause some displacement of the lateral malleolus and fibula when it is brought to a position of full dorsiflexion. This displacement was measured by Inman as being between 0 and 2 mm. Inman summarized his findings as follows:[20]

1. The trochlea of the talus, viewed from above, shows various degrees of wedging from individual to individual. The degree of the wedging may vary from no wedging ($\pm 5\%$) to marked wedging (the posterior width may be 25% or as much as 6 mm less than the anterior width).
2. The malleoli show a similar convergence posteriorly.
3. The articular surfaces of the malleoli closely approximate the sides of the trochlea in all positions from full plantar flexion to full dorsiflexion.
4. There is no appreciable lateral play of the talus within its mortise on full plantar flexion.
5. Some slight motion of the lateral malleolus (rotatory or lateral displacement or bending) can usually be perceived on dorsiflexion. The amount of this motion varies from zero to not more than 2 mm.
6. No definite relationship has been established between the movement of the lateral malleolus and the degree of wedging of the trochlea of the talus.
7. The curvature of the trochlea always closely approximates an arc of a circle on the lateral side and in the majority (80%) of specimens it is an arc of a circle on the medial side. The same is true of the curvature of the mortise.
8. The radius of curvature of the trochlea on its medial side is almost invariably shorter than on the lateral side. However, in spite of a shorter radius of curvature and a shorter arc on the

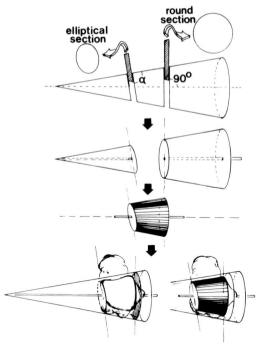

FIGURE 25–1. The trochlea of the talus as depicted by Inman. The articular surface of the talus is a *frustum*, a section of the surface of a cone. The medial and lateral borders usually converge posteriorly. (From Inman VT: The Joints of the Ankle. Baltimore, Williams & Wilkins, 1976. © 1976, The Williams & Wilkins Company, Baltimore.)

medial side, the subtended angles are the same in the medial and lateral sides of the trochlea.

9. For all practical purposes, motion of the ankle joint can be considered to be about a single axis (this is true in 80% of the specimens, and in 20% the axis may be a changing one of not more than 10 degrees of displacement in a transverse plane).
10. The axis of the ankle joint is obliquely oriented to the long axis of the leg.
   a. When projected on a transverse plane it is directed laterally and posteriorly.
   b. When projected on a coronal plane it is directed laterally and downward.
   c. The axis passes slightly distal to the distal tips of the malleoli.
   d. When projected upon the coronal plane, the axis bears no consistent relationship to the articular surfaces of the ankle joint.
11. The articular surfaces of the plafond and trochlea are more congruent than those of the other major articulations of the lower extremity.*

---

*From Inman VT: The Joints of the Ankle. Baltimore, Williams & Wilkins, 1976. © 1976, The Williams & Wilkins Company, Baltimore.

PRIMARY IMPORTANCE OF THE FIBULA

With an understanding of the normal anatomic findings as described by Inman, the role of the malleoli in maintaining the normal relationship of the talus to the plafond must be appreciated in preparation for a discussion of fractures and fracture-dislocations.

Historically, the medial malleolus was thought to be the critical component of ankle mortise disruptions,[19] but within the past 30 years, this emphasis has changed. Hughes clarified the importance of the medial malleolar fracture in two regards:[19] (1) fixation of the medial side is necessary to allow early motion and functional rehabilitation; and (2) osteochondral fragments from the medial axilla of the plafond are often loose within the joint, necessitating intra-articular inspection and débridement.

Yablon and colleagues have been largely responsible for our current appreciation of the role of the fibula in maintaining the congruity of the ankle.[45, 46] They showed that reduction of *medial malleolar* fractures is neither necessary nor sufficient to reduce the talus under the plafond of the tibia. This work was corroborated by Harper.[15] In contrast, anatomic reduction plus stable fixation of displaced *fibular* fractures accompanying talar displacement is both necessary and often sufficient to reduce the talus. This is especially true in patients with disruption of the anterior talofibular ligament accompanying the fibular fracture. Further, translational shifts of the talus as small as 1 mm are sufficient to severely decrease the contact area of the tibiotalar joint.[38, 43] With this decrease in congruity, the logical outcome is an acceleration of post-traumatic arthritis (Fig. 25–2).[14] The fibula also has a limited weight-bearing function.[39]

Reconstruction and maintainance of fibular length are also critical. Because of the sloping relationship of the fibula with the lateral face of the talus, proximal migration of the fibula will allow lateral talar displacement. Further, proximal displacement of the distal fibula leads to incongruity of the incisura of the distal tibia with the medial side of the distal fibula, making accurate repositioning of the fibula at the syndesmosis level impossible (Fig. 25–3).

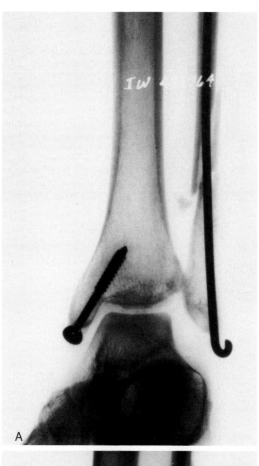

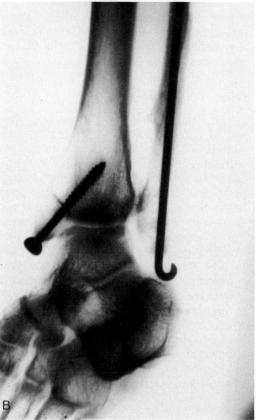

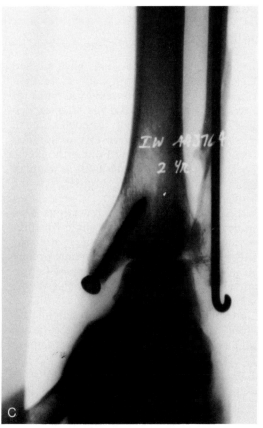

FIGURE 25–2. *(A)*, An AO type C fracture treated with Rush rod fixation for fibular fracture. Note the shortened fibula with the syndesmosis unreduced and the abnormal lateral joint space. *(B)*, An oblique view at 2 years shows loss of tibiotalar joint space. *(C)*, A mortise view at 2 years shows lateral migration of the talus and loss of joint congruity. The patient required an arthrodesis for pain relief.

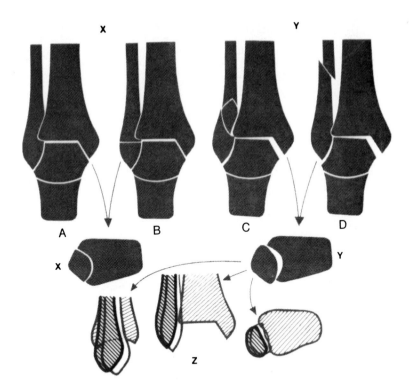

FIGURE 25–3. Incongruity resulting from fibular fractures: *(A and B)*, Intact fibula or AO type A fracture with syndesmosis preserved, as in X. *(C and D)*, Proximal fibular migration from unreduced AO type B or C fractures with incongruity of the fibula at the incisura, as in Y. The fibula cannot be reduced and remains displaced, as in Z. (From Hanke J: Luxationsfrakturen des oberen Sprunggelenkes. Berlin, Springer-Verlag, 1988, p 102.)

DISRUPTIONS OF THE ANKLE MORTISE

Classification of Injuries

In the modern era, physicians have studied and classified ankle fractures for more than 200 years. Lauge-Hansen reviewed most of this work in preparation for his later experiments,[25] and any historically minded surgeon may consult his exhaustive history to appreciate the great sophistication of our orthopaedic forebears. Certainly, the only fault in many of the early analyses of ankle injuries was the lack of Roentgen's invention.

Although a number of classifications have been devised for evaluation of ankle fractures involving the mortise and malleoli,[13] within the last 10 years, two systems have become preeminent in North America: the system of Lauge-Hansen[26] and the system of Danis and Weber as adopted by the AO.[34]

Lindsjö proposed three requirements for fracture classification systems:[29] (1) the system should be reproducible and permit comparisons between different case studies; (2) the system should be simple and easily applied in daily practice; and (3) the system should pro-

vide information of importance for treatment and research.

I agree with Lindsjö that neither the AO classification nor the Lauge-Hansen (L-H) system fulfills all of these ideals but that each provides some useful features.

Lauge-Hansen Decoded

The Lauge-Hansen (L-H) system is the result of careful studies performed on experimental, reproducible fractures with radiologic correlation. It describes fractures in terms of causative forces, naming the fracture by the position of the forefoot and hindfoot relative to the leg. Lauge-Hansen believed that a surgeon who was able to infer the deforming forces accurately from the history, physical examination, and radiographic findings would then be able to select and perform the proper countermaneuvers to reduce the fracture and correct the deformity. This would logically lead to improved closed reductions and improved results from nonsurgical treatment.

The L-H system, when fully understood, is a powerful tool for the closed treatment of ankle mortise fractures, but it is cumbersome to apply and teach, and its rigorous use results in as many as 15 subtypes of injuries. However, the greatest problem with the system is one of language.

I would argue that to most English-speaking surgeons, an injury caused by supination of the hindfoot is the result of an inversion force. Further, supination of the forefoot and adduction of the hindfoot are actually part of a continuum, a single event or motion. Because the native language of Lauge-Hansen was Danish, his work required translation into English. In the process, external rotation of the foot in the plane perpendicular to the long axis of the fixed leg became "eversion," and internal rotation of the foot in the plane perpendicular to the long axis of the fixed leg became "inversion." Many young residents, on first seeing a fracture described as a "supination-eversion" injury, fall into a nauseated state of unease: the terms are mutually contradictory for an English-speaking surgeon. This anxiety is heightened somewhat when these same surgeons encounter a "supination-adduction" injury and wonder why two words are being used to describe a motion that in English is one phenomenon. None of this is Lauge-Hansen's fault, because a careful reading of his original English-language article[26] reveals that although his terminology was confusing, he explained everything very clearly based on the nomenclature that he proposed.

I suggest the following changes in the terminology of the L-H system:

1. The terms *inversion* and *eversion*, which are now hopelessly confused by past usage, should be dropped completely when the L-H system is being used.

2. The terms *supination* and *pronation* are not necessary because they are applied to indicate the position of the forefoot at the time of injury, when in fact it is the position of the talus and hindfoot that transmits the injuring force to the malleoli and ligaments.[20, 35] The clear and universally understood terms *valgus* and *varus* may be substituted for *pronation* and *supination*, respectively.

The application of these simple changes to the terminology of Lauge-Hansen results in a useful simplification (Table 25-1).

Little is lost by these changes. All that the surgeon needs to remember is that in valgus ankle fractures, *both* the hindfoot and forefoot

TABLE 25–1. SUGGESTED CHANGES IN THE TERMINOLOGY OF THE LAUGE-HANSEN SYSTEM

OLD TERMINOLOGY	NEW TERMINOLOGY
Supination-adduction fracture	Varus ankle fracture
Pronation-abduction fracture	Valgus ankle fracture
Supination-eversion fracture	Varus–external rotation fracture
Pronation-eversion fracture	Valgus–external rotation fracture

are in a valgus position. Similarly, in a varus ankle fracture, *both* the hindfoot and forefoot are in a varus position. In fractures with external rotation forces, it is clear that the foot rotates externally on the fixed leg. Although this does not describe the actual relative frames of motion at the time of injury, when it is the foot that is fixed, it is again a useful change for the surgeon: corrective manipulations of ankle fractures based on this system are performed with the foot and ankle free to move on the leg, not with the foot fixed, as it would be at the time of injury.

With this clarification of the L-H system, following Lauge-Hansen's subdivision of the classification into subtypes or stages is the next step. Through his experimental reproduction of fractures, Lauge-Hansen deduced that for any of his four major types of malleolar fractures, a series of injuries occurred in a predictable order. He further inferred that for a given radiographic appearance of a bony injury, concomitant ligamentous injuries must have also taken place. Thus, for example, a stage III valgus–external rotation injury with a high fibular fracture presupposes a tear of the syndesmotic ligaments (Fig. 25–4). In some cases, only the history as given by the patient regarding the position of the foot at the time of injury allows the use of the L-H system. For example, the medial malleolar fracture in some L-H valgus stage I injuries will be radiographically similar to some varus stage II fractures associated with a lateral ligament avulsion rather than the more common fracture of the lateral malleolus.

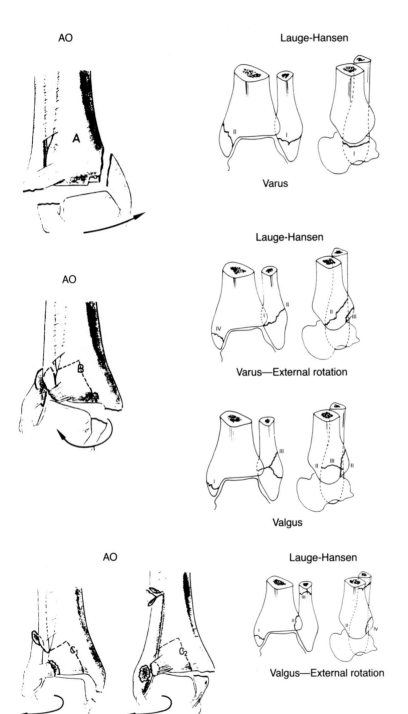

FIGURE 25–4. The relationship between the AO and the Lauge-Hansen classification systems for ankle fractures. The most confusing area is the AO type B fracture, which corresponds to two different fracture types and mechanisms of injury in the Lauge-Hansen system.

Danis-Weber AO System

Despite some overlap of the Danis-Weber AO classification system with the L-H system, there are major differences between the two, both philosophic and in application. The AO system (see Fig. 25–4) was conceived by orthopaedic surgeons with an aggressive philosophy of fracture fixation and early motion as the key to successful management of intra-articular injuries. Therefore, the AO system serves largely to categorize the surgical approach and fixation methods to be chosen for these fractures.

The AO system is based on the level of the fibular fracture relative to the tibiofibular syndesmosis, rather than purely on the mechanisms of injury as described by Lauge-Hansen. The AO system does schematically describe the mechanism of injury, but it generally ascribes fractures to somewhat simpler forces. In type C injuries, for example, the high fibular fracture is thought to be purely the product of external rotation of the foot on the fixed leg, whereas Lauge-Hansen would describe the cause as a combination of valgus (*pronation* in the old terminology) and external rotation. The areas of overlap of the systems are seen in Table 25–2.[32]

The obvious area of discordance or confusion is the AO type B group, which includes the most common type of fracture in the L-H system, the varus–external rotation injury, and the pure valgus injury as well. In actual practice, this is not a major problem, as long as the surgeon recognizes that about 50 percent of the B injuries will have disruption of the tibiofibular syndesmosis and addresses this injury as needed.

I suggest that the surgeon have a detailed knowledge of the L-H system and the wealth of information it provides about mechanisms of injury and anticipation of soft tissue disruptions but that the AO system be used for ease of communication in daily practice. Thus, to summarize: think L-H, but speak AO.

Management of Ankle Mortise Disruptions

The choice of treatment for fractures and fracture-dislocations of the ankle mortise must involve the answers to these questions:

1. Does the injury dislocate or subluxate the talus from its normal position in the mortise?
2. If the injury has not caused an appreciable shift of the talus, has it nevertheless destabilized the mortise so that later subluxation is likely?
3. If displaced, can the talus be repositioned in its normal location in the mortise? If so, is late subluxation likely to occur when splinting is discontinued?
4. What are the position and condition of the fibula? That is, has it shortened or displaced laterally or posteriorly?

Clearly, these queries may be resolved only by an accurate history taking and accurate physical examination findings, and most important, by good-quality conventional radiography. *The minimum acceptable studies for evaluation of any ankle fracture are the anteroposterior, true lateral, and mortise views* (Fig. 25–5). Fibular length relative to the medial malleolus may vary a good deal from one individual to another. Therefore, anteroposterior views, mortise views, or both views of the uninjured ankle may be needed to resolve questions of fibular length.

With clinical and radiographic information in hand, the surgeon may construct a simple algorithm for the management of ankle mortise disruptions:

- As with the terminology of spinal fractures, a *stable* injury is one that is not likely to progress to further deformity; *unstable* injuries are prone to late displacement or deformity.
- Injuries without dislocation of the talus that are stable with splinting are obviously to be treated closed, as are injuries with the talus dislocated or subluxated, which may be ren-

TABLE 25–2. AREAS OF OVERLAP OF THE AO AND LAUGE-HANSEN SYSTEMS	
DANIS-WEBER AO SYSTEM	**LAUGE-HANSEN SYSTEM**
A	Varus
B	Varus–external rotation Valgus
C	Valgus–external rotation

SYNDESMOSIS RADIOGRAPHIC CRITERIA

Mortise View

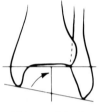

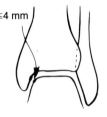

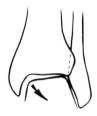

Talocrural Angle
(83° ± 4°)

Medial Clear Space
(≤4 mm)

Talar Tilt
(≤2 mm)

Anteroposterior View

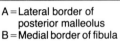

A = Lateral border of
posterior malleolus
B = Medial border of fibula
C = Lateral border of
anterior tibial
tubercle

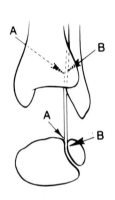

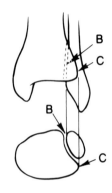

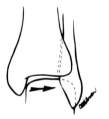

Syndesmosis A
(<5 mm)

Syndesmosis B
(≥10 mm)

Talar Subluxation

FIGURE 25–5. Radiographic criteria for abnormalities in ankle joint spaces, as suggested by Stiehl. (From Stiehl JB: Ankle fractures with diastasis. Instruct Course Lect 39:95, 1990.)

dered stable by closed reduction and splinting.

- Fracture-dislocations that cannot be adequately reduced by closed manipulation are obviously to be managed surgically. These tend to be unstable injuries.
- The injuries requiring the greatest skill and judgment are those that, although reducible by closed manipulation, are unstable and those that, although not initially causing talar displacement, are unstable and thus causes of late talar displacement and disability.

Because of wide variations in their experience and abilities, not all surgeons will agree in decisions between closed treatment and surgical management. Inescapably, the surgeon's skills and preferences must be factored into the "personality" of the fracture. The elements of judgment, skill, and philosophy separate

algorithms from cookbooks. This statement is certainly not intended to demean the talents of the skillful cook, because not every cook can successfully re-create every recipe. But the *chef* decides which recipe is appropriate for the occasion, and he or she is using an *algorithm*.

As befits this volume, the intent of this chapter is to outline *operative* management of ankle fractures. Charnley's classic work should be consulted regarding closed reduction and casting techniques.[7]

Techniques of Operative Treatment By Injury Type

AO Type A—Lauge-Hansen Varus-Type Fracture

The AO type A or L-H varus-type fracture is relatively uncommon, constituting 6 to 20

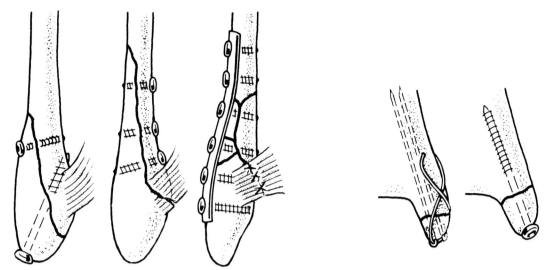

FIGURE 25–6. Fracture fixation constructs as suggested by the AO for varying (fibular type B) fracture patterns. (From Müller ME, Allgöwer M, Schneider R, Willenegger H: Manual of Internal Fixation, 2nd Ed. Berlin, Springer-Verlag, 1979.)

percent of ankle fractures in several series.[29] These injuries are characterized by a transverse fracture of the fibula below the level of the syndesmosis, which is in fact an avulsion or traction injury. An oblique fracture of the medial malleolus extending from the axilla of the plafond accompanies the fibular fracture when the force applied reaches L-H stage II. Although the fibular fracture may be stable with closed manipulation and splinting, the medial malleolar fracture may be a major concern for reasons outlined previously, thus leading to surgical treatment.

The fibula may be fixed with an AO 1/3 plate and 3.5-mm screws if fragment size and bone quality allow (Fig. 25–6), but small fragments may call for tension band wiring or for fixation with a single longitudinal lag screw (Fig. 25–7). Because the fibular fracture in this type of injury is transverse and not likely to shorten, intramedullary Rush pin or longitudinal screw fixation is sometimes possible. However, this fixation affords little rotational control of the fragment if early motion is anticipated. The Inyo nail,[33] a device with a V-shaped cross section, may give better rota-

FIGURE 25–7. Longitudinal screw fixation or tension band wiring may be needed for smaller fragments. (From Müller ME, Allgöwer M, Schneider R, Willenegger H: Manual of Internal Fixation, 2nd Ed. Berlin, Springer-Verlag, 1979.)

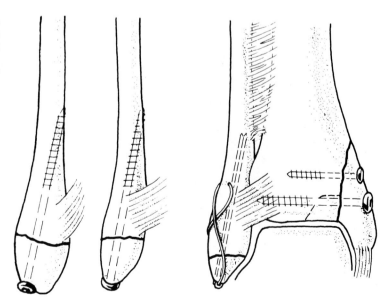

tional control than other intramedullary nails, but I have no experience with it.

On the medial side, two partially threaded 4.0-mm cancellous bone screws usually give good fixation (Fig. 25–8). These screws should not exceed 35 to 40 mm in length in order to gain purchase in the dense subchondral bone surmounting the tibial plafond. The use of the original AO "malleolar" screw should be discouraged: the head is too large and tends to cause undue skin tension, and the 4.5-mm screw diameter is also overlarge and may lead to iatrogenic fracture of the medial malleolar fragment. In cases involving small fragments or porotic bone, tension band wiring is also clinically useful and mechanically sound.[8, 36]

The L-H stage III varus ankle fracture involves a posterior lip or "posterior malleolar" fracture, generally of small size, that is usually reduced spontaneously when the lateral and medial fractures are reduced and fixed. A full discussion of the posterior lip fracture is found in the next section.

AO Type B—Lauge-Hansen Valgus and Varus–External Rotation Fractures

The AO type B or Lauge-Hansen valgus and varus–external rotation fractures constitute the largest group of ankle fractures, including about 60 to 80 percent of all malleolar fractures in large series.[29] Depending on the fracture pattern and the level of injury at the syndesmosis, the AO B fracture may involve complete disruption of the tibiofibular syndesmosis or may leave the syndesmosis intact (Figs. 25–9 and 25–10). This will be an important determination for the surgeon to make, since the disrupted syndesmosis must be reduced and stable for good long-term results.[22, 28, 40, 41]

The surgical treatment of the type B fracture should begin with the lateral malleolar fracture. This rule is to be followed in all ankle fractures with fibular involvement, because accurate reduction and stabilization of the fibula will reduce the tibiotalar joint and thus expedite the treatment of the medial or tibial component of the injury.

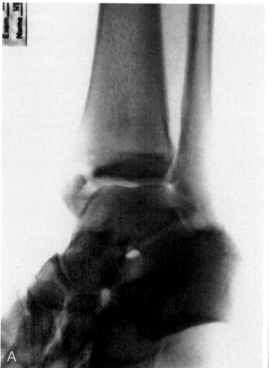
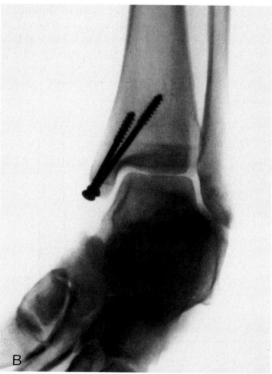

FIGURE 25–8. *(A),* Displaced medial malleolar fracture. *(B),* Results 1 year after lag screw fixation with partially threaded 4.0-mm cancellous bone screws.

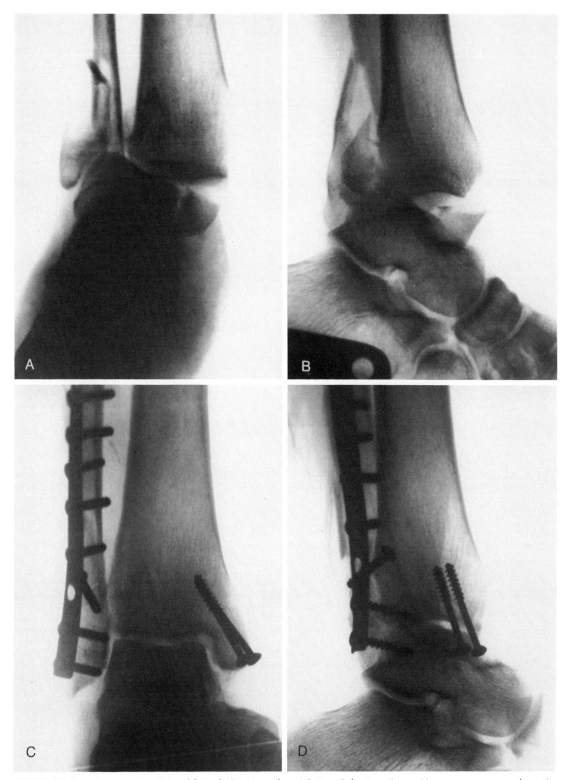

FIGURE 25–9. Anteroposterior *(A)* and lateral *(B)* views of an AO type B fracture (Lauge-Hansen varus–external rotation type). Note that the syndesmosis is not disrupted and that there is a small posterior margin fracture of the tibia. Mortise *(C)* and lateral *(D)* views after fixation. Note that the talus is reduced and that separate fixation of the posterior margin fracture and syndesmosis is not needed in this case.

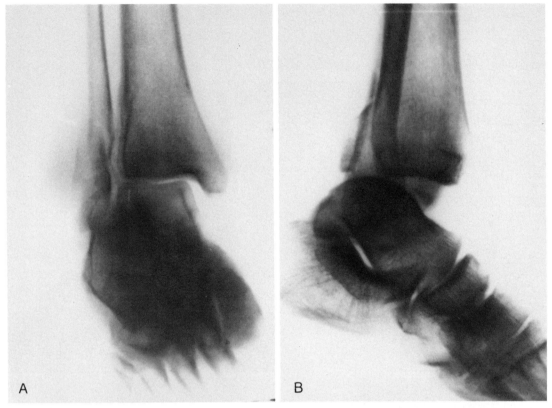

FIGURE 25–10. Anteroposterior *(A)* and lateral *(B)* views of an AO type B injury, in this case with slight widening of the tibiofibular space and posterolateral subluxation of the talus. The syndesmosis in this case required fixation.

In most cases, the fibula may be stabilized with an AO 1/3 tubular plate, which will maintain fibular length better than intramedullary devices; the oblique pattern of the fibular fracture increases the risk for shortening and

subsequent joint incongruity. In addition, the plate itself may be used as an aid to reduction (Figs. 25–11 and 25–12) with indirect reduction techniques described by Mast and colleagues.[30] Such methods tend to decrease soft tissue

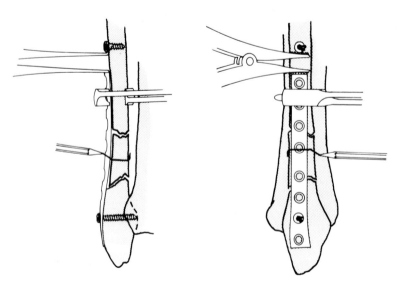

FIGURE 25–11. The plate fixed to the distal fragment may be used as an aid to reduction by a distraction maneuver. (From Mast J, Jakob R, Ganz R: Planning and Reduction Technique in Fracture Surgery. Berlin, Springer-Verlag, 1989.)

FIGURE 25–12. The 1/3 tubular plate used as a spring-buttress device, simultaneously effecting reduction and fixation. (From Mast J, Jakob R, Ganz R: Planning and Reduction Technique in Fracture Surgery. Berlin, Springer-Verlag, 1989.)

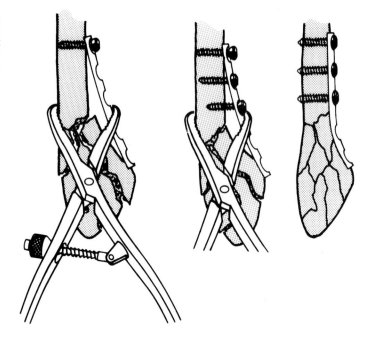

stripping of small bone fragments and to reduce operating time as well.

The patient should be positioned with a large roll under the ipsilateral hip to afford easy access to the posterolateral aspect of the ankle. Tourniquet control is appropriate in most cases.

Proper positioning of the fibular plate is essential. The plate should be twisted slightly to follow the contour of the distal fibula, with the most distal portion of the plate placed along the posterior surface of the fibula and the more proximal part rotating gently to a more lateral position (Figs. 25–13 and 25–14). Careful study of the lateral malleolus shows a flat surface ideal for placement of the plate in the area just described, curving from posterior caudad to lateral cephalad. The fibular plate should be posterior on the distal fibula for these reasons:

1. In the area in which the fibula is subcutaneous, the plate is rotated away from the most prominent part of the malleolus so as to minimize soft tissue tension.

2. In the majority of fibular fractures (AO type B or L-H varus–external rotation), the spike of the distal fragment is directed obliquely posterior. The slight posterior position of the plate allows the use of an "antiglide" plate, which is mechanically superior in

fixation of minimal size. In severely comminuted fractures, a spring-buttress plate as suggested by Mast and colleagues[30] may also be used.

3. Because of the direction of the fracture in the majority of cases, lag screw fixation of the oblique fracture through the plate enhances the mechanical stability of the construct.

4. The lateral malleolus is wider in the anteroposterior direction than in the mediolateral direction. Posterior placement of the distal part of the plate thus allows purchase in a larger amount of tissue, which in the cancellous bone of the lateral malleolus is a major advantage.

5. Screws directed posteroanteriorly in the lateral malleolus are pointing away from the ankle joint and the talus. This serves to minimize the chances for accidental injury from drill bits or overlong screws.

6. The fibula lies about 20 to 30 degrees posterior to the tibia. In cases requiring screw fixation of the syndesmosis, the syndesmotic screw must therefore be directed in a posteroanterior direction at an angle of approximately 20 degrees. It is frequently desirable to position the screw through the plate, and the posterior rotation of the plate expedites proper aiming of the syndesmotic screw.

7. If a posterolateral Volkmann fragment of

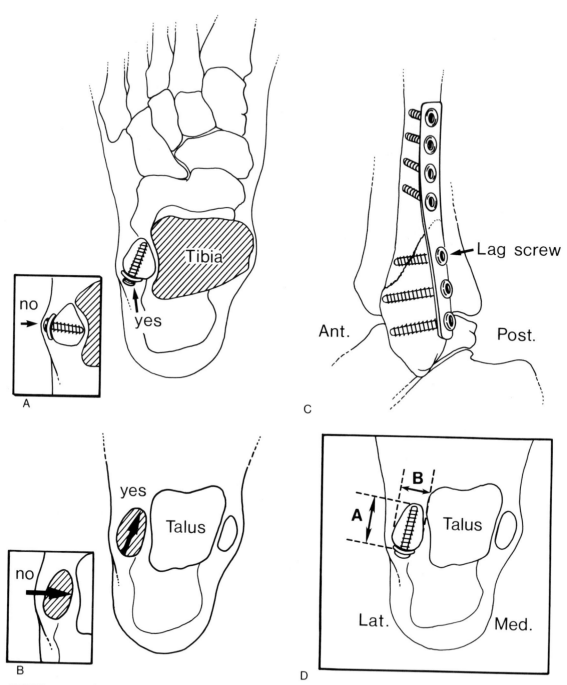

FIGURE 25–13. The positioning of the fibular plate on the posterolateral surface of the distal fibula has numerous advantages. (*A*), The plate and screws are less prominent and less likely to damage the overlying soft tissues. (*B*), Drilling in the posteroanterior direction for screw fixation aims away from the talus, minimizing the risk of joint penetration. (*C*), The most common fibular fracture pattern (oblique in the coronal plane) can often be fixed with a lag screw through the posteriorly positioned plate. (*D*), The distal fibula is broader in the posteroanterior (A) than in the mediolateral (B) dimension. This allows use of a longer screw in an area in which fixation may be tenuous because of small fragment size or soft cancellous bone.

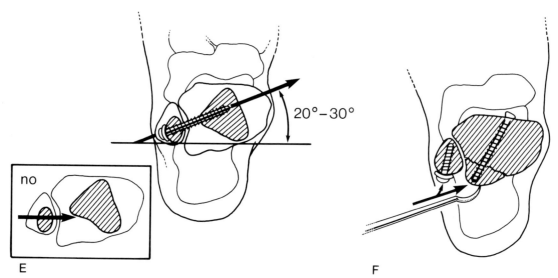

E   F

FIGURE 25–13 *Continued (E),* The posterior position of the fibula and the slope of the posterior tibial cortex conspire to make malposition of a syndesmotic screw all too easy. A posteriorly positioned plate allows proper direction of the syndesmotic screw through the plate, if needed. *(F),* In cases requiring direct reduction of Volkmann's fragment, the posterior dissection for the plate is easily extended to allow for manipulation of the fragment.

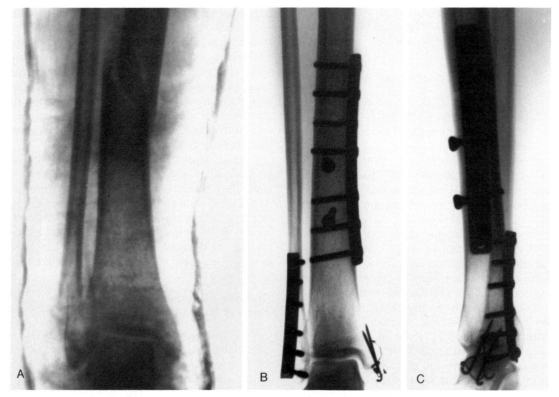

FIGURE 25–14. *(A),* An AO type C fracture combined with a tibial shaft fracture. *(B and C),* At 2-year follow-up, the ankle joint is normal. Note the posterior rotation of the fibular plate.

the tibia must be reduced and fixed, the initial posterior dissection for the plate may be easily extended from this approach (Fig. 25–15).

If treatment of the medial malleolus is indicated, screw or tension band wire fixation may be used, as described previously.

Concomitant Deltoid Ligament Injury

In patients who have deltoid ligament injury, rather than fractures of the malleolus, repair of the ligament not only is unnecessary but may actually produce inferior results.[2] Only patients in whom an incarcerated deltoid ligament seems to be preventing congruous reduction of the talus within the mortise require medial exploration for ligamentous injuries.

When these fractures are classified as AO type B injuries, about 50 percent of them will be accompanied by disruption of the syndesmosis. The presence of this lesion must therefore be suspected and tested for using a small bone hook to apply a distraction force. Ruptured syndesmotic ligaments may be sutured if their condition warrants, but screw fixation of the fibula should still be used. This technique is described in a later section.

Posterior "Malleolar"—Posterior Margin Fractures

Although some surgeons have been taught to call the posterior margin of the tibial plafond a malleolus, the functional anatomic facts probably do not bear this out. Both Harper[16, 17] and Yablon and Wasilewski[47] found that as long as the lateral malleolus and lateral ligamentous structures were intact, important subluxation of the talus did not occur, even with the medial or posterior margins of the plafond removed. The intuitive image of the posterior margin of the plafond as maintaining the position of the talus is thus in error. But incongruity of the weight-bearing surface of the plafond *is* likely to be important, especially if the fractured posterior fragment constitutes more than about 25 percent of the surface of the plafond.[12] Although Heim reported good long-term outcome in patients with posterior margin fractures that were fixed,[18] I have found that in many cases it is not necessary to address the posterior fragment separately, especially if it is a posterolateral Volkmann fragment (see Fig. 25–15). In most cases having a posterior

margin fragment of 25 percent or less, when the lateral malleolus is reduced and stably fixed in its anatomic position, the posterior fragment is satisfactorily reduced by ligamentotaxis. An intraoperative radiograph obtained after the bimalleolar component of the injury has been addressed should tell the surgeon if further treatment of the posterior margin is needed. In the process of preoperative planning, if the size and nature of the posterior fragment are in doubt, computed tomographic scans of the affected ankle should be obtained.

Postsurgical Care

In the operating room, a bulky dressing consisting of a layer of soft cotton wool followed by a sugar-tong plaster splint with a foot plate (Fig. 25–16) and an elastic bandage should be applied. This dressing provides gentle compression to control swelling and prevents equinus positioning of the foot. The limb should be elevated on several pillows, or better, on a Böhler-Braun frame. At 24 to 48 hours after surgery, when the suction drains are removed, active range-of-motion exercises are started. Cooperative patients may be treated with a removable splint or an orthosis, performing exercises several times per day and then donning the splint again. Graduated weight bearing can usually be started at about 6 weeks, along with resistive strengthening exercises for the peroneals and more aggressive active and passive range-of-motion exercises for the ankle.

Patients likely to be noncompliant with limited activities should be kept in the hospital until they have regained some active motion and should then be given a short-leg cast. For patients whose injuries require syndesmotic repair with screw fixation, weight bearing should be delayed until the screw has been removed to avoid the risk of screw breakage.

AO Type C—Lauge-Hansen Valgus– External Rotation Fracture

The AO type C or Lauge-Hansen valgus– external rotation fracture, which is characterized by a fracture of the fibula above the level of the plafond, invariably involves disruption of the syndesmosis. The syndesmotic injury may be purely ligamentous, or it may have a bony avulsion off the anterior fibula or the anterolateral tibia. In the latter case, the tibial

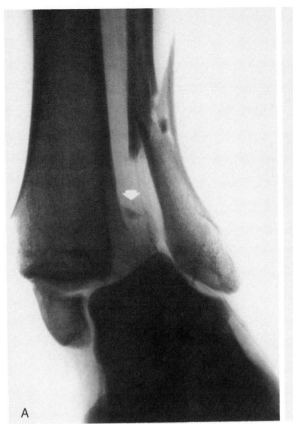

A

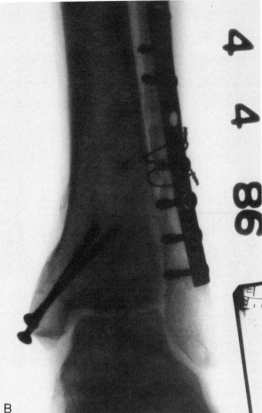

B

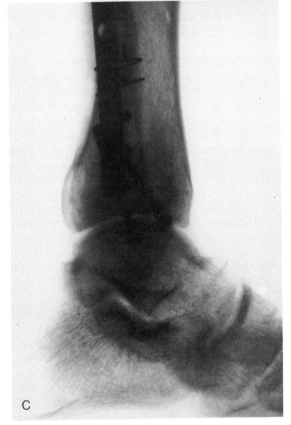

C

FIGURE 25–15. (A), An AO type C injury with comminuted fibular fracture and Volkmann's fragment (arrow). (B and C), At 2-year follow-up, the mortise is normal. The interosseous membrane is largely intact, and direct fixation of the syndesmosis has not been needed.

341

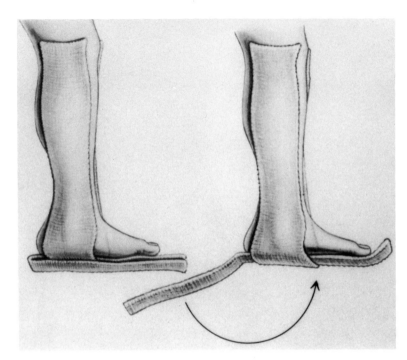

FIGURE 25–16. Plaster splint provides good support of the ankle and still allows some dorsiflexion. (From Müller ME, Allgöwer M, Schneider R, Willenegger H: Manual of Internal Fixation, 2nd Ed. Berlin, Springer-Verlag, 1979.)

bone fragment may be referred to as a Tillaux or a Chaput-Tillaux fragment, and it is sometimes large enough to be fixed as a separate fragment (Fig. 25–17). The medial malleolar fragment, when one exists, is a small, transverse avulsion that often requires tension band wiring due to its diminutive size.

Fractures of the fibula relatively close to the syndesmosis may leave much of the interosseous membrane intact (Fig. 25–17A). When this is true, direct repair of the syndesmosis or use of a syndesmotic screw may not be needed, as long as accurate reduction plus stable fixation of the fibula is possible.[40]

The importance of accurate and stable reduction of the syndesmosis should be clear, based on the conclusions of Leeds and Ehrlich.[28] They found a direct correlation between (1) the adequacy of reduction of the syndesmosis and late arthritis; (2) the adequacy of the initial reduction of the syndesmosis and the late stability of the syndesmosis; (3) the late stability of the syndesmosis and the final outcome; and (4) the adequacy of the reduction of the lateral malleolus and that of the syndesmosis. The relationship between the accuracy of reduction of the lateral malleolus fracture and the adequate reduction of the syndesmosis must be clearly understood (see Fig. 25–3).

Maisonneuve's Fracture

The Maisonneuve fracture is actually a variant of the AO type C2 in which the fibular fracture occurs in the proximal one-third of the fibula (Fig. 25–18). The patient may complain only of ankle pain and not be aware of the fibular fracture until it is palpated by the examining physician. The syndesmotic disruption that accompanies this injury may not be visible without the use of stress radiographs in which lateral translational force or valgus force, or both are applied to the ankle. This type of syndesmotic injury is not uncommonly missed by inexperienced emergency room personnel, with potentially disastrous long-term consequences for the patient's ankle function. Any patient evaluated for a severe ankle sprain should thus be examined with palpation of the proximal fibula and with radiographs of the proximal fibula as well.

Screw Fixation of the Syndesmosis

If radiographic (see Fig. 25–5) or clinical analysis indicates a need for syndesmotic fixation with transverse screws, the following points must be kept in mind: the syndesmotic screw is not a lag or compression screw but serves only to maintain position; to avoid dam-

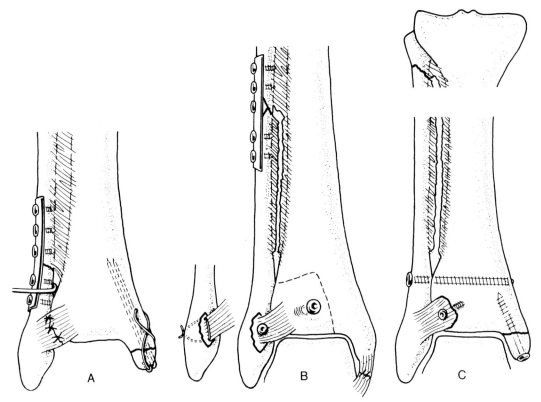

FIGURE 25–17. *(A),* Testing of the syndesmosis after fixation of the fractured fibula will determine whether repair is needed. *(B and C),* A Chaput-Tillaux fragment may be large enough to fix with lag screws. (From Müller ME, Allgöwer M, Schneider R, Willenegger H: Manual of Internal Fixation, 2nd Ed. Berlin, Springer-Verlag, 1979.)

age to the bony surfaces within the syndesmosis, screws should be placed at not less than 2 to 3 cm above the level of the plafond; because the screw will be subject to bending and shear forces with ordinary walking activities, there is a risk of screw breakage, and early removal of the screw at 6 to 8 weeks is recommended.

Technical Considerations. As described earlier, the fibula lies posterior to the tibia, and the drill for the transfixing screw must therefore be directed anteriorly about 25 to 30 degrees. Either a 3.5-mm or 4.5-mm cortical bone screw should be used, and each has some good and some bad features.

The 4.5-mm screw necessarily makes a sizable hole in the fibula, and if this screw is not inserted through a fibular plate, it may represent an unacceptable stress riser. However, the head of the screw is large, which makes the screw easy to retrieve without radiographic control under local anesthesia (see Fig. 25–18).

The modified AO 3.5-mm cortical screw has a 2.5-mm shank and is notably stronger than the older design with its 2.0-mm shank. It is probably strong enough for most cases, and if it is not, a second syndesmotic screw of the same size may be inserted. Although its 3.5-mm size makes it a smaller stress riser on removal, the screw is not so easily palpated or removed.

Author's Preferred Method. Although the syndesmotic screw is *not* to be used as a lag fixation, I prefer to drill a gliding hole in the fibula of appropriate (3.5-mm or 4.5-mm) size, with a threaded hole only in the lateral cortex of the tibia. The screw may then be inserted loosely, the ankle is brought into dorsiflexion, and the syndesmosis is reduced and held either by manual pressure or with a pointed reduction forceps applied with minimal tension. The screw is next tightened until its head contacts the surface of the fibular plate (or bone) *but no further.* At this point, an intraoperative mortise view radiograph will show the ade-

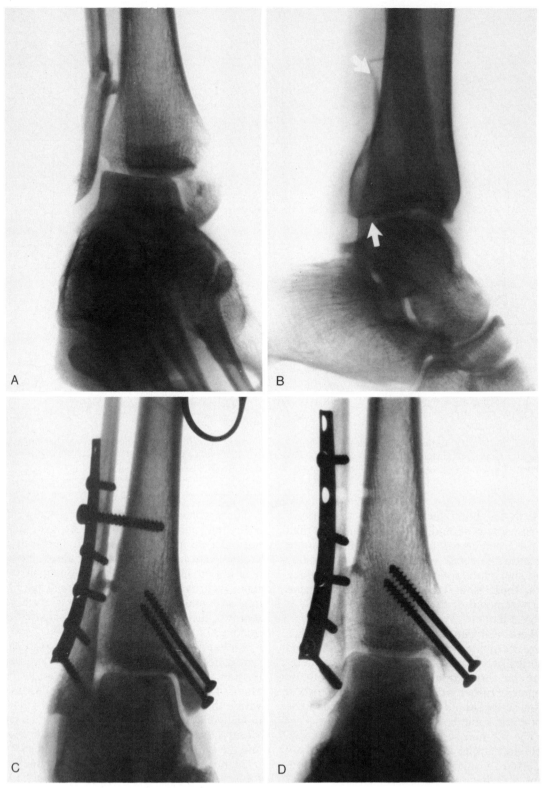

FIGURE 25–18. (A and B), An AO type C fracture with a long posterior spike on the fibular fragment and a small posterior margin fracture (arrows). (C), Syndesmosis fixation with a 4.5-mm cortical screw. The most distal screw in the fibular plate was too long and was exchanged. (D), Three months after syndesmosis screw removal, the defect left by the screw is still visible but is protected by the plate. A synostosis has formed distally.

quacy of reduction; if further closure of the mortise is required, the screw may be tightened one or two additional turns. Techniques that call for screw-thread purchase in the fibular cortices make such adjustment of the syndesmotic closure impossible without removal of the screw from the tibia and repositioning of the fibula.

The use of the gliding hole technique allows for slightly more toggle of the fibula on the screw and may thus reduce the bending forces applied to the screw. I have used this method for 10 years without failure of fixation or screw breakage.

FRACTURES OF THE TIBIAL PLAFOND

Two terms are frequently used interchangeably in describing fractures of the distal tibial articular surface, but they are different because one refers to the mechanism of injury and the other describes anatomic location. The pilon fracture was described by Destot. *Pilon* is the French term for the pestle of a mortar and pestle apparatus; the mechanism of injury is clearly one of impaction or compression.[1] *Plafond* is the French term for a roof or vault and therefore describes a location rather than a mechanism of injury. Logically, *plafond* should be used as a general term because all fractures of the distal tibial articular surface are by definition plafond fractures. The pilon fracture is a subtype of this injury caused by impaction of the talus on the tibia, and it is not present in every case. My choice is thus to describe the group of fractures as injuries of the plafond of the tibia.

These fractures, which constitute about 3 to 7 percent of all lower extremity fractures,[1, 3] have been a source of both interest and frustration for orthopaedic surgeons, as they require expert treatment for good long-term results but may have a disappointing outcome even in the best of hands.

Classification

Of several classifications that have been suggested,[1, 27] I prefer the approach of Mast and colleagues,[31] which refines and extends the previous AO system of Rüedi and Allgöwer (Table 25–3).[42] This classification clearly dif-

FRACTURE TYPE	DESCRIPTION AND MECHANISM
I	Severe malleolar fracture of AO type B (L-H varus–external rotation or valgus-dorsiflexion type) with large tibial plafond fragment; limited joint impaction
II	Distal tibial spiral fracture with extension of primarily nonarticular fracture to intra-articular level; little or no joint impaction
Pilon Fractures	
IIIA	Minimally displaced plafond fracture with two to three large fragments; caused by impaction
IIIB	Displaced plafond fracture with three to four large fragments; caused by impaction
IIIC	Severely comminuted, displaced plafond fracture; compressive bone loss in metaphysis often requires bone graft; caused by impaction

TABLE 25–3. **AO TIBIAL PLAFOND FRACTURE CLASSIFICATION AS MODIFIED BY MAST**

ferentiates between the fractures caused largely by torsional forces, combined with some component of axial load due to valgus, varus, or dorsiflexion (type I and II fractures), and the more purely compressive or impact injuries (type IIIA, IIIB, and IIIC fractures), which have a far worse prognosis.

In the majority of reviews of the plafond fracture, the results of treatment are similar: the type I, II, IIIA, and IIIB fractures do well when treated surgically by those skilled in the management of these injuries. The surgeon should expect 70 to 80 percent good results in these cases.[1, 4, 23] In the severely comminuted, displaced fractures, most surgeons report poor results in 40 to 55 percent of cases.[1, 3–5, 23, 31, 37] The reasons for failure of treatment in these cases are nonanatomic reduction, unstable fixation, infection, nonunion, and angulation.[4]

The challenges and risks of surgery are multiple, but in the most severely comminuted cases, nonoperative treatment usually fails.[1, 4]

Nevertheless, surgical treatment is carried out through some of the most limited soft tissues in the body, where the bone is largely subcutaneous. In displaced fractures, the skin is often damaged by the bone fragments, even when it has not been actually penetrated. The cortical bone of the tibial metaphysis is very thin, and the underlying cancellous bone is often crushed or "missing," making fixation with plates and screws tedious and sometimes undependable.

Author's Preferred Method of Treatment

I agree with Mast and colleagues[31] and others that if surgery is to be performed, it must either be accomplished within 10 to 12 hours of injury or be postponed for a week or more, until soft tissue swelling subsides and it can be certain that wound closure can be accomplished without undue skin tension. For injuries in which a long delay is inevitable, such as those with fracture blisters that form early, skeletal traction is advisable. Especially for type IIIB and IIIC fractures, calcaneal pin traction helps re-establish and maintain tibial

length before operation. The patient should always give permission for adjunctive bone grafting, although with many fracture types other than IIIC, it may not be needed.

The patient is positioned as for treatment of a malleolar fracture, with a large roller under the ipsilateral hip to allow easy access to the lateral side of the ankle. In almost all cases, tourniquet control is appropriate.

The surgical approach is that popularized by the AO,[34] with the fibula reached through an incision a bit posterior to the midline of the bone in order to maximize the skin bridge between the medial and lateral wounds (Fig. 25–19). In no case should the skin bridge be less than 7 cm in width. If the fibula is fractured, it should be fixed first in most cases to help maintain the length of the tibia and to stabilize the fracture (Figs. 25–20 and 25–21).

The tibia is exposed through an incision that begins proximally 1 cm lateral to the anterior tibial crest and curves gently over the anterior ankle joint, along the anterior edge of the medial malleolus to its tip. The paratenon of the anterior tibial tendon must be preserved so that if wound healing is delayed, the tendon will accept a skin graft.[31] The only major

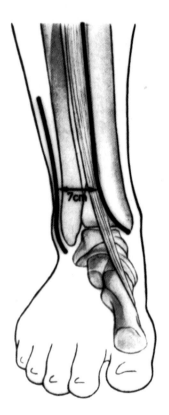
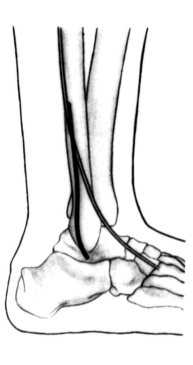

FIGURE 25–19. The suggested approach for many distal tibial fractures. If fibular dissection is needed, the skin bridge must not be less than 7 cm. (From Müller ME, Allgöwer M, Schneider R, Willenegger H: Manual of Internal Fixation, 2nd Ed. Berlin, Springer-Verlag, 1979.)

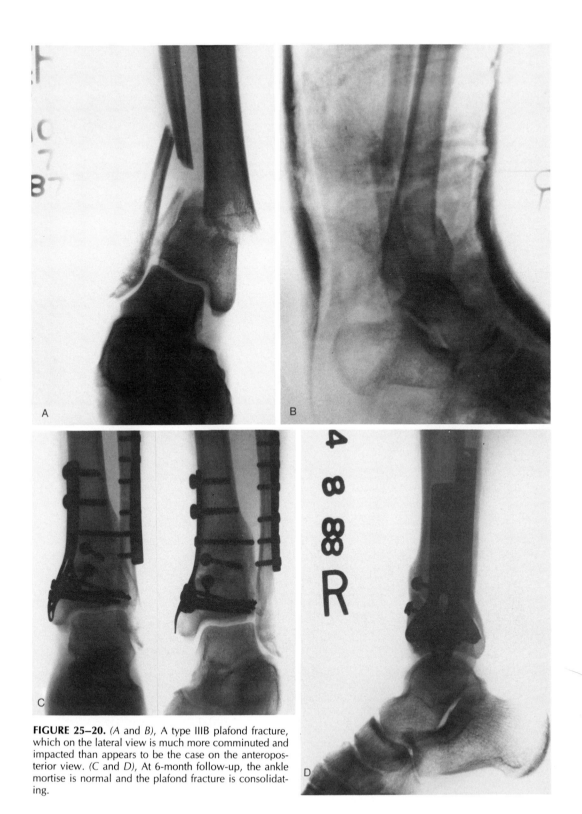

FIGURE 25–20. (A and B), A type IIIB plafond fracture, which on the lateral view is much more comminuted and impacted than appears to be the case on the anteroposterior view. (C and D), At 6-month follow-up, the ankle mortise is normal and the plafond fracture is consolidating.

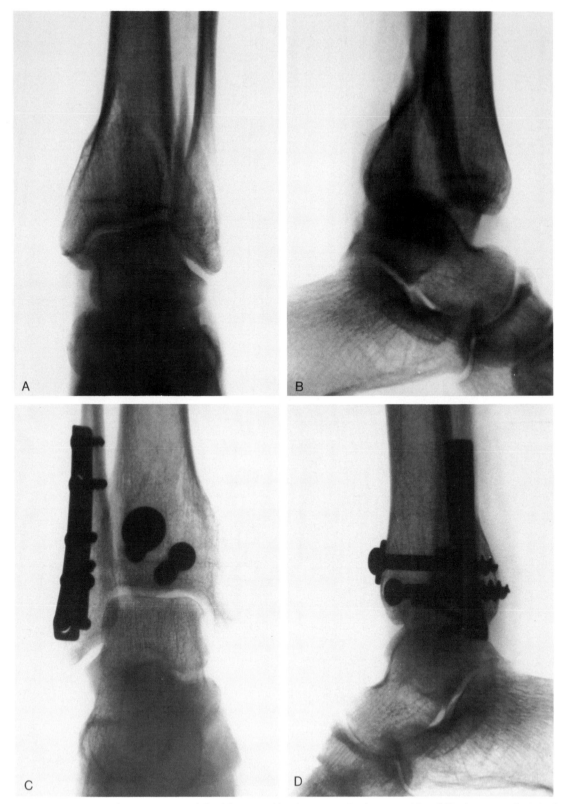

FIGURE 25–21. *(A and B)*, A type IIIA plafond fracture with a large posterior fragment. *(C and D)*, At 1 year, the joint is well preserved after lag screw fixation.

vascular structure crossing the incision, the greater saphenous vein, is isolated and tagged with a small rubber sling for manipulation during surgery. No undermining of the skin is tolerated in this area: full-thickness flaps down to the level of the periosteum are the rule, and

the extensor retinaculum is divided before any real exposure is accomplished.

A useful aid to reduction of these fractures during surgery is the application of an external fixator[23] or the AO femoral distractor[31, 34] spanning the tibia and talus (Fig. 25–22). The talus

FIGURE 25–22. *(A and B)*, The femoral distractor can simplify reduction of severely comminuted plafond fractures. (From Mast J, Jakob R, Ganz R: Planning and Reduction Technique in Fracture Surgery. Berlin, Springer-Verlag, 1989.)

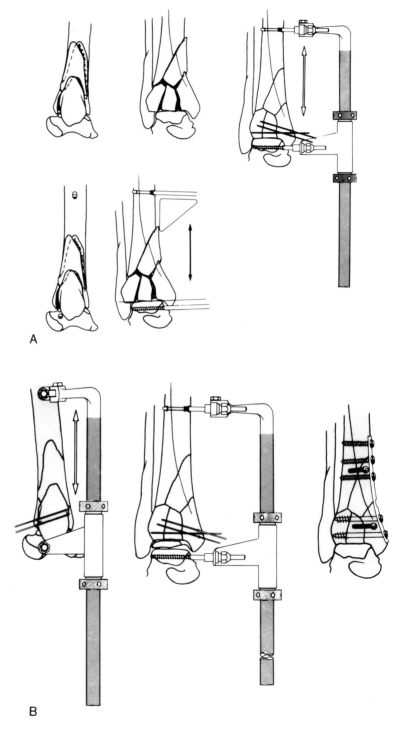

A

B

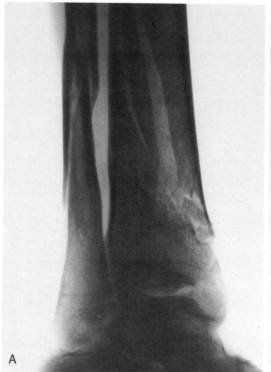

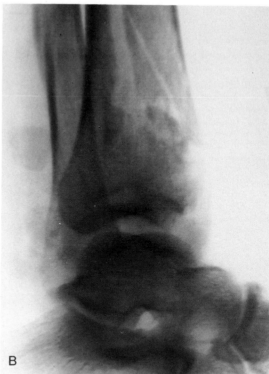

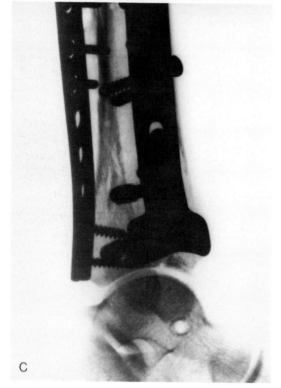

FIGURE 25–23. *(A* and *B)*, Comminuted, impacted fracture of the tibial plafond. *(C)*, After fixation, the ankle joint is well maintained. The hole used for anchoring the distractor pin in the talus is clearly visible.

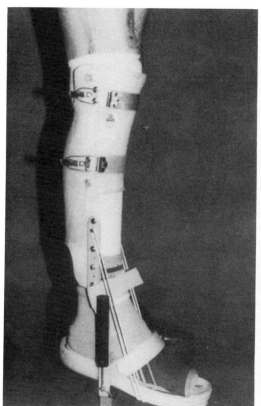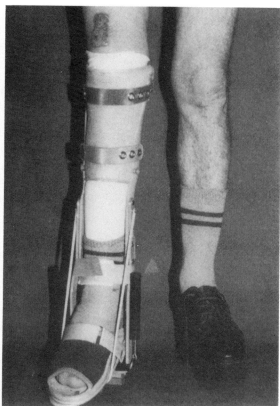

FIGURE 25–24. A caliper brace fitted for rehabilitation and ambulation after plafond fracture. This relieves the ankle joint of most weight-bearing stresses. (From Hanke J: Luxationsfrakturen des oberen Sprunggelenkes. Berlin, Springer-Verlag, 1989.)

may be safely transfixed from the medial side at a point just below the medial malleolus (Fig. 25–23).

Fixation hardware should be of minimum size to accomplish the task at hand and not increase skin tension. The surgeon must remember that in this area, fixation most often fails because of weak, comminuted, and sometimes necrotic bone, not because of screw or plate breakage. The lever arms acting in this area are small during non–weight-bearing range-of-motion exercises, in contrast to the more proximal parts of the extremity.

Postoperative care is as described previously for malleolar fractures, with elevation and early motion used to minimize swelling and stiffness. Continuous passive mobilization, when available, is likely to be a useful adjunct.

The patellar tendon–bearing caliper brace may be used to allow the patient to walk while relieving the injured joint of any axial load (Fig. 25–24). Because non–weight-bearing status may be protracted to 12 weeks or more in severe injuries, such braces, although rather costly, may be worth the expense in terms of increased patient mobility and improved psychological well-being.

OPEN FRACTURES AND FRACTURE-DISLOCATIONS

Open fractures and fracture-dislocations are devastating injuries. Occurring in an area of limited soft tissue coverage, they require the emergent treatment directed toward any open musculoskeletal injury, with urgent irrigation and débridement as the foundation of any other treatment.

Acute stabilization of the open fracture or fracture-dislocation may be with external fixation[3] or with immediate internal fixation,[6, 9] with delayed wound closure or skin grafting as indicated. The results of treatment vary with the severity of soft tissue injury, but stabilization of the injury at the earliest time appears to enhance the outcome in most cases. Non-salvageable limbs should be amputated early to spare the patient the physiologic and psychological burdens of long hospitalization and multiple surgical procedures (Fig. 25–25).[21, 24]

FUTURE DEVELOPMENTS: ALLOGRAFT RECONSTRUCTION

I am familiar with the results of allograft reconstruction for post-traumatic degeneration of the ankle joint from two surgeons[10, 11] with a minimum of 2 years of follow-up (Figs. 25–26 and 25–27). Although in many instances ankle arthrodesis may provide patients with excellent function and pain relief, preservation of joint function, if possible, is certainly preferable. Allograft reconstruction, which is mentioned by Hanke,[14] shows promise in carefully selected patients under the care of technically accomplished practitioners and is a logical extension of the increasing use of allograft reconstruction in nontumor cases.

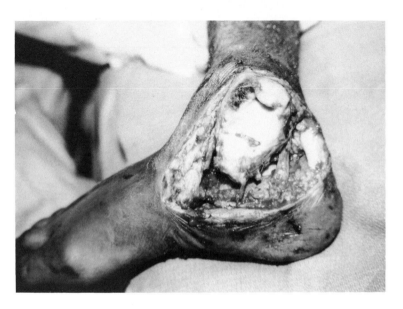

FIGURE 25–25. Open fracture-dislocation of the ankle joint, which was accompanied by severe neurovascular injuries. The patient accepted early amputation because his foot was insensate and dysvascular.

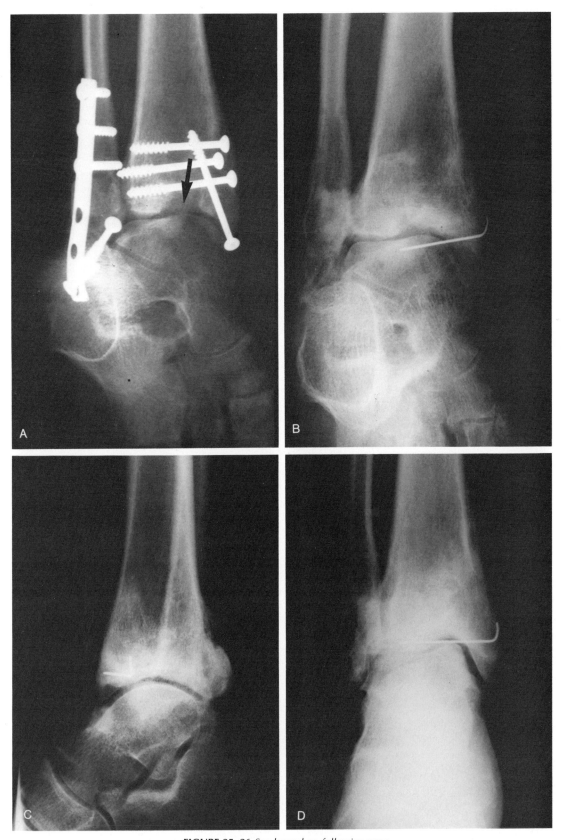

FIGURE 25–26 *See legend on following page*

Illustration continued on following page

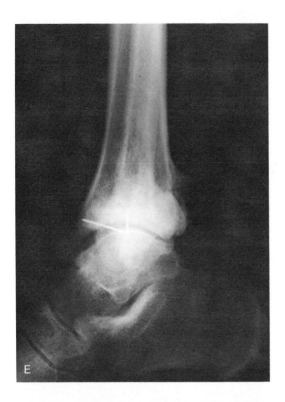

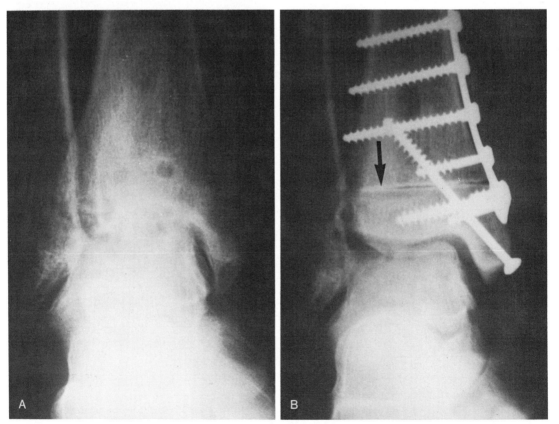

FIGURE 25–26. (A), Oblique view of a tibial plafond fracture treated with internal fixation. An osteocartilaginous defect is present *(arrow)*, and the ankle is symptomatic. *(B and C)*, After osteocartilage allografting to fill the defect, the joint space is preserved. *(D and E)*, At over 2 years, the joint space is still visible and the patient has painless weight-bearing function and moderate range of motion. (Courtesy of Christoph Geel, M.D., Syracuse, NY.)

FIGURE 25–27. (A), Severe posttraumatic arthritis in a young patient who has pain and decreased function. *(B)*, A large osteocartilage allograft at 2 years. Joint function is satisfactory, and the graft is incorporating on the lateral side of the plafond *(arrow)*. (Courtesy of John C. Garrett, M.D., Atlanta, GA.)

354

References

1. Ayeni JP: Pilon fractures of the tibia: A study based on 19 cases. Injury 19:109–114, 1988.
2. Baird RA, Jackson ST: Fractures of the distal part of the fibula with associated disruption of the deltoid ligament. Treatment without repair of the deltoid ligament. J Bone Joint Surg 69A:1346–1352, 1987.
3. Bone LB: Fractures of the tibial plafond. The pilon fracture. Orthop Clin North Am 18:95–104, 1987.
4. Bourne RB, Rorabeck CH, MacNab BA: Intra-articular fractures of the distal tibia: The pilon fracture. J Trauma 23:591–596, 1983.
5. Brennan MJ: Tibial pilon fractures. Instr Course Lect 39:167–170, 1990.
6. Chapman M, Mahoney M: The role of early internal fixation in the management of open fractures. Clin Orthop 138:120–131, 1979.
7. Charnley J: The Potts fracture. *In* The Closed Treatment of Common Fractures. Edinburgh, Churchill Livingstone, 1961, pp 250–269.
8. Chojnacki DJ, Wertheimer S: Internal fixation of malleolar fractures using the A.O. tension band wiring techniques. J Foot Surg 22:69–72, 1983.
9. Franklin JL, Johnson KD, Hansen ST Jr: Immediate internal fixation of open ankle fractures. Report of thirty-eight cases treated with a standard protocol. J Bone Joint Surg 66A:1349–1356, 1984.
10. Garrett JC, personal communication.
11. Geel C, personal correspondence. State University of New York Medical Center, Syracuse, NY.
12. Grantham SA: Trimalleolar ankle fractures and open ankle fractures. Instr Course Lect 39:105–111, 1990.
13. Hall H: A simplified workable classification of ankle fractures. *In* Bateman JE, Trott AW (Eds): The Foot and Ankle. New York, Thieme-Stratton, 1980, pp 5–10.
14. Hanke J: Diskussion. *In* Luxationsfrakturen des oberen Sprunggelenkes. Berlin, Springer-Verlag, 1988, pp 101–110.
15. Harper MC: An anatomic study of the short oblique fracture of the distal fibula and ankle stability. Foot Ankle 4:23–29, 1983.
16. Harper MC: Posterior instability of the talus: An anatomic evaluation. Foot Ankle 10:36–39, 1989.
17. Harper MC: Talar shift. The stabilizing role of the medial, lateral, and posterior ankle structures. Clin Orthop 257:177–183, 1990.
18. Heim UFA: Trimalleolar fractures: Late results after fixation of the posterior fragment. Orthopedic 12:1053–1059, 1989.
19. Hughes JL: The medial malleolus in ankle fractures. Orthop Clin North Am 11:649–660, 1980.
20. Inman VT: The Joints of the Ankle. Baltimore, Williams & Wilkins, 1976.
21. Johansen K, Daines M, Howey T, et al: Objective criteria accurately predict amputation following lower extremity trauma. J Trauma 30:568–572, 1990.
22. Kaye RA: Stabilization of ankle syndesmosis injuries with a syndesmosis screw. Foot Ankle 9:290–293, 1989.
23. Kellam JF, Waddell JP: Fractures of the distal tibia metaphysis with intraarticular extension—the distal tibia explosion fracture. J Trauma 19:593–601, 1979.
24. Lange RH, Bach AW, Hansen ST Jr, Johansen KH: Open tibial fractures with associated vascular injuries: Prognosis for limb salvage. J Trauma 25:203–208, 1985.
25. Lauge-Hansen N: Fractures of the ankle: Analytic historic survey as the basis of new roentgenologic and clinical investigations. Arch Surg 56:259–317, 1948.
26. Lauge-Hansen N: Fractures of the ankle: II. Combined experimental-surgical and experimental-roentgenologic investigations. Arch Surg 60:957–985, 1950.
27. Lauge-Hansen N: Fractures of the ankle: V. Pronation-dorsiflexion fractures. Arch Surg 67:813–820, 1953.
28. Leeds HC, Ehrlich MG: Instability of the distal tibiofibular syndesmosis after bimalleolar and trimalleolar ankle fractures. J Bone Joint Surg 66A:490–503, 1984.
29. Lindsjö U: Classification of ankle fractures: The Lauge-Hansen or AO system. Clin Orthop 199:12–16, 1985.
30. Mast J, Jakob R, Ganz R: Planning and Reduction Technique in Fracture Surgery. Berlin, Springer-Verlag, 1989.
31. Mast JW, Spiegel PG, Pappas JN: Fractures of the tibial pilon. Clin Orthop 230:68–82, 1988.
32. Mast JW, Teipner WA: A reproducible approach to fixation of adult ankle fractures: Rationale, technique and early results. Orthop Clin North Am 11:661–769, 1980.
33. McLennan JG, Ungersma J: Evaluation of the treatment of ankle fractures with the Inyo nail. J Orthop Trauma 2:272–276, 1988.
34. Müller ME, Allgöwer M, Schneider R, Willenegger H: Manual of Internal Fixation, 2nd Ed. Berlin, Springer-Verlag, 1979.
35. Olerud C, Molander H: Atypical pronation-eversion ankle joint fractures. Arch Orthop Trauma Surg 102:201–202, 1984.
36. Ostrum R, Litsky A: Unstable ankle fractures. Orthop Consultation June–July:5–12, 1990.
37. Ovadia DN, Beals RN: Fractures of the tibial plafond. J Bone Joint Surg 68A:543–551, 1986.
38. Ramsey PL, Hamilton W: Changes in tibio-talar area of contact caused by lateral talar shift. J Bone Joint Surg 58A:356, 1976.
39. Reuwer JH, Van Straaten TJ: Evaluation of operative treatment of 193 ankle fractures. Neth J Surg 36:98–102, 1984.
40. Riegels-Nielsen P, Christensen J, Greiff J: The stability of the tibio-fibular syndesmosis following rigid internal fixation for type C malleolar fractures: An experimental and clinical study. Injury 14:357–360, 1983.
41. Roberts RS: Surgical treatment of displaced ankle fractures. Clin Orthop Jan–Feb:164–170, 1983.
42. Rüedi TP, Allgöwer M: The operative treatment of intra-articular fractures of the lower end of the tibia. Clin Orthop 138:105–110, 1979.
43. Willenegger H, Weber BG: Malleolar fractures. *In* Müller ME, Allgöwer M, Willenegger H (Eds): Technique of Internal Fixation of Fractures. Berlin, Springer-Verlag, 1963, pp 112–145.
44. Wilson FC: Fractures and dislocations of the ankle. *In* Rockwood CA, Green DP (Eds): Fractures in Adults. Philadelphia, JB Lippincott, 1984, pp 1665–1702.
45. Yablon IG: Treatment of ankle malunion. Instr Course Lect 33:118–123, 1984.
46. Yablon IG, Heller FG, Shouse L: The key role of the lateral malleolus in displaced fractures of the ankle. J Bone Joint Surg 59A:169–173, 1977.
47. Yablon IG, Wasilewski S: Management of unstable ankle fractures. *In* Bateman JE, Trott AW (Eds): The Foot and Ankle. New York, Thieme-Stratton, 1980, pp 11–19.

26

Late Reconstruction of Complex Ankle Fractures and Dislocations

JAMES B. STIEHL

TRAUMATIC ARTHRITIS

The long-term complications of traumatic injury of the ankle joint are related to the degree of articular surface damage, the severity of the fracture, and the amount of actual disruption of the normal anatomy of the joint. Cartilage of the ankle joint will normally repair itself after certain impact loads, but exaggerated forces can kill cartilage cells at the microscopic level, leading to permanent joint damage.[50]

Fractures and ligamentous disruption alter the normal anatomic relationships, leading to stress overload of the joint surfaces. Ramsay and Hamilton found loss of normal articular congruity with 1 mm of lateral talar shift.[33] Macko and colleagues found significant experimental alteration in joint reaction forces with loss of a posterior malleolar fragment from simulated fracture.[21] Nepola investigated articular congruity with talar shift from fibular diastasis using pressure-sensitive film and did not identify the diminished joint surface contact suggested by Ramsay and Hamilton. Other factors, such as joint instability and altered joint mechanics, may be even more important in causing joint destruction.[29]

Numerous clinical reports have demonstrated that articular anatomy must be perfectly restored in order for a good result to be achieved. If that goal is not accomplished, traumatic arthrosis is the likely outcome.[44] The exact cause of degenerative arthritis at the microscopic level remains unclear, but structural changes are well recognized. There is a radiographic decrease in joint space and formation of sclerotic joint margins, peripheral osteophytes, and subchondral cysts.

A typical history includes morning stiffness or pain until the person has had a chance to "loosen up." Symptoms are aggravated by prolonged walking and standing. "Change of weather" aches are common.[23] Physical examination demonstrates localized joint line tenderness, and slight warmth may be detectable over the joint. There is pain at the extremes of range of motion, which becomes more restricted as time passes. Bony proliferation can be palpated and occasionally visualized along the malleoli.

Conservative Treatment

All patients should undergo conservative treatment initially, which should include anti-inflammatory medication and the judicious use of local corticosteroid injections. As stress overload and instability are the causes of progression, modification of activity should be encouraged. Overweight patients should be encouraged to lose weight, and those with jobs involving standing or walking should switch to more sedentary ones if possible.

Orthotic devices should be tried, including polypropylene ankle foot orthoses or double upright braces, with the axis fixed in the neutral position. Rocker-bottom shoes or SACH (solid-ankle, cushioned-heel) modifications reduce stress in the ankle.[22, 23]

356

Operative Management

Arthrodesis remains the treatment of choice for relief of pain and instability in patients with disabling tibiotalar arthritis. The vast majority of patients should wait at least 1 year before this operation is considered. Davis and Millis found the average time to fusion secondary to trauma was 12 months in 48 cases.[11] Morrey and Wiedeman similarly found that more than one-half of their post-traumatic arthrodesis patients required fusion within 12 months after injury.[27]

Certain post-traumatic injuries require very early or "primary" arthrodesis, but this should be considered only as a last resort. Such patients have bone loss, severe tissue injury, or comminution involving both the distal tibia articular surface and talus.[43]

Morrey and Wiedeman found a higher rate of complications in the post-traumatic arthrodesis group, including infection, nonunion, and malunion.[27] Davis and Millis noted an infection rate of 22 percent in their series, and 39 of 48 patients complained of persistent pain that originated in the subtalar joint.[11]

At least 30 different methods have been devised for ankle arthrodesis.[24] Because of the diversity of problems and evolving surgical techniques, future modifications are likely. However, any ankle arthrodesis should include the following components: (1) tibiotalar compression arthrodesis with internal or external fixation; (2) fibular osteotomy to shorten the relative length compared with the normal joint line and to narrow the distal fibula; (3) medial malleolar osteotomy to narrow the medial side of the ankle; (4) careful and appropriate surgical approach to avoid skin slough and damage to neurovascular structures; and (5) bone grafting to fill in defects in difficult situations. Whatever surgical technique is used, the optimum result depends on positioning the ankle arthrodesis in neutral to 5 degrees of plantar flexion and 5 to 10 degrees of external rotation. Slight heel valgus may be allowed, but varus and dorsiflexion should be meticulously avoided.[8, 22, 25–27, 36]

In traumatic cases, choice of surgical approach is multifactorial. Patients at high risk for complications are those with previous infection, severe soft tissue injury with tenuous skin or surgical scars, significant talar avascularity, spasticity, or neurotrophic joint. Any surgical technique should take the safest approach to limit the pseudarthrosis, infection, and reflex sympathetic dystrophy that can occur after these procedures. Total ankle arthroplasty has been investigated as an alternative to ankle arthrodesis, but most authors would recommend that this procedure be avoided in young healthy individuals with single joint involvement.[6, 47] Arthroscopic techniques for ankle arthrodesis have been attempted but remain experimental.

We recommend the following three basic techniques with possible modifications: (1) simple arthrodesis through an anterior approach with percutaneous three-screw internal fixation; (2) arthrodesis using medial and lateral incisions with medial and lateral malleolar osteotomy and internal fixation; (3) arthrodesis, using any of above methods, combined with external fixation; and (4) tibiocalcaneal arthrodesis, from an anterior or posterior approach, for salvage.

Anterior Arthrodesis

Anterior arthrodesis has become popular in recent years because of its limited exposure and the use of three screws directed from medial, lateral, and posterior. It is most appropriate in cases of limited soft tissue trauma and when there is no risk of potential skin slough from previous incisions. It may be contraindicated when previous screws and plates have been inserted or when fibular osteotomy may be required, because of shortening needed to compensate for joint loss. This approach should also be avoided in patients with suspected vascular damage to the posterior tibial artery or absent posterior pulse.[19]

Technique

The anterior approach described by Colonna is used (Fig. 26–1).[9, 15] After elevation of the tourniquet, the incision begins on the anterior aspect of the ankle and extends 6 cm proximal to and 5 cm below the joint line. Extreme caution should be used in identifying the superficial peroneal nerve branches. The deep fascia is divided in line with the skin incision. The approach is developed between the extensor hallucis longus and extensor digitorum longus. The anterior tibial artery and deep peroneal nerve are identified and protected medially. The capsule, synovium, and perios-

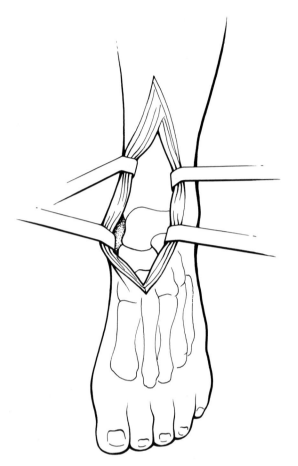

FIGURE 26–1. Anterior approach to the ankle joint. Extensor hallucis longus and anterior tibial tendons and neurovascular bundle are retracted medially. Extensor digitorum longus is retracted laterally. (Redrawn from Colonna PC, Ralston EL: Operative approaches to the ankle joint. Am J Surg 52:44, 1951.)

teum of the anterior ankle joint are exposed to gain full access to the articular surface exactly perpendicular to the long axis of the leg. A similar cut is made on the surface of the talus. Cartilage and subchondral bone are removed sparingly until viable cancellous bone is visualized; usually no more than 5 to 10 mm of shortening occurs. The abutting surfaces of the medial and lateral malleoli are removed, and adjustments are made until perfect apposition of articular surfaces is accomplished. At this point, foot position is assessed, seeking anatomic neutral or slight equinus angulation, neutral or slight valgus heel position, and 5 to 10 degrees of foot external rotation comparable to the contralateral normal side. The pos-

terior screw is the most difficult to insert; a cannulated 6.5-mm cancellous lag screw and image intensification may be helpful. Another method is an indirect one in which a 4.5-mm hole is drilled from the joint surface proximally and posteriorly. A suction tip is inserted through the distal hole to serve as a guide for a 3.2-mm drill inserted percutaneously through the skin and into the talus. A 6.5-mm screw is inserted into the dense talar bone, and 6.5-mm cancellous screws are inserted obliquely through the medial and lateral malleoli into the talus. Rigid stability should be achieved, and screws must not enter the subtalar joint (Fig. 26–2). To facilitate screw insertion, a large smooth Steinmann pin may be placed through the sole of the foot into the distal tibia. This can be removed after screw insertion but can be left if rigid stability is not present. Intraoperative radiographs assess foot position and ensure that screws have not entered the subtalar joint. Bone chips are used to fill any defects at the fusion site. The wound is closed routinely over a drain, and a bulky dressing with posterior plaster splint is applied. A modification of the above technique involves use of an anterior AO spoon plate instead of three screws (Fig. 26–3).[28]

Postoperative Care and Rehabilitation

The patient is kept non–weight bearing for 6 weeks, and the initial splint is taken off at 10 to 14 days and the sutures are removed. A new short-leg cast is applied for 4 weeks, and a short-leg walking cast is used for an additional 6 weeks. Once clinical and radiologic union are ensured, the patient is allowed unprotected weight bearing and encouraged to resume normal activities. An appropriate heel lift and rocker-bottom sole are indicated for all patients to increase comfort. If radiographic union is likely, but the patient has persistent discomfort, a removable ankle-foot orthosis may be used for an additional 6 to 12 weeks. The presence of reflex sympathetic dystrophy should not be overlooked and should be treated aggressively at this point.

Transmalleolar Arthrodesis

This approach has been utilized in ankle arthrodesis by numerous authors and has an

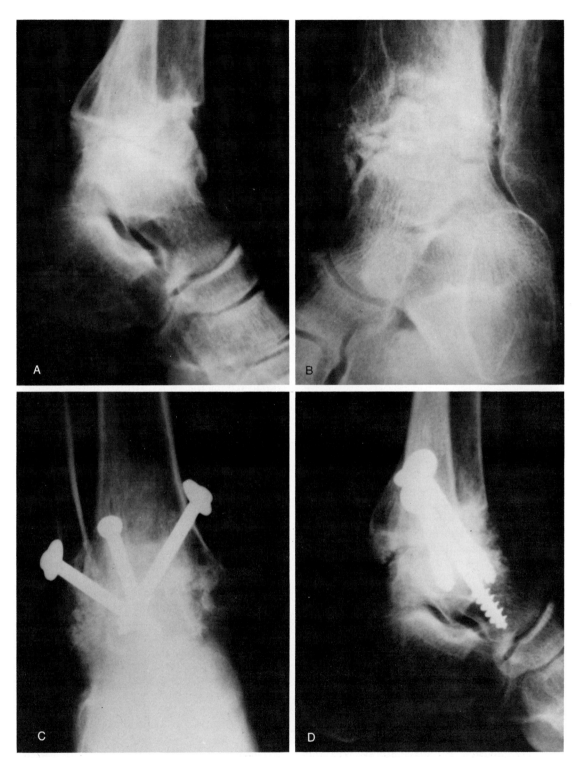

FIGURE 26–2. (*A* to *D*), Clinical example of the anterior approach for ankle arthrodesis using medial-, lateral-, and anterior-directed screws placed percutaneously for internal fixation.

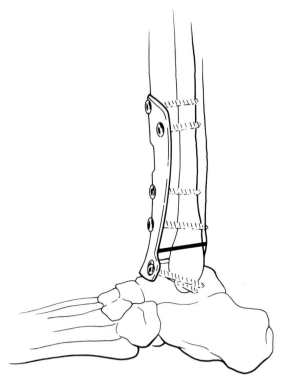

FIGURE 26–3. AO spoon plate for anterior internal fixation. (Redrawn from Müller ME, Allgöwer M, Schneider R, Willenegger H: Manual of Internal Fixation: Techniques Recommended by the AO Group. New York, Springer-Verlag, 1979.)

excellent rate of success.* The particular advantage in traumatic situations is the ability to use previous operative incisions and to gain access to previously placed hardware. Also, the foot can be narrowed by osteotomizing the medial malleolus and distal fibula. With greater articular loss, the fibula must be shortened to restore the normal relationship to the foot. If soft tissues are adequate, internal fixation is sufficient.[38] Otherwise, minimal internal fixation combined with external compression fixation is used (Fig. 26–4).

Several authors recommend excision of the distal fibula, but incorporating the fibula as a lateral bone plate may add strength to the fusion and allow for better peroneal tendon function.[34] Similarly, retaining the posterior beak of the medial malleolus may preserve the pulley for the posterior tibial tendon (Fig. 26–5).[39] The incision is anterolateral over the distal fibula and ankle joint, extending 8 cm

---

*See references 1, 2, 13, 19, 24, 26, 42, 45, and 48.

from the tip of the lateral malleolus proximally. The distal tibiofibular joint is identified, and the syndesmotic ligaments are removed. Osteotomy of the fibula is done 3 to 4 cm above the joint line. A second cut is made if shortening of the fibula is needed to restore the anatomic relation to the lateral talus. The medial one-third of the distal fibula is removed, and the lateral distal tibia and talus are decorticated and contoured to match the fibular surface. The distal fibula thus becomes a lateral bone plate or strut (Figs. 26–6 and 26–7).[42, 49] A second incision is made medially, starting over the tip of the medial malleolus and extending proximally for 8 cm. The periosteum of the medial aspect of the tibia and the deltoid ligaments are reflected (Fig. 26–8), and the medial malleolus is resected in line with the medial shaft of the distal tibia. It is possible to save the posterior one-third of the medial malleolus to protect the neurovascular structures and posterior tibial tendon. At this point, the distal tibial surface can be resected in a plane perpendicular to the long axis of the tibia and the superior articular surface of the talus resected in a line parallel to the longitudinal axis of the foot. Adjustments are made for the ideal neutral position of the ankle and heel, and external rotation of the foot is accomplished. Temporary fixation is obtained using Kirschner wires inserted from the tibia distally into the talus. The fibula is fixed using a 6.5-mm cancellous screw into the distal tibia, and a second 6.5-mm screw into the talus, avoiding the subtalar joint. A small T-plate is then applied to the medial side, using a tensioning device to gain compression prior to final screw fixation (Fig. 26–9).[34] Temporary fixation is removed, and bone grafting is done as needed. Final radiographs should confirm the desired foot position. Closure over a drain is done in the usual fashion, and a bulky dressing, with posterior splint, is applied. Modifications include using a large Steinmann pin through the sole of the foot for stability and a second T-plate laterally with excision of the fibula.

External Fixation in Arthrodesis

The Charnley compression technique for ankle arthrodesis has been standard for many years. Biomechanical improvements have created more stable reconstructions, using pins in

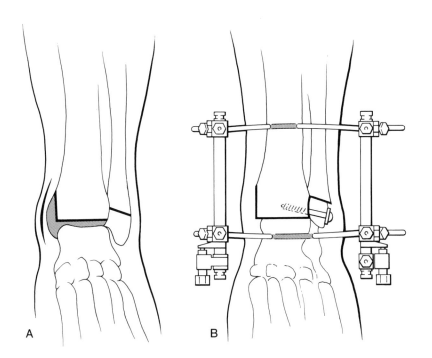

A   B

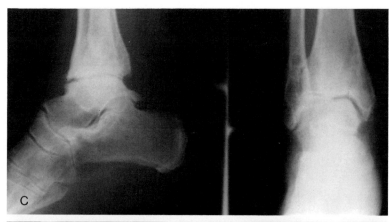

C

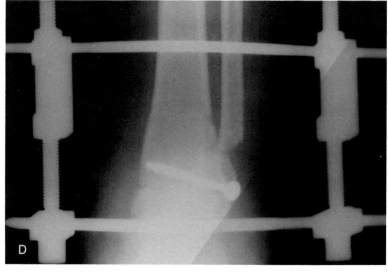

D

FIGURE 26–4. (A), Technique of ankle arthrodesis using medial and lateral incisions, osteotomy of medial malleolus, and osteotomy of fibula with shortening. (B), Minimal internal fixation of distal fibula and external fixation with AO external fixation clamps. (C to F), Clinical example of satisfactory arthrodesis using this technique.

Illustration continued on following page

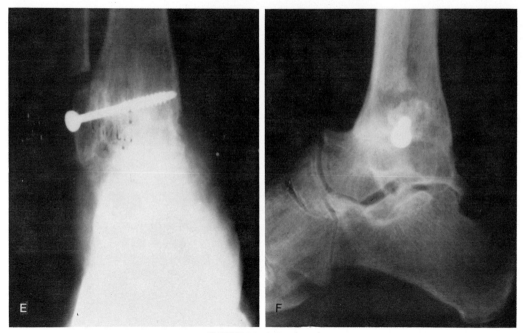

FIGURE 26–4 *Continued*

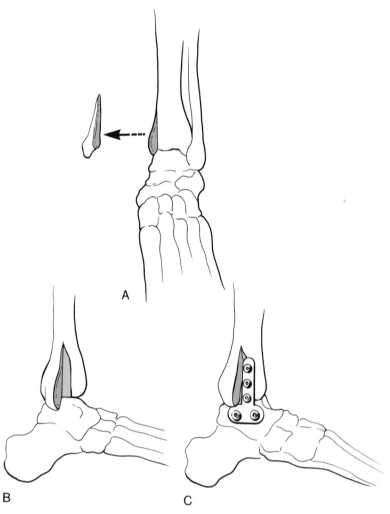

FIGURE 26–5. (*A* to *C*), Posterior beak of medial malleolus is maintained to protect posterior tibial tendon and neurovascular structures. Internal fixation with AO small fragment T-plate. (Redrawn from Scranton PE Jr: Use of internal compression in arthrodesis of the ankle. J Bone Joint Surg 67A:553, 1985.)

A

B   C

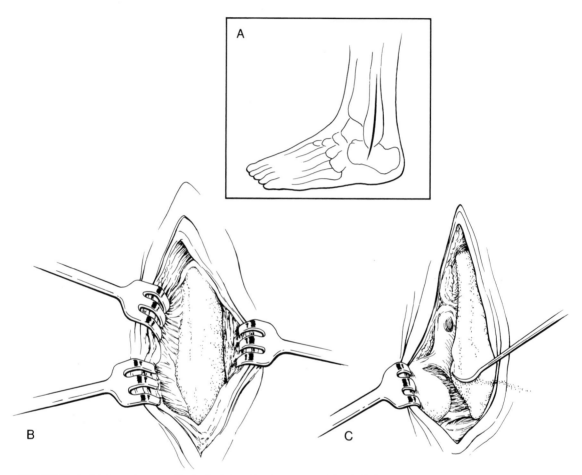

FIGURE 26–6. *(A)*, Lateral transmalleolar incision. *(B)*, Osteotomy of distal fibula and incision of anteroinferior tibiofibular ligament and syndesmosis. *(C)*, Exposure of lateral ankle joint.

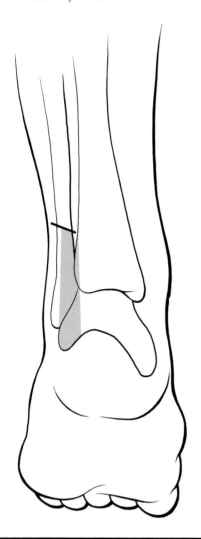

FIGURE 26–7. Removal of medial fibula and lateral distal tibia and lateral talus.

a triangular configuration (Figs. 26–10 and 26–11).[4, 14, 18, 28, 46] In addition to providing stability when internal fixation is inadequate, external frames are advantageous in certain traumatic cases. Previous sepsis, necrotic intra-articular fractures, and previous soft tissue trauma with resultant scarring are other indications for external fixation.

Severely comminuted fractures involving the distal tibia and talar dome may require fusion within the first 3 weeks of injury. The talar distal pin insertion is not possible in this situation, and a triangular frame is constructed using two pins through the calcaneus, away from the neurovascular bundle, with extension to the first metatarsal. Kenzora and associates

advise using slight distraction to avoid damage to the subtalar joint.[18] These frames can be left in place for up to 3 months (Fig. 26–12).

Technique

External fixation utilizes percutaneous pin fixation through separate 1-cm stab incisions. The neurovascular structures must be meticulously avoided. Predrilling of all pin sites is mandatory, especially in dense cortical bone. Appropriate pin guides are used to avoid soft tissue damage, and pins are inserted by hand through the predrilled holes. Compression across the exposed bone surfaces can be done, once the frame is applied. Further skin release is done after final adjustment to avoid tenting. Ointments and salves are avoided, and pin tracts are cleansed daily with hydrogen peroxide.

Tibiocalcaneal Arthrodesis

This fusion is indicated in salvage situations that may result from complex fracture-dislo-

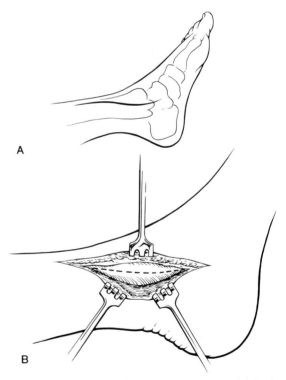

FIGURE 26–8. (A), Medial incision. (B), Incision of deltoid ligament and periosteum.

FIGURE 26–9. Medial and lateral tensioning device applied to small fragment T-plates. (Redrawn from Ross SK, Matta JM: Internal compression arthrodesis of the ankle. Clin Orthop 199:54, 1985.)

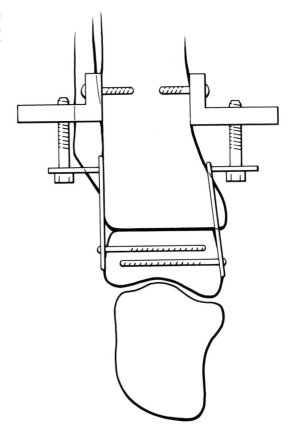

FIGURE 26–10. (*A* to *C*), Calandruccio frame demonstrates three-point fixation of the talus to the distal tibia.

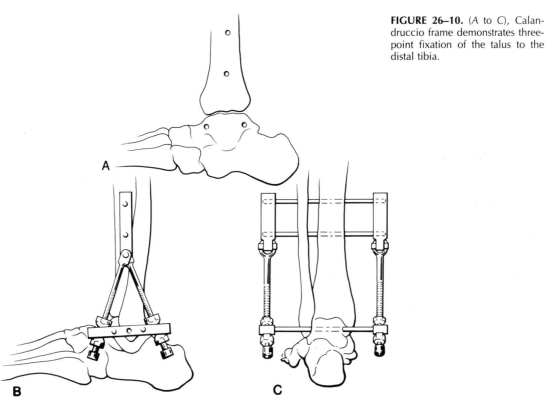

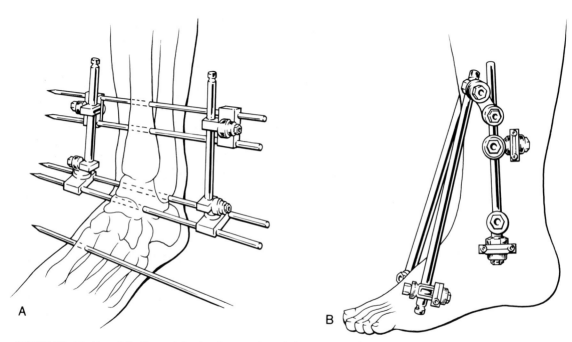

FIGURE 26–11. (*A* and *B*), External fixation frame using tubular system with triangular extension to position forefoot in neutral.

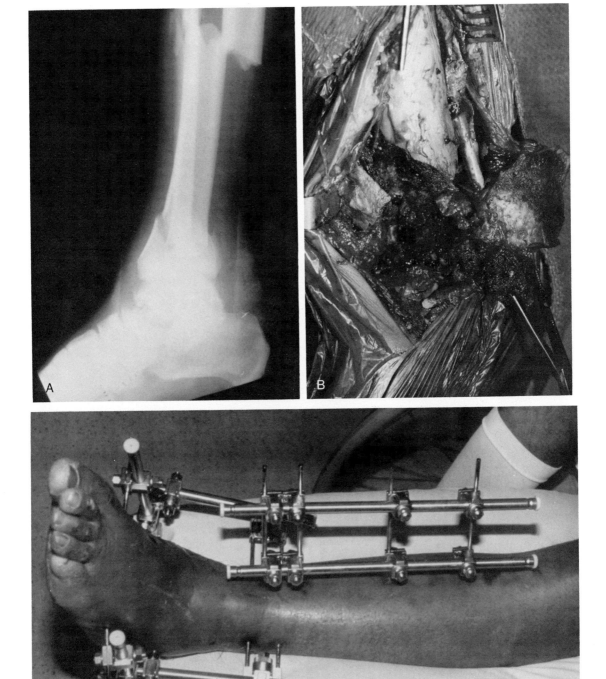

FIGURE 26–12. *(A)*, Lateral radiograpah of acute comminuted fracture of distal tibia articular surface and talar dome. *(B)*, Intraoperative photograph demonstrating complete articular destruction. *(C)*, Triangular frame engaging distal tibia, body of calcaneus, and first and fifth metatarsals.

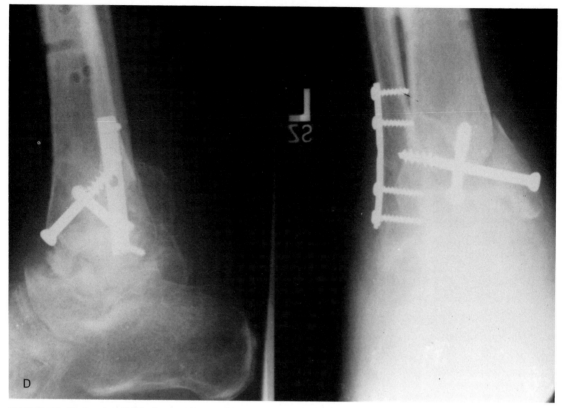

FIGURE 26–12 *Continued (D),* Six-month postoperative radiograph demonstrates solid ankle fusion and minimal internal fixation placed at initial procedure.

cations involving both the tibia and talus, avascular necrosis of the talus, and nonunion of a tibiotalar arthrodesis (Fig. 26–13).[5, 35] Avascularity of the body of the talus frequently leads to nonunion of ankle fusions. It is also possible to use this fusion in failed total ankle arthroplasty and neuropathic arthropathy. This operation is important primarily in cases in which both the ankle and the subtalar joints are involved, with severe deformity and degenerative arthritis. This procedure should be done only in those cases in which the only surgical option is tibiocalcaneal fusion. Either an anterior or a posterior approach can be used, depending on the need for hardware removal or status of the soft tissues. The posterior approach, described in the next section, offers the advantage of avoiding previous incisions and providing wide access to both joints of the hindfoot. External fixation is required and must be optimally placed for rigid fixation and compression of bone surfaces.

Fixators can safely be left in place for 9 to 12 weeks.

Technique

The patient is placed in the prone position, and iliac crest bone graft is taken from the ipsilateral iliac crest. A 20-cm posterolateral incision is made along the lateral border of the Achilles tendon (Fig. 26–14). The Achilles tendon is longitudinally split in half in its distal third and the halves are transected, one proximally and one distally. The flexor hallucis tendon is retracted medially to protect the neurovascular structures. The tibiotalar and subtalar joint capsules are removed subperiosteally. A trough is cut from the tibia into the body of the calcaneus, and articular cartilage from the joint surfaces is removed through the trough. Adjustments are made to obtain apposition of bone surfaces. The foot is then placed in the neutral plantigrade position, with

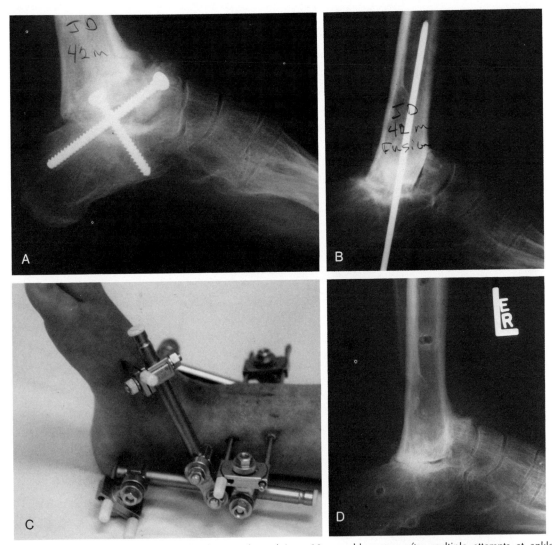

FIGURE 26–13. *(A)*, Tibiocalcaneal arthrodesis performed in a 30-year-old woman after multiple attempts at ankle arthrodesis for talar body dislocation. *(B)*, Anterior tibiocalcaneal fusion with intraoperative stabilization using a long Steinmann pin. *(C)*, Triangular external frame left in place for 12 weeks. *(D)*, Incomplete union at 8 months following attempted fusion.

Illustration continued on following page

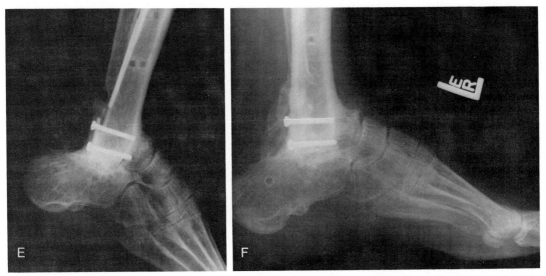

FIGURE 26–13 *Continued (E),* Refusion through the posterior approach using a sliding graft of posterior distal tibia. *(F),* Solid fusion after the second attempt of tibiocalcaneal fusion.

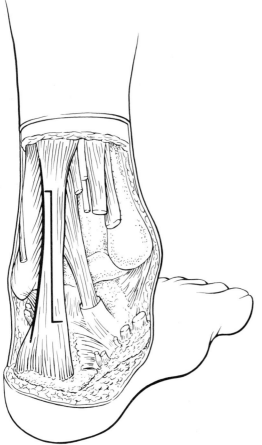

FIGURE 26–14. Tibiocalcaneal arthrodesis through posterolateral incision, splitting Achilles tendon longitudinally and transecting proximal and distal segments. Flexor hallicus longus muscle and tendon are retracted medially.

the heel in from neutral to 5 degrees of valgus. Approximately 5 degrees of external rotation of the foot are obtained, comparable to the opposite side. The external fixation device is applied, with the Steinmann pins placed posteriorly in the calcaneus to avoid the neurovascular structures. Cancellous bone graft is then inserted along the posterior trough to create an intra-articular and extra-articular arthrodesis. The flexor hallucis longus is returned to its normal position and sutured, and the Achilles tendon is resutured. The wound is closed over a drain, and a bulky compressive dressing is applied. Sutures are removed at 10 to 14 days, and pin care is explained. The frame is worn for 9 to 12 weeks, then a short-leg walking cast is applied for an additional 4 to 6 weeks.

FIBULAR MALUNION AND ANKLE DIASTASIS

Malunion after an ankle fracture most commonly results from inadequate reduction at the time of initial treatment. It is now understood that operative intervention is needed to restore the anatomic relations in most unstable ankle fractures, and this is particularly true if fibular fracture and diastasis of the syndesmosis are associated with disruption of either the deltoid ligament or the medial malleolus. Correction requires restoration of the short externally rotated fibula and reduction to its normal position in the fibular notch.[10, 12, 16, 30, 40, 48, 50]

Patients with this problem usually have a history of an ankle fracture that was treated by closed reduction and cast immobilization. If malunion has resulted, pain and swelling appear over the anterior aspect of the joint and are aggravated by strenuous physical activity. Younger active individuals develop symptoms much more quickly than older sedentary patients. Eventually, the symptoms become constant and are relieved only by cessation of weight bearing. Fibular malunion is best identified on the lateral radiograph, where displacement and posterior subluxation can be identified.

Radiographic Criteria

For preoperative planning and postoperative assessment, radiologic criteria of the normal joint are essential. The following criteria were derived from review of the literature (Fig. 26–15):

1. The talocrural angle is the superior medial angle of a line perpendicular to the distal tibial articular surface and a line joining the tips of both malleoli on the mortise view. The adult talocrural angle is 83 degrees ± 4 degrees and there is normally less than 2 degrees difference from the opposite side. Any difference over 5 degrees is abnormal.

2. The medial clear space is the distance from the lateral border of the medial malleolus to the medial border of the talus at the level of the talar dome on the mortise radiograph. A space of more than 4 mm is abnormal.

3. Talar tilt refers to any differences in the width of the joint spaces proximal to the medial and lateral talar ridges on the mortise radiograph. Two millimeters of difference is considered the upper limit of normal.

4. Syndesmosis A measures the tibiofibular clear space from the lateral border of the posterior tibial malleolus (point A) to the medial border of the fibula (point B) on the anteroposterior radiograph. This space is normally less than 5 mm and represents syndesmosis disruption if abnormal.

5. Syndesmosis B measures the tibiofibular overlap from the medial border of the fibula (point B) to the lateral border of the anterior tibial prominence (point C) on the anteroposterior radiograph. This is abnormal if less than 10 mm.

6. Talar subluxation is a subjective assessment of congruity of the tibial articular surface and talar dome on the anterior radiograph. Any incongruity is abnormal (see Fig. 26–15).[17, 31, 32, 37]

Conservative treatment, including anti-inflammatory medication, physical therapy, and rest, are of limited benefit but may be tried initially. Operative treatment is considered if the patient is young and intends to resume an active lifestyle. Contraindications include significant degenerative arthritis with joint space narrowing and osteophytes and osteochondral defects of the talus.

Yablon has had excellent results in 20 of 26 cases treated from 1 to 7 years after injury.[51] Weber had similar results in 17 of 23 cases and stated that the quality of reduction achieved, length of time to revision, and condition of the joint surface were the main factors determining

Mortise View

FIGURE 26–15. Syndesmotic radiographic criteria. (See text.)

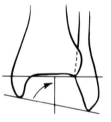

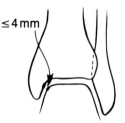

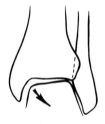

| Talo Crural Angle
(83° ± 4°) | Medial Clear Space
(≤ 4 mm) | Talar Tilt
(≤ 2 mm) |

Anterior Posterior View

A = Lateral border of
    posterior tibial malleolus
B = Medial border of fibula
C = Lateral border anterior
    tibial tubercle

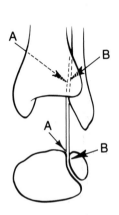

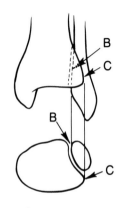

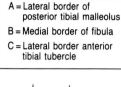

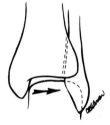

| Syndesmosis A
(<5 mm) | Syndesmosis B
(≥ 10 mm) | Talar
Subluxation |

outcome.[48] When arthritic changes are advanced, ankle arthrodesis is the primary treatment. Therapy must be individualized, although it is apparent from Yablon's studies that patients with occult fibular malunion with no talar subluxation are likely to have better results than those with gross fibular diastasis and talar subluxation.

Technique

The patient is placed supine with a sandbag under the ipsilateral hip. A 10-cm incision is made over the distal fibula, starting at the tip and extending proximally. The fibula is exposed, and the site of malunion is identified. Scar tissue must be removed from the fibular

notch to allow for reduction. Failure of the talus to reduce anatomically must be corrected by a separate medial incision to resect soft tissue from the medial clear space. If medial malleolar malunion is noted, osteotomy and re-osteosynthesis of the medial malleolus may be needed.

An oblique osteotomy is made in the fibula through the previous malunion site. If this cannot be identified, a transverse osteotomy is made 7 cm proximal to the tip of the lateral malleolus. A five- or six-hole AO/ASIF small fragment semitubular plate is selected and contoured with internal rotation to allow for the anatomic bend and twist of the distal fibula. The plate is applied to the fibula distal to the osteotomy site using two 3.5-mm cortical screws. An AO compression-distraction device is applied proximal to the plate, and the fibula is distracted to the appropriate level, which is reached when the most proximal articular cartilage is at the level of the joint line. The fibula is reduced into the fibular notch by forcibly inverting and internally rotating the foot and by applying direct thumb pressure from a posterolateral direction so that the fibula does not remain subluxed posteriorly. A radiograph confirms restoration of fibular length and joint space as per the syndesmotic radiographic criterion (see Fig. 26–15). The remaining screws are inserted into the plate and a transverse position screw or syndesmosis screw is inserted 2 cm above the joint line to hold the anatomic position of the fibula. If this is placed through the plate, the foot should be held in maximal dorsiflexion at insertion. Special care must be taken in those cases in which there is a prior posterior malleolar fracture that remains unreduced, which will allow the fibula to sublux posteriorly. Bone graft is added to the osteotomy site from the distal tibial metaphysis. The syndesmosis and surrounding ligaments are not sutured. Final radiographs are made, and the wound is closed over a drain. A posterior splint is applied after wound closure (Fig. 26–16).

Postoperative Care

The posterior splint is changed at 10 days, and the sutures are removed at that time. A short-leg removable ankle-foot orthosis (AFO) is applied, and the patient is kept non–weight bearing for an additional 4 weeks. During this period, the AFO is removed two or three times daily to allow for active range-of-motion exercises. Six weeks following surgery, the patient is allowed full weight bearing, within the confines of the AFO, for an additional 6 weeks. Removal of the syndesmosis screw can be done under local anesthesia at 12 weeks prior to unprotected weight bearing.

Complications

The two reasons for failure of this operation are (1) attempting to reconstruct joints that show significant degenerative arthritis and (2) technical failure to meet the criteria for anatomic reconstruction of the ankle joint. Both problems can be avoided if careful attention is paid to radiographs. Ankle arthrodesis remains the salvage procedure for failed cases.

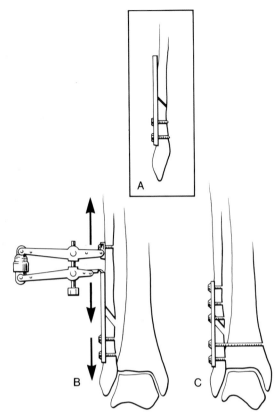

FIGURE 26–16. *(A)*, Fibular lengthening is accomplished by corrective osteotomy through an old fracture site, and the plate is secured distally. *(B)*, Tensioning device applied to proximal plate. *(C)*, The fibula is lengthened to the ideal position and a bone graft is applied. A syndesmotic screw may be added through the distal plate hole.

MEDIAL MALLEOLUS NONUNION

Failure of the medial malleolus to unite after fracture is occasionally seen, especially with displacement. Medial malleolar pseudarthrosis is interpreted as nonunion if not healed by 6 months. Treatment of these nonunions is difficult: Sneppen reported osseous union after surgical intervention in only 50 percent of cases.[41] However, Lindenbaum reported a case of traumatic loss of the medial malleolus that resulted in a stable ankle, with internal fixation of the lateral malleolus and simple reapproximation of the medial soft tissues.[3, 10, 20]

It is important to rule out other causes of pain, such as degenerative arthritis, before any attempt is made to treat these nonunions. Sneppen suggested that osteosynthesis should be attempted early, usually before 2 years. Surgical extirpation of a fragment may be done

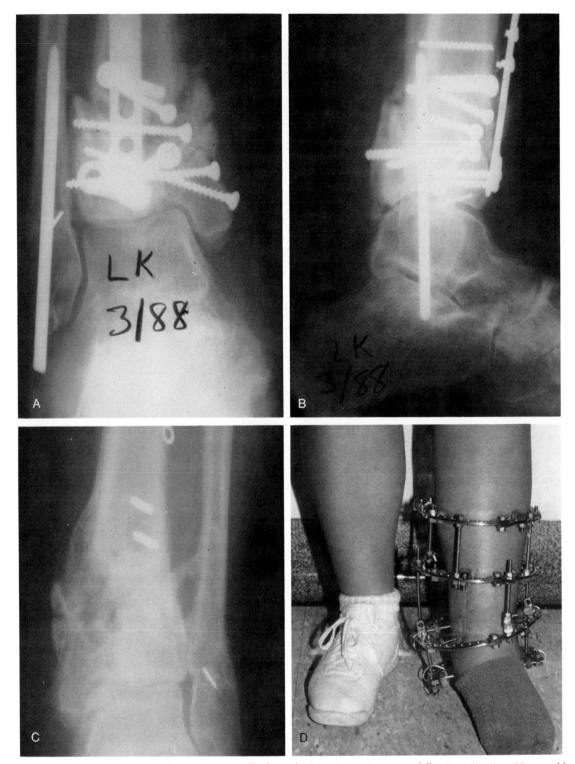

FIGURE 26–17. (A), Painful post-traumatic supramalleolar malunion or nonunion 1 year following injury in a 27-year-old woman. (B), Lateral radiograph. (C), Operative procedure consisted of hardware removal, osteotomy of the fibula, and application of Ilizarov device. (D), Sequential lengthening and correction of malunion is accomplished, and the bone is stabilized until union occurs.

if the remaining portion of the medial malleolus is large enough to preserve ankle joint stability. In those painful cases in which osseous union is sought, the operation should include excision of fibrous tissue, restoration of fracture surfaces, internal fixation of the fragment, and application of bone graft.

Technique

The medial malleolus is exposed by a 7-cm incision over the medial aspect of the ankle. The bone is dissected subperiosteally and the nonunion site is exposed. All fibrous tissue is removed from the nonunion site, except at the depth of the hole adjacent to the articular surface. Sclerotic bone is removed until cancellous surfaces are identified. The fragments are reduced with a towel clip, and two Kirschner wires are used to stabilize the fragment, supplemented with a figure-eight tension band wire. Autologous bone graft, obtained from a separate window in the distal tibia, fills any remaining defect in the nonunion site. The wound is closed over a drain, and a short-leg cast is applied.

Postoperative Care

The cast is changed at 2 weeks, and the patient is kept non–weight bearing for an additional 2 weeks. At that point, a walking heel is added, and the patient may walk with full weight bearing for an additional month. If radiographic union is demonstrated, the cast can be eliminated.

SUPRAMALLEOLAR MALUNION

Malunion of the distal tibia above the articular surfaces of the ankle joint is the result of angulation that occurs with closed treatment. Even a minor degree of varus or valgus produces an abnormal weight-bearing alignment. If traumatic arthritis has not developed and the patient has a symptomatic deformity, corrective osteotomy is considered. A valgus deformity can be repaired by creating an opening wedge laterally with fibular osteotomy. Varus deformity carries the added risk of damage to the medial neurovascular structures if done in a single stage. This situation optimally requires

the use of an external fixator, such as the Ilizarov device, that can be sequentially lengthened over a period of time and then compressed until union occurs (Fig. 26–17).[7]

Technique

For valgus malunion, a lateral incision is made over the distal fibula extending 7.5 cm. A long oblique osteotomy is made in the distal fibula, the lateral distal tibia is exposed, and a saw or osteotome is used to make a transverse osteotomy at the level of the malunion. Correction is made by manual osteoclasis. Iliac crest bone can be grafted to the osteotomy site. An external fixation device can be applied through the tibia and talus as described for ankle arthrodesis.

For varus malunion, a 5-cm medial incision is used for the distal tibia osteotomy and a lateral incision for the fibular osteotomy. An external fixation (Ilizarov) device is applied for staged distraction over a 2-week period. After correction has been achieved, the external fixation device can maintain compression for an additional 4 to 6 weeks. An alternative to this method is to use internal fixation with an AO/ASIF spoon plate on the distal tibia.

Postoperative Care

After the external fixation device is removed, a short-leg cast may be applied until the osteotomy has healed. Physical therapy is then initiated to restore normal function.

References

1. Adams JC: Arthrodesis of the ankle joint. J Bone Joint Surg 30B:506, 1948.
2. Baciu CC: A simple technique for arthrodesis of the ankle. J Bone Joint Surg 68B:266, 1986.
3. Banks SW: The treatment of non-union of fractures of the medial malleolus. J Bone Joint Surg 31A:658, 1949.
4. Berman DT, Bosacco SJ, Yanicko DR, et al: Compression arthrodesis of the ankle by triangular external fixation: An improved technique. Orthopedics 12:1327, 1989.
5. Bingold AC: Ankle and subtalar fusion by transarticular graft. J Bone Joint Surg 38B:862, 1956.
6. Boyd HB: Indications for fusion of the ankle. Orthop Clin North Am 5:191, 1974.
7. Brunner C, Weber BG: Special Techniques in Internal Fixation. New York, Springer-Verlag, 1982.

8. Buck P, Morrey BF, Chao EYS: The optimum position of arthrodesis of the ankle. J Bone Joint Surg 69A:1052, 1987.
9. Colonna PC, Ralston EL: Operative approaches to the ankle joint. Am J Surg 52:44, 1951.
10. Crenshaw AH: Campbell's Operative Orthopaedics. St. Louis, CV Mosby, 1987.
11. Davis RJ, Millis MB: Ankle arthrodesis in the management of traumatic ankle arthrosis: A long-term retrospective study. J Trauma 20:674, 1980.
12. Fogel GR, Sim FA: Reconstruction of ankle malunion. Orthopedics 5:1471, 1982.
13. Gallie WE: Arthrodesis of the ankle joint. J Bone Joint Surg 30B:619, 1948.
14. Hagen RJ: Ankle arthrodesis. Clin Orthop 202:152, 1986.
15. Hallock H: Arthrodesis of the ankle joint for old painful fractures. J Bone Joint Surg 27:49, 1945.
16. Heim U, Pfeiffer KM: Small Fragment Set Manual. Technique Recommended by the A.S.I.F. Group. New York, Springer-Verlag, 1982.
17. Joy G, Patzakis MJ, Harvey JP: Precise evaluation of severe ankle fractures: technique and correlation with end results. J Bone Joint Surg 56A:979, 1974.
18. Kenzora JE, Simmons SC, Burgess AR, et al: External fixation arthrodesis of the ankle joint following trauma. Foot Ankle 7:49, 1986.
19. Lance EM, Paval A, Fries I, et al: Arthrodesis of the ankle joint. Clin Orthop 142, 1979.
20. Lindenbaum BL: Loss of medial malleolus in a bimalleolar fracture. J Bone Joint Surg 65A:1184, 1983.
21. Macko VW, Zwirkoxki P, Goldstein SA, et al: Joint contacture of the ankle: Contribution of the posterior malleolus. Orthop Trans 11:326, 1987.
22. Mann RA: Surgical implications of biomechanics of the foot and ankle. Clin Orthop 146:111, 1980.
23. Mann RA: Surgery of the Foot, 5th Ed. St. Louis, CV Mosby, 1986.
24. Marcus RE, Balourdas GM, Heiple KG: Ankle arthrodesis by chevron fusion with internal fixation and bone grafting. J Bone Joint Surg 65A:833, 1983.
25. Mazur JM, Schwartz E, Simon S: Ankle arthrodesis. J Bone Joint Surg 61A:964, 1979.
26. Morgan CD, Henke JA, Bailey RW, et al: Long-term results of tibiotalar arthrodesis. J Bone Joint Surg 67A:546, 1985.
27. Morrey BF, Wiedeman GP: Complications and long-term results of ankle arthrodesis following trauma. J Bone Joint Surg 62A:777, 1980.
28. Müller ME, Allgöwer M, Schneider R, Willenegger H: Manual of Internal Fixation: Techniques Recommended by the AO Group. New York, Springer-Verlag, 1979.
29. Nepola J: Personal communication.
30. Offierski CM, Graham JD, Hall JH, et al: Late revision of fibular malunion in ankle fractures. Clin Orthop 171:145, 1982.
31. Pettrone FA, Gail M, Pee D, et al: Quantitative criteria for prediction of the results after displaced fractures of the ankle. J Bone Joint Surg 65A:667, 1983.
32. Phillips WA, Schwartz HS, Keller CS, et al: A prospective, randomized study of management of severe ankle fractures. J Bone Joint Surg 67A:67, 1985.
33. Ramsay PL, Hamilton W: Changes in tibiotalar area of contact caused by lateral talar shift. J Bone Joint Surg 58A:356, 1976.
34. Ross SDK, Matta J: Internal compression arthrodesis of the ankle. Clin Orthop 199:54, 1985.
35. Russotti GM, Johnson KA, Cass JR: Tibiocalcaneal arthrodesis for arthritis and deformity of the hindpart of the foot. J Bone Joint Surg 70A:1304, 1988.
36. Said E, Hunka L, Siller TN: Ankle fusions: A current study. *In* Bateman JE, Trott AW (Eds): The Foot and Ankle: A Selection of Papers from the American Orthopaedic Foot Society Meetings. Philadelphia, BC Decker, 1980, p 131.
37. Sarkisian JS, Cody SW: Closed treatment of ankle fractures: A new criterion for investigation—a review of 250 cases. J Trauma 16:323, 1976.
38. Scranton PE, Fu FH, Brown TD: Ankle arthrodesis: A comparative clinical and biomechanical evaluation. Clin Orthop 151:234, 1980.
39. Scranton PE Jr: Use of internal compression in arthrodesis of the ankle. J Bone Joint Surg 67A:550, 1985.
40. Sneppen O: Pseudarthrosis of the lateral malleolus. Acta Orthop Scand 42:187, 1971.
41. Sneppen O: Treatment of pseudarthrosis involving the malleolus. Acta Orthop Scand 42:201, 1971.
42. Stewart MJ, Beeler TC, McConnell JC: Compression arthrodesis of the ankle. J Bone Joint Surg 65A:219, 1983.
43. Stiehl JB, Dollinger B: Primary ankle arthordesis in trauma: Report of three cases. J Orthop Trauma 2:277, 1989.
44. Stiehl JB: Ankle fractures with diastasis. Instruc Course Lect 39:95, 1990.
45. Thomas FB: Arthrodesis of the ankle. J Bone Joint Surg 51B:53, 1969.
46. Velasco A, Fleming L: Compression arthrodesis of the knee and ankle withe the Hoffman external fixator. South Med J 11:1393, 1983.
47. Wagner FW: Ankle fusion for degenerative arthritis secondary to the collagen diseases. Foot Ankle 3:24, 1982.
48. Weber BG, Simpson LA: Corrective lengthening osteotomy of the fibula. Clin Orthop 199:61, 1985.
49. Wilson HJ: Arthrodesis of the ankle. J Bone Joint Surg 51A:776, 1969.
50. Woo SL-Y, Buckwalter JA: Injury and repair of the musculoskeletal soft tissues. AAOS Symposium, Savannah, Georgia, June, 1987, p 467.
51. Yablon IG: Occult malunion of ankle fractures—a cause of disability in the athlete. Foot Ankle 7:300, 1987.

27

Surgical Treatment of Fractures of the Talus

ROBERT S. ADELAAR

This chapter discusses the preferred treatment of fractures of the talus at the Medical College of Virginia Hospitals and compares it with current treatment proposed by other institutions. The chapter emphasizes the surgical management of talar injuries, specifically talar neck fractures, which make up more than 50 percent of all talar injuries.

ANATOMY OF THE TALUS

Certain anatomic features of the talus predispose it to complex injury (Fig. 27–1). There are seven articular surfaces of the talus, and 60 percent of the talus is cartilage. The talus has no muscular attachments. It is stabilized by the bone mortise of the ankle, the subtalar constraining ligaments, and the articular facets of the calcaneus. The posterior articular facet of the calcaneus maintains the body of the talus upright with the help of the interosseous ligaments. The talus is wider anteriorly than posteriorly; therefore, dorsiflexion gives increased stability.[5, 11, 23] The talar neck deviates in a medial direction and is shorter on the medial side than on the lateral side; biomechanical fixation of talar fractures from the medial side is thus difficult because of the very narrow limits of screw placement. Most screws placed in from the medial side exit on the lateral cortex, and there are also problems with impingement on the tubercle of the navicular, which varies in size. Bone density analyses in cadaver models have demonstrated increased density in the lateral aspect of the talar head and neck.[42]

The talocalcaneal ligament is important in stabilizing the talar neck and distal fragment of talar neck fractures. With destruction of this ligament, dorsal subluxation and varus displacement can occur. The posterior talocalcaneal ligament is usually the last supporting structure that is ruptured before complete dislocation of the body of the talus from the mortise.

Injuries to the posterior structures of the talus are difficult to demonstrate by normal radiographic techniques. The medial and lateral posterior processes contain the flexor hallucis longus (see Fig. 27–1). The lateral posterior process is larger than the medial and is the process associated with the accessory bone called the os trigonum. The os trigonum is often difficult to distinguish from a lateral process fracture. The lateral tubercle has many articular facets and important ligamentous attachments with the anterior talofibular and posterior talofibular ligaments.[21, 32] The lateral tubercle of the talus is a strong, dense portion that acts as a wedge to destroy the strut of Gissane in lateral calcaneal fractures.

The trochlea, or talar neck, is narrow and less dense to allow for dorsiflexion. With impingement on the tibia in dorsiflexion, the trochlea is more likely to fracture.

CIRCULATION OF THE TALUS

Osteonecrosis of the talus is the most morbid complication of talar injuries. The unique circulation to the body of the talus must be

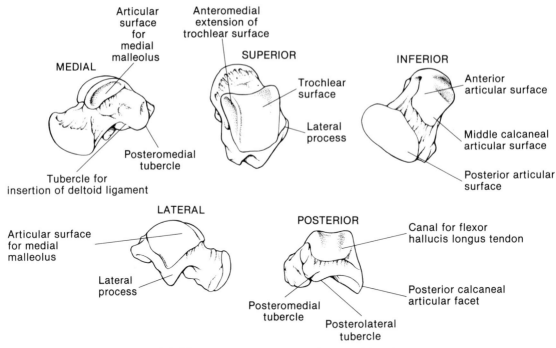

FIGURE 27–1. Important anatomic features of the talus.

recognized in order to avoid iatrogenic vascular injury to this area. The blood supply to the talus comes from two main sources: the extraosseous and the intraosseous circulation. The extraosseous circulation is composed of contributions from the anterior tibial, posterior tibial, and peroneal vasculature. A vascular extraosseous ring, described by Wildenauer,[44] forms around the talar neck and sinus tarsi (Fig. 27–2).[19, 24, 27, 33, 38, 44] The tarsal sinus artery forms from contributions of the anterior tibial artery and peroneal artery branches. The tarsal canal artery consistently arises from the posterior tibial artery within the deltoid ligament below the medial malleolus (Figs. 27–2 and 27–3). The tarsal canal artery branches to give the deltoid artery within the deltoid ligament. The deltoid artery is an important source of extraosseous circulation to the body of the talus. It is critical to preserve the deltoid artery when attempting to fix the talar neck and body.

With regard to the intraosseous circulation, 60 percent of talar anatomic specimens have demonstrated a complete intraosseous anastomosis between all regions of the talus (see Fig. 27–2).[44] Regional sections of the talus show differences in density of circulation. The talar head has an abundant vasculature supplied primarily by the anterior tibial artery. Multiple vascular foramina are seen in the superior and anterior portions of the talar head, and the incidence of osteonecrosis is low for talar head fractures. The deltoid artery is seen to make significant contributions to the interosseous circulation in the medial and proximal portions of the body of the talus. The relatively avascular areas of the talus are the anterolateral surface of the body and the posterior tubercles.[27]

HISTORY OF TALAR INJURIES

The first case of an isolated talar fracture was reported in 1608 by Fabricius of Hilden, who described a compound fracture of the talus from a 3-foot fall.[5, 11, 23] Anderson, in 1919, was the first to collect a series of cases on the talar neck fracture.[2] He reported on 18 cases of aviator injuries that were due to the position of the foot on the rudder at the time of impact. Coltart collected the first large series of cases when he reported on the Royal Air Force fractures between 1940 and 1945; there were 228 fractures of the talus of 25,000 fractures and dislocations.[8] Many investigators have reported on small series of talar injuries, including Bonnin,[5] Pennal,[36] Dunn and col-

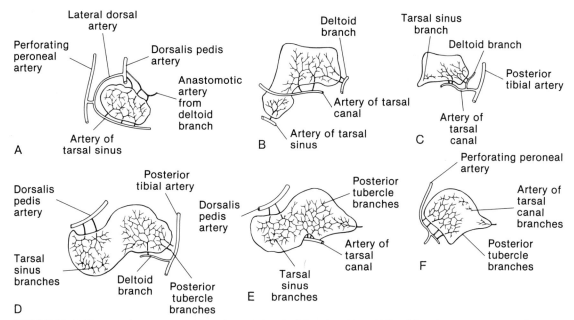

FIGURE 27–2. The vascular anatomy of the talus. (*A*), Head of the talus. (*B*), Middle of the talus. (*C*), Posterior talus. (*D*), Medial third of the talus. (*E*), Middle third of the talus. (*F*), Lateral third of the talus.

leagues,[15] Penny and Davis,[37] Gillquist and colleagues,[18] Mindell and colleagues,[31] Kenwright and Taylor,[25] and others.[7, 20, 26, 29, 35] In these series, fractures of the talus have accounted for approximately 1 percent of all fractures.

TALAR HEAD INJURIES

Talar head fractures account for 5 to 10 percent of all talar injuries. The mechanism of

injury is usually compressive forces secondary to hyperdorsiflexion.[11, 23] The talar head is well vascularized, and there is a low incidence of osteonecrosis (see Fig. 27–2). The key problems with this injury are difficulty in recognizing it, midtarsal instability, and future arthrosis, which can occur from improper reduction or instability.

On examination of the talar head fracture, tenderness and possible instability in the talonavicular area are often present. Instability of the talonavicular joint can be caused by a

FIGURE 27–3. (*A*), Intact blood supply to the talar head and body. (*B*), Dorsal disruption of the blood supply.

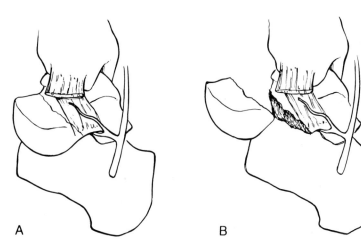

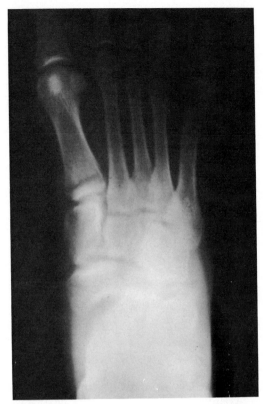

FIGURE 27–4. Radiographic view of a talar head fracture demonstrating an unstable midtarsal joint.

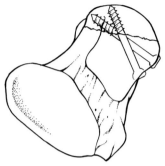

FIGURE 27–5. An oblique fracture of the talar head that has been fixed with two small screws that start on the medial aspect of the proximal talar fragment and extend into the head.

fracture fragment of greater than 50 percent (Fig. 27–4). It is often necessary to obtain special oblique radiographs in order to define the talonavicular joint and talar neck.

Talar head fractures that are unstable, and certainly those of greater than 50 percent, need fixation by rigid means (Fig. 27–5). A medial approach is used, with care being taken not to disturb the posterior tibial tendon attachment to the navicular or the spring ligament (Fig. 27–6A). A portion of the medial and anterior talonavicular capsule needs to be released. A blunt instrument such as a joker can be placed anterior to the capsule of the talonavicular area in order to retract the anterior tibial tendon and important neurovascular structures. The goal of reduction is rigid fixation in order to allow early motion after soft tissue healing. Long-term problems with arthrosis are totally dependent on anatomic articular fixation. Cancellous or lag screw fixation is appropriate, with two screws being used if possible, or a combination of screw and Kirschner wire (K-wire). Percutaneous K-wires do not provide a stable reduction, and they cause soft tissue problems.

The complications that can occur with talar head fractures are instability from nonunion

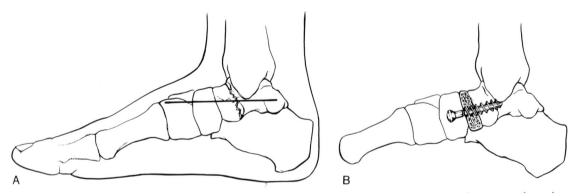

FIGURE 27–6. (*A*), Reduction of a talar head fracture can be obtained with 0.062-inch Kirschner wires from the anteromedial approach. Fixation can then occur from a posterolateral or anteromedial approach. (*B*), A talonavicular fusion can be performed for articular pain after talar head fracture. A wedge graft is taken from the top of the iliac crest, and fixation is with one or two lag screws.

FIGURE 27–7. The mechanism of injury for most talar neck fractures is hyperdorsiflexion with an axial load. After impingement of the trochlea (the talar neck) on the tibia, the posterior capsule is put under stretch and supination occurs, thus stabilizing the subtalar joint.

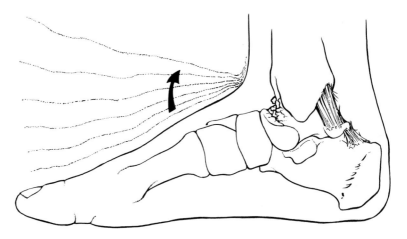

and missed fractures that do not unite. Arthrosis of the talonavicular joint can occur from poor articular reduction, and collapse can occur from vascular necrosis. Osteonecrosis is not common because of the excellent blood supply of the talar head. If these complications do occur and it is not believed that the fragment can be securely fixed, a talonavicular fusion should be considered. The fusion technique that we use at the Medical College of Virginia is screw fixation through the navicular with slotting of a corticocancellous wedge graft from the iliac crest into the talonavicular joint (Fig. 27–6B). Cancellous bone graft is also packed into any spaces prior to screw fixation. It is important when a fusion or fracture reduction is being attempted not to strip the blood supply entirely from the talar head and to approach it only from the anteromedial aspect.

TALAR NECK FRACTURES

Fractures of the talar neck represent 50 percent of all talar injuries. The principles that apply to the treatment of talar neck injuries also apply to talar body fractures, with some modification in exposure. The mechanism of injury is usually dorsiflexion with impingement of the talar neck, which is the weakest area of the talus on the tibial dome (Fig. 27–7). As the force continues, there is usually dorsal comminution of the talus, disruption of the talocalcaneal ligament, and disruption of the posterior and subtalar capsule. Finally, supination with subluxation of the subtalar joint occurs as in class II injuries, with eventual complete dislocation of the body as in class III injuries (Fig. 27–8B and C).[20] When the body dislocates, it is usually found on the posteromedial aspect adjacent to the Achilles tendon,

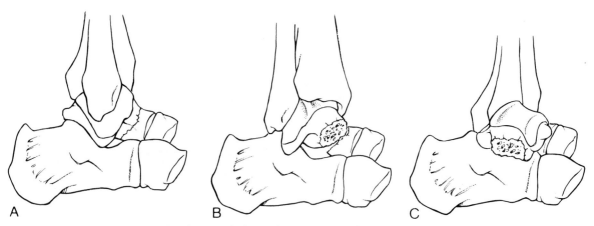

A   B   C

FIGURE 27–8. Hawkins-type classification of talar neck injuries. *(A)*, Class I. *(B)*, Class II. *(C)*, Class III. (See text for description.)

compressing the neurovascular structures. Therefore, care should be taken in approaching a dislocated body of the talus not to injure the neurovascular structures.[11, 23]

The goal of fracture treatment with talar neck fractures is to restore the anatomic talar neck. The deforming forces of varus and supination need to be corrected. Supination forces cause subluxation of the talar joint to occur in class II and class III injuries; therefore, it is important to reduce the subtalar joint (see Fig. 27–8B and C). Fractures of the medial malleolus and lumbar spine injuries have been found in association with talar neck injuries.[11, 23] In class III injuries, compound fractures have been associated with 50 percent of the reported cases.

The Medical College of Virginia uses a modified classification of Hawkins (see Fig. 27–8):[20] a class I injury is a nondisplaced vertical neck fracture with no subluxation; a class II injury has mild dorsal displacement of the talar neck fragment with subluxation of the subtalar joint (Fig. 27–9); and a class III injury has displacement of the talar body and associated subtalar subluxation and talar neck displacement (Fig. 27–10). As the displacement of the talar neck increases, the incidence of malunion, osteoarthritis, and osteonecrosis increases.[18, 25] The talocalcaneal ligament is rup-

tured when dorsal displacement of the distal fragment is present. With rupture of this ligament, it is difficult to control talar neck fractures by closed means because of the supination deformity or varus that occurs, and open techniques are recommended with failure to achieve anatomic reduction, with at least 3 to 5 mm of dorsal displacement and 5 degrees of varus.

Class I Injuries

Class I injuries occur when there is minimal displacement of the distal fragment. These injuries can usually be treated by closed means with an anatomic reduction that includes correction of the minimal dorsal displacement and talar neck supination. The incidence of osteonecrosis is low (10 percent) because the circulation is usually intact.[11, 23] If an anatomic reduction is obtained, as confirmed by appropriate radiographs, a cast can be used for treatment until trabeculation is demonstrated. Weight bearing is allowed only after trabeculation occurs across the talar neck because of the problem of shear forces with weight bearing before trabeculation, particularly without rigid fixation. If anatomic reduction cannot be obtained, open treatment with either the an-

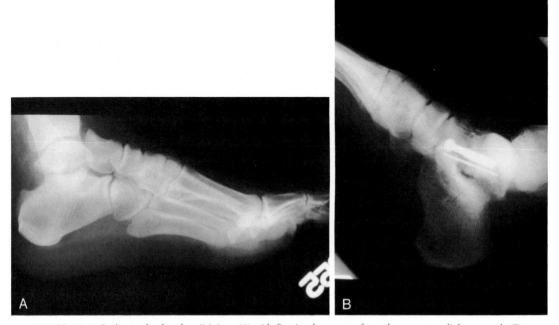

FIGURE 27–9. Radiograph of a class II injury *(A)* with fixation by screws from the anteromedial approach *(B)*.

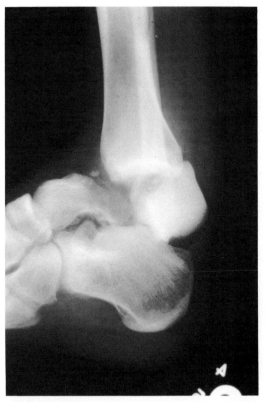

FIGURE 27–10. Radiograph of a class III injury with disruption of the talocalcaneal ligaments and subluxation or frank dislocation of the subtalar and ankle joints.

teromedial, anterolateral, or posterolateral approach can be used.

Surgical Approaches

Anteromedial. The classic approach to the talar neck fracture has been the anteromedial (Fig. 27–11). There is a safe interval between the extensor hallucis longus and the anterior tibial tendons. The incision needs to be extended to the ankle joint, and care should be taken in doing any periosteal stripping. The problem with this approach is the difficulty in obtaining a good biomechanical fixation at the fracture site because the talar neck is deviated and shortened in a medial direction. The threads of the screws usually exit the lateral cortex just proximal to the fracture and do not give adequate compression or an axis perpendicular to the fracture site. With open treatment, we do not believe that there is any place for K-wire fixation alone. K-wires (0.062 inch) can often be used in combination with an

appropriate threaded screw to supply some rotational stability (Fig. 27–12). At our institution, 4.5-mm or 6.5-mm cannulated screws have been very helpful, when used with the image intensifier. It is important to restate that lateral, anterior, and oblique radiographs should be obtained at the conclusion of treatment for each patient because the image intensifier may often not give an accurate picture of the reduction.

Anterolateral. In the anterolateral approach, an attempt is made to obtain a better biomechanical approach to the fracture (Fig. 27–13). The difficulty with this approach is the danger of causing damage to the anterior tibial vessels and the superficial peroneal nerve. The same methods of fixation are used as with the anteromedial approach. However, we have abandoned this approach with the development of a posterolateral approach because there are many vascular foramina in the anterolateral region to be avoided.

Posterolateral. A posterolateral approach, which was described by Trillat and colleagues

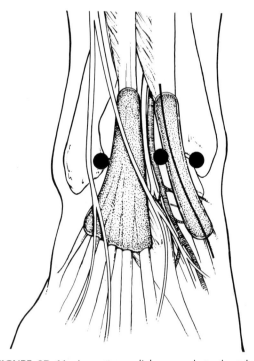

FIGURE 27–11. An anteromedial approach to the talar neck fracture through the interval between the anterior tibial and extensor hallucis longus tendons, avoiding neurovascular bundles. Care should be taken not to do a great deal of stripping on the talar neck.

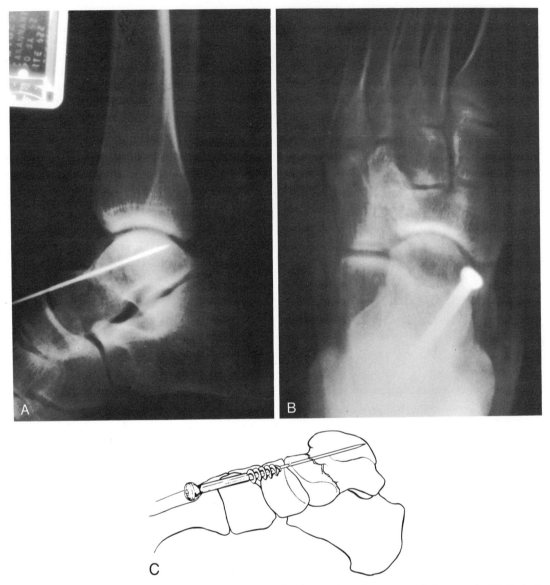

FIGURE 27–12. Fixation of a talar neck fracture with a cannulated screw from the anteromedial approach. *(A)*, Reduction and provisional fixation. *(B)*, Cannulated screw fixation. *(C)*, Artist's rendition of the technique.

in 1970,[43] has been used in combination with an anteromedial open or closed manipulation of the fracture site.[17, 28] In the posterolateral approach (Fig. 27–14), the patient is placed in the prone or lateral position, and an incision is made on the lateral portion of the heel cord. The enlarged lateral posterior process of the talus underneath the flexor hallucis muscle mass is identified, and with the use of cannulated screws and the image intensifier, K-wires are placed in position while an attempt is made to manipulate the fracture (Fig. 27–15). In our

experience, it is difficult to obtain a good closed reduction because this approach is usually used in class II or III injuries, in which a great deal of dorsal subluxation and supination of the distal fragment is present. Therefore, we do not hesitate to use a combined anteromedial and anterolateral approach to open the fracture and anatomically hold it while the K-wire is placed in from the lateral posterior aspect. With the patient in the prone position, the knee can be flexed. This anteromedial approach is difficult, and this is the reason to

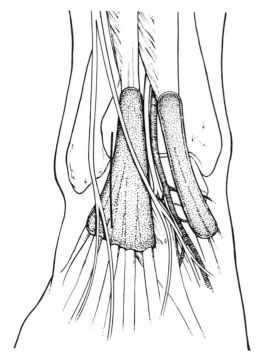

FIGURE 27–13. An anterolateral approach to the talar neck.

use the lateral patient position. We believe that no important blood supply is violated by the anteromedial approach or by the posterolateral approach. Once again, it is important to obtain good radiographs at the conclusion of treatment, particularly an oblique film as described by Canale and Kelly,[7] before accepting a closed or open reduction. Another technique used is opening the fracture and, with the patient in the lateral position and using the anteromedial approach, passing K-wires retrograde across the proximal fracture and out the posterolateral aspect. A posterolateral incision is made. The problem with this approach is that the cannulated K-wires are often not directed out the appropriate posterolateral tubercle.

The surgeon should also remember that portions of the talus are very firm, particularly the posterolateral aspect, and it is often difficult to use cannulated K-wires. We find no difference in the titanium and stainless steel alloy screws.

Summary. In summary, then, the principles of fixation are that we do not use K-wires as the sole means of fixation.[42] Rigid anatomic reduction with a large cancellous screw, mal-

leolar screw, or cannulated screw is recommended. The approach used is dependent on fracture location and type.

Class II Injuries

In class II injuries, there is disruption of the talocalcaneal ligament, and it is therefore difficult to obtain a closed anatomic reduction (see Figs. 27–8 and 27–9). The indication for open reduction is the inability to obtain an accurate closed anatomic reduction. We use the guidelines of 3 to 5 mm of dorsal displacement or any rotational deformity.

The anteromedial and posterolateral approaches have been used for exposure. The combination of both approaches has been used successfully, with the initial approach being posterolateral. Swanson and Bray performed histomorphometric analysis of the bone density

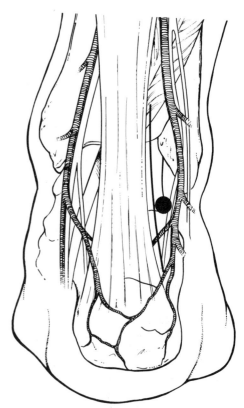

FIGURE 27–14. A posterolateral approach to the talus. A lateral approach adjacent to the Achilles tendon is carried out down to the posterolateral tubercle after reflection of the flexor hallucis longus. Cannulated screws can be placed from this approach at a biomechanical advantage for fracture fixation. Dot indicates the interval described.

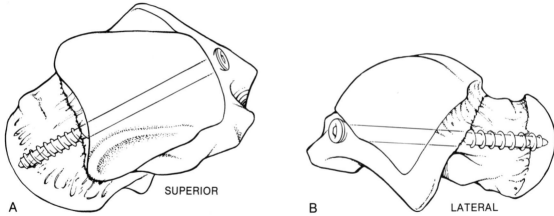

FIGURE 27–15. (A and B), Fixation from the posterolateral approach provides the best biomechanical fixation for fractures of the talar neck and body. The screws are usually firmly fixed in the talar head at an angle between 90 and 45 degrees to the fracture.

within the talus.[42] The greatest bone density was in the lateral portion of the head and neck. Their study also demonstrated that K-wire fixation was inferior biomechanically to the use of cancellous screws and that the posterolateral approach gave the best biomechanical fixation.

The postoperative care of patients with class II injuries is directly related to the biomechanical rigidity of fixation. With rigid fixation, a short-leg cast can be used for approximately 6 weeks, after which an initial period of early active and passive motion is initiated. The important aspect is that no weight bearing be allowed for at least 3 months, or until trabeculation is demonstrated. There are shear forces across the talus just by the action of the extensor tendon and anterior tibial muscles; therefore, we believe that an initial 6-week period in a cast despite fixation is important.

Class III Injuries

In class III talar neck fractures, the talar body and subtalar joint subluxate or dislocate (see Figs. 27–8 and 27–9). A large percentage of these injuries are open (50 percent). There is a high incidence of osteonecrosis, which has been reported to be as low as 25 percent in the nondisplaced talar body and greater than 50 percent in those with dislocation.[11, 15, 23] With a dislocation of the talar body in a class III injury, it is important to reduce the body of the talus as soon as possible to decrease the

stress on the medial neurovascular bundle. It is important not to injure the deltoid vessels. The closed manipulation method requires the use of a traction pin in the os calcis. The hindfoot is pulled into equinus, and after distraction occurs, the hindfoot is supinated and pronated to reduce the body of the talus (Fig. 27–16). The soft tissues associated with these injuries are usually débrided and left open if they do not violate a joint space or tendons.

The surgical approach used for class III injuries is usually more extensive than that for class II injuries because of the magnitude of the injury and displacement of the talus. If the talar body cannot be relocated from its displaced position, a medial incision is required, with care taken to preserve the neurovascular bundle. This bundle is retracted, and direct manipulation of the body of the talus is attempted. K-wires can be used to temporarily hold the body of the talus in the mortise and the distal portion of the talar neck. A femoral distractor is also helpful in cases that resist closed attempts (Fig. 27–17).

The treatment of talar neck fractures is directed to reduction anatomically with no subtalar dislocation or varus malrotation. Rigid anatomic fixation is required to allow early mobilization after bone trabeculation has been observed by radiography. Gastrocsoleus muscle contractures should be avoided by limiting the immobilization in the equinus position. With open reduction, it is critical to preserve the vascularity of the fracture, particularly the deltoid branch of the tarsal canal

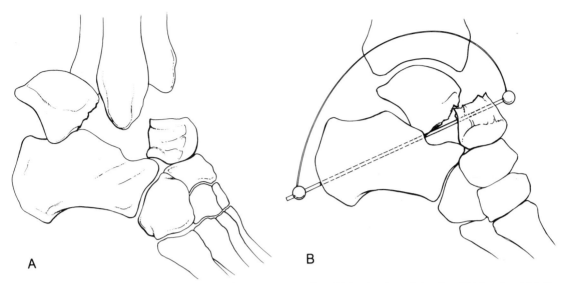

FIGURE 27–16. *(A* and *B),* Closed reduction techniques are used for initial reductions of the class III injury in which the talus has been dislocated, usually in the medial direction. Traction is usually applied with a pin through the os calcis in combination with equinus positioning and rotation to allow the talar body to be relocated in the subtalar joint. Getting the body over the posterior articular process is sometimes difficult, and a femoral distractor may be necessary.

artery. The complications that occur with talar neck fractures are delayed union, nonunion, subtalar and ankle arthritis, and osteonecrosis. The most accurate reports of long-term complications from this injury are from the Scandinavian literature.[9, 18, 29, 35] The work of these investigators demonstrated that osteonecrosis occurred in only 10 percent of nondisplaced fracture cases but that the incidence approached 70 percent when there was significant displacement. Delayed unions occurred primarily in class II and class III injuries, and the incidence of subtalar arthritis was also higher as the grade of injury increased. The major morbid complication of talar neck fractures is avascular necrosis.

OSTEONECROSIS

Osteonecrosis has been demonstrated to increase with the severity of injury.[18] In the minimally displaced class I fractures, the incidence of osteonecrosis is approximately 10 percent. As the class III injury with dislocation is approached, the incidence can be as high as 70 percent. Hawkins' sign is described as evidence of revascularization of the talar body (Fig. 27–18).[20] This sign of patchy subchondral osteoporosis usually occurs from 6 to 8 weeks after injury. If this sign is present, the talar body usually has enough blood supply to allow remodeling and revascularization.

Magnetic resonance imaging (MRI) has been used to diagnose and quantify osteonecrosis in patients who have suspicious findings on anteroposterior radiographs. Lateral radiographs are difficult to interpret because of the overlying shadows of the medial malleolus and lateral malleolus.[4] Once the physician suspects osteonecrosis, MRI should be performed to determine the extent of the involvement of the talar body (Fig. 27–19). The determination of when to put weight on the talus is made when trabeculation is evident on the lateral radiographs. The method of weight bearing, whether it is foot flat, associated with a patellar tendon–bearing brace, or associated with some type of ankle orthosis, is determined by the extent of osteonecrosis. The goal of treatment of osteonecrosis is to limit the amount of shear forces from inversion and eversion stresses about the ankle. The length of time that the forces are limited depends on the judgment of the treating physician and the needs of the patient. Osteonecrosis has taken up to 2 years to declare itself. It is also important to make sure that patchy osteopenia from disuse is not being mistaken for a revascularization sign.

For involvement of a small avascular seg-

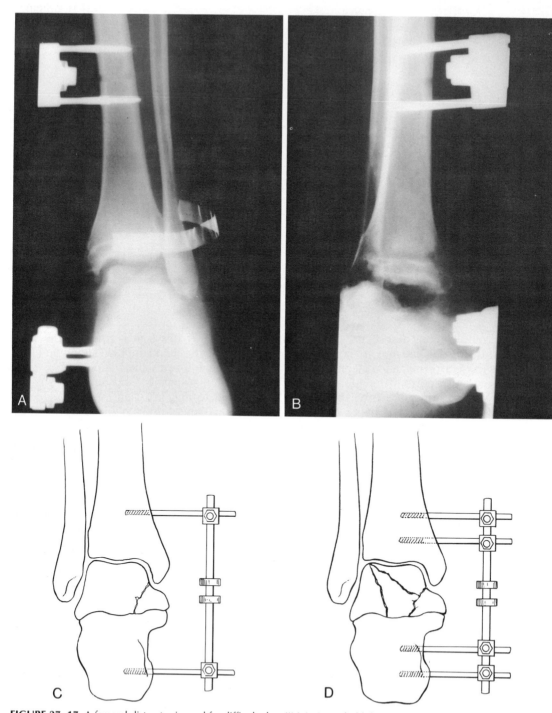

FIGURE 27–17. A femoral distractor is used for difficult class III injuries to hold the anatomic height of the hindfoot. It can be used whether the talar body is available for reinsertion into the mortise or not. *(A and B),* Clinical use of the femoral distractor. *(C and D),* Artist's rendition.

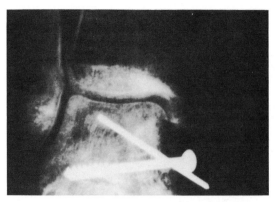

FIGURE 27–18. A mortise view of the ankle between 6 and 10 weeks after injury can show evidence of some resorption of bone, which indicates revascularization of the body of the talus (Hawkins' sign).

degrees of segmental collapse and deformity. Class I is osteonecrosis with some condensation and no bone deformity; class II is healed condensation with mild to moderate deformity of the trochlea; class III is healed condensed bone with a severely deformed trochlea; and class IV is sequestration of the trochlea.[4, 27, 40] We believe that no more than 1 cm of revascularization of the body of the talus is obtained by attempting a subtalar arthrodesis with bone grafting; therefore, I do not believe that this procedure will give sufficient revascularization to the entire bone. Core decompressions have not been attempted when the disease is diagnosed prior to collapse, but they may be of some consideration in the future. Therefore, at this time we do not recommend any invasive procedures for avascular necrosis.

TALAR SALVAGE PROBLEMS

It is important to discuss the severely traumatized avascular or completely detached body of the talus. Our goal is to preserve the body of the talus when it can be reasonably reimplanted. The body of the talus is used in maintaining the architecture of the foot until soft tissue healing allows the best reconstructive procedure. The best reconstructive procedure is the Blair tibiotalar arthrodesis (Fig. 27–20).[12, 29] A femoral distractor can be used to preserve length and gain soft tissue healing (Fig. 27–21; see also Fig. 27–17). The Blair

ment documented by MRI, unconstrained weight bearing with limitation of activity is important (see Fig. 27–19B). For a large avascular segment, more restraint may be appropriate (e.g., with a patellar tendon–bearing brace) and follow-up MRI studies can be obtained to determine the revascularization process after hardware is removed. In addition, many patients with avascularity of the talus can continue to function with some limitation in activity. These patients are restricted from activities of recreation that create increased shear forces, such as running. A bone scan can be used to screen for an avascular talus.

Osteonecrosis can be classified into various

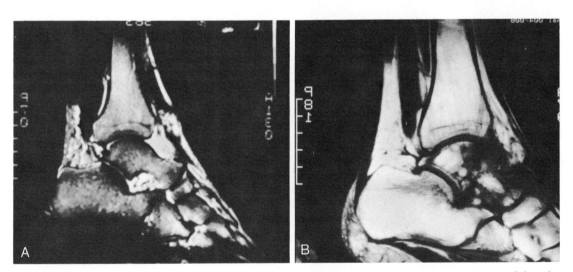

FIGURE 27–19. (A), A magnetic resonance image of the normal talus. (B), A magnetic resonance image of the talus demonstrating evidence of segmental avascular necrosis 3 months after a talar neck class II fracture.

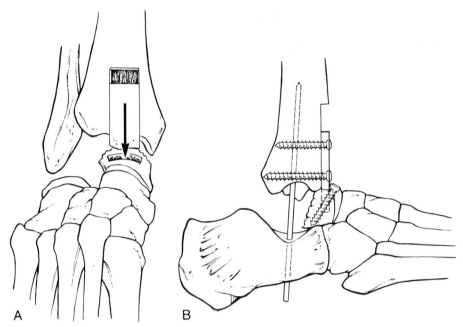

FIGURE 27–20. A Blair-type arthrodesis. (*A*), A slot graft from the tibia is fitted into the vascularized talar head and small portion of the neck. (*B*), Fixation with screws is recommended.

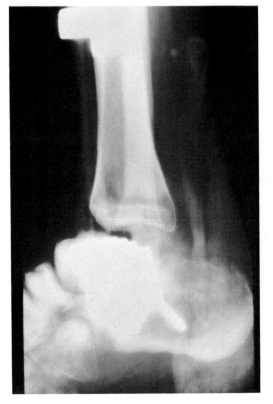

FIGURE 27–21. A femoral distractor for an external fixator can maintain the height of the heel in the absence of the body of the talus until a secondary reconstructive procedure can be done, which is usually 6 to 8 weeks after injury, unless there is severe soft tissue compromise.

procedure seems to be the best salvage procedure. With this procedure, tibia is fused, after excision of the body of the talus, to the live distal portion of the talar neck. An attempt is made to leave the subtalar joint free to allow some minimal motion in that area. Reconstructive procedures have also been done with large corticocancellous autogenous or allogeneic grafts, which are placed in the body of the talus space and secured with cannulated screws to maintain hindfoot height (Fig. 27–22). The use of good fixation screws with appropriate bone grafts can maintain the anatomic architecture. The rigidity of the fixation helps with revascularization.

If it is not possible to save the body of the talus, a tibiocalcaneal fusion can be done after soft tissue healing. A talectomy is the last choice of salvage procedure. A talectomy gives a severely unstable and uncosmetic shortened hindfoot, which is not tolerated well by the neurologically intact adult patient.

TALAR BODY FRACTURES

Fractures of the talar body are less common than talar neck fractures, and they are classi-fied into five groups. These fractures constitute about 20 percent of all talar fractures (Fig. 27–23). The most common talar body fractures are located in the posterior process and lateral tubercle.[11, 23] Talar fractures have been classi-fied into group I, osteochondral fractures; group II, fractures of the body of the talus, including coronal, sagittal, horizontal, and shear fractures; group III, posterior process fractures of both the medial and the posterior tubercle; group IV, lateral tubercle fractures; and group V, crush or compression injuries of the talar body. The group II and V fractures of the body of the talus have an osteonecrosis incidence of 25 percent when no dislocations occur. With dislocation, they have a greater than 50 percent incidence of osteonecrosis and take an average of 3 to 4 months for bone union. Nonunion and osteoarthritis are common with these injuries. Group II fractures are body fractures without significant commi-nution. They are classified with respect to the direction of the fraction: vertical, horizontal, or coronal (see Fig. 27–23).[1, 41] The commi-nuted fractures are classified, and it is often necessary to use computed tomography to de-fine the fracture (Fig. 27–24). Because these

FIGURE 27–22. Reconstruction for loss of the body of the talus when there is insufficient talar head for a Blair fusion is accomplished with a tibiocalcaneal fusion with a cor-ticocancellous graft and cancellous screw fixation from heel to tibia.

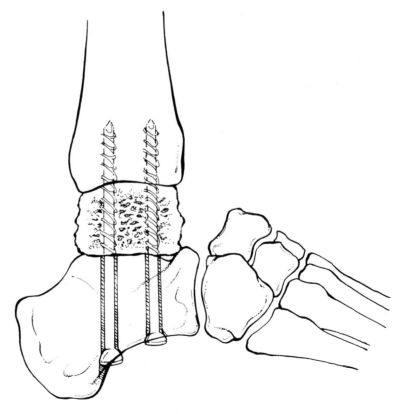

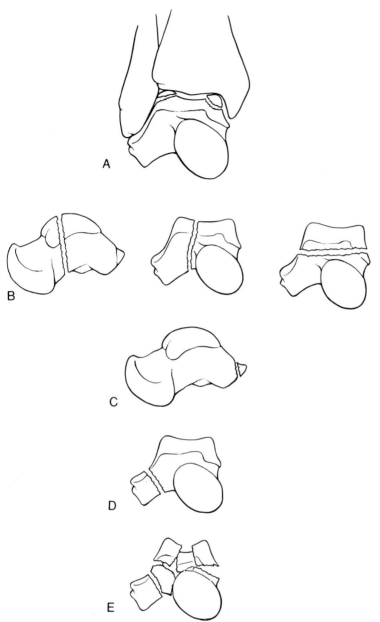

FIGURE 27–23. Classification of talar body fractures. (*A*), Osteochondral fracture (group I). (*B*), Sagittal, vertical, and horizontal talar body injuries (group II). (*C*), Posterior process fracture (group III). (*D*), Lateral tubercle fracture (group IV). (*E*), Crush injury (group V).

fractures occur underneath the ankle mortise, it is often necessary to perform medial or lateral malleolar osteotomy to gain sufficient exposure (Fig. 27–25).[13] The principles of fixation for talar body fractures are the same as with talar neck fractures, involving temporary fixation with K-wires, débridement of fracture portions that cannot be fixed, and cannulated screw or lag screw fixation to allow early motion and stability. The screws used for the

comminuted body of the talus fractures are the 3.5-mm cannulated screws.

Osteochondral Lesions

Osteochondral lesions of the talus were described by Monroe in 1738, by König in 1887, and by Rendu in 1932.[3, 6, 23, 34, 39] Such lesions are often included in the category of osteo-

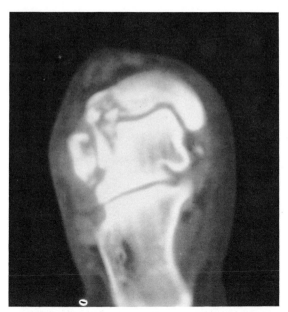

FIGURE 27–24. A computed tomographic scan of a crushed or comminuted body of the talus (fracture type V).

ing the depth of involvement and detachment. MRI also helps by showing the degree of devascularization of the fragment (Fig. 27–27).

The approach to these lesions depends on their location. Medial lesions, which are usually posterior, cannot be approached by an arthrotomy and require an osteotomy of the medial malleolus for open evaluation. Lateral lesions are usually anterior and require an anterolateral arthrotomy. The best initial treatment for osteochondral lesions is arthroscopy and arthroscopic débridement (Fig. 27–28). Anterior and posterior arthroscopic portals are used for the evaluation of osteochondral lesions. A posterior approach is often necessary to see a posteromedial lesion. Most of the lesions can be treated by débridement, drilling, or pinning, all of which can be performed under arthroscopic control. Pinning of a detached or partially detached lesion has a poor

chondrosis. Diagnosis is often delayed, and symptoms include ankle pain, recurrent swelling, and giving way. In addition, joint laxity may coexist with osteochondral fractures. The types of lesions that have been described fall into two major categories. The medial lesions are more typical of osteochondrosis and have a correlation with degenerative cystic disease (Fig. 27–26).[3] The lateral lesions are probably secondary to trauma (see Fig. 27–26). The medial and lateral lesions have been characterized as stage I, compression of subchondral bone without a break in the cartilage; stage II, lesions that are present but are not complete; stage III, partially detached lesions; and stage IV, lesions with total detachment.[3, 6, 10, 39]

Traumatic lesions are usually secondary to inversion with or without dorsiflexion.[3, 6, 30, 45] Long-term results show that few lesions unite when treated surgically, and the ankles go on to develop osteoarthritis regardless of the type of treatment used.[6, 34, 39] Surgical treatment consists of applications of a short-leg cast with some type of patellar tendon–bearing brace or a brace to avoid full weight bearing on the ankle for 3 months. Lateral lesions appear to cause more degenerative changes than do medial lesions. All lateral lesions were wafer shaped; medial lesions were cup shaped.[3, 40] Computed tomography is helpful in determin-

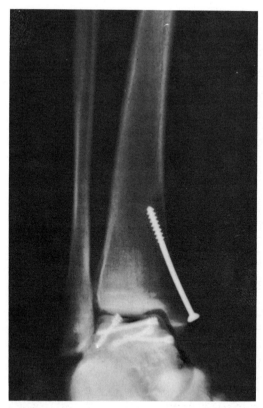

FIGURE 27–25. Osteotomy of the medial malleolus is often needed to treat comminuted fractures of the body of the talus. Care should be taken not to destroy the deltoid ligament.

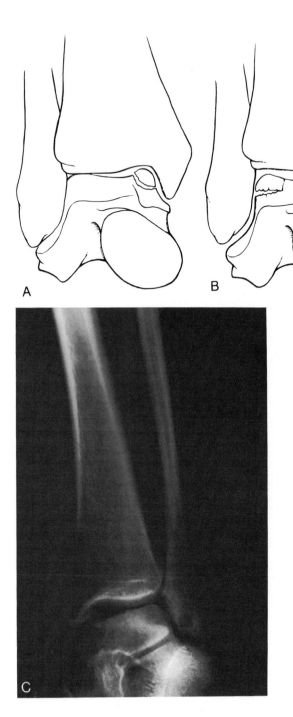

A   B

C

FIGURE 27–26. Osteochondral lesions of the talus. (*A*), A medial defect is usually in the postero-medial position and is difficult to approach except by arthroscope. (*B*), Lateral lesions are usually secondary to trauma and are usually located in the anterolateral area, which can be approached by the arthroscope or by an arthrotomy. (*C*), Radiograph of a lateral osteochondral lesion.

FIGURE 27-27. A magnetic resonance image is helpful in finding the extent of the osteochondral lesion in a 30-year-old patient. This image demonstrates approximately 20 percent involvement of the medial portion of the talus. At arthroscopy, the cartilage was found to be attached and somewhat soft, and it was drilled at the time.

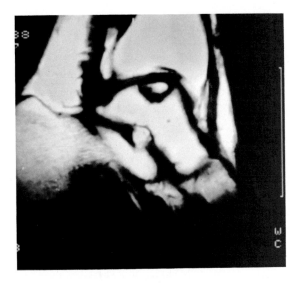

prognosis. Absorbable nails may be helpful to secure these lesions through the arthroscope.

Posterior Facet Fractures

Posterior facet fractures account for 20 percent of talar body fractures (see Fig. 27–14).[14] The lateral posterior process is larger than the medial process (see Fig. 27–1). The os trigonum, which is usually an accessory bone of the lateral posterior process, has been reported to have an incidence that varies from 3 to 20 percent. A posterior process injury can be differentiated from an accessory bone by a bone scan. The medial and lateral posterior processes form a groove for the flexor hallucis longus tendon (see Fig. 27–1). Injuries to the posterior process may involve entrapment of the flexor hallucis longus tendon. Treatment of the lateral process usually requires casting in mild equinus, excision for small fractures, or fixation of the larger lesions. To approach these lesions, a posterolateral incision near the Achilles tendon is used. The sural nerve is located medially (see Fig. 27–14). The flexor hallucis muscle and tendon can be easily found, and excision of the lateral process or release of the tendon can be performed.

Lateral Tubercle Fractures

Fractures of the lateral tubercle constitute 24 percent of all talar body fractures (Fig. 27–29). The talofibular and talocalcaneal ligaments are often involved.[21, 22] The most common mechanism of injury is compression by dorsiflexion and external rotation[32] or inversion, which can cause an avulsion.[16] Treatment depends on the symptoms and on the size of the fragment. If the fragment is small, the patient is placed in a cast in slight equinus and kept non–weight bearing for 6 weeks. A larger fragment may require open reduction and internal fixation. Débridement may be necessary for large crush injuries. It is important to note that the lateral tubercle has many articular surfaces and may be a source of arthrosis if the fracture is not treated. This injury is often mistaken for a lateral ankle sprain.

CONCLUSIONS

In summary, talar neck fractures are the most common talar injuries, and their treatment serves as a model for other talar fractures. Displacement is the key, and fixation should always be anatomic and rigid to allow for early motion with or without varus or valgus stress. Osteonecrosis is a serious problem, and its treatment depends on how much of the talar body is involved, which can be determined by MRI. Controlled weight bearing is allowed as soon as trabecular union occurs. The vascular status of the talus determines the method of weight bearing. When a large avascular segment is present, only mild

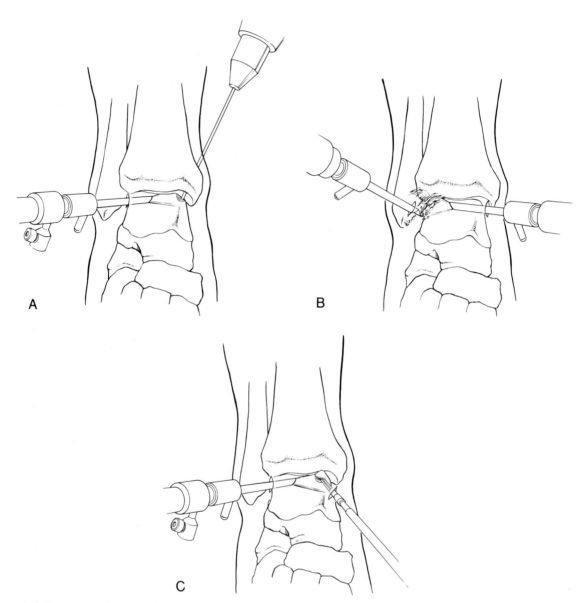

FIGURE 27–28. Arthroscopic portals used for the treatment of osteochondral lesions of the talus. (*A*), Drilling of a medial osteochondral lesion. (*B*), Débridement of an osteochondral lesion of the lateral talus. (*C*), A flap tear of a medial osteochondral lesion is being débrided.

FIGURE 27–29. *(A),* Fracture of the lateral process is often mistaken for a sprain. It can be treated by fixation through a lateral approach. *(B),* The compression mechanism is depicted by the arrows.

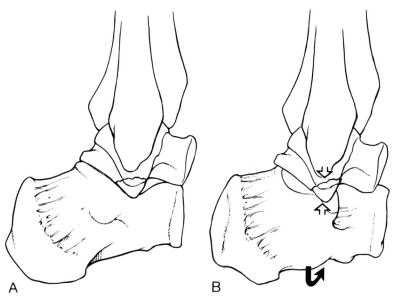

dorsiflexion and plantar flexion are allowed, with no varus or valgus shear stresses.

The approach for fixation should give the best mechanical fixation without the destruction of important blood supply. The approach to the talus should not injure the deltoid artery. MRI and computed tomography can help define the extent of the fracture and the presence of vascular collapse or osteochondral injury. Bone scans are helpful with posterior process injury. A high index of suspicion is needed for lateral tubercle fractures in these painful inversion injuries that do not improve. The image intensifier is useful, but complete fracture visualization requires obtaining anteroposterior, lateral, and oblique radiographs before leaving the operating room.

References

1. Alexander AH, Lichtman DM: Surgical treatment of transchondral talar-dome fractures; Osteochondritis dissecans; Long term follow-up. J Bone Joint Surg 62A:646, 1980.
2. Anderson HG: The medical and surgical aspects of aviation. London, Oxford Medical Publications, 1919.
3. Berndt AL, Harty M: Transchondral fractures (osteochondritis dissecans) of the talus. J Bone Joint Surg 41A:988, 1959.
4. Bobechko WP, Harris WR: The radiographic density of avascular bone. J Bone Joint Surg 42B:626, 1960.
5. Bonnin JG: Dislocations and fracture-dislocations of the talus. Br J Surg 28:88, 1940.
6. Canale ST, Belding RH: Osteochondral lesions of the talus. J Bone Joint Surg 62A:97, 1980.
7. Canale ST, Kelly FB Jr: Fractures of the neck of the talus: Long term evaluation of seventy one cases. J Bone Joint Surg 60A:143, 1977.
8. Coltart WD: Aviator's astragalus. J Bone Joint Surg 34B:545, 1952.
9. Comfort TH, Behrens F: Long term results of displaced talar neck fractures. Clin Orthop 199:81, 1985.
10. Davidson AM, Steele HD, MacKenzie DA et al. A review of twenty-one cases of transchondral fracture of the talus. J Trauma 7:378, 1967.
11. Delee JC: Fractures and dislocations of the foot. *In* Mann RA (Ed): Surgery of the Foot, 5th Ed. St. Louis, CV Mosby, 1986, p 656.
12. Dennis MD, Tullos HS: Blair tibiotalar arthrodesis for injuries to the talus. J Bone Joint Surg 62A:103, 1980.
13. Deyerle WM, Burkhardt B, Comport T: Diplaced fractures of the talus: An aggressive approach. Orthop Trans 5:465, 1981.
14. Dimon JH III: Isolated displaced fracture of the posterior facet of the talus. J Bone Joint Surg 43A:275, 1961.
15. Dunn AR, Jacobs B, Campbell RD Jr: Fractures of the talus. J Trauma 6:443, 1966.
16. Fjeldborg O: Fracture of the lateral process of the talus: Supination dorsiflexion fracture. Acta Orthop Scand 39:407, 1968.
17. Gatellier J: The juxtoretro-peritoneal route in the operative treatment of fracture of the malleolus with posterior marginal fragment. Surg Gynecol Obstet 52:67, 1931.
18. Gillquist J, et al: Late results after vertical fracture of talus. Injury 6:173.
19. Haliburton RA, Sullivan CR, Kelly PJ: The extra-osseous blood and intra-osseous supply of the talus. J Bone Joint Surg 40A:1115, 1958.
20. Hawkins LG: Fractures of the neck of the talus. J Bone Joint Surg 52A:991, 1970.
21. Hawkins LG: Fracture of the lateral process of the talus: A review of thirteen cases. J Bone Joint Surg 47A:1170, 1965.

22. Heckman JD, Mclean MR: Fracture of the lateral process of the talus. Clin Orthop 199:108, 1985.
23. Heckman JD: Fractures and dislocations of the foot. *In* Rockwood CA Jr, Green DP (Eds): Fractures in Adults, 2nd Ed. St. Louis, CV Mosby, 1987, p 1703.
24. Kelly PJ, Sullivan CR: Blood supply of the talus. Clin Orthop 30:37, 1963.
25. Kenwright J, Taylor RG: Major injuries of the talus. J Bone Joint Surg 52B:36, 1970.
26. Kleiger B: Fractures of the talus. J Bone Joint Surg 30A:735, 1948.
27. Larson RL, Sullivan CR, James JM: Trauma, surgery and circulation of the talus—what are the risks of avascular necrosis. J Trauma 1:13, 1961.
28. Lemaire RG, Bustin W: Screw fixation of fractures of the neck of the talus using a posterior approach. J Trauma 20:669, 1980.
29. Lorentzen JE, Christensen SB, Krogsoe O: Fractures of the neck of the talus. Acta Orthop Scand 48:115, 1977.
30. McCullough CJ, Venugopal V: Osteochondritis dissecans of the talus; The natural history. Clin Orthop 144:264, 1979.
31. Mindell ER, Cisek EE, Kartlaliam G: Late results of injuries of the talus; Analysis of forty cases. J Bone Joint Surg 45A:221, 1963.
32. Mukherjee SK, Pringle RM: Fracture of the lateral process of the talus. J Bone Joint Surg 56B:263, 1974.
33. Mulfinger GL, Trueta J: The blood supply of the talus. J Bone Joint Surg 52B:160, 1970.
34. O'Farrell TA, Costello BG: Osteochondritis dissecans of the talus. The late results of surgical treatment. J Bone Joint Surg 64B:494, 1982.
35. Pantazopoulos Th, Galanos P, Vayanos E: Fractures of the neck of the talus. Acta Orthop Scand 45:296, 1974.
36. Pennal GF: Fractures of the talus. Clin Orthop 30:53, 1963.
37. Penny JN, Davis LA: Fractures and fracture-dislocations of the neck of the talus. J Trauma 20:1029, 1980.
38. Peterson L, Goldie IF, Irstam L: Fractures of the talus. Acta Orthop Scand 48:696, 1977.
39. Ray RB, Coughlan EJ Jr: Osteochondritis dissecans of the talus. J Bone Joint Surg 29:697, 1947.
40. Scharling M: Osteochondritis dissecans of the talus. Acta Orthop Scand 49:89, 1978.
41. Sneppen O, Christensen SB, Krogsoe O: Fractures of the body of the talus. Acta Orthop Scand 48:317, 1977.
42. Swanson TV, Bray TJ: Talar neck fractures: A mechanical and histomorphometric study of fixation. Orthopedic Trauma Association Annual Meeting. Dallas, Texas, October 1988.
43. Trillat A, Bousquet G, Lapeyre B: Les fractures-separations totales du col ou de corps de l'astraglae. Interet du vissage par vole posterleure. Rev Chir Orthop 56:529, 1970.
44. Wildenauer E: Die Blutversorgung des talus. J Anat 115:32, 1950.
45. Yvars MF: Osteochondral fractures of the dome of the talus. Clin Orthop 114:185, 1976.

28

Metatarsal Fractures and Dislocations and Lisfranc's Fracture-Dislocations

NAOMI N. SHIELDS
RAY R. VALDEZ
MICHAEL J. BRENNAN
JEFFREY E. JOHNSON
JOHN S. GOULD

METATARSAL FRACTURES

Metatarsal fractures are a common injury of the foot. Most are nondisplaced, requiring only immobilization and protected weight bearing to heal without sequelae. Others are more complicated and frequently lead to impaired foot function and chronic problems.[13] Complications often follow those injuries with marked fracture displacement, multiple fractures, intra-articular extension, open fractures, and significant soft tissue injuries.[18]

Metatarsal fractures result either from direct trauma, including crush injuries, or from indirect trauma, such as a twisting injury that causes a myriad of fractures and dislocations in the foot and ankle.[2, 29, 58] Metatarsal stress or fatigue fractures also occur. Anatomically, fractures may involve the metatarsal base (often associated with tarsometatarsal fracture-dislocations, or Lisfranc's injury), shaft, neck, or head. All regions must be examined because it is common to have multiple areas of involvement.[2] Fractures occur in all five metatarsals. The fifth is the most commonly injured, if fractures of the base of the fifth metatarsal are included; the third is the second most commonly injured, followed by the second, first, and fourth metatarsals.[26, 29]

Evaluation

The history is as important in the evaluation of metatarsal fractures as it is in any injury. Direct trauma from a heavy object falling on a foot, a motor vehicle or machinery crush injury, and injuries from similar causes are often associated with significant soft tissue damage, compartment syndrome, open fractures, and multiple fractures. Indirect trauma often leads to oblique fractures, tendon disruption, joint dislocations, or injuries that span the length of the metatarsal region. Stress fractures occur with a history of increased or changed activity level, with a variation in an athlete's or worker's walking or running surface, or after a change in the biomechanical properties of the foot following injury or surgery.[6, 17, 33] Peripheral neuropathy is associated with Charcot's fractures, which may involve the metatarsals as well as the midfoot and hindfoot.[9]

Physical examination usually reveals an area of localized pain, swelling, discoloration, crepitus, or motion at the fracture site and an antalgic gait. Pain, motion, or crepitus at the fracture site may be elicited by grasping the metatarsal head and passively plantarflexing or dorsiflexing the metatarsal.[58, 59] Palpation of

399

the metatarsal head may reveal increased or decreased prominence on the plantar surface of foot associated with angulation at the fracture site. Rotational alignment is assessed by checking digital and toenail position.

A thorough neurovascular evaluation should be performed. Vascular evaluation begins with palpation of the dorsalis pedis and posterior tibial pulses. If these cannot be palpated, Doppler examination or even angiography may be necessary to determine the nature and extent of vascular injury. Capillary refill time may assist in the evaluation of digital vascularity. A neurologic examination should incorporate an examination of motor function, which may be limited by the extent of injury, and a sensory evaluation of the major sensory regions of the foot and digits.

Suspicion of a compartment syndrome must be high, especially with crush or multiple injuries.[6, 44] Compartment syndrome may occur even with open injuries because the injury may not adequately decompress all compartments. Pain out of proportion to the injury, especially unrelenting pain unresponsive to adequate immobilization, is highly suggestive of compartment syndrome. Pain with passive stretch of the toes (dorsiflexion) is also suggestive. Compartment pressure measurements may be taken with various techniques (using the Whitesides infusion technique, the Wick catheter, or the slit catheter). Pressure measurements greater than 30 mm Hg are abnormal. Myerson recommends that decompression be considered in acute injuries with pressures greater than 30 mm Hg, especially if these pressures are associated with clinical signs of compartment syndrome.[44, 45] Some patients may tolerate higher pressures without having severe pain. Other patients, particularly those with poor peripheral perfusion and clinical signs of compartment syndrome, may require fasciotomy at lower pressures.[7, 44, 45]

Initial radiographic evaluation includes anteroposterior, lateral, and oblique views of the foot with proper exposure technique.[2] Technetium bone scans, especially with enhanced digital techniques, are helpful for stress fracture evaluation. Computed tomography or planar tomography assists with evaluation of the tarsometatarsal joints to confirm suspicion and provide details of intra-articular fractures. Stress radiographs, which often require anesthesia, may be obtained to determine ligamentous involvement.

Treatment

The treatment of metatarsal fractures must apply the same principles used in the treatment of fractures elsewhere in the body. The best clinical outcome is achieved by obtaining proper alignment and length, with fixation as needed, and by good management of the concomitant soft tissue injury. Treatment goals include obtaining a plantigrade, flexible, stable foot with maximal function and sensibility.[38]

Isolated Metatarsal Shaft Fracture

Most minimally displaced or nondisplaced isolated metatarsal shaft fractures are treated with immobilization and protected weight bearing. Because of the strong ligamentous connection between adjacent metatarsals, this may be achieved with taping (strapping), wooden-soled shoes, and arch supports.[38, 42] Myerson recommends a firm metatarsal pad under the involved metatarsal, with 1-inch adhesive tape wrapped circumferentially about the forefoot and changed weekly.[46] However, many patients are initially more comfortable in a short-leg walking cast for up to 4 to 6 weeks,[2, 29, 41] followed by a wooden-soled shoe until the fracture is clinically and radiologically healed. First metatarsal shaft fractures should be treated with a short-leg non–weight-bearing cast for 2 weeks, followed by a walking cast for 4 weeks or until healing is clinically complete.[25] Radiographs 1 or 2 weeks after injury to confirm maintenance of position, especially in the sagittal plane, are important in treating nondisplaced or minimally displaced fractures. Sagittal displacement can be seen best on the lateral view. Dorsal angulation of the distal first metatarsal may lead to various problems, including a dorsal bunion and transfer metatarsalgia.[11]

Displaced Metatarsal Shaft Fracture

Closed treatment will reduce most displaced fractures of the metatarsal shaft. This is achieved by hanging the anesthetized foot from finger traps with a counterweight at the ankle and applying digital pressure to the shaft. Fractures that have angulation of the distal fragment in either plane that is greater than 10 degrees or displacement that is greater than 3 or 4 mm should have attempted reduction.[58, 59] If the fracture is stable after reduction, a short-leg cast is applied.[2] If the reduction cannot be maintained after discontinuation of traction, consideration must be given to surgical stabilization. The more distal the fracture, the more likely that reduction and fixation will be needed. Isolated metatarsal shaft fractures are more likely to be stable, whereas multiple shaft fractures often require stabilization.

Closed reduction with percutaneous crossed (0.045-inch) Kirschner wire (K-wire) fixation is often possible. If it is not, open reduction and internal fixation, with either K-wires, interfragmentary screws,[27, 41] or plating,[27] or external fixation[33] is indicated.

To approach an isolated metatarsal shaft fracture, a dorsal longitudinal incision centered over the fracture with retraction of the appropriate extensor tendon and subperiosteal dissection will expose the fracture site. Multiple fractures, especially open ones, require placement of the incisions to allow access to multiple metatarsals.[2] Often, incisions between the first and second metatarsals, between the third and fourth metatarsals, and laterally for the fifth metatarsal are required. Internal fixation may then be accomplished using basic fracture principles. K-wires are removed after evidence of osseous union, usually at about 6 weeks. Fractures of the first metatarsal frequently occur in the middle third of the bone. Displaced fractures of the first metatarsal shaft may be fixed with plates (a one-third semitubular or small T-plate) and screws through a dorsolateral approach. Bone grafting may be indicated, especially when there is comminution or segmental bone loss. The dorsal aspect of the first metatarsal is not the tension side, and placing the plate more laterally improves the stabilizing effect but does not create a true tension band action.[27] Displaced fractures of the fifth metatarsal shaft may require open reduction and internal fixation with plate fixation.[27] The middle metatarsals rarely require plate fixation but are amenable to fixation with cross-pins, both smooth and threaded, and to screw fixation with either mini or small fragment cortical screws.

Metatarsal Neck Fracture

Metatarsal neck fractures are often multiple and are associated with plantar angulation and displacement as a result of the strong plantar-flexing forces from the lumbricals, interossei, and extrinsic flexors.[2, 38, 46] Closed reduction may be successful, but the fracture is rarely stable, and fixation with intramedullary K-wires (0.062 inch) is recommended. It is possible, but difficult, to direct a K-wire obliquely from the condyle of the metatarsal head just proximal to the articular surface across the neck and into the shaft. However, this is the preferred method because it avoids violation of the metatarsophalangeal joint and the volar plate and results in less postoperative joint stiffness (Fig. 28–1).

Percutaneous fixation may be attempted, but

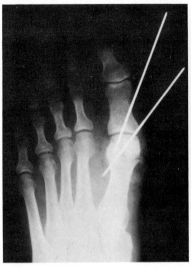
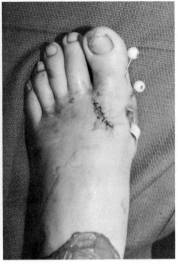

A   B

FIGURE 28–1. (*A* and *B*), Metatarsal neck fracture, repaired with Kirschner wires.

intramedullary K-wire fixation frequently requires a longitudinal dorsal incision placed midway between and parallel to the metatarsal shafts. The K-wire is passed retrograde through the metatarsal head, with the toe held in extension, and is then passed antegrade into the metatarsal shaft. The wires are removed at 3 to 4 weeks, and weight bearing is begun with a postoperative shoe or a short-leg walking cast. A stiff-soled shoe is used after 6 weeks if there is clinical and radiographic union.

An alternate technique that buries the K-wire permanently within the metatarsal avoids the potential complications of a protruding K-wire and violation of the metatarsophalangeal joint. A limited dorsal incision is made, and a K-wire is passed into the shaft of the metatarsal until resistance is felt at the base. The wire is then cut off with enough remaining to engage the distal fragment. The fracture ends are pressed together.[46] Protected weight bearing with a postoperative shoe is begun.

Ballet dancers frequently sustain a spiral fracture of the fifth metatarsal neck due to an inversion injury.[21, 56] This may be treated with a short-leg cast for 6 to 8 weeks. Grossly malaligned or displaced fractures should be reduced with distal traction and fixed with a heavy intramedullary K-wire.[21]

Metatarsal Head Fractures

Metatarsal head fractures usually result from direct trauma.[26] They have also been reported to be due to shear force on the metatarsal head.[16] The fracture produces a distal intra-articular fragment without capsular attachments.[26] A typical injury involves the shorter lateral metatarsals in association with medial metatarsal neck fractures. They are minimally displaced, with plantar and lateral angulation. Manipulation and traction usually reduce these fractures, and because they are said to be stable, they can be treated with a short-leg walking cast with an ample toe plate for 6 weeks.[16, 26] However, because there are no capsular attachments, stability may not be inherent, and open reduction and K-wire fixation may be necessary (Fig. 28–2). If excessive comminution is present, fragment removal and even metatarsal head resection may have to be considered.[24] This is unfortunate because metatarsal transfer lesions will result. However, good total contact inserts for the shoes may help distribute the weight bearing more evenly and decrease symptoms.

Freiberg's infraction (avascular necrosis) involves the metatarsal head in adolescents (particularly the head of the second metatarsal) and is believed to be produced by ischemia and fatigue fracture. This leads to a progressive osteochondral deformity of the metatarsal head.[19, 47, 56] (Avascular necrosis has not been reported as a complication of metatarsal head fracture in adults.[16, 24, 26]) Freiberg's infraction may often be treated with simple surgical joint debridement. More complicated cases require excisional arthroplasty, usually of the base of the proximal phalanx, to relieve synovitis and preserve metatarsal head weight bearing.[47] Dorsiflexion osteotomy of the metatarsal head[19] is an alternate treatment.

Intra-articular Fractures

Intra-articular fractures should be evaluated closely for joint incongruity. If this has occurred, the components should be reduced and stabilized or the fracture fragment should be débrided. K-wires are useful in stabilizing both the fracture and the joint. Intra-articular fractures damage the articular hyaline cartilage and may lead to post-traumatic degenerative arthritis and joint stiffness.

Stress Fractures

The common underlying mechanism for stress fractures is repetitive stress applied to a bone that does not have the structural strength to withstand that stress.[22, 34, 37, 48] Most patients with metatarsal stress fractures have normal bone, a history with no direct trauma but usually with an inciting event, and a history of prodromal aching or pain with activity. These fractures are seen in patients with a history of a change in their level of physical activity or other factors that increase the stresses applied to the foot (see Chapter 47). The most common sites of stress fractures are the second and third metatarsal necks and the base of the fifth metatarsal.[4, 34, 46, 48, 49, 56] Stress fractures of the fourth metatarsal occur near the middle or distal diaphysis, and those of the first metatarsal occur at the medial base.[11, 46] Proximal second metatarsal stress fractures involving Lisfranc's joint occur in ballet dancers.[39] Drez and colleagues noted that the relative length

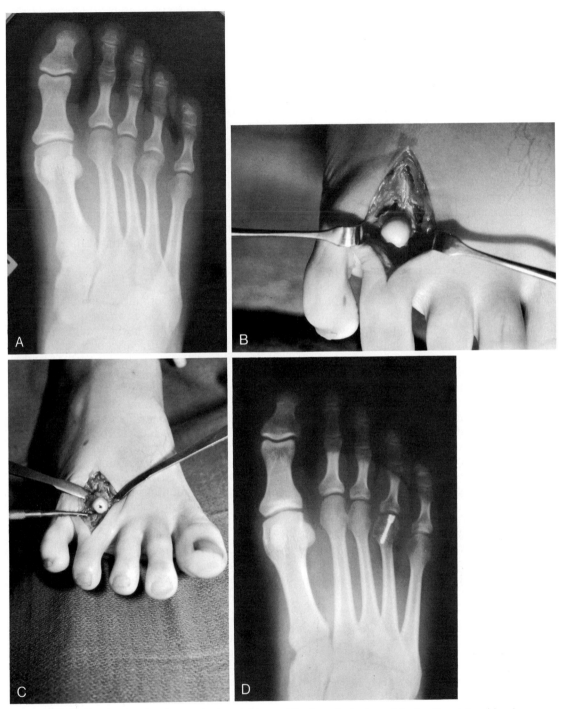

FIGURE 28–2. (*A* to *D*), Open reduction and internal fixation of a fracture of the fourth metatarsal head.

of the first metatarsal was not significant when they compared a control group with a metatarsal stress fracture group.[15] Harris and Beath studied more than 3000 soldiers and found no disability related to a short first metatarsal.[23] Metatarsal stress fractures are commonly seen in athletes and military trainees.* A military prospective study from Israel noted a higher incidence of metatarsal stress fracture in patients with low-arched feet.[61] Sullivan and colleagues reported on 19 runners with pes planus who developed stress fractures.[63] These fractures have also been reported to occur after corrective surgery for hallux valgus or hallux rigidus deformities that altered the weight-bearing mechanics of the foot.[5, 17, 33] Patients with recurrent stress fractures, especially those without a history of excessive repetitive stress, may have an underlying metabolic bone disease.[13, 22]

Although radiographic findings are normal in 10 to 30 percent of patients with stress fractures, changes may include a hairline fracture through one cortex, reactive bone or localized periostitis, endosteal thickening, intramedullary sclerosis, and resorption at the fracture line.[63] The most sensitive method of detecting stress fractures remains the technetium bone scan, which demonstrates focal uptake within 24 hours of fracture.[40, 63]

The majority of stress fractures can be treated with a combination of decreased activities, limited weight bearing, and possibly the use of a well-molded arch support with or without taping (strapping).[37] The use of a short-leg walking cast for 4 to 6 weeks, followed by wearing of a well-molded arch support, should be reserved for patients with severe pain and an inability to ambulate.[11] Return to activities should be gradual and within discomfort limits. Stress fractures of the base of the fifth metatarsal behave differently than other metatarsal fractures and are discussed separately.

Fracture of the Base of the Fifth Metatarsal

Proximal fractures of the fifth metatarsal can be divided into two primary groups. The first group, fractures of the tubercle (styloid), are thought to occur after an inversion injury. These fractures represent either an avulsion of

*See references 4, 14, 37, 40, 48, 49, 61, and 63.

the peroneus brevis tendon[36] or traction by the lateral cord of the plantar fascia aponeurosis, and they usually heal with conservative therapy.[10, 31, 66] The second group, fractures of the proximal diaphysis distal to the tuberosity (within 1.5 cm), tend to occur in the athletic patient.[31] These fractures may be stress fractures,[55] are usually not due to inversion, and have a high rate of nonunion.

The proximal fifth metatarsal base is bound to the base of the fourth metatarsal and to the cuboid by strong interosseous ligaments. The lateral aspect of the base of the fifth metatarsal is a tuberosity that protrudes beyond the lateral aspect of the fifth metatarsal shaft. The peroneus brevis tendon inserts on the dorsal surface of the tuberosity at the broadest portion of the base, and the strong lateral cord of the plantar fascia aponeurosis inserts at the tip, proximal to the insertion of the peroneus brevis.[8]

Pearson, using a cadaver model, found that an avulsion fracture of the base of the fifth metatarsal alone (without a lateral malleolar fracture) occurred only when the foot was forcibly inverted while in the equinus position and concluded that the peroneus brevis was responsible.[50] However, Richli and Rosenthal surmised that the lateral cord of the plantar aponeurosis, rather than the peroneus brevis tendon, provided the resistance that caused the fracture.[54] Kavanaugh and colleagues evaluated the force mechanism for proximal fifth metaphyseal fracture and found that the fracture results from vertical and mediolateral forces concentrated over the fifth metatarsal of the planted foot and not from inversion at all.[31] This situation occurs clinically when an athlete turns suddenly on a foot that is firmly planted on the ground.

Carp, in 1927, believed that the difficulty with healing of fractures of the fifth metatarsal base was related to the blood supply.[7] Sheriff and colleagues described the vascular supply to the fifth metatarsal and found that the greatest concentration of extraosseous vessels lies at the medial aspect of the bone.[60] The extrinsic vascular supply emanates from proximal to the articulation between the bases of the fourth and fifth metatarsals, with a nutrient artery penetrating the fifth metatarsal at the medial aspect of the shaft at the junction of the proximal and middle thirds. Intraosseous metaphyseal and epiphyseal arteries originate from extracapsular branches to the base and head but not to the proximal diaphysis. This anatomic finding may help to explain the high rate of delayed union and nonunion of these fractures.

In 1902, Sir Robert Jones described six cases of proximal metatarsal fracture, including his own, all of which healed with closed treatment.[30] The term *Jones fracture* has since been used to describe fractures involving the proximal metatarsal diaphysis and has been applied to both acute and stress fractures. Jones' original description, "whilst dancing, I trod on the outer side of my foot, my heel at the moment being off the ground . . . and the fifth metatarsal was found fractured approximately three-fourths of an inch from its base,"[30] is assumed to apply to the acute and not to the stress fracture.

Various classifications for fractures of the base of the fifth metatarsal have been provided[10, 62, 64, 68] and reviewed.[35, 65] DeLee[13] uses a classification system that combines those of Stewart[62] and Zelko and colleagues.[68] Type 1 fractures are acute fractures at the junction of the shaft and the base. Type 1A fractures are nondisplaced, and type 1B fractures are displaced or comminuted. Type 2 fractures are fractures at the junction of the metatarsal shaft and base with clinical evidence (prodromal symptoms) and radiographic evidence (radiolucent fracture line, periosteal reaction, callus on the lateral cortical margin, and intramedullary sclerosis) of previous injury. Type 3 fractures are fractures of the tuberosity (styloid) that are extra-articular (type 3A) or intra-articular involving the fifth metatarsal-cuboid joint (type 3B).[13]

Treatment of the type 1A fractures is a non–weight-bearing cast from toes to knee for up to 12 weeks.[11, 13, 35, 64, 69] In most of these patients, union of the fracture occurs. Seitz and Grantham treated nonathletes with a short-leg walking cast until union. Patients whose fractures do not unite may undergo surgical treatment, as described later.[64]

Type 1B fractures have the potential for delayed union or nonunion. Open reduction internal fixation, and early bone grafting (in high-performance athletes) are recommended[62] to decrease motion and accelerate healing. A frequently recommended technique, however, is closed reduction with cross-pinning for stability.[3, 13]

Treatment of type 2 fractures is relatively controversial. Many authors treat these frac-

tures with a non–weight-bearing cast, but the time to union may be lengthy.[1] Most authors agree that athletes, both young and recreational, and those patients with delayed union should have surgical treatment.[10] Surgical treatment options include inlay bone grafting,[28, 64] medullary curetting and bone grafting, and intramedullary screw fixation with or without bone grafting.[12, 43]

Our recommended treatment for type 2 fractures is to begin with a short-leg cast. If the radiographs show evidence of progressive union, casting is continued until union is achieved. In high-level athletes or in patients who do not progress toward union after 6 to 8 weeks of casting, surgical treatment with intramedullary screw fixation is recommended. A modification of DeLee's surgical technique is used (Fig. 28–3). DeLee did not use bone grafting in any of the fractures he fixed with the axial intramedullary screw technique.[12, 13] We approach the fracture through a lateral incision and curet the fracture or nonunion site. A bone graft is taken from either the lateral calcaneus or the iliac crest and is packed around and between the fracture fragments. The incision is extended proximally to the tuberosity, parallel to the plantar aspect of the foot. The interval between the peroneus longus and the peroneus brevis is located, and the tuberosity is identified. A guide wire is then inserted into the tuberosity to locate the axis of the medullary canal. The position is verified

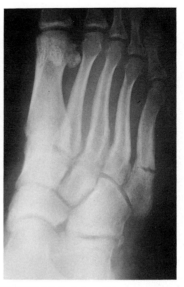

FIGURE 28–3. A type 2 Jones fracture.

by fluoroscopy or plain radiography. A cannulated drill for the 4.0- or 4.5-mm malleolar screw is then passed over the guide wire. The position is again verified by radiography or other imaging. The malleolar screw is then inserted after countersinking is performed for the head. The screw should be long enough that all threads are distal to the fracture site but short enough that the screw does not exit the medullary canal distally. Postoperatively, the patient is protected in a short-leg non–weight-bearing cast for 2 to 4 weeks and then begins weight bearing with either a postoperative shoe or a short-leg walking cast. Removal of the screw should be considered when the fracture is healed, if the activity level of the patient decreases, or if the screw is painful. A total contact insert with a relief over the screw head may alleviate symptoms if they are a problem.

Treatment of type 3A fractures may be with taping,[10] a shoe with an arch support, or a short-leg walking cast. With initially displaced fractures, a short-leg walking cast is used until the patient is asymptomatic. In patients who develop a painful nonunion or malunion, excision of the fracture fragment with advancement of the peroneus brevis tendon may be performed.[38]

Type 3B fractures may be treated with a short-leg walking cast, as described for type 3A fractures. If, after healing, these fractures are symptomatic, excision of the fragment with

peroneus brevis tendon advancement may be required. In athletes, particularly, consideration of open reduction and internal fixation to restore articular congruity is recommended. Fixation may be achieved with K-wires or small intrafragmentary screws through a lateral approach (Fig. 28–4).[51, 62]

Open Fractures

The principles of open fracture management must be applied to the management of open metatarsal fractures of the foot.[42] Thorough emergency department evaluation, cultures, administration of antibiotics, and tetanus prophylaxis should be standard. Irrigation and debridement should be accomplished in the operating room as soon as possible. All devitalized soft tissue should be removed. Internal or external fixation is also important to provide both bone and soft tissue stability. Fractures with segmental bone loss should have length maintained and may need delayed bone grafting. This is particularly true of the first metatarsal.[41] The surgeon should redébride every 24 to 48 hours after initial débridement until the wounds are clean.[58] The soft tissue wound may undergo delayed primary closure, secondary closure, split-thickness skin grafting if there is an appropriate tissue bed, or need a free vascularized tissue flap. Rotational flaps are usually contraindicated in the management of open fractures of the foot because of the

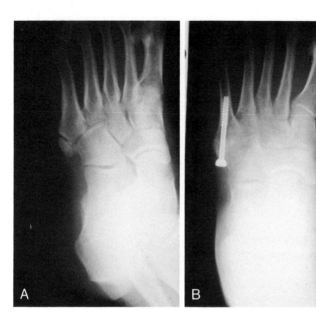

FIGURE 28–4. (*A* and *B*), Clinical example of a type 3 Jones fracture with open reduction and internal fixation.

localized foot trauma and the increased risk of flap necrosis (see Chapters 24 and 32).

Multiple Metatarsal Fractures

Multiple metatarsal fractures are typically caused by a direct blow to the dorsum of the foot or result from a high-energy injury. Falls from heights, motor vehicle accidents, injuries caused by high-velocity or close-range gunshots, and injuries caused by power equipment, such as lawn mowers, frequently result in these fractures. The soft tissue, neurovascular, and associated ligamentous and bony injuries need to be considered. Many of these injuries will be open. In patients with polytrauma, the foot has historically been considered after other injuries were addressed. Kenzora and Burgess recommend treating the foot of the patient with polytrauma aggressively to avoid many of the long-term complications.[32] They stress the need for bony stabilization, particularly in patients with closed head injuries to avoid late displacement of seemingly benign fractures. Basic objectives in the se-

verely injured foot include preserving circulation, preserving sensation (particularly plantarward), maintaining plantigrade position of the foot, preventing infection, preserving gross motion, achieving bony union, and finally, preserving fine motion.[26]

Treatment of multiple metatarsal fractures is often complicated by associated soft tissue conditions. Fractures should be treated with appropriate fixation (internal fixation with K-wires, interfragmentary screws, or plates, or external fixation) for the specific type of fracture (Fig. 28–5). The fixation should allow access for soft tissue management. Simple longitudinal intramedullary pinning, which does not firmly stabilize the bone in all parameters, is typically insufficient to achieve the stated goals.

Rehabilitation

After metatarsal fractures, especially multiple injuries, patients may experience aching, swelling, and fatigue, especially with activity.

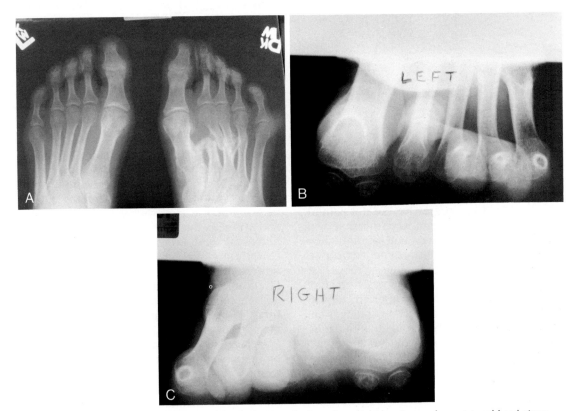

FIGURE 28–5. (*A to C*), Multiple metatarsal fractures. Note the irregular weight bearing on the metatarsal head views.

Illustration continued on following page

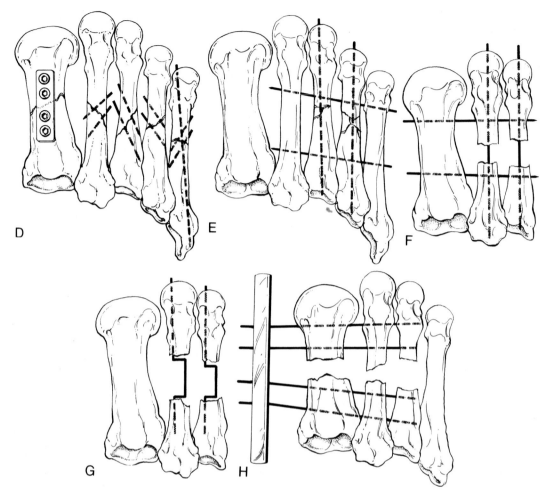

FIGURE 28–5 *Continued* (*D* to *H*), Management options for multiple metatarsal fractures.

Casting is discontinued as soon as bone stability is achieved. The foot should be protected with adequately shock-absorbing shoes and orthotics with well-molded arches. Return to activity should be progressive but not painful. Mobilization should begin when possible with active assistive and active range-of-motion exercise (joint mobilization techniques also apply), progress to strengthening exercises, develop proprioception, and use desensitization methods and massage. Control of edema with exercise, elevation, elastic wrapping, and pumping devices apply throughout the rehabilitation period. Heat and cold modalities may be used judiciously but should be discontinued if increased edema or stiffness ensues.

Complications

An acute complication of metatarsal fractures of the foot is a compartment syndrome; chronic complications of metatarsal fractures include nonunion, malunion, digital nerve entrapment, and reflex sympathetic dystrophy. In a crush injury to the lower extremity, muscle necrosis may occur, with subsequent fibrosis and stiffness. Increased serum creatine phosphokinase and urine myoglobin levels from crush injury may have renal effects.[58] Arthrofibrosis of joints may also be a sequela. Delayed union and nonunion are seen frequently with metatarsal shaft and neck fractures, fractures of the proximal diaphysis of the fifth metatarsal, and some stress fractures.

Delayed unions or nonunions may be treated by immobilization, bone grafting and internal fixation, or excision of the fracture fragment.[39, 49] Refractures may also occur.[67] Malunion of the metatarsal fracture can occur in the sagittal plane, leading to abnormal plantar load distribution. Plantar flexion of the fracture fragment may lead to a prominent plantar metatarsal head and an intractable plantar keratosis. Dorsiflexion of the metatarsal fracture may lead to transfer lesions under the compensating metatarsal heads. Coronal plane malunion may lead to entrapment of the common digital nerve between adjacent metatarsal heads. The sural nerve has been entrapped by avulsion fractures of the fifth metatarsal base. The symptoms are resolved with resection of the avulsion fragment.[20]

Treatment of symptomatic malunions begins with appropriate shoewear that has accommodative total contact inserts with metatarsal pads as needed. Surgical correction of the malunion may be necessary.[38] Hallux valgus has also been reported as a complication of metatarsal fracture after a crush injury and gunshot wound.[18] Medial or lateral bony prominence may result in shoe-fitting difficulties and can be resolved with simple excision.

Intra-articular involvement can lead to joint stiffness and post-traumatic arthritis. Compartment syndrome, if untreated, will result in fibrosis of the intrinsic musculature. This presents as a fixed intrinsic palsy with clawtoes. An intrinsic release with metatarsophalangeal dorsal capsulotomy and tenotomy and a flexor-to-extensor transfer may be needed for reconstruction. Reflex sympathetic dystrophy is potentially the most devastating sequela of a crush injury, with chronic pain, swelling, stiffness, and deformity.

Summary

The treatment of metatarsal fractures must consider the mechanism of injury and the extent of both the soft tissue and bone injuries. Although the majority of metatarsal fractures are simple to treat, many are complex and can result in impaired foot function and chronic problems. For the best clinical outcome, metatarsal fractures should be treated with adequate reduction, immobilization, and fixation as needed for each fracture type.

TARSOMETATARSAL FRACTURE-DISLOCATIONS

The significance of fracture-dislocations of the tarsometatarsal joint complex lies in the frequency of missed diagnoses and the great potential for chronic disability, even with accurate treatment.[97, 134] Injury through these

articulations bears the name of Lisfranc, who served as a surgeon in the Napoleonic army and described amputation through the tarsometatarsal joint.[112] In bygone days, this injury was usually caused by an equestrian mishap. Today, most Lisfranc's joint injuries are incurred in motorcycle,[73, 81] motor vehicle,[73, 81] industrial[85] accidents or during athletic[103, 122] events. They are recognized with increasing frequency as a manifestation of a neuropathic disorder, particularly diabetes mellitus.[94, 97, 120] The clinical presentation varies, but the recognition of injury to the tarsometatarsal joint is essential for proper treatment.

Mechanism of Injury

The forces responsible for injuries to the tarsometatarsal articulations may be broadly classified as direct or indirect (Fig. 28–6).* Direct trauma represents blows or crushing-type injuries on the foot. Although these injuries are the least common, this mechanism of injury is the most easily recognized. Application of a direct force may result in plantar dislocation, with secondary displacement dependent on the direction of the remaining forces. No definite pattern of disruption can be attributed to these injuries. The physician must be aware of associated injuries, including other fractures, soft tissue avulsions or lacerations, and elevated compartment pressures, all of which are secondary to the crushing effect.[73, 78, 85, 97, 117] In contrast, indirect trauma represents a force applied distant to the tarsometatarsal articulation, and these injuries are the most common. There are numerous proposed mechanisms. However, a longitudinal force combined with bending, torsion, or compression is involved in producing various patterns of tarsometatarsal fracture-dislocation. The foot commonly assumes a plantar-flexed position at the time of injury, with the metatarsals usually displaced dorsally and laterally. Whatever the mechanism of injury, spontaneous reduction may occur, more often with dislocation than with fracture.

Anatomy

The bony anatomy of the tarsometatarsal joint consists of five metatarsals, three cunei-

---

*See references 71, 85, 97, 102, 106, 110, 115, 119, 131, and 134.

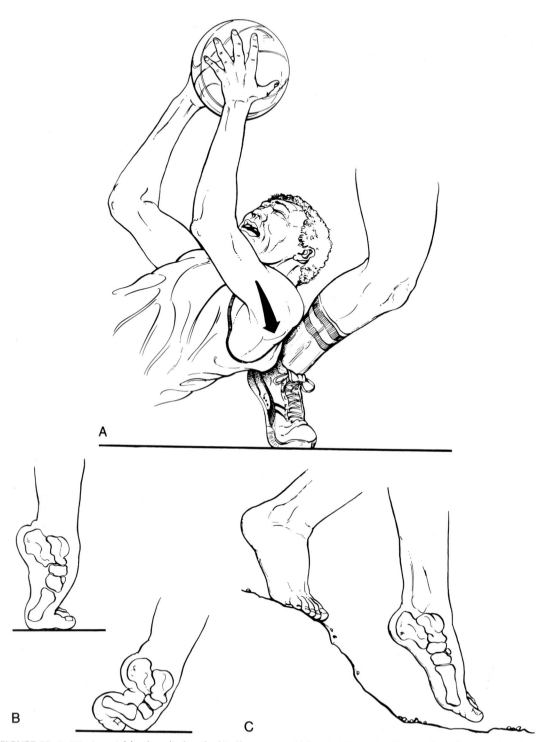

FIGURE 28–6. (*A*), An axial load applied to the hindfoot creates Lisfranc's injury. (*B*), The usual mechanism of Lisfranc's injury. (*C*), A misstep leading to Lisfranc's injury. (Modified from Rockwood CA Jr, Green DP: Fractures in Adults, 3rd Ed. Philadelphia, JB Lippincott, 1992, p 2143.)

forms, and the cuboid. The second metatarsal-cuneiform joint is recessed between the adjacent metatarsal-cuneiform joints and is the key to stability of the tarsometatarsal joint.[126] The bases of the metatarsals and cuneiforms are wedge shaped, being wider dorsally, and resemble the keystone of a Roman arch in shape, position, and function.[75, 111] Because of the intrinsic support of this architecture, either fracture or dislocation of the second metatarsal-cuneiform joint must precede the dislocation of an adjacent metatarsal or cuneiform.[72, 76, 81, 92, 104, 110] In addition, the tarsometatarsal joint line is oblique and directed posterolaterally, which, combined with the bony anatomy, may contribute to the most common pattern of disruption—dorsal and lateral displacement.[71, 75, 82, 97, 126, 131]

The ligamentous and tendinous structures provide stability equal to that of the bony anatomy.[97, 110, 111] There are no ligaments between the first and second metatarsal bases. Instead, Lisfranc's ligament courses dorsally from the medial cuneiform to the second metatarsal base and serves as the primary attachment of the four lesser metatarsal bases to the first ray. Intermetatarsal stability between the second through fifth metatarsal bases is provided by both plantar and dorsal transverse ligaments (Fig. 28–7), with the former being the strongest.[71, 83, 111, 131] The first metatarsal-cuneiform joint ligament is directed longitudinally, which permits marked abduction; therefore, a greater force is required to disrupt its attachment.[83, 85] Interosseous ligaments are present between the bases of the metatarsals; however, they provide no significant stability to these articulations.[106, 127] The insertion of the tibialis anterior and peroneus longus to the proximal aspect of the first metatarsal adds stability to the first metatarsal-cuneiform joint.[72, 131] The remaining structures on the sole of the foot, including the plantar fascia and the intrinsic muscles, resist plantar dislocation of the tarsometatarsal joint.[71, 72, 106, 131]

The dorsalis pedis artery and deep peroneal

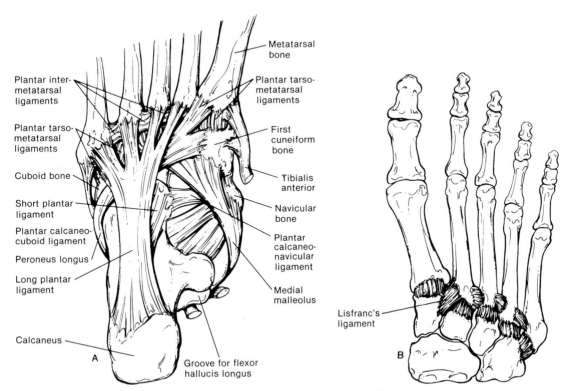

FIGURE 28–7. (*A*), Plantar ligaments involving the tarsometatarsal joints. (Modified from Rockwood CA Jr, Green DP: Fractures in Adults, 3rd Ed. Philadelphia, JB Lippincott, 1992, p 2050.) (*B*), Dorsal ligaments of the tarsometatarsal joints. (Modified from Mann RA: Surgery of the Foot and Ankle, 6th Ed. St. Louis, CV Mosby, 1993, p 1677.)

nerve are at risk for injury because of their proximity to the tarsometatarsal joint.* The dorsalis pedis artery passes between the first and second metatarsals. The communicating branch then enters the plantar aspect of the foot through the proximal 1–2 metatarsal interval to form the plantar arterial arch. The deep peroneal nerve courses from beneath the extensor retinaculum onto the dorsum of the foot between the first and second metatarsals.

*See references 75, 76, 82, 83, 85, 86, 95, 97, 100, and 134.

Injury to these neurovascular structures may occur with fracture or dislocation of Lisfranc's joint or with open reduction and internal fixation.

Classification

Although new classification systems have been proposed, the most accepted system is based on incongruity of the tarsometatarsal joints (Fig. 28–8).[73, 85, 102, 123]

1. Total incongruity. This injury type is in-

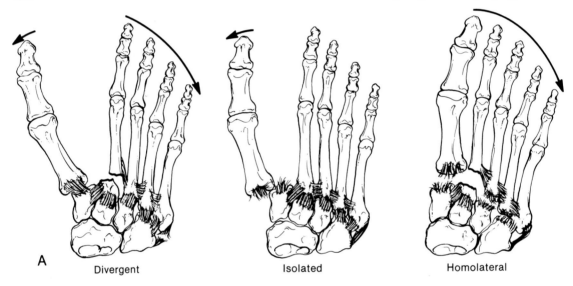

A
Divergent   Isolated   Homolateral

Type A: Total Incongruity

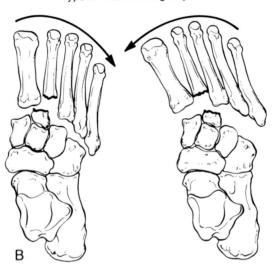

B

Type B: Partial Incongruity

FIGURE 28–8. (*A*), Typical Lisfranc's fracture-dislocations. (Modified from Rockwood CA Jr, Green DP: Fractures in Adults, 3rd Ed. Philadelphia, JB Lippincott, 1992, p 2144.) (*B*), The Hardcastle classification of Lisfranc's fracture-dislocation. (*C*), Fractures noted at the base of the second metatarsal and cuboid are frequently a component of the Lisfranc injury. (Modified from Mann RA: Surgery of the Foot and Ankle, 6th Ed. St. Louis, CV Mosby, 1993, p 1678.)

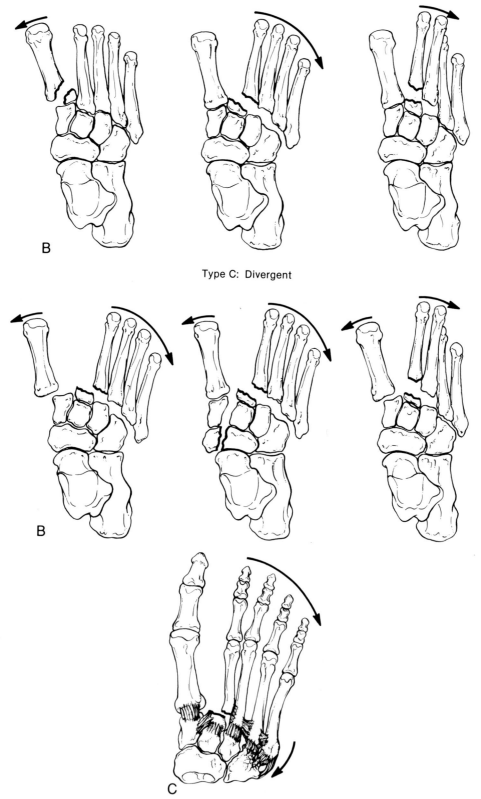

B

Type C: Divergent

B

C

FIGURE 28–8 *See legend on opposite page*

congruity of the entire tarsometatarsal joint and may be directed either medially or laterally. Displacement is in one plane: sagittal, coronal, or combined.

2. Partial incongruity. This injury type is incongruity of only part of the tarsometatarsal joint. Intermetatarsal disruption is possible, thereby varying the number of involved metatarsals. Dislocation may be either medial or lateral. Medial dislocations affect the first metatarsal–cuneiform junction, either in isolation or combined with one or more adjacent metatarsals. Lateral dislocations do not involve the first metatarsal. Displacement is in one plane: sagittal, coronal, or combined.

3. Divergent incongruity. This injury type may be a partial or total incongruity. The sine qua non of this injury, which is shown on an anteroposterior radiograph, is medial displacement of the first metatarsal and lateral displacement of any combination of the second through fifth metatarsals. Both sagittally and coronally displaced segments can occur.

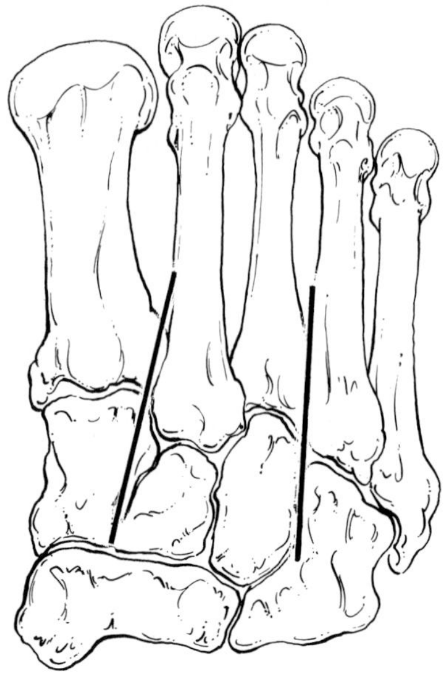

FIGURE 28–9. The proper alignment of the tarsometatarsal joint.

Evaluation

Although reported to be an uncommon entity,[71, 91, 102, 135] injury to the tarsometatarsal congruity of the entire tarsometatarsal joint is most commonly overlooked in patients with either multiple trauma or "simple" sprains.* Recognition of the injury is further complicated by varied clinical presentations, which are dependent on the degree of displacement.[72] Although the diagnosis is obvious for gross displacement, spontaneous reduction can occur.[76] The deformity, if present, is that of forefoot abduction and prominence of the medial tarsal area. However, if no deformity is present, the injury should be suspected in patients who report midfoot pain. Clinically, these patients exhibit an inability to tiptoe, and they experience marked pain at the tarsometatarsal joint with passive motion, especially forced abduction.

Radiographic evaluation of the tarsometatarsal articulation requires a complete understanding of the spatial relationship of the metatarsal bases with the cuneiforms and cuboid.[92, 121, 128] This allows assessment of both the initial displacement and the accuracy of the reduction. A complete evaluation requires a trauma series including dorsal-plantar, 30-degree me-

dial oblique, and lateral-view radiographs, all of which should be extended to include the foot and ankle because associated injuries, both proximal and distal to the tarsometatarsal joint, are common.* Intermetatarsal disruptions are not unusual; therefore, each tarsometatarsal articulation requires critical analysis. Extensive reviews have indicated common radiographic findings (Fig. 28–9).[92, 96, 101, 121, 128]

1. The first metatarsal base aligns with the lateral edge of the medial cuneiform but can vary with the diameter of the metatarsal. In general, offsets do not occur at this joint.

2. The most consistent relationship is that of the second tarsometatarsal joint, where the metatarsal base aligns with the medial edge of the middle cuneiform (see Fig. 28–9). Moreover, the second metatarsal base displaces or fractures in most injuries of Lisfranc's joint.

3. The third metatarsal base aligns with the medial and lateral margin of the lateral cuneiform at the third tarsometatarsal joint. Because of the wedge shape of the metatarsal and cuneiform, numerous well-defined borders are present that assist in accurate assessment of alignment. Offsets do not occur at this articulation.

4. The fourth and fifth tarsometatarsal artic-

---

*See references 72, 75, 85, 97, 107, 119, 129, and 132.

*See references 72, 73, 85, 92, 96, 102, and 121.

ulations are the most difficult to assess radiographically. The medial border of the fourth metatarsal should be in alignment with the medial border of the cuboid (see Fig. 28–9). Usually, they dislocate as a unit, which assists in their evaluation. Offsets of 1 to 2 mm can occur normally. However, any offset of greater than 3 mm or the presence of an avulsion fracture at the metatarsal bases should be considered an abnormal finding.[92, 121]

5. Lateral radiographs are useful in evaluating the first three metatarsal articulations only. Dorsal offset of the metatarsal bases is never seen without injury to the Lisfranc joint complex.

An injury to the tarsometatarsal joint may be obscured by a spontaneuos reduction. Radiographic findings (Fig. 28–10) that suggest an injury to the tarsometatarsal joint complex include (1) fracture at the base of the second metatarsal (fleck sign),[118] (2) compression frac-

ture of the cuboid,[71, 72, 85] (3) avulsion fracture of the medial pole of the navicular,[81, 85] (4) cuneiform subluxation or dislocation,[71, 79, 81, 105, 127] and (5) metatarsophalangeal joint dislocation.[91] Computed tomography is the procedure of choice for evaluation of these subtle injuries.[76, 96] The optimal scanning plane is along the metatarsal shafts as they articulate with the tarsals.[96] If reduction is not possible, magnetic resonance imaging can be used to determine if tendons are trapped between fragments.[76] Stress radiographs are useful but require anesthesia, and usually the decision to treat the fracture-dislocation surgically has already been made.[73, 76, 85]

Treatment

The goal of treatment is to achieve and to maintain accurate anatomic reduction, which provides the best prognosis for a painless plan-

FIGURE 28–10. Stigmata of the Lisfranc injury. (*A*), Fleck sign. (*B*), Malalignment of the tarsometatarsal joint. (*C*), Dorsal displacement on the lateral view of the tarsometatarsal joint.

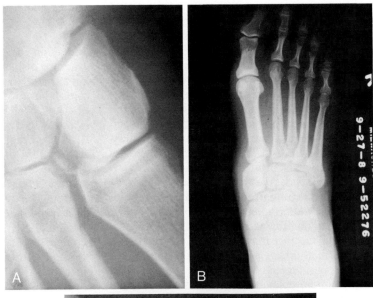

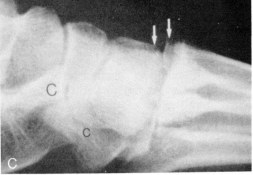

tigrade foot.[73] Whether this reduction should be achieved by open or closed methods is subject to debate. The initial attempt should be a closed reduction, with the reducing forces applied longitudinally through the use of woven wire cablegrip fingertraps. Radiographic evaluation is then performed to evaluate the reduction at each metatarsal base with the respective cuneiform or cuboid. Percutaneous smooth K-wire fixation is performed at each injured segment, even if reduction has occurred. Casting alone after reduction is not recommended because reduction without fixation does not necessarily produce stability.[74, 85, 116, 119, 135, 136]

The indications for open reduction are less controversial. An incomplete or unreducible dislocation is frequently seen in treating these injuries and is most often due to infolded ligament or capsule,[86, 93, 116, 119] bony fragments,[77, 83, 86, 111] a displaced tibialis anterior* or peroneus longus,[90] and intercuneiform injury.[71, 79, 81, 87, 105, 127] An offset of greater than 3 mm at any tarsometatarsal articulation should not be accepted.[92, 121] Most Lisfranc's injuries are closed unless they are associated with crushing forces. Open injuries require irrigation and débridement before reduction if no neurovascular compromise is present. Thereafter, principles for treating open injuries should be used, including stabilization of the injury, culture-directed antibiotic therapy, and delayed wound closure. Ischemia is rare unless the tarsometatarsal injury is accompanied by damage to the posterior tibial artery. A compartment syndrome should always be suspected, and compartment pressures should be measured when indicated.[78, 117]

Open reduction requires the use of longitudinal dorsal incisions between the first and second metatarsals and between the third and fourth metatarsals as necessary (Fig. 28–11). The neurovascular structures should always be protected. On visualization of the tarsometatarsal articulation, the bony fragments should be reduced if possible. Small fragments should be removed, especially if they interfere with reduction. If the first tarsometatarsal articulation is displaced, it should be aligned under direct visualization first, recreating the recessed articulation of the second tarsometatarsal joint. The base of the second metatarsal is then reduced and stabilized. This facilitates

---

*See references 77, 84, 87, 103, 105, 114, and 133.

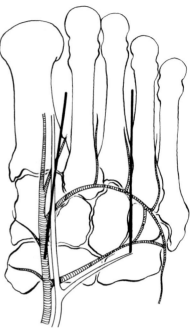

FIGURE 28–11. The approach for reduction of a Lisfranc fracture-dislocation.

reduction of the remaining tarsometatarsal fracture-dislocations. Each unstable tarsometatarsal joint should be stabilized. Stabilization has most commonly been provided with K-wires,[93, 113, 129] but temporary internal fixation with AO screws has been proposed (Fig. 28–12).[73] Internal fixation should remain in place a minimum of 12 weeks and be kept beneath the skin.[73] Repair of the ligaments is not required, and primary arthrodesis is not supported. If elevated compartment pressures are present, fasciotomies are required to release the medial, interosseous, central, and lateral compartments. These procedures can be performed through the longitudinal dorsal incisions.[78, 117] Delayed closure or split-thickness skin grafting may then be necessary. Initially, a non–weight-bearing cast is applied, then a partial–weight-bearing cast is worn for 6 to 8 weeks, after which the patient progresses to ambulation in a stiff-soled shoe. The orthopaedic hardware should be retrieved before unrestricted weight bearing.

Prolonged discomfort is always present, regardless of treatment. Secondary arthrodesis is reserved for patients who have persistent symptoms.[73, 108] Patients with a tarsometatarsal injury without antecedent trauma should be evaluated for sensory neuropathy.[94] These in-

FIGURE 28–12. (A and B), Open reduction and internal fixation of a Lisfranc fracture-dislocation.

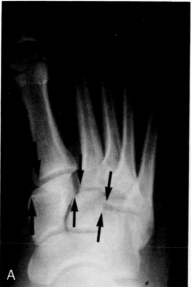
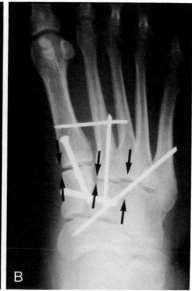

juries differ in their treatment from those secondary to trauma, and their management is discussed elsewhere in this text. Obtaining and maintaining precise anatomic reduction of the tarsometatarsal articulations provide the best prognosis for a stable, painless foot in the patient with a traumatic injury to Lisfranc's joint and anticipates an eventual return to both vocational and recreational activities without restrictions.

References

Metatarsal Fractures and Dislocations

1. Acker JH, Drez D: Nonoperative treatment of stress fractures of the proximal shaft of the fifth metatarsal (Jones' fracture). Foot Ankle 7:152–155, 1986.
2. Anderson LD: Injuries of the forefoot. Clin Orthop 122:18–27, 1977.
3. Arangio GA: Proximal diaphyseal fractures of the fifth metatarsal (Jones fracture): Two cases treated by cross-pinning with a review of 106 cases. Foot Ankle 3:293–296, 1983.
4. Bernstein A Stone JR: March fracture: A report of three hundred and seven cases and a new method of treatment. J Bone Joint Surg 26:743–750, 1944.
5. Black JR: Second metatarsal stress fracture secondary to Keller arthroplasty: Case report. Milit Med 148:747–749, 1983.
6. Bonutti PM, Bell GR: Compartment syndrome of the foot. J Bone Joint Surg 68A:1449–1451, 1986.
7. Carp L: Fracture of the fifth metatarsal bone with special reference to delayed union. Ann Surg 86:308–320, 1927.
8. Christopher F: Fractures of the fifth metatarsal. Surg Gynecol Obstet 37:190–194, 1923.
9. Cundy RF, Edmonds ME, Watkins PJ: Osteopenia and metatarsal fractures in diabetic neuropathy. Diabetic Med 2:461–464, 1985.
10. Dameron TB: Fractures and anatomical variations of the proximal portion of the fifth metatarsal. J Bone Joint Surg 57A:788–792, 1975.
11. Davis AW, Alexander IJ: Problematic fractures and dislocations in the foot and ankle of athletes. Clin Sports Med 9:163–181, 1990.
12. DeLee JC, Evans P, Julian J: Stress fractures of the fifth metatarsal. Am J Sports Med 11:349–353, 1983.
13. DeLee JC: Fractures and dislocations of the foot. *In* Mann RA (Ed): Surgery of the Foot. St. Louis, CV Mosby, 1986.
14. Devas MB: Stress fractures in athletes. Proc R Soc Med 62:933–937, 1969.
15. Drez D, Young J, Johnson RD, Parker WD: Metatarsal stress fractures. Am J Sports Med 8:123–125, 1980.
16. Dutkowsky J, Freeman BL: Fracture-dislocation of the articular surface of the third metatarsal head. Foot Ankle 10:43–44, 1989.
17. Ford LT, Cilula LA: Stress fractures of the middle metatarsals following the Keller operation. J Bone Joint Surg 59A:117–118, 1977.
18. Ganel A, Israeli A, Horoszowski H: Posttraumatic, development of hallux valgus. Orthop Rev 16:79–82, 1987.
19. Gauthier G, Elbaz R: Freiberg's infraction: A subchondral bone fatigue fracture. Clin Orthop 142:93–95, 1979.
20. Gould N, Trevino S: Sural nerve entrapment by avulsion fracture of the base of the fifth metatarsal bone. Foot Ankle 2:153–155, 1981.
21. Hardaker WT: Foot and ankle injuries in classical ballet dancers. Orthop Clin North Am 20:621–627, 1989.
22. Harper MC: Metabolic bone disease presenting as multiple recurrent metatarsal fractures: A case report. Foot Ankle 9:207–209, 1989.

23. Harris RI, Beath T: The short first metatarsal: Its incidence and clinical significance. J Bone Joint Surg 31A:553–565, 1949.

24. Harrison M: Fractures of the metatarsal head. Can J Surg 11:511–514, 1968.

25. Heck CV: Fractures of the bones of the foot (except the talus). Surg Clin North Am 45:103–117, 1965.

26. Heckman JD: Fractures and dislocations of the foot. *In* Rockwood CA, Green DP (Eds): Fractures in Adults, 2nd Ed. Philadelphia, JB Lippincott, 1984.

27. Heim U, Pfeiffer KM: The foot. *In* Small Fragment Set Manual. New York, Springer-Verlag, 1981.

28. Hens J, Martens M: Surgical treatment of Jones fractures. Arch Orthop Trauma Surg 109:277–279, 1990.

29. Irwin CG: Fractures of the metatarsals. Proc R Soc Med 31:789–793, 1938.

30. Jones R: Fracture of the base of the fifth metatarsal bone by indirect violence. Ann Surg 35:697–700, 1902.

31. Kavanaugh J, Brower T, Mann R: The Jones fracture revisited. J Bone Joint Surg 60A:776–782, 1978.

32. Kenzora JE, Burgess AR: The neglected foot and ankle in polytrauma. Adv Orthop Surg 7:89–98, 1983.

33. Kitaoka HB, Cracchiolo A: Stress fractures of the lateral metatarsals following double-stem silicone implant arthroplasty of the hallux metatarsophalangeal joint. Clin Orthop 239:211–216, 1989.

34. Leavitt DG, Woodward HW: March fracture: A statistical study of forty-seven patients. J Bone Joint Surg 26:733–742, 1944.

35. Lehman RC, Torg JS, Pavlov H, DeLee J: Fractures of the base of the fifth metatarsal distal to the tuberosity: A review. Foot Ankle 7:245–252, 1987.

36. Lichtblau S: Painful nonunion of a fracture of the 5th metatarsal. Clin Orthop 59:171–175, 1968.

37. McBryde AM: Stress fractures in athletes. J Sports Med 3:212–217, 1975.

38. McKeever FM: Fractures of tarsal and metatarsal bones. Surg Gynecol Obstet 90:735–745, 1950.

39. Micheli LJ, Sohn RS, Solomon R: Stress fractures of the second metatarsal involving Lisfranc's joint in ballet dancers. J Bone Joint Surg 67A:1372–1375, 1985.

40. Milgrom C, Giladi M, Stein M, et al: Stress fractures in military recruits: A prospective study showing an unusually high incidence. J Bone Joint Surg 67B:732–735, 1985.

41. Morrison GM: Fracture of the bones of the feet. Am J Surg 38:721–726, 1937.

42. Morrissey EJ: Metatarsal fractures. J Bone Joint Surg 28:594–602, 1946.

43. Munro T: Fractures of the base of the fifth metatarsal. J Assoc Can Radiol 40:260–261, 1989.

44. Myerson M: Acute compartment syndromes of the foot. Bull Hosp Jt Dis Orthop Inst 47:251–261, 1987.

45. Myerson MS: Experimental decompression of the fascial compartments of the foot—the basis for fasciotomy in acute compartment syndromes. Foot Ankle 8:308–314, 1988.

46. Myerson MS: Injuries to the forefoot and toes. *In* Jahss MH (Ed): Disorders of the Foot and Ankle, 2nd Ed. Philadelphia, WB Saunders, 1991.

47. Omer GE: Primary articular osteochondroses. Clin Orthop 158:33–40, 1981.

48. Orava S, Puranen J, Ala-Ketola L: Stress fractures caused by physical exercise. Acta Orthop Scand 49:19–27, 1978.

49. Orava S, Hulkko A: Delayed unions and nonunions of stress fractures in athletes. Am J Sports Med 16:378–382, 1988.

50. Pearson JR: Combined fracture of the base of the fifth metatarsal and the lateral malleolus. J Bone Joint Surg 43A:513–516, 1961.

51. Pritsch M, Heim M, Tauber H, Horoszowski H: An unusual fracture of the base of the fifth metatarsal. J Trauma 20:530–531, 1980.

52. Rao J, Banyon M: Irreducible dislocation of the metatarsophalangeal joints of the foot. Clin Orthop 145:224–226, 1979.

53. Richardson EG: Fractures and dislocations of the foot. *In* Crenshaw AH (Ed): Campell's Operative Orthopaedics. St. Louis, CV Mosby, 1991.

54. Richli WR, Rosenthal DI: Avulsion fracture of the fifth metatarsal: Experimental study of pathomechanics. AJR Am J Roentgenol 143:889–891, 1984.

55. Roca J, Roure F, Fairen MF, Yunta A: Stress fractures of the fifth metatarsal. Acta Orthop Belg 46:630–636, 1980.

56. Sammarco GJ, Miller EH: Forefoot conditions in dancers. Foot Ankle 3:85–98, 1985.

57. Seitz WH, Grantham SA: The Jones fracture in the non athlete. Foot Ankle 6:97–100, 1985.

58. Shereff MJ: Complex fractures of the metatarsals. Orthopedics 13:875–882, 1990.

59. Shereff MJ: Fractures of the forefoot. Instr Course Lect 39:133–140, 1990.

60. Shereff MJ, Yang QM, Kummer FJ, et al: Vascular anatomy of the fifth metatarsal. Foot Ankle 11:350–353, 1991.

61. Simkin A, Leichter I, Giladi M, et al: Combined effect of foot arch structure and an orthotic device on stress fracture. Foot Ankle 10:25–29, 1989.

62. Stewart IM: Jones's fracture: Fracture of base of fifth metatarsal. Clin Orthop 16:190–198, 1969.

63. Sullivan D, Warren RF, Pavlov H, Kelman G: Stress fractures in 51 runners. Clin Orthop 187:188–192, 1984.

64. Torg JS, Baldwine F, Zelko R, et al: Fractures of the base of the fifth metatarsal distal to the tuberosity. Classification and guidelines for non-surgical and surgical management. J Bone Joint Surg 66A:209–214, 1984.

65. Torg JD: Fractures of the base of the fifth metatarsal distal to the tuberosity. Orthopedics 13:731–737, 1990.

66. Wharton HR: Fracture of the proximal end of the fifth metatarsal bone. Ann Surg 47:824–826, 1908.

67. Whitesides JA, Fleagle SB, Kalenak A: Fractures and refractures in intercollegiate athletes. Am J Sports Med 9:369–377, 1981.

68. Zelko R, Torg JS, Rachum A: Proximal diaphyseal fractures of the fifth metatarsal—treatment of the fractures and their complications in athletes. Am J Sports Med 7:95–101, 1979.

69. Zogby R, Baker B: A review of nonoperative treatment of Jones' fracture. Am J Sports Med 15:304–307, 1987.

Tarsometatarsal Fracture-Dislocations

70. Adelaar RS: The treatment of tarsometatarsal fracture-dislocation. Instr Course Lect 39:141–145, 1990.

71. Aitken AP, Poulson D: Dislocations of the tarso-metatarsal joint. J Bone Joint Surg 45A:246–260, 1963.
72. Anderson LD: Injuries of the forefoot. Clin Orthop 122:18–27, 1977.
73. Arntz CT, Veith RG, Hansen ST: Fractures and fracture-dislocations of the tarsometatarsal joint. J Bone Joint Surg 70A:173–181, 1988.
74. Ashhurst APC: Divergent dislocaiton of the metatarsus. Ann Surg 83:132–136, 1926.
75. Bassett FH: Dislocations of the tarsometatarsal joints. South Med J 57:1294–1302, 1964.
76. Berquist TH, Johnson KA: Trauma. *In* Berquist TH (Ed): Radiology of the Foot and Ankle. New York, Raven Press, 1989.
77. Blair WF: Irreducible tarsometatarsal fracture-dislocation. J Trauma 21:988–990, 1981.
78. Bonutti PM, Bell GR: Compartment syndrome of the foot. J Bone Joint Surg 68A:1449–1450, 1986.
79. Brown DC, McFarland GB: Dislocation of the medial cuneiform bone in tarsometatarsal fracture-dislocation. J Bone Joint Surg 57A:858–859, 1975.
80. Brunet JA: The late results of tarsometatarsal joint injuries. J Bone Joint Surg 69B:437–440, 1987.
81. Cain PR, Seligson D: Lisfranc's fracture-dislocation with intercuneiform dislocation: Presentation of two cases and a plan for treatment. Foot Ankle 2:156–160, 1981.
82. Cassebaum WH: Lisfranc fracture-dislocations. Clin Orthop 30:116–128, 1963.
83. Collett HS, Hood TK, Andrews RE: Tarsometatarsal fracture dislocations. Surg Gynecol Obstet 106:623–626, 1958.
84. DeBenedetti MJ, Evanski PM, Waugh TR: The unreducible Lisfranc fracture. Clin Orthop 136:238–240, 1978.
85. DeLee JC: Fractures and dislocations of the foot. *In* Mann RA (Ed): Surgery of the Foot. St. Louis, CV Mosby, 1986.
86. DelSel JM: The surgical treatment of tarso-metatarsal fracture-dislocations. J Bone Joint Surg 37B:203–207, 1955.
87. Denton JR: A complex Lisfranc fracture-dislocation. J Trauma 20:526–529, 1980.
88. Dunn AW: Injuries of the tarsometatarsal joints. J La State Med Soc 127:125–128, 1975.
89. Easton ER: Two rare dislocations of the metatarsals at Lisfranc's joint. J Bone Joint Surg 20:1053–1056, 1938.
90. Engber WD, Roberts JM: Irreducible tarsometatarsal fracture-dislocation. Clin Orthop 168:102–104, 1982.
91. English TA: Dislocations of the metatarsal bone and adjacent toe. J Bone Joint Surg 46B:700–704, 1964.
92. Foster SC, Foster RR: Lisfranc's tarsometatarsal fracture dislocation. Radiology 120:79–83, 1976.
93. Geckeler EO: Dislocations and fracture-dislocations of the foot: Transfixation with Kirschner wires. Surgery 25:730–733, 1949.
94. Giesecke SB, Dalinka MK, Kyle GC: Lisfranc's fracture dislocation: A manifestation of peripheral neuropathy. AJR Am J Roentgenol 131:139–141, 1978.
95. Gissane W: A dangerous type of fracture of the foot. J Bone Joint Surg 33B:535–538, 1951.
96. Goiney RC, Connell DG, Nichols DM: CT evaluation of tarsometatarsal fracture-dislocation injuries. Am J Radiol 144:985–990, 1985.
97. Goossens M, De Stoop N: Lisfranc's fracture-dislocations: Etiology, radiology, and results of treatment. Clin Orthop 176:154–162, 1983.
98. Gopal-Krishnan S: Dislocation of medial cuneiform in injuries of tarsometatarsal joints. Int Surg 58:805–806, 1973.
99. Graham J, Waddell JP, Lenczner E: Tarso-metatarsal (Lisfranc) dislocation. J Bone Joint Surg 55B:666, 1973.
100. Granderry WM, Lipscomb PR: Dislocation of the tarsometatarsal joints. Surg Gynecol Obstet 114:467–469, 1962.
101. Hall MC: The trabecular patterns of the normal foot. Clin Orthop 16:15–20, 1960.
102. Hardcastle PH, Reschauer R, Kutscha-Lissberg E, Schoffman W: Injuries to the tarsometatarsal joints. J Bone Joint Surg 64B:349–356, 1982.
103. Heckman JD Jr: Fractures and dislocations of the foot. *In* Rockwood CA Jr, Green DP (Eds): Fractures, Vol 2. Philadelphia, JB Lippincott, 1984.
104. Hesp WLEM, Van der Werken C, Goris RJA: Lisfranc dislocations: Fractures and/or dislocations through the tarso-metatarsal joints. Injury 15:261–266, 1984.
105. Holstein A, Joldersman RD: Dislocation of first cuneiform in tarsometatarsal fracture-dislocation. J Bone Joint Surg 32A:419–421, 1950.
106. Jeffreys TE: Lisfranc's fracture-dislocation. J Bone Joint Surg 45B:546–551, 1963.
107. Johnson GF: Pediatric lisfranc injury: "Bunkbed" fracture. Am J Radiol 137:1041–1044, 1981.
108. Johnson JE, Johnson KA: Dowel arthrodesis for degenerative arthritis of the tarsometatarsal (Lisfranc) joints. Foot Ankle 6:243–253, 1986.
109. King RE: Dislocation of the tarsometatarsal joints. Bull Hosp Jt Dis Orthop Inst 47:190–202, 1987.
110. LaTourette G, Perry J, Patzakis JS, et al: Fractures and dislocations of the tarsometatarsal joint. *In* Bateman JE, Trott AW (Eds): The Foot and Ankle. New York, Thieme-Stratton, 1980.
111. Lenczner EM, Waddell JP, Grahan JD: Tarsal-metatarsal (Lisfranc) dislocation. J Trauma 14:1012–1020, 1974.
112. Lisfranc J: Nouvelle Methode Operatoire pour l'Amputation Partielle du Pied dans son Articulation Tarso-Metatarsienne: Methode Precedee des Nombreuses Modifications qu'a Subies Celle de Chopart. Paris, Gabon, 1815.
113. London PS: Major injuries of the foot. J Bone Joint Surg 58B:385, 1976.
114. Lowe J, Yosipovitch Z: Tarsometatarsal dislocation: A mechanism blocking manipulative reduction. J Bone Joint Surg 58A:1029–1030, 1976.
115. Manter JT: Distribution of compression forces in joints of the human foot. Anat Rec 96:313–321, 1946.
116. Markowitz HD, Chase M, Whitelaw GP: Isolated injury of the second tarsometatarsal joint. Clin Orthop 248:210–212, 1988.
117. Myerson MS: Experimental basis for fasciotomy in acute compartment syndromes of the foot. Foot Ankle 8:308–314, 1988.
118. Myerson MS: The diagnosis and treatment of injuries to the Lisfranc joint complex. Orthop Clin North Am 20:655–664, 1989.

119. Myerson MS, Fisher RT, Burgess AR, Kenzora JE: Fracture dislocations of the tarsometatarsal joints: End results correlated with pathology and treatment. Foot Ankle 6:225–242, 1986.

120. Newman JH: Spontaneous dislocation in diabetic neuropathy. J Bone Joint Surg 61B:484–488, 1979.

121. Norfray JF Geline RA, Steinberg RI, et al: Subtleties of Lisfranc fracture-dislocations. Am J Radiol 137:1151–1156, 1981.

122. O'Donoghue DH: Treatment of Injuries to Athletes, Vol 1, 4th Ed. Philadelphia, WB Saunders, 1984.

123. Quenu E, Kuss G: Etude sur les luxations du metatarse. (Luxations metatarso-tarsiennes.) Rev Chir 39:281–336, 720–791, 1093–1134, 1909.

124. Resch S, Stenstrom A: The treatment of tarsometatarsal injuries. Foot Ankle 11:117–123, 1990.

125. Sangeorzan BJ, Veith RG, Hansen ST: Salvage of Lisfranc's tarsometatarsal joint by arthrodesis. Foot Ankle 10:193–200, 1990.

126. Sarrafian SK: Anatomy of the Foot and Ankle. Philadelphia, JB Lippincott, 1983.

127. Schiller MG, Day RD: Isolated dislocation of the medial cuneiform bone—a rare injury of the tarsus. J Bone Joint Surg 52A:1632–1636, 1970.

128. Stein RE: Radiological aspects of the tarsometatarsal joints. Foot Ankle 3:286–289, 1983.

129. Turco VJ, Spinella AJ: Tarsometatarsal dislocation—Lisfranc injury. Foot Ankle 2:362, 1982.

130. van der Werf GJIM, Tonino AJ: Tarsometatarsal fracture-dislocation. Acta Orthop Scand 55:647–651, 1984.

131. Wiley JJ: The mechanism of tarso-metatarsal joint injuries. J Bone Joint Surg 53B:474–482, 1971.

132. Wiley JJ: Tarso-metatarsal joint injuries in children. J Pediatr Orthop 1:255–260, 1981.

133. Wilppula E: Tarsometatarsal fracture-dislocation. Acta Orthop Scand 44:335–345, 1973.

134. Wilson DW: Injuries of the tarso-metatarsal joints. J Bone Joint Surg 54B:677–686, 1972.

135. Wilson PD: Fractures and dislocations of the tarsal bones. South Med J 26:833–845, 1933.

136. Wynne AT, Southgate GW: Delayed tarsometatarsal joint dislocation following forefoot injury. Orthopedics 9:52–54, 1986.

29 *Fractures of the Calcaneus*

DROR PALEY

The calcaneus is the most common tarsal bone fractured. Calcaneal fractures can be subdivided into intra-articular and extra-articular fractures of the subtalar joints. Intra-articular fractures make up 70 to 75 percent of all calcaneal fractures, whereas extra-articular fractures make up 25 to 30 percent.[12, 22] Intra-articular fractures are the fractures that usually come to mind when calcaneal fractures are being discussed, and they are the most controversial fractures to treat.[15] These fractures are known for their significant socioeconomic impact on a patient's ability to work and for their effect on long-term disability. On the other hand, extra-articular fractures are usually much more benign and treatable and lead to far less disability.

EXTRA-ARTICULAR FRACTURES

Extra-articular fractures (Fig. 29–1) have been grouped into five different types: (1) anterior process, (2) tuberosity, (3) medial process, (4) sustentaculum, and (5) body. The sustentacular and body fractures are probably not truly separate entities and have the same mechanism of injury as intra-articular fractures.

Anterior Process Fractures

Anterior process fractures have been reported to make up 15 percent of fractures in a large series of calcaneal fractures.[5] The two reported types of anterior process fractures are (1) avulsion and (2) compression. The avulsion type is the most common. This fracture is usually small and extra-articular. The mechanism of injury is thought to be an avulsion by either the bifurcate ligament or the extensor digitorum brevis following an inversion stress to an adducted plantarflexed foot.[42] This injury is most common in women wearing high heels. The compression fracture was reported by Hunt to be a larger fragment that is usually displaced superiorly and posteriorly, with significant calcaneocuboid joint involvement and incongruity.[25] It is thought to result from a forced abduction injury, which causes an impaction of the calcaneocuboid joint and thus a compression fracture of the anterior process.

Treatment for the avulsion type is usually a cast for immobilization if no displacement is present and the fragment is small. When the fragment is larger and there is displacement, open reduction and internal fixation should be considered to reduce the calcaneocuboid joint incongruity. Degan and colleagues reported on seven patients who required late excision.[9] Six of them had an ununited fragment and secondary pain. The investigators reported that although not all of these fractures healed, not all nonunions are painful. Late excision relieved symptoms in five of the seven patients.

Tuberosity Fractures

Tuberosity fractures were previously subdivided into beak or avulsion fractures.[34, 53] These two types are now considered to be the same entity. Tuberosity fractures result from avulsion of the superior tuberosity of the calcaneus by the tendo Achillis. They are most common in osteoporotic older women.

421

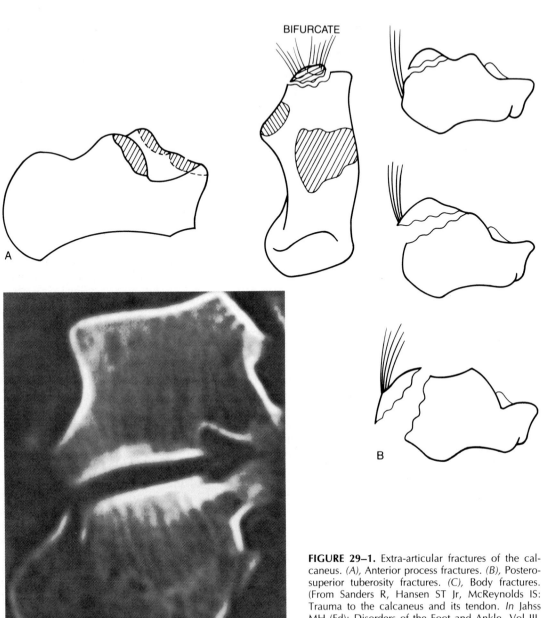

FIGURE 29–1. Extra-articular fractures of the calcaneus. *(A)*, Anterior process fractures. *(B)*, Posterosuperior tuberosity fractures. *(C)*, Body fractures.
(From Sanders R, Hansen ST Jr, McReynolds IS:
Trauma to the calcaneus and its tendon. *In* Jahss
MH (Ed): Disorders of the Foot and Ankle, Vol III,
2nd Ed. Philadelphia, WB Saunders, 1991, p 2239.)

If the fracture is minimally displaced or undisplaced, it can be treated by a cast in equinus. On the other hand, if it is displaced, an attempted closed reduction can be tried but is usually unsuccessful. Open reduction with fixation using a tension band technique over Kirschner wires (K-wires) is the preferred method of treatment.

Medial Calcaneal Process Fractures

Fractures of the medial calcaneal process are rare. Watson-Jones attributed these to shear injuries from a direct blow.[65] Bohler believed that they were avulsion injuries of the plantar fascia.[2] The medial calcaneal process is also the site of origin of the abductor hallucis longus and part of the flexor digitorum longus.

Treatment is not required if the fracture is minimally displaced or undisplaced. In significantly displaced fractures, closed reduction may be attempted. Open treatment should be considered only if the fracture cannot be reduced manually and threatens to create a bothersome exostosis.

INTRA-ARTICULAR FRACTURES

Intra-articular fractures make up the majority of calcaneal fractures, as noted earlier. Eighty to 90 percent of these fractures are secondary to a fall, and an increasing number seem to be due to high-energy motor vehicle accidents.[30, 56] Five to 9 percent are bilateral. Ten percent have associated compression fractures in the lumbar spine. Other associated injuries are reported in 60 percent of cases by Lance and colleagues[30] and in 70 percent of cases by Slatis and colleagues.[60] Although some controversy exists about modalities of treatment, there is generalized agreement on the pathoanatomy and pathomechanics of injury. Knowledge of both is essential to understanding the pathology of this fracture and options for treatment.

Pathoanatomy and Pathomechanics

Intra-articular calcaneal fractures occur following eccentric axial loading of the talus on the calcaneus (Fig. 29–2).[4] This produces a primary shear fracture line that is parallel to the posterolateral edge of the talus and passes through the posterior calcaneal facet. The primary fracture line separates the calcaneus into two parts: (1) body (posterolateral) and (2) sustentaculum (anteromedial) (see Fig. 29–2). Each part contains a portion of the posterior facet. The amount of posterior facet belonging to each fragment depends on how medial or lateral the split occurs.[55] This, in turn, is related to the position of the foot at the time of impact (inversion or eversion position). The more medial the split, the larger the articular component on the body fragment, and vice versa. The body fragment displaces laterally and proximally toward the fibula while the sustentacular fragment stays home, anatomically fixed to the undersurface of the talus by the capsule and ligaments of the middle facet (Fig. 29–3).

If the injurious force continues to be applied, secondary fracture lines develop off the primary shear line. The posterior secondary fracture line creates the "thalamic fragment" (also known as semilunar, comet, or superolateral fragment),[57] which is the depressed portion of the posterior subtalar facet (see Fig. 29–3).[61] The size of the thalamic fragment depends on the posterior exit point of the secondary fracture line. When the line exits superiorly, this fracture is called a central depression type, and when the line exits posteriorly, the fracture is called a tongue type.[12] As the body of the talus drives the thalamic fragment into the spongy, cancellous bone of the calcaneal body fragment, it usually shears the attachment of the thalamic fragment from the lateral wall[10, 54, 57] and causes a blow-out fracture, leading to the well-recognized lateral bulge. Together with the lateral displacement of the body fragment, the lateral bulge impinges on the fibulocalcaneal space, predisposing the patient to fibulocalcaneal impingement and peroneal tendon entrapment.[27] The eccentric loading causes the thalamic fragment's articular facet to rotate medially as it is impacted into the calcaneal body fragment.

The fracture lines on the medial side are therefore sharp, well defined, and relatively uncomminuted because they were produced by a shearing force. In contrast, the fracture lines on the lateral side are comminuted and poorly defined because they were produced secondary to the axial impaction and lateral expansion (see Fig. 29–2). The body fragment, having been released from its attachment anteriorly,

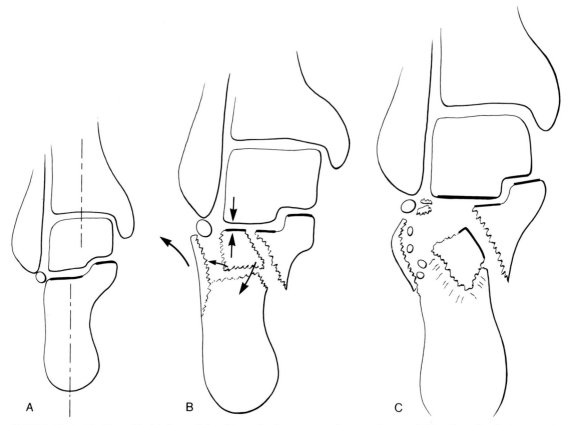

FIGURE 29–2. *(A),* The midaxial lines of the tibia and calcaneus are shown to be parallel but laterally displaced with respect to each other.

(B), As the primary fracture line develops, the body of the calcaneus displaces laterally and proximally. This impacts the lateral portion of the posterior facet against the posterior lateral edge of the talus, leading to the shearing off of the lateral wall and the development of the posterior secondary fracture line.

(C), As the body of the calcaneus progresses proximally and laterally, it causes the thalamic fragment to rotate medially and to impact into its cancellous bone. This explodes out the sheared-off lateral wall fragment and results in several comminuted fragments impinging into the peroneal tendon space against the fibula. A bone defect is left above the thalamic fragment and adjacent to the lateral wall fragment from the depression.

FIGURE 29–3. Multiple views of the calcaneus demonstrating the primary and secondary fracture lines.

(A), Superior view of the calcaneus demonstrating the primary fracture line dividing the calcaneus into anteromedial and posterolateral segments, also known as the sustentacular and body fragments, respectively. The posterior secondary fracture line parallels the posterolateral rim of the subtalar joint. The anterior secondary fracture line extends into the calcaneocuboid joint.

(B), A view of the calcaneus from its plantar (inferior) aspect demonstrates the primary fracture line across the waist of the calcaneus and the anterior secondary fracture line, which splits the calcaneus in a transverse plane and may enter the calcaneocuboid joint. The posterior secondary fracture line cannot be seen from this view.

(C), From the lateral view, the secondary fracture lines are clearly seen to emanate off the primary fracture line. The posterior secondary fracture line can extend even more posteriorly, becoming a tongue-type fracture instead of the central depression–type fracture illustrated. The anterior secondary fracture line may extend into the plantar aspect of the calcaneus or may enter into the calcaneocuboid joint, as illustrated.

(D), Medial view of the calcaneus demonstrates the medial extension of the posterior secondary fracture line along the posterior rim of the posterior facet. The anterior secondary fracture line goes under the sustentaculum.

(E), An axial view of the calcaneus shows how the primary fracture line splits the medial wall. The level of this split is important in deciding on the operative approach. The posterior secondary fracture line can be seen to shear away the lateral wall of the calcaneus and to have a compression front to it on its inferior aspect. An anterior secondary fracture line is not appreciated from this view.

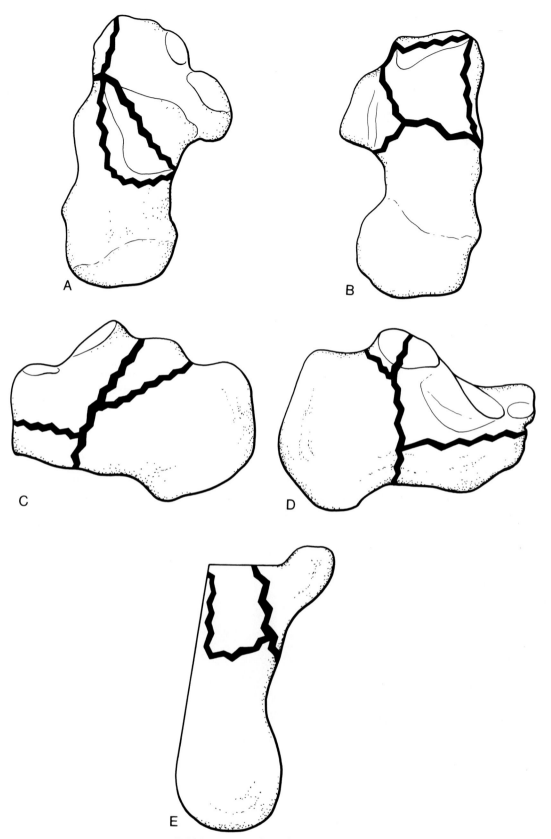

FIGURE 29–3 *See legend on opposite page*

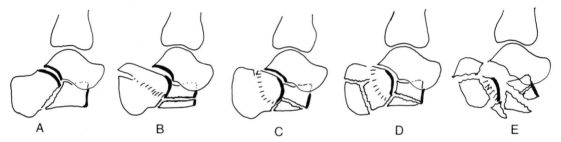

FIGURE 29–4. Classification of intra-articular fractures of the calcaneus. *(A)*, Shear. *(B)*, Tongue type. *(C)*, Central depression type. *(D)*, B or C with comminution. *(E)*, Comminuted. (From Paley D, Hall H: Calcaneal fracture controversies: Can we put Humpty Dumpty together again? Orthop Clin North Am 20:667, 1989.)

loses its alignment and pitch as it tilts into varus and is plantarflexed proximally by the tendo Achillis. As the calcaneal pitch collapses, the calcaneal length and tendo Achillis fulcrum shorten. At the same time, secondary fracture lines extend anteriorly, entering into the plantar aspect of the calcaneus anteriorly or penetrating into the calcaneocuboid joint. This fracture line extension allows the arch to further collapse.

The shearing compression and angular forces take their toll on the surrounding soft tissues, leading to a stretch, shearing injury on the medial side and a compression injury on the plantar aspect. The lateral soft tissues suffer impingement from the expanding lateral wall and translation of the calcaneal body, but they are relatively spared compared with the plantar and medial sides. For this reason, fracture blisters are more commonly seen on the medial side, and hemorrhage is more commonly seen on the plantar aspect, indicating the maximal areas of tissue disruption.

The pathoanatomy of the calcaneus and foot

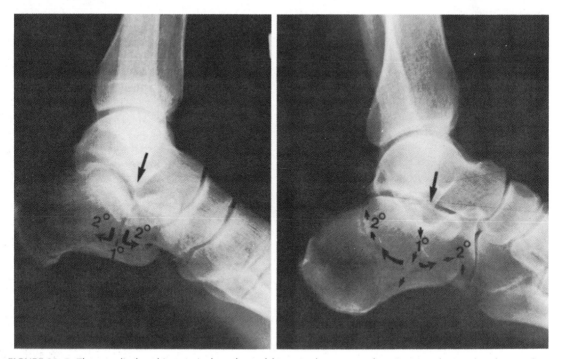

FIGURE 29–5. These undisplaced intra-articular calcaneal fractures demonstrate the primary and secondary fracture lines. The primary line (1°) is a shear line extending from the lateral process of the talus plantarward. The secondary lines develop off this primary line anteriorly and posteriorly. The extension is either tongue type *(left)* or central depression type *(right)*. The anterior extension is either "calcaneocuboid" or "plantar." (From Paley D, Hall H: Calcaneal fracture controversies: Can we put Humpty Dumpty together again? Orthop Clin North Am 20:667, 1989.)

has measurable and predictable changes.[46] Böhler's angle becomes flattened. The talocalcaneal angle, which indicates varus or valgus malalignment of the heel, decreases in magnitude, indicating varus malalignment. The bony longitudinal arch formed by the base of the calcaneus and the first metatarsal is decreased. The length of the calcaneus shortens posterior to the lateral talar process. This portion of the calcaneal length is called the tendo Achillis fulcrum. The heel height decreases, and the fat pad height slightly increases. The width of the calcaneus increases at the level of the blowout, encroaching into the fibulocalcaneal space.[27] The subtalar joint becomes incongruous, and extension into the calcaneocuboid joint may also lead to incongruity of the calcaneocuboid joint. This constellation of displacement is fairly constant,[19] and the variability seen between fractures is related more to degree than to variations in pathoanatomy.

Classification (Figs. 29–4 to 29–6)

The classic categorization of intra-articular calcaneal fractures was described by Essex-Lopresti in 1952.[12] He divided intra-articular fractures into two main groups: tongue and central depression types. Stephenson incorporated the Essex-Lopresti classification with a consideration for the number of fracture parts, subdividing fractures into two- and three-part types.[63] Soeur and Remy included a comminuted group in their classification.[61] Rowe and colleagues categorized tongue-type and central depression–type fractures into those with and those without comminution.[56]

Based on the examination of more than 100 calcaneal radiographs, I have noted that just as consistently as a posterior secondary fracture line occurs, there is also an anterior secondary fracture line, which extends forward off the primary shear line. As noted in the

FIGURE 29–6. Axial radiograph showing the depressed "thalamic" (TH) posterior facet fragment. The "body" (B) of the calcaneus, the posterolateral fragment, is displaced laterally and proximally, and impinges on the fibula and peroneal tendon space. The "sustentaculum" (ST), the anterior fragment, remains anatomically reduced to the talus. The fracture between the thalamus and the sustentaculum is the primary fracture line, and the fracture between the thalamus and the body is the secondary fracture line. (From Paley D, Hall H: Calcaneal fracture controversies: Can we put Humpty Dumpty together again? Orthop Clin North Am 20:666, 1989.)

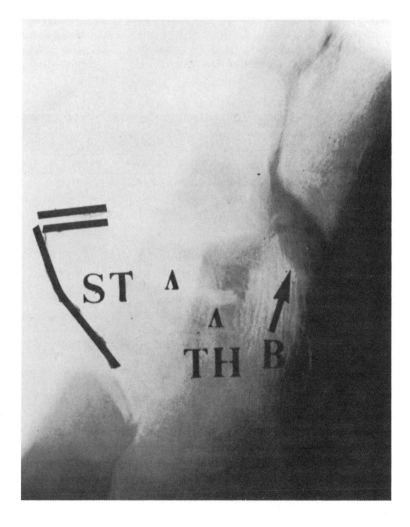

description of the pathomechanics, the anterior secondary fracture line may extend into the plantar aspect of the calcaneus, just posterior to the calcaneocuboid joint, or into the calcaneocuboid joint itself. I have called these lines plantar and calcaneocuboid types.[46, 47] In order to grade the degree of comminution of calcaneal fractures from plain radiographs, these anterior secondary fracture lines are useful. Comminution can be defined as the presence of more than one posterior and one anterior secondary fracture line. Therefore, central depression and tongue-type fractures can be subdivided into those with and those without comminution.

When comminution and displacement are so significant that the fracture pattern cannot be readily classified into a central depression or tongue type, the fracture is subclassified as *comminuted*. Displaced intra-articular calcaneal fractures can therefore be subclassified into the following four groups: (1) shear fracture (two-part fracture); (2) tongue-type fracture (A, no comminution; B, with comminution); (3) central depression fracture (A, no comminution; B, with comminution); and (4) comminuted fracture.

Certainly, comminution is best defined using computed tomography (CT). Unfortunately, CT is not always readily available, especially at night. Therefore, a classification based on plain radiographs remains useful.

Recently, CT classifications have been reported.[8, 10, 57] These provide more objective criteria on which to define comminution and the size of the joint fragments. Crosby and Fitzgibbons[8] divided fractures by displacement and comminution: type I, undisplaced; type II, displaced; type III, displaced and comminuted. Although this is a simple system to follow, there is no definition of location or amount of comminution. Eastwood and colleagues divided fractures according to the lateral wall of the calcaneus because this is the first part seen on lateral exposure and thereby affects treatment.[10, 11] In type I, the lateral wall is formed by the lateral joint fragment; in type II, the lateral wall is formed by both the lateral joint proximally and the lateral wall distally. In type III, the body fragment makes up the entire lateral wall.

TABLE 29–1. LONG-TERM RESULTS OF TREATMENT OF CALCANEAL FRACTURES		
TREATMENT	**SATISFACTORY RESULTS (%)**	**UNSATISFACTORY RESULTS (%)**
No Reduction		
Pozo et al[51]	67	33
Rowe et al[56]	58	42
Lance et al[30]	50	50
Essex-Lopresti[12]	63	37
Closed Reduction		
Cotton et al[7]	50	50
Hermann[23]	73	27
Rowe et al[56]	47	53
Primary Arthrodesis		
Lindsay et al[33]	60	40
Hall et al[18]	75	25
Zayer[66]	46	54
Thompson et al[64]	84	16
Percutaneous Reduction		
Essex-Lopresti[12]	60	40
Open Reduction		
Essex-Lopresti[12]	59	41
Rowe et al[56]	56	44
Maxfield et al[35]	70	30
Hazlett[21]	86	14
McReynolds[36]	70	30
Letournel[31]	76	24
Stephenson[63]	77	23
Harding et al[20]	75	25

Sanders proposed what appears to be the most useful classification using CT criteria (Fig. 29–7).[57, 58] Based on the coronal cuts, fractures are classified by the number and location of intra-articular fracture lines. The posterior subtalar joint facet is divided into three columns: lateral, central, and medial. The sustentaculum is a separate entity. This classification correlated with the results after operative treatment.

Natural History of Operative and Nonoperative Treatment of Calcaneal Fractures

The results of nonoperative and operative treatment of intra-articular calcaneal fractures are listed in Table 29–1. In general, nonoperative treatment results reported in the literature were unsatisfactory in 30 to 50 percent of cases. In comparison, operative treatment results were reportedly unsatisfactory in 25 to 40 percent of cases.

Following calcaneal fracture, usually a gradual improvement in painful symptomatology occurs over a 2- to 6-year period (Table 29–2). More than half of patients reach a plateau in their symptomatology within the first 2 years, with more than 75 percent having a plateau within 4 years. Only a very small percentage (usually between 5 and 10 percent) actually show worsening symptoms. Therefore, recorded results in the literature with only short-term follow-up of 2 to 4 years actually underestimate rather than overestimate suc-

cessful results. This is fortunate because few long-term studies of calcaneal fractures are available.

The major shortcoming of all of the studies noted in Tables 29–1 and 29–2 is that the clinical evaluation of results was based on completely different criteria and evaluation protocols from author to author. This lack of standardization makes it difficult to compare results. In addition, the fracture classification used varied from author to author.

Standardized Protocol for Evaluating Calcaneal Fracture Outcome

Factors Related to Outcome

The literature is not clear about which factors are significant for or prognostic of final outcome.[39, 46] Tables 29–3 and 29–4 list factors that are reported to be associated or not to be associated, respectively, with poor outcome. As noted in these tables, some factors are significant in some studies and not significant in others.

In a personally and independently conducted external review of patients with intra-articular calcaneal fractures, I reviewed the cases of 45 patients with 52 heel fractures who were followed up for 4 to 14 years.[47] All patients had been treated by the medial approach by one surgeon (H. Hall) between 1972 and 1982. The purpose of this study was not only to evaluate the results of treatment but also to make a determination of anatomic and nonanatomic

TABLE 29–2. SYMPTOM STABILIZATION AFTER FRACTURE

STUDY	CHANGE IN SYMPTOMS	PATIENTS (%)	PERIOD
Essex-Lopresti[12]	Plateau	88	18 mo
	Worse	0	6 mo–7 yr
Lindsay et al[33]	Plateau	57	1 yr
		15	3–8 yr
	Improving	few	10 yr
	Worse	7	8.8 yr
	Temporarily worse	6	4.7 yr
Pozo et al[51]	Plateau	66	2–3 yr
		24	3–6 yr
	Worse	0	>6 yr
Paley et al[47]	Plateau	60	2 yr
		20	2–4 yr
		10	4–6 yr
	Worse	10	>6 yr

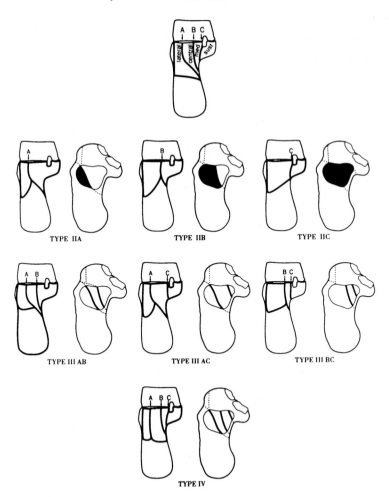

FIGURE 29–7. CT scan classification of intra-articular calcaneal fractures. It is important that the coronal section analyzed include the widest point of the articular surface: that is, it must include the sustentaculum. (From Sanders S: Intra-articular fractures of the calcaneus: Present state of the art. J Orthop Trauma 6:254, 1992.)

factors that were significantly related to patient outcome. Similar to a previously published ankle fracture score,[43] we developed a calcaneal fracture score.[47] A result was determined for each patient and for each heel using this score. In the 44 patients with unilateral fractures, the opposite, uninjured foot was radiographed, and 11 measurable parameters of calcaneal anatomy or pathoanatomy were determined and compared between sides. Not only was the absolute value of each measured parameter compared, but the ratio and the difference between sides were statistically analyzed.

According to this critical study,[47] the factors found to be significantly associated with an unsatisfactory result were (1) increased patient weight; (2) decreased patient height; (3) increased time off work; (4) heavy labor occupation; (5) increased heel width; (6) decreased fibulocalcaneal space; (7) subtalar and calca-

neocuboid joint incongruity; (8) subtalar and calcaneocuboid joint arthrosis; (9) ankle arthrosis; (10) fracture type (comminuted was worst, central depression was second worst, and tongue type was best); (11) fracture comminution; and (12) decreased Böhler's angle ratio of the injured to the normal side. The factors that were not associated with an unsatisfactory result included (1) height of the fall, (2) workmen's compensation status, (3) heel height, (4) heel alignment, (5) arch angle, (6) tendo Achillis fulcrum length, and (7) calcaneal length.

No significant age difference was found between result groups. However, patients older than 50 years of age did have a more unsatisfactory outcome. Similarly, there was no difference in the proportion of female patients in each result group, but four of six female patients sustained a satisfactory result. Thus, age and sex are probably related to prognosis. The

nant of an unsatisfactory result. The potential sources of pain are numerous. Aside from fibulocalcaneal impingement, peroneal tendon space stenosis, heel pad pain, and subtalar joint pain, pain sources also included the medial side of the foot in the sustentacular region (possible tarsal tunnel syndrome); the midfoot apex of the flattened longitudinal arch of the foot; the forefoot (metatarsalgia); the tendo Achillis (tendonitis); and the calcaneocuboid, talonavicular, and ankle joints (arthritis). Another occasional source of pain is a plantar exostosis from a protruding fracture fragment. Some sources of pain, such as incisional neuromas, protuberant hardware, and reflex sympathetic dystrophy, are related to surgery.

Further examination of the data revealed that the average number of painful clinical problem areas in the satisfactory-result group was one, compared with an average of two clinical problem areas in the unsatisfactory-result group. In a smaller group of nonoperatively treated calcaneal fractures with similar follow-up time that were evaluated by the same protocol, we found an average of seven painful clinical problem areas per foot in the unsatisfactory-result group.[47]

Review of the literature, including the overall results from our series, shows that the results following open reduction and internal fixation are not much better than those following conservative treatment. This has been the basis of the long-standing treatment controversy. Our operative results were 62 percent satisfactory and 38 percent unsatisfactory. The nonoperative results were 60 percent satisfactory and 40 percent unsatisfactory. The difference is that a patient with an unsatisfactory result in this operatively treated group had fewer painful problem areas per foot than a

TABLE 29–3. FACTORS ASSOCIATED WITH POORER OUTCOME

FACTOR	STUDY
Age >50	
Lateral impingement	Lindsay et al[33]
Peroneal entrapment	Slatis et al[60]
	Pozo et al[57]
Heel pad pathology	Lindsay et al[33]
Subtalar arthritis	Pridie[52]
Subtalar incongruity	Essex-Lopresti[12]
	Lance et al[30]
	Gaul et al[14]
	Hammersfahr[19]
	Stephenson[62]
Subtalar stiffness	Lance et al[30]
	Pozo et al[51]
Decreased Böhler's angle	Slatis[60]

anatomic factors in this analysis that proved most significant were increase in calcaneal width, decrease in fibulocalcaneal space, subtalar incongruity, and subtalar arthrosis. The first two factors are measurable manifestations of clinical problems frequently seen following malunion of calcaneal fractures. Increase in calcaneal width and decrease in fibulocalcaneal distance lead to fibulocalcaneal impingement and peroneal tendon space encroachment. These are some of the more common sources of pain following calcaneal fracture. Subtalar joint incongruity leads to subtalar arthrosis, another important cause of pain and of an unsatisfactory outcome.

The most common primary clinical problems were heel pad pain and fibulocalcaneal impingement pain, which were equally frequent. The difference between the patients who suffered from fibulocalcaneal pain and those who suffered from heel pad pain was that the majority of heels with the fibulocalcaneal area as the primary painful area had a satisfactory outcome, whereas the majority of heels with the heel pad as the primary painful area had an unsatisfactory outcome. The most common secondary painful area was the subtalar joint; for patients with pain at this site, results were equally divided between satisfactory and unsatisfactory outcomes. All patients who had no painful area had a satisfactory result. Similarly, the majority of patients who had no secondary painful area also had a satisfactory result. Thus, pain seems to be the primary determi-

TABLE 29–4. FACTORS NOT ASSOCIATED WITH POORER OUTCOME

FACTOR	STUDY
Age	Lindsay et al[33]
Sex	Lindsay et al[33]
Arch flattening	Lindsay et al[33]
Subtalar arthritis	Lindsay et al[33]
	Pozo et al[51]
Decreased Böhler's angle	Gaul et al[14]

patient in the nonoperatively treated group (two versus seven).[45]

Radiographic Assessment

Radiographic evaluation of the fractured os calcis should include plain radiography and, whenever possible, CT. Plain radiography should include four standard views of the fractured side and the same views of the uninjured side.

The lateral view of the foot allows evaluation of Böhler's angle and is useful in classifying the type of fracture (joint depression versus tongue). It also shows anterior fracture lines extending into the calcaneocuboid or plantar aspect of the foot. The lateral radiograph can be used to assess the decrease in the calcaneal pitch and arch angle; the shortening of the tendo Achillis fulcrum; the talocalcaneal angle, which is a measure of heel alignment; the loss of heel height; and the protrusion of bony fragments, which may act as exostoses, into the soft tissues. The lateral view in a weight-bearing position gives a good evaluation of the fat pad.

The anteroposterior view of the ankle is useful in assessing the fibulocalcaneal space. This space is usually greater than 15 mm. Extrusion of bone fragments into this space can easily be seen. Normally, it should be possible to place a dime between the shadow of the fibula and the calcaneus (dime sign).

The axial view shows the lateral displacement of the body of the calcaneus toward the fibula, as well as the step at the medial cortex. It should show the posterior facet with the depression in its articular surface. Widening of the heel can be appreciated, and varus malalignment can be noted. To improve the assessment of the malalignment, the standard 45-degree axial radiograph should be taken with a long tibial x-ray plate under both the heel and the tibia. The alignment of the tibia should normally be parallel to that of the calcaneus, although the midaxial line of the calcaneus lies lateral to that of the tibia. Any angulation on the midaxial line of these two bones demonstrates a malalignment. This view has been termed the long axial view.

Finally, an anteroposterior external oblique view of the foot shows the calcaneocuboid joint and any fracture line extension into it. These same radiographs should be taken of the uninjured side for reference. For purposes of

reconstruction, the uninjured side can serve as a template. In addition to these standard views, a medial oblique axial projection gives an excellent view of the middle and posterior facets of the subtalar joint and often shows the fracture line in its best projection. The interval between the lateral malleolus and the calcaneus is also best evaluated on this view.

CT has greatly improved our understanding of the pathoanatomy of each individual fracture. Positioning of the foot is important when this technique is being used.[16] The patient lies supine in the scanner, with both ankles in 30 degrees of plantar flexion, the knees and hips flexed, and the feet 30 degrees off the flat surface of the table. The gantry should be oriented to provide semicoronal sections at 90-degree orientation to the table, 60-degree orientation to the sole of the foot, and 90-degree orientation to the posterior facet plantar aspect of the foot.[59] This gives axial CT cuts of the calcaneus and its posterior facet. The orientation can be checked on the scout view. A second angle of tomographic cut should be parallel to the sole of the foot to assess the calcaneocuboid joint.

Nonoperative Treatment

The foot should be examined for its neurovascular status, and the degree of swelling should be assessed. Attention should be paid to the possibility of a tarsal tunnel or compartment syndrome. The clinical signs and symptoms include pain above and beyond that expected from the injury, severe degrees of swelling, and decreased sensation in the distribution of the plantar nerves, with intact sensation in the distribution of the calcaneal branch of the posterior tibial nerve and in the adjacent sural and saphenous nerves. Stretch pain on passive abduction or adduction of the toes may be elicited. In the face of these signs or symptoms, compartment pressure may be measured in the interosseous compartments, or fasciotomies may be performed on a prophylactic basis, without any further objective evidence. These fasciotomies are performed thorough two dorsal intermetatarsal longitudinal incisions, either with or without a medial incision in the region of the abductor hallucis muscle. If a tarsal tunnel syndrome is present, the tarsal tunnel should be exposed from the posterior to the medial malleolus, to the point where the nerve enters the abductor hallucis muscle. The treatment of compartment syndrome in the foot is independent of the surgeon's choice of operative or nonoperative treatment.

Fortunately, in the majority of cases, especially those due to a fall from a height, there is no compartment syndrome. Treatment begins in the emergency room with immediate elevation of the foot and packing of the foot in ice, with sufficient protection to prevent an ice burn of the skin. The icing should be performed for 15 minutes on and 10 minutes off routinely for the first several hours and should then be performed intermittently over the next 24 hours. The foot should be wrapped in an elastic bandage. Many surgeons prefer to wrap the foot in a thick cotton wad dressing with a posterior plaster slab. I see no advantage to this because it prevents the ice from working through all of the layers and provides no significant additional compression over that provided by a simple tensor bandage. The foot should be kept strictly elevated for several days.

At this point, a plaster cast can be applied and the patient can start walking with crutches, with full weight bearing as tolerated. Because the foot will tend to swell, walking should be performed for short periods only (20 minutes), followed by elevation for 1 to 2 hours. The cast should be changed after 1 week to accommodate for the decreased amount of swelling. The skin needs to be inspected, and fracture blisters must be kept sterile. Walking should be encouraged, mixed with appropriate periods of elevation, until the vasomotor edema period is over (approximately 2 to 3 weeks). The patient should be encouraged to bear weight to desensitize the heel and thus decrease the chance of late pain. The patient must be made aware that modified shoewear may become necessary because of the widened heel and the flattened arch. After 6 weeks, the cast can usually be discontinued in favor of shoewear. Physical therapy can be started for ankle and subtalar range of motion.

Operative Treatment

Several operative techniques have been used to treat displaced intra-articular calcaneal fractures. These include percutaneous elevation of

the tongue fragment,[12] and open reduction and internal fixation and primary arthrodesis.[18, 41, 64]*

Percutaneous elevation is primarily used in the treatment of tongue-type fractures. A Steinmann pin or Gissane spike is inserted into the posterior aspect of the tongue fragment and then levered distally to improve Böhler's angle and reduce the tongue fragment. The Steinmann pin is then driven across into the rest of the calcaneus to immobilize this fragment. A slipper cast may be incorporated around the protruding Steinmann pin. This procedure does not address anatomic joint congruity or the problems of heel width or heel alignment. Recently, indirect dynamic and closed reduction methods have been described.[40, 44]

Open Reduction

Several different open reduction techniques have been popularized: the medial approach, the lateral approach, and the combined medial and lateral approach.

The medial approach described by McReynolds has the advantages of using a very small incision and exposing the side of the fracture where the fracture lines are best delineated because the least amount of comminution is present.[36] This makes reduction of the body fragment to the sustentacular fragment relatively accurate. It is also easier to judge heel alignment medially. This side has good bone available for fixation in the arch under the sustentaculum. The disadvantages of this approach are its proximity to the neurovascular bundle, which limits the extensibility of the incision. Furthermore, with this approach, the reduction of the subtalar joint is performed in a blind fashion. This approach offers very limited room for hardware, and for this reason, the staple has been chosen as the simplest device for the limited exposure. There is poor access for bone grafting and no accessibility to the calcaneocuboid joint. The medial approach is contraindicated when the sustentacular fragment is very small.

The lateral approach described by Palmer gives excellent access to the subtalar joint and is an extensile approach.[49] There is no proximity to a significant neurovascular bundle, with the exception of the sural nerve. Ample

---

*See references 19, 31, 36, 46, 61, and 63.

room is present for bone grafting and for fixation. In addition, the lateral bulge and fibulocalcaneal space can be decompressed easily. This incision may be extended to include exposure of the calcaneocuboid joint if necessary. The disadvantages of this approach are that it exposes the more comminuted side and thus makes judging the alignment and reduction of the body fragment more difficult, with the most common error being that of nonreduction of the lateral shift of the body. Laterally, there is poor bone for fixation. This approach involves greater soft tissue dissection, and closure of the incision may be difficult.[17]

Medial Approach (Figs. 29–8, 29–9)

An incision is made two fingerbreadths below the medial malleolus, starting at the posterior aspect of the calcaneus and continuing anteriorly. The neurovascular bundle is palpated; it is usually located within one fingerbreadth behind the medial malleolus. The incision may be extended just to that point, avoiding exposure of the structure, but is preferably extended anterior to this point, with careful dissection and identification of these structures for their protection. Care should be taken to identify the calcaneal branch of the posterior tibial nerve. It is sometimes necessary to sacrifice one of the branches of this calcaneal nerve because it crosses the middle of the operative field. However, the main branch should be spared at all costs, both because of its important innervation of the heel pad and because of the risk of a painful neuroma if it is injured. Decompression of the tarsal tunnel may be considered prophylactically in association with this procedure.

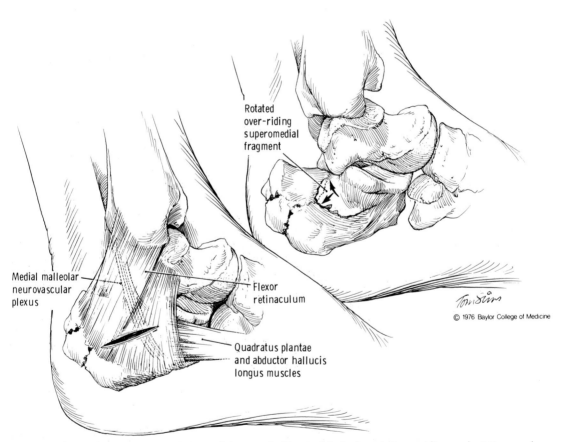

FIGURE 29–8. Operative treatment using a medial approach. The medial displacement, overriding, and rotation are drawn from the roentgenogram of this tongue-type fracture *(arrows)*. The approximate location of the incision, fascia, and vascular plexus is shown. (© 1976 Baylor College of Medicine.)

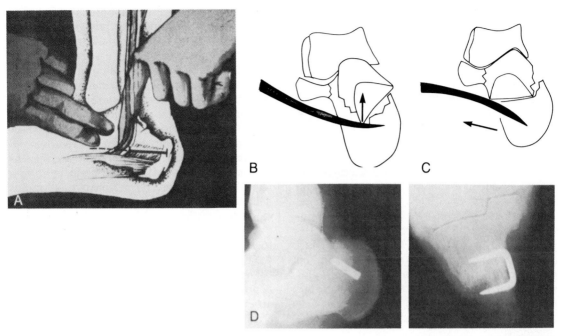

FIGURE 29–9. Medial approach. *(A),* Incision: Two fingerbreadths below and one fingerbreadth behind the medial malleolus extending posteriorly. *(B),* The facet is depressed and rotated medially. The instrument is inserted and the facet is elevated and rotated laterally. *(C),* The laterally displaced body fragment is levered over medially and reduced to the sustentaculum. *(D),* Fixation is achieved with a staple. (From Paley D, Hall H: Calcaneal fracture controversies: Can we put Humpty Dumpty together again? Orthop Clin North Am 20:672, 1989.)

The dissection is carried through the abductor hallucis longus muscle down to bone. The primary shear fracture line is easily identified: it lies posterior to the sustentaculum fragment. Dissection can be extended proximally to identify the sustentaculum. The extensor hallucis longus tendon is easily identified in this location and may on occasion be caught in the fracture line. A blunt-tipped elevator is inserted into the fracture line and used to elevate the depressed posterior facet fragment or fragments. The surgeon performs this maneuver in a completely blind fashion, guided only by touch. On decompression of this fragment, a loud cracking sound may be heard. This does not represent formation of a new fracture but simply disimpaction of the depressed fragment from the body of the calcaneus. As this fragment is elevated from the medial approach, it spontaneously rotates laterally. This assists in its reduction because it is rotated medially when it is depressed. This fact is important to recognize and can be seen on a CT scan. The articular surface of the depressed fragment usually faces the sustentacular fragment. After this fragment is elevated, it needs to be pushed up as high as possible against the overlying talar portion of the posterior subtalar joint. The articular surface of the talus acts as a template for the reduction of this fragment.

After this fragment has been elevated, the elevator is turned around and is used to lever the body fragment medially. To assist in this reduction, it is worthwhile to insert one Steinmann pin axially and one transversely into the body fragment of the calcaneus. While the surgeon performs the levering maneuver, an assistant can use these two pins to correct the equinus position of the calcaneus, thus restoring Böhler's angle, and to assist in shifting the calcaneus medially and out of varus. The fracture line on the medial side is usually quite crisp and sharp, and an accurate reduction of the body fragment to the medial wall of the sustentacular fragment can easily be achieved. An anterior extension fracture is often seen also, and this fracture may need to be reduced as well as possible from the medial side. The reduction of the body fragment should not be attempted before elevation of the posterior facet because this facet would block the medial repositioning.

Once the body fragment has been reduced, an assistant should keep it in place using the two Steinmann pins. Two small drill holes are made at a distance apart equal to that of the prongs of a staple. The staple is then driven into the calcaneus, with one prong in the sustentacular fragment and one prong in the body fragment. If a third split is easily seen and reachable, a three-prong staple can be inserted, as described by McReynolds.[36] This fixes part of the anterior extension of the fracture line. The lateral wall of the calcaneus is then pushed in manually to reduce the lateral bulge.

Additional fixation can be provided by insertion of one or two axial pins from the posteroinferior surface of the calcaneus, just above the weight-bearing surface and in the direction of the posterior facet. The pins should not extend across the joint. Another pin can be inserted in line with the calcaneo-cuboid joint to give longitudinal support to the calcaneus.

Lateral Approach (Figs. 29–10 to 29–13)

The lateral approach to the calcaneus should extend from the base of the fifth metatarsal to the superior posterior corner of the tuberosity of the calcaneus. This incision can be extended more proximally by a longitudinal incision parallel to the tendo Achillis. This incision is made at the junction between the smooth and the rough skin felt just anterior to the tendo Achillis.

After incision of the skin and subcutaneous tissues, the sural nerve should be identified and retracted proximally. The dissection should continue perpendicular to the os calcis, with care taken not to skive the anterior proximal flap. The peroneal tendons are identified, and the incision is carried down distal to them straight to bone. The fibulocalcaneal ligament is incised at its attachment to the bone and is elevated together with the periosteum on the surface of the calcaneus, the periosteum under the peroneal tendons, and the rest of the soft tissues anterior to the incision and elevated flap. This prevents skin vascularity problems because the skin is not dissected off of this flap. The flap is retracted proximally and anteriorly and is held in the retracted position by two small Steinmann pins drilled into the talus and fibula and bent back to support the flap. The body of the calcaneus is thus exposed,

and the dissection is carried out in the direction of the fibula to expose the posterior subtalar joint.

Distally, the exposure is carried out to the calcaneocuboid joint if necessary. During the dissection, it may become evident that there is a sheared off fragment of lateral wall that will be completely stripped and devoid of its vascularity if the periosteum is removed. A decision must be made whether to remove the periosteum off this fragment or whether to elevate this fragment with the periosteum as a flap. The latter may be performed as long as it does not interfere with the more important exposure of the subtalar joint. In either case, this fragment will need to be deroofed in order to expose the underlying depressed facet of the calcaneus.

On initial inspection, the location of the depressed facet is often unclear because no articular cartilage is seen. Because of the crushed cancellous bone, a bone defect is evident. An elevator may be inserted to search for the depressed fragment.[4] This fragment is not evident because its articular surface has been rotated medially and is facing away from the lateral exposure.

Once this fragment has been identified, first by irrigating and removing all of the surrounding clot and then by probing with a blunt instrument, the fragment is elevated and reoriented so that it can be reduced into place. Not infrequently, this fragment is noted to be completely devoid of soft tissue attachments and must therefore be avascular. The depressed articular fragment can be elevated and left in place or can actually be removed temporarily from the wound and placed in a dish. I remove the fragment from the os calcis and put it safely into a bone dish covered with a blood clot to keep it well nourished and moist. Usually, the fragment is left within the wound. A headlamp may be useful to see into the cavity to inspect the undersurface of the talus and the remaining impacted posterior facet of the os calcis.

The amount of intact, undisplaced os calcis posterior facet will depend on how medially or laterally the primary fracture line occurred. In some cases, the primary fracture line is very medial, leaving no articular facet connected to the sustentaculum. In all cases, however, the exposed lateral aspect of the sustentacular fragment can be seen, and a sharp vertical fracture line can be identified below the un-

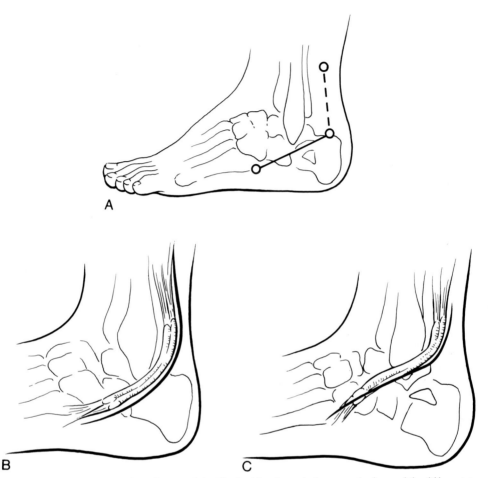

FIGURE 29–10. *(A),* Lateral approach to the os calcis. The incision is made between the base of the fifth metatarsal and the posterosuperior corner of the calcaneus.

(B), The incision can be extended proximally just anterior to the tendo Achillis at the junction between the rough and smooth skin. The sural nerve should be identified and kept with the anterior flap.

(C), The incision should be carried down perpendicular to bone without skiving. The peroneal tendons should be elevated with the subperiosteal flap, exposing them as little as possible. The calcaneofibular ligament may or may not be identified before it is cut and is elevated with the subperiosteal dissection. A flap of sheared-off lateral cortex may be identified and can be elevated or simply stripped and excised. The bony defect beneath the subtalar joint is identified after this lateral cortex is elevated. The depressed facet fragment is difficult to identify because it is medially rotated. Its articular surface is facing away from the incision. A cortical margin of bone may be noted facing up. This is the lateral cortex of the depressed facet fragment. The incision can be used to expose the calcaneocuboid joint. The incision should be extended proximally or distally, as needed, for additional exposure.

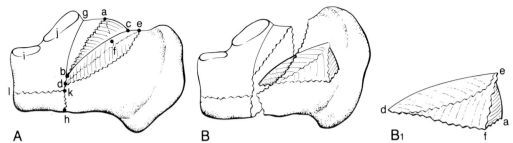

FIGURE 29–11. *(A)*, The calcaneus with its primary and secondary fracture lines. The primary fracture line is line **ah;** the posterior secondary fracture line is line **de;** the anterior secondary fracture line is line **lk;** the posterior facet is identified between the points **b, c,** and **g;** the middle facet is identified as **j;** and the anterior facet is identified as **i.** The primary fracture line component running through the posterior facet is **ab.** The extension of the primary fracture line on the medial aspect of the calcaneus is **af.** The extension of the secondary fracture line component on the medial aspect of the calcaneus is **ef.** The undersurface of the thalamic fragment and the direction to which it will displace is along line **df.** The thalamic fragment is a wedge-shaped piece with the following sides to it: a superior aspect consisting of the lateral part of the posterior facet **abca;** a lateral aspect consisting of the lateral cortex cancellous surface **bcedb;** a purely cancellous surface facing inferiorly, **defd;** another cancellous surface facing inferomedially, **abfa;** and finally, an articular and cortical surface facing medially, **acef.**

(B), With displacement, the thalamic fragment is depressed into the calcaneus, as shown. The thalamic fragment has been removed and is shown in a 90-degree medially rotated position *(B1)*. The body fragment has plantarflexed and shifted laterally into varus. The anterior secondary fracture line, which extends into the calcaneocuboid joint, remains undisplaced.

(C), After exposure of the fracture region, a 2-mm Kirschner wire (K-wire) is inserted into the center of the sustentaculum immediately beneath the subchondral bone of the subtalar joint.

(D), The wire is withdrawn from the medial side until only the tip of the wire is seen protruding from the lateral side of the sustentacular fragment.

(E), The depressed fragment is elevated, rotated, and reduced anatomically to the sustentacular fragment. The K-wire is then advanced from the medial side to fix the thalamic fragment in place. A second K-wire is inserted to hold the reduction.

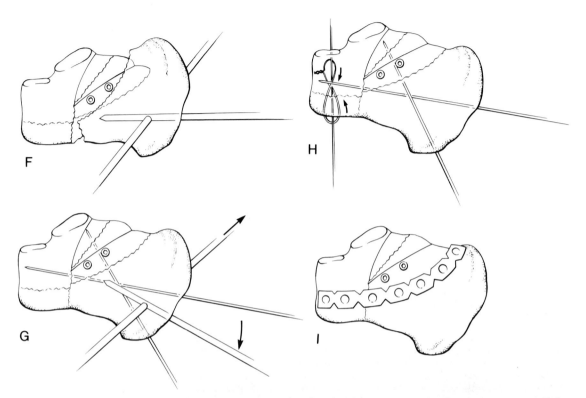

FIGURE 29–11 *Continued (F),* The first K-wire is removed and replaced by an appropriate-length 4-mm screw. If the cannulated screw system is being used, a screw is introduced over the K-wire. In this manner, both K-wires are replaced with 4-mm cancellous screws. A Steinmann pin is inserted transversely into the body of the calcaneus, and the second one is inserted axially into the body fragment.

(G), These two heavy pins are used to manipulate the body fragment back into position. The transverse pin is used to restore the calcaneal length and to shift the calcaneus medially, whereas the axial pin is used to dorsiflex the calcaneus and restore its pitch and Böhler's angle. With the reduction being maintained by means of these two pins, two K-wires can be inserted, one longitudinally and the other axially, to stabilize the reduction of the body fragment. The surgeon must ensure that the calcaneal body has been shifted medially far enough and dorsiflexes far enough. A common error is to reduce the body fragment insufficiently in these two directions. Radiographs can be taken or the image intensifier can be used to obtain a spot check of the reduction on the lateral and axial views.

(H), The split in the calcaneocuboid joint can be fixed by a figure-of-eight technique. A K-wire is inserted from the plantar to the dorsal aspect. A figure-of-eight wire is placed around the K-wire and tightened to close the split and maintain the reduction.

(I), A 3.5 reconstruction plate is molded to the lateral side of the calcaneus. The topmost hole is bent at about 60 to 90 degrees to go over the top of the calcaneus posteriorly. A screw is drilled and fixed into the body of the calcaneus at this point. The posterior half of the plate should parallel the subtalar posterior facet to the level of the primary split. At this point, the plate is bent in line with the longitudinal axis of the anterior calcaneus to end just proximal to the calcaneocuboid joint, and 4-mm cancellous screws are inserted along the whole length of the plate, except in the region of the subthalamic bone defect. The plate acts as a buttress for the calcaneus.

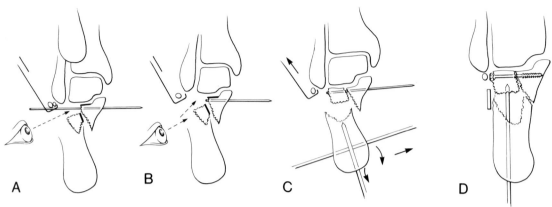

FIGURE 29–12. (A), After bone defect described above is exposed by elevation of the sheared-off lateral wall and by retraction of the superior flap that contains the peroneal tendons, a K-wire is inserted into the sustentacular fragment subchondrally, as shown. (B), The K-wire is backed out the medial side until only its tip is seen within the bone defect. The thalamic fragment is elevated and reduced to the sustentacular fragment, and the K-wire is advanced to fix it in place. A Steinmann pin is introduced transversely and axially into the body fragment to facilitate the reduction. (C), The body fragment is reduced by dorsiflexing it and medially translating it so that its medial wall is now in line with the medial wall of the sustentacular fragment. Two K-wires are used to maintain this alignment, one axial and one longitudinal. (D), The K-wires fixing the thalamic fragment have been replaced by lag screws. A reconstruction plate has been applied along the lateral side of the calcaneus.

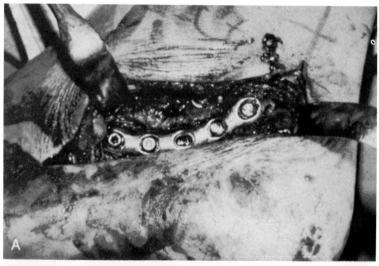

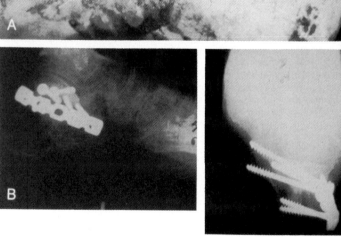

FIGURE 29–13. (A), The lateral approach to the calcaneus with fixation using lag screws and a 3.5 reconstruction plate. (B), The radiograph shows the plate to run parallel to the subtalar joint and curve distally to reach the calcaneocuboid joint and proximally over the tuberosity. (From Paley D, Hall H: Calcaneal fracture controversies: Can we put Humpty Dumpty together again? Orthop Clin North Am 20:673, 1989.)

dersurface of the talus. A thin blunt elevator should be used to probe into the remaining posterior subtalar facet of the sustentacular fragment and the talus. The surgeon can also probe in the direction of the middle facet between the sustentaculum and the talus. To allow for this inspection, the depressed fragment must either be removed or redepressed. The moment this fragment is elevated, it obliterates the view of the sustentacular fragment. It is therefore preferable to first drill a subchondral 2-mm K-wire under the posterior facet in the direction of the sustentaculum for fixation. This is a safe direction to exit medially because the neurovascular bundle runs posterior and inferior to the sustentaculum. After the wire exits through the bone, it should be tapped out the medial side to minimize the amount of spinning that it must do in the soft tissues, thus decreasing the risk of wrapping up any important structures.

A second wire is inserted in a similar manner from the lateral side in another portion of the sustentacular fragment. Both wires are then backed up until only their tips are protruding from the lateral aspect of the sustentacular fragment. The depressed joint fragment can now be re-elevated and carefully reduced into place so that it is congruous with the overlying talar articular surface and with the sustentacular fragment fracture line. The latter can be better appreciated by reinserting the thin elevator to ensure that there is no step-off across this fracture line. The K-wire is then drilled from the medial side back into the sustentacular fragment to hold it in place. The same is done with the second K-wire. One of the K-wires can be backed out medially and replaced with a 4-mm AO cancellous screw. The length of the screw is first determined using a depth gauge. A washer is used under the head of the screw, and the screw is inserted to gain interfragmentary compression into the sustentacular fragment. This procedure is repeated for the second K-wire. This provides stable fixation of the depressed fragment in its anatomic position. If cannulated screws are available, the appropriately sized K-wire for the screw is used instead of the 2-mm wire.

The next step is to reduce the body fragment. This is perhaps the most difficult step. Again, I prefer to use one Steinmann pin across the body of the calcaneus and one axially into the body of the calcaneus. Traction is placed on the transverse Steinmann pin. The calcaneus is then shifted medially. An elevator may be inserted from lateral to medial into the primary fracture line to help lever the body fragment medially. It is often quite difficult to get the calcaneal body out to length and height despite the Steinmann pin maneuver.[20, 22] The use of a femoral distractor or even an external fixator can facilitate this maneuver. Once the body is sufficiently medial, the axial pin is used to dorsiflex the body of the calcaneus out of its equinus position. This Steinmann pin should be pushed distally as hard as possible because in my experience it is not possible to overcorrect. Once the body reduction has been achieved, a second axial Steinmann pin can be inserted, and a longitudinal Steinmann pin can be inserted toward the calcaneocuboid joint. These pins provide temporary stability but can also be left in place throughout the duration of treatment.

Next, attention should be given to the anterolateral aspect of the calcaneus, including the calcaneocuboid joint. Any displaced fracture in this region should be reduced. If a displaced fracture line extends into the calcaneocuboid joint, the dissection should be carried out to expose this joint and reduce the displacement. Because the split into the joint is usually in a transverse plane, fixation should be from dorsal to plantar. Two forms of fixation may be used. If it does not involve too much increased dissection and if the bone stock allows, an interfragmentary screw with a washer should be inserted from dorsal to plantar. Most of the time, however, there is too much comminution and not enough bone for fixation for this screw to be effective. I find tension band wiring to be the best way to fix this fracture. A K-wire is inserted from dorsal to plantar. A figure-of-eight wire is then placed around the K-wire where it exits dorsally and where it exits on the plantar surface. Twisting this wire leads to interfragmentary compression, which maintains the reduction of the calcaneocuboid joint split.

Once the entire calcaneus has been reduced as well as possible, a reconstruction plate extending from the body fragment all the way to the anterior portion of the calcaneus can be attached. This step is carried out by first shaping the plate. The proximal-most hole should be bent around the top of the calcaneus. The next three holes are usually parallel to the posterior facet of the subtalar joint. The plate is then bent again to follow the lateral contour of the anterior half of the calcaneus distal to the joint. A screw needs to be placed through the proximal-most hole into the body fragment and into the distal fragment. Fixation into the comminuted portion between these fragments is not essential. One or two screws may be added for support in this region. If a sheared-off lateral wall fragment is present, it should be put back into place before plating. Furthermore, if bone grafting of the bone defect is planned, it should be performed before the plate is applied because the lateral wall fragment will close off the opening and make it difficult to insert a bone graft. A Y-plate can also be used, with the upper arm of the Y following the direction described for the reconstruction plate and the lower arm of the Y gaining fixation to the body of the calcaneus.

If bone grafting is chosen, the graft should be taken from the iliac crest. Only cancellous bone should be used. The use of allograft or bone from a bone bank should be avoided if possible because of the risk of infection. When the bone graft is inserted, the pieces should be kept to a maximum of 5 mm in diameter. The bone should be packed in, but care should be taken not to pack it too tightly and to avoid extrusion of this bone into the plantar aspect of the foot. There is disruption and often bone loss on the cortical surface of the plantar aspect of the foot, and packing in too much bone will lead to extrusion into the heel pad. The tourniquet times should be limited to a total of 2 hours in one session or two 1 1/2-hour periods separated by a 15-minute interval.

The last maneuver, which must not be forgotten, is to feel under the fibula in the peroneal tendon space. Small bone fragments may have been extruded into this region and are often attached to soft tissues in that region. This will lead to exostosis with calcaneofibular impingement or peroneal tendon stenosis. These fragments should be excised and used as bone grafts. The skin flap is closed over a suction drain in two layers. Repair of the calcaneofibular ligament is unnecessary. The ligament can usually be left to heal on its own. A sterile dressing is applied with a bulky wrap. The foot should be supported in a neutral position using a posterior slab. If this adds undue tension to the incision, the foot is best left alone to lie in equinus.

Combined Medial and Lateral Approach

For the combined medial and lateral approach, the patient is best positioned prone.

Again, one Steinmann pin is introduced axially into the heel and one is introduced transversely across the body of the heel posteriorly and in its midportion. It is easiest to approach the heel through the lateral incision described earlier, and after the depressed fragment is reduced, a small medial incision is made to assist in the reduction and to ensure the accuracy of reduction of the body fragments. The Steinmann pins in the heel are used to assist in the reduction, as described previously. With the patient in the prone position, there is less difficulty with the management of the axial pin because it does not get in the way. It may take some reorientation to get used to the upside-down appearance of the anatomy because of the prone position. One of the big advantages is that if any bleeding occurs, the blood does not accumulate; thus, the operative field is kept relatively dry. Fixation is with a plate and screws on the lateral side and a staple on the medial side.

Open Reduction and External Fixation
(Fig. 29–14)

For open reduction and external fixation, the circular external fixator of Ilizarov is applied as the first step. Application of this device includes certain reduction maneuvers using the wires of the apparatus. Once the maximum possible reduction by ligamentotaxis has been achieved, a limited lateral incision is made, directly over the subtalar joint, and open reduction with internal fixation is carried out. A preconstructed two-ring frame with an anterior and a posterior threaded rod is applied to two wires on the tibia. The rings are parallel to each other. They are connected to these two wires, which are perpendicular to the tibia. They are fixed to the wires with wire fixation bolts. The rings are centered around the soft tissues of the leg to ensure at least a finger-breadth of space circumferentially. The threaded rod anteriorly should be parallel to the crest of the tibia on both anteroposterior and lateral inspection of the tibia. The wires are then fixed and tensioned to 130 kg. With the rings used as guides, two olive wires are then inserted from anteromedial to posterolateral on the tibia in the direction of the fibula or two half-pins are added perpendicular to the wires. Two additional threaded rods are added medially and laterally to complete the tibial fixation.

Using the image intensifier, the surgeon inserts a smooth wire into the cuboid and across into the cuneiforms. This wire should not cross into the metatarsals or into the navicular. Insertion of this wire should start on the dorsal aspect of the cuboid so that the wire is not at too great an inclination. A half-ring is fixed onto this wire, roughly centered on the foot. This half-ring is then connected to the distal tibial ring, with the forefoot placed in a plantigrade position at a 90-degree angle to the tibia. This locks the position of the foot. The reduction maneuver of the heel can now be performed because any downward shift on the calcaneus will result in movement of the body

of the heel, not the foot. If the forefoot were not fixed, any downward push on the calcaneus would result only in dorsiflexion of the ankle.

A smooth wire is inserted into the body of the calcaneus so that it is situated posteriorly and proximally in the body. This wire should be inclined from distally on the lateral side to proximally on the medial side to help correct the varus deformity. A half-ring is connected to the distal tibial ring with three threaded rods, one at each end of the half-ring and one in the middle. The half-ring is connected to the wire in the heel. The wire in the heel is arched posteriorly by one hole to aid in lengthening of the heel. Two tensioners are placed

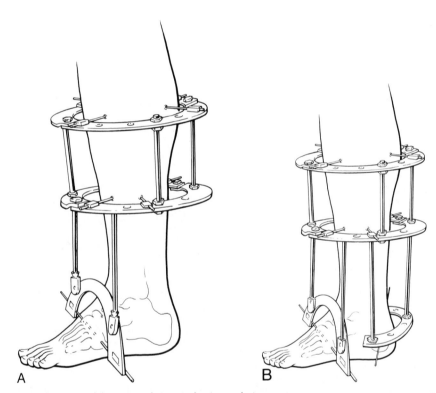

A   B

FIGURE 29–14. Circular external fixation and open reduction technique.

(A), A two-ring fixator is applied to the tibia with anterior, posterior, medial, and lateral threaded rods. These are applied from the midtibia down, with a separation of approximately 10 cm between the upper and lower rings. The wires are inserted perpendicular to the tibia. First, one wire is inserted proximally and one is inserted distally in the tibia, spaced apart the distance of the rings. The frame is then centered on these wires, and the rings are fixed and tensioned to these wires. The other two wires are then inserted. The first wire is an olive wire inserted from the lateral side, aiming for the posteromedial tibia. This is called a medial-face wire. The second reference wire is one from the lateral side going in the midfrontal plane. These two act as the reference wires, and the frame is centered around them to the limb. Once these are fixed and tensioned, the other two wires are inserted. On the proximal ring, a wire goes through the tibia at an angle of approximately 60 degrees to the first wire, and on the second ring, a wire with an olive goes posteriorly in the same direction as the medial face of the tibia, posteromedial to anterolateral. These two are fixed and tensioned to 130 kg. The foot is brought to 90 degrees, and a wire is inserted across from the cuboid through the cuneiforms. This is connected to a half-ring, as shown. The half-ring is then connected to the tibial rings to maintain the foot at 90 degrees.

Illustration continued on following page

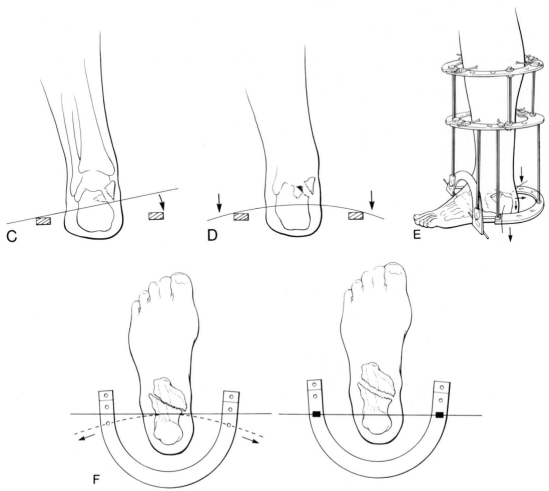

FIGURE 29–14 *Continued*

(B), With the foot fixed in 90 degrees, one wire is inserted into the body of the calcaneus, taking into consideration its varus tilt. A half-ring is connected by three threaded rods, two from the ends of the half-ring and one in its midline. This is connected to the distal tibial ring, as shown. The wire is located in the posterior midbody of the calcaneus.

(C), On the axial view, this wire is inclined to take into account the varus tilt of the calcaneus. It should pass only through the body fragment and should not go into the sustentacular fragment. The position of this wire can be confirmed using the image intensifier on an axial view. The wire is brought down to the ring, which is shown in cross section, thus correcting the varus tilt acutely.

(D), The wire is tensioned to the ring, correcting the varus tilt.

(E), The wire is arced by moving the fixation point posteriorly, thus correcting the calcaneal length at the same time.

(F), The wire is shown the way it lies on a cross-sectional view of the calcaneus. The wire is displaced one hole posteriorly and arced. Tensioning the wire will pull the calcaneus posteriorly as well as downward and out of varus. The heel ring is then pulled distally to correct Böhler's angle. The tensioning of this wire needs to be performed from both sides simultaneously. The wire in the heel must be a smooth wire (i.e., no olive).

(G), Reduction of the lateral shift of the calcaneus. After Böhler's angle and varus have been restored, a limited open reduction from the lateral approach is performed. It is necessary to elevate the posterior facet in order to reduce the lateral shift because the thalamic fragment acts as a wedge between the body and sustentacular fragments. Once this wedge is elevated, either by open surgical means or percutaneously, the body fragment can be shifted medially. This is performed by inserting a transverse olive wire from the lateral side with a stainless steel washer on the olive. This wire is tensioned from the medial side to pull the body fragment over. The reduction is judged by image intensification or by plain radiography.

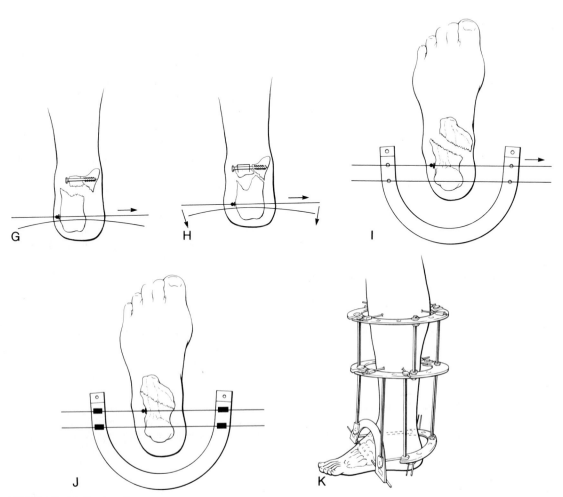

FIGURE 29–14 *Continued*

(H), The final position on the axial view is shown with the forces that are acting on the body fragment. On the olive wires, there is a lateral-to-medial force holding the reduction of the primary fracture line. On the smooth wire, there is a force pulling distal and out of varus, maintaining alignment of the body fragment.

(I), The position of this wire on the cross-sectional view of the calcaneus is shown.

(J), After reduction of the body fragment, the olive wire is fixed and tensioned with wire fixation bolts.

(K), The final maneuver is to connect the posterior heel half-ring to the anterior half-ring in the midfoot by medial and lateral threaded rods. This can be facilitated by preapplying connection points to the threaded rods on the anterior ends of the half ring. The calcaneus is shown in its reduced position maintained by the triangle of fixation. This triangle consists of fixation points in the tibia, midfoot, and hindfoot. The crushed zone in between is thus prevented from collapse. In fact, both the ankle and subtalar joints can be distracted and thus prevented from experiencing any pressure during treatment. This fixation, therefore, allows for full weight bearing, as tolerated, by the patient without fear of loss of reduction. The counterbalanced forces are shown: the force of the tendo Achillis pulling upwards is balanced by the strut between the tibia and the calcaneus. The force of collapse of the arch through the plantar fascia is counterbalanced by the strut between the midfoot and the hindfoot, and the force of the hindfoot distraction between the tibia and calcaneus is balanced by the solid strut between the midfoot and the tibia.

onto this wire and tensioned simultaneously from either side. This assists in the reduction of the heel. Once this wire is fixed and tensioned, the half-ring is pulled distally while the nuts in the threaded rod are loosened. The half-ring is then fixed in place by tightening of all of its nuts, which thus holds the heel in the reduced position. The position should now be checked with an image intensifier, and as the heel height has been reduced, no more distal traction should be applied. A No. 11 blade should be used to release the skin distal to the heel wire. This step is extremely important, and if it is not performed, the skin tension will lead to necrosis proximal to the wire.

The next step must be to reduce the depressed subtalar facet. This must be achieved before the heel can be shifted medially. First, a small incision is made on the lateral side. The peroneal tendons are not in the way as much because the height of the heel has been restored. The incision is parallel to the subtalar joint just below the fibula. Operating through the fracture lines, the surgeon elevates the posterior facet. It can be fixed into place using a 4-mm cancellous screw. Reduction and fixation with the temporary K-wires are done in the same manner as that described for the lateral approach.

Next, an olive wire with a small fragment washer is applied from the lateral side. It is used to pull the heel medially. When this wire is pulled on from the medial side, the entire body of the calcaneus is shifted over medially. The first wire in the heel does not impede this shift because it is a smooth wire. This reduction should be carried out under image intensifier control. The image intensifier is placed in an axial position so that it is at a 45-degree angle to the heel. The surgeon can then determine if the medial side has been sufficiently reduced.

Once the medial translation has been completed, the open reduction is treated in the same manner as described previously. This includes addressing the calcaneocuboid joint and bone grafting if needed. The fragments in the fibulocalcaneal space should be excised, and those in the lateral wall should be reduced or removed. The wound is then closed. If there is any significant tension on the wound, the one advantage of this system is that longitudinal traction on the heel wires, and thus the tension on the wound, can be decreased. The height of the heel can be relengthened gradually, starting 7 to 10 days later at 1 mm/day.

In some cases, it may be advisable to insert one wire into the depressed subtalar fragment in its reduced position, instead of adding a second screw. This will support the fragment from potential collapse during weight bearing.

The frame is completed by connecting the anterior half-ring to the posterior half-ring. This is performed medially and laterally. Once this has been completed, sterile sponges are applied to the pin sites, together with clips that hold the sponges in place. Lateral and axial radiographic views of the heel should be used to confirm reduction. It should be noted that reduction in this case is much easier than in all of the above-described approaches because it is not necessary to fight the pull of the soft tissues, which tends to collapse the body fragment in. The fixator holds the reduction while the surgeon is free to work. The frame is usually not found to be in the way. Because of the wire's flexibility with distraction, the half-ring on the heel lies distal to the wire insertion site and is thus out of the way.

Postoperative Management

Whether operative or nonoperative treatment is chosen, one principle of management has been early range of motion. Early range of motion of the subtalar joint adheres to the principles of treatment of intra-articular fractures. Non–weight bearing for 8 to 12 weeks is recommended to prevent collapse of the surgically fixed and reduced calcaneus and subtalar joint. Current methods of internal fixation are not strong enough to allow earlier weight bearing. On the other hand, some nonoperative treatment methods allow early weight bearing.[24, 37, 50] Does early weight bearing desensitize the heel pad? The magnitude of injury to the heel pad cannot be underestimated, and its tendency toward fibrosis and dystrophic changes of the soft tissues around the heel is well recognized.[37] Would the stimulation from partial or complete early weight bearing reduce this soft tissue dystrophy? This important question remains to be answered.

I have begun treating calcaneal fractures by first applying the Ilizarov external fixator and achieving as anatomic a ligamentotaxis reduction as possible.[1, 13, 48] This is followed by a lateral approach to the fracture and anatomic open reduction of the remaining displacement and deformity. I fix the depressed thalamic fragment in its anatomically reduced position using a screw. The rest of the fixation is carried out with the external fixator. The base of fixation is the apparatus on the tibia, extending to the midfoot and hindfoot to bypass the crushed midpart of the calcaneus. This non-collapsible triangle of fixation allows the patient to begin weight bearing within 24 hours of the surgery. This resulted in a painless heel and foot in seven of eight patients treated in this manner with more than 2 years of follow-up.[48] These preliminary results of early weight-bearing treatment of anatomically reduced calcaneal fractures are encouraging. I do not believe that immobilization of the subtalar joint with early weight bearing interferes with the prognosis for this joint. In the case illustrated (Fig. 29–15), there is a 75 percent return of subtalar function; the patient returned to work as a roofer. These early results remain anecdotal but promising and add to the existing questions about calcaneal controversies.

Results of Open Reduction and Internal Fixation of Intra-Articular Calcaneal Fractures

A summary of the long-term results of numerous studies of calcaneal fractures treated by a variety of operative and nonoperative means is given in Table 29–1. It is worth highlighting the published results and complications of some studies reporting on open reduction and internal fixation by different approaches.

We reported on 52 calcaneal fractures, all of which were treated by the medial approach by one surgeon (H. Hall).[47] The results were excellent in 19, good in 13, fair in 13, and poor in seven.[47] There were 17 complications: superficial wound infection in one, bone graft donor site infection in one, calcaneal nerve hypoesthesia in 11, calcaneal nerve neuroma in one, exostosis requiring removal in two, and a protuberant staple requiring removal in one.

Letournel reported on 83 cases; all patients were treated by the lateral approach using his multiple-H plate.[31] He reported eight wound necroses and three wound infections. His results were normal in 27 percent, good in 31 percent, fair in 33 percent, and poor in 9 percent. The normal-, and good-result groups were considered to have no functional disability. Subtalar motion was normal in only three cases. It was greater than 50 percent normal

in 47 percent of cases. In the rest, it was less than 50 percent normal.

Harding and Waddell reported on 52 fractures, all of which were treated by the lateral approach.[20] They used an external fixator to aid in the reduction and then fixed the fragments using minimal internal fixation with a threaded pin or screw. Fifty percent of heels had greater than 50 percent subtalar range of motion. Complications included three pin track infections from the Roger Anderson device, two superficial infections, and one deep infection, which required a ring sequestrectomy. One patient developed a nonunion of the calcaneus. Thirty-nine of the patients were considered to have a satisfactory result.

Stephenson reported on 22 feet treated by a combined medial and lateral approach.[63] He had six cases of superficial skin necrosis but no deep infections. Twenty of 22 feet had normal restoration of the medial border. Nineteen of 22 had congruent subtalar reduction. The average subtalar motion was 75 percent normal (range, 30 to 100 percent). Based on these criteria, the final result was rated as good in 77 percent, fair in 4 percent, and poor in 19 percent.

Sanders and associates reported on 120 fractures using their CT classification and with a follow-up averaging 29 months.[58] All fractures were treated using a lateral approach, lag screw and H-plate fixation, and no bone grafting. Postoperative reduction of heel height, length, and width were 98 percent, 100 percent, and 110 percent of normal, respectively, irrespective of fracture type. A radiographic anatomic reduction was achieved in 86 percent of type II, 60 percent of type III, and 0 percent of type IV fractures. The clinical outcome in the 79 type II fractures was 73 percent good or excellent, 10 percent fair, and 17 percent poor. The clinical outcome in the 30 type III fractures was 70 percent good or excellent, 10 percent fair, and 20 percent poor. Seven of these fractures required later fusion. The clinical outcome in the 11 type IV fractures was 9 percent excellent or good, 18 percent fair, and 73 percent poor. Sanders identified a learning curve in which the number of good or excellent results improved with each year of experience of the surgeon for types II and III fractures but not for type IV fractures, even after 4 years of experience.

Leung and colleagues[52] compared operative with nonoperative treatment in 44 operated and 19 nonoperated intra-articular calcaneal

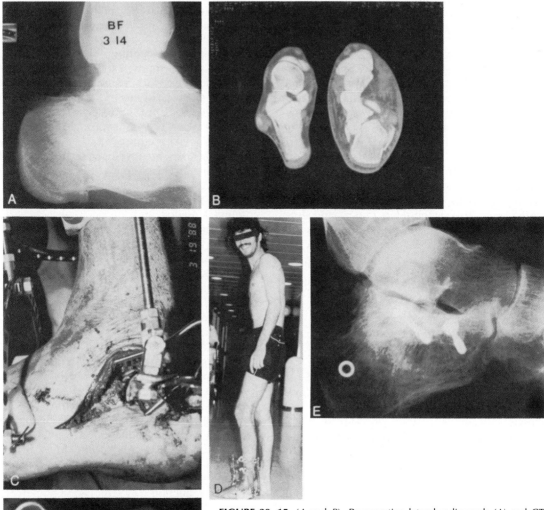

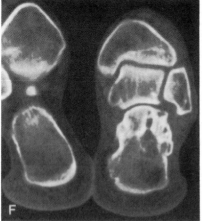

FIGURE 29–15. (A and B), Preoperative lateral radiograph (A) and CT scan (B) of an intra-articular calcaneal fracture, central depression type. Note the depression and medial rotation of the posterior facet. The facet faces away from a lateral incision. (C), The Ilizarov apparatus was applied and the heel height restored. The Seligson modification of the lateral incision was then made. One can see the cartilaginous edge of the medially rotated facet. The undersurface of the talus is also seen. Between the two is seen the cartilage of the undepressed portion of the posterior facet on the sustentacular fragment. The thalamic fragment was elevated and fixed with screws and suspended with an Ilizarov wire. (D), After anatomic restoration of the calcaneus, the patient is seen ambulating, with full weight bearing as tolerated 2 days after surgery. The fixator was removed after 8 weeks. (E), The 1-year follow-up lateral radiograph. (F), CT scan of the subtalar joint after 1 year shows anatomic restoration and normal heel height and width. The result is a painless heel with 75 percent normal range of motion. (From Paley D, Hall H: Calcaneal fracture controversies: Can we put Humpty Dumpty together again? Orthop Clin North Am 20:674, 1989.)

fractures. All surgery was through a lateral approach. There were 17 excellent, 23 good, four fair, and zero poor results in the operative group compared with zero excellent, 10 good, six fair, and three poor results in the nonoperative group. There was more pain, more limited walking distance, less subtalar range of motion, and a lower rate of return to work in the nonoperative group. The only complications of surgery were irritation of the peroneal tendons by hardware in two patients.

Buckley and Meek also compared open reduction with closed treatment. They used a cohort matched for fracture type, age, occupation, and year of injury. Seventeen patients were operated on by the lateral approach, and 17 were treated nonoperatively. There was no significant difference in heel pain, subtalar motion, and return to work between the two groups. However, in those fractures treated operatively, the overall clinical result was better when an anatomic reduction was achieved. Conversely, when the reduction was less than perfect, the overall clinical score was the same as that with no operation. This study highlights the persistent unsolved controversy.[3a]

The most severe fractures (Sanders type IV) remain an unsolved problem. These may be best treated by combined internal and external fixation. The role and need for bone grafting remain controversial. Palmer recommended its use as a means of fixation.[49] Letournel believed it was unnecessary because lag screws were sufficient to hold the articular surface together.[31] Stephenson, using no bone graft, had only one late collapse.[63] Leung used bone graft in all cases.[32] Sanders does not recommend bone grafting and believes it can block articular reduction.[58] Hall used bone graft in 10 cases and had a 67 percent satisfactory result. In the other 42 cases, in which bone grafting was not used, a 62 percent satisfactory result was achieved. There is no significant difference between these results.[47] The literature does not support the need for bone grafting even in the presence of a large bone defect. The only late collapse in my most recent series was the only patient in the group who had had bone grafting.[48]

Salvage of the Painful Calcaneal Fracture Malunion

The painful foot following a calcaneal fracture malunion presents a formidable challenge.

In the majority of cases, there is not just one source of pain. There has been distortion of the calcaneal anatomy, subtalar joint, foot biomechanics, and pericalcaneal soft tissues. It is no wonder that simply excising the protuberant bone on the lateral side of the foot or fusing the arthritic subtalar joint frequently does not relieve the patient's chronic pain.[3, 52] Braly and colleagues reported only a 46 percent satisfactory result rate after late subtalar fusion for calcaneal malunion.[3] When combined with lateral wall excision, the results were 75 percent satisfactory.[3] Johansson and colleagues reported a 95.6 percent satisfactory result rate after in situ modified Grice fusion for malunited calcaneal fractures.[28] However, 15 of 23 patients continued to have problems with shoewear, and 18 of 23 had heel widening, valgus, and loss of heel height.

These approaches might be more successful in the previously operated foot in which a restoration of part of the anatomy was carried out, leaving only one or two painful problem areas. In less fortunate patients with multifactorial sources of chronic pain refractory to all other modes of therapy, amputation was the occasional final solution.[26] Even then, only 62 percent of patients had relief after the ablative procedure.

In 1988 Carr and colleagues described a new salvage procedure for calcaneal fracture malunion (Fig. 29–16).[6] This procedure was first described in 1977 by Koshkareva and Zhitnitskiĭ in the Soviet Union.[29] This is the first procedure that addresses the majority of the painful calcaneal problem areas simultaneously, with one operation. Through a posterior operative approach to the subtalar joint, the calcaneus is distracted away from the overlying talus hinging on the anterior talocalcaneal articulations. A tricortical iliac crest bone graft is inserted between the calcaneus and the talus. This simultaneously increases the calcaneal height, eliminates the limb length discrepancy, fuses the subtalar joint, decompresses the fibulocalcaneal impingement and peroneal tendon space entrapment, corrects the heel malalignment, restores the longitudinal foot arch, and decompresses tibiotarsal impingement. Carr and colleagues reported satisfactory results in 13 of 16 patients with chronic pain.

Myerson and Quill reported on the salvage of 43 painful calcaneal fractures that had been previously treated by open or closed techniques to union.[38] They tried to identify the focus of pain and treat such foci selectively.

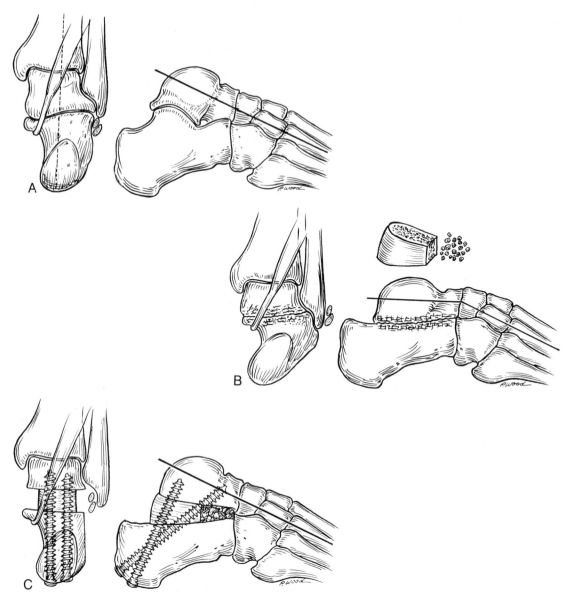

FIGURE 29–16. (A), The normal alignment of the hindfoot in relation to the midfoot and forefoot is shown on the lateral view. Note the declination of the anterior talus: a straight line can be drawn through the midline of the body, through the midfoot, and into the midline of the first metatarsal. Viewed from behind, the varus-valgus alignment of the heel is neutral and the mid–weight bearing line from the tibia lies slightly toward the medial wall of the os calcis. (B), This composite picture of an old os calcis fracture demonstrates that the talus is crushed down into the body of the os calcis and has lost its normal anterior declination. This is a common situation following a comminuted intra-articular fracture of the os calcis and places the tibiotalar joint in 15° ± 10° of dorsiflexion with the foot plantigrade. The hindfoot loses 1 to 2 cm of height and the malleoli ride low, where they often impinge on the shoe counter. As a result, the leg is also shortened from 1 to 2 cm, and this causes a pelvic tilt. The lateral wall of the os calcis is exploded outward, where it impinges under the lateral malleolus, often causing the perioneal tendons to dislocate.

Note that although the heel is tilted into varus in the sagittal plane, it may be laterally displaced in relation to the leg. The inset shows fragments of iliac crest and the block graft that resolves much of this anatomic distortion.

(C), Leg length, hindfoot height, and malleolar position are corrected in an old os calcis fracture using the distraction bone block technique. In addition, the heel is narrowed by removing the lateral wall. The peroneals can now be replaced under the decompressed end of the fibula. Two fully threaded screws prevent rotation and maintain exact position and height without further compressing the heel. Proper talocalcaneal angles in both the sagittal and the transverse planes must be achieved before the screws are inserted so that the hindfoot does not end up in varus. Although this correction results in loss of subtalar motion, cosmetic appearance and function are markedly improved and pain is significantly reduced. (From Sanders R, Hansen ST Jr, McReynolds IS: Trauma to the calcaneus and its tendon. *In* Jahss MH (Ed): Disorders of the Foot and Ankle, Vol III, 2nd Ed. Philadelphia, WB Saunders, 1991, p 2351.)

The subtalar distraction bone block arthrodesis was used in patients with subtalar osteoarthritis, with a decreased talar declination angle indicating loss of heel height. In situ fusion was used when there was no loss of heel height. Lateral ostectomy was part of both procedures as needed. Lateral ostectomy on its own was used when there was no evidence of subtalar joint arthritis or pain on selective injections of local anesthetic. Subtalar distraction bone block arthrodesis yielded seven good, three fair, and four poor results. The results of in situ arthrodesis were good in 11, fair in two, and poor in two cases. Triple arthrodesis produced fair results in two cases and poor results in three. Ostectomy alone yielded results that were good in one, fair in two, and poor in four. In addition to these bony procedures, Myerson and Quill identified and treated a group of patients with tarsal tunnel decompression, reflex sympathetic dystrophy blocks, and neuroma exploration and excision. Tibial nerve decompression yielded two good results, two fair results, and one poor result. Sural nerve resection relieved symptoms in six of seven patients. They concluded that distraction bone block arthrodesis is the most useful salvage procedure. Ostectomy alone yielded poor results despite patient selection owing to osteoarthritis that was not detected preoperatively.[38]

CONCLUSIONS

Numerous controversies surround our understanding of the treatment of intra-articular calcaneal fractures. These controversies include the basic issue of operative versus nonoperative treatment, prognostic factors, the surgical approach, the use of bone graft, and the method of fixation. In attempting to resolve some of these issues, I have tried to clarify the question of prognostic factors while adding to the existing list of controversies by questioning the role of early subtalar range of motion versus early weight bearing. The solution to many of these controversial issues lies in better standardization of classification and evaluation methods so that better comparisons can be made, and in better understanding of the pathoanatomy so that anatomic reconstruction can be better carried out.

References

1. Besmertny PC, Vitrik BD: Compression treatment of calcaneal fractures. Ortop Travmatol Protez 4:66, 1973.
2. Böhler L: Diagnosis, pathology, and treatment of fractures of the os calcis. J Bone Joint Surg 13:75–89, 1931.
3. Braly W, Bishop J, Tullos H: Lateral decompression for malunited os calcis fractures. Foot Ankle 6:90, 1985.
3a. Buckley RE, Meek RN: Comparison of open versus closed reduction of intraarticular calcaneal fractures: A matched cohort in workmen. J Orthop Trauma 6:216, 1992.
4. Burdeaux BD: Reduction of calcaneal fractures by the McReynolds medial approach technique and its experimental basis. Clin Orthop 177:87, 1983.
5. Carey EJ, Lance EM, Wade PA: Extra-articular fractures of the os calcis. J Trauma 5:362–372, 1965.
6. Carr J, Hansen S, Benirschke S: Subtalar distraction bone block fusion for late complications of os calcis fractures. Foot Ankle 9:81, 1988.
7. Cotton FJ, Wilson LT: Fractures of the os calcis. Boston Med J 159:559, 1908.
8. Crosby LA, Fitzgibbons T: Computerized tomography scanning of intra-articular fractures of the calcaneus. A new classification system. J Bone Joint Surg 72A:852, 1990.
9. Degan TJ, Morey BF, Braun DP: Surgical excision for anterior process fractures of the calcaneus. J Bone Joint Surg 64A:519–524, 1982.
10. Eastwood DM, Gregg PJ, Atkins RM: Intra-articular fractures of the calcaneum. Part I: Pathologic anatomy and classification. J Bone Joint Surg 75B:183, 1993.
11. Eastwood DM, Gregg PJ, Atkins RM: Intraarticular fractures of the calcaneum. Part II: Open reduction and internal fixation by the extended lateral transcalcaneal approach. J Bone Joint Surg 75B:189, 1993.
12. Essex-Lopresti P: The mechanism, reduction technique, and results of the os calcis. Br J Surg 39:395, 1952.
13. Fishkin IV: The treatment of calcaneal fractures. Ortop Travmatol Protez 8:61, 1986.
14. Gaul JS Jr, Greenberg BG: Calcaneus fractures involving the subtalar joint: A clinical and statistical survey of 98 cases. South Med J 59:605, 1966.
15. Giachino AA, Uthoff HK: Intra-articular fractures of the calcaneus. Current concepts review. J Bone Joint Surg 71A:784–787, 1989.
16. Gilmer D, Herzenberg J, Frank J, et al: Computerized tomographic analysis of acute calcaneal fractures. Foot Ankle 6:184, 1986.
17. Gould N: Lateral approach to the os calcis. Foot Ankle 4:218, 1984.
18. Hall MC, Pennal GF: Primary subtalar arthrodesis in the treatment of severe fractures of the calcaneus. J Bone Joint Surg 42B:336, 1960.
19. Hammersfahr JF: Surgical treatment of calcaneal fractures. Orthop Clin North Am 20:679–689, 1989.
20. Harding D, Waddell JP: Open reduction in depressed fractures of the os calcis. Clin Orthop 199:124–131, 1985.
21. Hazlett JW: Open reduction of the calcaneum. Can J Surg 12:310, 1969.

22. Heckman JD: Fractures and dislocations of the foot. *In* Rockwood C, Green D (Eds): Fractures in Adults, Vol 1 and 2, 2nd Ed. Philadelphia, JB Lippincott, 1984.

23. Hermann OJ: Conservative therapy for fracture of the os calcis. J Bone Joint Surg 19:709, 1937.

24. Houghton GR: Weight relieving cast for comminuted os calcis fractures. A preliminary report.

25. Hunt DD: Compression fracture of the anterior articular surface of the calcaneus. J Bone Joint Surg 52A:1637–1642, 1970.

26. Hunter GA, James ETR: The dilemma of painful old os calcis fractures. Clin Orthop 177:112, 1983.

27. Isbister J: Calcaneo-fibular abutment following crush fracture of the calcaneus. J Bone Joint Surg 56B:274, 1974.

28. Johansson JE, Harrison J, Greenwood F: Subtalar arthrodesis for adult traumatic arthritis. Foot Ankle 2:294, 1982.

29. Koshkareva ZV, Zhitnitskiĭ RE: Modification of subtalar arthrodesis in the treatment of deformities of the talus and calcaneus. Ortop Travmatol Protez 3:70–72, 1977.

30. Lance EM, Carey EJ, Wade PA: Fractures of the os calcis: A followup study. J Trauma 4:15, 1964.

31. Letournel E: Open reduction and internal fixation of calcaneal fractures. *In* Spiegel P (Ed): Topics in Orthopaedic Trauma. Baltimore, University Park Press, 1984, pp 173–192.

32. Leung KS, Yuen KM, Chan WS: Operative treatment of displaced intra-articular fractures of the calcaneum. J Bone Joint Surg 75B:196, 1993.

33. Lindsay W, Dewar F: Fractures of the os calcis. Am J Surg 95:555, 1958.

34. Lowy M: Avulsion fractures of the calcaneus. J Bone Joint Surg 51B:494–497, 1969.

35. Maxfield JE, McDermott FJ: Treatment of calcaneal fractures by open reduction. J Bone Joint Surg 45A:868, 1963.

36. McReynolds IS: The case for operative treatment of fractures of the os calcis. *In* Leach RE, Hoaglund FT, Riseborough EJ (Eds): Controversies in Orthopedic Surgery. Philadelphia, WB Saunders, 1982, pp 232–254.

37. Miller WE: Pain and impairment considerations following treatment of disruptive os calcis fractures. Clin Orthop 177:82, 1983.

38. Myerson M, Quill G: Late complications of fractures of the calcaneus. J Bone Joint Surg 75A:331, 1993.

39. Nade S, Monahan P: Fractures of the calcaneum: A study of the long-term prognosis. Injury 4:201, 1971.

40. Nakaima N, Yamashita H, Tonogai R, Ikata T: A technique of dynamic reduction for displaced fractures of the thalamus of the calcaneum. Int Orthop 7:185, 1983.

41. Noble J, McQuillan N: Early posterior subtalar fusion in treatment of fractures of the os calcis. J Bone Joint Surg 61A:90, 1979.

42. Norfray JF, Rogers LF, Adamo GP: Common calcaneal avulsion fractures. AJR Am J Roentgenol 134:119–123, 1980.

43. Olerud C, Molander H: A scoring scale for symptom evaluation after ankle fracture. Arch Orthop Trauma Surg 103:190, 1984.

44. Omoto H, Sakurada K, Sugi M, Nakamura K: A new method of manual reduction for intraarticular fractures of the calcaneus. Clin Orthop 177:104, 1983.

45. Paley D: Radiologic assessment and factors in evaluating results. Symposium presentation at the Foot and Ankle Society Meeting, San Francisco, CA, Jan 1987.

46. Paley D, Hall H: Calcaneal fracture controversies: Can we put Humpty Dumpty together again? Orthop Clin North Am 20:665–677, 1989.

47. Paley D, Hall H: Intra-articular fractures of the calcaneus. A critical analysis of results and prognostic factors. J Bone Joint Surg 75A:342, 1993.

48. Paley D, Fischgrund J: Open reduction and circular external fixation of intraarticular calcaneal fractures. Clin Orthop 290:125–131, 1993.

49. Palmer I: The mechanism and treatment of fractures of the calcaneus. Open reduction with the use of cancellous grafts. J Bone Joint Surg 30A:2, 1948.

50. Parkes J: The nonreductive treatment for fractures of the os calcis. Orthop Clin North Am 4:193, 1973.

51. Pozo JL, Kirwan E, Jackson AM: The long-term results of conservative management of severely displaced fractures of the calcaneus. J Bone Joint Surg 66B:386, 1984.

52. Pridie KH: A new method of treatment for severe fractures of the os calcis. A preliminary report. Surg Gynecol Obstet 82:671, 1946.

53. Protheroe K: Avulsion fractures of the calcaneus. J Bone Joint Surg 51B:118–122, 1969.

54. Romash M: Calcaneal fractures: Three dimensional treatment. Foot Ankle 8:180, 1988.

55. Ross S, Sonerby M: The operative treatment of fractures of the os calcis. Clin Orthop 199:132, 1985.

56. Rowe CR, Sakellarides HT, Sorbie C, Freeman PA: Fractures of the os calcis: A long-term followup study of 146 patients. JAMA 184:920, 1963.

57. Sanders R, Hansen ST, McReynolds IS: Trauma to the calcaneus and its tendon in disorders of the foot and ankle. *In* Jahss MH (Ed): Disorders of the Foot and Ankle. Philadelphia, WB Saunders, 1992, p 2326.

58. Sanders R: Intra-articular fractures of the calcaneus: The present state of the art. J Orthop Trauma 6:252, 1992.

59. Segal D, Marsh J, Leiter B: Clinical application of computerized axial tomography (CAT) scanning of calcaneus fractures. Clin Orthop 199:114, 1985.

60. Slatis MD, Kiviluoto O, Santavirta S, Laasonen M: Fractures of the calcaneus. J Trauma 19:939, 1979.

61. Soeur R, Remy R: Fractures of the calcaneus with displacement of the thalamic portion. J Bone Joint Surg 57B:413, 1975.

62. Stephenson JR: Displaced intra-articular fractures of the os calcis involving the subtalar joint: The key of the superomedial fragment. Foot Ankle 4:91, 1983.

63. Stephenson JR: Treatment of displaced intra-articular fractures of the calcaneus using medial and lateral approaches, internal fixation, and early motion. J Bone Joint Surg 1:115, 1987.

64. Thompson KR, Friesen CM: Treatment of comminuted fractures of the calcaneus by primary triple arthrodesis. J Bone Joint Surg 41A:1423–1436, 1959.

65. Wilson JN (Ed): Watson-Jones Fractures and Joint Injuries, 5th Ed. Edinburgh, Churchill Livingstone, 1976.

66. Zayer M: Fractures of the calcaneus: A review of 110 fractures. Acta Orthop Scand 40:530–542, 1969.

30

Late Reconstruction of Calcaneal Fracture Problems

JEFFREY E. JOHNSON

Fractures of the calcaneus represent only 2 percent of all fractures. However, the calcaneus is the most commonly fractured of all the tarsal bones,[72] and calcaneal fractures constitute 60 percent of all major tarsal injuries.[14] Historically, the results of all forms of treatment for intra-articular fractures of the calcaneus have been considered dismal, with unsatisfactory results in an average of 35 to 40 percent of cases.* Statistics from the New York Workers Compensation Board indicate that the average disability rating for calcaneal fractures is a 22-percent loss of function of the foot.[23]

More attention has been placed on anatomic reduction and rigid internal fixation of these fractures.† Although a significant number of unsatisfactory results still occur, it has been shown that final outcome is improved when the shape of the calcaneal bone is restored.[4, 36, 60]

Of all patients with calcaneal fractures, approximately 10 to 25 percent have associated fractures of the spine or extremities.[50, 69] However, it is often the calcaneal fracture that contributes to long-term disability.

Calcaneal fractures are of significant economic importance because the majority occur in middle-aged industrial workers.[1, 5, 70, 79] The economic impact becomes even more apparent in view of the fact that 20 percent of patients may be incapacitated for up to 3 years after

fracture, and many are partially incapacitated for as long as 5 years after fracture.[59]

Regardless of treatment, most patients who have had a calcaneal fracture do not reach a healing plateau until at least 1 year after injury.[57] More than half of patients reach a plateau in their symptomatology within the first 2 years, and more than 75 percent reach a plateau within 4 years.[60] However, time seems to have a positive effect on late symptoms. Only a small percentage of patients show worsening of symptoms over time,[60] and in a review of industrial cases of calcaneal fracture, Deyerle found that pain was almost nonexistent after 3 to 5 years, regardless of the type of treatment.[23]

Given the length of disability and associated economic consequences, the patient and the surgeon may be compelled to undertake a course of early reconstructive surgery to salvage a presumedly poor result of initial treatment. However, in view of the natural history of calcaneal fracture, an early salvage procedure may be unnecessary. In general, nonoperative treatment should be maintained as long as improvement continues.[57] Once the condition of the foot has stabilized, surgical solutions may be indicated for specific and continuing sources of pain.

NONOPERATIVE TREATMENT

Nonoperative management of the healed calcaneal fracture that is painful may include nonsteroidal anti-inflammatory medications,

---

*See references 17, 25, 34, 38, 40, 50, 51, 56, 58, 62, 69, and 76.

†See references 4, 10, 11, 30, 35, 36, 60, 66–68, 75, and 76.

prescription footwear with a custom insert, an ankle-foot orthosis, local steroid injections, and walking aids, depending on the source of disability.

Proper shoe selection and fitting are important when any significant loss of motion or deformity of the hindfoot is present. Shoes with firm heel counters and cushion soles will offer the best support and shock absorption.[80] Impingement of the malleoli on the shoe counter from shortening of the calcaneus can be treated by modification of the shoe counter or by a cushioned heel lift inside the shoe. A widened or prominent calcaneal tuberosity can be relieved by a cushioning and supportive custom-molded total contact insert made of a closed-cell polyethylene foam such as Plastizote.

For patients with degenerative arthritis of the subtalar joint who are not surgical candidates, a UCBL (University of California Biomechanics Laboratory)–type orthosis may help to support the foot and limit subtalar joint motion and pain. If this is not satisfactory, a leather lace-up ankle-foot orthosis built into the shoe insole[80] or a custom-made polypropylene ankle-foot orthosis may be symptom relieving. These orthoses limit motion and weight-bearing load at the involved joints and can be made to fit into a shoe. For the severe deformity with pain, a double-upright calf lacer or patellar tendon–bearing brace attached to an extra-depth shoe may be necessary.

FRACTURES NOT INVOLVING THE SUBTALAR JOINT

Although most of the long-term morbidity of calcaneal fractures is secondary to fractures involving the subtalar joint, a few fractures not involving the subtalar joint deserve mention.

Anterosuperior Process Fracture

Fracture of the anterosuperior process of the calcaneus is more common than appreciated, is often misdiagnosed as an ankle sprain,[6, 29, 42, 61] and can lead to long-term disability.[19, 29, 61]

The mechanism of injury is usually an avulsion fracture by the bifurcate ligament during forceful inversion and plantar flexion of the foot (Fig. 30–1). Most patients achieve a satisfactory result with a solid union or an asymp-

tomatic nonunion; however, time to full recovery may average 2 years.[19] Symptomatic nonunion of the avulsed fragment can occur despite initial treatment and is more common when the diagnosis is missed.[19]

Evaluation

Pain symptoms are usually located to the anterior sinus tarsi area. Radiographic evaluation consists of foot radiographs, including an oblique view. If a fracture nonunion is not visualized, a technetium bone scan can be helpful to localize the pathology. If increased technetium uptake is found in the anterior calcaneus, computed tomography (CT) of that area allows the best visualization of the fracture pattern.

Surgical Treatment

The indication for surgical excision of a symptomatic nonunion following anterior process fracture is pain with disability persisting for at least 9 to 12 months after injury.[19, 20] Surgery is delayed in an effort to allow complete recovery before surgical intervention.

The ununited anterosuperior process fracture is excised through a longitudinal dorsal incision overlying the fragment. Care is taken to avoid injury to the lateral branch of the superficial peroneal nerve medially and to the sural nerve lateral to the incision. The extensor digitorum brevis muscle is retracted medially, and the anterosuperior process is exposed. The fragment is excised using a small osteotome or rongeur. A compression dressing is used postoperatively, and early range-of-motion exercises are begun. Weight bearing is allowed as tolerated.

After surgical excision, Degan and colleagues reported that five of seven patients achieved satisfactory results; however, three of seven patients required more than 1 year to become asymptomatic or to reach a healing plateau.[19] When considering surgical excision, both patient and surgeon should be aware of the sometimes-prolonged healing time.

Anterior Calcaneal Fractures Involving the Calcaneocuboid Joint

Isolated intra-articular fractures involving the anterior process of the calcaneus, although rare, may cause late disability. The mechanism

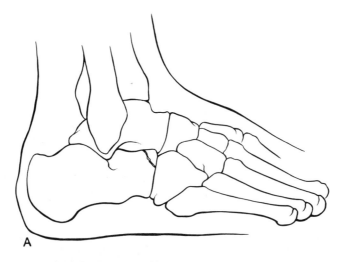

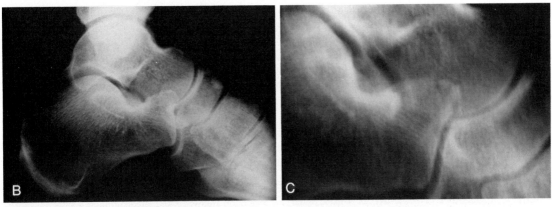

FIGURE 30–1. *(A)*, Avulsion fracture of the anterosuperior process of the calcaneus. *(B)*, Lateral radiograph showing a nondisplayed anterosuperior process fracture. *(C)*, Magnified view of the same radiograph demonstrating fracture of the anterosuperior process.

is usually forceful abduction of the forefoot producing a compression fracture of the anterior calcaneus (Fig. 30–2). These injuries may be associated with subluxation of the tarsometatarsal joints or a "nutcracker" compression fracture of the cuboid. Late symptoms may develop from direct injury of the articular surfaces or joint incongruity from a displaced fracture that leads to degenerative arthritis.

Evaluation

Anteroposterior, lateral, and oblique radiographs of the foot usually demonstrate degenerative changes in the calcaneocuboid joint from a displaced intra-articular anterior process fracture. If the findings of plain radiography are equivocal, or if surgery is considered, CT of the hindfoot (using 3-mm cuts in two

planes) is helpful. CT demonstrates the extent of degenerative changes at the calcaneocuboid joint and also evaluates the talonavicular and subtalar joints for associated injury.

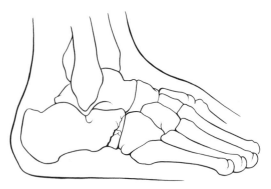

FIGURE 30–2. Compression fracture of the anterior process of the calcaneus.

Surgical Treatment

Pain localized to the calcaneocuboid joint following an intra-articular fracture of the anterior process of the calcaneus can be treated by an isolated calcaneocuboid arthrodesis when the post-traumatic degenerative arthritis is limited to that joint. If the radiograph or CT scan shows degenerative changes at the subtalar joint also, triple arthrodesis is indicated. If the changes involve only the transverse tarsal joints (calcaneocuboid and talonavicular joints), a double arthrodesis[55] of these joints is indicated.

Calcaneocuboid Arthrodesis: Author's Preferred Method

The surgical technique for an isolated calcaneocuboid arthrodesis involves a longitudinal incision centered over the calcaneocuboid joint. The surgeon carries the dissection through the subcutaneous tissue, avoiding the sural nerve and retracting it laterally. With a small straight osteotome, the opposing joint surfaces are denuded of cartilage to expose bleeding subchondral bone. If there has been significant comminution of the anterior calcaneus with shortening of the lateral column of the foot, an intercalary corticocancellous bone graft from the iliac crest is inserted to restore length (Fig. 30–3). The graft is fixed with screws or crossed Steinmann pins driven from the cuboid into the calcaneus while the arthrodesis site is compressed. Fixation can be augmented with power-driven wire staples, but these staples are not sufficient fixation alone for the intercalary graft. If no significant lateral column shortening is present, morselized iliac crest bone graft is placed into the calcaneocuboid space and internally fixed, as described previously.

A short-leg non–weight-bearing cast is worn for 6 weeks, at which time any percutaneous pins are removed. If the arthrodesis site is healing, weight bearing is allowed in a short-leg cast, which is removed 3 months after surgery.

INTRA-ARTICULAR FRACTURES INVOLVING THE SUBTALAR JOINT

The majority of late problems following calcaneal fracture are caused by intra-articular

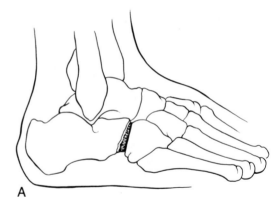

A

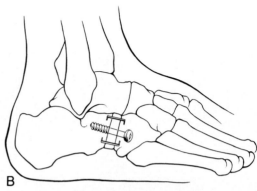

B

FIGURE 30–3. *(A)*, Shortening of the lateral column of the foot and degenerative changes at the calcaneocuboid joint after anterior calcaneal fracture. *(B)*, Arthrodesis of the calcaneocuboid joint with interposition of a corticocancellous bone graft to restore lateral column length.

fractures involving the subtalar joint. The calcaneus has three major functions: providing a foundation for the transmission of weight-bearing loads, serving as a pedestal for support and proper function of the talus, and acting as a lever for increasing the mechanical advantage of the gastrocnemius-soleus muscle group. A fracture may disrupt some or all of these functions of the calcaneus (Fig. 30–4).

Displacement of an intra-articular fracture from an axial load occurs along the line of shear or the primary fracture line.[25] The tuberosity fragment of the calcaneus, including the lateral wall, shifts superiorly and laterally in relation to the sustentacular fragment, which remains with the talus. This displacement along the primary fracture line, as well as the outward buckling of the lateral wall of the calcaneus, is the major cause of the late problems following this fracture.

Problems leading to disability after intra-

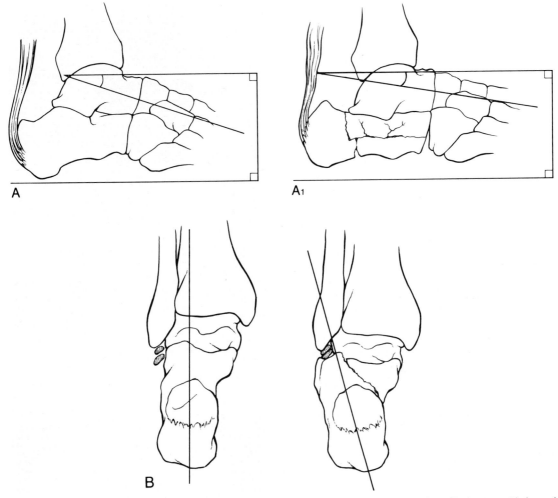

FIGURE 30–4. (A), Lateral view of deformities after calcaneal fracture. Note the posterior facet depression with loss of Böhler's angle, shortening and flattening of the calcaneus, extension of the primary fracture line into the calcaneocuboid joint, and a decrease in the angle of talar declination (A1). (B), Axial view of deformities after calcaneal fracture. Note the widening of the calcaneus with protrusion of the lateral wall, calcaneofibular abutment, decreased space available for peroneal tendons, and varus heel malalignment.

articular calcaneal fracture include the following:

1. Subtalar joint incongruity and degenerative arthritis
2. Loss of calcaneal height and length, with shortened Achilles tendon lever arm
3. Dorsiflexion of the talus with loss of the normal angle of talar declination
4. Varus or valgus malalignment of the heel
5. Flatfoot deformity
6. Increased heel width
7. Calcaneofibular abutment
8. Impingement or dislocation of the peroneal tendons

9. Neuroma or entrapment neuropathy of the sural nerve

Because these problems often coexist, they do not have easy salvage solutions, and many require more than simply a subtalar arthrodesis. Perhaps one of the most compelling arguments for open anatomic reduction and rigid internal fixation of acute calcaneal fractures is the difficulty in restoring the shape and alignment of a malunited calcaneus.[37, 39, 45] Although some of the late problems of calcaneal fractures are secondary to a previous surgical attempt at fracture treatment, it is usually easier to salvage a painful hindfoot when the shape and alignment of the calcaneus are re-stored as part of the treatment of the acute fracture. The challenge for the surgeon is to sort out what component or components of the postfracture pathology are causing the pain symptoms so that the appropriate salvage pro-cedure can be performed.

Physical Examination

Careful history taking and physical exami-nation are necessary to determine the etiology of the symptoms. The description of the pain as burning, tingling, stabbing, or radiating may point to a sural nerve neuroma, as opposed to the aching, activity-related pain of subtalar degenerative arthritis. Careful palpation for points of tenderness as well as for the position and strength of the peroneal tendons is impor-tant. Range of motion of the ankle and hind-foot joints should be measured, and any sen-sory nerve deficits should be documented. Malalignment of the hindfoot in relation to the mechanical axis of the leg should be measured with the patient in the standing position. The patient's skin condition and the location of previous incisions should be noted for preop-erative planning. Local diagnostic injections of a local anesthetic can be helpful in differen-tiating between the various causes of hindfoot pain.

Radiographic Evaluation

Anteroposterior, lateral, and oblique foot radiographs with an axial calcaneal view may demonstrate protrusion of the lateral wall of the calcaneus (Fig. 30–5), incongruity or de-generative changes in the subtalar joint, and changes in the overall alignment of the body of the calcaneus. Standing anteroposterior radiographs of both ankles (on the same film) will demonstrate calcaneofibular abutment (Fig. 30–6), although these imaging findings are occasionally difficult to interpret because of the positioning of the foot in excessive external rotation. This view will also rule out the ankle as an associated cause of hindfoot malalignment. The standing hindfoot align-ment view (Figs. 30–7 and 30–8) allows accu-rate measurement of the amount of hindfoot varus in relation to the long axis of the tibia.[9, 15] The hindfoot alignment view is helpful

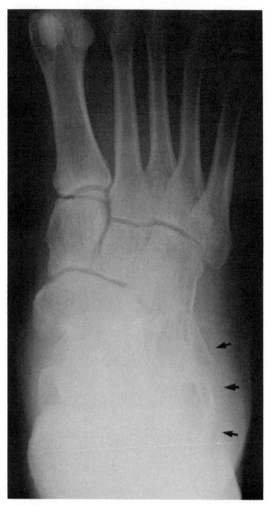

FIGURE 30–5. Anteroposterior radiograph of a foot with previous calcaneal fracture demonstrating protrusion of the lateral wall of the calcaneus *(arrows)*.

for preoperative planning as well as for post-operative evaluation.

Broden's[8] or Athmonsen's[2] views of the cal-caneus and the Isherwood[43] series of radio-graphs to visualize the subtalar joint articular surfaces are helpful, but they are highly de-pendent on proper patient positioning. Since the advent of CT, their greatest use is for the intraoperative evaluation of fracture reduction during treatment of the acute fracture.

When performed in two planes (coronal and axial; 3-mm cuts), CT of the entire calcaneus, including the transverse tarsal joints, yields the greatest amount of information, and the proper views are consistently reproducible (Fig. 30–9). CT demonstrates the height,

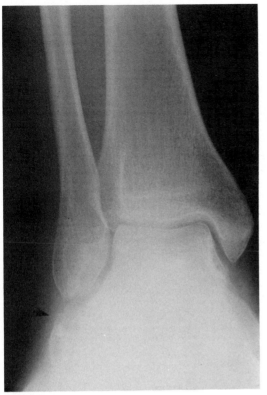

FIGURE 30–6. Anteroposterior standing radiograph of the ankle demonstrating a displaced lateral wall of the calcaneus *(arrow)* abuting the distal fibula.

width, and length of the calcaneus, and because both feet are scanned simultaneously, it allows easy comparison with the normal side. CT has been shown to be critical in the evaluation of acute calcaneal fractures.[71] In addi-

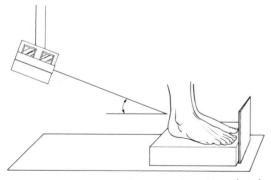

FIGURE 30–7. Hindfoot alignment view. Note that the beam is angled 20 degrees caudad and a portion of the cassette is placed below the level of the standing platform. (Modified from Buck P, Morrey BF, Chao EYS: The optimum position of arthrodesis of the ankle. J Bone Joint Surg 69A:1052–1062, 1987.)

tion, in the evaluation of late calcaneal fracture problems, it readily demonstrates the location and extent of degenerative changes, including the status of the calcaneocuboid joint. The peroneal tendons are visualized and can be evaluated for dislocation or impingement in the subfibular area, and the space between the tip of the lateral malleolus and the lateral wall of the calcaneus can be evaluated for calcaneofibular abutment. Often the primary fracture line is visible, which may aid in the planning of a corrective osteotomy.

Subtalar Joint Incongruity and Degenerative Arthritis

Most calcaneal fractures that involve the subtalar joint result in some amount of radiographically detectable degenerative change (Fig. 30–10). Commonly, this fracture presents as lateral hindfoot and sinus tarsi pain with decreased subtalar joint range of motion. However, sural nerve neuropathy, subfibular impingement, and peróneal tendon entrap-

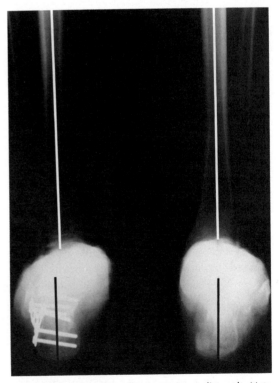

FIGURE 30–8. Hindfoot alignment view radiograph. Note the satisfactory postfracture heel alignment compared with the noninjured side.

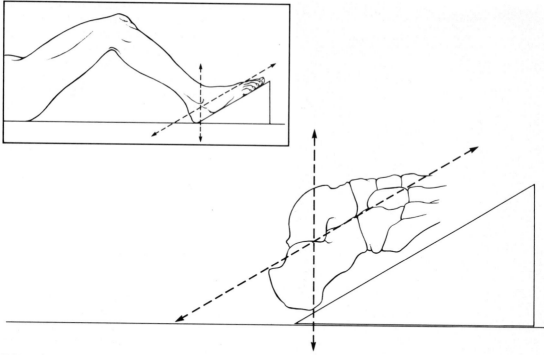

FIGURE 30–9. Computed tomography of the calcaneus is done in two planes, semicoronal (perpendicular to the posterior facet) and transverse, using 3-mm cuts.

ment may all present with similar lateral hind-foot pain. The presence of subtalar joint stiffness is not helpful in differentiating between these various post-traumatic conditions because stiffness is common after calcaneal fracture. The diagnosis of subtalar joint degenerative arthritis is confirmed by significant improvement in pain symptoms following an injection of local anesthetic into the subtalar joint. Because usually the posterior facet is most involved, the needle is placed into the posterior facet from a posterolateral or an anterolateral approach under fluoroscopic guidance, and a small amount of contrast is injected first to confirm needle placement (Fig. 30–11).[64] The anterior and middle facets are injected by injecting the talonavicular joint that communicates with them. The posterior facet does not normally communicate with the anterior and middle facets.[64]

Surgical Treatment

Isolated subtalar arthrodesis is the treatment of choice when symptoms are localized to the subtalar joint. If CT shows significant degen-erative changes at the calcaneocuboid joint, subtalar fusion combined with fusion of the transverse tarsal joints (i.e., triple arthrodesis) is recommended. Associated problems such as calcaneofibular abutment or peroneal tendon impingement are addressed at the time of fusion, as described later.

Many techniques have been described for subtalar arthrodesis.* The most useful techniques for this purpose use a lateral approach, bone grafting, and some type of internal fixation with pins, screws, or staples. A lateral approach gives access to the sural nerve, distal fibula, peroneal tendons, and lateral wall of the calcaneus for any additional procedures. It also allows removal of any hardware used for a previous open reduction and internal fixation. Care is taken to avoid producing sub-fibular impingement with a misplaced bone graft or by overcorrection of the heel alignment. The sural nerve is carefully protected from iatrogenic injury.

Techniques that remove significant amounts of bone should be avoided because the height

---

*See references 21, 28, 32, 33, 44, 46, and 77.

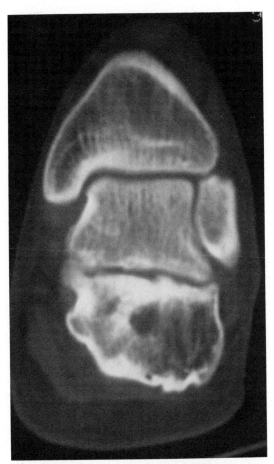

FIGURE 30–10. Semicoronal computed tomographic scan of the posterior facet of the subtalar joint showing incongruity and post-traumatic degenerative arthritis.

over the sinus tarsi area, from the tip of the fibula to the calcaneocuboid joint (Fig. 30–12). If a previous lateral incision is present, it is used, and any lateral hardware is removed. The extensor digitorum brevis muscle insertion on the neck and lateral aspect of the talus is incised, and the muscle belly is retracted distally to expose the subtalar joint. The articular surfaces of the posterior and middle facets are removed with osteotomes and curettes. If mild heel varus exists, enough bone is removed to position the heel in a slightly valgus position. Exposure of the joint surfaces is greatly aided by the use of a small lamina spreader placed into the sinus tarsi. Morselized autogenous iliac crest bone graft is inserted to fill the dead space, but it is not packed tightly until the position of the heel is fixed.

A small longitudinal dorsal incision is made between the anterior tibial and extensor hallucis longus tendons to expose the dorsal neck of the talus and to avoid the anterior neurovascular bundle. A cannulated 6.5-mm cancellous screw or a large Steinmann pin is inserted obliquely across the neck of the talus into the tuberosity of the calcaneus while the heel is held in proper alignment (Fig. 30–13). The head of the screw is countersunk to prevent impingement by the anterior tibia with ankle dorsiflexion. The remaining bone graft is packed into the subtalar joint and sinus tarsi, and the extensor digitorum brevis muscle is closed over the graft. A short-leg cast is used without weight bearing for 6 weeks, followed

of the calcaneus is usually somewhat shortened already. Similar to the situation with acute calcaneal fractures, symptoms tend to improve for at least 1 year following fusion.

Although other authors have achieved good results with a modification of Grice's extra-articular arthrodesis in adults with traumatic arthritis,[44, 77] I have had no experience with this technique in adults.

Author's Preferred Method of Treatment

For isolated post-traumatic subtalar degenerative arthritis, I prefer an intra-articular arthrodesis using autogenous bone graft.[46] Internal fixation is placed in a manner similar to the technique of Dennyson and Fulford,[21] except that the bone graft is placed intra-articularly. A slightly curving lateral incision is made

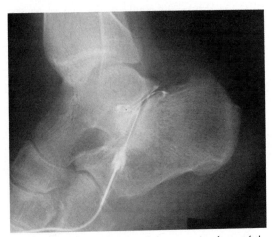

FIGURE 30–11. Arthrogram of the posterior facet of the subtalar joint to document accurate needle placement before diagnostic injection of local anesthetic.

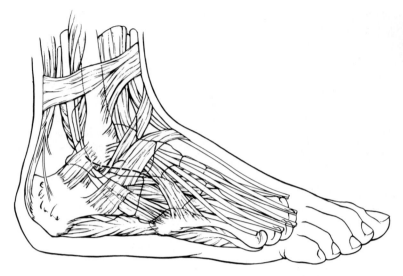

FIGURE 30–12. Preferred lateral incision for subtalar fusion. The incision is modified if a previous incision is present or a calcaneal osteotomy is required.

by a walking cast for 6 weeks. A supportive lace-up shoe with a cushioned sole is then recommended. If a Steinmann pin is used, it is removed under local anesthetic 6 weeks postoperatively.

Loss of Calcaneal Height and Talar Declination Angle

Normally, the angle between the neck of the talus and the floor in the weight-bearing stance ranges from 14 to 36 degrees, with a mean angle of 24.5 degrees.[74] Loss of support for the body of the talus by a calcaneal fracture allows the talus to subside into the calcaneus and loss of the normal talar declination angle (see Fig. 30–4A). When the angle is decreased to less than 15 degrees, painful impingement of the

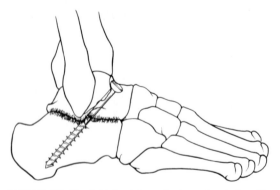

FIGURE 30–13. Subtalar intra-articular arthrodesis with internal fixation.

dorsal neck of the talus on the anterior tibia may occur; this is associated with a loss of ankle dorsiflexion. Loss of height and length of the calcaneus reduces the mechanical advantage of the gastrocnemius-soleus muscle group by shortening the Achilles lever arm. Associated problems of subtalar arthritis, peroneal tendon impingement, or calcaneofibular abutment may also be present.

Subtalar Distraction Bone Block Fusion

Carr and colleagues described the technique of subtalar distraction bone block fusion for restoration of the height of the calcaneus, arthrodesis of the subtalar joint, and correction of the talar declination angle.[13] When the height of the heel is raised, the calcaneofibular abutment, peroneal tendon impingement, and tibiotalar neck impingement are also simultaneously relieved, and the Achilles tendon lever arm is restored.

This surgical technique[13] is modified from the Gallie posterior subtalar fusion,[28, 47] and according to Paley and Hamilton, it was initially described by Koshkareva and Zhitnitskiĭ in the Soviet Union.[49] The patient is placed in the lateral decubitus position. A longitudinal posterolateral Gallie approach to the subtalar joint is used (Fig. 30–14). The femoral distractor is applied medially, with one pin along the subcutaneous border of the tibia and the other in the calcaneal tuberosity. The lateral wall of the calcaneus is subperiosteally exposed, and a portion of bone is excised to ensure adequate

FIGURE 30–14. Posterolateral approach for subtalar bone block arthrodesis.

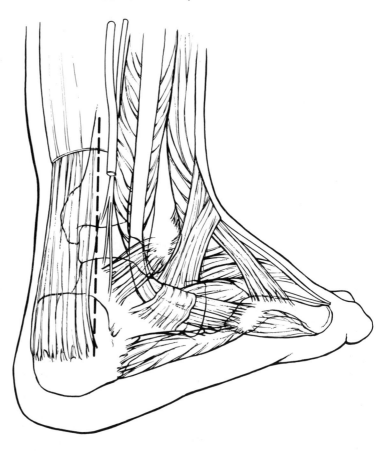

peroneal tendon decompression. The subtalar joint is distracted and denuded of articular cartilage. Any hindfoot malalignment is corrected, and a bone block taken from the posterior iliac crest is placed in the subtalar joint to maintain the hindfoot height. The remaining subtalar joint area is packed with cancellous bone graft. Two fully threaded 6.5-mm cancellous screws are placed through stab wounds in the heel to fix the calcaneus to the talus (Fig. 30–15). A short-leg cast is used without weight bearing for the first 6 weeks, followed by a short-leg walking cast for 6 weeks.

Complications have occurred with healing of the incision, nonunion, screw breakage, tenderness at the screw insertion site, and persistent heel varus.[13, 27, 63] A straight incision, careful handling of the skin and sural nerve, the use of two countersunk screws (instead of one), the use of additional bone graft, and a slight valgus positioning of the heel at the time of screw insertion should help avoid these problems.

Preliminary results on the first 16 feet were satisfactory in 13 of the feet.[13] Although no large experience has been reported with this method by others, Quill and Myerson reported good results in 10 of 14 patients with this technique at an average follow-up of 2 years.[63] Two poor results occurred because of heel varus, which required corrective osteotomy, and five patients required removal of a painful screw.

Fortin and colleagues reported on 30 patients (31 feet) who underwent subtalar fusion for salvage after calcaneal fracture.[27] The subtalar bone block technique was used in 15 feet, and an in situ fusion was used in 16 feet. Overall, 60 to 65 percent of patients had a good or excellent rating according to the Maryland foot score, but subjectively, only 36 to 40 percent of patients considered themselves to be in the good and excellent category. No statistically significant difference was found in the overall results of subtalar fusion between those who had prior surgical treatment and those who had nonoperative treatment of their calcaneal fractures. However, postoperative

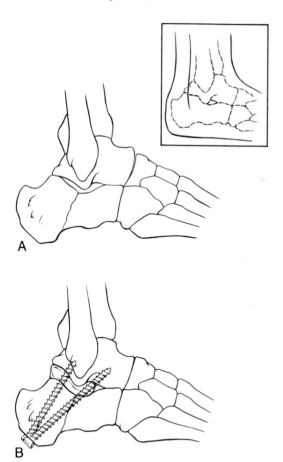

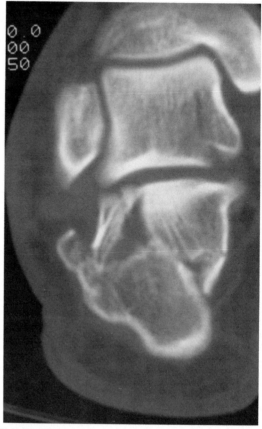

FIGURE 30–15. Subtalar bone block arthrodesis. *(A),* Preoperative deformity with loss of the talar declination angle and tibiotalar abutment. *(B),* Postoperative view with restoration of calcaneal height and the talar declination angle, relief of tibiotalar abutment, and fusion of the subtalar joint. (Redrawn from Carr JB, Hansen ST Jr, Benirschke SK: Subtalar distraction bone block fusion for late complications of os calcis fractures. Foot Ankle 9:81–86, 1988. Courtesy of Bruce J. Sangeorzan, M.D. © American Orthopaedic Foot and Ankle Society 1988.)

tioned earlier. Careful attention should be given to heel alignment intraoperatively. Significant complications that require additional surgery may occur, and healing time postoperatively may be prolonged for a year or more.

Varus or Valgus Malalignment of the Heel

With many intra-articular fractures of the calcaneus, in addition to the loss of calcaneal height and length that occurs, the tuberosity fragment displaces into varus or valgus. Varus malalignment is more common because of the varus position of the heel at the time of fracture, the obliquity of the primary fracture line (from posteromedial to anterolateral), and the direction of pull of the Achilles tendon on the tuberosity fragment (Fig. 30–16). If left unreduced, a varus heel will cause difficulty with shoe fitting, lateral ankle pain or instability

heel height was higher in the subgroup of patients who had had previous surgical treatment of their calcaneal fractures. Complications included varus heel alignment in five feet, all of which required osteotomy and eventually obtained good results. There were two nonunions and one infection. Seventy percent of the patients had workers' compensation injuries; of this group, 35 percent returned to work.[27]

Although additional experience with this procedure is needed, the concept of the reconstruction is sound, and this procedure should be considered in cases of significant loss of heel height with the associated problems men-

FIGURE 30–16. Intra-articular calcaneal fracture with varus displacement of the tuberosity fragment.

symptoms, and forefoot supination with increased weight bearing on the lateral border of the foot. CT is the best imaging modality for defining the shape of the calcaneal bone, but it is not performed in the weight-bearing stance. The hindfoot alignment view allows direct measurement of the weight-bearing axis of the calcaneus in relation to the axis of the tibia.[9, 15]

Calcaneal Osteotomy

When symptomatic heel varus exists alone, without subtalar arthritis or other problems, a Dwyer lateral closing wedge osteotomy will correct the alignment (Fig. 30–17).[24] If more correction is needed or if the heel is already significantly shortened, a lateral displacement osteotomy alone[16] or a closing wedge osteotomy combined with a displacement osteotomy will correct the alignment. Symptomatic heel valgus may be treated with a medial displacement osteotomy of the calcaneus by Coleman's technique.[16]

Subtalar Arthrodesis

Often a varus heel is associated with other problems that may require subtalar arthrodesis. If the heel is in less than 5 to 10 degrees of varus, this can usually be corrected at the time of arthrodesis by either the intra-articular morselized bone graft technique[46] or the posterior subtalar bone block technique[13] described previously. Additional bone graft is placed medially or a bone block is fashioned to wedge the heel back into a neutral or slightly valgus position, and the talus is rigidly fixed to the calcaneus.

Subtalar Arthrodesis plus Calcaneal Osteotomy

When there is marked heel varus of greater than 10 degrees associated with subtalar arthritis, it is difficult to realign the heel adequately in a neutral or slightly valgus position with subtalar arthrodesis alone. In this case, subtalar fusion combined with a calcaneal osteotomy may be required.

Author's Preferred Technique

The subtalar arthrodesis is performed through a lateral L-shaped incision.[41] The peroneal tendons are removed from their retinaculum along the lateral border of the calcaneus and are retracted superiorly during the exposure. An exostectomy of the lateral wall is performed, and if there is calcaneofibular abutment or peroneal tendon impingement, the peroneal tendon sheath is opened.

The intra-articular portion of the arthrodesis is performed as described earlier; it is followed by a Dwyer lateral closing wedge osteotomy or a lateral displacement osteotomy as needed to correct hindfoot alignment to neutral or slight valgus (see Fig. 30–17). The arthrodesis site and the calcaneal osteotomy are fixed with a cancellous screw or a percutaneous Steinmann pin augmented by power-driven staples (Fig. 30–18). The fixation can be placed either from the neck of the talus across the subtalar joint and osteotomy into the tuberosity fragment or from the opposite direction. There appear to be fewer problems with screw head symptoms postoperatively when the screw is inserted through the neck of the talus. A cannulated screw system is helpful in this situation because provisional fixation can be obtained with the guide pin, and after a satisfactory position is confirmed radiographically, the screw can be inserted without a loss of position. A screw with a low-profile head is used so that it will not impinge on the anterior aspect of the ankle joint or cause a painful prominence on the heel. Aftercare is similar to that used with a subtalar arthrodesis.

Alternative Technique (Romash's Technique)

Romash described an alternative technique of subtalar arthrodesis combined with calcaneal osteotomy in which the osteotomy is performed along the original primary fracture line.[65] The tuberosity fragment is then displaced downward and medially to correct the loss of heel height and varus alignment. When this is done, the calcaneofibular abutment and talar declination angle are also improved. I have had no experience with this technique, but the preliminary results are satisfactory in a small group of patients.

An oblique lateral incision is made over the sinus tarsi area, bounded inferiorly by the peroneal tendons. The posterior facet of the subtalar joint is exposed and denuded of articular cartilage. The lateral wall of the calcaneus is subperiosteally exposed by elevating the

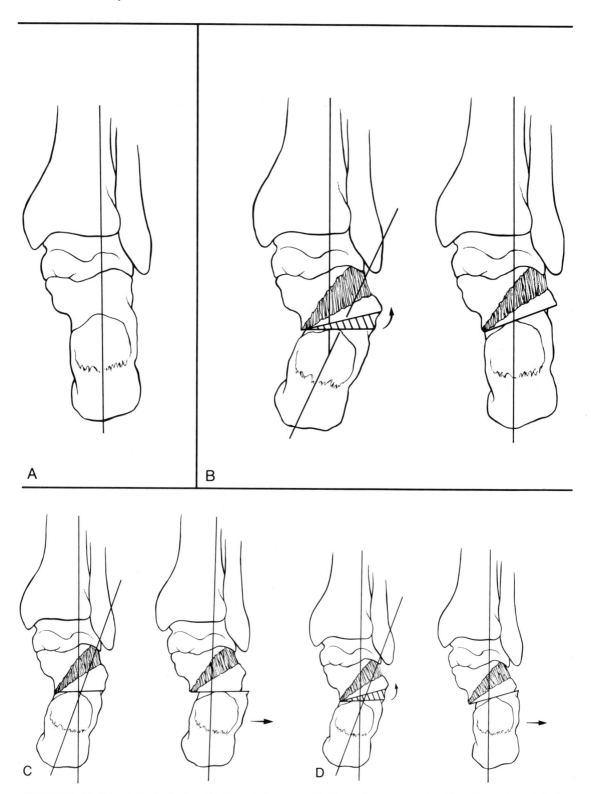

FIGURE 30–17. Calcaneal osteotomies. *(A)*, Normal alignment. *(B)*, Varus alignment corrected by a Dwyer lateral closing wedge osteotomy. *(C)*, Varus alignment corrected by lateral displacement osteotomy. *(D)*, Varus alignment corrected by a closing wedge osteotomy combined with a lateal displacement osteotomy for a severe deformity.

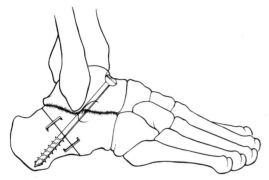

FIGURE 30–18. Subtalar arthrodesis combined with a calcaneal osteotomy fixed with a single cannulated cancellous screw and augmented with staples.

calcaneofibular ligament and the peroneal tendon sheaths. The primary fracture line is identified laterally, and a smooth Steinmann pin is driven obliquely from superolateral to inferomedial along the healed fracture line. An axial radiograph of the calcaneus is obtained to confirm proper placement of the pin. The osteotomy is then performed across the neck of the calcaneus along the guide pin from superolateral to inferomedial, exiting below the neurovascular bundle on the medial side and proximal to the calcaneocuboid joint laterally (Fig. 30–19A).

Provisional fixation of the talus to the sustentacular fragment is performed with a malleolar screw (later removed) before distraction of the osteotomy. An external fixator or AO distractor is placed medially, and the tuberosity fragment is shifted inferiorly and medially along the line of the osteotomy (Fig. 30–19B). With 4.0-mm cancellous lag screws, the lateral side (tuberosity fragment) is fixed to the medial side (sustentacular fragment), and proper positioning is confirmed by intraoperative radiography. The distractor and the provisional screw across the talus into the sustentacular fragment are then removed. Cancellous bone graft is packed into the subtalar joint and lateral osteotomy site. A countersunk 6.5- or 7.0-mm cannulated cancellous screw is placed across the neck of the talus into the calcaneus, further stabilizing the reconstruction (Figs. 30–19C and 30–20).

A short-leg cast is used in the gravity equinus position, without weight bearing, for 1 month, followed by casting in a plantigrade position until union is achieved at approximately 8 to 10 weeks. Touch weight bearing is allowed at 4 weeks, and progression to full weight bearing is allowed by 8 to 10 weeks, at which time ankle range-of-motion exercises and muscle strengthening are begun.

Flatfoot Deformity

Isolated fixed flatfoot deformity secondary to calcaneal fracture occurs secondary to the upward displacement of the posterior half of the os calcis.[57] It is usually treated nonoperatively with a custom-molded total contact insert and a supportive shoe with a cushioned sole. If this is not effective or if the flatfoot is associated with other postfracture deformities, the subtalar bone block arthrodesis technique will plantarflex the calcaneal tuberosity and help restore the longitudinal arch. The osteotomy described by Romash may also be useful to correct the flatfoot deformity.[65]

Increased Heel Width

As an isolated entity, increased heel width causes problems primarily with shoe fitting. This can be treated by modifying the heel counter of the shoe and adding a moldable foam heel cup.

However, increased heel width may cause secondary problems of calcaneofibular abutment or of impingement or dislocation of the peroneal tendons.

Calcaneofibular Abutment

Calcaneofibular abutment, when associated with symptomatic subtalar traumatic arthritis (Fig. 30–21), may be managed as outlined earlier, with either subtalar fusion with ostectomy of the lateral wall of the calcaneus; subtalar distraction bone block arthrodesis[13]; or subtalar arthrodesis with calcaneal osteotomy, as described previously (Romash's technique).[65] The associated symptoms and type of postfracture deformity of the calcaneus will determine which of these procedures to use for a given case.

Because of the difficulty in delineating whether subtalar arthritis, peroneal tendon impingement, or calcaneofibular abutment is re-

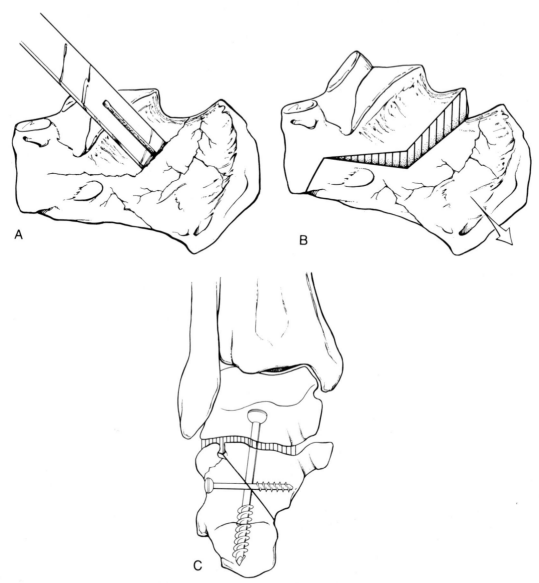

FIGURE 30–19. *(A)*, A reconstructive osteotomy is made along the original primary fracture line from superolateral to inferomedial. *(B)*, Distraction shifts the tuberosity fragment inferior and medial along the line of the osteotomy. *(C)*, Lag screws fix the tuberosity fragment to the sustentacular fragment, bone graft is inserted, and a large cannulated cancellous screw is used to fix the subtalar arthrodesis and the reduced osteotomy. (Redrawn from Romash MM: Reconstructive osteotomy of the calcaneus with subtalar arthrodesis for malunited calcaneal fractures. Presented at the Sixth Annual American Orthopaedic Foot and Ankle Society Meeting. Banff, Canada, June 1990.)

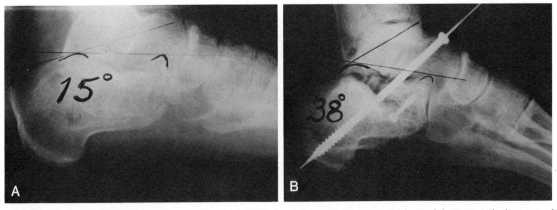

FIGURE 30–20. *(A)*, Preoperative lateral radiograph following joint depression–type calcaneal fracture with decrease of the talar declination angle and decrease of Böhler's angle to 15 degrees. *(B)*, Following reconstructive osteotomy and subtalar arthrodesis, the talar declination angle has been improved and Böhler's angle has been restored to 38 degrees. (Courtesy of Michael M. Romash, M.D. From Romash MM: Reconstructive osteotomy of the calcaneus with subtalar arthrodesis for malunited calcaneal fractures. Presented at the Sixth Annual American Orthopaedic Foot and Ankle Society Meeting. Banff, Canada, June 1990.)

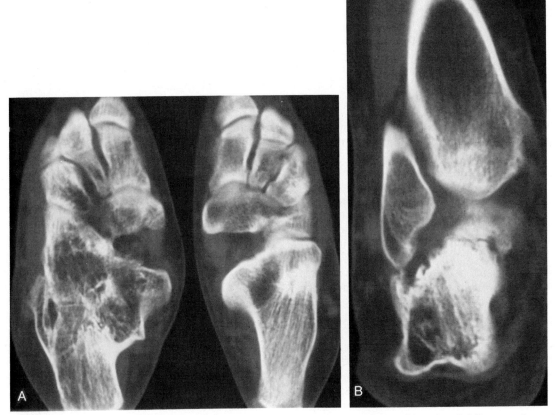

FIGURE 30–21. *(A)*, Transverse computed tomographic scan demonstrating a displaced lateral wall following calcaneal fracture. This patient had previously undergone a triple arthrodesis for post–calcaneal fracture pain, but a failure to decompress lateral wall impingement caused continued pain. *(B)*, Semicoronal computed tomographic scan of the same patient demonstrating calcaneofibular abutment.

sponsible for lateral pain following calcaneal fracture, DeLee states that Mann performs a lateral calcaneal wall decompression at the time of subtalar fusion.[20] The lateral cortical wall of the calcaneus is removed intact from beneath the peroneal tendons. The underlying cancellous bone is removed and used for grafting. The cortical wall is then replaced to decrease the potential for scarring between the exposed cancellous bone and the peroneal tendons.

Treatment of isolated lateral hindfoot pain secondary to abutment of the inferior tip of the fibula on the lateral wall of the calcaneus by subtalar fusion alone has a poor success rate.[7] Significantly improved results have been obtained by excision of the displaced lateral wall bone to decompress the space between the fibula and calcaneus.[7, 12, 18, 54] Braly and colleagues reported on a decompression procedure consisting of a lateral calcaneal wall ostectomy, sural nerve release or neurectomy, peroneal tendon release with relocation or lengthening as needed, and repair or reconstruction of the peroneal retinaculum. Satisfactory results were reported in 75 percent of eight patients who had previously undergone subtalar arthrodesis and in 82 percent of 11 patients who underwent lateral decompression as an alternative to subtalar fusion.[7] Lateral decompression is technically simpler and may be an effective alternative to late subtalar fusion in carefully selected patients with lateral pain and subfibular impingement symptoms.

Distal Fibula Resection

Isbister advocated resection of a small portion of the distal tip of the fibula to relieve calcaneofibular abutment.[73] Approximately 1 cm of the distal fibula is removed subperiosteally through a longitudinal lateral incision. The line of the ostectomy avoids the articular surface in contact with the talus. Satisfactory lateral pain relief was obtained at short-term follow-up in all five patients reported on.[73]

Patient selection for the lateral decompression procedure was primarily by history and physical examination in the series of Braly and colleagues.[7] However, when the surgeon is choosing between a lateral decompression procedure alone or subtalar fusion plus lateral decompression, it is very helpful to use differential diagnostic injections of local anesthetic to determine the pain contribution from the various potential sources on the lateral aspect of the hindfoot. These injections may need to be performed at sequential office visits, at the first visit blocking the sural nerve and at the next visit injecting the peroneal tendon sheath or subtalar joint, depending on the symptoms.

Technique of Lateral Decompression (Braly's Technique)

A Kocher incision is made over the lateral hindfoot just inferior to the course of the peroneal tendons and extending from the level of the ankle joint to the calcaneocuboid joint. Attempts are made to use a previous lateral incision. The sural nerve is identified and released from surrounding scar tissue. If a neuroma is present, the nerve is transected in the proximal end of the wound. The peroneal sheath is opened, and a tenolysis is performed. If the peroneal tendons are found dislocated, they are relocated and Z-lengthened as necessary, and the peroneal retinaculum is repaired or reconstructed. Before relocation of the tendons, the lateral wall of the calcaneus is subperiosteally exposed, and a lateral calcaneal ostectomy is performed to decompress the space beneath the tip of the fibula (Fig. 30–22). The ostectomy surface is rasped, and bone wax is applied.

Aftercare consists of application of a soft compression dressing followed by early range-of-motion exercises and weight bearing as tolerated at 2 to 3 days postoperatively. In cases requiring tendon lengthening, relocation, and retinacular repair, a short-leg non–weight-bearing cast is used for 3 weeks, after which a walking cast is used for another 3 weeks. Range-of-motion and strengthening exercises are begun after immobilization. Full activity is allowed 8 to 12 weeks postoperatively.

Impingement or Dislocation of the Peroneal Tendons

Flattening and widening of the calcaneus during fracture causes the blown-out lateral wall to encroach on the fibulocalcaneal space. Deyerle noted that in some patients, spreading of the os calcis actually pushed the peroneal tendons out of the tunnel behind the fibula, and they became dislocated anterior to the fibula.[23] Patients with dislocated peroneal tendons have an inability to resist inversion and

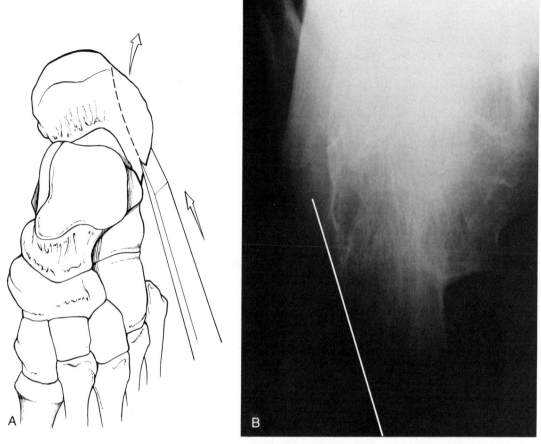

FIGURE 30–22. *(A),* Ostectomy of the lateral wall of the calcaneus. *(B),* Postoperative axial radiograph of the same patient as in Figure 30–20 after lateral wall ostectomy *(along white line).*

complain of instability and lack of control of the foot.[23] Impingement of the peroneal tendons causes symptoms of tenosynovitis with an antalgic gait, limited subtalar motion, and point tenderness at the inferior peroneal retinaculum.[26] The diagnosis is further substantiated by an injection of local anesthetic into the tendon sheath or by peroneal tenography findings showing a complete or partial block of contrast agent at the level of the inferior peroneal retinaculum.[26]

Surgical Treatment

Treatment of tenosynovitis and impingement is by surgical decompression of the subfibular space, either by longitudinal incision of the peroneal tendon sheath (leaving sufficient retinaculum intact to prevent subluxation),[57]

lateral calcaneal wall ostectomy,[7, 26, 63] or excision of the tip of the distal fibula.[73] The few published reports of results that are available have small patient numbers and were discussed earlier.[7, 62, 73]

Peroneal tendon dislocation is treated by lateral wall decompression followed by rerouting of the tendons behind the fibula with repair of the retinaculum.[7, 23] Deyerle reported "significant improvement" in all nine patients in his series who were treated with this technique.[23] Braly and colleagues did not separate the results obtained after tendon dislocation from those obtained after treating the other causes of lateral pain, but they had satisfactory results with this procedure in approximately 75 to 82 percent of a group of 19 patients, three of whom had relocation of dislocated peroneal tendons.[7]

Author's Preferred Method of Treatment

I favor the lateral decompression procedure as described by Braly and colleagues for peroneal tendon impingement or dislocation and for calcaneofibular abutment.[7] Although it is often difficult to determine preoperatively exactly which of the various potential sources of pain is causing the disability, surgery is preceded by careful physical examination, radiography, CT, and diagnostic injections of anesthetic to define as closely as possible the source or sources of the lateral pain. Resection of only the tip of the fibula, as advocated by Isbister,[73] may not fully decompress all peroneal tendon impingement, would not be helpful in cases in which tendon relocation was required, and does not address sural nerve pathology.

Neuroma or Entrapment of the Sural Nerve

Injury to the sural nerve resulting in a neuroma or nerve entrapment by surrounding scar tissue usually occurs in patients who have had prior surgical treatment of their fracture using a lateral incision.[7, 34] Symptoms consist of lateral hindfoot pain, a positive Tinel sign at a point along the sural nerve, paresthesias, and possibly decreased or absent sensation along the lateral border of the foot. Other causes of lateral hindfoot pain, as previously discussed, may make the diagnosis difficult. Marked improvement in symptoms following local anesthetic block of the nerve at a level above the ankle joint confirms the diagnosis.

Nonoperative Treatment

Nonoperative treatment is based on the known pathophysiologic mechanisms of pain generation by injured peripheral nerves.[22] The treatment program consists of desensitization physical therapy maneuvers, trial of a transcutaneous electrical nerve stimulation unit, local anesthetic injections with or without a corticosteroid, and a trial of a sympathetic nerve block, possibly followed by a series of blocks if the trial is effective.[78] Oral medications that may be helpful include tricyclic antidepressants, anticonvulsants, and antiarrhythmics. If these measures fail, prolonged local anesthetic blockade provided by a continuous epidural infusion may be helpful.[78]

Surgical Treatment

Surgical treatment of sural nerve entrapment (spindle neuroma) consists of exploration of the nerve and neurolysis. In the case of an amputation neuroma (bulb neuroma), a more proximal transection of the nerve is performed (Fig. 30–23).[48] Nerve transection may be combined with a nerve graft repair, fascicular ligation,[3, 52] autologous transplantation,[31] wandering nerve grafting (the distal end of the graft is left unrepaired),[53] or burying the cut nerve end into a vessel, muscle, or bone. Quill and Myerson reported relief of neuritic symptoms in all seven patients who underwent transection and proximal transposition of the sural nerve after calcaneal fracture treatment.[63] Kenzora reported good results in 13 of 23 patients with neuromas of cutaneous nerves

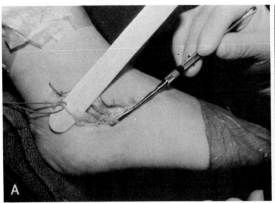 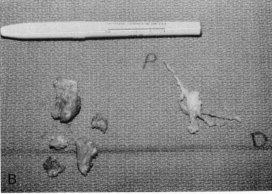

FIGURE 30–23. *(A)*, Symptomatic neuroma-in-continuity of the sural nerve after operative treatment of a displaced calcaneal fracture. *(B)*, Neuroma specimen following resection showing proximal (P) and distal (D) ends of the nerve. Note the bone fragments from ostectomy of the lateral wall of the calcaneus.

about the foot and ankle who were treated by proximal resection with or without burial of the stump in muscle.[48] Although the results of sural nerve treatment were not reported separately, Braly and colleagues had overall satisfactory results in 75 to 82 percent of 19 patients who underwent the lateral decompression procedure, 10 of whom had sural nerve neurolysis and two of whom underwent neurectomy.[7] However, DeLee has found this problem to be extremely recalcitrant to treatment.[20]

Author's Preferred Method of Treatment

If the symptoms and physical examination findings indicate a localized neuropathy of the sural nerve, an initial attempt at nonoperative treatment is made, regardless of whether complete transection of the nerve, a neuroma-in-continuity, or entrapment from scar tissue is present. The nonoperative regimen is that described earlier and is ideally carried out in the setting of a pain management center. Trials of the various treatments can be time consuming, and it is difficult to predict which patients will respond to which modalities.

On failure of a trial of these modalities that lasts at least 3 to 6 months, sural nerve exploration is recommended, but the surgeon must make it clear to the patient that relief of symptoms is not predictable. If the nerve appears normal except for surrounding scar tissue, a neurolysis is performed. If there is an amputation stump neuroma or a neuroma-in-continuity, the nerve is transected in the proximal end of the wound so that the inevitable stump neuroma that forms will not be in an area subject to external compression by footwear. Desensitization therapy is resumed immediately after the procedure.

The sural nerve is of sufficient size that adjunctive techniques to help prevent neuroma formation may be considered. The groups of fascicles, of which there are usually three, can be dissected out under magnification and sutured to each other by the technique of centro-central nerve union with autologous transplantation.[31] The wandering nerve graft technique can be used on the sural nerve by transecting it proximally and then repairing it at the same site. The painful distal end of the nerve is then buried in muscle or fat in an area in which mechanical irritation would be minimized. Although I have had no personal experience with these adjunctive techniques, the autologous transplantation technique[31] and the wandering nerve graft technique[53] have been used successfully in the hand and may likewise be of benefit for treating sural nerve neuromas.

SUMMARY

Late problems following calcaneal fracture are a dilemma for both patients and physicians. Reconstructive procedures should be timed with the knowledge that most patients' conditions continue to improve after initial treatment of their calcaneal fracture for up to 2 to 5 years. However, postfracture deformity may lead to multiple sources of pain and disability. The key to a successful salvage procedure is understanding the postfracture pathology and how it contributes to the symptoms exhibited by each patient. To achieve a satisfactory result, the procedures performed must address all the identified sources of postfracture pain and disability.

References

1. Aaron DAR: Intra-articular fractures in the calcaneus. J Bone Joint Surg 56B:567, 1974.
2. Athmonsen W: An oblique projection for roentgen examination of the talo-calcaneus joint, particularly regarding intraarticulation fracture of the calcaneus. Acta Radiol 24:306, 1943.
3. Battista AF, Cravioto H: Neuroma formation and prevention by fascicle ligation in the rat. Neurosurgery 8:191–204, 1981.
4. Benirschke SK, Mayo KA, Sangeorzan BJ, Hansen ST Jr: Results of operative treatment of os calcis fractures. Presented at the AAOS meeting. New Orleans, LA, February 1990.
5. Bohler L: Diagnosis, pathology, and treatment of fractures of the os calcis. J Bone Joint Surg 13:75–89, 1931.
6. Bradford CH, Larsen I: Sprain-fractures of the anterior lip of the os calcis. N Engl J Med 244:970–972, 1951.
7. Braly WG, Bishop JO, Tullos HS: Lateral decompression for malunited os calcis fractures. Foot Ankle 6:90–96, 1985.
8. Broden B: Roentgen examination of the subtaloid joint in fractures of the calcaneus. Acta Radiol (Diagn) 31:84, 1949.
9. Buck P, Morrey BF, Chao EYS: The optimum position of arthrodesis of the ankle. J Bone Joint Surg 69A:1052–1062, 1987.
10. Burdeaux BD: Calcaneus fractures: Rationale for the medial approach technique of reduction. Orthopedics 10:177–187, 1987.
11. Burdeaux BD: Reduction of calcaneal fractures by the McReynolds medial approach technique and its experimental basis. Clin Orthop 177:87–103, 1983.

12. Cabot H, Binney H: Fractures of the os calcis and astragalus. Ann Surg 45:51–68, 1907.
13. Carr JB, Hansen ST Jr, Benirschke SK: Subtalar distraction bone block fusion for late complications of os calcis fractures. Foot Ankle 9:81–86, 1988.
14. Cave EF: Fracture of the os calcis—the problem in general. Clin Orthop 30:64–66, 1963.
15. Cobey JC: Posterior roentgenogram of the foot. Clin Orthop 118:202–207, 1976.
16. Coleman SS: Equinavarus congenita. *In* Complex Foot Deformities in Children. Philadelphia, Lea & Febiger, 1983, p 93.
17. Cotton FJ: Fractures. Ann Surg 64:480, 1916.
18. Cotton FJ: Old os calcis fractures. Ann Surg 74:294–303, 1921.
19. Degan TJ, Morrey BF, Braun DP: Surgical excision for anterior-process fractures of the calcaneus. J Bone Joint Surg 64A:519–524, 1982.
20. DeLee JC: Fractures and dislocations of the foot. *In* Mann RA (Ed): Surgery of the Foot, 5th Ed. St. Louis, CV Mosby, 1986, pp 592–808.
21. Dennyson WG, Fulford GE: Subtalar arthrodesis by cancellous graft and metallic internal fixation. J Bone Joint Surg 58B:507–510, 1976.
22. Devor M: The pathophysiology of damaged peripheral nerves. *In* Wall PD, Melzack R (Eds): Textbook of Pain. New York, Churchill Livingstone, 1989, pp 63–81.
23. Deyerle WM: Long term follow-up of fractures of the os calcis. Orthop Clin North Am 4:213–227, 1973.
24. Dwyer FC: Osteotomy of the calcaneum for pes cavus. J Bone Joint Surg 41B:80, 1959.
25. Essex-Lopresti P: The mechanism, reduction technique, and results in fractures of the os calcis. Br J Surg 39:395–419, 1952.
26. Fitzgerald RH Jr, Coventry MB: Post-traumatic peroneal tendonitis. *In* Bateman JE, Trott AW (Eds): The Foot and Ankle. New York, Brian C. Decker, 1980.
27. Fortin PT, Walling AK, Sanders RW: Subtalar arthrodesis following calcaneal fractures. Presented at the Sixth Annual American Orthopaedic Foot and Ankle Society Meeting. Banff, Alberta, Canada, June 1990.
28. Gallie WE: Subastragalar arthrodesis in fractures of the os calcis. J Bone Joint Surg 25:731–736, 1943.
29. Gellman M: Fracture of the anterior process of the calcaneus. J Bone Joint Surg 33A:382–386, 1951.
30. Giachino AA, Uhthoff HK: Current concepts review: Intra-articular fractures of the calcaneus. J Bone Joint Surg 71A:784–787, 1989.
31. Gorkisen K, Boese-Landgraf J, Vaubel E: Treatment and prevention of amputation neuromas in hand surgery. Plast Reconstr Surg 73:293–296, 1984.
32. Grice DS: An extra-articular arthrodesis of the subastragalar joint for correction of paralytic flat feet in children. J Bone Joint Surg 37A:246, 1952.
33. Gross RH: A clinical study of the Batchelor subtalar arthrodesis. J Bone Joint Surg 58A:343, 1976.
34. Hall MC, Pennal GF: Primary subtalar arthrodesis in the treatment of severe fractures of the calcaneus. J Bone Joint Surg 42B:336, 1960.
35. Hammesfahr JFR: Surgical treatment of calcaneal fractures. Orthop Clin North Am 20:679–689, 1989.
36. Hammesfahr R, Fleming LL: Calcaneal fractures: A good prognosis. Foot Ankle 2:161–171, 1981.
37. Harding D, Waddell JP: Open reduction in depressed

fractures of the os calcis. Clin Orthop 199:124–131, 1985.
38. Hazlett JW: Open reduction of the calcaneum. Can J Surg 12:310, 1969.
39. Heckman JD: Fractures and dislocations of the foot. *In* Rockwood CA Jr, Green DP (Eds): Fractures in Adults, 2nd Ed. Philadelphia, JB Lippincott, 1984, pp 1703–1832.
40. Hermann OJ: Conservative therapy for fracture of the os calcis. J Bone Joint Surg 19A:6709, 1937.
41. Hoppenfeld S, deBoer P: Lateral approach to the posterior talocalcaneal joint. *In* Surgical Exposures in Orthopaedics. Philadelphia, JB Lippincott, 1984, pp 504–506.
42. Hunt DD: Compression fracture of the anterior articular surface of the calcaneus. J Bone Joint Surg 52A:1637–1642, 1970.
43. Isherwood I: A radiological approach to the subtalar joint. J Bone Joint Surg 43B:366, 1966.
44. Johansson JE, Harrison J, Greenwood FA: Subtalar arthrodesis for adult traumatic arthritis. Foot Ankle 2:294, 1982.
45. Johnson EW Jr, Peterson HA: Fractures of the os calcis. Arch Surg 92:848–852, 1966.
46. Johnson KA: Arthrodeses of the foot and ankle. *In* Surgery of the Foot and Ankle. New York, Raven Press, 1989, pp 151–208.
47. Kalamchi A, Evans JG: Posterior subtalar fusion: A preliminary report on a modified Gallie's procedure. J Bone Joint Surg 59B:287–289, 1977.
48. Kenzora JE: Sensory nerve neuromas—leading to failed foot surgery. Foot Ankle 7:110–117, 1986.
49. Koshkareva ZV, Zhitnitskiĭ RE: Modification of subtalar arthrodesis in the treatment of deformities of the talus and calcaneus. Ortop Travmatol Protez 3:70–72, 1978. As referenced in Paley D, Hamilton H: Calcaneal fracture controversies. Can we put Humpty Dumpty together again? Orthop Clin North Am 20:665–677, 1989.
50. Lance EM, Carey EJ, Wade PA: Fractures of the os calcis: A followup study. J Trauma 4:15, 1964.
51. Lindsay WRN, Dewar FP: Fractures of the os calcis. Am J Surg 95:555–576, 1958.
52. Lusskin R, Battista A: Evaluation and therapy after injury to peripheral nerves. Foot Ankle 7:71–81, 1986.
53. Mackinnon SE: Wandering nerve graft technique for management of the recalcitrant painful neuroma in the hand: A case report. Microsurgery 9:95–101, 1988.
54. Magnuson PB: An operation for relief of disability in old fractures of os calcis. JAMA 80:1511–1513, 1923.
55. Mann RA: Miscellaneous afflictions of the foot. *In* Mann RA (Ed): Surgery of the Foot, 5th Ed. St. Louis, CV Mosby, 1986, p 232.
56. Maxfield JE, McDermott FJ: Treatment of calcaneal fractures by open reduction. J Bone Joint Surg 45A:868, 1963.
57. McLaughlin HL: Treatment of late complications after os calcis fractures. Clin Orthop 30:111–115, 1963.
58. McReynolds IS: The case for operative treatment of fractures of the os calcis. *In* Leach RE, Hoaglund FT, Riseborough EJ (Eds): Controversies in Orthopedic Surgery. Philadelphia, WB Saunders, 1982, pp 232–254.
59. Nade SML, Monahan PRW: Fractures of the calcaneum: A study of the long term prognosis. Injury 4:200–207, 1973.
60. Paley D, Hamilton H: Calcaneal fracture controver-

sies. Can we put Humpty Dumpty together again? Orthop Clin North Am 20:665–677, 1989.

61. Piatt AD: Fracture of the promontory of the calcaneus. Radiology 67:386–390, 1956.

62. Pozo JL, Kirwan E, Jackson AM: The long-term results of conservative management of severely displaced fractures of the calcaneus. J Bone Joint Surg 66B:386, 1984.

63. Quill G, Myerson M: Late treatment after calcaneal fracture. Presented at the Sixth Annual American Orthopaedic Foot and Ankle Society Meeting. Banff, Alberta, Canada, June 1990.

64. Resnick D: Radiology of the talocalcaneal articulations. Radiology 111:581–586, 1974.

65. Romash MM: Reconstructive osteotomy of the calcaneus with subtalar arthrodesis for malunited calcaneal fractures. Presented at sixth annual AOFAS meeting, June 1990, Banff, Alberta, Canada.

66. Romash MM: Calcaneal fractures: Three-dimensional treatment. Foot Ankle 8:180–197, 1988.

67. Ross DK, Sowerby RR: Operative treatment of fractures of the os calcis. Clin Orthop 199:132–143, 1985.

68. Ross DK: Operative treatment of complex os calcis fractures. Techniques Orthop 2:55–70, 1987.

69. Rowe CR, Sakellarides HT, Sorbie C, et al: Fractures of the os calcis: A long-term followup study of 146 patients. JAMA 184:920, 1963.

70. Schofield RO: Fractures of the os calcis. J Bone Joint Surg 18:566–580, 1936.

71. Segal D, Marsh JL, Leiter B: Clinical application of computerized axial tomography (CAT) scanning of calcaneus fractures. Clin Orthop 199:114–123, 1985.

72. Sisk TD: Fractures. *In* Edmonson AS, Crehshaw AH (Eds): Campbell's Operative Orthopaedics, Vol 1, 6th Ed. St. Louis, CV Mosby, 1980.

73. Isbister JF: Calcaneo-fibular abutment following crush fracture of the calcaneus. J Bone Joint Surg 56B:274–278, 1974.

74. Steel MW, Johnson KA, Dewitz MA, Ilstrup DM: Radiographic measurements of the normal adult foot. Foot Ankle 1:151–158, 1980.

75. Stephenson JR: Surgical treatment of displaced intra-articular fractures of the calcaneus. Surg Rounds Orthop Dec:19–32, 1987.

76. Stephenson JR: Treatment of displaced intra-articular fractures of the calcaneus using medial and lateral approaches, internal fixation, and early motion. J Bone Joint Surg 69A:115–130, 1987.

77. Thomas FB: Arthrodesis of the subtalar joint. J Bone Joint Surg 49B:93, 1967.

78. Vidger D: Peripheral neuralgias. *In* Abram SE (Ed): The Pain Clinic Manual. Philadelphia, JB Lippincott, 1990, pp 137–141.

79. Whittaker AH: Treatment of fractures of the os calcis by open reduction and internal fixation. Am J Surg 74:687–696, 1947.

80. Winkler W: The role of orthotics in the rehabilitation of patients with fracture of the calcaneum. Prosthet Orthot Int 13:70–75, 1989.

31

Principles of Foot Deformity Correction: Ilizarov Technique

DROR PALEY

The Ilizarov technique lends itself well to correction of foot deformities because of the three-dimensional nature of the foot and of the apparatus. The two approaches to the correction of foot deformities are (1) soft tissue distraction of the deformity and (2) distraction of an osteotomy. In the former, the deformity is corrected by eliminating pre-existing contractures and by distracting across joints in an attempt to bring them into a new congruous relationship to a plantigrade position.[3, 5, 8, 18] In the second, the distraction occurs through osteotomies, regenerating new bone and eliminating deformities by opening wedge–type corrections.[7, 8, 15, 18] The joints remain undisturbed with osteotomy distraction techniques. The decision as to which approach to use depends on several factors: (1) age, (2) the presence or absence of fixed bony deformities, and (3) the stiffness of the deformity.

The decision for nonosteotomy treatment depends primarily on the age of the patient. Essentially, any deformity can be treated without osteotomy in patients younger than 8 years of age. In patients older than 8, the presence of fixed bony deformities is generally a contraindication to nonosteotomy treatment. An exception to this rule is when the joints to be distracted are so stiff that there is significant risk of physeal disruption rather than joint distraction. In these cases, osteotomy treatment may be preferable. The indications for nonosteotomy treatment are similar to those for soft tissue release by conventional means.[17] Soft tissue release relies on biologic plasticity and remodeling of cartilaginous bones. Dis-

traction is thought to reshape bones by activation of the circumferential physis of these bones.[15] Nonosteotomy treatment may still be considered in the presence of fixed bony deformity if limited arthrodeses are planned to maintain the correction that is obtained by joint distraction. This reduces the amount of bone that needs to be resected at the time of arthrodesis.

Therefore, osteotomy treatment is indicated for fixed bony deformity in patients older than 8 years of age in whom sufficient incongruity of the joints, which could not be expected to remodel, would result from the soft tissue distraction or release. This treatment may also be indicated in patients with neuromuscular imbalance in whom soft tissue correction would obtain but not maintain the correction. An osteotomy in such patients provides a lasting correction through bone instead of joints.

NONOSTEOTOMY FOOT DEFORMITY CORRECTION

There are two approaches to the correction of contractures by the Ilizarov method: constrained and unconstrained. In the constrained system, it is necessary to find the axis of rotation of the joint contracture and to perform the correction around this axis. In the unconstrained system, one allows the contracture to correct itself around soft tissue hinges and natural axes of rotation of joints.

The advantage of the constrained system is that the uniaxial hinge allows disconnection of

476

the distraction rod with active and passive range of motion of the joint being treated. With the unconstrained system, the fixation is relatively unstable the moment the distraction rods are removed. Therefore, the system must remain under distraction at all times, without any joint mobilization. The advantage of the unconstrained system is that it is simpler to apply and allows for errors in application. The constrained system, on the other hand, is very precise, and the hinges must be aligned to the joint axis within a narrow range of tolerance to avoid jamming of the joint. Incorrect hinge placement can also inadvertently lead to joint compression. The unconstrained method is advantageous for the treatment of the multiple foot joints that do not have a known simple single axis of rotation and is less advantageous for the treatment of joints such as the ankle, which do have an easy-to-locate axis.

Equinus Deformity

The ankle joint lends itself well to both constrained and unconstrained methods of treatment. The axis of rotation of the ankle lies approximately at the level of the lateral process of the ankle. Its axis extends laterally through the tip of the lateral malleolus and medially below the tip of the medial malleolus. The ankle joint surface has the curvature of a frustum, which is a section of a cone. The center of rotation of a cone is not parallel to its edges. Therefore, the center of rotation of the ankle is not parallel to the tibial plafond. Rather, the center of rotation is higher on the medial side than on the lateral side. This is easily remembered according to the levels of the two malleolei.

Constrained Method (Figs. 31–1 and 31–2)

The image intensifier is used to locate the axis of rotation of the ankle. Preoperatively, Mose circles are applied to a true lateral image of the ankle to identify the level of the axis of rotation. The center is usually within the lateral process of the ankle. The image intensifier is used to obtain a true lateral image of the ankle such that the lateral malleolus is centered

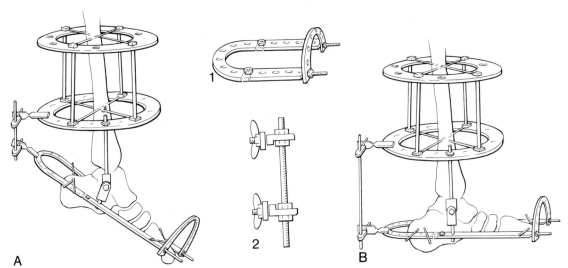

A   2   B

FIGURE 31–1. Correction of ankle equinus deformity: constrained method. *(A)*, The apparatus is shown applied to the tibia and foot. The apparatus consists of a two-ring frame on the tibia and a foot ring on the foot. The two are articulated using a threaded rod and hinges. The hinges are applied medially and laterally so that they overlie the center of rotation of the ankle. The ankle joint can be distracted apart by the threaded rod end of the hinge so as to avoid crushing the joint cartilage. The foot ring consists of a half-ring and two plates with threaded rod extensions connected by an anterior half-ring perpendicular to the rest *(inset 1)*. The distraction apparatus posteriorly consists of two twisted plates with a threaded rod distracting between them connected by a post or hinge. The post or hinge is fixed to the twisted plate with wing nuts *(inset 2)*. This allows removal and reapplication with ease. Two wires are fixed on each of the tibial rings, with an important olive wire placed anteriorly. Two wires are fixed to the calcaneus and two are fixed to the metatarsals. *(B)*, The distraction is performed at 1 to 2 mm/day to the patient's tolerance level. Overcorrection of the equinus is achieved. The patient maintains range of motion during the distraction.

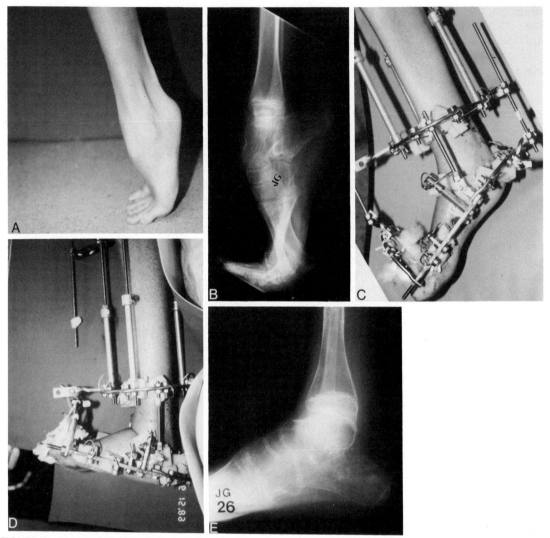

FIGURE 31–2. (*A* and *B*), Lateral photograph and radiograph of the ankle before correction. (*C* and *D*), The apparatus is shown from the lateral view during correction and at the end of overcorrection. Note that in this example, a wire was inserted across the axis of rotation of the ankle joint and connected to the hinges. This is another modification of the constrained technique. (*E*), The lateral radiograph after correction. (Courtesy of Dror Paley, M.D.)

over the midlateral tibia. A wire is used to point to the center of rotation. Once the wire overlaps the region of the lateral process, this spot is marked on the skin. The same process should be repeated for both the medial and lateral sides. The image intensifier must be perpendicular to the tibia.

Step 1. Apply a preconstructed two-level frame to the tibia. Use four wires to fix the tibial frame to the leg. For equinus correction, use one anterior olive medial-face wire on the distal of the two rings and one transverse wire on this ring.

Step 2. Suspend hinges from threaded rods off the distal tibial ring. Overlap the hinge with the center of rotation of the ankle joint.

Step 3. Apply the foot frame to the hinges. Adjust the foot frame so that it is parallel to the plantar aspect of the foot. This can be done by placing a board on the plantar aspect of the foot and making sure the foot frame is parallel to the board. A distraction rod off two pivot points such as a twisted plate is connected posteriorly in the central hole between the two hinges. Wing nuts are used to connect the posts at either end of the distraction rod. This allows quick application and removal. The patient can combine distraction with removal of the distraction rod for exercise and rehabilitation.

Unconstrained Method (Figs. 31–3 to 31–5)

The same tibial base of fixation is used for the unconstrained method as for the constrained method, but the foot frame is much simpler. This consists of a half-ring suspended off three threaded rods that are locked by a nut at their distal end and by conical washers at their proximal end. The maximum posterior tilt of these washers is 7.5 degrees. The half-ring is locked in place at that angle. Two smooth wires are inserted through the heel and fixed and tensioned to this half-ring. Deformity correction is performed by distraction on all three rods in order to pull the heel distally.

The reason for the posterior tilt of these rods is that the ankle capsule in equinus runs in a straight line from the back of the talus to the posterior lip of the tibia. When the foot is in the plantigrade position, the line of the ankle capsule is tilted 5 to 7 degrees posteriorly. This is because the posterior lip of the talus protrudes posterior to that of the tibia. If the rods were not tilted back but were parallel to the tibia, distraction along that line would pull the ankle capsule directly distally. This would force the talus forward, out of the mortise. When the rods are tilted posteriorly, the talus is pulled back into the mortise.

Varus Deformity (Figs. 31–6 and 31–7)

Heel varus deformity is corrected by the same type of construct as that used in an unconstrained correction of equinus deformity. The difference is that an olive is used on the medial side. The threaded rods are connected via hinges. The posterior threaded rod is connected to a two-, three-, or four-hole hinge so that the hinge point is proximal to the level of

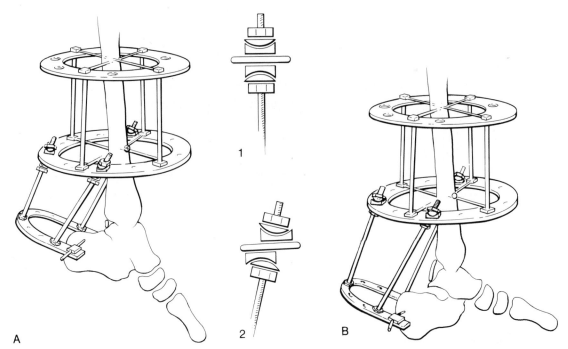

A

2

B

FIGURE 31–3. Correction of ankle equinus deformity: unconstrained method. *(A)*, The unconstrained apparatus consists of two rings in the tibia and a half-ring in the heel. One- or two-wire fixation is used in the heel, and two wires are used on each of the tibial rings, with an olive anteriorly on the distal ring. Three threaded rods are used to suspend the half-ring. These are fixed with nuts directly to the half-ring but are fixed with interposing conical washers on the distal tibial ring. This allows the half ring to be tilted posteriorly by approximately 7 degrees *(insets 1 and 2)*. *(B)*, At the end of the correction, the foot has been distracted downward and posteriorly at a 7-degree tilt. This keeps the ankle in the mortise. Notice that the ankle capsule in the uncorrected position runs vertically from the posterior lip of the tibia to the back of the talus. In the corrected position, the ankle capsule is oriented with a posterior slope to it. This slope parallels the 7-degree direction of distraction. Note also that the ankle and subtalar joints are overdistracted. This method does not allow removal of the rods for exercise of the joints; therefore, the overdistraction is important in maintaining a loose joint.

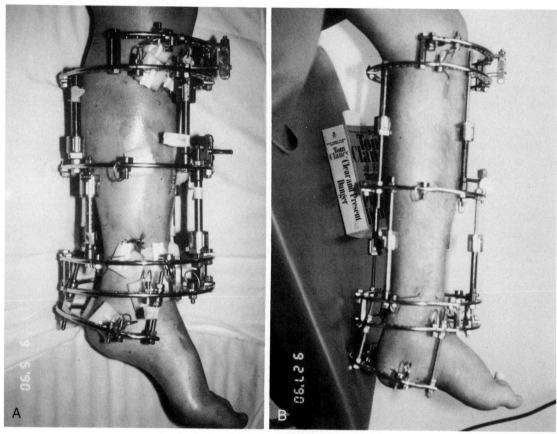

FIGURE 31–4. *(A),* A patient at the beginning of unconstrained equinus deformity correction combined with a two-level tibial lengthening. Note that the posterior heel rods are not parallel to the tibia. *(B),* Toward the end of correction, note the position of the heel ring. It is posteriorly displaced relative to the distal tibial ring. This keeps the talus in the mortise. (Courtesy of Dror Paley, M.D.)

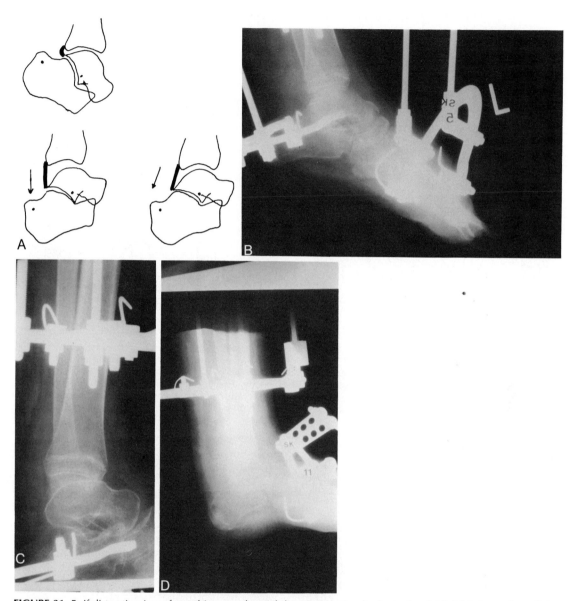

FIGURE 31–5. If distraction is performed in a purely axial direction, perpendicular to the distal tibial ring and parallel to the tibia, the ankle will tend to sublux forward *(A, left)*. If distraction is performed in a posteriorly inclined direction, the ankle does not sublux *(A, right)*. A clinical example of this phenomenon is shown at the beginning of distraction *(B)*, when the posterior heel rods are parallel to the tibia, during distraction *(C)*, demonstrating anterior subluxation, and after correction of subluxation *(D)*. (Courtesy of Dror Paley, M.D.)

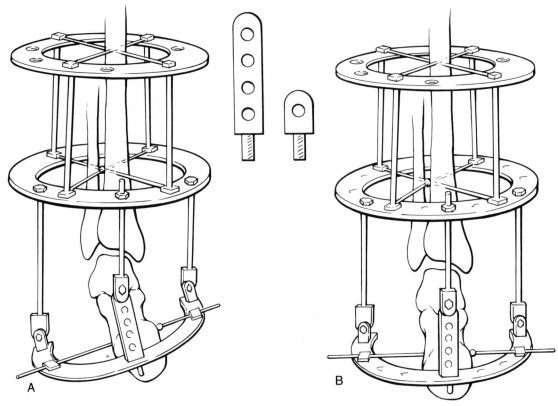

FIGURE 31–6. *(A)*, The drawing of the construct for correction of varus deformity is shown from the posterior view. This construct uses the standard two-ring fixation on the tibia, with two wires at each level and one with an olive placed laterally. One wire uses one hinge medially and one laterally on the half-ring. The main hinge is posterior and uses a three- or four-hole post *(inset)* to raise it above the level of the other two so that it is closer to the center of rotation of the subtalar joint. The level of this hinge also serves to force the olive on this half-ring against the body of the calcaneus to correct the varus deformity. *(B)*, At the end of correction, the rings are parallel and the contracture of the subtalar joint is reduced.

the heel wire. In this way, as the medial side is distracted, because it has to pivot around the hinge, it will translate laterally, forcing the heel out of varus. The rods medially and laterally are connected with a hinge distally and conical washers proximally, or with twisted plates that have pivot points at both ends, or with a mixture of the two. The choice depends on the degree of deformity. Conical washers can adapt only to a 7.5-degree tilt in either direction. The correction is produced by asymmetrical distraction of all three rods. The medial rod is lengthened at five 0.25-mm adjustments per day, the middle rod at three 0.25-mm adjustments per day, and the lateral rod at one 0.25-mm adjustment per day. In this manner, there is no risk of crushing of the joint surfaces.

Equinovarus Deformity

Correction of equinovarus deformity is essentially performed with a combination of the two previous constructs. The olive wires in the tibial construct must resist the equinus distraction as well as the varus distraction. Therefore, an anterolateral olive wire is used distally as a medial-face wire, and a posteromedial olive wire is used proximally as a medial-face wire.[11] If a hybrid construct using half-pins and wires is used, olive wires are not necessary. Smooth wires are used instead. An olive wire is used in the heel to pull the foot out of varus. The heel ring is tilted 7 degrees for the equinus to resist the anterior translation and is tilted the number of degrees of varus, as needed. The varus tilt is on the distal half-ring, whereas the

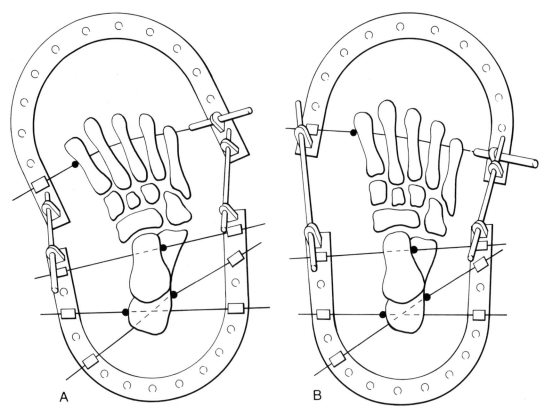

FIGURE 31–7. *(A)*, Adductus deformity correction is performed using a half-ring for the forefoot and one for the hindfoot, which are articulated by threaded rods suspended off posts. Two olive wires are fixed into the calcaneus with olives on either side; one olive wire is fixed into the talus with an olive on the lateral side; and one olive wire is fixed into the metatarsals with an olive on the medial side. This forms a three-point bending mechanism in which the midfoot and forefoot are distracted away from the fixed hindfoot. The distraction is produced by the threaded rods connecting the two half-rings and by a translation mechanism in the form of a slotted threaded rod that is connected to the distal wire. Note that the medial edge of the distal wire is fixed using a buckle onto the half-ring so as to allow it to slide as the translation of the metatarsals is carried out. *(B)*, At the end of the correction, the metatarsals are realigned and even overcorrected into abductus. The fifth metatarsal lies closer to the ring. The distal wire passes through only the first and fifth metatarsals and goes under the second, third, and fourth metatarsals.

equinus tilt is on the conical washers on the tibial ring. The distraction rate chosen is five 0.25-mm adjustments per day on the medial rod, four 0.25-mm adjustments per day on the posterior rod, and three 0.25-mm adjustments per day on the lateral rod.

Alternatively, a constrained construct can be used for equinovarus. This would involve application of a foot construct with hinges medially and laterally for the equinus, as described earlier, centered on the center of rotation of the ankle joint. The varus complicates the application of the hinges. The physician can accommodate for the varus by conical washers proximally if the amount of varus is not very large. For a larger amount of varus,

a biplanar hinge is used. This is made up of two half-hinges, which are at a 90-degree angle to each other. Alternatively, if universal hinges are available, they are much easier to use. They will accommodate for both the varus and the equinus. They need to be oriented for the varus. A distraction rod is placed posteriorly, with a biplanar hinge distally and a uniplanar pivot proximally.

Adductus Deformity (Figs. 31–7 and 31–8)

Adductus deformity can be corrected by a simple oval frame from the hindfoot to the

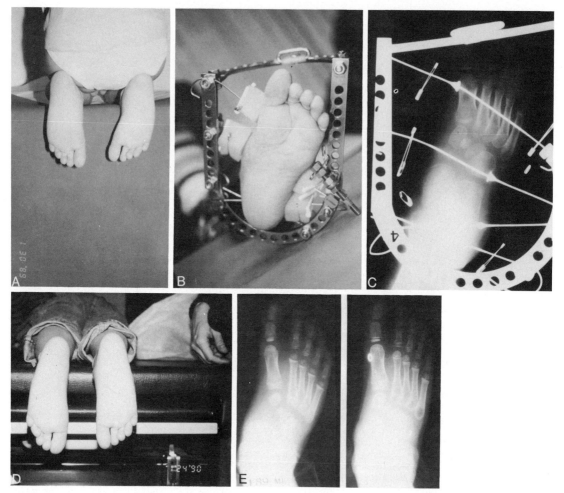

FIGURE 31–8. *(A)*, A 4-year-old boy with a persistent metatarsus adductus and a skewfoot despite previous casting. *(B)*, The foot is shown in the apparatus during treatment. *(C)*, The radiograph at the end of treatment showing overcorrection. *(D)*, The clinical appearance of the foot at 1-year follow-up. *(E)*, The standing radiograph of the foot at the end of treatment *(right)* compared with before. (Courtesy of Dror Paley, M.D.)

forefoot. The oval is made up of two half-rings connected by plates. The correction is a three-point bending one, locking the calcaneus with two olive wires. One lateral olive wire goes across the neck of the talus or the navicular and cuboid, and one comes from the medial aspect of the first metatarsal into the fifth metatarsal. This metatarsal wire goes under the second, third, and fourth metatarsals. A slotted, threaded rod is connected to the distal wire, which slowly transports the forefoot laterally. Together with this, the medial column can be distracted from the lateral column. Instead of two plates being used to connect the two half-rings to form an oval, threaded rods are used.

Cavus Deformity (Figs. 31–9 to 31–11)

There are numerous types of constructs for cavus deformity correction. The simplest consists of a half-ring anteriorly and one posteriorly, with distraction between them. Fixation is by one wire in the heel and one in the forefoot. For overcorrection of cavus, one wire is placed at the apex of the deformity, which is either the neck of the talus or the navicular-cuboid row. If there is a base of fixation on the tibia, it can be used to pull up the forefoot relative to the hindfoot. Because cavus is frequently associated with equinus, the surgeon should first correct the equinus deformity and then correct the forefoot cavus deformity or

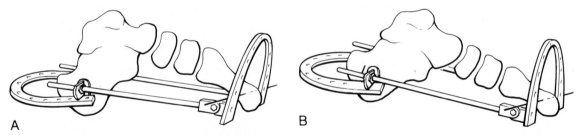

FIGURE 31–9. *(A),* The apparatus for the correction of cavus deformity. This apparatus may be very simple, including only a half-ring posteriorly and a half-ring anteriorly, with one- to two-wire fixation of the forefoot and hindfoot. The half-rings are distracted with threaded rods on hinges. *(B),* The appearance at the end of the distraction.

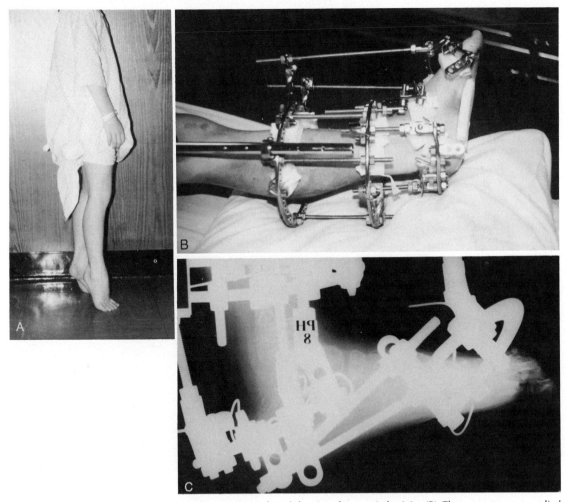

FIGURE 31–10. *(A),* A boy with a bilateral equinocavus foot deformity of congenital origin. *(B),* The apparatus was applied for the correction of the hindfoot equinus, followed by correction of the forefoot cavus. *(C),* The lateral radiograph during treatment. *(A to C courtesy of Dror Paley, M.D.)*

Illustration continued on following page

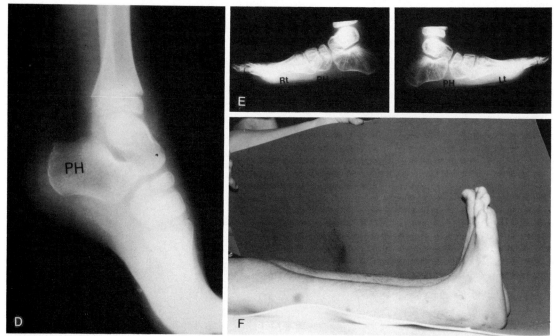

FIGURE 31–10 *Continued (D),* A lateral standing radiograph of the foot before the correction. *(E),* Radiographs of both feet at the end of the correction. Note the overcorrection achieved in the flattening of the arch on one of the sides, with plantar subluxation of the talonavicular joint on the left (Lt). One wire was placed in each navicular to act as a fulcrum for the correction. *(F),* The final clinical appearance shows no equinus or cavus deformity.

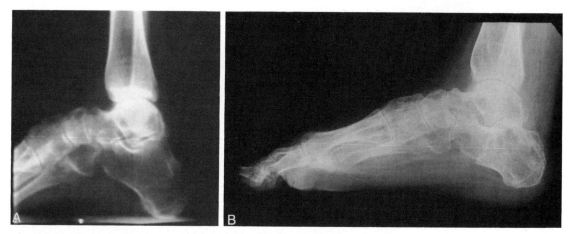

FIGURE 31–11. Combined forefoot and hindfoot cavus due to poliomyelitis. *(A),* The preoperative radiograph. Correction was performed using a posterior calcaneal osteotomy to decrease the calcaneal pitch and simultaneous distraction of the forefoot from the hindfoot, as well as elevation of the forefoot upward by pulling from the tibial ring. It should be noted that the rate of distraction of the forefoot upward should be approximately two times the rate of distraction of the forefoot away from the hindfoot. This is based on a mathematical calculation. *(B),* The final radiograph demonstrating the correction of the hindfoot and the forefoot equinus. (Courtesy of Dror Paley, M.D.)

should perform both corrections simultaneously.

Clubfoot (Figs. 31–12 and 31–13)

Clubfoot correction involves all of the previously mentioned constructs combined. In this correction, the use of a strong base on the tibia with the olive pattern described for equinovarus deformity is the first step. The heel ring is placed as it is for an equinovarus deformity. The distraction pattern for the hindfoot is as that described for equinovarus. The forefoot is fixed using a single wire through the first and fifth metatarsals with the olive medially. This is connected to a half-ring. A threaded rod medially connects the forefoot and hindfoot rings. It is preferable to have a universal joint, either of the commercially available type or one that can be created by putting three hinges together. This joint should be articulated between the hindfoot and forefoot rings. The forefoot ring is further attached to a vertical threaded rod that connects the tibial frame via a pivot point and twisted plate. This rod controls elevation of the forefoot, as well as supination and pronation. To this rod, I connect a push rod off a post. The push rod goes right to the vertical forefoot rod. Its function is to push the vertical rod laterally, thus helping to correct the adductus deformity. The pivot point is the base of the twisted plate on the tibial ring.

The order of correction is very important. Correction starts with distraction posteriorly in an asymmetrical fashion at a rate of 1 mm/day, as described for the equinovarus deformity. Simultaneously, the forefoot is pulled up at 1 mm/day. Because the forefoot ring is further from the center of ankle rotation than is the hindfoot ring, an opening wedge of the ankle joint will occur, thus stretching the posterior capsule more. This is the desired outcome. If pulling up is performed too quickly anteriorly, crushing of the anterior joint cartilage may occur. Therefore, radiographic monitoring of the lateral ankle is needed.

The medial and lateral rods, which are for the correction of the adductus deformity and the cavus deformity, are lengthened at 1 mm/day on the medial side and at 0.5 mm/day on the lateral side. If there is no cavus deformity, lengthening is at 1 mm/day on the medial side and at 0.25 mm/day on the lateral side. A

purely cavus correction would require approximately half the rate of distraction of the plantar aspect of the foot, as in pulling up on the foot. Once the equinus varus and adductus deformities have been corrected, the frame is converted for the correction of supination. Supination and pronation are corrected with two anterior rods. The surgeon pulls up more on the lateral side than on the medial side if simultaneous cavus correction is being performed. If no cavus correction is being performed, the surgeon can actually push down on the medial side and pull up on the lateral side. This can be done at a rate of 0.5 to 1 mm/day. The adductus push rod is also lengthened at 1 to 2 mm/day.

Each of the deformities treated should be overcorrected beyond the neutral level. If rebound occurs, it will only bring the foot to a neutral level, not into a nonplantigrade position.

Pain during distraction should be treated by titrating the dose of distraction. Because there is no risk of bony consolidation, there is no hurry. The surgeon can slowly distract to a level that the patient can tolerate.

Obviously, the younger the patient, the greater the expected growth and therefore the more potential for recurrence of the deformity. The less fixed bony deformity present, the smaller the chance for recurrence. The factors that the surgeon can alter that will decrease the risk of recurrence include the degree of overcorrection and the length of time in the fixator. Overcorrection of 20 to 30 percent can minimize the recurrence due to the rebound effect of the stretched soft tissues. After removal of the apparatus, the foot should be splinted with an ankle-foot orthosis or a total contact orthosis. The splint should be maintained full-time for at least 6 months and should then be used only at night for an extended period. Once the patient has reached skeletal maturity, splinting can be discontinued.

The length of time the apparatus is left in place after deformity correction is also important. In children, the apparatus should be removed approximately 6 weeks after the deformity has been fully distracted and corrected. In adults, a wait of 3 to 6 months after deformity correction is achieved may be necessary to prevent recurrence.

Recurrence can also be prevented by tendon transfer or selective arthrodeses after the dis-

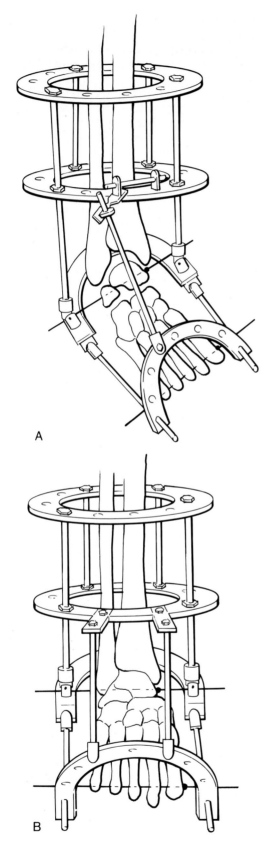

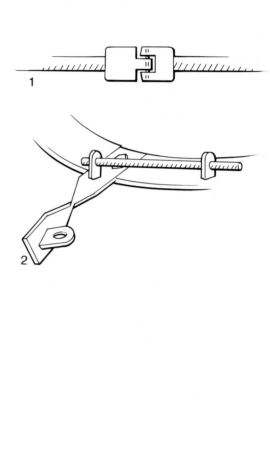

FIGURE 31–12. Clubfoot correction. *(A)*, The apparatus used is demonstrated. It consists of two rings on the tibia, a half-ring on the heel, and a half-ring on the forefoot. The forefoot and hindfoot half-rings are connected with threaded rods. Because the deformity is so complex, it requires specialized hinges called universal joints *(inset 1)*. The connection between the forefoot ring and the tibia anteriorly is via a single threaded rod initially, suspended off a twisted plate and hinge *(inset 2)*. This twisted plate and hinge assembly pushes the forefoot laterally by means of the medially placed olive. The push force comes from a threaded rod assembly, which attaches to the twisted plate on the tibial ring occurring medially *(inset 2)*. *(B)*, At the end of correction, the foot is overcorrected. Two threaded rods are attached anteriorly to correct the supination deformity.

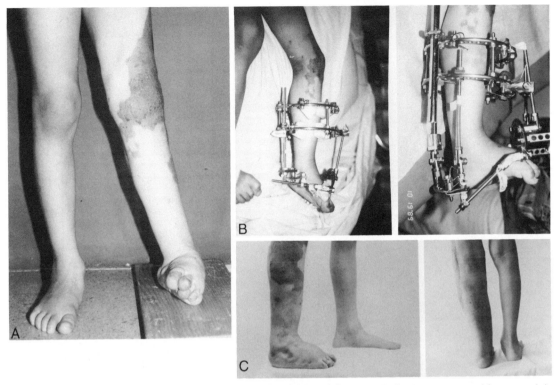

FIGURE 31–13. *(A)*, This 6-year-old boy had an untreated clubfoot deformity. His foot went untreated because of the extensive hemangiomatous involvement of his lower leg and foot. Note that he is standing on the lateral border of his foot. *(B)*, The apparatus is applied to mimic equinovarus, cavus, adductus, and supination deformities *(left)* and is shown at the end of correction *(right)*. *(C)*, The appearance of his foot from the side and from the back at the end of correction. This photograph was taken 3 months after removal of the apparatus, and there was still persistent edema. He has remained splinted using an ankle-foot orthosis since then, without any evidence of recurrent deformity after 3 years. (Courtesy of Dror Paley, M.D.)

traction correction is complete. For example, in Charcot-Marie-Tooth syndrome, the deformity can be eliminated by distraction, which converts a rigid, deformed foot into a flexible foot. A tendon transfer can then be performed to maintain the correction. Alternatively, a limited arthrodesis to maintain the foot position after soft tissue distraction is complete can be performed either by the Ilizarov method or by conventional means. The advantage of this technique is that it allows the surgeon to minimize the amount of bone resection, and a simple arthrodesis is carried out rather than a deformity-correcting one.

FOOT DEFORMITY CORRECTION WITH OSTEOTOMY

Distraction osteotomies of the foot are classified according to the level of the osteotomy. The osteotomy levels are supramalleolar, hind-foot, forefoot, and combined hindfoot and forefoot.

Supramalleolar (Figs. 31–14 to 31–16)

The indications for correction at the supramalleolar level are deformities of the metaphyseal or juxta-articular region of the distal tibia; deformities at the level of a previous ankle arthrodesis; and deformities at the level of the talus or subtalar joint in the presence of ankle ankylosis. The deformities that can be corrected through the supramalleolar region are equinus, calcaneal, varus, and valgus deformities; tibial torsion; and leg length discrepancy. The ability to lengthen the tibia and derotate it are two significant advantages of the supramalleolar osteotomy. Its other major advantage is its simplicity. This level is a relatively easy one at which to perform an osteotomy and correction. The supramalleolar os-

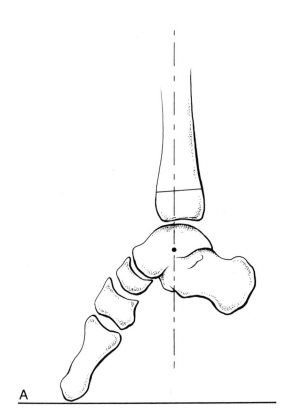

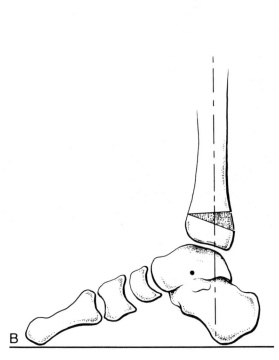

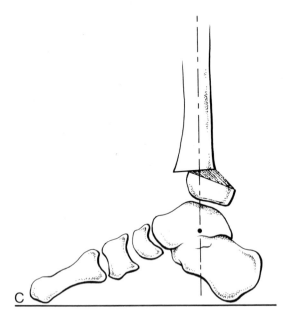

FIGURE 31–14. *(A),* An equinus deformity with a flat-top talus and stiff ankle. The center of rotation of the talus is marked *(point). (B),* An opening wedge osteotomy in the supramalleolar region corrects the equinus but translates the foot forward. *(C),* Combining an opening wedge with posterior translation realigns the foot.

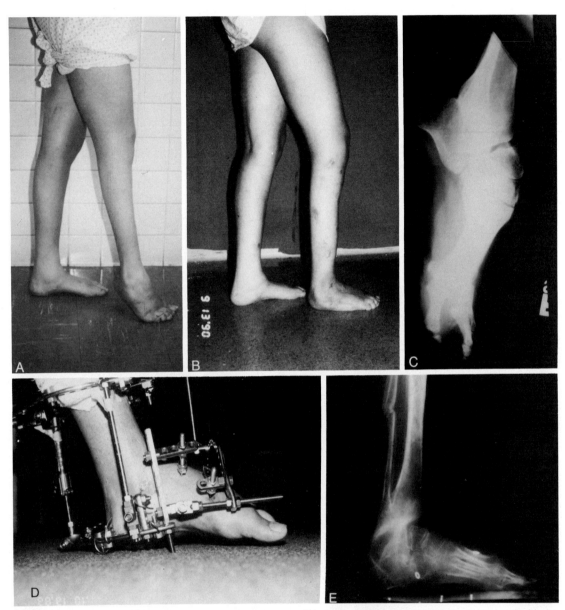

FIGURE 31–15. *(A)*, A 16-year-old girl with a fixed equinovarus deformity of the hindfoot and forefoot cavus and adductus due to a clubfoot deformity. *(B)*, After correction of the hindfoot by a supramalleolar osteotomy and nonosteotomy distraction of the forefoot cavus. *(C)*, Preoperative lateral radiograph of the foot demonstrating 65 degrees of equinus. There had been a previous talectomy and tibial calcaneal fusion. Note the forefoot cavus and the short heel. *(D)*, The lateral view of the apparatus is shown. The hinge lies below the level of the osteotomy so as to create a translation effect. *(E)*, After correction, the heel is more prominent because the foot was translated posteriorly. A 2.5-cm lengthening was performed through the distal tibia. With the use of a translation hinge, the regenerated new bone was translated back. Note that the forefoot equinus is eliminated. This was carried out by distraction through the joint and soft tissues. The leg was also simultaneously widened for cosmesis. (Courtesy of Dror Paley, M.D.)

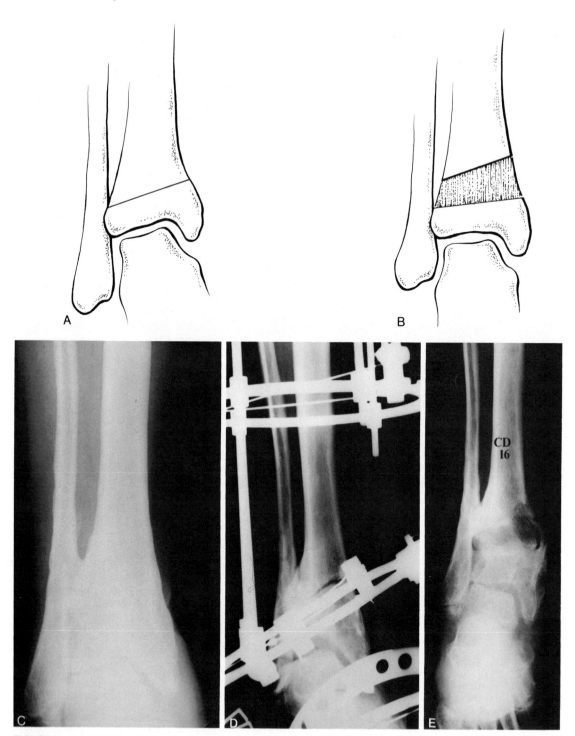

FIGURE 31–16. *(A),* Varus deformity of the distal tibia with shortening relative to the fibula. *(B),* Supramalleolar osteotomy with distraction and correction of the varus deformity and differential lengthening of the tibia relative to the fibula. *(C),* A post-traumatic varus deformity of the distal tibia with shortening of the tibia relative to the fibula, as in *B.* *(D),* A supramalleolar osteotomy was performed. *(E),* The final radiographic appearance after correction of the varus deformity and lengthening of the tibia relative to the fibula by 1.5 cm. *(C* to *E* courtesy of Dror Paley, M.D.)

teotomy offers rapid and reliable bone consolidation. It avoids surgery on a foot that has already had multiple operations in cases in which the deformity is below the level of the ankle joint. Its main limitation is the inability to correct deformities between the hindfoot and forefoot.

The most common pitfall of supramalleolar osteotomies is translational malalignment. This occurs when an angular deformity at one level is corrected at another level. For example, if a distal tibial deformity is at the level of the plafond (juxta-articular) rather than the metaphysis, a metaphyseal osteotomy will lead to a translational deformity. It is necessary to translate the metaphyseal osteotomy in addition to performing the angular correction.

It is preferable to use the supramalleolar osteotomy to correct only malalignment of the distal tibial articular surface. It can be used to correct deformities at the level of the talus when the ankle joint is very stiff. This leads to a tilt of the plafond, which is insignificant when the ankle is very stiff. Because the apex of the deformity is distal to the osteotomy, the supramalleolar osteotomy must be translated, as mentioned previously.

U-Osteotomy (Figs. 31–17 to 31–19)

The U-osteotomy[2] passes under the subtalar joint and through the superior part of the calcaneus posteriorly, and across the sinus tarsi and the neck of the talus anteriorly. It is indicated in cases in which the deformity is in the talus, such as in a flat-top talus. In the flat-top talus, there is a limited range of painless ankle motion. Because the joint is not spherical, it would not be congruous in any other position and is therefore not amenable to soft tissue distraction or release. The alternatives are either osteotomy or arthrodesis. With the U-osteotomy, the foot can be repositioned into a plantigrade position while the ankle mortise is left undisturbed. This preserves the limited range of ankle motion available.

Because the osteotomy crosses the sinus tarsi, an absolute prerequisite is a stiff subtalar joint. If the U-osteotomy is performed in the presence of a normal subtalar joint, subtalar motion will be blocked and lost. Fortunately, the majority of patients who have a flat-top talus have a pre-existing stiff subtalar joint or

even a talocalcaneal coalition or fusion. This osteotomy is able to correct equinus, calcaneal, varus, valgus, and foot height deformities. It is unable to correct deformities between the hindfoot and forefoot.

The U-osteotomy correction may be performed either rapidly or gradually. For rapid corrections, a percutaneous Achilles tendon lengthening is first carried out. If a gradual correction is performed, the bone ends should first be distracted apart in order to disimpact them and avoid a premature consolidation and failure of separation of the bone surfaces. Once the osteotomy has been separated, the deformity can be corrected gradually using a hinge. If lengthening is to be performed, the hinge should be centered more anteriorly. To avoid anterior translation of the foot, the hinge should be at or distal to the center of rotation of the ankle joint.

V-Osteotomy (Figs. 31–20 to 31–23)

The V-osteotomy[2] is a double osteotomy: one osteotomy is across the body of the calcaneus posterior to the subtalar joint, and one osteotomy is across the neck of the talus and the anterior calcaneus, through the sinus tarsi. The two osteotomies converge on the plantar aspect of the calcaneus. This leaves a triangular wedge of calcaneus and subtalar joint connected by the posterior facet to the body of the talus. The V-osteotomy is indicated for deformities between the hindfoot and forefoot. A prerequisite for this osteotomy is a stiff subtalar joint. Essentially all foot deformities can be corrected through the V-osteotomy, including hindfoot and forefoot equinus or calcaneal deformities, rocker-bottom deformities, cavus deformities, abductus and adductus deformities, and even deformities of length and bony deficiency of the hindfoot or forefoot.

Posterior Calcaneal Osteotomy (Figs. 31–24 to 31–26; see also Fig. 31–11)

The posterior calcaneal osteotomy[6, 7] is the same as the posterior limb of the V-osteotomy and the Dwyer osteotomy. It is used in deformities of the hindfoot when no forefoot deformity is present. It can also be used for bony

Text continued on page 501

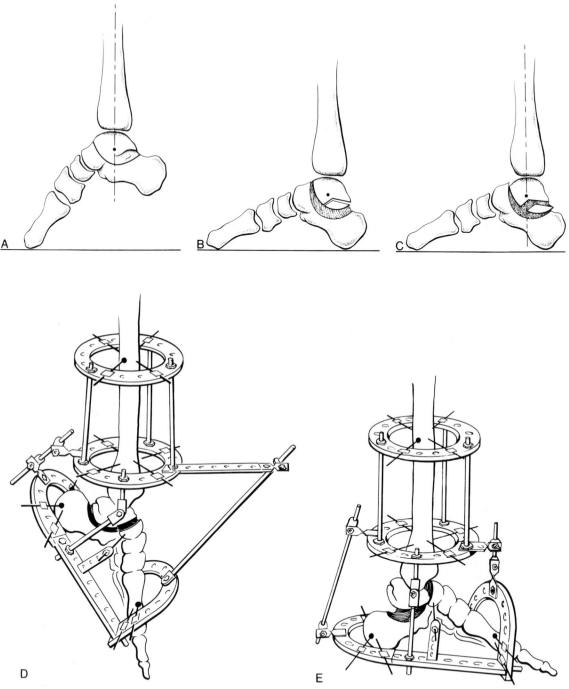

FIGURE 31–17. U-osteotomy. *(A),* Equinus deformity with flat-top talus. The U-osteotomy passes across the neck of the talus, through the sinus tarsi, and under the subtalar joint to exit posteriorly in the calcaneus. *(B),* Correction of the equinus is performed by slight distraction followed by rotation around the center of rotation of the ankle. *(C),* For acute corrections through the dome-shaped U-osteotomy, the head of the talus translates proximally in front of the ankle joint. *(D),* The apparatus at the onset of treatment. Note the location of the hinge. The head of the talus is fixed with a wire. There is a wire through the hinges to fix the body of the talus. *(E),* At the end of correction (acute), the head of the talus rides proximally.

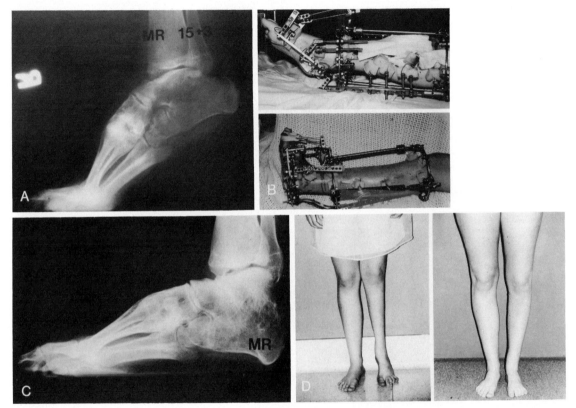

FIGURE 31–18. *(A),* A 15-year-old girl with postclubfoot flat-top talus and 8 cm of discrepancy. There is a subtalar congenital coalition. *(B),* The apparatus at the onset of treatment *(top)* and at the end of the deformity correction *(bottom).* This leg was also lengthened and widened. *(C),* The final radiograph demonstrates a plantigrade foot with restoration of foot height through the U-osteotomy. The correction was performed gradually. *(D),* At the onset of treatment *(left),* note the extremely thin calf and the fixed equinus deformity. At the end of treatment *(right),* note the widening and reshaping of the calf. The foot is now plantigrade. (Courtesy of Dror Paley, M.D.)

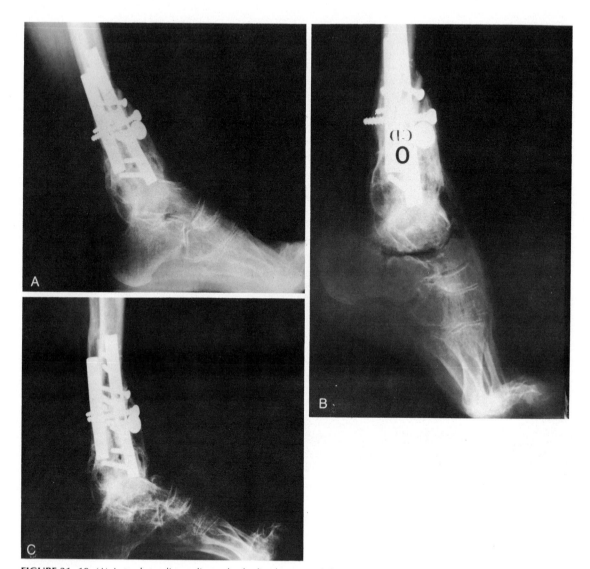

FIGURE 31–19. *(A)*, Lateral standing radiograph of a fixed equinus deformity in a woman with juvenile rheumatoid arthritis and a triangular-top talus. *(B)*, The U-osteotomy. *(C)*, The lateral radiograph after correction, demonstrating the acute correction around a U-osteotomy. Note the step in the neck of the talus. (Courtesy of Dror Paley, M.D.)

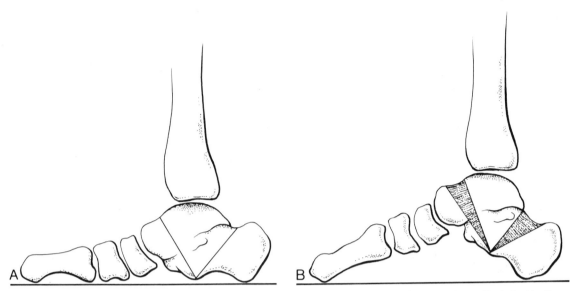

FIGURE 31–20. V-osteotomy. *(A)*, V-osteotomy for rocker-bottom foot. *(B)*, Opening wedge corrections of both the hindfoot and forefoot, recreating the longitudinal arch.

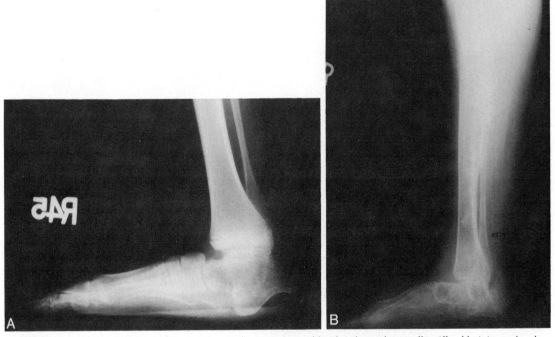

FIGURE 31–21. *(A)*, A rocker-bottom foot deformity in an 11-year-old girl with an abnormally stiff ankle joint and a short hindfoot and forefoot. *(B)*, Both the hindfoot and forefoot deformities were corrected by opening wedges using the V-osteotomy, recreating the longitudinal arch of the foot. (Courtesy of Dror Paley, M.D.)

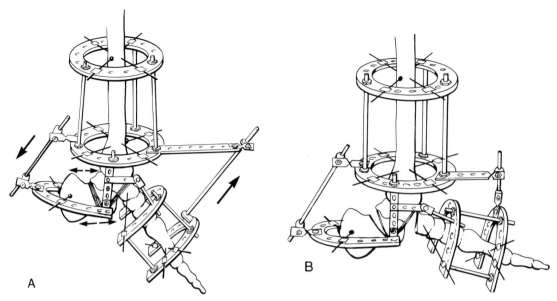

FIGURE 31–22. (A), The apparatus is used for a correction through a V-osteotomy. The deformity is similar to that in Figure 31–23. Note the position of the hinges at the apex of the deformities at the convex end of each osteotomy. (B), The apparatus after distraction of a V-osteotomy.

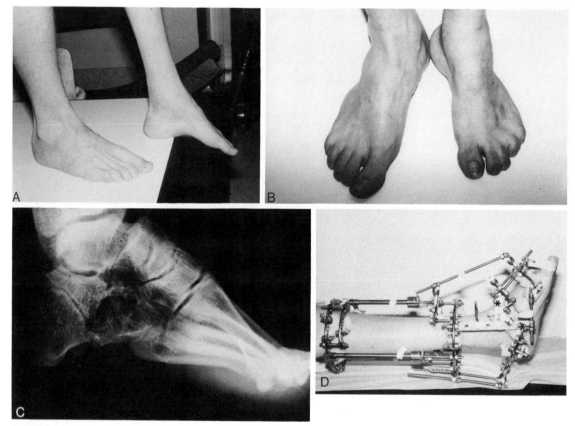

FIGURE 31–23. (A), A 16-year-old boy with residual clubfoot deformity; he has hindfoot equinus and forefoot cavus to different degrees. (B), His foot also has an adductus deformity. (C), The lateral radiograph demonstrates a flat-top talus. A V-osteotomy was performed to correct the hindfoot and forefoot deformities independently. The V-osteotomy can be seen on the radiograph before application of the apparatus. (D), The apparatus is quite complex. The anterior and posterior hinges are marked with asterisks. The tibia was simultaneously lengthened.

498

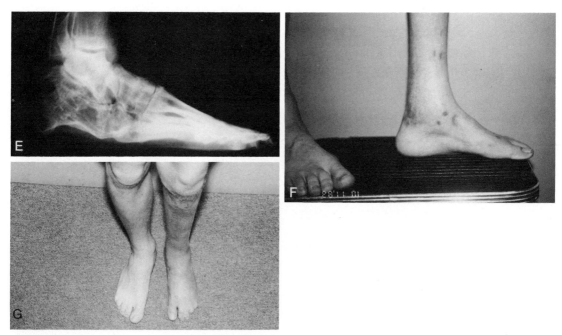

FIGURE 31–23 *Continued (E),* The lateral standing radiograph after distraction demonstrates that the foot is plantigrade. Opening wedges of new bone were generated anteriorly and posteriorly in the talus and calcaneus. *(F),* The foot is plantigrade postoperatively. The normal longitudinal arch is restored, and the equinus deformities of both the hindfoot and forefoot are eliminated. *(G),* The adductus deformity has also been corrected through the talocalcaneal neck portion of the V-osteotomy. (Courtesy of Dror Paley, M.D.)

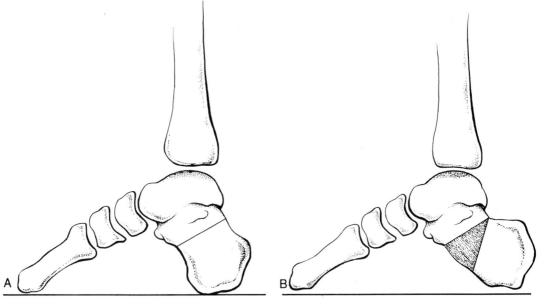

FIGURE 31–24. *(A),* The posterior calcaneal osteotomy is applied to a calcaneal cavus deformity. *(B),* A plantar opening wedge osteotomy is performed for the correction of this deformity. A clinical example is shown in Figure 31–11.

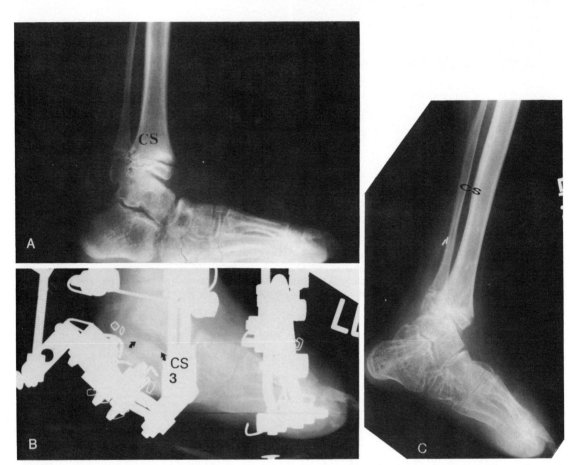

FIGURE 31–25. *(A)*, Lateral radiograph of a 7-year-old girl with a varus rocker-bottom heel secondary to Streeter's syndrome. Her insensate foot was developing an area of breakdown under the prominent rocker-bottom apex. *(B)*, A posterior calcaneal osteotomy was performed with simultaneous tibial lengthening and opening wedge correction of the calcaneal deformity. The calcaneal osteotomy prematurely consolidated due to lack of fixation of the anterior portion of the calcaneus. The path of least resistance was for distraction of the subtalar joint rather than the osteotomy. Note the diastasis of the subtalar joint *(arrows)*. A repeated osteotomy was necessary to complete the treatment. *(C)*, The final lateral radiograph demonstrates a plantigrade appearance to the plantar aspect of the foot. The heel ulcer promptly healed. (Courtesy of Dror Paley, M.D.)

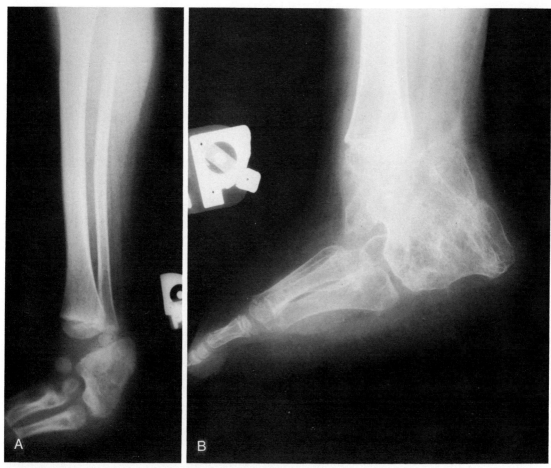

FIGURE 31–26. *(A)*, Congenital deficiency of the calcaneus and supinated forefoot. *(B)*, A posterior calcaneal osteotomy was used to regenerate a heel. The forefoot was demonstrated by distraction alone. (Courtesy of Dror Paley, M.D.)

correction of the hindfoot deformity while soft tissue correction is carried out on the forefoot deformity. Specifically, it is used for varus, valgus, equinus, and calcaneal deformities of the hindfoot, as well as for treating bone defects and deficiencies of the calcaneus.

Talocalcaneal Neck Osteotomies and Midfoot Osteotomies (Figs. 31–27 to 31–30)

The talocalcaneal neck osteotomy[6, 7, 9, 16] is essentially the anterior limb of the V-osteotomy without the posterior calcaneal limb. This is used for the correction of forefoot deformities, including abductus, adductus, cavus, rocker-bottom, supination, and pronation deformities and shortening of the forefoot. The

talocalcaneal neck osteotomy is carried out when the subtalar joint is stiff. When the subtalar joint is mobile, I prefer to use the midfoot osteotomy across the cuboid and navicular or the cuboid and cuneiforms. The cuboid and navicular essentially form one fixed unit and have minimal to no mobility between them. This is therefore a safe plane with large, wide bony surfaces for bone regeneration.

Metatarsal Osteotomies (Fig. 31–31; see also Fig. 31–2)

Metatarsal osteotomies[6] are most commonly used when individual metatarsals are shortened or deformed. Multiple-metatarsal osteotomies are generally not used for lengthening of the foot because of disturbance of the inter-

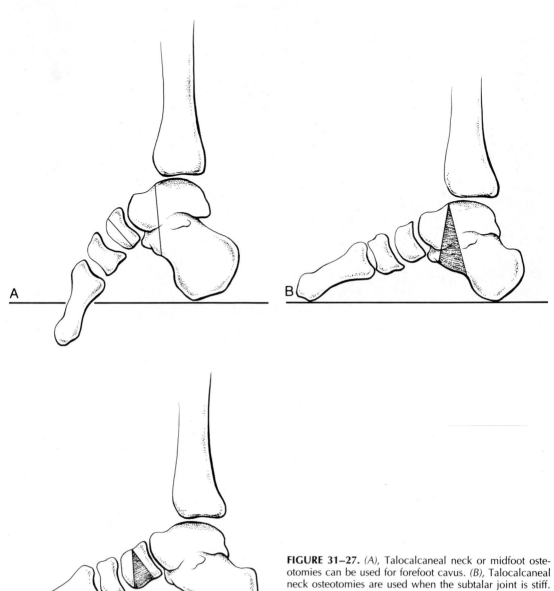

FIGURE 31–27. *(A)*, Talocalcaneal neck or midfoot osteotomies can be used for forefoot cavus. *(B)*, Talocalcaneal
neck osteotomies are used when the subtalar joint is stiff.
(C), Midfoot osteotomies across the navicular and cuboid
or cuboid and cuneiforms are used when the subtalar joint
is mobile.

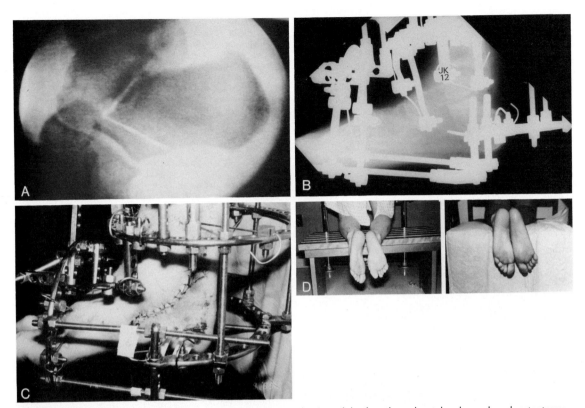

FIGURE 31–28. *(A),* Talocalcaneal neck osteotomy. *(B),* Lengthening of the foot through a talocalcaneal neck osteotomy. Note the regenerated bone between the anterior and posterior portions of the calcaneus. This boy had a ball-and-socket ankle joint and subtalar coalition in addition to a short foot. The foot was lengthened 3 cm. *(C),* He developed a postoperative tarsal tunnel syndrome, which was treated by an emergent release. *(D),* The appearance of the foot before *(left)* and after *(right)* lengthening. Note that the foot length discrepancy has been eliminated. (Courtesy of Dror Paley, M.D.)

ossei and the higher risk of injury to the neurovascular structures. Furthermore, stability and the healing rate are major factors with these bones and are less of a problem with the tarsal bones. Theoretically, there would be a significant risk of metatarsalgia if disruption of the arch were to occur. Therefore, the only indication for multiple-metatarsal lengthening or deformity correction is in cases in which there is a contraindication or significant absence or deficiency of the tarsal bones.

SURGICAL METHODS

Supramalleolar Osteotomy
(see Fig. 31–12)

The preconstructed Ilizarov apparatus consists of proximal and distal blocks of two rings each: one at the proximal tibia and one just proximal to the planned supramalleolar oste-

otomy. The distal block consists of one supramalleolar ring and sometimes of a calcaneal half-ring, in the case of a stiff or fused ankle joint. The two blocks are connected with a hinge. The hinge level is planned according to the level of the apex of the deformity. In true metaphyseal-level deformities, the hinge is proximal to the distal block, whereas in true juxta-articular deformities, the hinge lies at the level of the ankle joint below the ring and acts as a translation hinge. The osteotomy is performed either at the level of the apex of the deformity, if this is possible, or as distal as possible in the supramalleolar region, allowing adequate room for two levels of fixation. A distraction rod is connected to two twisted plates on the concave side. The twisted connections allow for a pivot point at either end of the distraction rod for self-adjustment of its alignment. Lengthening is accomplished by distracting the two hinge rods and the distraction rod.

Text continued on page 508

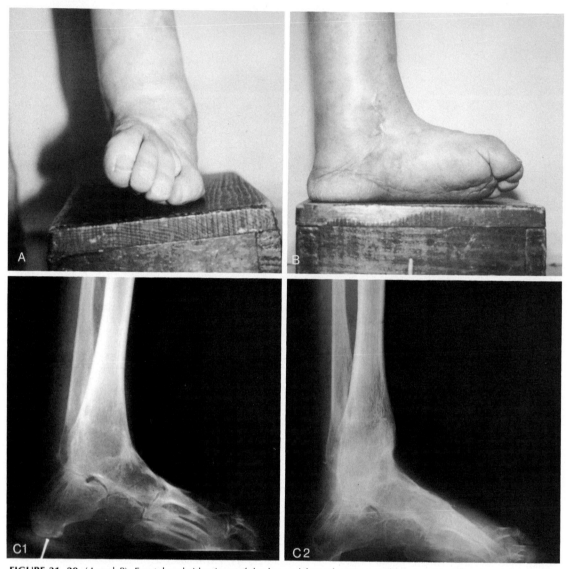

FIGURE 31–29. (*A* and *B*), Frontal and side views of the leg and foot of a 63-year-old man who suffered an injury at the age of 6. He was previously told that nothing could be done to correct the very severe supination deformity of the forefoot and equinovarus malunion of his ankle arthrodesis. *(C1),* Note the anteroposterior forefoot appearance on this lateral preoperative radiograph. *(C2),* At the end of correction, the lateral radiograph appears normal.

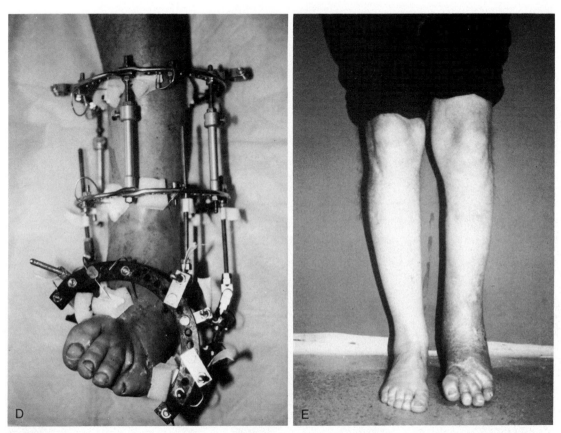

FIGURE 31–29 *Continued (D),* The deformity was corrected through a midfoot osteotomy and a supramalleolar osteotomy in combination. The foot was lengthened and derotated through the forefoot osteotomy, which went across the cuboid and cuneiforms. The equinovarus deformity was corrected and lengthening of 4 cm was achieved through the supramalleolar osteotomy. *(E),* The final clinical appearance of this man's foot, demonstrating the complete correction of the varus and the supination. (Courtesy of Dror Paley, M.D.)

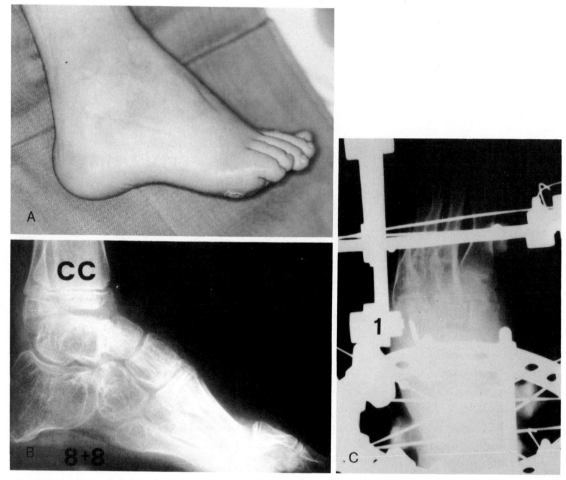

FIGURE 31–30. (*A* and *B*), Preoperative photograph and radiograph demonstrating forefoot cavus secondary to a previously treated clubfoot deformity. (*C*), An osteotomy was performed across the cuboid and cuneiforms. Because of the lack of constraint, the distraction force led to separation of the adjacent joints. The osteotomy never separated.

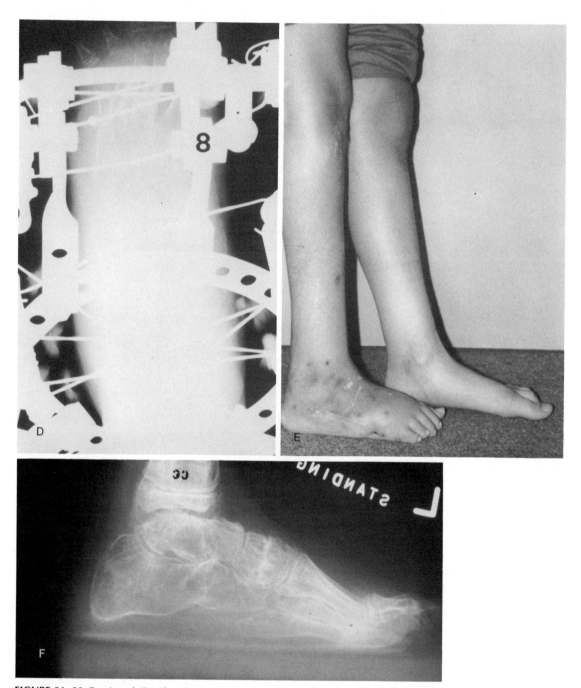

FIGURE 31–30 *Continued (D),* Therefore, one wire on each side of the osteotomy was inserted to concentrate the forces across the osteotomy and to lock the adjacent joints. *(E),* At the end of the correction, the foot is plantigrade and longer. *(F),* Because of the abnormal growth in this foot from previous arthrodeses and surgery, the patient developed a supination deformity of his foot 3 years later. (Courtesy of Dror Paley, M.D.)

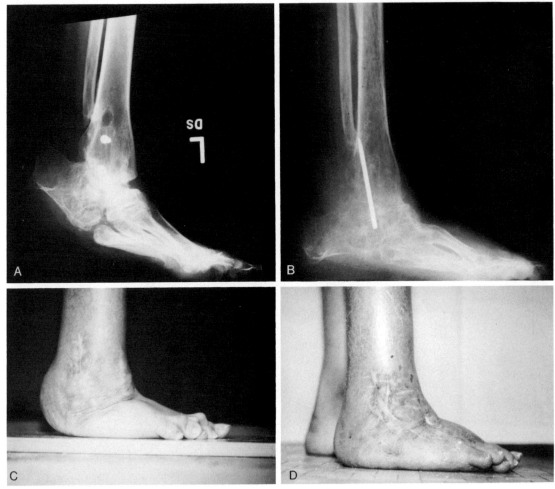

FIGURE 31–31. *(A),* Severe shortening of the foot following talectomy for a clubfoot deformity. Note the equinus deformity of the heel and the painful nonunion of the tibia and navicular. *(B),* The foot was osteotomized across the calcaneus and metatarsals. The nonunion was débrided and compressed. The final radiograph after correction of the foot deformity demonstrates the plantigrade foot with re-establishment of the heel and a longer forefoot. *(C and D),* The appearance of the foot before and after the correction of deformity. This patient also had a simultaneous leg lengthening and widening procedure. (Courtesy of Dror Paley, M.D.)

The corticotomy is performed through two separate incisions. Through a posterolateral incision, the fibula can be cut either by exposing it subperiosteally through a 1- to 2-cm incision or percutaneously using an osteotome. The tibia is cut in a standard corticotomy fashion through a 5-mm anterior tibial crest incision with protection of the medial and lateral periosteum. The osteotomy is completed with a rotational osteoclasis. It is important to ensure that the osteotomy is complete. The osteotomy can be distracted 5 mm to see if it separates. It is easy to mistakenly leave an intact posterior hinge of bone, which would lead to nonseparation of the bone ends.

U-Osteotomy (see Fig. 31–15)

Before the apparatus is applied to the leg, the osteotomy should be performed. Before the osteotomy, a percutaneous Achilles tendon lengthening should be performed for equinus correction. Under tourniquet control, the image intensifier is used to mark the line of the osteotomy on the skin. The anterior half of this line is used for the incision. Care should be taken to identify the sural nerve and to protect it. The peroneal tendons are encountered and can be retracted, or in the case of a rigid foot with no subtalar function and a stiff forefoot, they may be cut. The osteotomy may be performed using a special curved osteotome or gouge. Alternatively, a 1/2-inch osteotome may be used. Before the cut is made, the position of the osteotome is checked with the image intensifier. Intermittent hammering on the osteotome with radiographic checks is performed. The surgeon must be careful to listen and feel as the osteotome penetrates deeper and must use the image intensifier as needed to confirm if it has exited on the medial side. Alternatively, an incision may first be made on the medial side to decompress the tarsal tunnel and a finger may be placed to feel the osteotome exiting on the medial side. The posterior portion of the osteotomy is performed with a curved osteotome. The overlying soft tissues are elevated only with a periosteal elevator around the lateral wall. Care must be taken as the cut is extended medially. This may be performed partially open as a prophylactic measure for the neurovascular structures. The osteotome is twisted 90 degrees to spread the osteotomy apart. This completes the osteotomy. At the end of the procedure, the surgeon should be able to shift the foot from side to side, thus demonstrating that the osteotomy is completely mobile. If the foot does not shift, the osteotomy is probably incomplete. After the osteotomy has been completed, the incision is closed in a standard fashion. Because the incision was carried straight down to bone, there are no soft tissue flaps, which is important in a foot that has had multiple operations.

The apparatus consists of a proximal block of two rings, as described for the supramalleolar osteotomy. This apparatus is modified if a proximal tibial lengthening is to be performed concomitantly. A foot plate is constructed using a half-ring, two plates with threaded extensions, and another half-ring at 90 degrees to these plates. The angular deformity of the foot should be resolved into one plane and, therefore, one hinge.[13] Once this hinge direction has been determined, the foot plate can be connected to the tibial ring with a single hinge. Alternatively, the surgeon can ignore one plane of deformity and correct first the equinus deformity and then the varus deformity. The former method allows simultaneous correction of the equinus and varus deformities through the true oblique plane of the deformity. Fixation to the tibia is accomplished with two wires on each ring, with olives appropriately placed relative to the type of angular

correction. Because the majority of corrections are for equinovarus deformity, an olive wire is required anterolaterally on the tibia. An additional olive wire should be placed posteromedially to permit posterior translation of the foot on the tibia if needed. The foot fixation consists of two wires in the calcaneus, two wires in the metatarsals, and, most importantly, one wire in the head or neck of the talus distal to the osteotomy. One wire is needed in the body of the talus, and one wire is needed in the floating fragment of calcaneus. If these bone segments are not transfixed on distraction, the joints (subtalar, talonavicular, and tibiotalar) will separate instead of the osteotomy. To ensure that the path of least resistance is through the osteotomy and not through the joints, the joints must be locked with these wires.

V-Osteotomy (see Fig. 31–18)

As in the U-osteotomy, the first step is to perform the osteotomy before application of the apparatus. For equinus heel corrections, a percutaneous Achilles tendon lengthening is performed. In a fashion similar to that used for the U-osteotomy, the image intensifier is used to mark the osteotomy line on the skin. The osteotomy parallels the anterior cut more than the posterior cut. An Ollier-type incision is generally used. The anterior cut is performed across the calcaneus, the sinus tarsi, and the talar neck. The posterior cut is performed so as to meet with the anterior cut on the plantar surface of the calcaneus. The surgeon may elect to prophylactically decompress the posterior tibial nerve and feel for the osteotome as it exits medially. The osteotome is twisted to complete the osteotomies and spread the osteotomy surfaces apart. A radiograph is obtained at the completion of the osteotomy and before application of the hardware. A temporary Kirschner wire can be inserted into the calcaneus to decrease the bleeding. The apparatus is then applied, with the hinges centered in the right places. It is usually very crowded around the foot and very difficult to connect all the wires and hinges because of the tight spaces. The V-osteotomy requires the maximum in apparatus efficiency to allow for fixation and hinge placement.

The proximal block of fixation on the tibia is prepared in a manner similar to that described for the U-osteotomy. Hinges are used between a posterior half-ring, which is connected to the calcaneus, and an anterior half-ring for the forefoot. The forefoot may have a second half-ring over the midfoot. Alternatively, the second level of fixation for the forefoot can be off posts. The hinges are placed relative to the apex of deformity posteriorly and anteriorly. Two transverse wires and one axial half-wire are used in the calcaneus for fixation. Two metatarsal wires and one talar neck wire are used for fixation in the forefoot. The body of the talus and the floating fragment of calcaneus must be transfixed to the tibial ring.

Other Osteotomies

The posterior calcaneal and talocalcaneal neck osteotomies, when used alone, are performed as described for each limb of the V-osteotomy.

The midfoot osteotomy may be performed through one dorsal incision or through one medial incision and one lateral incision. Care must be taken to follow the arch of the foot so as not to exit on the plantar side and risk injuring the neurovascular structures. A subperiosteal elevator may be inserted dorsally and on the plantar aspect of the foot to protect the osteotome. The construct is similar to that used with the talocalcaneal neck osteotomy. One technical pearl is to insert one wire on either side of the osteotomy to lock the talonavicular and calcaneocuboid joints and the midfoot tarsometatarsal joints. If this is not done, distraction will occur through the adjacent joints rather than through the osteotomy. Joints, rather than osteotomies, are usually the paths of least resistance to distraction.

RESULTS

Grill and Franke reported on 10 clubfoot deformities in patients ranging from 8 to 15 years of age.[3] The etiologies included neglected or relapsed congenital clubfoot, post-traumatic equinovarus deformity, arthrogryposis, spastic diplegia, and Charcot-Marie-Tooth disease. All of the feet were stiff preoperatively. All were treated by the nonosteotomy distraction technique of Ilizarov. A plantigrade foot was

achieved in all patients, with satisfactory radiographic and clinical results. All of the feet had subtalar stiffness pre- and postoperatively, and the average range of movement at the ankle was 20 degrees. The complications were mostly minor ones, such as pin track infections. One patient required a tendon lengthening for clawtoe. Another patient with an arthrogrypotic foot had a relapse because of the lack of postoperative immobilization. The treatment was repeated, and a good result was achieved. All patients were satisfied with their results and were for the first time able to wear normal shoes. The period of distraction ranged from 4 to 10 weeks. The device was then maintained in place for an additional 8 to 10 weeks, after which patients were put into below-knee plaster casts for 3 to 4 months. The mean time to follow-up in this study was 3.3 years (range, 6 months to 6 years).

I reported the results of osteotomy treatment in 23 patients with 25 severely deformed feet who were treated with Ilizarov distraction osteotomies.[15] Nineteen of the 25 feet had had multiple operations for recalcitrant leg and foot deformities. Pre-existing foot stiffness was present in all cases. There were 10 males and 13 females. The patients' ages ranged from 6 to 63 years, with a mean age of 25 years. A wide range of foot deformities of different etiologies were treated. The corrective osteotomies included 13 supramalleolar osteotomies, two U-osteotomies, two V-osteotomies, two talocalcaneal neck osteotomies, five posterior calcaneal osteotomies, two midfoot osteotomies, and one panmetatarsal osteotomy. The treatment included lengthening of the leg in 20 of the limb segments. Lengthening of the foot was carried out in five cases. Other associated treatments included leg widening for cosmesis in seven cases, distraction of forefoot deformities in four cases, and tibial or femoral mechanical axis realignment (or both) in three cases.

The mean treatment time was 6.4 months (range, 3 to 11.3 months). In most cases, the treatment time was dependent on the consolidation of the tibial limb lengthening segment rather than on the foot osteotomy. All but seven patients experienced one or more minor to major complications (20 complications in 18 feet). Pin track infection of a superficial nature occurred in at least one pin in every patient at some time during their treatment. This rarely caused problems and was easily treated by local measures and oral antibiotics. Three patients had deep soft tissue infections of their pin sites, requiring pin removal and operative intervention for wire insertion or débridement. One patient developed osteomyelitis and septic arthritis of the fifth metatarsophalangeal joint after a pin cut out of the metatarsal shaft into the joint. This required two serial débridements and healed uneventfully. This patient simultaneously developed an abscess on the lateral wall of the calcaneus in a pin track. Débridement and the use of antibiotics led to complete resolution of both infections.

The next most common problem was failure of separation of the osteotomy. This occurred in nine cases. The cause was incomplete surgical osteotomy in three cases and premature consolidation due to an incorrect mechanical construct in six cases. The typical example that led to an incorrect construct was lack of one of the locking wires. The distraction led to diastasis of the adjacent joint instead of the osteotomy.

Acute tarsal tunnel syndrome developed within 24 hours of the surgery in two patients. In one, it was discovered in the recovery room. The patient was immediately returned to the operating room, and the tarsal tunnel was decompressed. The patient reawoke with completely normal sensation. The second case of tarsal tunnel syndrome did not develop until the first postoperative day and was treated by immediate decompression. Full recovery of neuromuscular function occurred over the next 3 months. In both cases, there was edema but no hemorrhage in the tarsal tunnel.

Toe contractures were common, especially with corrections of equinus and cavus deformities and with foot lengthenings. Most toe contractures resolved, with the exception of three cases. Two of these were treated with percutaneous release during or at the end of treatment. In one case, the patient refused further treatment, although he remained symptomatic with clawed toes. This patient was the one whose tarsal tunnel syndrome took 3 months to resolve. Possibly an element of neuromuscular dysfunction contributed to the toe clawing, in addition to the abnormal muscle tension of the foot lengthening. Prophylaxis of toe contractures is carried out with toe slings and elastic bands. More recently, I have been using a 1-mm wire inserted across the base of the distal phalanx and connected to the apparatus to prevent contracture of the toes. Since

I started using this method, I have not had any further difficulty with toe contractures during foot lengthening.

There were several wire problems not related to pin track infections. In one patient, the wires began to cut out of the heel, and insertion of an additional wire was required. In another patient, several wires broke at different times. This patient was paraparetic and had an anesthetic foot. Because the usual instructions are for weight bearing as tolerated to and including full weight bearing, this patient literally walked full weight bearing without support throughout the treatment. This led to repeated wire fractures. Fortunately, reinsertion of wires was facilitated by his anesthetic leg and foot and did not require a return to the operating room.

One patient with a supramalleolar lengthening and deformity correction developed a buckle fracture due to premature removal of the apparatus. Because the treatment was bilateral and the buckle fracture occurred on only one side, this patient was left with a 1.5-cm leg length discrepancy.

One patient with multiple osteochondromas developed a nerve injury due to the proximal tibial osteotomy. The distal tibial supramalleolar osteotomy did not lead to any complications. Fortunately, the nerve injury resolved.

There was one case of skin breakdown from a talocalcaneal neck re-osteotomy following a premature consolidation. This healed uneventfully after the wound was left open.

None of the previously mentioned complications, with the exception of the one persistent toe contracture and the minor leg length discrepancy, led to any permanent residual effect on the patient, and although they complicated the treatment, they did not obstruct the treatment goals. In total, 19 secondary surgical procedures were carried out in 13 patients to treat problems and complications that arose secondary to the foot deformity correction, and two additional secondary procedures were carried out to treat complications of the proximal tibial osteotomy.

At the time of fixator removal, 24 feet were plantigrade. At follow-up, only 22 feet were plantigrade. One foot was not plantigrade at the time of fixator removal; this problem was due to an unrecognized varus deformity (5 degrees) of the heel. The leg length discrepancy and midfoot cavus were treated successfully; only the untreated varus remained. A supramalleolar osteotomy through the ankle arthrodesis malunion was performed to correct the varus. There was one recurrent deformity due to an unrecognized ball-and-socket ankle joint. This patient had a preoperative post-traumatic ball-and-socket ankle joint with a varus heel deformity, which was treated by a posterior calcaneal osteotomy. With valgus distraction, the deformity corrected by eversion of the unconstrained ball-and-socket ankle joint instead of by the opening of a wedge in the calcaneal osteotomy. This could have been avoided by the use of wires in the talus. This patient will require a second osteotomy.

These two patients were considered to have unsatisfactory results despite the significant improvement in pain and gait in both because of persistent foot deformity at follow-up. Both had successful elimination of length discrepancy and leg deformity. Finally, one boy who was treated successfully for postclubfoot cavus developed a mild supination of the forefoot due to previous arthrodeses of the foot. This secondary deformity was unrelated to the distraction treatment, and the result was graded as satisfactory.

Pain was a preoperative complaint in only eight patients. Postoperatively, three patients complained of pain: the patient with a partial recurrence of deformity complained of pain; one patient with successful resolution of equinovarus complained of arch pain; and one patient with a rocker-bottom deformity complained of ankle pain.

Gait was improved in all patients. The patient with a stiff rocker-bottom foot (mentioned earlier) complained of a stiff foot gait at follow-up. This patient had insisted on a foot lengthening in addition to the deformity correction. The final result was feet of equal length and a stiff plantigrade foot with a longer platform to step over. Although a plantigrade foot was achieved, her flatter, longer forefoot applied more stress to her abnormal ankle than was applied preoperatively, resulting in pain. The result was therefore graded as unsatisfactory despite her successful foot deformity correction and 9 cm of lengthening. In total, there were 21 satisfactory (84 percent) and four unsatisfactory (16 percent) results at the time of follow-up. It should be noted that foot stiffness was difficult to assess in this group of patients because the majority had had significantly stiff feet before correction (19 of 25 feet). Pre-existing ankle, subtalar, and midfoot range of motion was preserved when it was present preoperatively; however, toe motion was decreased in two patients who had foot lengthening. Radiologic loss of joint space was noted in the midfoot joints of two asymptomatic patients. Its significance remains unclear.

DISCUSSION

The Ilizarov method is well known for its limb lengthening and correction of long-bone deformities. The correction of complex foot deformities using specialized distraction osteotomies is less well recognized.[12, 13, 14] Conventional treatment of complex foot deformities has many limitations. First and foremost is the limitation imposed by the presence of neurovascular structures, which are acutely placed on stretch. The exposure needed places important collaterals at risk in an already compromised circulation. Re-exploration and osteotomy of these feet is therefore fraught with complications and is a high-risk procedure. The second limitation is that of length. Conventional osteotomies need to sacrifice foot and leg length to achieve correction of significant angular deformities. This further shortens an already short leg or foot. Conventional osteotomies often resect, arthrodese, or cross normal foot joints.[4, 10] This further stiffens an already stiff foot.

The Ilizarov method offers the advantages of being minimally invasive and using minimal dissection; therefore, it carries a decreased risk of neurovascular and soft tissue injury and infection. This is particularly advantageous in the foot that has had multiple operations. The Ilizarov method is also not limited by the magnitude of the deformity, and it relies on bone regeneration rather than bone resection. Therefore, there is no need to shorten the leg or foot. Correction can be performed either through the bone, joint, or arthrodesis. The choice of method depends on the location and type of deformity. The Ilizarov method allows a comprehensive approach to foot deformity correction by treating not only the foot deformity but also the associated tibial deformities, length discrepancies, and even thin calves. Foot lengthening, although it is rarely indicated, can be combined with some of the foot osteotomies.[6, 7, 16] Because no length is sacrificed in deformity correction, a significant amount of foot length is regained simply by deformity correction with an opening wedge technique. Although conventional surgery relies on three-dimensional methods that must be accomplished within the time frame of the operation, the Ilizarov technique is four dimensional because time is one of the variables that can be adjusted. The manipulation of the three-dimensional deformity in time, therefore, provides a safer method of foot deformity correction in many instances.

The disadvantages of the Ilizarov technique are obviously those of an external fixation device and in particular those of pin site problems. In addition, the Ilizarov method requires a lengthy treatment time with prolonged joint immobilization and is frequently associated with mild to moderate pain during the distraction period.

Functional loading, including full weight bearing as tolerated, is permitted during treatment. This helps counteract the prolonged joint immobilization. The patients reported on in both my[15] and Grill and Franke's[3] series had some of the most difficult and complex foot deformities that present to the orthopaedic surgeon. Whereas complex problems demand complex solutions, simple problems demand more simple solutions. Therefore, for more simple foot deformities, conventional methods may be preferable. Nevertheless, even for simple foot deformities, the Ilizarov solution offers the advantage of minimal invasiveness.

Furthermore, the Ilizarov method offers one major advantage over standard conventional treatments in that it is adjustable even after an acute correction is performed. Achieving a perfectly plantigrade foot in the operating room is not a simple task, whether with an osteotomy or an arthrodesis. With the circular external fixator, the desired correction can be obtained either rapidly in the operating room, or gradually postoperatively, and the surgeon can ensure that the patient is comfortable with the foot position before accepting it as the final position. With greater adjustability, there is little excuse for not achieving an absolutely plantigrade foot that the patient is happy with.

Despite all these advantages, the main limitation of this technique is still the foot with which one starts. A stiff equinovarus foot that is corrected into a plantigrade position becomes a stiff plantigrade foot. Frequently, patients' expectations do not take this into consideration, and patients may be disappointed

that their foot, which is now aesthetically more pleasing and functionally plantigrade, does not perform like a normal foot. Therefore, before the treatment of any complex foot deformity is started, it is important to convey to the patient a realistic sense of what the foot deformity correction will accomplish, what the foot will be like in the corrected position, and what its limitations will be. Careful attention to the indications for treatment and an appropriate choice of construct and osteotomy are essential. Compared with the application of the Ilizarov method to other limb segments, the application to the foot has a much steeper learning curve. Application to the foot should probably be undertaken only by surgeons who have experience with this method on long bones. When properly planned and applied, this method, although associated with frequent complications, can still accomplish the goals of treatment in almost all cases.[14]

References

1. Carroll N: Clubfoot. *In* Morrissey R (Ed): Lovell and Winter's Pediatric Orthopedics, 3rd Ed. Philadelphia, JB Lippincott, 1990, pp 927–956.
2. Grant AD, Atar D, Lehman WB: Ilizarov technique in correction of foot deformities: A preliminary report. Foot Ankle 11:1–5, 1990.
3. Grill F, Franke J: The Ilizarov distractor for the correction of relapsed or neglected clubfoot. J Bone Joint Surg. 69B:593–597, 1987.
4. Herold HZ, Torok G: Surgical correction of neglected clubfoot in the older child and adult. J Bone Joint Surg 55A:1385–1395, 1973.
5. Ilizarov GA, Shevtsov VI, Kuzmin NV: Results of treatment of equinus foot deformity. Ortop Travmatol Protez 5:46–48, 1983.
6. Ilizarov GA, Shevtsov VI, Kalyakina VI, Okutov GV: Foot form shaping and lengthening methods. Ortop Travmatol Protez 1:49–51, 1983.
7. Ilizarov GA, Shevtsov VI, Shestakov VA, Kuzmin NV: The Treatment of Foot Deformities in Adults by the Ilizarov Transosseous Osteosynthesis. Methodological Recommendation Book. Kurgan, Russia: Kurgan Internal Publication, 1987.
8. Istomina IS, Kuzmin VI: Treatment of equino-excavato-varus deformation of the foot in adults with a hinge distraction apparatus. Ortop Travmatol Protez 3:19–22, 1990.
9. Kovalev YV, Gorlov GA: Bone and musculotendinous surgery for treatment of recurrent and residual congenital clubfoot. Ortop Travmatol Protez 7:37–40, 1986.
10. Lambrinudi C: New operations on drop foot. J Bone Joint Surg 15:193–200, 1927.
11. Lehman WB, Paley D, Atar D: Operating Room Guide to Cross Sectional Anatomy of the Extremities and Pelvis. New York, Raven Press, 1989.

12. Paley D: Current techniques of limb lengthening. J Pediatr Orthop 8:73–92, 1988.
13. Paley D: The Principles of Deformity Correction by the Ilizarov Technique. Technical Aspects. Tech Orthop 4:15–29, 1989.
14. Paley D: Problems, obstacles, and complications of limb lengthening by the Ilizarov technique. Clin Orthop 250:81–104, 1990.
15. Paley D: The correction of complex foot deformities using Ilizarov's distraction osteotomies. Clin Orthop 1993, in press.
16. Rojkov AV, Startzev TE, Batenkova GI, et al: Methodology of reconstruction of short foot stumps with the help of distraction methods. Ortop Travmatol Protez 5:48–52, 1983.
17. Umhanov HA: Method of apparatus correction in orthopedic treatment of children with the cerebral spastic palsies.
18. Zavialov PV, Stabskaya EA: Treatment of the congenital clubfoot by the distraction-compression method. Ortop Travmatol Protez 2:41–44, 1978.

32

Tendon, Vascular, Nerve, and Skin Injuries

MICHAEL D. ROOKS

The intern suffers not only from inexperience, but also from over-experience. He has in his short term of service responsibilities which are too great for him; he becomes accustomed to act without preparation and he acquires a confidence in himself and a self-complacency which may be useful in times of emergency, but which tend to blind him to his inadequacy and to warp his career.

William Stewart Halsted*
(1852–1922)

TRAUMATIC TENDON INJURIES OF THE FOOT AND ANKLE

Tendon injuries involving the foot and ankle commonly occur through one of three general mechanisms. The most common cause by far is related to overuse syndromes in competitive and recreational athletes. Most of these present as tendinitides and usually respond to conservative measures. Ruptures can also be associated with unusual forces or, more commonly, with chronic attrition. Direct lacerations of tendons can occur secondary to injuries with sharp objects. This occurs in particular with stepping on or dropping glass. Avulsions and lacerations of tendons can also

---

*From Halsted WS: Bull Johns Hopkins Hosp 15:267, 1904.

occur with major forces such as falls from heights, motor vehicle accidents, industrial machinery injuries, and lawn mower injuries.

Approximately 17 percent of competitive athletic exertion injuries involve the ankle, foot, or heel.[171] A similar figure, 24 percent, is seen in recreational athletes.[170] Fifty-two percent of these injuries are incurred during track-and-field activities, and another 17 percent occur during playing of ball sports.[171] The vast majority of these injuries are tendinitides and will respond to conservative measures, as discussed in Part V of this book. Tendon dislocations, ruptures, or both commonly involve the tendo Achillis, tibialis posterior, peroneus longus, or flexor hallucis longus. These injuries are discussed in a later section.

Compared with the voluminous literature on lacerations of the hand and wrist, the literature on foot and ankle tendon lacerations is quite limited. This problem is further compounded by conflicting recommendations for treatment of these injuries. These injuries commonly occur after stepping on or kicking sharp objects, particularly glass, or after dropping the same type of objects on the foot. Up to 50 percent of these injuries are seen in children.[51, 244] Sixteen to 30 percent of these lacerations occur at or above the ankle, approximately 8 percent occur at the midfoot, and approximately 75 percent occur in the

515

forefoot.[51, 244] Fifty[244] to 70[51] percent of these injuries involve the flexor tendons. Multiple tendons are involved in 12 to 44 percent of these injuries.[51, 244]

Lacerations and avulsions of tendons can occur with more violent injuries to the foot, such as those incurred in motor vehicle accidents, falls, lawn mower accidents, and industrial accidents. These injuries tend to involve an older group and show a predominance for the extensor tendons, compared with lacerations caused by sharp objects. Fifty-eight percent of these injuries may have associated bone, joint, or nerve injuries, compared with only 14 percent of lacerations caused by sharp objects.[51]

Flexor Hallucis Longus

Diagnosis of flexor hallucis longus (FHL) lacerations or avulsions generally does not present a dilemma as long as an examination for the injury is undertaken. The absence or weakness of interphalangeal flexion of the great toe is presumptive evidence of injury. Associated injuries to the plantar digital nerves, the terminal branch of the saphenous nerve, or the flexor hallucis brevis should also be defined.

Review of the Literature

Griffiths reported on 19 patients with tendon injuries about the ankle.[66] He reported satisfactory results in 11 of the 19 patients who underwent early repair. Although none of his patients suffered flexor tendon injuries, he recommended repair of all tendon injuries except those of the extensor hallucis longus.

Frenette and Jackson reported on 10 cases of FHL lacerations involving young athletes.[53] Six of the injuries had primary repair, and three were not repaired. All patients returned to athletics, but one of the patients who did not undergo repair later developed a hyperextension deformity of the great toe interphalangeal joint, necessitating arthrodesis. The authors recommended primary repair of FHL lacerations.

Floyd and colleagues reported 13 FHL lacerations.[51] Ten had primary repair, two had secondary repair, and one was not repaired. Three of the 12 "repaired tendons" ruptured after discontinuance of cast immobilization, one at 4 weeks and two at 6 weeks. The nine cases of successful repair all went on to have good results. The nonrepaired tendon and the three ruptured tendons all had fair results. Floyd and colleagues located five FHL lacerations that were not repaired through a review of the literature. In this group, only three of the five nonrepaired tendons went on to have good results. These authors also recommended early repair of FHL lacerations (Fig. 32–1).

Krackow reported a single case of traumatic FHL rupture in a 34-year-old man.[112] This patient was treated with surgical repair, and an "excellent result" was obtained. Sammarco and Miller reported partial ruptures in two dancers that responded well to retinacular release for associated tendinitis.[197]

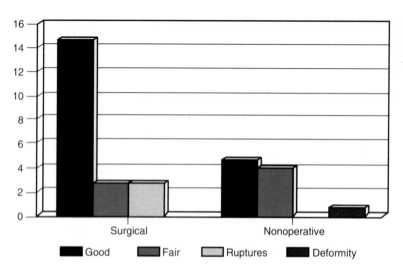

FIGURE 32–1. Treatment results for 27 cases of flexor hallucis longus disruption. (Data from references 51, 58, 66, and 112.)

Author's Preferred Treatment

The chance of producing a good result without repair of the FHL tendon when it is lacerated is approximately 50 percent (four good results and four fair results were obtained, based on the review of the literature). There is also a risk of developing a great toe interphalangeal hyperextension deformity. Surgical repair, if successful, can be expected to produce good results almost 100 percent of the time (in 16 of 16 cases, based on the review of the literature). The risk of producing a painful scar on the sole of the foot with tendon repair is reported to be approximately 20 percent[51] although this complication has not specifically been related to FHL repair. Primary or delayed primary repair of an FHL tendon in a satisfactory wound environment is thus recommended whenever practical. There is a 25-percent risk of subacute FHL rupture after repair (three of 12 cases in the review of the literature). The repair should use a grasping suture technique (Kessler-type or Bunnell) with 3–0 permanent suture material (Fig. 32–2). Migration of the proximal tendon stump in forefoot lacerations is prevented by interconnections between the FHL and flexor digitorum longus in the midfoot, making a second, more proximal, incision rarely necessary. If possible, the foot should be immobilized for 8 weeks in a short-leg cast in a protective position. If the consequences of repair rupture are consequential (e.g., in a competitive athlete), immobilization for 8 weeks with gradual resumption of unlimited activity over 3 to 4 weeks should be advised. A rocker sole or non–weight-bearing should be used to prevent terminal toe-off.

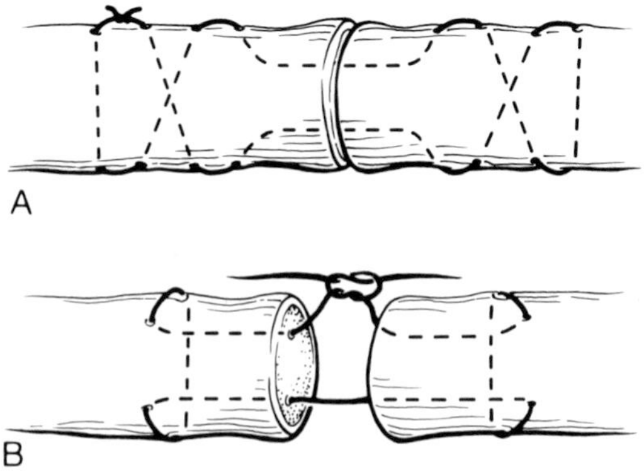

FIGURE 32–2. The Bunnell *(A)* and modified Kessler *(B)* sutures.

Extensor Hallucis Longus

As with diagnosis of FHL injuries, diagnosis of extensor hallucis longus (EHL) injuries should present little difficulty. The EHL tendon is palpable over the forefoot with great toe extension. Inability to palpate the tendon in the forefoot on attempted great toe extension with weakness of great toe interphalangeal extension is diagnostic of injury. Structures at risk for associated injury include the terminal branches of the saphenous, superficial peroneal, or deep peroneal nerves; the dorsalis pedis artery; the extensor hallucis brevis tendon; and the great toe metatarsophalangeal and interphalangeal joints.

Review of the Literature

As noted previously, Griffiths reported on 19 patients with tendon injuries about the ankle.[66] Eight of the 19 patients did not have repair. Included in this group were three peroneal tendon lacerations, two tibialis posterior lacerations, one EHL laceration, and one extensor digitorum longus laceration. Both the EHL and the extensor digitorum longus injuries had satisfactory results without repair, and Griffiths deemed EHL repair unnecessary. (The five EHL and the three extensor digitorum longus tendons that were repaired also did satisfactorily.) This single case has been the source for the common statement that EHL lacerations do not require repair.

Floyd and colleagues reported 13 EHL lacerations in 1983.[51] Eleven underwent primary repair, one underwent secondary repair, and one was not repaired. Two of the 12 repairs ruptured. There were seven good, six fair, and no poor results. None of the fair results were directly related to failed repair or lack of repair. Five of the six fair results were secondary to painful scars, and the sixth was associated with an open joint and subsequent stiffness. Floyd and colleagues recommended early EHL tendon repair (Fig. 32–3). Sim and Deweerd[212] and Langenberg[118] reported on two spontaneous EHL ruptures.

Author's Preferred Treatment

The potential for spontaneous repair of extensor injuries of the foot is generally conceded and is acknowledged by Floyd and colleagues.[51] The real potential for developing a

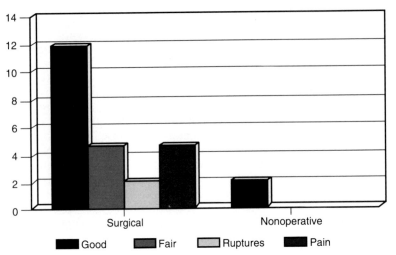

FIGURE 32–3. Treatment results for 19 cases of extensor hallucis longus disruption. (Data from references 51 and 66.)

Legend: ■ Good   ■ Fair   ☐ Ruptures   ■ Pain

painful scar (38 percent[51]) must be weighed against the theoretical advantages of surgical repair. If the tendon of the EHL can be repaired without extension of the wound or with minimal extension, I favor this approach. I would counsel against surgically doubling the wound size to realize EHL repair. Short-leg cast immobilization in a protected position should be employed in either event to minimize the risk of great toe extensor weakness. The immobilization span should be at least 6 weeks, and discontinuance of immobilization should be determined by the propensity for extensor lag rather than based on any rigid time interval (e.g., 6 weeks). If surgical repair is undertaken, attention should also be directed toward lacerated nerves. If possible, they should be repaired. If a lacerated nerve cannot be repaired, it should be dissected proximally to remove the neuroma from the superficial scar region.

(*Editor's note:* I prefer primary or delayed repair of the EHL from my experience as a reconstructive surgeon. Many patients with EHL lag or dysfunction complain of frequent toe stubbing or dragging. Late reconstruction is more problematic. I use either the grasping suture or a locking horizontal mattress stitch with the author's postoperative management. I fully concur with the author's emphasis on looking for adjacent injuries, particularly of the sensory nerves, which he noted.)

Flexor Digitorum Longus

Diagnosis of flexor digitorum longus (FDL) lacerations can present more difficulty than

anticipated. Most patients have very poor individual control of the lesser toes and a limited arc of distal interphalangeal motion. Diagnosis can usually be confirmed by holding the distal interphalangeal joint in full hyperextension and asking the patient to flex ("pull") all of his or her toes down (Fig. 32–4). Associated injuries include those of the flexor digitorum brevis and the digital neurovascular bundles.

Review of the Literature

The literature contains little information on FDL lacerations. Griffiths advocated repair of FDL lacerations but offered no specific data.[66] Similarly, Wicks and colleagues recommended early repair.[244] They noted symptomatic hyperextension deformities of the metatarsophalangeal joints in two of eight cases of FDL

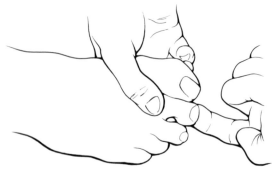

FIGURE 32–4. Intact function in the flexor digitorum longus or flexor hallucis longus tendon can be determined by stabilizing the more proximal joints and asking the patient to flex the tip of the toe against resistance.

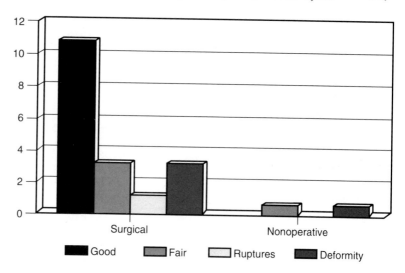

FIGURE 32–5. Treatment results for 15 cases of flexor digitorum longus disruption. (Data from references 51 and 244.)

repair. Floyd and colleagues reported on seven patients with 10 FDL lacerations.[51] Six of the seven underwent repair. One patient suffered a repair rupture. The patient with the ruptured repair and the patient with the nonrepaired FDL each developed a fair result because of asymptomatic but mild proximal interphalangeal joint hyperextension. Fifteen percent of the plantar wounds had unsuspected nerve or tendon lacerations at exploration (Fig. 32–5).

Author's Preferred Treatment

The loss of long toe flexor function after a plantar laceration implies a deep wound to the plantar foot. There is a 15-percent incidence of associated injuries and a real possibility of late foot deformity. The chances of producing a painful plantar scar (20 percent in the series of Floyd and colleagues[51]) should be appreciated. A formal wound débridement and exploration procedure is indicated in these injuries. Although the necessity for repair of FDL lacerations is far from proven, I recommend repair, when it can easily be achieved, following the guidelines set forth for flexor hallucis longus lacerations. My concerns over the loss of minor toe flexor strength and young patients' complaints about this motivate me more than the proximal interphalangeal joint hyperextension. Associated digital nerve injuries should be repaired to prevent neuroma formation on a weight-bearing surface.

Extensor Digitorum Longus

Diagnosis of extensor digitorum longus (EDL) lacerations is similar to that of extensor

hallucis longus lacerations. Inability to palpate the tendon in the forefoot and weakness of metatarsophalangeal extension are diagnostic. Injuries to the extensor digitorum brevis, the superficial peroneal or sural nerve, or the dorsal arterial arch should be ruled out.

Review of the Literature

Akhtar and Levine reported the only case of EDL dislocation of which I am aware.[3] They recommended surgical repair for symptomatic complaints. As noted earlier, Griffiths reported satisfactory results in a single extensor hallucis longus laceration and a single EDL laceration, each of which was treated without repair.[66] He implied that surgical repair of extensor tendons was not essential to a satisfactory result. This recommendation was contested by Lipscomb and Kelly 4 years later.[131] They reported 11 of 13 fair to good results with surgical repair of extensor tendon lacerations of the distal leg and ankle. Lipscomb and Kelly recommended surgical repair of these injuries.

Floyd and colleagues had eight cases of EDL injury in their series.[51] Seven cases were treated by primary surgical repair, and a single injury was treated without repair. There were three good, four fair, and one poor result. The poor result was in the single patient who did not have repair. This patient was a 57-year-old man who developed symptomatic progressive clawing in the fourth and fifth toes adjacent to the nonrepaired tendons within 5 years. The investigators also noted that scar complaints were more common after dorsal wounds than after plantar wounds. Sixty per-

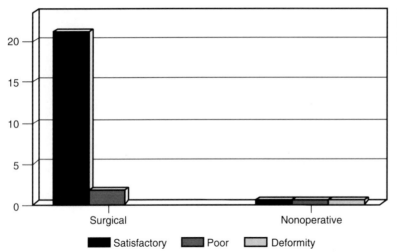

FIGURE 32–6. Treatment results for 26 cases of extensor digitorum longus disruption. (Data from references 51, 66, and 244.)

■ Satisfactory   ■ Poor   □ Deformity

cent of their dorsal wounds (six of 10) had scar complaints, compared with 20 percent of the plantar wounds (three of 15). Floyd and colleagues recommended surgical repair of EDL lacerations. This recommendation was echoed by Wicks and colleagues,[244] who treated four EDL lacerations surgically (Fig. 32–6).

Author's Preferred Treatment

My feelings regarding EDL repairs are similar to those regarding repair of extensor hallucis longus injuries. I believe that these wounds can be successfully treated by closed means and cast immobilization for 6 to 8 weeks. Lack of treatment can be expected to lead to a tendon imbalance in the toes. This may lead to patient complaints of toe "catching," particularly that the toes tend to roll up when patients are putting on hose or sliding into a shoe. I advise surgical repair if it can be accomplished with minimal extension of the wound, especially in children. Whether or not the tendon is repaired, I believe cast immobilization for 6 to 8 weeks is indicated. I advise careful attention to associated nerve injuries, as noted previously for extensor hallucis longus lacerations.

Intrinsic Muscles of the Foot

Isolated injuries to the intrinsic muscles of the foot, particularly the extensor and flexor digitorum brevis muscles, can present a diagnostic dilemma. As noted earlier, the flexor digitorum brevis, although possessing separate muscle bellies, lacks the individual actions demonstrated by the flexor digitorum sublimis of the hand. Interphalangeal flexion contractures associated with adult clawtoe deformities can only worsen this problem. Weakness of flexion in one toe relative to another or the presence of an associated flexor digitorum longus laceration may be the only clue to this injury. The same problem exists with the extensor digitorum brevis. Most individuals also have difficulty with abduction of the great and lesser toes. Abductor hallucis function is best demonstrated by having the patient extend all toes. With the lesser toes extended, the great toe is passively flexed and adducted. The patient is asked to straighten the great toe, and abduction can usually be demonstrated (Fig. 32–7). Associated injuries include those to nearby neurovascular structures and tendons, as discussed previously.

Review of the Literature

By far the most common cause of injury to intrinsic muscles of the foot reported in the literature is the reconstructive surgeon.* The extensor hallucis brevis muscle is commonly incorporated with the dorsalis pedis pedicle and free flap.[63] The extensor digitorum brevis and the flexor digitorum brevis have both been used as local flaps,† as have the abductor hallucis, flexor hallucis brevis, and abductor digiti minimi.[56, 57, 251] Each of these studies

---

*See references 56, 57, 61, 63, 81, 117, 122, 206, 213, 220, and 251.

†See references 61, 81, 117, 122, 206, 213, and 220.

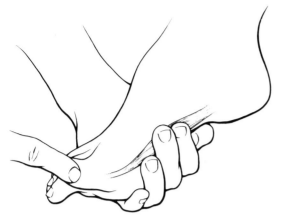

FIGURE 32–7. The action of the abductor hallucis muscle can be tested by asking the patient to flex and adduct all the toes. The patient is then asked to extend and abduct the great toe against the resistance of one hand while the physician palpates the muscle with the other hand.

reports that the muscle is expendable and can be sacrificed without significant deficit to the foot. However, long-term follow-up of these patients that specifically examines this point seems lacking. Floyd and colleagues reported three flexor digitorum brevis lacerations in their study.[51] All were repaired, and one developed a repair rupture. The result in the ruptured flexor digitorum brevis was rated fair, whereas the results in the other two were rated good.

Author's Preferred Treatment

I have personal long-term experience with several patients who have no extensor hallucis brevis secondary to its incorporation in a dorsalis pedis flap. I can detect no deficit in foot or toe function secondary to this muscle loss and believe this muscle is indeed expendable. I embrace similar scientifically unsupported beliefs about the expendability of the extensor digitorum brevis. My concerns about painful scars over the dorsum of the foot further underline my advice to avoid any added dissection or risks in order to restore the function of these two muscles.

My beliefs about the expendability of the plantar intrinsic muscles are less cavalier, especially with regard to the flexor digitorum brevis. There is a high prevalence of clawtoe deformity in the US population. I fear that the propensity to develop or to show progression of these deformities would be worsened by the

loss of a significant toe flexor. I recommend repair of this tendon when possible and believe that its function is as crucial to normal painless foot function as is the function of the flexor digitorum longus. If repair is not undertaken, I still recommend a formal wound exploration and débridement. Fear of hallux valgus deformity leads me to the same recommendation regarding the abductor hallucis. However, I have not seen this problem as yet in patients in whom I have used this muscle as a reconstructive flap. Despite its size, I believe that the abductor digiti minimi is expendable if the intrinsic flexors to the small toe are intact.

Muscles of the Ankle-Subtalar-Tarsal Complex

Motion and dynamic stability of the ankle, subtalar, and tarsal joints is accomplished through the coordinated actions of five separate muscles, with lesser contributions from the flexors and extensors of the toes. These five muscles are the gastrocnemius-soleus complex acting through the tendo Achillis, the tibialis anterior and posterior, and the peroneus longus and brevis. The tendo Achillis is the major plantar flexor of the ankle joint and exerts a slight inversion force. The plantar flexion of the ankle is assisted by the peroneus longus and brevis, the tibialis posterior, the flexor hallucis longus, and the flexor digitorum longus to a much lesser extent. The tibialis anterior serves primarily to provide dorsiflexion of the ankle and is seated almost directly along the inversion-eversion plane of the subtalar joint. The extensor digitorum longus and the extensor hallucis longus assist in this dorsiflexion moment to a lesser extent. The tibialis anterior and the peroneus longus both insert at the base of the first metatarsal–medial cuneiform. They provide an opposing, balanced supination-pronation moment to the forefoot. The tibialis posterior forms a sling under the navicular and performs the dual function of dynamic support of the arch and hindfoot inversion. Hindfoot eversion is accomplished primarily through the peroneus brevis, whose function is only poorly duplicated by the peroneus longus. None of these five tendons are expendable in normal foot function (Fig. 32–8).

These tendons can be disrupted by laceration, by traumatic avulsion, or through the

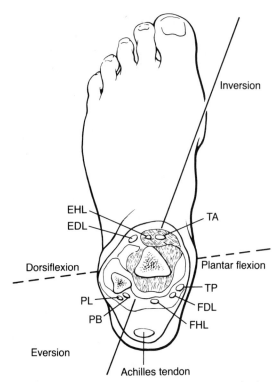

FIGURE 32–8. The moment of action of the various tendons acting across the ankle and subtalar joint. EHL, extensor hallucis longus; EDL, extensor digitorum longus; PL, peroneus longus; PB, peroneus brevis; FHL, flexor hallucis longus; FDL, flexor digitorum longus; TP, tibialis posterior; TA, tibialis anterior.

overuse-associated attrition of chronic tendinitis. The peroneals and the tibialis posterior are also subject to dislocations and subluxations that are often painful. The Achilles tendon is involved in sports-related overuse syndromes such as tendinitis or rupture at an incidence of 7.4 to 9 percent of all athletic exertional injuries.[170, 171] The tendo Achillis is by far the most commonly ruptured tendon in the leg or foot. As many as one-third of the lacerations about the foot and ankle in children may involve the tendo Achillis.[244] Sixteen[51] to 45[244] percent of lacerations of the foot occur at or above the ankle and involve one of these five tendons. Not unexpectedly, traumatic ruptures are well recognized at this level, although they are rare in the foot except for ruptures of the flexor hallucis longus. The recommendations for treatment in this area are less controversial than those for treatment of tendon injuries in the foot. Diagnosis can often be more difficult, as can be treatment, because of the predominance of atretic lesions.

Tendo Achillis

The gastrocnemius–soleus–tendo Achillis complex is the largest and most powerful musculotendinous structure below the knee. As many as 35 percent of all tendon ruptures in the body occur at the tendo Achillis,[94] and up to one-third of all lacerations in the foot involve this tendon.[244] Despite the frequency of injury to this tendon and a voluminous literature on treatment, with follow-up often exceeding 4 to 5 years, there is an amazing amount of controversy about the treatment of this injury. This controversy is fired by the complications associated with the two major conflicting treatment options and a lack of clear evidence for superiority of function with one treatment over the other. These two treatment options are, of course, surgical repair and closed equinus cast immobilization. The major arguments against closed treatment, which are often cited, are weakness of function after repair and a high incidence of rerupture. The major arguments against surgical repair are the risks of surgery and anesthesia.

Diagnosis of tendo Achillis ruptures can be problematic (Fig. 32–9). Plantar flexion of the ankle is possible secondary to tibialis posterior, flexor digitorum longus, flexor hallucis longus, and peroneal function. Furthermore, the weakness of plantar flexion can be mistaken for a partial rupture or simple tendinitis of the Achilles tendon. The patient's gait can appear amazingly normal to the untrained eye. Diagnosis is thus confirmed most commonly by the technique of Thompson and Doherty (Fig. 32–10).[227] With the patient lying prone on a table, the foot relaxed and positioned at neutral over the end of the table, the calf is squeezed above the suspected rupture or laceration. Failure of plantar flexion of the ankle on squeezing of the calf is considered diagnostic for tendo Achillis disruption. O'Brien[168] described a technique using percutaneous placement of a needle in the tendo Achillis that can be useful in situations in which Thompson and Doherty's technique is not thought to be definitively diagnostic (Fig. 32–11). In O'Brien's test, a 25-gauge needle is inserted at a right angle into the tendo Achillis just medial to the midline of the posterior calf at a point 10 cm proximal to the superior border of the calcaneus. The foot is alternately plantarflexed and dorsiflexed, and the needle hub is observed for swiveling. Only slight movement or the absence of movement is diagnostic of a disrup-

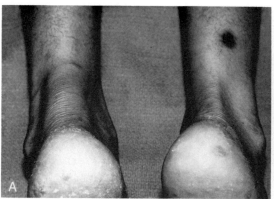
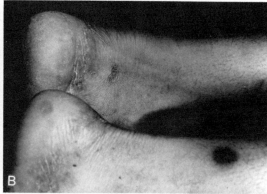

FIGURE 32–9. (A and B), Patient with a complete disruption of the left Achilles tendon. Hematoma and edema mask the defect. Active plantar flexion of the ankle is present.

tion. If the diagnosis is still in question, both ultrasonography[22, 43, 52, 116, 121, 136] and magnetic resonance imaging[97, 139, 181, 185] have been well substantiated as diagnostically reliable techniques.

Review of the Literature

Lacerations of the tendo Achillis can involve any age group but are very common in children. Ruptures classically occur in sedentary individuals in the third decade of life who are involved in recreational sports.[78, 94] Rupture characteristically occurs in the distal tendinous portion, where the blood supply is the most tenuous. There is a higher incidence of hyperuricemia in patients who experience tendo Achillis ruptures. Beskin and colleagues reported a 14-percent incidence of gout in 42

consecutive ruptures.[17] Dodds and Burry noted a significant increase in uric acid levels in 30 patients with ruptures of the tendo Achillis versus 30 age- and sex-matched cohorts.[44] Bilateral and unilateral ruptures have been associated with systemic steroid therapy,[15, 72, 107, 180] as well as with local steroid injections.[17, 93] Beskin and colleagues reported a 7-percent incidence of local injection in their patients.[17]

The advocacy for closed treatment of Achilles tendon ruptures over the last three decades has held a relatively lonely position in the literature. Approximately 10 to 11 articles in the English literature between 1959 and 1989 have advocated closed treatment of Achilles tendon ruptures, whereas more than 30 articles have advocated surgical treatment. The major arguments against closed treatment have been a fear of reduced function and an increased rerupture rate. The argument against surgery has been the increased complication risk. The risks of surgery are those associated with the use of anesthesia, skin slough over

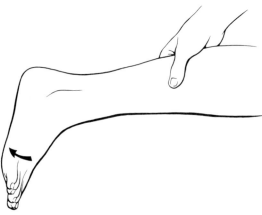

FIGURE 32–10. Thompson and Doherty's test for continuity of the Achilles tendon.

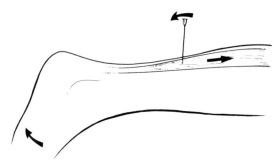

FIGURE 32–11. O'Brien's test for continuity of the Achilles tendon.

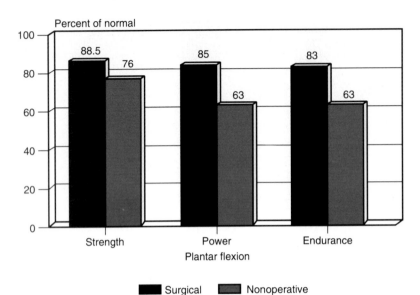

FIGURE 32–12. Isokinetic testing of surgical versus equinus casting repair of Achilles tendon ruptures. The pooled results of three studies include 190 subjects tested for strength, 98 tested for power, and 61 tested for endurance. All tests were done using a Cybex isokinetic dynamometer. (Data from references 82, 164, and 211.)

the repair, infection, tendon adhesion to the overlying skin, sural nerve injury, the formation of suture granulomas, deep venous thrombosis, pulmonary embolism, and death.

Carlstedt and colleagues compared surgical and conservative care in an elegant study on rabbits with transverse tenotomies of the plantaris.[28] Biochemical and biomechanical evaluation of the two groups revealed no difference between them. This study lends scientific credence to the concept that these injuries can be treated closed with expectations of a return of function. Tension spring, isometric, and isokinetic dynametric testing have been used to test surgical and nonsurgical groups. Comparison of surgically and nonsurgically treated patient groups has consistently shown slightly superior results with surgery.* Compared with the normal leg, the postoperative strength in the injured leg has returned to approximately 75 to 100 percent of normal for surgical groups and approximately 50 to 84 percent of normal for nonsurgical groups (Fig. 32–12).

However, none of these studies have indicated a greater return of functional strength in the surgical group, and the results of several studies lacked statistical significance. Carden and colleagues compared surgically and nonsurgically treated patients and noted a significant decrease in plantar flexion strength only in nonsurgical patients who were treated more than 1 week after injury.[27] Hiyashi reported a

98-percent return to the preinjury activity level after nonsurgical treatment in 100 patients.[75] The reported percentages of return to preinjury level after surgery have been 68,[106] 71,[147] 86,[175] 88,[17] and 90[174] percent. Nistor compared surgically and nonsurgically repaired Achilles tendon injuries.[164] Six of six competitive athletes returned to the same level of activity after closed treatment. Only one of three competitive athletes returned to the same level of activity after operative treatment. Inglis and colleagues, in contrast, noted in a similar study that only six of 23 competitive athletes returned to the same level of activity after closed treatment, whereas 37 of 39 returned to this level after surgical treatment.[82]

Rerupture rates in nonsurgically treated groups range from 0 to 45 percent and average 12 percent (42 of 339 cases) for the cumulative results of 10 articles reported since 1970.[27, 100, 245] For surgically treated groups, reported on in 21 articles, the average is less than 2 percent (17 of 1055 cases) and the range is from 0 to 5 percent.*

The major argument against surgery has been the risk of anesthetic and surgical complications. A review of 20 articles since 1959 that had good reporting of complication rates reveals an incidence of 17 percent (173 of 1017 cases).† These complications, in order of decreasing incidence, are primarily scar-related

---

*See references 60, 71, 82, 83, 88, 164, 179, and 211.

*See references 17, 27, 99, 106, 128, 232, and 245.
†See references 4, 17, 27, 99, 106, 232, and 245.

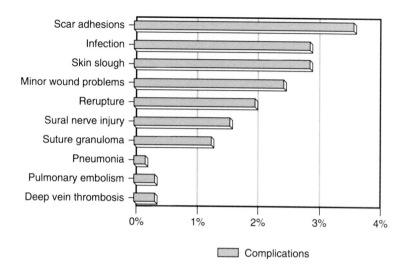

FIGURE 32–13. The complication rate for surgical repair of Achilles tendon disruptions obtained by pooling the results of a review of the literature is 19 percent for 1055 cases. (Data from references 4, 17, 27, 99, 106, 232, and 245.)

complaints, wound infections, skin slough, sural nerve injury, deep venous thrombosis, and pulmonary embolism. Complications of closed therapy are primarily deep venous thrombosis and pulmonary embolism. The incidence of these complications is 5 percent (five of 96 cases) for the combined results of Carden and colleagues[27] and Persson and Wredmark[179] (Figs. 32–13 and 32–14).

Author's Preferred Treatment

Enough evidence shows that function is more likely to be returned to normal after surgery to make me advocate surgery for an Achilles tendon disruption in a child or young athlete, as well as in a high-performance athlete. However, the majority of these occur in middle-aged weekend athletes. The risk of complications from surgery (17 percent) and a questionably significant increase in function should be weighed against the risk of rerupture with closed therapy (12 percent). The period of immobilization and the percentage of patients who return to unlimited activity are nearly identical for closed or open treatment groups. The risks and options should be discussed with the patient, and treatment should be individualized in this situation. If surgery is elected and the injury is less than 1 week old, I would advise percutaneous repair as described by Ma and Griffith.[135] A sedentary lifestyle, chronic tobacco use, diabetes melli-

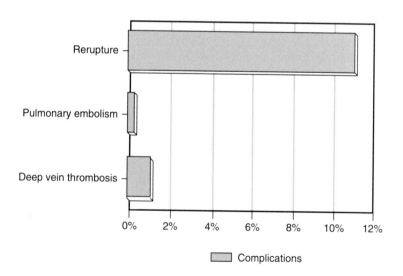

FIGURE 32–14. The complication rate for nonoperative treatment (equinus casting) of Achilles tendon disruptions obtained by pooling the results of a review of the literature is 13 percent for 339 cases. (Data from references 27, 100, 179, and 245.)

tus, or systemic diseases would lead me to advise closed treatment. I recommend surgical treatment for injuries older than 1 week.

Closed treatment should consist of initial equinus cast immobilization in a long-leg cast for 4 weeks. Immobilization should be continued for another 4 weeks in a short-leg cast with the ankle at neutral to slight equinus. Weight bearing during this period can be safely allowed with a rocker-bottom sole or cast shoe.[16] After 8 weeks, I would allow ambulation with a 1/4-inch heel lift. Unlimited sports activity should not be allowed for 5 months after injury.

I advocate surgical repair using either a modified Kessler or a Bunnell-type technique with a No. 2 braided polyester suture. There are a variety of techniques recommended to give a more secure repair. These include the use of the plantaris tendon or fascia lata as a graft or the transfer of the peroneus brevis.[231, 232] Techniques using Dacron vascular,[127, 128] carbon fiber,[79, 174, 175] and Marlex[172] grafts are also described. I do not believe that the theoretical advantages of these techniques justify the added dissection in the majority of cases. For late cases, I think any of these techniques can be used to advantage. I recommend the same postoperative protocol as that used without surgery, except for the exchange of the initial long-leg cast for a short-leg non–weight-bearing cast. I would allow weight bearing in the short-leg cast as soon as wound healing is evident.

Tibialis Posterior

In tendon injuries about the ankle, the incidence of tibialis posterior (TP) tendon injury is second only to that of tendo Achillis injury. Problems with tendinitis, dislocation, rupture, and laceration can all present with the TP. The critical role of the TP in stabilizing the tarsal-subtalar complex against hindfoot valgus and forefoot pronation has become evident over the last few decades. This critical function in running and walking accounts for the frequency of TP injury. The specific problem of tendinitis is discussed in Part V of this text. It is notable that posterior tibial tendinitis and planovalgus are the two overuse syndromes that are most responsive to orthotic foot management.[38]

The ability of the flexor digitorum longus to mimic the inversion and supination of the TP

can make the diagnosis of a rupture or laceration difficult. Localized tenderness along the course of the TP, weakness and pain on active resisted inversion and supination, and pain on passive pronation and eversion all point to pathology in the TP. An actual disruption of the TP can be confirmed by the inability to invert and supinate the foot while simultaneously wiggling the toes (Fig. 32–15).[32] Further radiographic confirmation can be obtained in chronic injuries by the presence of a cutoff on a TP tenogram. Computed tomography can also be quite useful in evaluating suspected tendon injuries about the ankle.[190–193]

Review of the Literature

Johnson and Strom[92] classified the stages of TP dysfunction, and D'Ambrosia[38] discussed the treatment principles. This problem is discussed further in Part V of this book. Larsen and Lauridsen described two cases of traumatic symptomatic TP dislocation.[119] These injuries occurred in both a 36-year-old woman and an 18-year-old man during running activities. The mechanism of injury was inversion and dorsiflexion. Both patients obtained good results after suturing of the flexor retinaculum to the posterior margin of the medial malleolus. Stanish and Vincent[218] and Mittal and Jain[154] have each added another single case of TP dislocation.

Progression to painful planovalgus deformity after disruption of the TP is well documented in the literature, with at least six reported cases by four different authors involving both

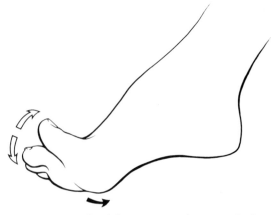

FIGURE 32–15. The ability to invert and supinate the foot while simultaneously wiggling the toes denotes an intact posterior tibial tendon.

children and adults. Griffiths reported two nonrepaired TP lacerations in children.[66] Both resulted in progressive deformity and poor results. He noted a spontaneous rupture in a 35-year-old individual that went on to have a satisfactory result without repair. A primary repair was carried out in one child (10 years of age) and one adult (42 years of age). A late repair was also performed in another child 3 years after the injury. Both of the repairs in children produced unsatisfactory results, whereas the repair in the adult had a satisfactory result. Kettlekamp and Alexander reported four cases of spontaneous rupture of the TP.[104] These cases were all in adult patients. One of the four patients was treated without surgery and had persistent medial arch pain. Of the three operated on, only one became asymptomatic. The other two had persistent pain with the persistence of some planovalgus.

Jahss reported 10 cases of spontaneous rupture of the TP.[89] Disappointed with the results of repair in the literature, he treated the first five patients nonsurgically. All had unsatisfactory results, with persistence or progression of their planovalgus. He subsequently treated the next five patients with transfer of the flexor digitorum longus by side-to-side suture. He had "consistently excellent results" in each of these patients, although all had some residual planovalgus. Floyd and colleagues reported two TP lacerations.[51] One was repaired and did well. The second, nonrepaired TP laceration led to a progressive planovalgus deformity. Johnson reported another case of spon-

taneous rupture.[91] Citron noted two painful planovalgus foot deformities in children after initially missed TP lacerations.[32] Kerr reported on an adult with a missed TP rupture that progressed to a painful unilateral planovalgus deformity over a period of weeks.[103] TP ruptures and entrapments have also been reported to be associated with ankle fractures[58, 98, 198, 238] and can produce a treacherous pitfall in the treatment of these injuries (Fig. 32–16).

Author's Preferred Treatment

Any individual who suffers medial ankle pain after a running injury should be examined to rule out a TP dislocation or rupture. The same edict applies to anyone who suffered a laceration behind the medial malleolus. A dislocating TP tendon is palpable with resisted active inversion and supination of the foot. Tenderness, ecchymosis, or edema along the course of the TP implies a disruption. Weakness of foot inversion and supination should be present, but a lack of weakness does not reliably rule out TP disruption masked by flexor digitorum longus activity. The inability to wiggle the toes while holding the foot in inversion and supination is confirmatory. Late cases are easier to diagnose because patients are unable to do a single side toe rise on the affected foot, bringing the heel from valgus to varus as the heel leaves the floor. Rarely, contrast tenography, computed tomography, or magnetic resonance imaging is necessary.

If a disruption is present, repair should be

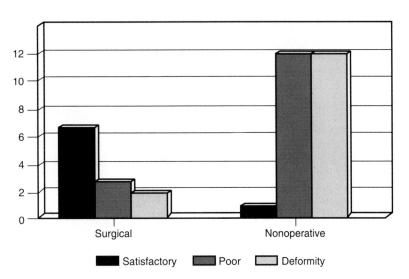

FIGURE 32–16. Treatment results for 24 cases of tibialis posterior disruption. (Data from references 51, 66, 89, and 104.)

carried out before a planovalgus deformity develops. I recommend repair with 3–0 permanent suture material in a grasping technique, as advised for flexor hallucis longus lacerations, if repair is possible. When primary repair is not possible, as with many ruptures, the reconstruction can be accomplished by transfer of the distal TP stump to the flexor digitorum longus, as advocated by Jahss.[89] A portion of the flexor retinaculum should be left intact behind the medial malleolus in the repair of disruptions to prevent postoperative dislocations. The repaired TP should be protected in a short-leg cast, with the foot held in slight inversion with a carefully molded arch. Immobilization should be for a least 8 weeks and should probably be followed by the use of a well-molded arch orthosis for another month or more based on the propensity for repair rupture of the long tendons of the foot and the tendency for recurrence of the planovalgus. I advise repair of dislocations as advocated by Larsen and Lauridsen.[119] Mann recommended bony reconstructive procedures for failed symptomatic repairs.[138]

Tibialis Anterior

The tibialis anterior (TA) is the major dorsiflexor of the ankle. Disruption of this tendon predictably produces a drop foot deformity. Surprisingly, this tendon is rarely involved with tendinitis but is subject to injury and rupture. Rupture of the TA is a peculiar entity reported in diabetics older than 45 years of age and is usually associated with minor trauma.[95] The major differential diagnosis for TA disruption is peroneal nerve palsy. Intact extensor hallucis longus and extensor digitorum longus function associated with palpation of TA muscle contraction proximal to the rupture helps rule out peroneal nerve palsy.

Review of the Literature

In view of the fact that the TA is a subcutaneous tendon in an exposed position, relatively few reports have appeared on its injury and treatment. Griffiths reported three TA lacerations in his series.[66] The two lacerations repaired less than 4 months after injury obtained satisfactory results. One patient, a 10-year-old, had repair more than 2 years after the injury and obtained an unsatisfactory response. Lipscomb and Kelley reported nine

cases of TA laceration.[131] Floyd and colleagues reported four TA lacerations in their series.[51] Three were repaired, and a fourth was not. The nonrepaired tendon produced a poor result, with deformity requiring reconstruction. Mensor and Ordway reported two cases of spontaneous rupture of the TA and noted 10 others in their review of the literature.[150] Kashyap and Prince reported a single case of spontaneous rupture of the TA in a 65-year-old diabetic man with minor trauma.[95] Surgical treatment produced a good result (Figs. 32–17 and 32–18).

Author's Preferred Treatment

TA function is crucial for normal gait. A lacerated tendon should be repaired using a grasping technique and 3–0 permanent suture material. Augmentation with the peroneus tertius or a lesser toe extensor should be planned with ruptures. Cast immobilization in a protective position for 6 to 8 weeks is indicated, followed by a therapy program that initiates range-of-motion exercises and then begins progressive resistance exercises. Late injuries require Z-lengthening or free tendon grafting and need longer protection to prevent recurrence of footdrop with stretching secondary to remodeling of the repair.

Peroneus Longus

The peroneus longus (PL) performs forefoot pronation, the function complementary to that of the tibialis anterior, and assists in hindfoot eversion. The function of the PL is partially but incompletely duplicated by the peroneus brevis. The PL is subject to many of the same problems as the tibialis posterior. These include peroneal tendon dislocation, tendinitis, and rupture. Ruptures can occur through fracture of the os peroneum. The differential diagnosis for PL rupture includes chronic lateral ligamentous ankle sprain, avulsion of the bony insertion of the peroneus brevis tendon, peroneal tendon dislocation, trauma to a congenitally multipartite os peroneum, and calcific tendinitis of the PL.[177] Peroneal tendinitis and dislocation are discussed in Part V of this text.

Review of the Literature

Griffiths reported three lacerations of the PL, all of which involved children.[66] All of

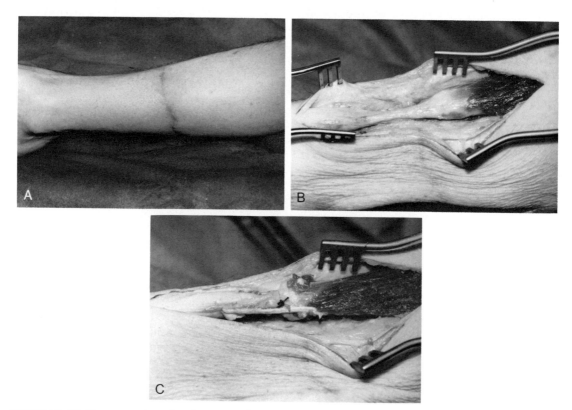

FIGURE 32–17. The expected results of nonsurgical treatment of a tibialis anterior laceration. *(A),* Four months after a chain saw laceration to his anterior and lateral compartments, the patient complains of a footdrop. *(B),* Spontaneous attempted repair with an elongated scar. *(C),* Late reconstruction with excision of the scar and repair with a plantaris muscle and a No. 1 braided suture.

FIGURE 32–18. Treatment results for seven cases of tibialis anterior disruption. (Data from references 51, 66, 131, and 150.)

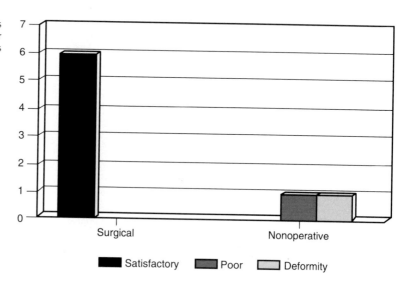

these tendons, which were treated without repair, progressed to deformity and poor results. This deformity consisted of forefoot supination and a failure of the first metatarsal to reach the ground when the patient was standing. He reported on two other peroneal tendon injuries treated with surgical repair, both of which had satisfactory results. DeLuca and Banta reported a case of pes cavovarus deformity in a child that was a late consequence of an isolated PL laceration that had not been repaired.[42]

Peacock and colleagues reported a PL disruption through an os peroneum fracture.[177] The injury resulted from forced eversion of a supinated inverted foot in an attempt to prevent a fall. A positive result was obtained from repair of the os peroneum. Cachia and colleagues reported two cases of PL rupture and os peroneum fracture (one was complete and the other was partial).[26] Each occurred with an inversion stress with an audible snap. The complete disruption occurred in a 64-year-old man who had a painful prodrome for 2 weeks. He responded to surgical excision of the os peroneum and repair of the PL. An incomplete injury occurred in a 39-year-old woman, who responded to physical therapy. Thompson and Patterson reported three PL ruptures (Fig. 32–19).[226]

Author's Preferred Treatment

In a child, the peroneus brevis cannot be expected to replace the function of the PL. Progressive deformity can be expected; accord-

ingly, the PL should be repaired. The treatment principles discussed previously, in the section on treatment of the TP, should be followed. Augmentation of the tendon by suture to the peroneus brevis is indicated in late repair or with attrition of the tendon.

Eversion of the hindfoot is largely the function of the peroneus brevis. However, the peroneus brevis cannot be expected to reestablish forefoot pronation or to maintain normal weight bearing on the first ray. I recommend repair of an isolated PL disruption in an athletic or active adult, with suture to the peroneus brevis when necessary.

Peroneus Brevis

The peroneus brevis (PB) provides hindfoot eversion and is a dynamic protector of the lateral ankle ligament complex against inversion sprains. There is little literature on the natural history of nonrepaired, isolated PB disruption secondary to avulsion or laceration. The PB has been used for augmentation of the tendo Achillis after rupture[231, 232] and for lateral ankle ligament reconstructions, with no reported untoward effects.

Review of the Literature

Stiehl reported a concomitant rupture of the PB tendon and a bimalleolar ankle fracture.[221] The same year, Cross and colleagues reported a PB rupture in a classical ballet dancer in the absence of a peroneus longus muscle.[37] LeMelle and Janis[123] reported eight cases of PB

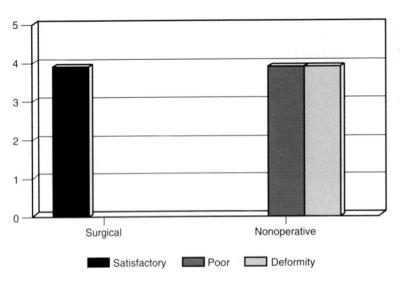

FIGURE 32–19. Treatment results for eight cases of peroneus longus disruption. (Data from references 26, 66, and 177.)

rupture.[123] These authors recommended surgical repair.

Author's Preferred Treatment

My convictions regarding an isolated PB injury are the same as those regarding an isolated peroneus longus injury. I believe that the PB is a relatively nonexpendable tendon and advocate repair in children and in athletic or active adults. Augmentation with the peroneus longus is available when necessary.

TRAUMATIC VASCULAR INJURIES OF THE FOOT AND ANKLE

As many as 6.5 percent of orthopaedic injuries are associated with vascular injuries.[21] These vascular injuries can be due to penetrating or blunt trauma.* Most vascular injuries around the knee are associated with blunt trauma, and the lower extremity as a whole sustains most of its vascular injuries from penetrating trauma (more than 80 percent).[11, 50] Reports of injuries below the knee list penetrating causes from 14[207] to 67[96] percent of the time. Penetrating trauma most commonly consists of single-gunshot wounds, stabbings, and shotgun wounds, in order of decreasing frequency.[176] Blunt trauma is generally associated with motor vehicle accidents and falls from heights. The complications of a missed vascular injury include loss of a limb from ischemia secondary to injury or late arterial occlusion; compartment syndromes of the leg, foot, or both; pseudoaneurysm and later rupture; and arteriovenous fistulas and possible cardiac failure.† Appreciation of the signs of vascular injury and early appropriate intervention are thus critical in lower extremity injuries.

Just under 5 percent of vascular injuries involve vessels below the knee.[101, 178] During World War II, the amputation rate without repair after single-vessel tibial artery injuries was 14 percent, and it was 65 percent after double-vessel injuries.[40] Ligation for single-vessel injuries of the tibial vessels during the Vietnam conflict produced a 75-percent amputation rate.[186] Shah and colleagues reported 29 isolated tibial artery injuries over a 4-year

---

*See references 11, 21, 50, 96, 176, 207, 215, and 216.

†See references 10, 11, 21, 41, 46, 159, 176, 207, 215, 243, 249, and 252.

period.[207] Twenty of these patients had a viable foot; therefore, the artery was not repaired. Three patients underwent primary amputation, and two more required later amputation. Eighty-eight percent of these patients required later angiographic evaluation for arterial reconstruction 2 to 12 months after injury for nonhealing of wounds, fracture malunion, and soft tissue defects. The significance of early diagnosis and treatment is self-evident.

Vascular Anatomy

It is critical to understand the vascular anatomy, common anatomic variations, and the relative importance of the various vessels in the leg, ankle, and foot before any decisions regarding treatment of these injuries can be made. Among primates, humans are unique in the respect that the major blood supply to the foot comes from the popliteal artery. In other primates, the femoral artery gives rise to a large saphenous artery, which sends a branch to the dorsalis pedis artery and a second, posterior branch to the sole of the foot. The popliteal branches end in muscular branches.[30] In humans, the major arterial contributions to the foot come from popliteal branches, the peroneal artery being a constant finding in the human leg.[225] Taylor and colleagues defined the arterial anatomy of the leg in normal young individuals.[225] These authors examined 66 cadavers and reviewed the arteriograms of 100 young, healthy individuals being studied for free fibula transfers. They noted the "normal pattern" of an anterior tibial, posterior tibial, and peroneal artery in 80 percent of individuals. Fourteen percent had no posterior tibial vessel. Three percent had no anterior tibial vessel, and 2 percent had neither an anterior nor a posterior tibial artery. Arterial anastomoses between these vessels do not occur to a significant extent after initial branching until the level of the ankle and distal tibia. The peroneal artery anastomoses to the posterior tibial artery just above the ankle in most individuals.[67, 160, 250] The peroneal artery also sends a relatively constant branch between the fibula and tibia just above the joint line that anastomoses with the dorsal foot circulation (Figs. 32–20 and 32–21).[18, 120, 140, 142]

Anatomic arterial variations occur whenever a point is reached in the arterial tree where major anastomoses between vessels are pres-

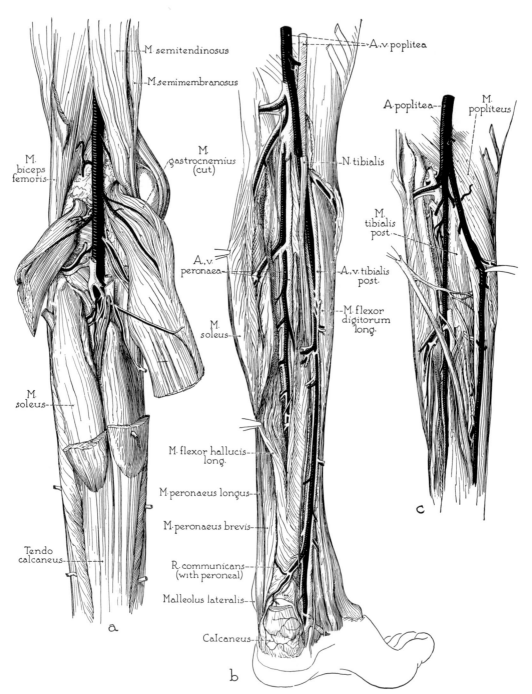

FIGURE 32–20. Vessels and nerves of the posterior crural region at successively deep levels. *(A),* The popliteal artery in the popliteal fossa and in the space distal to it; the latter continuation of the fossa is opened by reflection of the gastrocnemius muscle. *(B),* The posterior tibial vessels and the tibial nerves, revealed by reflection of the soleus muscle. *(C),* The arterial pattern clarified by excision of the veins. (From Anson BJ: Atlas of Human Anatomy. Philadelphia, WB Saunders, 1950, p 479.)

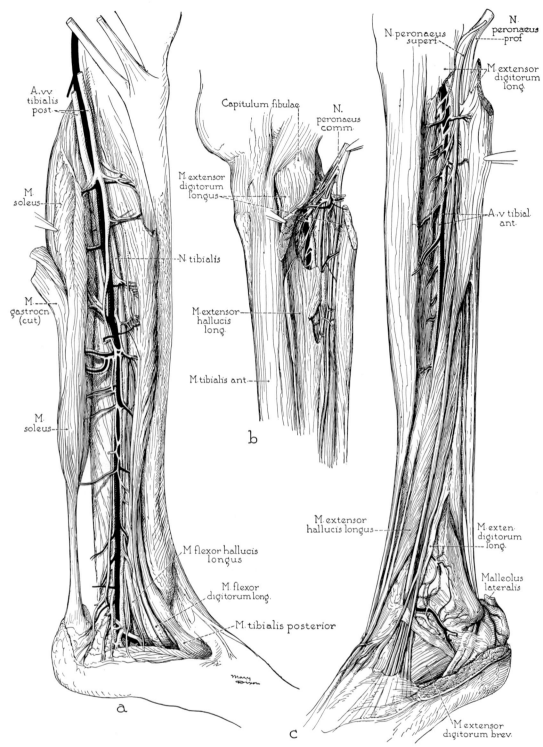

FIGURE 32–21. Vessels and nerves of the crural regions (medial and lateral views). *(A)*, The vessels and nerves of the posterior crural region, shown by retraction of the soleus muscle. *(B)*, The vessels and nerves of the lateral crural region, deep to the peroneus longus. *(C)*, Those of the anterior crural region, deep to the extensor digitorum longus. (From Anson BJ: Atlas of Human Anatomy. Philadelphia, WB Saunders, 1950, p 480.)

ent. This occurs in the leg at the knee, the ankle, and the forefoot. The variations associated with branching at the knee were just discussed. With respect to the arterial supply from the ankle to the forefoot, the "normal pattern" is a dorsalis pedis artery formed as an extension of the anterior tibial vessel, and medial and lateral plantar vessels formed as extensions of the posterior tibial vessel. Anastomoses between the peroneal and posterior tibial vessels occur within the distal 10 cm above the ankle.[67, 250] In 16 percent of individuals, the posterior tibial vessel is absent, and the plantar vessels receive their supply through this branch from the peroneal artery. The dorsalis pedis forms a dorsal arch that connects with the peroneal artery laterally (through the dorsal tarsal artery, dorsal arch, or both) through the peroneal's branch between the distal tibia and fibula. In 5 percent of individuals, the anterior tibial vessel is absent, and the dorsal circulation is from this peroneal branch. The dorsalis pedis artery is absent in approximately 3 to 14 percent of individuals.[30, 80, 157, 184] The lower percentages are associated with anatomic dissections and Doppler ultrasonography, and the higher percentages with clinical palpation of pulses. The posterior tibial pulse behind the ankle is nonpalpable in 2 to 9 percent of feet.[223]

Bailleul and colleagues carried out an anatomic dissection of 67 feet to define the dorsal arterial network of the foot.[13] In 9 percent of their study group, the dorsalis pedis artery was absent or insignificant, and the dorsal circulation was from the peroneal artery laterally. Sixty-six percent of the time, the "classic description" prevailed, with a single dorsalis pedis artery originating from the anterior tibial vessel and connecting with the deep plantar arch of the lateral plantar artery through the first metatarsal interspace. Three percent of the time, the dorsalis pedis connected with the deep plantar arch through the second metatarsal interspace. Twenty-two percent of the time, the dorsalis pedis artery branched into two terminal branches (Fig. 32–22).

The next level of anastomoses is at the forefoot. "Normally," the dorsal and volar arches connect through small branches at the intermetatarsal and metatarsophalangeal regions, providing significant dorsal (variably present in descending frequency from the great to third toes) and volar digital arteries to the toes. The relative significance of the dorsalis

pedis circulation to the toes is greater than would be expected. Lippert illustrated that in more than 50 percent of his study material, the main blood supply to the plantar aspect of the toes was derived from the dorsal circulation of the foot through intermetatarsal branches.[130] In contrast, the dorsal circulation to the third, fourth, and fifth toes is often supplied through the plantar arch through intermetatarsal connections. Palm and Husum studied the blood pressure of the great toe in 100 healthy individuals using strain gauge plethysmography with alternating and simultaneous digital compression of the dorsalis pedis and posterior tibial arteries.[173] In 50 percent of their 200 examinations, the great toe pressure was significantly dependent on the dorsalis pedis artery, and in 41 percent, the toe pressure was significantly dependent on the posterior tibial artery.

Diagnosis of Arterial Injuries

Specific clinical signs are considered indicative of extremity vascular injury (Table 32–1). These include a distal circulatory deficit manifested by diminished or absent pulses and capillary refill of greater than 6 seconds. A bruit or thrill implies an arteriovenous fistula. Bright red hemorrhage, an expanding or pulsatile hematoma, unexplained shock, and a small to moderate-sized stable hematoma imply arterial injury. Adjacent nerve injury or close proximity of a penetrating wound to a major artery is also suggestive. Arteriography remains the gold standard for evaluating arterial injuries and is indicated if the patient is hemodynamically stable.

Menzoian and colleagues reviewed 165 civilian vascular injuries.[151] Vascular injuries were

TABLE 32–1. SIGNS OF ARTERIAL INJURY
Diminished or absent pulse
Prolonged capillary refill
Bruit or thrill
Bright red hemorrhage
Expanding or pulsatile hematoma
Unexplained shock
Adjacent nerve injury
Arterial proximity of wound

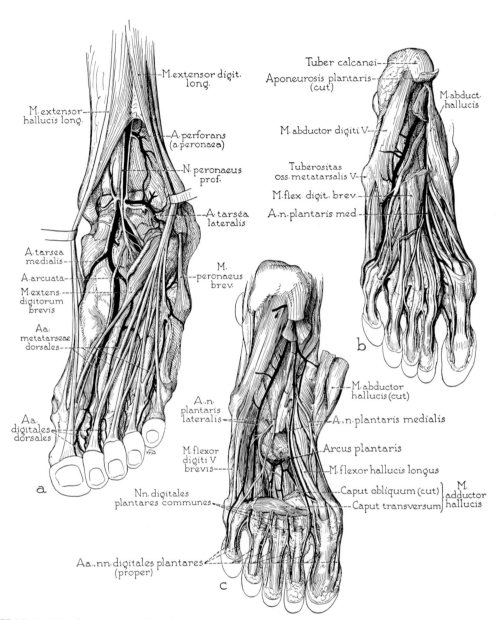

FIGURE 32–22. Vessels and nerves of the foot (dorsal and plantar surfaces). *(A)*, The vessels and nerves of the dorsum of the foot, shown by retraction of the long extensor tendons and by excision of the short extensors. *(B)*, The vessels and nerves of the plantar surface of the foot at intermediate levels. *(C)*, The vessels and nerves of the plantar surface of the foot at deep levels. (From Anson BJ: Atlas of Human Anatomy, Philadelphia, WB Saunders, 1950, p 481.)

associated with clinical findings at a rate of 100 percent for signs of acute ischemia, 100 percent for a bruit or thrill, 91 percent for absent pulse, 89 percent for shock, 78 percent for neurologic deficit, and 55 percent for hematoma. Arteriography for proximity of a penetrating wound alone showed abnormal findings in 16 percent of cases (Fig. 32–23). Early aggressive therapy resulted in an amputation rate of only 1.5 percent. Snyder and colleagues reported the results of arteriography in 177 civilian vascular injuries, in which they obtained only one false-negative finding.[216]

Treatment of Arterial Injuries

A preponderance of evidence shows that arterial repair is indicated when feasible and that ligation has some serious complications, both potential and real. Our abilities in the management of these injuries have advanced to the point that arterial repair is now practical. DeBakey and Simeone reported 2471 arterial injuries among US soldiers during World War II.[40] Of the 81 arteries sutured during this war, only three remained patent. During the Korean and Vietnam conflicts, repair of larger vessels became the standard of care, and the amputation rate after arterial injury dropped from 50 percent during World War II to 13 percent during the Vietnam conflict.[186] Nevertheless, in 1967 the reported success rate for arteries of less than 2 mm in diameter with standard vascular techniques was 0 percent (0

of 67 patients).[23] With the advent of microsurgical techniques, the success rate for the same injury type (forearm radial and ulnar artery repairs) was 93 percent for critical vessels.[55]

Occasionally, concern arises over the sequencing of repair for unstable fractures of the foot, ankle, or leg when they are associated with vascular injuries. Shah and colleagues showed that the risk of damage to a repaired vessel around the knee with reduction is approximately 10 percent.[208] When the extremity is not ischemic or is noncritically so, initial expedient fracture stabilization seems prudent. In an ischemic extremity, the restoration of circulation should be of paramount importance because of the risk of ischemic damage and compartment syndrome. However, the repair often impedes a thorough débridement and increases the risk of limb loss secondary to infection. This problem can be overcome by the initial use of a vascular shunt,[90, 105, 163] followed by débridement, stabilization, and vascular repair.

Venous Injuries

The venous drainage of the lower extremity is much more dependent on the deeper veins than is drainage of the upper extremity. Ligation of associated venous injuries of the thigh region is associated with a higher incidence of chronic edema (50 versus 7 percent after repair) and a higher incidence of compartment syndrome (37 versus 5 percent).[2] If not pres-

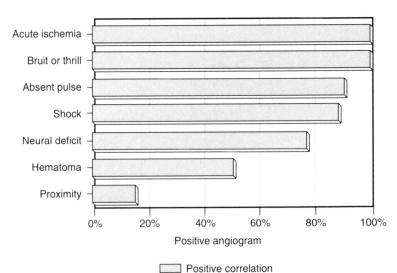

FIGURE 32–23. The incidence of positive angiographic findings for arterial injury based on the presence of a given clinical finding. (Data from reference 151.)

ent, a deep venous system should be restored for injuries below the knee, although this is unnecessary with all but major injuries.

Replantations

After 26 years of replantation surgery, a great deal of controversy remains about lower extremity replantation in the medical community. Although lower extremity replantations are relatively common in China, reports of it are rare in the West.[25] A brief review of the literature from the last 10 years reveals reports of more than 40 lower extremity replantations, less than half of which are found in the US literature.* Most of these reports list only one or two cases (more than half list only one). Of interest, a 1983 report from Louisville listed nine cases.[115] It is difficult to ascertain the actual success rate for lower extremity replantations because most of the reports are limited to single successful replantations.

Kutz and colleagues reported 44-percent tissue survival for their nine cases.[115] Good to excellent functional results have been reported at levels above the knee,[137, 235] through the tibia,† and through the foot.[115, 155, 230] A successfully replanted forefoot can be expected to produce a near-normal extremity.[230] For successful replantations through the tibia, the

*See references 19, 25, 31, 36, 54, 62, 113–115, 125, 137, 152, 155, 204, 219, 230, 234, 235, and 237.

†See references 25, 62, 113–115, 125, 204, 234, and 237.

results are still quite good. Shortening of 3.5 to 7.5 cm has been reported.[25, 114, 125] Ambulation without support can be expected by 9 months to 1 year.[25, 54, 114, 237] Return to work can be expected by 1 to 1 1/2 year.[62, 114, 237] The results that can be expected for successful replantations above the knee are not as good. Mamakos reported a replantation just above the knee in an 11-year-old.[137] Follow-up at 2 1/2 years revealed the patient ambulating without crutches, with a brace for ankle instability and a 5.5-cm shoe lift. Chronic edema does not appear to be a problem, and when the nerve can be repaired, protective sensation to the sole appears to be the rule.

The majority of patients with lower extremity amputation will not be candidates for replantation because of associated trauma and unsuitable wounds secondary to crush and contamination. I would agree with Seiler and colleagues that the only good candidates for lower extremity replantation in the United States are children with guillotine-type injuries in the absence of polytrauma that involve the distal one-third of the leg and occasionally patients with bilateral cases (Fig. 32–24).[204] Forefoot and toe replantation should be considered an aesthetic procedure. I would advise against replantation after lawn mower injuries of the foot and leg because of the risk of failure or invalidism associated with chronic osteomyelitis. Recovery from a replantation of the distal one-third of the leg requires 1 to 1 1/2 years. Failure will occur and reamputation will be necessary at a significantly higher

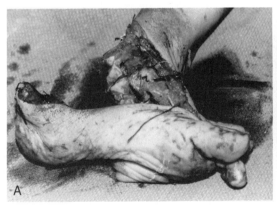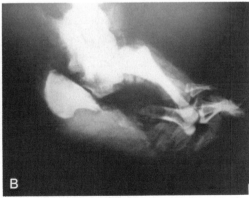

FIGURE 32–24. *(A and B),* An incomplete amputation in a young woman that is secondary to a riding lawn mower injury. The forefoot and heel pad are without circulation, and there are multilevel injuries to the nerves and vessels of the foot and ankle. Severe comminution, contamination, and devascularization of the bony elements of the midfoot are present. Attempted salvage by microvascular techniques would be ill-conceived. The patient was well serviced by immediate conversion to a below-knee amputation and immediate prosthetic fitting.

rate than for upper extremity replantations. Shortening often occurs, and later use of a shoe lift is commonly necessary. The decision for replantation should be carefully weighed against the advantages of revision amputation and early prosthetic fitting and against the risks of phantom pain and the psychological trauma of amputation. The prosthetically fitted patient can be expected to be ambulatory without aids within 3 months. Users of Syme and below-knee prosthetics will have gait velocities approaching 90 percent of normal for these patients.

TRAUMATIC NERVE INJURIES OF THE LOWER EXTREMITY

The peripheral nervous system of the foot and leg is no less intricate in anatomy and end-organ diversity than is that of the hand and forearm. However, the compulsion for nerve repair in the foot has never gained the momentum of that for repair in the hand. Wallenfang and Rudigier reported 390 nerve repairs over a 15-year period.[239] The incidence of repair for upper extremity nerve injuries was 20 times that for injuries of the lower extremity. Furthermore, nerve repairs were found in less than 1 percent of major lower extremity injuries. This is far out of proportion to the expected incidence of major nerve injury with this type of lower extremity injury. The incidence of major nerve injury in the lower extremity associated with arterial injuries is 40 to 50 percent.[49, 188, 241] The reasons for this rather laissez faire attitude to the lower extremity are multiple.[5] A primary factor is delegation of the foot to the lowly, often-unappreciated job of ambulation. Compared with the haughty jobs of environmental manipulation, feeding, caressing, and acquisition of income reserved for the hands, it is no wonder the attentions of the nerve surgeon are more often directed to the upper extremity. The more reliable reconstructions offered by tendon transfer, joint fusion, or prosthetic rehabilitation for lower extremity nerve injuries have also added to this uninspired attitude. The greater lengths of regeneration for nerve repair in the lower extremity and the poor results of nerve repairs of the lower extremity during World War II further add to this ambivalence toward lower extremity nerve repair. However, with the principles of microsurgery

and interfascicular nerve grafting firmly founded over the last 20 years, this attitude needs re-evaluation.

Anatomy and Principles of Repair

The motor, sensory, pain, and proprioceptive functions of the foot are controlled through the peripheral nervous system. The major element of this system is a single nerve cell extending from either the anterior horn of the spinal cord (motor fibers) or the dorsal root ganglia (sensory fibers) for up to a meter to its end-organ. These individual cell fibers exist in the hundreds of thousands in an organ that we call the nerve. Inside this nerve are also blood vessels, connective tissues, lymphatics, and a host of supporting cellular elements, including Schwann's cells, fibroblasts, and macrophages. It is important to remember that a nerve repair is an attempt to restore a complex organ with multiple elements rather than the relatively simpler retubing associated with vascular repair or the restringing associated with tendon repair.

The major areas of attention in nerve repair are the connective tissue elements. The endoneurium is a loose connective tissue layer surrounding each nerve fiber or axon and its associated Schwann's cell population. Nerve fibers in the tens and hundreds of thousands are grouped in bundles called fascicles. Each individual fascicle is surrounded by a second connective tissue tube, the perineurium. The association of multiple fascicles, their respective blood vessels, and lymphatics, surrounded by an epineurium, constitutes the nerve organ. The attention in nerve repair is directed toward the epineurium and perineurium, although it is the restoration of the endoneurial sheaths and their respective axons on which successful repair depends (Fig. 32–25).

Because of the complexity of the nerve, it is necessary to classify a nerve injury before any logical approach to repair can be formulated. Two such classifications of nerve injury are popular today. The simpler is that described by Seddon.[201, 202] Seddon classified nerve injuries as neurapraxia, axonotmesis, or neurotmesis. With neurapraxia, the axon and its surrounding tissues are anatomically intact, and the principal effect is physiologic. No surgical intervention is indicated, and complete recovery within a few weeks is to be expected.

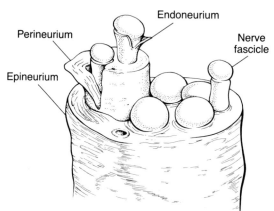

FIGURE 32–25. The cross-sectional microanatomy of a peripheral nerve fiber. (Modified from Kutz JE, Shealy G, Lubbers L: Interfascicular nerve repair. Orthop Clin North Am 12:281, 1981.)

Axonotmesis, in contrast, describes a nerve injury in which the axons undergo wallerian degeneration. The connective tissue components (i.e., endoneurium, perineurium, and epineurium) will be intact to varying degrees. Recovery is dependent on axonal regrowth down the individual endoneurial sheaths, and the quality of recovery depends on the degree of disorganization of the endoneurial tubes, intervening scar, and degree of regrowth. Possibly the only intact structure will be the epineurial sheath, and no useful spontaneous recovery can be expected. If anatomic disruption of the entire nerve structure, including the epineurium, occurs, the lesion is called a neurotmesis. Recovery without repair in a human will not occur to a functional extent.

The ambiguity of injury present in Seddon's axonotmesis category is rectified by the classification of Sunderland.[224] Sunderland described five classes of nerve injury. Sunderland's first-degree nerve injury is equivalent to Seddon's neurapraxia. His fifth-degree injury is equivalent to Seddon's neurotmesis. However, Sunderland's classification allows a more precise delineation of Seddon's axonotmesis. It is useful to think of Sunderland's injury classes in relation to the axons and the various connective sheaths. A first-degree injury is a physiologic conduction defect without any anatomic disruption, although demyelination of the axons may occur. Anatomic disruption of the axon with wallerian degeneration occurs in second- to fifth-degree injuries. The endoneurium is intact in the second-degree injury. The

third-degree injury is an injury at the fascicular level. The endoneurium is no longer intact, but the perineurium is. In the fourth-degree injury, the perineurium is also disrupted, but the epineurium is intact. The entire nerve, including the epineurium, is disrupted in a fifth-degree injury.

Sunderland's classification allows a better definition of the nerve injury in regard to prognostic and surgical considerations. The defect is physiologic in a first-degree injury, and spontaneous recovery without surgical intervention can be expected within weeks. In a second-degree injury, axonal death has occurred; however, the connective tissue scaffold is intact, and surgical intervention is not expected to help or to be necessary. Full recovery may not occur. Chemotherapeutic modalities may one day prove useful in treating these lesions. A second-degree injury can be differentiated from a first-degree injury by the extended time to recovery and the presence of a distally progressive Tinel-Hoffmann sign, denoting a sprouting axon. In the third-degree injury, the perineurium is intact, but the endoneurium is not. Complete spontaneous recovery is less likely, although significant functional return is still probable. In the fourth-degree injury, the nerve is intact at the epineural level only. A significant gap may exist between the individual axons. Fibrosis in this gap may prevent any sprouting of axons across the injury site, resulting in a neuroma-in-continuity. Failure of distal progression of the Tinel-Hoffmann sign suggests this lesion, and resection and repair of the nerve are indicated. The nerve is completely divided with a fifth-degree injury, and recovery without surgery is not to be expected. In practice, varying degrees of injury may be present in the same nerve (Table 32–2).

Nerve injuries to the lower extremity may result from an incision, a laceration, a crush, or a traction mechanism. Specific factors relative to individual nerves are noted in the following sections. General treatment principles are noted here. In lacerations, incisions, and puncture wounds caused by sharp objects, a fifth-degree Sunderland injury should be expected. A complete injury or a significant partial injury deserves surgical exploration, preferably within 72 hours. Significant spontaneous recovery is not to be expected. Peripheral nerves contain elastin fibers and retract when divided. The ability to coapt the

TABLE 32–2. CLASSIFICATIONS OF NERVE INJURY (SUNDERLAND VERSUS SEDDON)

SUNDERLAND	STRUCTURAL DAMAGE	SEDDON
First-degree injury	Physiologic	Neurapraxia
Second-degree injury	Axon	Axonotmesis
Third-degree injury	Endoneurium	Axonotmesis
Fourth-degree injury	Perineurium	Axonotmesis
Fifth-degree injury	Epineurium	Neurotmesis

divided nerve ends can decrease with time because of edema and fibrosis in the nerve, necessitating extensive mobilization of the nerve or interfascicular grafting. Furthermore, early repair allows use of the vasa neurvosum for fascicular alignment. For crush, traction, and penetrating injuries caused by blunt projectiles (i.e., bullets), a period of observation for spontaneous recovery is recommended. The absence of an advancing Tinel-Hoffmann sign indicates a Sunderland fourth- or fifth-degree injury, and surgical exploration is indicated. Early surgical intervention in the lower extremity is particularly important because of the distances the axon must grow to reach its end-organ. Axon growth is only 1 to 2 mm/day, and if reinnervation of the motor end-plates does not occur within 18 months, useful function will not occur. A careful clinical examination should allow the clinician to determine if the Tinel-Hoffmann sign is progressing within 1 to 3 months at the most (advance of 2 to 8 cm). Repair should be carried out under microscopic magnification of at least 10×. A 9–0 or 10–0 suture on a needle no larger than 135 μm in diameter is appropriate. The superiority of a group fascicular repair over an epineural repair remains unproven. However, with mixed nerves and distal lesions, in which the motor and sensory fascicles are more apt to be segregated in the nerve, an attempt at group fascicular repair seems prudent.

Peroneal Nerve

The peroneal nerve is the most commonly injured nerve in the lower extremity.[5] This is in part because of its outward lateral location in the leg and in part because of the particularly vulnerable nature of its anatomy. The peroneal nerve separates from the sciatic nerve

either just above or just below the piriform muscle. Proximally, the superior and inferior gluteal nerves arise from the peroneal division of the sciatic nerve and innervate the tensor fascia lata and the three gluteal muscles (i.e., the gluteus medius, gluteus minimis, and gluteus maximus). In the proximal thigh, the peroneal nerve lies on top of the short external rotators beneath the gluteus maximus. More distally the nerve passes under the origin of the long head of the biceps femoris. It then runs along the medial border of the short head of the biceps femoris to the knee. The only thigh muscle receiving innervation from the peroneal nerve is the short head of the biceps femoris. At the knee, the common peroneal nerve passes superficially around the neck of the fibula and under the origin of the peroneus longus, branching into the superficial peroneal and deep peroneal nerves. The deep peroneal nerve almost immediately gives off multiple branches to the muscles of the anterior and lateral compartments of the leg (the peroneus longus and brevis, extensor digitorum longus, tibialis anterior, extensor hallucis longus, and peroneus tertius, when present). The superficial peroneal nerve runs between the peroneal muscles and the extensor digitorum longus in the lateral compartment, piercing the compartment fascia several inches above the ankle. It then travels in the subcutaneous tissues of the distal leg and foot to provide sensation to the dorsal foot.

In the foot, the superficial peroneal nerve branches into the medial and intermediate dorsal cutaneous nerves of the foot. The dorsum of the foot (exclusive of the first web space, the lateral-most aspect, occasionally the medial aspect, and the dorsum of the toes distal to the proximal interphalangeal joints) is supplied by these two nerves. The lateral aspect of the foot is supplied by the lateral dorsal cutaneous nerve, a distal branch of the sural nerve. The medial aspect of the foot is often supplied to a large extent by the distal branch of the saphenous nerve. The first web space is supplied by the deep peroneal nerve. The dorsal innervation of the toes is analogous to that of the hand. The medial three and one-half toes are covered by the medial plantar nerve, and the lateral one and one-half toes are covered by the lateral plantar nerve.

Proximally, the deep peroneal nerve lies in the anterior compartment between the exten-

sor digitorum longus and the tibialis anterior. Distally, the deep peroneal nerve lies between the extensor hallucis longus and the tibialis anterior. The nerve passes under and lateral to the extensor hallucis longus and the extensor hallucis brevis in the ankle and foot. In the foot, this nerve usually provides the innervation to the extensor digitorum brevis, the extensor hallucis brevis, and the first dorsal interosseous muscle (Figs. 32–26 to 32–28; see also Figs. 32–20 and 32–21).

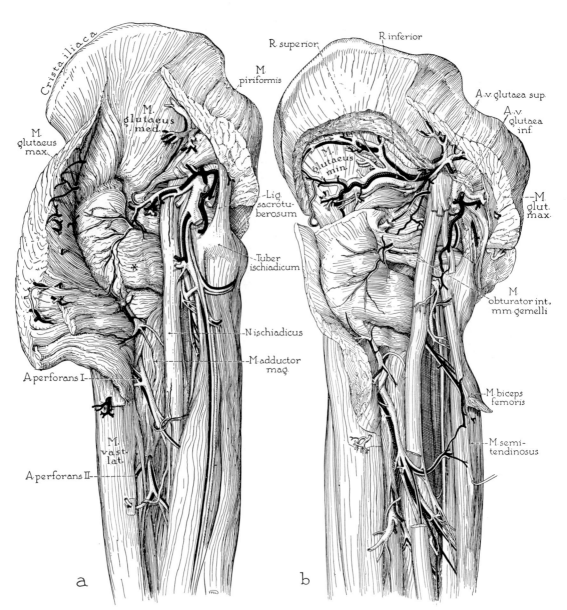

FIGURE 32–26. *(A and B),* Neural anatomy of the buttock and posterior thigh. (From Anson BJ: Atlas of Human Anatomy, Philadelphia, WB Saunders, 1950, p 477.)

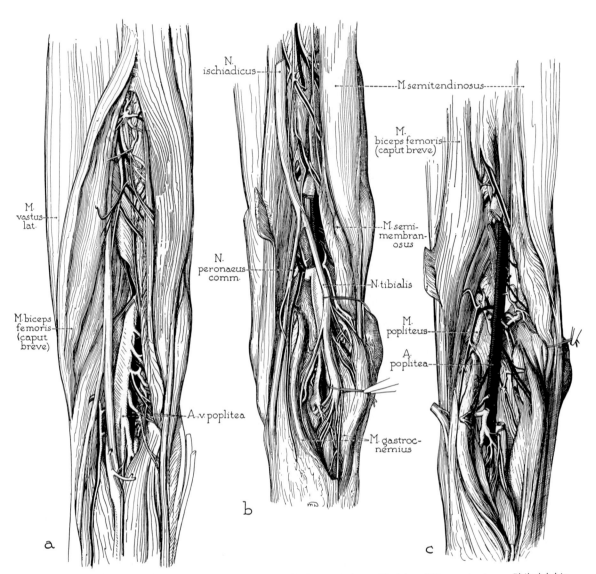

FIGURE 32–27. *(A to C)*, Neural anatomy of the posterior thigh. (From Anson BJ: Atlas of Human Anatomy, Philadelphia, WB Saunders, 1950, p 478.)

Mechanisms of Injury

The peroneal nerve may be injured at any point along its course, but it is particularly vulnerable as it courses around the neck of the fibula. Peroneal nerve injuries occur in up to 18 percent of knee dislocations.[169] Shelbourne and colleagues described four superior dislocations of the fibular head.[210] One of these patients developed a permanent peroneal nerve palsy. Acute injury to the peroneal nerve can also occur from wearing ski boots.[129] Entrapment of the superficial peroneal nerve in

fibular fracture callus has also been described after combined tibial and fibular fracture.[153]

A relatively common but unappreciated cause of peroneal nerve injury is inversion ankle sprains. At least 13 cases of clinically demonstrable peroneal nerve injuries after ankle inversion injuries have been described.[124, 148, 222] Several of these were severe enough to require footdrop bracing. Nitz and colleagues examined 66 consecutive ankle sprains with electromyography 2 weeks after injury to define the incidence of peroneal nerve injury.[165]

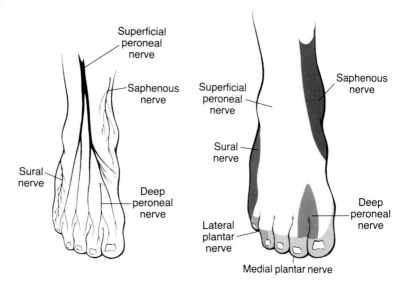

FIGURE 32–28. Sensory nerves of the foot dorsum.

Seventeen percent of grade II and 86 percent of grade III ankle sprains showed evidence of peroneal nerve injury. All the ankles with grade II lesions demonstrated normal peroneal nerve function by 2 weeks after injury. Ankle active range-of-motion and heel-toe walking were impaired for an average of 5 weeks in the grade III injury group. This recognition is particularly important in considering patients with recurrent ankle sprains for ligament reconstruction.

The major disability resulting from peroneal nerve injury is the footdrop associated with a loss of foot dorsiflexion. This palsy produces a steppage gait and often requires a brace for efficient ambulation. The ability to run or to walk with any increased speed is significantly hindered. The functional impairment to the lower extremity from a complete peroneal nerve palsy can be up to 38 percent.[7]

Treatment

Very little information is available on the results to be expected after peroneal nerve repair. It is known that lacerations have better results than do traction injuries. The largest series of peroneal nerve repairs, 72 common peroneal nerve repairs, was reported by Seddon.[203] Seventy-four percent obtained sensory recovery. Only 35 percent of the repairs resulted in correction of the footdrop. However, better results with recent microsurgical techniques have been described in small series.[85, 109] Early repair within 72 hours for complete fifth-degree Sunderland injuries is recommended for young individuals.

Tibial Nerve

The tibial nerve makes up the other half of the sciatic nerve and is also known as the medial popliteal nerve. In the hip region, the tibial component of the sciatic nerve innervates the obturator internus and the quadratus femoris. It follows a course in the thigh just medial to the peroneal nerve in the same muscle plane. It innervates all of the hamstring muscles coming from the ischial tuberosity (the long head of the biceps femoris, the semitendinosus, and the semimembranosus), as well as the adductor magnus. The tibial nerve lies just under the popliteal fascia in the knee, passing superficial to the plantaris and popliteus below the knee. It then passes beneath the soleus arch with the popliteal vessels. The tibial nerve lies in the deep posterior compartment of the leg superficial to the tibialis posterior and between the flexor digitorum longus and the flexor hallucis longus. In the leg, the tibial nerve innervates all of the muscles of the deep posterior compartment (popliteus, tibialis posterior, flexor digitorum longus, and flexor hallucis longus) and the superficial posterior compartment (plantaris, gastrocnemius, and soleus).

The tibial nerve again becomes superficial at the ankle, where it passes around the medial malleolus just under the skin. The nerve then travels under the flexor retinaculum and over the calcaneus (the tarsal canal) until it enters the foot passing under the origin of the abductor hallucis muscle. Just proximal to or within the tarsal canal, the tibial nerve sends a medial calcaneal branch to the sole of the foot. The tibial nerve then branches into the medial and lateral plantar nerves within the tarsal canal. The medial and lateral plantar nerves lie in the midfoot deep to the flexor digitorum brevis, abductor hallucis, and abductor digiti minimi but superficial to the quadratus plantae and long toe flexors (flexor digitorum longus and flexor hallucis longus). More distally in the foot, the flexor hallucis brevis, adductor hallucis, and flexor digiti minimi lie just deep to these nerves. All of the plantar muscles (including the interosseous muscles, with the exception of the first) are innervated by the tibial nerve. The medial plantar nerve innervates the abductor hallucis, flexor digitorum brevis, flexor hallucis brevis, and second toe lumbrical muscle. The lateral plantar nerve generally innervates the rest. Most sensory supply to the sole of the foot is provided by the tibial nerve. Additional innervation is provided medially by the saphenous nerve and laterally by the sural nerve (see Fig. 32–20, 32–21, and 32–26 to 32–28).

Mechanisms of Injury

The tibial nerve is superficial and vulnerable to injury at three places in the lower extremity. It is superficial just distal to the gluteal fold before it passes under the hamstrings. It is superficial in the popliteal fossa and again at the medial ankle and hindfoot. The nerve is further at risk because of its plantar location and the risk of plantar laceration. In addition to being vulnerable to trauma, the tibial nerve and its branches are vulnerable to iatrogenic injury associated with ankle and hindfoot surgery.

The major disability with tibial nerve injury is its combined sensory and motor effects on the sole of the foot. Loss of tibial innervation results in an asensate sole aggravated by the loss of support and padding secondary to paralysis and atrophy of the intrinsic muscles of the foot. This can be further aggravated by an intrinsic foot deformity (clawtoes with prominent metatarsals secondary to the clawing and loss of the transverse arch). Added to this may be a progressive planovalgus deformity secondary to an associated tibialis posterior palsy. The final result may be chronic ulceration, infection, and eventual amputation. Seddon reported that 14 percent of his patients with tibial palsies developed foot ulcers, most of which appeared within 2 years.[203] The lower extremity impairment for a complete tibial nerve injury above the knee is 45 percent, and it is 28 percent for a complete injury below the midcalf.[7] A medial or lateral plantar nerve injury alone has a 10-percent impairment.

Treatment

As is the case with peroneal nerve repair, there is a paucity of information on the results of tibial nerve repair. Seddon reported the results of tibial nerve repair in 47 patients.[203] Sixty-two percent had sensory recovery, and 79 percent had functional motor recovery. The results after replantation of the foot imply that even better results are being obtained with present techniques. However, the hyperesthesias often seen with reinnervation can be a particular problem with repair of the tibial nerve. This problem has been noted by Seddon,[203] Kline and Kahn,[110] and Aldea and Shaw.[5] Seddon noted this problem in 67 percent of his ankle-level nerve injuries and warned that the sole hyperesthesias associated with repair might be more incapacitating than the anesthesia of the injury. Kline and Kahn warned against the risk of converting a relatively asymptomatic ambulatory patient into a nonambulatory patient with a hyperesthetic sole. Aldea and Shaw noted a tendency for this hyperesthesia to abate within 1 to 2 years after replantation. A careful examination to delineate the depth of the sensory defect after tibial nerve injury with intact saphenous and sural nerves is mandatory. The risks of no repair probably outweigh the risks of surgery in the young. However, the decision for surgery must be entertained more cautiously in a patient older than 30 years of age who has injuries at and above the ankle.

Sciatic Nerve

With respect to both sensory and motor functions, the sciatic nerve is the major nerve for the leg and foot. The function of all muscles below the knee and the sensation of the entire leg and foot are dependent on the sciatic nerve, with the exception of the medial foot and shin. This area is innervated by the saphenous branch of the femoral nerve. The anatomy of this nerve was discussed previously in the section on the peroneal and tibial nerves.

Mechanisms of Injury

The sciatic nerve remains at risk throughout an individual's life. In infancy, it is at risk secondary to gluteal injections. At least 93 cases of sciatic nerve injury in children secondary to gluteal injections have been reported in the literature.[20, 187, 229] Untreated, these injuries can lead to cavovarus, calcaneocavus, and ankle equinus deformities of the foot.[20] Robert emphasized the importance of early neurolysis in the treatment of these lesions.[187] Of 23 sciatic paralyses secondary to injection, he obtained satisfactory results in 78 percent after neurolysis. In the 22 percent in whom neurolysis failed, three of five had a direct needle prick injury to the nerve. These results contrast with 29-percent full recovery and 58-percent partial recovery in patients treated with reconstructive efforts directed at late-occurring deformities secondary to sciatic nerve injection injuries in childhood.[229] In the young adult, the sciatic nerve is mainly at risk for injury from traumatic hip injuries, which are usually associated with motor vehicle accidents. Sciatic nerve palsies can be seen in 13 percent of posterior hip dislocations and fracture-dislocations.[169] In older groups, the sciatic nerve is again at risk with total hip arthroplasty. This risk has been reported to be 0.6 percent.[217] The lower extremity impairment for complete sciatic nerve palsy is 81 percent.[7]

Treatment

The results of sciatic nerve repair are not unexpectedly poor relative to the results of repair of the other peripheral nerves. Anticipated useful recovery is estimated at 30 percent for the peroneal portion and at 50 percent for the tibial portion of the sciatic nerve.[109] The results for clean-cut, or guillotine-type, injuries are somewhat better. Kline and Kahn reported the return of useful tibial motor and sensory functions after primary repair of complete sciatic transections.[110] Partial recovery of foot dorsiflexion was noted in two of the four patients.

For complete sciatic palsies, the disability is severe and the prognosis poor. I recommend early surgical intervention for all complete sciatic palsies. I advocate neurolysis for complete lesions-in-continuity. The surgeon should be prepared to evaluate the nerve with intraoperative electrodiagnostic techniques when surgical intervention is delayed. Resection and primary repair or grafting should be carried out for nonfunctioning fascicles.

Sensory Nerves of the Foot Dorsum

Sensation to the dorsum of the foot is supplied by the superficial and deep peroneal nerves, the terminal saphenous nerve, and the sural nerve (see Fig. 32–28). A separate note regarding injuries to these nerves seems warranted. As noted earlier in the discussion of tendon injuries to the dorsum of the foot, Floyd and colleagues noted a 60-percent incidence of scar complaints with dorsal traumatic lacerations. The sensory superficial peroneal and sural nerves have also been described in entrapment syndromes secondary to encasement in fracture callus.[64, 153] The same nerves are subject to boot injuries with entrapment-type syndromes.[129, 200]

The foot dorsum is also subject to iatrogenic nerve injury with reconstructive foot surgery. Kliman and Freiberg reported a 14-percent incidence of cutaneous nerve injury with the excision of foot ganglia in 21 cases.[108] Meier and Kenzora reported a 30-percent incidence of cutaneous nerve injury with 72 bunion procedures; more than one-half of these injuries were highly symptomatic.[149] Noyez and Martens reported a 32-percent incidence of sural nerve injury with Chrisman-Snook lateral ligament reconstruction of the ankle.[166] The superficial location of these nerves, as well as the lack of intervening muscle between these nerves and the underlying bone, makes them particularly prone to symptomatic neuroma formation. This is aggravated by the social custom of wearing shoes and the resultant added pressure over these nerves, particularly with the more fashionable women's shoes.

Kenzora emphasized the point that neuromas are easier to prevent than to treat.[102] He reviewed 27 surgical procedures in 37 patients who had 55 symptomatic sensory neuromas of the foot. Neurolysis for neuromas-in-continuity was successful in only two of four neuromas. Twenty-three neuromas were treated with proximal resection. Only 13 of the 23 (56 percent) obtained good results, and another four (17 percent) obtained fair results. Sensory nerves of the foot should be repaired with fine microsutures using the same meticulous techniques and magnification recommended in the hand.

TRAUMATIC INJURIES TO THE INTEGUMENT OF THE FOOT AND ANKLE

Coverage problems about the foot and ankle may arise because of the limited mobility of the overlying integument, the weight-bearing requirements of this structure, and the absence of intervening muscle between the skeletal elements and the integument over much of this structure. This lack of intervening muscle means that wounds often result in exposure of tendons, bone, or nerves where loss of the respective peritenon, periosteum, or epineurium precludes skin grafting. Coverage can be further complicated by vascular disease, peripheral neuropathies, or both involving the lower extremities. High-energy injuries with associated open fractures can also complicate the treatment of foot and ankle coverage problems.

Avulsion injuries of the foot and ankle are commonly associated with motorcycle injuries. These injuries are usually associated with the rider's catching a foot, usually the right, in the rear-wheel assembly while using poor protective footwear.[39] Major open injuries to the foot and ankle can result from motor vehicle accidents, falls, attempted suicidal leaps, gunshot wounds, lawn mower injuries, and industrial crush injuries. More than 40 separate procedures are recommended for treating wounds of the foot and ankle not amenable to primary closure or skin grafting. These include local, distant, and free tissue transfers. These transfers can be of muscle, myocutaneous, fasciocutaneous, or fascial flaps. Both random- and axial-pattern flaps are described, and the transferred flap can be innervated or denervated. Before the appropriate procedure can be chosen, several factors regarding the wound and the patient must be delineated. A useful classification of the potential flaps based on the size of the wound, the difficulty and complications of the procedure, the reliability of the graft, coverage of donor defects, the potential

TABLE 32–3. WOUND CLASSIFICATION BY ANATOMIC SITE
Forefoot
Heel pad and calcaneus
Achilles tendon and posterior calcaneus
Ankle

for providing sensate coverage, and anatomic location then assists in the flap choice.

Wound Classification

The first stage in planning the reconstructive procedure is defining the wound. Anatomically, the wound should be defined as involving the ankle, distal Achilles tendon and posterior calcaneus, heel pad and calcaneus, dorsal or plantar forefoot, or a combination of these areas (Table 32–3). Anatomic localization defines the weight-bearing status of the area as well as available local transfer options.

The next step is defining the size of the wound (Table 32–4). This size is that portion of the wound that can not be managed by skin grafting and should be expressed in centimeters. A very small wound is less than 2×2 cm. A small wound is from 2×2 to 4×5 cm. A medium wound is from 4×5 to 7×7 cm. A large wound is from 7×7 to 10×20 cm, and a very large wound is from 10×20 to 15×40 cm.

The arterial, neurologic, and skeletal status of the foot should then be defined. Does the patient have protective sensation in the posterior tibial nerve over the weight-bearing portions of the foot if they are present? If not, is the nerve reconstructible? Are the other major nerves of the foot intact (i.e., the superficial peroneal, saphenous, and sural nerves)? The

TABLE 32–4. WOUND CLASSIFICTION BY SIZE	
Very small	$< 2 \times 2$ cm
Small	2×2–4×5 cm
Medium	4×5–7×7 cm
Large	7×7–10×20 cm
Very large	10×20–15×40 cm

arterial status of the foot proper can be determined most readily by ultrasonic Doppler examination using an 8-MHz vascular probe. Examination of the dorsalis pedis pulse with Doppler ultrasonography while the dorsalis pedis artery is occluded manually proximal to the Doppler probe will detect posterior tibial artery flow with patent communications between the deep arches of the foot and the dorsal circulation. The dorsalis pedis pulse should be followed into the forefoot with manual occlusion of the posterior tibial artery. Similarly, a good posterior tibial artery pulse with occlusion of the posterior tibial artery proximal to the Doppler probe implies good circulation through the forefoot communications. Capillary refill should be observed in the toes with sequential occlusion of the posterior tibial and dorsalis pedis arteries. Occasionally, contrast arteriography is necessary. The skeletal injury, the likelihood of loss of normal motion with resultant changes in foot biomechanics, and the need for future bone grafting or fusion procedures, as well as the expected duration of immobilization, should then be defined. The degree of crush or secondary injury to related areas of the foot should also be estimated to determine if local tissues will be suitable for transfer.

The infectious status of the wound should also be defined. Is the wound sterile, grossly infected, contaminated, or colonized? Is osteomyelitis present or likely to occur? Basic principles of treatment include radical débridement of nonviable tissues, appropriate antibiotic coverage based on culture results and sensitivities from the wound, and effective dead-space management. Dead-space management may be by obliteration with viable muscle, by implantation of antibiotic-impregnated polymethyl methacrylate beads, or by grafting of cancellous bone.

Patient Classification

Once the wound problem has been adequately identified, several factors regarding the patient must be delineated (Table 32–5). Associated injuries and medical illnesses (in particular, diabetes mellitus and significant atherosclerosis) should be noted. The age of the patient is a significant factor. Although reconstructive microsurgical procedures can be used in children,[87] they are less reliable in this group

TABLE 32–5. PATIENT CLASSIFICATION
Age
Systemic compromise
Local compromise
Occupation
Cosmetic concerns
Tobacco use
Rehabilitation potential
Vascular disease

because of their smaller vessel size (especially under 2 years of age) and their increased potential for postoperative vasospasm. However, children are able to tolerate immobilization without serious threat of contracture development.[161] The functional results after free tissue transfer are also better in patients younger than 40 years of age. Gidumal and colleagues, in reviewing the functional results in 16 patients with nonsensate free flap coverage of weight-bearing portions of the foot, found good results in 70 percent. However, in patients younger than 40 years of age, 92 percent (12 of 13) had good or excellent results.

The patient's occupation and tolerance for lost time from work associated with rehabilitation, further surgery, and healing should also be delineated. The feelings of the patient and his or her family about amputation should be explored, and realistic expectations of the projected cosmesis and function should be discussed. The patient's use of tobacco products and willingness to give them up are significant factors in planning elective microsurgery.

Classification of Coverage Options

General Considerations

For non–weight-bearing areas of the foot and ankle where there is no exposure of tendons, nerves, or bone, skin grafting is the usual procedure of choice. Local random-pattern transposition flaps have limited value in the foot and ankle, particularly over the plantar surface.[133] When this type of flap is used, it should be proximally based, and the width-to-length ratio should be equal to or greater than 1:1. Care should be taken in designing any local random-pattern flap to avoid sacrificing the potential for other procedures if the local transpositional flap fails. It is generally agreed that skin grafts are inadequate for weight-bearing areas and will be subject to chronic breakdown. The possible exception to this general belief is in the treatment of children (Fig. 32–29). Children are relatively resistant to breakdown over skin grafts.[77] Furthermore, in a small child, skin grafting can serve as a temporizing procedure. Contracture in the graft will decrease the size of the soft tissue defect in time.

There is some debate about whether well-vascularized flaps in weight-bearing areas require sensation to prevent chronic breakdown. Wood and colleagues stated that reinnervation is not necessary for success.[247] May and colleagues performed clinical and gait analyses of nine individuals who had weight-bearing surfaces of the foot covered with free muscle flaps, which were covered with split-thickness skin grafts.[146] They had ulceration in two patients, only one case of which was chronic. They attributed the chronic ulceration to flap redundancy. Their mean follow-up was more than 19 months. Gidumal and colleagues reviewed 16 of 27 patients who had nonsensate free flaps transferred to the sole of the foot.[59] These individuals had a variety of flaps, including groin, tensor fascia lata, and latissimus flaps. Sixty-three percent of their patients had a history of skin ulceration, and 33 percent had ulceration at the time of follow-up examination. Given these data, it appears that when practical, a sensate or reinnervated flap is preferable over weight-bearing wounds. This is particularly true when a patient has little or no access to good protective orthotic devices.

The potential function of the extremity with free tissue reconstruction should also be considered.[59, 146, 205] It is to be expected that well over 90 percent of patients with traumatic below-knee amputations will ambulate with prosthetic rehabilitation. May and colleagues studied 18 patients with free flaps over their feet, nine of which were over weight-bearing areas, with footprint Harris mat analysis and footprint force plate analysis.[146] Mean follow-up was 19.3 months. Analysis of this subgroup revealed several factors. All patients were ambulatory without aids, although they walked slower than normal. The amount of time spent on the resurfaced foot equalled that spent on the contralateral, normal foot. The amounts of vertical and shear force were also approximately the same. The rate of rise and the peak amount of vertical force, as well as the maximum fore-aft and medial-lateral shear forces, were less than normal in both feet.

A similar study was performed by Gidumal and colleagues with detailed gait analysis.[59] They used an objective and a subjective rating scale to evaluate 16 patients with nonsensate free flap coverage of weight-bearing surfaces. They reported good functional results in 70 percent of the whole group and excellent and good results in 92 percent of patients under 40 years of age. Combined ankle and forefoot problems were associated with poorer results. Gait velocity for the whole group (68.6 m/min)

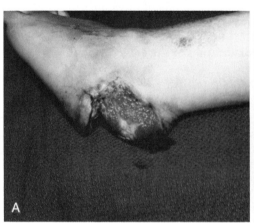
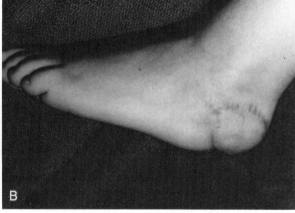

FIGURE 32–29. *(A)*, A 4-year-old boy suffered this large heel pad avulsion in a motor scooter injury. *(B)*, Coverage with full-thickness skin grafts has provided stable coverage with a Plastizote insert for 2 years. Contracture of the graft has decreased the wound size and expanded other coverage options.

was slightly less than that for patients with traumatic below-knee amputations (71 m/min). Normal gait velocity is 83 m/min. Thirty-one percent of the patients returned to their original job. Forty-four percent changed to a new job because of their injury. Twenty-five percent were unemployed, retired, or disabled.

Reported success rates for free tissue transfers to the foot and ankle are 92 percent (12 flaps),[12] 90 percent (10 flaps),[247] 100 percent (five flaps),[1] 100 percent (seven flaps),[194] and 100 percent (18 flaps).[146] For a total of 52 flaps, this represents a 96-percent success rate. This rate is comparable to the 92-percent success rate (11 of 12 flaps with one partial loss) reported for cross-leg fasciocutaneous flaps.[14]

Coverage Options

It is useful to classify flap options according to the difficulty of the procedure and the surgical expertise necessary (Table 32–6). Other considerations are the potential to provide sensate coverage, donor defects, the necessity of skin grafting in the donor defect, the need for immobilization, and the potential for neuromata formation at the donor site. Flaps are thus classified as local transpositional flaps (Table 32–7); island pedicle flaps, either proximally or distally based (Table 32–8); distant pedicle flaps (Table 32–9); or free flaps (Table 32–10). Flaps are further subclassified as muscle, fascial, fasciocutaneous, or myocutaneous. These subdivisions are discussed in the appropriate sections.

Distant pedicle and free flaps are indicated when local flap options are not available because of the size of the wound or because of associated local wound injuries. Free flaps[111] are usually preferred to distant pedicle flaps because of the required immobilization and

TABLE 32–6. **FLAP TYPES**
Local transpositional
Local island pedicle
Distant pedicle
Free tissue

risk of contracture development with use of the latter. This preference is sometimes overridden in children and in patients in whom free flap coverage is inappropriate.

The list of available donors for free flaps is limited only by the surgeon's imagination. However, every surgeon has a set of flaps with which he or she is proficient. This proficiency should take precedence over any theoretical advantage of one flap over another. The only rational exceptions are those made to obtain reinnervation potential, as discussed earlier, or to meet size requirements. Accordingly, several free flap options are listed in Table 32–10 with a brief description of their size limits and their potential for reinnervation.

Specific Flap Options

Forefoot

Most integumental problems in the forefoot result from neuropathic diseases and foot malalignments. Only a small proportion of these problems are secondary to trauma. Fortunately, the prognosis for those secondary to trauma is much better. Preferred flap options for this area are listed in Table 32–11.

Very Small to Small Lesions

Very small (less than 2 × 2 cm) and small (2 × 2 to 4 × 5 cm) lesions frequently occur

TABLE 32–7. **LOCAL TRANSPOSITIONAL FLAPS**		
FLAP	**SITE**	**SIZE**
V-Y transpositional	Forefoot, heel	Very small to small
Flexor hallucis brevis	Forefoot	Very small
Abductor hallucis	Forefoot, ankle	Very small
Abductor digiti minimi	Forefoot, ankle	Very small
Flexor digitorum brevis	Forefoot, heel	Very small to small
Soleus (distally based)	Ankle, Achilles tendon	Very small to small
Lateral calcaneal	Heel, Achilles tendon, lateral ankle	Very small to small
Peroneus brevis	Lateral ankle	Very small to small

TABLE 32–8. LOCAL ISLAND PEDICLE FLAPS

FLAP	SITE	SIZE
Neurovascular toe	Forefoot, heel	Very small to small
Extensor digitorum brevis	Forefoot, ankle	Very small to small
Dorsalis pedis	All	Small to medium
Lateral supramalleolar	Ankle, heel, Achilles tendon	Small to medium
Lateral plantar	Forefoot	Very small to medium
Medial plantar	Forefoot, heel	Small to medium
Peroneal artery	Ankle, Achilles tendon, heel	Small to very large

over the plantar surfaces of the metatarsals. Local transpositional (see Table 32–7) and pedicle island options (see Table 32–8) exist for this level. Distant pedicle and free flaps are usually contraindicated for lesions of this size at this location.

Local transpositional options for this area include double V-Y fasciocutaneous flaps, the distally based abductor digiti quinti flap, and the distally based flexor hallucis brevis flap. The V-Y flap procedure is the simplest and can be used for any metacarpal head or the calcaneus. Colen and colleagues reported 100-percent survival in 38 cases involving 34 diabetics.[34] Twenty-seven percent of their patients had pinprick sensation. This was retained in all flaps after transposition. They had three recurrences. This flap is based on the plantar fascial skin perforators and is mobilized by division of the plantar fascia. Defects of 1.5 to 4.0 cm can be closed with this technique.

A distally based abductor digiti quinti muscle flap was described by Yoshimura and colleagues for coverage over the fifth metatarsal region.[251] This flap requires division of the proximal lateral plantar artery for mobilization. The authors described the use of this flap

for thermal injury secondary to frostbite. Ger described a similar flap for the first metatarsal head that uses a distally based flexor hallucis brevis.[56, 57] He has used this flap successfully in diabetics. The medial plantar artery is not divided.

Island pedicle options for injuries of this size include distally based medial and lateral plantar artery fasciocutaneous flaps[33] and digital neurovascular fillet flaps. Morain described the use of eight plantar island toe flaps for the treatment of neurotrophic ulcers of the foot and ankle.[156] Wounds from 2 × 2 cm to 6 × 8 cm were covered with these flaps. The skeletal elements of the donor toe are excised, and the dorsal skin is used for coverage of the

TABLE 32–9. DISTANT PEDICLE FLAPS

FLAP	SENSATE	SIZE
Cross-leg sural	+	Small to medium
Cross-leg tensor fascia lata	+	Medium to large
Cross-leg fasciocutaneous	−	Small to large
Cross-leg thigh	−	Small to large

+, yes; −, no.

TABLE 32—10. SELECT FREE FLAPS

FLAP	SENSATE	SIZE
Medial plantar	+	Small to medium
Dorsalis pedis	+	Small to medium
Posterior brachial	+	Small to medium
Peroneal artery	−	Small to large
Lateral brachial	+	Small to medium
Saphenous	+	Small to large
Gracilis	−	Small to medium
Radial forearm	+	Small to large
Latissimus	−	Small to very large
Groin	−/+	Medium to very large
Scapular	−	Small to large
Deltoid	+	Small to very large
Posterior calf fasciocutaneous	−	Small to very large
Temporoparietal	−	Small to large
Tensor fascia lata	−/+	Medium to very large

+, yes; −, no; −/+, potential for reinnervation is variable.

TABLE 32–11. FOREFOOT FLAPS (AUTHOR'S PREFERENCE)	
SIZE	**FLAP**
Very small	V-Y transpositional
Small	Flexor digitorum brevis
Medium	Medial plantar artery
Large	Free tissue
Very large	Free tissue

donor defect. The greatest arc of rotation and the largest flap are unfortunately obtained from the great toe. A distally based lateral plantar artery island flap incorporating the flexor digitorum brevis muscle was described by Sakai and colleagues for coverage of a 3 × 5-cm lateral metatarsal head defect.[196] Amarante and colleagues described the use of a distally based medial plantar artery island pedicle fasciocutaneous flap for coverage over the first metatarsophalangeal joint.[6] They previously used the same type of flap, but proximally based, as a cross-foot flap.

Both the V-Y flap and the distally based flexor hallucis brevis flap can be elevated simply, without risk to the remaining vasculature of the foot. The V-Y flap is more reliable, but the flexor hallucis brevis has the advantage of bringing muscle into the area and allowing dead-space obliteration. The distally based abductor digiti quinti, medial plantar,[33] and lateral plantar[33] flaps all require division of one of the plantar vessels. However, they may be more reliable than the flexor hallucis brevis flap. The plantar island toe flaps provide good sensate, stable coverage, as well as revascularization of the wound, without any risk to the vasculature of the foot but at the loss of a toe.

Medium-Sized Lesions

Medium-sized wounds are 4 × 5 to 7 × 7 cm in size. No local transpositional options are available for wounds of this size at this level. The distally based medial and lateral plantar artery flaps discussed previously usually cover defects of this size, but they are often inappropriate because of possible disruption of the distal arterial arches. Creating another large defect on the plantar surface is also relatively contraindicated. If the dorsalis pedis artery still has good retrograde flow from the poste-

rior tibial artery, a distally based dorsalis pedis island myofasciocutaneous flap or extensor digitorum brevis muscle flap[122] can be used. The dorsalis pedis flap has the advantage of reinnervation potential. If the use of these pedicle flaps is not possible or is inappropriate, reconstruction with distant tissue is necessary. These options are discussed in the following section.

Large to Very Large Lesions

Large (7 × 7 to 10 × 20 cm) to very large (10 × 20 to 15 × 40 cm) wounds of the forefoot as well as many medium-sized (4 × 5 to 7 × 7 cm) wounds require distant tissues for reconstruction. In children and in patients in whom free flaps are inappropriate or rejected, there are several distant pedicle flap staged reconstruction options (see Table 32–9).[8, 14, 47, 86, 162, 233] All of these procedures require two operations. The cross-leg sural flap[8] is limited in size (approximately 3.5 × 9.5 cm) but allows reinnervation by division of the sural nerve at the time of flap division (generally 3 weeks) and suture to a recipient nerve in the foot. The tensor fascia lata cross-leg flap[162] also allows reinnervation with the lateral femoral cutaneous nerve. This flap covers defects up to 14 × 25 cm. The cross-leg fasciocutaneous[14] and the cross-leg thigh[86] pedicle flaps allow coverage of defects similar in size to those covered with the tensor fascia lata flap but without the potential for reinnervation in most cases. The cross-leg thigh and the cross-leg tensor fascia lata flaps are relatively contraindicated in adults because of the immobilization in acute knee flexion required with their use.

In considering free tissue transfer options, the best substitute should approximate the tissues lost as closely as possible. This is particularly important over the weight-bearing areas of the plantar surface of the foot (i.e., the metatarsal heads, heel pad, and lateral midfoot). When possible, sensate coverage should be considered if weight-bearing areas are involved. The only tissue that meets all of these requirements is a medial plantar artery free flap from the arch of the contralateral foot.[158] This flap is limited to medium-sized defects. It reproduces the specialized septate configuration of the plantar integument and has the potential for reinnervation. However, use of this flap requires sacrificing the tibialis posterior artery of the uninjured foot in most instances. The intraneural dissection necessary to separate the digital nerve supply from that to the flap can be tedious. The contralateral foot requires skin grafting and immobilization, adding to the initial disability of the patient. It can be argued that this flap should be limited to areas in which chronic ulceration has been demonstrated after other techniques. The dorsalis pedis free flap[48] offers easier nerve dissection with a considerable pedicle but has many of the same drawbacks of the medial plantar artery flap.

Other free flaps with which reinnervation is possible include the radial forearm,[73, 74, 214] deltoid,[195] posterior arm,[141] saphenous,[69, 167] lateral arm,[132, 199] and lateral intercostal[12] free flaps. The saphenous and posterior arm flaps are limited to medium-sized wounds. The groin[205] and the medial arm[167] flaps are omitted from this list because of the variable vascular anatomy. For a surgeon accustomed to these flaps, this omission is of course inappropriate. Other nonsensate free flap options are listed in Table 32–10.[84, 134, 182, 189, 246]

Forefoot Dorsum

The dorsal forefoot can present some unexpected problems. Very small to small defects over the dorsum can be covered by the distally based extensor digitorum brevis muscle flap, and small to medium defects can be covered by the distally based dorsalis pedis myofasciocutaneous flap. However, both of these flaps become useless if the dorsalis pedis collateral circulation from the deep arch to the flap is disrupted. Very small wounds, if laterally situated, can be covered by the distally based abductor digiti quinti muscle flap discussed earlier. Similar wounds, if medially situated, can be covered by the distally based abductor hallucis muscle flap. Both of these flaps require division of the respective pedicle proximally, but otherwise they have minimal effects on the plantar foot. The applicable wound size can be increased to include small wounds and wounds on the lower end of the medium range (up to 5 × 7 cm) by incorporating the flexor digitorum brevis muscle with one of these pedicles.[81] The distally based medial and lateral plantar artery fasciocutaneous flaps allow coverage up to 7 × 13 cm but with a loss of plantar skin that might well be considered inappropriate relative to other options. Very proximal small to medium-sized wounds can

be covered by the lateral supramalleolar flap[45, 140, 142] discussed in the later section on ankle wounds.

For most medium to very large dorsal forefoot wounds requiring flap coverage, the dorsalis pedis artery is no longer functional through the forefoot. Distant pedicle or free flap coverage is necessary, as discussed previously, for large to very large forefoot lesions. A sensate flap is not generally believed to be necessary over the dorsal forefoot. A flap with the capability of carrying live bone might be indicated. This could include the radial forearm,[73, 74, 214] groin,[167] or peroneal artery[67, 68, 250] flap.

Heel Pad and Calcaneus

The heel pad and calcaneus represent an area of great concern with regard to coverage problems of the foot. The integument is highly specialized and difficult to replace. Normal ambulation cannot occur without significant stresses being placed across this area, and chronic ulceration is a well-recognized problem. Furthermore, the risk of impending calcaneal osteomyelitis and its inherent problems forever looms over the scene. This area is commonly injured in trauma and neuropathic conditions. The need for sensate coverage was discussed earlier under the section on general considerations. Preferred flap options are listed in Table 32–12.

Very Small to Small Lesions

Very small (less than 2 × 2 cm) to small (2 × 2 to 4 × 5 cm) lesions of the plantar hindfoot are most frequently a problem with neuropathic diseases, particularly diabetes mellitus. For defects of up to 4 cm, a V-Y

TABLE 32–12. HEEL FLAPS (AUTHOR'S PREFERENCE)	
SIZE	**FLAP**
Very small	Flexor digitorum brevis transpositional
Small	Medial plantar artery
Medium	Medial plantar artery
Large	Free tissue or peroneal artery
Very large	Free tissue or peroneal artery

local transpositional flap[34, 35] provides stable coverage. Durability should be good, and sensation, if present, should be retained. The procedure is technically easy, but revascularization of the wound is relatively absent, as is the potential to obliterate any real dead space. An alternative transpositional muscle flap that gives good potential for dead-space management as well a revascularization of the wound is the flexor digitorum brevis muscle flap.[81, 144, 220] This flap covers defects of up to 5 × 7 cm but requires skin grafting and provides no sensation. In an asensate foot, this of course is not a consideration. The skin graft may not be as durable as the plantar skin used for the V-Y transpositional flap or some of the pedicle flaps listed later. Either of these flaps provides technically simple coverage of a smaller defect.

A neurovascular island toe flap[156] using either the great toe or a small toe allows coverage of defects approaching 2 × 2 to 6 × 8 cm in this area. The great toe island flap is raised on the medial plantar artery and can cover defects of up to several centimeters. Elevation of the small toe flap requires division of the plantar artery distally in the deep arterial arch. Either procedure results in the loss of a toe. Either provides a well-vascularized and durable reconstruction in which sensation, if present, is retained. An alternative that provides reconstruction of a similar quality (i.e., a reconstruction of a similar integumental structure that is sensate, durable, and well vascularized) is the proximally based medial plantar artery fasciocutaneous flap.[29, 126, 183, 209, 213] This flap is elevated as an island and is rotated 180 degrees to cover the defect. The nerves to the flap can be separated from the digital nerves and included for immediate sensation. If needed, the flexor digitorum brevis muscle can be incorporated in the flap. The donor defect will require skin grafting. Defects of up to 7 × 13 cm can be covered with this flap. The flap margins, however, should leave intact coverage over the metatarsal heads and lateral midfoot.

Medium-Sized Lesions

Medium-sized lesions of the heel pad region are from 4 × 5 to 7 × 7 cm in size. There are no transpositional options. The ideal transfer for this area, when possible, is the medial plantar artery fasciocutaneous flap (Fig. 32–30).[29, 126, 183, 209, 213] If this option is not possible, a proximally based dorsalis pedis island pedicle fasciocutaneous flap[63, 70] is another option that can provide sensate coverage. Of course, the tibialis anterior circulation to the foot is lost, and this flap would be inappropriate if the tibialis posterior artery was damaged. Nonsensate coverage can be obtained from a peroneal artery[67, 68, 250] or lateral supramalleolar[45, 140, 142] island pedicle flap. The peroneal artery flap has the greatest range of transfer, but the arterial anatomy is variable enough that preoperative evaluation with arteriography is mandatory.[225]

Large to Very Large Lesions

Lesions over the heel pad of greater than 7 × 7 cm can rarely be managed by local flap options. The statements regarding distant pedicle flaps and free flaps under the earlier sections on general considerations and large to very large lesions of the forefoot apply to this area.

Distal Achilles Tendon and Posterior Calcaneus

Wound coverage problems in the area of the distal Achilles tendon and posterior calcaneus are generally traumatic or iatrogenic and are often associated with surgery for Achilles tendon ruptures. Lesions are rarely larger than a few centimeters. Reconstruction can nevertheless often be elusive. Delay in coverage can result in desiccation of the Achilles tendon; necrosis; and infection, rupture, or both. Prompt attention to wounds in this area is a key point in any successful reconstructive effort. Preferred flap options are listed in Table 32–13.

TABLE 32–13. ACHILLES TENDON FLAPS (AUTHOR'S PREFERENCE)	
SIZE	**FLAP**
Very small	Lateral calcaneal transpositional
Small	Lateral calcaneal transpositional
Medium	Peroneal artery
Large	Free tissue or peroneal artery
Very large	Free tissue or peroneal artery

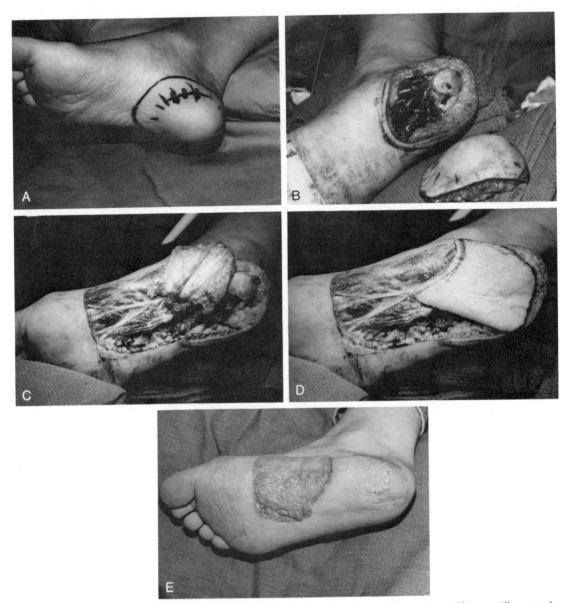

FIGURE 32–30. *(A),* A 20-year-old woman with a symptomatic recurrent sclerosing hemangioma. This case illustrates the potential of a medial plantar artery flap. *(B),* The medium-sized to large defect after excision. *(C),* Dissection of a medial plantar artery fasciocutaneous pedicle flap with inclusion of the nerves to the flap through intraneural dissection. *(D),* A 180-degree rotation of the flap. *(E),* The 6-month follow-up. The patient wears normal shoes and ambulates without a limp or breakdown. The sensation is equal to that of the opposite, normal heel.

Very Small to Small Lesions

Most lesions of the distal Achilles tendon and posterior calcaneus will be very small to small lesions (i.e., less than 4 × 5 cm). The use of distally based soleus and hemisoleus muscle flaps[9, 143, 228] has been suggested as a way of dealing with these problems. The intramuscular vascular anatomy is variable, and the viability of this procedure is difficult if not impossible to predict preoperatively. Partial muscle loss can occur in up to 50 percent of transfers.[228] Skin grafting should probably be delayed until muscle survival is ensured, thus necessitating two procedures.

A flap specifically suited for this area is the lateral calcaneal flap.[65, 76, 248] This flap can be raised as a local transpositional flap (Fig. 32–31) or as an island pedicle flap. Sensation is preserved, the flap is thin, and coverage is durable. Lesions of up to 4.5 cm wide can be covered with this flap. The final option is a distally based peroneal artery island fasciocu-

taneous flap.[67, 68, 250] As mentioned previously, the use of this flap should be preceded by arteriography. The flap is asensate, but coverage is durable and the donor site can often be closed without skin grafting.

Medium-Sized Lesions

Lesions in the 4 × 5- to 7 × 7-cm region require island pedicle or distant flap coverage. Injury of the tibialis posterior artery, nerve, or both can be a complicating factor. Both the lateral supramalleolar island pedicle[45, 140, 142] and the peroneal artery island pedicle[67, 68, 250] fasciocutaneous flaps allow asensate but thin, durable coverage (Fig. 32–32). Again, arteriography is indicated before a peroneal island flap is used. Either of these flaps can be used in the presence of a tibialis posterior artery injury.

If the tibialis posterior artery is intact, the dorsalis pedis island pedicle flap[63, 70] is a reconstructive option (Fig. 32–33). Extensor ten-

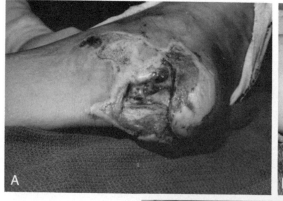
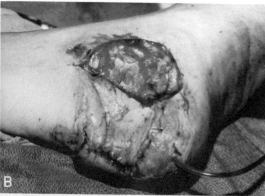
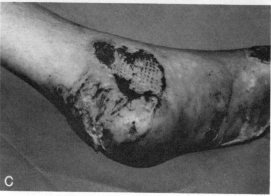

FIGURE 32–31. *(A)*, The results of a motorcycle injury in a young man with exposure of the Achilles tendon and posterior calcaneus. *(B)*, The defect is covered with a lateral calcaneal artery fasciocutaneous transpositional flap. *(C)*, Healing is complete 2 weeks later.

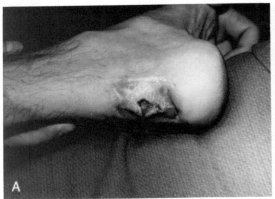
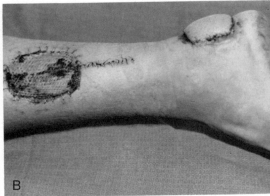

FIGURE 32–32. *(A)*, A 35-year-old man with a 20-year-old chronic wound ulceration secondary to unstable split-thickness skin graft coverage. The original wound was incurred in a bicycle accident. *(B)*, The results 2 weeks after wound excision and coverage with a distally based peroneal artery fasciocutaneous pedicle flap.

dons from the dorsum of the foot can be incorporated in this flap for Achilles tendon reconstruction, if needed.[236] Smaller defects (up to 5 × 7 cm) can be covered with a medial plantar artery–based flexor digitorum brevis muscle flap. This could be particularly useful for osteomyelitis over the posterior calcaneus. Although division of the medial plantar artery contribution to the foot is necessary, the tibialis posterior artery can generally be saved.

Large to Very Large Lesions

Large lesions (i.e., in the 7 × 7- to 10 × 20-cm range) can often be covered with a distally based peroneal artery island pedicle

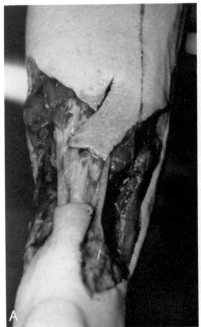
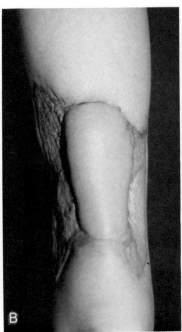
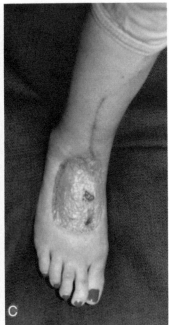

FIGURE 32–33. *(A)*, A 43-year-old woman sustained this injury through an accidental shooting with a high-velocity deer rifle. The deep compartment musculature and tendons were obliterated, as was the distal peroneal artery. *(B)*, The defect (9 × 5 cm) was closed with a proximally based dorsalis pedis pedicle flap and split-thickness skin grafts after assurance of adequate tibialis posterior blood flow with Doppler examination. *(C)*, The donor site 2 months later. The small area of skin graft loss healed without regrafting.

flap. However, larger lesions generally require a distant pedicle or free flap. Thin flaps, either skin or fascial,[24, 240] are indicated to prevent interference with normal shoewear. An aponeurosis-skin composite free groin flap[242] allows Achilles tendon and integument reconstruction. Distant and free flap considerations are discussed under the sections on general considerations and large to very large forefoot lesions.

Ankle

Soft tissue coverage problems about the ankle are usually associated with fractures, dislocations, or both of the distal tibia, tibial pilon, ankle, or tarsus. Open injuries or wound closure problems after open reduction and internal fixation of skeletal injuries usually account for the wounds. Osteomyelitis is frequently an additional problem, and local flap options are often inappropriate or impossible because of the degree of local injury. Preferred flap options for this area are listed in Table 32–14.

Very Small Lesions

Very small wound problems (less than 2 × 2 cm) about the ankle are frequent and often follow open reduction and internal fixation of tibial pilon fractures. The soleus and hemisoleus options were discussed earlier. The lack of reliability of these grafts offsets the relative ease of these procedures. Exposure of the fibula or a fibular plate can be treated proximally by use of a peroneus brevis local transpositional muscle flap.[145] Ankle function is not altered, and the flap is usually within the surgical wound. The distal metaphysis and epiphysis of the fibula are often not amenable

TABLE 32–14. ANKLE FLAPS (AUTHOR'S PREFERENCE)

SIZE	FLAP
Very small	Lateral calcaneal transpositional, peroneus brevis transpositional, or abductor hallucis transpositional
Small	Extensor digitorum brevis pedicle
Medium	Free tissue or peroneal artery
Large	Free tissue or peroneal artery
Very large	Free tissue or peroneal artery

to peroneus brevis coverage. Both the abductor digiti minimi muscle flap[144] and the lateral calcaneal flap[65, 76, 248] will cover this area. The dissection is about as easy in one as in the other. The extended coverage provided more proximally by the lateral calcaneal flap make this a more attractive choice in most instances. The peroneus brevis and abductor digiti minimi flaps are preferable in dealing with osteomyelitis.

The medial malleolar region has fewer coverage options. The abductor hallucis muscle[144] can be used to cover the more distal malleolus (Fig. 32–34). A proximally based island pedicle extensor digitorum brevis muscle flap[61, 117, 122] will cover the medial or lateral malleolus as well as the distal tibia.

Small to Medium-Sized Lesions

The local toe abductor flaps as well as the peroneus brevis muscle flap are inadequate for larger lesions (2 × 2 to 4 × 5 cm). The lateral calcaneal flap is applicable for lateral malleolar and anterior problems, and the extensor digitorum brevis island pedicle flap (Fig. 32–35) will cover anterior, lateral, and medial wounds.

Wounds in the medium range (4 × 5 to 7 × 7 cm) can be covered by any of three island pedicle flaps, all of which can be used for small wounds. The dorsalis pedis island pedicle flap[63, 70] is elevated on the tibialis anterior artery and will cover defects up to 7 × 7 cm (Fig. 32–36). The peroneal artery island pedicle flap[67, 68, 250] is based on the peroneal artery. Unlike the situation with the dorsalis pedis flap, evaluation for transfer of this flap requires arteriography. However, the donor defect for the peroneal island flap is a much simpler problem with which to deal. The lateral supramalleolar flap[45, 140, 142] can be elevated based on the peroneal perforator or retrograde circulation through the dorsal arch of the distal tibialis anterior artery.

Large to Very Large Lesions

The peroneal artery island pedicle flap can be used to cover defects up to 14 × 16 cm,[250] although some of this potential size can be lost because of pedicle length. The lateral supramalleolar flap can be used to cover defects up to 9 × 15 cm.[140, 142] However, the potential use of these two flaps is often lost because of

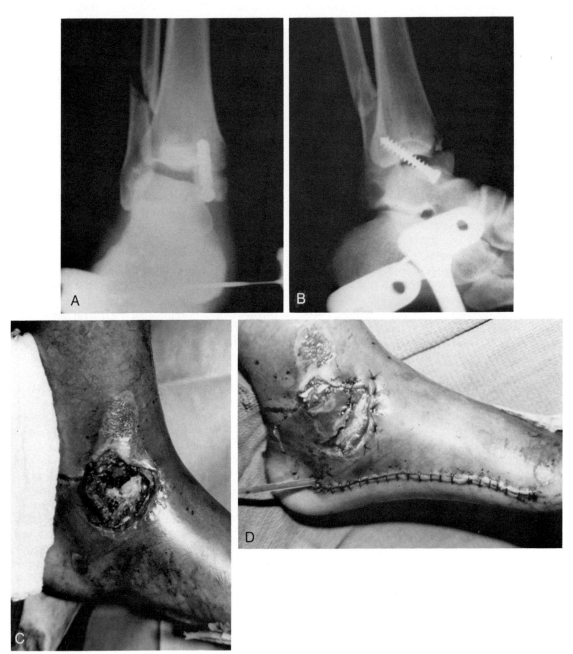

FIGURE 32–34. A middle-aged man was transferred for definitive care from another facility after sustaining an open unstable ankle fracture. Limited internal fixation *(A and B)* was used at the time of débridement several days before transfer. Inadequate coverage secondary to trauma and edema is present, with exposure of the medial malleolus and cancellous screw *(C)*. The fracture was stabilized with a lateral fibular plate and tension band fixation of a comminuted medial malleolus. The wound was covered with an abductor hallucis transpositional muscle flap and a split-thickness skin graft *(D)*.

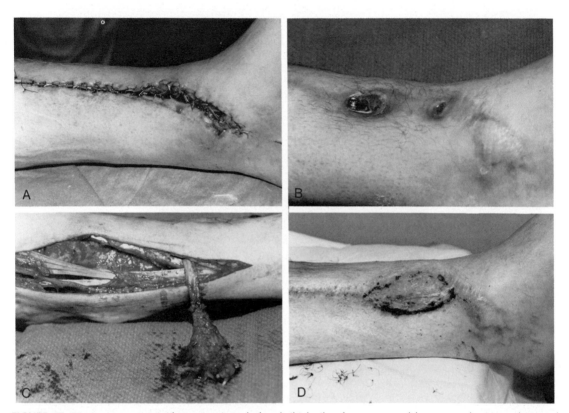

FIGURE 32–35. A young man with a comminuted closed tibial pilon fracture treated by open reduction and internal fixation using standard AO techniques. Wound closure could not be obtained at the time of surgery, and gradual closure was accomplished over 2 weeks using vessel loops *(A)*. The resultant wound was unstable; it broke down approximately 6 weeks postoperatively and progressed to fracture healing with superficial osteomyelitis *(B)*. This case illustrates the use of an extensor digitorum brevis muscle pedicle flap that, if used initially, could have prevented the secondary osteomyelitis *(C and D)*.

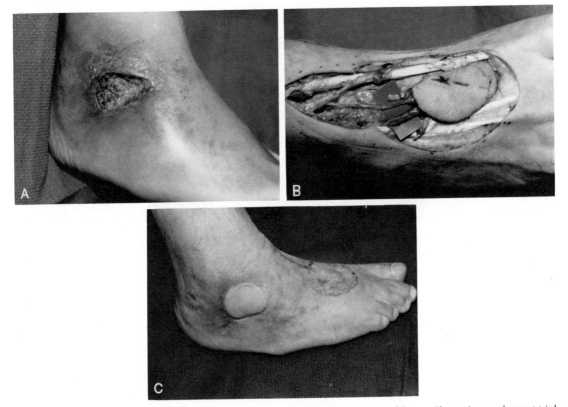

FIGURE 32–36. *(A),* A chronic recurrent ulcer on the lateral dorsal foot in a 20-year-old man. The patient underwent triple arthrodesis as an early adolescent for a cavovarus foot deformity. He received multiple split-thickness grafts, as well as one full-thickness graft, all of which healed and all of which later reulcerated. *(B),* A dorsalis pedis pedicle flap elevated, with incorporation of the superficial peroneal nerve. *(C),* At 1-year follow-up, the patient has good sensation in the transferred flap and no recurrent ulceration.

local arterial injury or, in the case of the lateral supramalleolar flap, because of involvement of the flap territory. In these instances and in cases in which muscle is needed (i.e., osteomyelitis), free tissue or distant pedicle flaps are necessary (Fig. 32–37). Distant and free flap considerations are discussed under the sections on general considerations and large to very large forefoot lesions. For technique descriptions and illustrations of soft tissue reconstructions of the foot and ankle, see Chapter 24.

Summary

Difficult wound coverage problems about the foot and ankle can occur secondary to trauma, osteomyelitis, foot deformities, tumors, or neuropathies (particularly diabetes mellitus). Coverage can be difficult because of the special weight-bearing properties of the foot, the lack of intervening muscle between the skeletal elements and the integument, and the limited mobility of the overlying integument. Sorting out the 40 to 50 flap options for the foot and ankle requires a classification that describes the wound, the patient, and the available surgical options. The wound is classified based on size, anatomic location, and the presence or absence of infection. The anatomic location also describes the weight-bearing characteristics of the wound. Associated arterial, nerve, and skeletal injuries are noted. Patient considerations include age and the presence of systemic or local compromise. Tobacco use, cosmetic concerns, occupation, rehabilitation potential, and amputee prejudices should be ascertained.

Flap options can be classified as local transpositional, island pedicle, distant pedicle, and free tissue transfers. The flaps may or may not

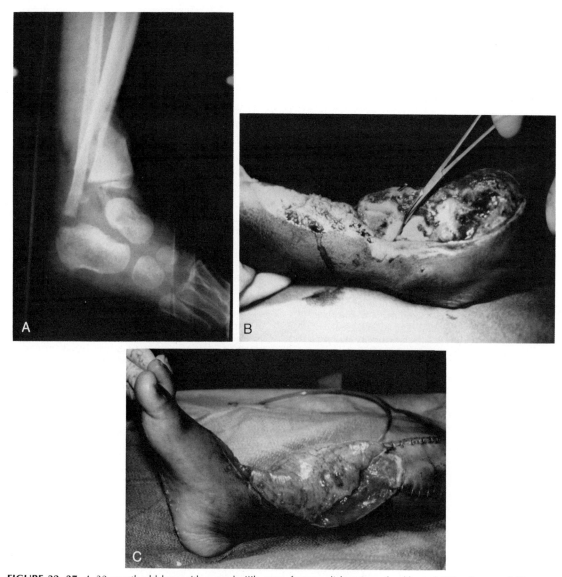

FIGURE 32–37. A 32-month-old boy with a grade IIIb open fracture-dislocation of ankle and tibia after a neighbor ran over the child backing out of the driveway. *(A)*, The skeletal injury. *(B)*, Exposure of the fracture, distal tibia, and tibiotalar joint. *(C)*, The wound was débrided and covered with a free latissimus muscle graft and a split-thickness skin graft.

incorporate muscle that may be needed for revascularization and dead-space management in osteomyelitis. Some flaps are inappropriate because of local artery or nerve injuries. Some flaps provide sensate coverage, and others can provide reinnervation potential. The potential to create new neuromas, ease of dissection, flap reliability, and cosmesis of the donor site are all important considerations.

References

1. The dorsalis pedis free flap: Technique of elevation, foot closure and flap application. Plast Reconstr Surg 77:93, 1986.
2. Agarwal N, Shah PM, Clauss RH, et al: Experience with 115 civilian venous injuries. J Trauma 22:827, 1982.
3. Akhtar M, Levine J: Dislocation of extensor digitorum longus tendons after spontaneous rupture of the inferior retinaculum of the ankle; Case report. J Bone Joint Surg 62A:1210, 1980.
4. Aldam CH: Repair of calcaneal tendon ruptures. A safe technique. J Bone Joint Surg 71B:486, 1989.
5. Aldea PA, Shaw WW: Management of acute lower extremity nerve injuries. Foot Ankle 7:82, 1986.
6. Amarante J, Martins A, Reis J: A distally based median plantar flap. Ann Plast Surg 20:468, 1988.
7. American Medical Association: Guides to the Evaluation of Permanent Medical Impairment, 6th Ed. Chicago, American Medical Association, 1977.
8. Angelats J, Albert LT: Sural nerve neurocutaneous cross-foot flap. Ann Plast Surg 13:239, 1984.
9. Arnold PG, Irons GB: Lower-extremity muscle flaps. Orthop Clin North Am 15:441, 1984.
10. Ascer E, Strauch B, Calligaro KD, et al: Ankle and foot fasciotomy: An adjunctive technique to optimize limb salvage after revascularization for acute ischemia. J Vasc Surg 9:594, 1989.
11. Ashworth EM, Dalsing MC, Glover JL, Reilly MK: Lower extremity vascular trauma: A comprehensive, aggressive approach. J Trauma 28:329, 1988.
12. Badran HA, El-Helaly MS, Safe I: The lateral intercostal neurovascular free flap. Plast Reconstr Surg 73:17, 1984.
13. Bailleul JP, Olivez PR, Mestdagh H, et al: Descriptive and topographical anatomy of the dorsal artery of the foot. Bull Assoc Anat (Nancy) 68:15, 1984.
14. Barclay TL, Sharpe DT, Chisholm EM: Cross-leg fasciocutaneous flaps. Plast Reconstr Surg 72:843, 1983.
15. Baruah DR: Spontaneous rupture of bilateral achilles tendon of a patient on long-term systemic steroid therapy. Unfallheilkunde 87:35, 1984.
16. Benum P, Berg V, Fretheim OJ: The strain on sutured Achilles tendons in walking cast. An EMG analysis. Eur Surg Res 16:14, 1984.
17. Beskin JL, Sanders RA, Hunter SC, Hughston JC: Surgical repair of Achilles tendon ruptures. Am J Sports Med 15:1, 1987.
18. Beveridge J, Masquelet AC, Romana MC, Vinh TS: Anatomic basis of a fascio-cutaneous flap supplied by the perforating branch of the peroneal artery. Surg Radiol Anat 10:195, 1988.

19. Biemer E, Stock W, Duspiva W: Replantations of the lower extremity. Chirurg 54:361, 1983.
20. Bigos SJ, Coleman SS: Foot deformities secondary to gluteal injection in infancy. J Pediatr Orthop 4:560, 1984.
21. Bishara RA, Pasch AR, Lim LT, et al: Improved results in the treatment of civilian vascular injuries associated with fractures and dislocations. J Vasc Surg 3:707, 1986.
22. Blei CL, Nirschl RP, Grant EG: Achilles tendon: US diagnosis of pathologic conditions. Work in progress. Radiology 159:765, 1986.
23. Boswick J: Injuries of the radial and ulnar arteries (abstract). *In* Proceedings of the American Society for Surgery of the Hand. J Bone Joint Surg 49A:582, 1967.
24. Brent B, Upton J, Acland RD, et al: Experience with the temporoparietal fascial free flap. Plast Reconstr Surg 76:177, 1985.
25. Buckley JR, Dunkley P: Successful reimplantation of both feet: Brief report. J Bone Joint Surg 70B:667, 1988.
26. Cachia VV, Grumbine NA, Santoro JP, Sullivan JD: Spontaneous rupture of the peroneus longus tendon with fracture of the os peroneum. J Foot Surg 27:328, 1988.
27. Carden DG, Noble J, Chalmers J, et al: Rupture of the calcaneal tendon. The early and late management. J Bone Joint Surg 69B:416, 1987.
28. Carlstedt CA, Madsen K, Wredmark T: Biomechanical and biochemical studies of tendon healing after conservative and surgical treatment. Arch Orthop Trauma Surg 105:211, 1986.
29. Carwell GR: Heel reconstruction using the medial plantar fasciocutaneous flap. Contemp Orthop 12:41, 1983.
30. Chavatzas D: Revision of the incidence of congenital absence of dorsalis pedis artery by an ultrasonic technique. Anat Rec 178:289, 1974.
31. Chen ZW, Zeng BF: Replantation of the lower extremity. Clin Plast Surg 10:103, 1983.
32. Citron N: Injury of the tibialis posterior tendon: A cause of acquired valgus foot in childhood. Injury 16:610, 1985.
33. Colen LB, Buncke HJ: Neurovascular island flaps from the plantar vessels and nerves for foot reconstruction. Ann Plast Surg 12:327, 1984.
34. Colen LB, Replogle SL, Mathes SJ: The V-Y plantar flap for reconstruction of the forefoot. Plast Reconstr Surg 81:220, 1988.
35. Congdon GC, Altman MI, Aldridge J: A comparison of transpositional neurovascular skin flaps for reconstruction of diabetic heel ulcers. J Foot Surg 27:127, 1988.
36. Costecalde M, Gaubert J, Durand J, et al: Subtotal traumatic amputation of the limb in young children; Analysis of 2 successful repairs. Chir Pediatr 29:184, 1988.
37. Cross MJ, Crichton KJ, Gordon H, Mackie IG: Peroneus brevis rupture in the absence of the peroneus longus muscle and tendon in a classical ballet dancer; A case report. Am J Sports Med 16:677, 1988.
38. D'Ambrosia RD: Orthotic devices in running injuries. Clin Sports Med 4:611, 1985.
39. Das De S, Pho RW: Heel flap injuries in motorcycle accidents. Injury 15:87, 1983.

40. DeBakey ME, Simeone FA: Battle injuries of the arteries in World War II. Ann Surg 123:534, 1946.
41. Dedichen H: Late sequelae after arterial injuries. Tidsskr Nor Laegeforen 109:324, 1989.
42. DeLuca PA, Banta JV: Pes cavovarus as a late consequence of peroneus longus tendon laceration. J Pediatr Orthop 5:582, 1985.
43. Dillehay GL, Deschler T, Rogers LF, et al: The ultrasonographic characterization of tendons. Invest Radiol 19:338, 1984.
44. Dodds WN, Burry HC: The relationship between Achilles tendon rupture and serum uric acid level. Injury 16:94, 1984.
45. Donski PK, Fogdestam I: Distally based fasciocutaneous flap from the sural region. A preliminary report. Scand J Plast Reconstr Surg 17:191, 1983.
46. Dorrler J, Lanta M, Mix C, et al: Functional results following complicated injuries of the extremities—how can they be improved? Langenbecks Arch Chir 372:667, 1987.
47. Drabyn GA, Avedian L: Ipsilateral buttock flap for coverage of a foot and ankle defect in a young child. Plast Reconstr Surg 63:422, 1979.
48. Duncan MJ, Zuker RM, Manktelow RT: Resurfacing weight bearing areas of the heel. The role of the dorsalis pedis innervated free tissue transfer. J Reconstr Microsurg 1:201, 1985.
49. Evans WE, King DR, Hayes JP: Arterial trauma in children: Diagnosis and management. Ann Vasc Surg 2:268, 1988.
50. Feliciano DV, Herskowitz K, O'Gorman RB, et al: Management of vascular injuries in the lower extremities. J Trauma 28:319, 1988.
51. Floyd DW, Heckman JD, Rockwood CA Jr: Tendon lacerations in the foot. Foot Ankle 4:8, 1983.
52. Fornage BD: Achilles tendon: US examination. Radiology 159:759, 1986.
53. Frenette JP, Jackson DW: Lacerations of the flexor hallucis longus in the young athlete. J Bone Joint Surg 59A:673, 1977.
54. Fukui A, Inada Y, Sempuku T, Tamai S: Successful replantation of a foot with satisfactory recovery: A case report. J Reconstr Microsurg 4:387, 1988.
55. Gelberman RH, Nunley JA, Koman LA, et al: The results of radial and ulnar arterial repair in the forearm—experience in three medical centers (abstract). J Bone Joint Surg 64A:383, 1982.
56. Ger R: Muscle transposition in the management of perforating ulcers of the forefoot. Clin Orthop 175:186, 1983.
57. Ger R: The clinical anatomy of the intrinsic muscles of the sole of the foot. Am Surg 52:284, 1986.
58. Giblin MM: Ruptured tibialis posterior tendon associated with a closed medial malleolar fracture. Aust N Z J Surg 50:59, 1980.
59. Gidumal R, Carl A, Evanski P, et al: Functional evaluation of nonsensate free flaps to the sole of the foot. Foot Ankle 7:118, 1986.
60. Gillies H, Chalmers J: The management of fresh ruptures of the tendo Achillis. J Bone Joint Surg 52A:337, 1970.
61. Giordano PA, Argenson C, Pequignot JP: Extensor digitorum brevis as an island flap in the reconstruction of soft-tissue defects in the lower limb. Plast Reconstr Surg 83:100, 1989.
62. Girot J, Marin-Braun F, Merle M, Xenard J: Cross replantation in a case of bilateral amputation of the legs. Rev Chir Orthop 74:259, 1988.
63. Gould JS: The dorsalis pedis island pedicle flap for small defects of the foot and ankle. Orthopedics 9:867, 1986.
64. Gould N, Trevino S: Sural nerve entrapment by avulsion fracture of the base of the fifth metatarsal bone. Foot Ankle 2:153, 1981.
65. Grabb WC, Argenta LC: The lateral calcaneal artery skin flap (the lateral calcaneal artery, lesser saphenous vein and sural nerve flap). Plast Reconstr Surg 68:723, 1981.
66. Griffiths JC: Tendon injuries around the ankle. J Bone Joint Surg 47B:686, 1965.
67. Gu YD, Wu MM, Li HR: Lateral lower leg skin flap. Ann Plast Surg 15:319, 1985.
68. Gu YD, Wu MM, Li HR: Lower leg lateral skin flap. Report of 7 cases. Chin Med J [Engl] 100:260, 1987.
69. Guan WS, Jin YT, Huang WY, et al: Experiences in the clinical use of the medial genicular flap. J Reconstr Microsurg 1:233, 1985.
70. Gulyas G, Mate F, Kartik I: A neurovascular island flap from the first web space of the foot to repair a defect over the heel: Case report. Br J Plast Surg 37:398, 1984.
71. Haggmark T, Liedberg H, Eriksson E, Wredmark T: Calf muscle atrophy and muscle function after non-operative vs operative treatment of achilles tendon ruptures. Orthopedics 9:160, 1986.
72. Haines JF: Bilateral rupture of the Achilles tendon in patients on steroid therapy. Ann Rheum Dis 42:652, 1983.
73. Hallock GG: Simultaneous bilateral foot reconstruction using a single radial forearm flap. Plast Reconstr Surg 80:836, 1987.
74. Hallock GG, Rice DC, Keblish PA, Arangio GA: Restoration of the foot using the radial forearm flap. Ann Plast Surg 20:14, 1988.
75. Hayashi M: Conservative treatment of Achilles tendon rupture. Nippon Seikeigeka Gakkai Zasshi 62:471, 1988.
76. Holmes J, Rayner CR: Lateral calcaneal artery island flaps. Br J Plast Surg 37:402, 1984.
77. Horowitz JH, Nichter LS, Kenney JG, Morgan RF: Lawnmower injuries in children: Lower extremity reconstruction. J Trauma 25:1138, 1985.
78. Hosey T, Wertheimer S: A retrospective study on surgical repair of the Achilles tendon. J Foot Surg 23:112, 1984.
79. Howard CB, Winston I, Bell W, et al: Late repair of the calcaneal tendon with carbon fibre. J Bone Joint Surg 66B:206, 1984.
80. Huber JF: The arterial network supplying the dorsum of the foot. Anat Rec 80:373, 1941.
81. Ikuta Y, Murakami T, Yoshioka K, Tsuge K: Reconstruction of the heel pad by flexor digitorum brevis musculocutaneous flap transfer. Plast Reconstr Surg 74:86, 1984.
82. Inglis AE, Scott WM, Sculco TP, Patterson AH: Rupture of the tendo Achillis. An objective assessment of the surgical and non-surgical treatment. J Bone Joint Surg 58A:990, 1976.
83. Inglis AE, Sculco TP: Surgical repair of ruptures of the tendo-Achillis. Clin Orthop 156:160, 1981.
84. Inoue G, Maeda N: Arterialized venous flap coverage for skin defects of the hand or foot. J Reconstr Microsurg 4:259, 1988.
85. Ionescu D, Ionescu A: Results of microsurgical suture in 200 nerves. Acta Chir Plast 26:166, 1984.

86. Irons GB, Verheyden CN, Peterson HA: Experience with the ipsilateral thigh flap for closure of heel defects in children. Plast Reconstr Surg 70:561, 1982.

87. Iwaya T, Harii K, Yamada A: Microvascular free flaps for the treatment of avulsion injuries of the feet in children. J Trauma 22:15, 1982.

88. Jacobs D, Martens M, Van Audekercke R: Comparison of conservative and operative treatment of Achilles tendon rupture. Am J Sports Med 6:107, 1978.

89. Jahss MH: Spontaneous rupture of the tibialis posterior tendon: Clinical findings, tenographic studies, and a new technique of repair. Foot Ankle 3:158, 1982.

90. Johansen K, Bandyk D, Thiele B, Hansen ST Jr: Temporary intraluminal shunts: Resolution of a management dilemma in complex vascular injuries. J Trauma 22:395, 1982.

91. Johnson KA: Tibialis posterior tendon rupture. Clin Orthop 177:140, 1983.

92. Johnson KA, Strom DE: Tibialis posterior tendon dysfunction. Clin Orthop 239:196, 1989.

93. Jones JG: Achilles tendon rupture following steroid injection (letter). J Bone Joint Surg 67A:170, 1985.

94. Jozsa L, Kvist M, Balint BJ, Reffy A: The role of recreational sport activity in Achilles tendon rupture. A clinical, pathoanatomical and sociological study of 292 cases. Am J Sports Med 17:338, 1989.

95. Kashyap S, Prince R: Spontaneous rupture of the tibialis anterior tendon. A case report. Clin Orthop 216:159, 1987.

96. Keeley SB, Snyder WH III, Weigelt JA: Arterial injuries below the knee: Fifty-one patients with 82 injuries. J Trauma 23:285, 1983.

97. Keene JS, Lash EG, Fisher DR, De Smet AA: Magnetic resonance imaging of Achilles tendon ruptures. Am J Sports Med 17:333, 1989.

98. Kelbel M, Jardon OM: Rupture of tibialis posterior tendon in a closed ankle fracture. J Trauma 22:1026, 1982.

99. Kellam JF, Hunter GA, McElwain JP: Review of the operative treatment of Achilles tendon rupture. Clin Orthop 201:80, 1985.

100. Keller J, Rasmussen TB: Closed treatment of Achilles tendon rupture. Acta Orthop Scand 55:548, 1984.

101. Kelly GL, Eiseman B: Civilian vascular injuries. J Trauma 15:507, 1975.

102. Kenzora JE: Sensory nerve neuromas—leading to failed foot surgery. Foot Ankle 7:110, 1986.

103. Kerr HD: Posterior tibial tendon rupture. Ann Emerg Med 17:649, 1988.

104. Kettlekamp SW, Alexander HH: Spontaneous rupture of the posterior tibial tendon. J Bone Joint Surg 51A:759, 1969.

105. Khalil IM, Livingston DH: Intravascular shunts in complex lower limb trauma. J Vasc Surg 4:582, 1986.

106. Kiviluoto O, Santavirta S, Klossner O, et al: Surgical repair of subcutaneous rupture of the Achilles tendon. Arch Orthop Trauma Surg 104:327, 1985.

107. Kleinman M, Gross AE: Achilles tendon rupture following steroid injection. Report of three cases. J Bone Joint Surg 65A:1345, 1983.

108. Kliman ME, Freiberg A: Ganglia of the foot and ankle. Foot Ankle 3:45, 1982.

109. Kline DG, Hudson AR: Surgical repair of acute peripheral nerve injuries: Timing and technique. In Morely TP (Ed): Current Controversies in Neurosurgery. Philadelphia, WB Saunders, 1976, pp 184–198.

110. Kline DG, Kahn EA: The surgery of peripheral nerve injuries. In Schneider RC, Kahn EA (Eds): Springfield, IL, Charles C Thomas, 1982, pp 506–527.

111. Koman LA: Free flaps for coverage of the foot and ankle. Orthopedics 9:857, 1986.

112. Krackow KA: Acute, traumatic rupture of a flexor hallucis longus tendon: A case report. Clin Orthop 150:261, 1980.

113. Krylov VS, Milanov NO, Peradze TY, et al: Lower leg replantation in children: Railroad amputation. J Reconstr Microsurg 3:321, 1987.

114. Kusunoki M, Toyoshima Y, Okajima M: Successful replantation of a leg—a 7-year follow-up. Injury 16:118, 1984.

115. Kutz JE, Jupiter JB, Tsai TM: Lower limb replantation. A report of nine cases. Foot Ankle 3:197, 1983.

116. Laine HR, Harjula AL, Peltokallio P: Ultrasonography as a differential diagnostic aid in achillodynia. J Ultrasound Med 6:351, 1987.

117. Landi A, Soragni O, Monteleone M: The extensor digitorum brevis muscle island flap for soft-tissue loss around the ankle. Plast Reconstr Surg 75:892, 1985.

118. Langenberg R: Spontaneous rupture of the tendon of the musculus extensor hallucis longus. Zentralbl Chir 114:400, 1989.

119. Larsen E, Lauridsen F: Dislocation of the tibialis posterior tendon in two athletes. Am J Sports Med 12:429, 1984.

120. Le Huec JC, Midy D, Chauveaux D, et al: Anatomic basis of the sural fascio-cutaneous flap: Surgical applications. Surg Radiol Anat 10:5, 1988.

121. Leekam RN, Salsberg BB, Bogoch E, Shankar L: Sonographic diagnosis of partial Achilles tendon rupture and healing. J Ultrasound Med 5:115, 1986.

122. Leitner DW, Gordon L, Buncke HJ: The extensor digitorum brevis as a muscle island flap. Plast Reconstr Surg 76:777, 1985.

123. LeMelle DP, Janis LR: Longitudinal rupture of the peroneus brevis tendon: A study of eight cases. J Foot Surg 28:132, 1989.

124. Lerman BI, Gornish LA, Bellin HJ: Injury of the superficial peroneal nerve. J Foot Surg 23:334, 1984.

125. Lesavoy MA: Successful replantation of lower leg and foot, with good sensibility and function. Plast Reconstr Surg 64:760, 1979.

126. Leung PC, Hung LK, Leung KS: Use of medial plantar flap in soft tissue replacement around the heel region. Foot Ankle 8:327, 1988.

127. Levy M, Velkes S, Goldstein J, Rosner M: A method of repair for Achilles tendon ruptures without cast immobilization. Preliminary report. Clin Orthop 187:199, 1984.

128. Lieberman JR, Lozman J, Czajka J, Dougherty J: Repair of Achilles tendon ruptures with Dacron vascular graft. Clin Orthop 234:204, 1988.

129. Lindenbaum BL: Ski boot compression syndrome. Clin Orthop 109, 1979.

130. Lippert H: Variability of hand and foot arteries. Handchir Mikrochir Plast Chir 16:254, 1984.

131. Lipscomb PR, Kelly PS: Injuries of the extensor tendons in the distal part of the leg and in the ankle. J Bone Joint Surg 37A:1206, 1969.

132. Lister G, Scheker L: Emergency free flaps to the upper extremity. J Hand Surg 13:22, 1988.

133. Lombardo M, Aquino JM: Local flaps for resurfacing foot defects: A vascular perspective. J Foot Surg 21:302, 1982.

134. Lukash FN: Microvascular free muscle reconstruction of a large plantar defect. Ann Plast Surg 15:252, 1985.

135. Ma GWC, Griffith TG: Percutaneous repair of acute closed ruptured achilles tendon: A new technique. Clin Orthop 128:247, 1977.

136. Maffulli N, Regine R, Angelillo M, et al: Ultrasound diagnosis of Achilles tendon pathology in runners. Br J Sports Med 21:158, 1987.

137. Mamakos MS: Lower extremity replantation—two and a half-year follow-up. Ann Plast Surg 8:305, 1982.

138. Mann RA: Rupture of the tibialis posterior tendon. Instr Course Lect 33:302, 1984.

139. Marcus DS, Reicher MA, Kellerhouse LE: Achilles tendon injuries: The role of MR imaging. J Comput Assist Tomogr 13:480, 1989.

140. Masquelet AC, Beveridge J, Romana C, Gerber C: The lateral supramalleolar flap. Plast Reconstr Surg 81:74, 1988.

141. Masquelet AC, Rinaldi S, Mouchet A, Gilbert A: The posterior arm free flap. Plast Reconstr Surg 76:908, 1985.

142. Masquelet AC, Romana MC: External supramalleolar flap in the reconstructive surgery of the foot. J Chir (Paris) 125:367, 1988.

143. Mathes SJ, Nahai F: Section three: Medial leg. *In* Mathes SJ, Nahai F (Eds): Clinical Atlas of Muscle and Musculocutaneous Flaps. St. Louis, CV Mosby, 1979, pp 133–198.

144. Mathes SJ, Nahai F: Section five: Foot. *In* Mathes SJ, Nahai F (Eds): Clinical Atlas of Muscle and Musculocutaneous Flaps. St. Louis, CV Mosby, 1979, pp 263–308.

145. Mathes SJ, Nahai F: Section four: Lateral leg. *In* Mathes SJ, Nahai F (Eds): Clinical Atlas of Muscle and Musculocutaneous Flaps. St. Louis, CV Mosby, 1979, pp 199–262.

146. May JW Jr, Halls MJ, Simon SR: Free microvascular muscle flaps with skin graft reconstruction of extensive defects of the foot: A clinical and gait analysis study. Plast Reconstr Surg 75:627, 1985.

147. Mayer M, Donner U, Strosche H: Surgical treatment of fresh subcutaneous rupture of the Achilles tendon and results of its treatment. Aktuel Traumatol 19:6, 1989.

148. Meals RA: Peroneal-nerve palsy complicating ankle sprain. Report of two cases and review of the literature. J Bone Joint Surg 59:966, 1977.

149. Meier PJ, Kenzora JE: The risks and benefits of distal first metatarsal osteotomies. Foot Ankle 6:7, 1985.

150. Mensor MC, Ordway GL: Traumatic subcutaneous rupture of the tibialis anterior tendon. J Bone Joint Surg 35A:675, 1953.

151. Menzoian JO, Doyle JE, Cantelmo NL, et al: A comprehensive approach to extremity vascular trauma. Arch Surg 120:801, 1985.

152. Milanov NO, Krylov VS, Peradze TI, et al: Leg replantation in children after amputation in traffic accidents (in Russian). Khirurgiia (Mosk) 8:97, 1987.

153. Mino DE, Hughes EC Jr: Bony entrapment of the superficial peroneal nerve. Clin Orthop 185:203, 1984.

154. Mittal RL, Jain NC: Traumatic dislocation of the tibialis posterior tendon. Int Orthop 12:259, 1988.

155. Mitz V, Menard P, Vilain R: Replantation of a complete section of the foot. Ann Chir Plast 27:194, 1982.

156. Morain WD: Island toe flaps in neurotrophic ulcers of the foot and ankle. Ann Plast Surg 13:1, 1984.

157. Morrison H: A study of the dorsalis pedis and posterior tibial pulses in 1000 individuals without symptoms of circulatory affection of the extremities. N Engl J Med 208:438, 1933.

158. Morrison WA, Crabb DM, O'Brien BM, Jenkins A: The instep of the foot as a fasciocutaneous island and as a free flap for heel defects. Plast Reconstr Surg 72:56, 1983.

159. Myerson M: Acute compartment syndromes of the foot. Bull Hosp Jt Dis Orthop Inst 47:251, 1987.

160. Nakashima H, Araki Y, Nishikido E, et al: Free peroneal flap for wide skin defects of the foot and volar scar contracture of the hand. J Reconstr Microsurg 3:105, 1987.

161. Nappi JF, Drabyn GA: External fixation for pedicle-flap immobilization: A new method providing limited motion. Plast Reconstr Surg 72:243, 1983.

162. Nappi JF, Ruberg RL, Berggren RB: Innervated cross-leg tensor fascia lata fasciocutaneous flap for foot reconstruction. Ann Plast Surg 10:411, 1983.

163. Nichols JG, Svoboda JA, Parks SN: Use of temporary intraluminal shunts in selected peripheral arterial injuries. J Trauma 26:1094, 1986.

164. Nistor L: Surgical and non-surgical treatment of Achilles tendon rupture. J Bone Joint Surg 63A:394, 1981.

165. Nitz AJ, Dobner JJ, Kersey D: Nerve injury and grades II and III ankle sprains. Am J Sports Med 13:177, 1985.

166. Noyez JF, Martens MA: Secondary reconstruction of the lateral ligaments of the ankle by the Chrisman-Snook technique. Arch Orthop Trauma Surg 106:52, 1986.

167. Nunley JA: Donor site selection for cutaneous and myocutaneous free flaps. Instr Course Lect 33:417, 1984.

168. O'Brien T: The needle test for complete rupture of the Achilles tendon. J Bone Joint Surg 66:1099, 1984.

169. Omer GE Jr: Results of untreated peripheral nerve injuries. Clin Orthop 163:15, 1982.

170. Orava S: Overexertion injuries in keep-fit athletes. A study of overexertion injuries among non-competitive keep-fit athletes. Scand J Rehabil Med 10:187, 1978.

171. Orava S, Puranen J: Athletic exertion injuries. Ann Chir Gynaecol 67:58, 1978.

172. Ozaki J, Fujiki J, Sugimoto K, et al: Reconstruction of neglected Achilles tendon rupture with Marlex mesh. Clin Orthop 238:204, 1989.

173. Palm T, Husum B: Blood pressure in the great toe with simulated occlusion of the dorsalis pedis artery. Anesth Analg 57:453, 1978.

174. Parsons JR, Rosario A, Weiss AB, Alexander H: Achilles tendon repair with an absorbable polymer-carbon fiber composite. Foot Ankle 5:49, 1984.

175. Parsons JR, Weiss AB, Schenk RS, et al: Long-term follow-up of achilles tendon repair with an absorba-

ble polymer carbon fiber composite. Foot Ankle 9:179, 1989.

176. Pasch AR, Bishara RA, Lim LT, et al: Optimal limb salvage in penetrating civilian vascular trauma. J Vasc Surg 3:189, 1986.

177. Peacock KC, Resnick EJ, Thoder JJ: Fracture of the os peroneum with rupture of the peroneus longus tendon. A case report and review of the literature. Clin Orthop 202:223, 1986.

178. Perry MO, Thal ER, Shires GT: Management of arterial injuries. Ann Surg 173:403, 1971.

179. Persson A, Wredmark T: The treatment of total ruptures of the achilles tendon by plaster immobilization. Int Orthop 3:149, 1979.

180. Price AE, Evanski PM, Waugh TR: Bilateral simultaneous achilles tendon ruptures. A case report and review of the literature. Clin Orthop 249, 1986.

181. Quinn SF, Murray WT, Clark RA, Cochran CF: Achilles tendon: MR imaging at 1.5 T. Radiology 164:767, 1987.

182. Ramasastry SS, Tucker JB, Swartz WM, Hurwitz DJ: The internal oblique muscle flap: An anatomic and clinical study. Plast Reconstr Surg 73:721, 1984.

183. Reading G: Instep island flaps. Ann Plast Surg 13:488, 1984.

184. Reich RS: The pulses in the foot. Their value in the diagnosis of peripheral circulatory disturbances. Ann Surg 99:613, 1934.

185. Reinig JW, Dorwart RH, Roden WC: MR imaging of a ruptured Achilles tendon. J Comput Assist Tomogr 9:1131, 1985.

186. Rich NM, Baugh JH, Hughes CW: Acute arterial injuries in Vietnam: 1,000 cases. J Trauma 10:359, 1970.

187. Robert H: The value of neurolysis following sciatic paralysis due to intrabuttock injections in children. Chir Pediatr 26:197, 1985.

188. Romanoff H, Goldberger S: Prognostic factors in peripheral vascular injuries. J Cardiovasc Surg (Torino) 18:485, 1977.

189. Rosen HM: Double island latissimus dorsi muscle-skin flap for through-and-through defects of the forefoot. Plast Reconstr Surg 76:461, 1985.

190. Rosenberg ZS, Cheung Y, Jahss MH, et al: Rupture of posterior tibial tendon: CT and MR imaging with surgical correlation. Radiology 169:229, 1988.

191. Rosenberg ZS, Feldman F, Singson RD: Peroneal tendon injuries: CT analysis. Radiology 161:743, 1986.

192. Rosenberg ZS, Feldman F, Singson RD, Kane R: Ankle tendons: Evaluation with CT. Radiology 166:221, 1988.

193. Rosenberg ZS, Jahss MH, Noto AM, et al: Rupture of the posterior tibial tendon: CT and surgical findings. Radiology 167:489, 1988.

194. Roth JH, Urbaniak JR, Koman LA, Goldner JL: Free flap coverage of deep tissue defects of the foot. Foot Ankle 3:150, 1982.

195. Russell RC, Guy RJ, Zook EG, Merrell JC: Extremity reconstruction using the free deltoid flap. Plast Reconstr Surg 76:586, 1985.

196. Sakai S, Soeda S, Kanou T: Distally based lateral plantar artery island flap. Ann Plast Surg 21:165, 1988.

197. Sammarco GJ, Miller EH: Partial rupture of the flexor hallucis longus tendon in classical ballet dancers: Two case reports. J Bone Joint Surg 61A:149, 1979.

198. Sballe K, Kjaersgaard-Andersen P: Ruptured tibialis posterior tendon in a closed ankle fracture. Clin Orthop 231:140, 1988.

199. Scheker LR, Lister GD, Wolff TW: The lateral arm free flap in releasing severe contracture of the first web space. J Hand Surg [Br] 13:146, 1988.

200. Schuchmann JA: Isolated sural neuropathy: Report of two cases. Arch Phys Med Rehabil 61:329, 1980.

201. Seddon HJ: Classification of nerve injuries. Br Med J 2:237, 1942.

202. Seddon HJ: Three types of nerve injuries. Brain 66:237, 1943.

203. Seddon HJ: Surgical Disorders of the Peripheral Nerves. Baltimore, Williams & Wilkins, 1972.

204. Seiler H, Braun C, Op Den W, et al: Macro- and microreplantations of the lower leg and foot. Langenbecks Arch Chir 369:625, 1986.

205. Seyfer AE, Lower R: Late results of free-muscle flaps and delayed bone grafting in the secondary treatment of open distal tibial fractures. Plast Reconstr Surg 83:77, 1989.

206. Shah A, Pandit S: Reconstruction of the heel with chronic ulceration with flexor digitorum brevis myocutaneous flap. Lepr Rev 56:41, 1985.

207. Shah DM, Corson JD, Karmody AM, et al: Optimal management of tibial arterial trauma. J Trauma 28:228, 1988.

208. Shah DM, Leather RP, Corson JD, Karmody AM: Polytetrafluoroethylene grafts in the rapid reconstruction of acute contaminated peripheral vascular injuries. Am J Surg 148:229, 1984.

209. Shanahan RE, Gingrass RP: Medial plantar sensory flap for coverage of heel defects. Plast Reconstr Surg 64:295, 1979.

210. Shelbourne KD, Pierce RO, Ritter MA: Superior dislocation of the fibular head associated with a tibia fracture. Clin Orthop 160:172, 1981.

211. Shields CL, Kerlin RK, Jobe FW, et al: Cybex II evaluation of surgically repaired Achilles tendon ruptures. Am J Sports Med 6:369, 1978.

212. Sim FH, Deweerd JH Jr: Rupture of the extensor hallucis longus tendon while skiing. Minn Med 60:789, 1977.

213. Skef Z, Ecker HA Jr, Graham WP III: Heel coverage by a plantar myocutaneous island pedicle flap. J Trauma 23:466, 1983.

214. Small JO, Millar R: The radial artery forearm flap: An anomaly of the radial artery. Br J Plast Surg 38:501, 1985.

215. Snyder WH III, Watkins WL, Whiddon LL, Bone GE: Civilian popliteal artery trauma: An eleven year experience with 83 injuries. Surgery 85:101, 1979.

216. Snyder WH III, Thal ER, Bridges RA, et al: The validity of normal arteriography in penetrating trauma. Arch Surg 113:424, 1978.

217. Solheim LF, Hagen R: Femoral and sciatic neuropathies after total hip arthroplasty. Acta Orthop Scand 53:531, 1980.

218. Stanish WD, Vincent N: Recurrent dislocation of the tibialis posterior tendon—a case report with a new surgical approach. Can J Appl Sport Sci 9:220, 1984.

219. Stepanov GA, Datiashvili RO, Oganesian OV: Complete traumatic amputation of the leg: Replantation of the foot with subsequent elongation of the crural bones (in Russian). Khirurgiia (Mosk) 4:135, 1988.

220. Stevenson TR, Kling TF Jr, Friedman RJ: Heel reconstruction with flexor digitorum brevis musculocutaneous flap. J Pediatr Orthop 5:713, 1985.

221. Stiehl JB: Concomitant rupture of the peroneus brevis tendon and bimalleolar fracture. A case report. J Bone Joint Surg 70A:936, 1988.
222. Stoff MD, Greene AF: Common peroneal nerve palsy following inversion ankle injury: A report of two cases. Phys Ther 62:1463, 1982.
223. Sun YQ, Zhu DL: Absent dorsalis pedis and posterior tibial pulsations in normal young Chinese. A survey of 1,728 young people. Chin Med J [Engl] 96:643, 1983.
224. Sunderland S: A classification of peripheral nerve injuries producing loss of function. Brain 74:491, 1951.
225. Taylor GI, Wilson KR, Rees MD, et al: The anterior tibial vessels and their role in epiphyseal and diaphyseal transfer of the fibula: Experimental study and clinical applications. Br J Plast Surg 41:451, 1988.
226. Thompson FM, Patterson AH: Rupture of the peroneus longus tendon. Report of three cases. J Bone Joint Surg 71A:293, 1989.
227. Thompson TC, Doherty GH: Spontaneous rupture of tendon of Achilles: A new clinical diagnostic test. J Trauma 2:126, 1962.
228. Tobin GR: Hemisoleus and reversed hemisoleus flaps. Plast Reconstr Surg 76:87, 1985.
229. Trubacheva LP, Ivashko LM: The clinical course of injection injuries to the peripheral nerves in young infants and their rehabilitation. Vestn Khir 125:111, 1980.
230. Tsai TM: Successful replantation of a forefoot. Clin Orthop 139:182, 1979.
231. Turco V, Spinella AJ: Team physician #2. Peroneus brevis transfer for Achilles tendon rupture in athletes. Orthop Rev 17:822, 1988.
232. Turco VJ, Spinella AJ: Achilles tendon ruptures—peroneus brevis transfer. Foot Ankle 7:253, 1987.
233. Uhm KI, Shin KS, Lew JD: Crane principle of the cross-leg fasciocutaneous flap: Aesthetically pleasing technique for damaged dorsum of foot. Ann Plast Surg 15:257, 1985.
234. Usui M, Minami M, Ishii S: Successful replantation of an amputated leg in a child. Plast Reconstr Surg 63:613, 1979.
235. Vagner EA, Sukhanov SG: Replantation of the lower extremity at the level of the thigh (in Russian). Khirurgiia (Mosk) 8:26, 1988.
236. Vila-Rovira R, Ferreira BJ, Guinot A: Transfer of vascularized extensor tendons from the foot to the hand with a dorsalis pedis flap. Plast Reconstr Surg 76:421, 1985.
237. Vilkki SK: Replantation of a leg in an adult with 6-years' follow-up. Acta Orthop Scand 57:447, 1986.
238. Walker RH, Farris C: Irreducible fracture-dislocations of the ankle associated with interposition of the tibialis posterior tendon: Case report and review of the literature of a specific ankle fracture syndrome. Clin Orthop 160:212, 1981.
239. Wallenfang T, Rudigier J: Therapeutic concepts in neurologic damage following severe soft tissue and bone injuries of the distal lower leg and foot (in German). Langenbecks Arch Chir 369:629, 1986.
240. Walton RL, Matory WE Jr, Petry JJ: The posterior calf fascial free flap. Plast Reconstr Surg 76:914, 1985.
241. Weaver FA, Rosenthal RE, Waterhouse G, Adkins RB: Combined skeletal and vascular injuries of the lower extremities. Am Surg 50:189, 1984.
242. Wei FC, Chen HC, Chuang CC, Noordhoff MS: Reconstruction of Achilles tendon and calcaneus defects with skin-aponeurosis-bone composite free tissue from the groin region. Plast Reconstr Surg 81:579, 1988.
243. White RA, Scher LA, Samson RH, Veith FJ: Peripheral vascular injuries associated with falls from heights. J Trauma 27:411, 1987.
244. Wicks MH, Harbison JS, Paterson DC: Tendon injuries about the foot and ankle in children. Aust N Z J Surg 50:158, 1980.
245. Wills CA, Washburn S, Caiozzo V, Prietto CA: Achilles tendon rupture. A review of the literature comparing surgical versus nonsurgical treatment. Clin Orthop 207:156, 1986.
246. Withers EH, Bishop JO, Tullos HS: Microvascular free flap transfer to foot and ankle: Report of 45 patients. Orthop Rev 14:540, 1985.
247. Wood MB, Irons GB, Cooney WP III: Foot reconstruction by free flap transfer. Foot Ankle 4:2, 1983.
248. Yanai A, Park S, Iwao T, Nakamura N: Reconstruction of a skin defect of the posterior heel by a lateral calcaneal flap. Plast Reconstr Surg 75:642, 1985.
249. Yeager RA, Hobson RW II, Lynch TG, et al: Popliteal and infrapopliteal arterial injuries. Differential management and amputation rates. Am Surg 50:155, 1984.
250. Yoshimura M, Shimada T, Imura S, et al: Peroneal island flap for skin defects in the lower extremity. J Bone Joint Surg 67A:935, 1985.
251. Yoshimura Y, Nakajima T, Kami T: Distally based abductor digiti minimi muscle flap. Ann Plast Surg 14:375, 1985.
252. Ziv I, Mosheiff R, Zeligowski A, et al: Crush injuries of the foot with compartment syndrome: Immediate one-stage management. Foot Ankle 9:185, 1989.

33

Compartment Syndrome of the Foot

MICHAEL M. HECKMAN
SCOTT R. GREWE
THOMAS E. WHITESIDES, Jr.

The late complications of ischemic contracture of the lower extremity have been well documented by Jepson,[31] Seddon,[50, 51] and Owen and Tsimboukis.[46] Retrospectively, these authors advised of the necessity of early recognition of ischemia and recommended therapy, including fasciotomy of the affected limbs. They noted that the classic signs of pain, pallor, paralysis, paresthesias, and pulselessness associated with ischemic changes could not be entirely relied on in evaluating patients with suspected compartment syndrome. Their descriptions of the catastrophic results of an unrecognized compartment syndrome are well known.

In the last 25 years, further investigations by Whitesides and colleagues,[57–59] Heppenstall and colleagues,[26, 27] Matsen and colleagues,[35–37] Mubarak and coworkers,[39–43] Hargens and coworkers,[22] and Szabo and associates[52] have established the histology and biochemical changes associated with tissue ischemia in acute conditions. Their research has been aimed at evaluating patients with suspected compartment syndromes, and their findings have been used to establish the parameters regarding the timing of and necessity for fasciotomy.

This condition, as initially described by von Volkmann in 1872,[55] was believed to most commonly involve the upper extremity.[13, 34] As understanding of the syndrome has improved, lower extremity involvement, including involvement of the foot, has been more frequently recognized.[14, 45] Compartment syndromes have been documented to occur following arterial injury,[17, 29] burns,[33] crush injuries,[1, 15, 48] arterial injections,[23] osteotomy,[32] embolectomy,[7, 17] snakebite,[9] drug overdose,[10, 49] acute and chronic exertional states,[12] gunshot wounds,[17] and both open[11] and closed[14, 21, 24, 28, 34, 45] fractures. Any patient sustaining injury to the foot, or more proximally to the leg or thigh, deserves critical evaluation for elevated tissue pressure and ischemia, which may lead to the diagnosis of a compartment syndrome.

PATHOGENESIS OF COMPARTMENT SYNDROME

Although compartment syndrome has not been commonly documented in the foot, the pathogenesis of the condition is identical to that of compartment syndromes elsewhere.[18, 19] Compartment syndromes result from an injury to the muscle that leads to swelling. In areas in which damage to the tissues is most severe, swelling and pressure within the tissue are the greatest. In patients sustaining fractures, the coinciding formation of a fracture hematoma adds to the problem of increased pressure because it has the effect of increasing volume within a closed space. The extremities, including the hand and foot, are anatomically arranged in unyielding fascial compartments. As tissue pressure within an extremity increases,

568

there is no compensatory manner in which the pressure can be released. This situation ultimately results in circulatory embarrassment, ischemia, and compartment syndrome.

Arterial injury deprives tissue of its blood supply, resulting in ischemia. Reanastomosis or re-establishment of circulation produces swelling within the tissues and elevation of tissue pressures. The extent to which the tissues are damaged depends on the degree of ischemia to which they were subjected and, more importantly, on the duration of the ischemic event.[27, 58, 59]

Nerve tissue conducts impulses for 1 hour after the onset of total ischemia and has been documented to survive up to 4 hours with only neurapraxic damage. Axonotmesis usually occurs after 8 hours of total ischemia, with irreversible changes in the nerve. In patients sustaining trauma, ischemia may not be the cause of underlying nerve damage because neurapraxia or axonotmesis of the nerve may have occurred at the time of injury. The prognosis associated with ischemia of the nerve is variable.[52, 58]

TISSUE PRESSURE AND ITS RELATIONSHIP TO ISCHEMIA

A number of methods for measuring tissue pressure have been described and are currently in use. These methods include (1) the infusion technique[58]; (2) the use of the Wick catheter[40]; (3) the use of the slit catheter[47]; and (4) the use of the Stryker Stic device.[24] Properly used, each of these methods is documented to be accurate in the measurement of interstitial tissue pressure.

Debate to establish the parameters regarding the critical tissue pressure at which ischemia occurs continues in the research community, but opinion on the issue is solidifying. Currently, it is believed that ischemia is related to the perfusion gradient of the tissue. This gradient is directly related to the patient's blood pressure. Tissue perfusion within a compartment diminishes as the tissue pressure approaches these critical values. Ischemia generally occurs in healthy tissue at 10 mm Hg below the diastolic pressure or at 30 mm Hg below the mean arterial pressure.[26, 52, 58, 59]

In tissue that has been damaged by injury, the resistance to ischemia from increasing tissue pressure is decreased. This is because perfusion of these injured tissues may not be as effective in preventing ischemia. In injured tissues, a pressure of 40 mm Hg below the mean arterial pressure, or of 20 to 30 mm Hg below the diastolic pressure, has been documented to significantly decrease tissue perfusion,[26, 27, 57–59] resulting in ischemia.

Because ischemia is based on the perfusion gradient of the tissues, patients with higher diastolic pressures will be able to withstand higher tissue pressures without ischemic damage than will patients with lower diastolic pressures. With ischemia occurring at 10 mm Hg below the diastolic blood pressure, we recommend that fasciotomy be performed at 20 to 30 mm Hg below diastolic pressure in any patient with a worsening clinical condition, a documented rising tissue pressure, significant tissue injury, or a history of 6 hours of total ischemia of an extremity.[26, 57–59]

EVALUATION OF THE PATIENT WITH A SUSPECTED COMPARTMENT SYNDROME

Pain, pallor, pulselessness, paresthesias, and paralysis have been classically described as the clinical hallmarks in a patient presenting with a compartment syndrome.[20, 36, 41, 58] Although such findings may be present, the examiner must be aware of the significance of each finding as it relates to making the diagnosis. It is important to understand that the examiner should not expect to document all of these findings in every patient diagnosed as having compartment syndrome.

Pain is the most important feature of a compartment syndrome, and pain aggravated by passive stretch of the affected tissues is the most reliable physical finding in making the diagnosis of an impending compartment syndrome. For example, in a normotensive patient with a diastolic blood pressure of 70 mm Hg, an increase in tissue pressure from the normal resting value of 0 to 4 mm Hg to a value of 30 to 40 mm Hg will result in significant discomfort with passive stretch of the tissues.[38, 54] Paresthesias, paralysis, and sensory changes are noted only after ischemia has been present for a longer time.[55] Capillary perfusion and refill will diminish as tissue pressure approaches diastolic pressure. A lack of distal pulses and pallor rarely occur unless there is arterial injury or the artery passes through a compartment subjected to tissue pressures approaching the patient's systolic blood pressure.[58, 59]

Because the physical findings and the patient's response to examination are important in making the diagnosis of a compartment syndrome, it is imperative that the patient undergoing evaluation be able to respond to the examiner. In unconscious patients or those with mental status changes, a close examination to rule out compartment syndrome is warranted. Tissue pressure measurements should be performed in any suspicious case and may supply the only objective criteria for diagnosis. In patients who are in shock or in a hypotensive state, there is a decreased ability to perfuse the tissues, and findings of only a slightly elevated tissue pressure may be significant enough to make the diagnosis of an impending compartment syndrome when these pressures are compared with the diastolic or mean arterial pressure.

UNDERSTANDING TISSUE PRESSURE MEASUREMENTS

Tissue pressure measurements should be obtained in any patient sustaining an injury who has the potential for developing a compartment syndrome. These measurements should be used in conjunction with the patient's history and physical examination findings to establish the diagnosis. If obtained properly, these measurements will help by providing objective information regarding the patient's condition.

Regardless of the technique used, tissue pressures need to be measured throughout the lower extremity to document that the area of highest pressure and greatest tissue damage has been recorded. In studies of patients sustaining lower extremity injuries, differences in tissue pressure over distances as small as 5 cm were found to be both clinically and statistically significant in making the diagnosis.[24] Palpation alone is not reliable for choosing the site of highest pressure for measurement; multiple sampling sites are needed within a compartment.[24] Proximal vascular injury in the extremity produces a diffuse ischemic process with uniform elevation of tissue pressure. However, trauma to the limb usually results in the development of a pressure gradient throughout the tissues. Compartment syn-

drome can exist in remaining muscle even in the presence of an open fracture.[11] After trauma, localized ischemic involvement may result, producing irreversible segmental injury to nerve or muscle and resulting in dysfunction of the more distal limb.

When tissue pressures approach the critical level for fasciotomy, careful follow-up is required. Repeated pressure readings should be performed every 1 to 2 hours, along with monitoring of other vital signs and symptoms. Pressure can be measured by reinserting the measuring device or rechecking an indwelling monitor. Tissue pressures have been documented to remain elevated as long as 48 to 72 hours following injury.[21] Readings should be continued until decreased pressure or a stabilization in pressure is noted or produced by fasciotomy.

THE WHITESIDES INFUSION TECHNIQUE

The equipment for tissue pressure measurements with the Whitesides technique is inexpensive and readily available. The equipment needed includes (1) a mercury manometer, (2) two plastic intravenous extension tubes, (3) two 18-gauge needles, (4) one 20-mL syringe, (5) one three-way stopcock, and (6) one vial of bacteriostatic normal saline.

1. The extremity to be evaluated should be clean and should be prepared so that measurements can be performed both proximal and distal to the level of injury.

2. An 18-gauge needle is inserted into the sterile saline to break the vacuum so that fluid can be easily withdrawn.

3. The 20-mL syringe is attached to the three-way stopcock, and an intravenous extension tube is attached to one port of the stopcock. The second 18-gauge needle is placed at the end of the extension tubing, and the third, unused port of the three-way stopcock is closed off.

4. The 18-gauge needle at the end of the extension tubing is inserted into the saline, which is aspirated without bubbles into approximately one-half the length of the extension tubing. The second 18-gauge needle should act as a vent in the saline bottle to prevent a vacuum from forming (Fig. 33–1). The three-way stopcock is turned to close off

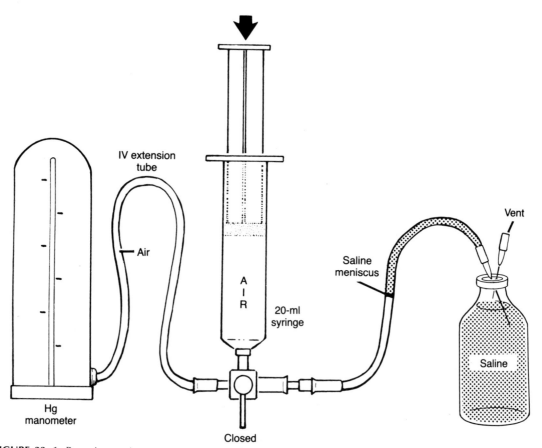

FIGURE 33–1. Preparing equipment to measure compartment pressure with the Whitesides technique. (From Smith R: Operative Surgery. London, Butterworths, 1991. By permission of Butterworth-Heinemann.)

the extension tubing so that the saline is not lost during the transfer of the needle into the tissue.

5. The second extension tube is connected to the three-way stopcock at its remaining open port. The other end of this tube is connected to the hose from the mercury manometer.

6. With the stopcock closed to the extension tubing containing the saline, the syringe is removed, and approximately 15 mL of air is aspirated. The syringe is reattached to the three-way stopcock, and the needle is inserted through the skin and fascia and into the muscle at the site of a compartment to be measured.

7. The stopcock is turned so that the syringe is open to both extension tubes, forming an open system between the compartment, the syringe, and the mercury manometer (Fig. 33–2). This creates a system that allows air from the syringe to flow into both extension tubes equally as pressure within the system is increased.

8. The entire apparatus should be at the same level as the compartment to be measured so that a fluid column does not artificially elevate the true pressure. A minute amount of saline is injected to clear the system of any soft tissue. The column of saline in the tubing, by capillary action, forms a convex meniscus away from the patient. Slow depression of the syringe gradually raises the air column pressure, increasing the pressure in the system. The saline meniscus flattens when the air pressure in the system equals the interstitial pressure of the tissue. If the air pressure is raised higher than the interstitial tissue pressure, the meniscus will reverse so that it is convex toward the patient. A pressure measurement should be taken from the manometer just as the meniscus flattens; this measurement is recorded in millimeters of mercury (Fig. 33–3). The meniscus can be visualized better if the tubing is placed over a white background. The pressure should not be read as saline is begin-

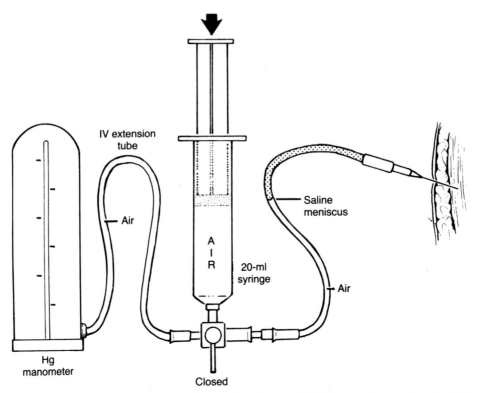

FIGURE 33–2. Measuring pressure with the Whitesides technique. (From Smith R: Operative Surgery. London, Butterworths, 1991. By permission of Butterworth-Heinemann.)

ning to infuse into the muscle because this will result in an erroneously high reading.

9. The pressure is reduced to 0 and the stopcock is closed before additional measurements are obtained to prevent loss of saline from the column.

Alternatives to the Whitesides infusion technique include the use of the Wick catheter, the slit catheter, and the Stryker Stic device. Each of these requires specialized electronic equipment. Each is accurate if used correctly. The examiner should be familiar with their use

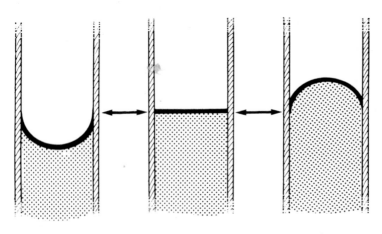

Plastic tubing   Measure at this point

FIGURE 33–3. Reading the meniscus. (From Smith R: Operative Surgery. London, Butterworths, 1991. By permission of Butterworth-Heinemann.)

before basing a clinical decision on a pressure reading and should not ignore the clinical findings.

TREATMENT

In any patient diagnosed as having a compartment syndrome of the foot or in any patient with a documented increase in tissue pressure in the lower extremity, a set of guidelines regarding initial treatment must be observed. All circumferential dressings need to be split or removed immediately, and the affected extremity must be raised or lowered to the level of the heart to maximize perfusion without compromising venous drainage. If resolution of the signs of ischemia does not occur and the tissue pressures remain elevated, surgical decompression is advised.

Compartment syndromes proximal to the foot are beyond the scope of this chapter. However, a more proximal process should be ruled out as a contributing factor to the development of this condition in the foot. In patients with documented compartment syndrome of the thigh or leg, the guidelines previously described should be followed. If fasciotomy is required, a mediolateral[2, 4, 8, 53] technique above the knee and a perifibular[36, 44] approach below the knee should be used.

Isolated compartment syndromes of the foot do occur.[6] Careful evaluation should be carried out in any patient sustaining a crush injury, a tarsal or metatarsal fracture or dislocation,[30] or vascular ischemia. Anatomically, the foot is divided into four compartments: the medial, central, lateral, and interosseous (Fig. 33–4).[6, 37, 41] The medial compartment contains the abductor hallucis and flexor hallucis brevis muscles. The central compartment contains the adductor hallucis, the quadratus plantae, the

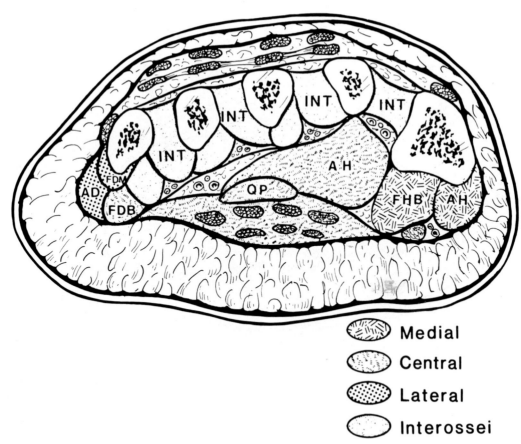

Medial

Central

Lateral

Interossei

FIGURE 33–4. Compartments of the foot. AD, abductor digiti; AH, abductor hallucis; FDB, flexor digitorum brevis; FDM, flexor digiti minimi; FHB, flexor hallucis brevis; INT, interossei; QP, quadratus plantae. (From Smith R: Operative Surgery. London, Butterworths, 1991. By permission of Butterworth-Heinemann.)

flexor digitorum brevis, and the tendons of the flexor digitorum longus and flexor hallucis longus. The lateral compartment contains the flexor digiti minimi and the abductor digiti muscles. The interosseous compartment contains the interossei of the foot and the plantar digital arterial arches and digital nerves. An additional, fifth compartment has been reported that includes the quadratus plantae muscle and is in connection with the deep posterior compartment of the calf.[38]

Tissue pressures should be recorded in the foot in each of the compartments plantarly (medial, central, and lateral) and in each of the interossei dorsally (Fig. 33–5). Decompression of the foot may be carried out through three separate incisions: two dorsal, with each incision releasing two of the interossei (Fig. 33–6), and a single medial incision using Henry's approach to the plantar structures of the foot (Fig. 33–7).[3, 25]

Henry divides the muscles of the foot into four distinct layers.[25] Through a medial incision overlying the first metatarsal and the navicular tuberosity, the skin and subcutaneous tissues are divided. The abductor hallucis is then identified and dissected plantarly from the first metatarsal, navicular, and underlying fibers of the flexor hallucis brevis. The knot of Henry is exposed and incised, with care taken to note the medial and lateral plantar neurovascular bundles (Fig. 33–8). The medial incision can then be extended proximally to inspect the neurovascular bundle and release the tarsal tunnel if needed. Through release of the master knot of Henry, the entire plantar aspect of the deep foot anatomy can be exposed. The first, second, and third layers of the foot may be retracted plantarly enough to trace the paths of the medial and lateral plantar nerves and arteries on the dorsal side of the third layer. With plantar retraction of the third layer, the plantar fascia of the interossei may be visualized and decompressed if the surgeon desires. We have found that decompression of the interossei may be performed more simply

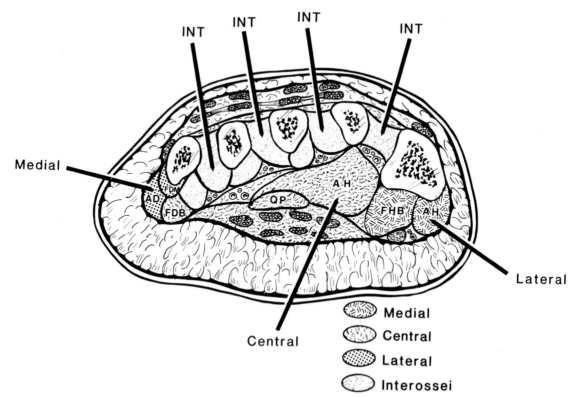

FIGURE 33–5. Location of tissue pressure measurements. AD, abductor digiti; AH, abductor hallucis; FDB, flexor digitorum brevis; FDM, flexor digiti minimi; FHB, flexor hallucis brevis; INT, interossei; QP, quadratus plantae. (From Smith R: Operative Surgery. London, Butterworths, 1991. By permission of Butterworth-Heinemann.)

FIGURE 33–6. Location of dorsal incisions. (From Smith R: Operative Surgery. London, Butterworths, 1991. By permission of Butterworth-Heinemann.)

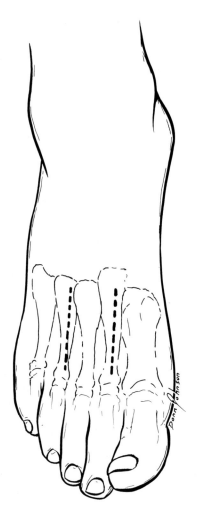

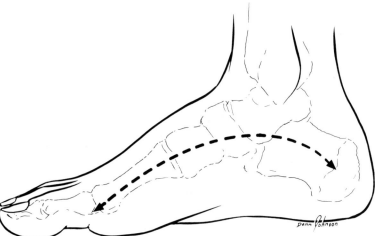

FIGURE 33–7. Location of medial incision. (From Smith R: Operative Surgery. London, Butterworths, 1991. By permission of Butter-worth-Heinemann.)

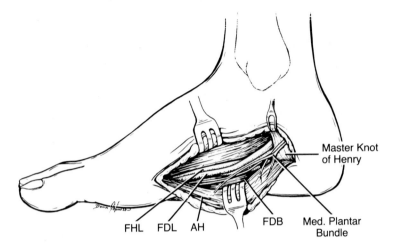

FIGURE 33–8. Medial exposure. AH, abductor hallucis; FDB, flexor digitorum brevis; FDL, flexor digitorum longus; FHL, flexor hallucis longus. (From Smith R: Operative Surgery. London, Butterworths, 1991. By permission of Butterworth-Heinemann.)

Master Knot of Henry

FHL   FDL   AH   FDB   Med. Plantar Bundle

and effectively through two dorsal incisions on the foot, allowing direct visualization and release of each of the four muscles.

In traumatic open injuries, débridement of the foot should be performed before decompression. Existing traumatic incisions may be used in fasciotomy. If there is a concern regarding flap viability in such injuries, a split-thickness skin excision technique may be performed intraoperatively.[61] Although it is described as a primary wound coverage procedure,[60] we use split-thickness excision initially only for diagnosis of flap viability and perform split-thickness skin grafting secondarily.

Postoperatively, the foot is splinted in a bulky dressing, with the ankle maintained in a neutral or dorsiflexed position. The extremity should be elevated to the level of the heart, and the evaluation of neurovascular status should be continued. Delayed primary skin closure or split-thickness skin grafting is then carried out after 48 to 72 hours to provide soft tissue coverage.

LATE COMPLICATIONS OF COMPARTMENT SYNDROMES

Richard von Volkmann's work on ischemic muscular paralysis and contractures in the leg was first published in 1872,[55] and his descriptions of findings in upper and lower extremities were reported in 1881.[56] He noted the difference in the onset of paralysis and contracture as they related to ischemic injury. He documented that there was some possibility for muscle regeneration after ischemia but that the prognosis for recovery was dependent on

the extent of muscle and nerve damage present. There was a greater tendency for fibrotic replacement of the muscle and accentuation of contractures than for resolution of the condition.

Residual deformity in the foot may result from compartment syndromes and ischemic contracture involving the leg. The extent of the involvement depends on the compartment involved and the extent of the ischemic event. In cases involving the deep posterior compartment of the leg, involvement in the foot may range from mild clawing of the toes to more extensive deformities with severe cavus of the foot, dorsiflexion of the talus, forefoot adduction and equinus, and a tendency for heel varus. More important, there can be a sensory loss to the sole of the foot and a loss of innervation to the intrinsic musculature (Fig. 33–9).

Ischemic contracture involving the anterior compartment of the leg may result initially in wasting of the compartment and a footdrop. Interestingly, as contracture of the affected muscles increases with time, the footdrop may actually diminish. If the deep peroneal nerve is damaged, there will be a resultant loss of sensation of the dorsum of the foot and the first web space and a loss of foot and ankle dorsiflexion power.

In cases in which damage has occurred in the superficial posterior compartment, an equinovarus deformity may result, with soleus and gastrocnemius muscle contracture. The lateral side of the foot may become asensate with sural nerve involvement.

Involvement of the lateral compartment of the leg results in no apparent clinical deformity

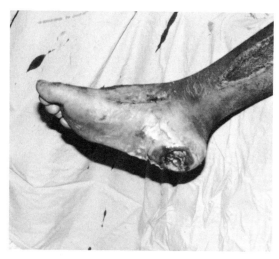

FIGURE 33–9. Foot ulcer complication of the deep posterior compartment of the calf.

within the foot with contracture of the peroneal muscles. If injury to the superficial peroneal nerve occurs, it may result in a loss of sensation to the dorsum of the foot.

Residual deformities from compartment syndrome of the foot occur and correspond to the specific muscles involved. Medial compartment ischemia can cause contracture in the abductor hallucis and flexor hallucis brevis muscles. The central compartment may have contracture of the adductor hallucis and flexor digitorum brevis. Quadratus plantae contracture primarily involves the medial toes supplied by the more muscular portion, compared with the lateral portion, which is more tendinous.[35] Lateral compartment involvement can be seen by contracture in the flexor digiti minimi and abductor digiti minimi muscles. Interosseous compartment involvement can result in contracture of the intrinsic muscles of the foot and may decrease sensation in the sensory distribution of the digital nerves.

Treatment of Volkmann's contracture of the lower leg or foot, as in the upper extremity, initially involves splinting and daily stretching.[19] Residual foot deformities may require braces, orthotics, and shoe modifications to allow the patient greater mobility. After 3 months,[41] if reconstruction is deemed necessary to improve function, surgical exploration is required. Exploration of all involved compartments is carried out, and areas of necrotic or fibrotic muscle are excised in their entirety. Tendon releases or lengthening should be per-

formed when necessary, and neurolysis of all involved nerves should be performed. Additional procedures in the foot may include the correction of fixed hammer toe or lesser toe deformities, plantar fasciotomy if appropriate, arthrodesis, and intrinsic muscular reconstruction by tendon transfer. Amputation may be indicated in cases of compartment syndrome that have resulted in severe uncorrectable deformities or an insensate foot.

References

1. Adams JP, Fowler FD: Wringer injuries of the upper extremity: A clinical, pathological and experimental study. South Med J 52:798, 1959.
2. An HS, Simpson JM, Gale S, Jackson WT: Acute anterior compartment syndrome of the thigh: A case report and review of the literature. J Orthop Trauma 1:180, 1987.
3. Ascer E, Strauch B, Calligaro KD, et al: Ankle and foot fasciotomy: An adjunctive technique to optimize limb salvage after revascularization for acute ischemia. J Vasc Surg 9:594–597, 1989.
4. Bass RR, Allison EJ Jr, Reines HD, et al: Thigh compartment syndrome without lower extremity trauma following application of pneumatic antishock trousers. Ann Emerg Med 12:382, 1983.
5. Bate JT: A subcutaneous fasciotomy. An instrument for relief of compressions in anterior, lateral, and posterior compartments of the leg from trauma and other causes. Clin Orthop 83:235, 1972.
6. Bonutti PM, Bell GR: Compartment syndrome of the foot: A case report. J Bone Joint Surg 68A:1449, 1986.
7. Chandler JG, Knapp RW: Early definitive treatment of vascular injuries in the Vietnam conflict. JAMA 202:136, 1967.
8. Clancey GJ: Acute posterior compartment syndrome in the thigh: A case report. J Bone Joint Surg 67A:1278, 1985.
9. Clement JF, Pietrukso RG: Pit viper snakebite in the United States. J Fam Pract 6:269, 1978.
10. Conner AN: Prolonged external pressure as a cause of ischemic contracture. J Bone Joint Surg 53B:118, 1971.
11. DeLee JCU, Stiehl JB: Open tibia fracture with compartment syndrome. Clin Orthop 160:175, 1981.
12. Detmer DE, Sharpe K, Sufit FL, Girdley FM: Chronic compartment syndromes: Diagnosis, management, and outcomes. Am J Sports Med 13:162, 1985.
13. Eaton RG, Green WT: Volkmann's ischemia—a volar compartment syndrome of the forearm. Clin Orthop 113:58, 1975.
14. Ellis H: Disabilities after tibial shaft fractures with special reference to Volkmann's ischaemic contracture. J Bone Joint Surg 40B:190, 1958.
15. Entin MA: Roller and wringer injuries: Clinical and experimental studies. Plast Reconstr Surg 15:290, 1955.
16. Ernst CB, Kaufer H: Fibulectomy-fasciotomy. J Trauma 11:365, 1971.

17. Gaspar MR, Treiman RL, Payne JH, et al: Principles of treatment and special problems in vascular trauma. Surg Clin North Am 48:1355, 1968.
18. Gelberman RH, Zakaib GS, et al: Decompression of forearm compartment syndromes. Clin Orthop 134:225, 1976.
19. Goldner JL: *In* Flynn JE (Ed): Hand Surgery. Baltimore, Williams & Wilkins, 1975.
20. Halpern AA, Mochizuki RM: Compartment syndrome of the interosseous muscles of the hand. A clinical and anatomic review. Orthop Rev 9:121, 1980.
21. Halpern AA, Nagel DA: Anterior compartment pressures in patients with tibia fractures. J Trauma 20:786, 1980.
22. Hargens AR, Schmidt DA, Evans KL, et al: Quantitation of skeletal muscle necrosis in a model compartment syndrome. J Bone Joint Surg 63A:631, 1981.
23. Hawkins LG, Loscher CG: The main line accidental intraarterial injection. Clin Orthop 94:268, 1973.
24. Heckman MM, Whitesides TE, Grewe SR: Spatial relationships of compartment syndromes in lower extremity trauma. Orthopaedic Transactions, J Bone Joint Surg 11:537, 1987.
25. Henry AK: Extensile Exposure, 2nd Ed. New York, Churchill Livingstone, 1982.
26. Heppenstall RB, Sapega AA, Scott R, et al: The compartment syndrome: An experimental and clinical study of muscular energy metabolism using phosphorus nuclear magnetic resonance spectroscopy. Clin Orthop 226:138–155, 1988.
27. Heppenstall RB, Scott R, Sapega AA, et al: A comparative study of the tolerance of skeletal muscle to ischemia: Tourniquet application compared with acute compartment syndrome. J Bone Joint Surg 68A:820, 1986.
28. Holden CEA: Compartment syndromes following trauma. Clin Orthop 113:95, 1975.
29. Hughes CS: Vascular injuries in the orthopaedic patient. J Bone Joint Surg 40A:1271, 1958.
30. Jahss MH: Disorders of the Foot. Philadelphia, WB Saunders, 1982, p 1201.
31. Jepson PN: Ischemic contracture. Ann Surg 84:785–795, 1926.
32. Kikuchi S, Hasue M, Watanabe M: Ischemic contracture in the lower limb. Clin Orthop 134:125–192, 1978.
33. Kingsley NW, Stein JM, Levenson SM: Measuring tissue pressure to assess the severity of burn induced ischemia. Plast Reconstr Surg 63:404, 1979.
34. Lipscomb PR, Burleson RJ: Vascular and neural complications in supracondylar fractures of the humerus in children. J Bone Joint Surg 37A:487, 1955.
35. Matsen FA III: Compartmental Syndromes. New York, Grune & Stratton, 1980, pp 86–93.
36. Matsen FA III, Winquist RA, Krugmire RB: Diagnosis and management of compartment syndromes. J Bone Joint Surg 62A:286, 1980.
37. Matsen FA, Clawson DK: The deep posterior compartmental syndromes of the leg. J Bone Joint Surg 57A:34, 1975.
38. Meyerson MD: Experimental decompression of the fascia compartments of the foot—the basis for fasciotomy in acute compartment syndromes. Foot Ankle 6:308–314, 1988.
39. Mubarak SJ, Owen CA, Hargens AR, et al: Acute compartment syndromes: Diagnosis and treatment with the aid of the Wick catheter. J Bone Joint Surg 60A:1091, 1978.
40. Mubarak SJ, Hargens AR, Owen CA, et al: The Wick catheter technique for measurement of intramuscular pressure. J Bone Joint Surg 58A:1016, 1976.
41. Mubarak SJ, Hargens AR: Compartment Syndromes and Volkmann's Contracture. Philadelphia, WB Saunders, 1981, pp 68, 100–101.
42. Mubarak SJ, Carroll NC: Volkmann's contracture in children—etiology and prevention. J Bone Joint Surg 61A:285, 1979.
43. Mubarak SJ, Owen CA: Double incision fasciotomy of the leg for decompression in compartment syndromes. J Bone Joint Surg 59A:184, 1977.
44. Nghiem DD, Boland JP: Four compartment fasciotomy of the lower extremity without fibulectomy: A new approach. Am Surg 46:414, 1980.
45. Nicoll EA: Fractures of the tibial shaft: A survey of 705 cases. J Bone Joint Surg 46B:373, 1964.
46. Owen R, Tsimboukis B: Ischaemia complicating closed tibial and fibular shaft fractures. J Bone Joint Surg 49B:268, 1967.
47. Rorabeck CH, Castle GSP, Hardie R, Logan J: Compartmental pressure measurements: An experimental investigation using the slit catheter. J Trauma 21:446, 1981.
48. Rowland SA: Fasciotomy. *In* Green DP (Ed): Operative Hand Surgery. New York, Churchill Livingstone, 1982, pp 565–581.
49. Schreiber SN, Liebowitz MR, Bernstein LH: Limb compression and renal impairment (crush injury) following narcotic and sedative overdose. J Bone Joint Surg 54A:1683, 1972.
50. Seddon HJ: Volkmann's ischemia in the lower limb. J Bone Joint Surg 48B:627–636, 1966.
51. Seddon HJ: Volkmann's contracture: Treatment by excision of the infarct. J Bone Joint Surg 38B:152, 1956.
52. Szabo RM, Gelberman RH, Williamson RV, Hargens AR: Effects of increased systemic blood pressure on the tissue fluid pressure threshold of peripheral nerve. J Orthop Res 1:172–178, 1983.
53. Tarlow SD, Achterman CA, Hayhurst J, Ovadia DN: Acute compartment syndrome in the thigh complicating fracture of the femur. A report of three cases. J Bone Joint Surg 8A:1439, 1986.
54. Tsuage K: Treatment of established Volkmann's contracture. J Bone Joint Surg 57A:925, 1975.
55. von Volkmann R: Von Verletzungen und Krankheiten der Bewegungsorgane. Handbuch der Allgemeinen und Speziellen Chirurgie, 1872.
56. von Volkmann R: Die ischaemischen Muskellamungen and Kuntraktunen. Zentralbl Chir 51:801, 1881.
57. Whitesides TE Jr, Hanley TC, Morimoto K, Harada H: Tissue pressure measurements as a determinant for the need of fasciotomy. Clin Orthop 113:43, 1975.
58. Whitesides TE Jr, Harada H, Morimoto K: Compartment syndromes and the role of fasciotomy, its parameters and techniques. Instr Course Lect 26:179, 1977.
59. Whitesides TE Jr, Harada H, Morimoto K: The response of skeletal muscle to temporary ischemia: An experimental study. Proc J Bone Joint Surg 53A:1027, 1971.
60. Ziv I, Mosheiff R, Zeligowksi A, et al: Crush injuries of the foot with compartment syndrome: Immediate one-state management. Foot Ankle 9:185–189, 1989.
61. Ziv I, Zeligowksi A, Mosheiff R, et al: Split-thickness skin excision in severe open fractures. J Bone Joint Surg 70B:23–26, 1988.

PART **IV** *PROBLEMS OF THE*

PEDIATRIC FOOT

Editor
GEORGE W. SIMONS

34

Congenital Malformations of the Feet and Toes

JOHN S. GOULD

INTRODUCTION AND CLASSIFICATION

Congenital malformations of the feet and toes occur from disturbances in the development of the limb bud of the embryo between the fourth and eighth weeks of gestation. Occasionally, genetic inheritance plays a role, and in some fetuses (e.g., those with congenital constriction band syndrome), the event may occur later in the pregnancy. Environmental or exogenous factors such as an anoxic episode, febrile illness of the mother, or drug use may play a role in some disturbances of the limb mesenchyma, but in many instances, the etiology is simply unknown.

The classification of anomalies has evolved from the complex meticulous categorization by Frantz and O'Rahilly[14] in 1961 and a myriad of terms with Greek and Latin roots to the rather simplistic but easily remembered categories proposed by Swanson[41] in 1976 and adopted for use in the hand by the American Society for Surgery of the Hand and the International Federation of Societies for Surgery of the Hand. I have adopted this classification for use in the foot. The following groupings are proposed:

1. Failure of formation of parts (arrest of development)
2. Failure of differentiation of parts (segmentation)
3. Duplication
4. Overgrowth (hyperplasia, macrodactyly or gigantism)
5. Undergrowth (hypoplasia)
6. Congenital constriction band syndrome
7. Other malformations, including angular deformities

PHILOSOPHY OF MANAGEMENT

Congenital anomalies involving the toes and feet have long been neglected. They could easily be concealed in footwear, and reconstruction allegedly did not improve function. In many cases, there was simply a reluctance to attempt "plastic" procedures on the foot, which was thought to have less tolerance for shifting and manipulation of tissue than did the hand. Hence, classic orthopaedic texts and well-known authorities frequently advised against surgical procedures.[15, 42]

As orthopaedists and other reconstructive surgeons developed increased skills in tissue handling, used magnification and better tools, and became familiar with traditional plastic methodologies, more interest in surgical solutions evolved.[16] Simultaneously, however, improved pedorthics, with better shoe modifications and new materials for inserts, has made nonoperative solutions more satisfactory as treatments for deformities or as adjuncts to surgery.

The appropriate indications and goals for surgical intervention include increased functional capacity, easier shoe fitting, and improved appearance. The psychological factors are very important for normal behavior patterns and social development. At age 6, a child is carefully scrutinized and criticized by his or

581

her peers. Minute variations from the norm are cause for ridicule. The adolescent is devastated by a lack of conformity. Even the adult alters normal activities because of congenital variations: for example, the adult will not go barefoot, go to the beach, wear open-toed shoes or sandals, or even go to bed without stockings. Social development and interactions are therefore distorted and disturbed.

Decision making for the orthopaedic surgeon for congenital anomalies of the feet and toes is influenced by all these factors. The timing for surgery is also affected by practical considerations. As soon as the child is walking, he or she wears hard-soled leather footwear. Surgical correction to allow fitting into such a shoe must precede this age (12 to 18 months). Operations to stabilize the foot are also done before the child reaches this age, and operations for appearance are done before age 6. Parents often want reconstructive surgery because they feel guilty about the plight of their

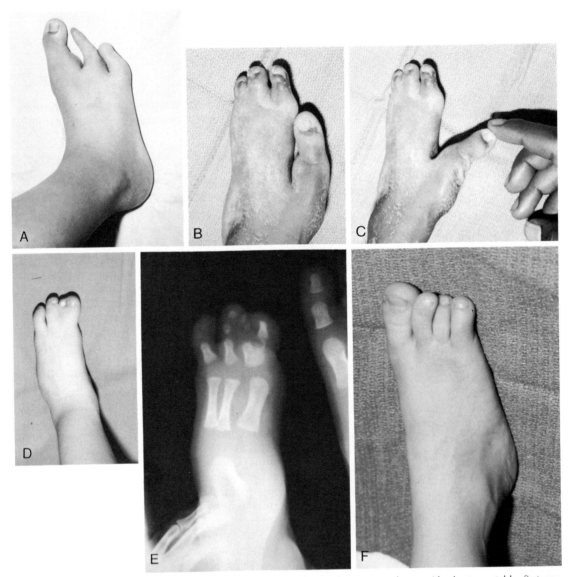

FIGURE 34–1. Failure of formation. *(A)*, Absent toes. *(B* and *C)*, Absent second ray with short, unstable first ray. Reconstruction included lengthening of the first metatarsal, arthrodesis of the cuneiform-metatarsal joint, and closure of the cleft. *(D* and *E)*, Two absent rays with incomplete formation of the toe adjacent to the great toe. *(F)*, Absence of the fifth ray only.

child and want him or her to be as normal as possible; they will shop until they find a "seller."[22] Clearly, responsible surgeons with a knowledge of functional requirements and psychological factors should respond appropriately to these needs.[5]

CATEGORIES OF DEFORMITIES

Failure of Formation of Parts

The category of failure of part formation includes innumerable variations and permutations, from longitudinal deficits such as the absence of a toe or ray to transverse arrests such as the absence of all toes, deficits at the midtarsal level, and the like (Fig. 34–1).[3, 10] Some longitudinal deficits of the fifth ray, for example, may include deficits of mid- and hindfoot structures, among them the fibula (Fig. 34–2). The absent fibula may be associ-

ated with ankle instability and tibial bowing (anteriorly, but not associated with congenital pseudarthrosis).

The treatment of most minor defects does not require the use of special appliances, but significant deficits can be nicely managed by pedorthic inserts. These devices are molded to the entire sole of the foot to balance weight bearing, with the deficient area filled in with insert material (e.g., Plastizote or Pelite) to keep the foot from shifting about and to fill out the shoe, thus allowing a matched pair of shoes to be worn.

The central longitudinal defect, or cleft foot, requires special attention (see Chapter 35). The cleft may be closed by flap shifts and syndactylization; splayed first and fifth metatarsals may require basilar osteotomies, and unstable first rays may need stabilization (Fig. 34–3). I use simple syndactylization techniques, with transpositional flaps as needed.

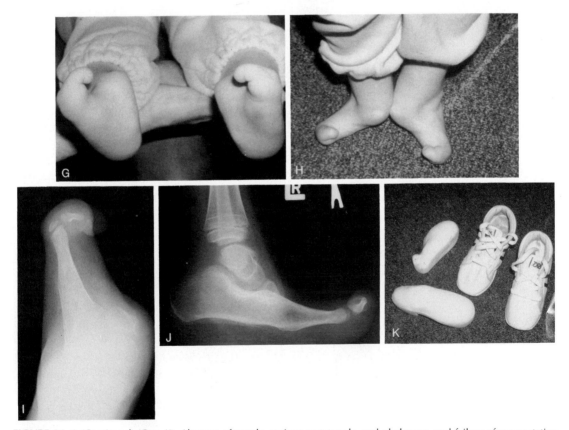

FIGURE 34–1 *(Continued) (G to K)*, Absence of tarsals, various metatarsals, and phalanges, and failure of segmentation. Recurrent painful bursae formed over the prominent talonavicular bone. An ostectomy was performed to remove this prominent tissue, the posterior tibial tendon was advanced to the lateral bone to better stabilize the subtalar joint, and molds of the feet were taken and cushioning orthoses were made to decrease shear and fill out the normal contours of the foot.

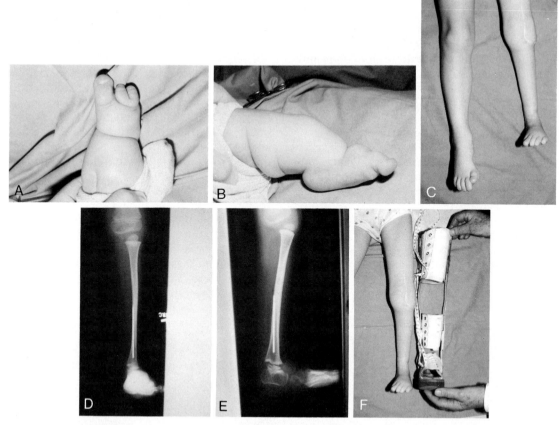

FIGURE 34–2. Longitudinal defects with proximal involvement. (*A* and *B*), Ray deficiencies with an absent fibula. The anterior bowing in this tibia is not associated with congenital pseudarthrosis. In this bilateral condition, an anterior wedge osteotomy of the tibia and a posterior soft tissue release and Achilles tendon lengthening, including a Z-plasty of the skin, aligned the tibia and brought the feet to about 45 degrees of equinus. A subsegment osteotomy (concentric with a distal wedge) through the unsegmented subtalar joint area produced plantigrade feet. (*C* to *F*), First ray and absent tibia (tibial hemimelia). Realignment of the ankle and knee was required. Note the fibular hypertrophy. This child continues to wear a brace with an extension to equalize leg length. Although bone lengthening is a consideration, the conventional approach would be the use of a below-knee prosthesis with a knee stabilizer and disarticulation of the foot at the ankle.

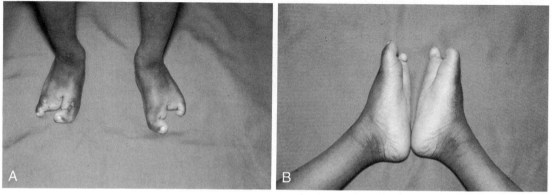

FIGURE 34–3. (*A* and *B*), Central ray deficiency (lobster claw).

Skin grafting is occasionally necessary for a donor flap site defect. For a short first or fifth ray, lengthening has been performed with the Matev[26] method. The Ilizarov device and technique will supersede the more traditional lengthening methods (see Chapter 31). Total contact inserts have been used to balance the foot, especially when the first ray is unstable. In the older child, I usually await first metatarsal growth plate closure, at bone age 13 in girls and at bone age 14 to 15 in boys, before arthrodesing the first metatarsal–cuneiform joint to gain a stable first ray. Occasionally, because of marked instability in a younger child, arthrodesis has been performed before maturity, preserving the epiphyseal plate and maintaining position with smooth pins and casting (see Chapter 36 for medial cuneiform–first metatarsal fusion techniques).

Failure of Segmentation

The typical representative of the category of failure of segmentation is syndactyly, and although its true incidence is unknown, syndactyly has a relatively frequent occurrence. Genetics plays a larger role in this category than in most of the other areas.[49] As in the hand, the webbing may be complete or incomplete, and the condition may be described as simple (skin only) or complex (synostosis or some other bone anomaly such as concealed polydactyly, either fully developed or partial). Dobyns and colleagues have referred to conditions in the complex category other than synostosis as "complex-complicated."[8] The vast majority of syndactylies involve the second and third toes or the second interspace, where they are usually simple (Fig. 34–4), or the fourth and fifth toes or fourth interspace, where they are frequently associated with a concealed or not-so-concealed polydactyly (Fig. 34–5). When the great toe is involved, polydactyly may also exist. The disturbed appearance is very deforming, and women, particularly, have difficulty with shoe fitting. Sandals and thongs often cannot be worn without prior reconstructive surgery. The 2–3 recon-

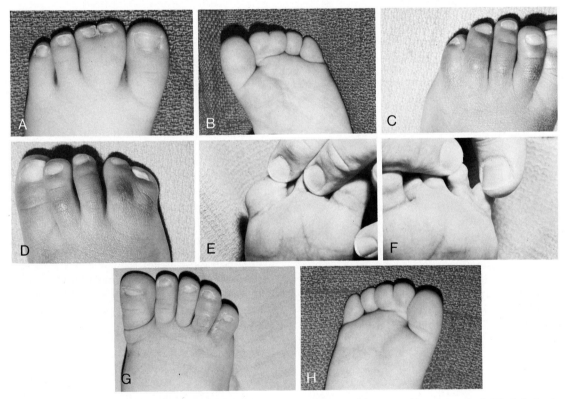

FIGURE 34–4. *(A and B),* 2–3 simple complete syndactyly. Reconstruction of the eponychium is required. *(C),* 4–5 simple incomplete syndactyly. *(D),* 4–5 simple complete syndactyly. *(E),* 4–5 simple complete syndactyly. *(F),* 4–5 simple incomplete syndactyly. *(G and H),* Postoperative reconstruction of a simple incomplete 4–5 syndactyly with the flap and graft technique described in the text.

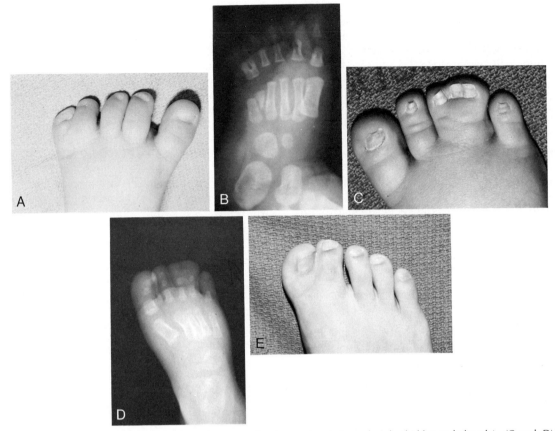

FIGURE 34–5. *(A* and *B),* Photograph and x-ray study of complex 4–5 syndactyly (hidden polydactyly). *(C* and *D),* Photograph and x-ray study of 3–4 complex syndactyly with polydactyly. Removal of the duplicated skeleton actually leaves more soft tissue in the reconstruction of the new web. Distal S-shaped flaps are necessary for the eponychial reconstruction. *(E),* 1–2 simple complete syndactyly.

structions are often performed around 1 year of age but should be done before 6 years of age, whereas the 1–2 and 4–5 reconstructions are performed before 1 year of age because of shoe-fitting problems, and sometime after the child doubles his or her birth weight (at age 3 months, at least).

In Apert's syndrome, which has a complex syndactyly involving all of the toes and a spade-like forefoot with a narrow heel and which often has a depressed second metatarsal head protruding on the plantar surface, several procedures may be necessary to allow comfortable wearing of standard footwear (Fig. 34–6).[25] I narrow the foot, evening the width of the forefoot and hindfoot, by excising the second ray (saving Lisfranc's joint). This also eliminates the plantar bump. The first web is easily reconstructed with the deletion of the second toe and metatarsal, allowing better wearing of sandals. When deformity of the first toe is

significant, osteotomies are used to narrow and align it. Dell and Sheppard have also excised the first toe and ray and hallucized the second (Figs. 34–7 to 34–9).[7] I have not reconstructed the minor toe webs.

My syndactyly reconstruction technique is significantly different from that used with the fingers[2, 28] for several reasons. First, the toes do not have to splay, and sensibility of the web is not a significant issue. Second, preservation of normal skin and sensibility on the plantar and dorsal surfaces is necessary for both protection and better appearance. Accordingly, the commissure is reconstructed with a combination of dorsal and plantar flaps (rectangular flaps with oblique distal margins or triangular side-to-side flaps), and the sides of the toes are covered with skin graft (Fig. 34–10). Although some surgeons use glabrous skin from the adjacent great toe and longitudinal arch, I use inguinal crease skin as a full-

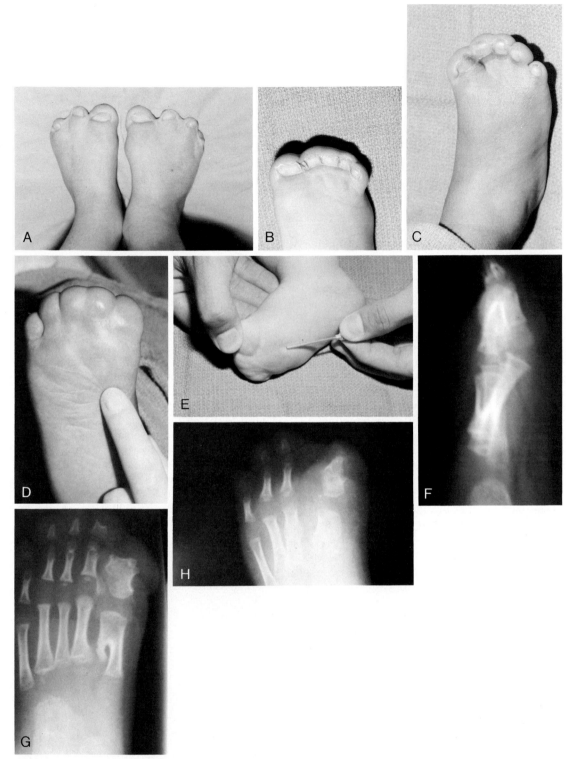

FIGURE 34–6. *(A to C),* Various presentations of the complex syndactylies of the Apert syndrome foot. *(D and E),* Prominence of the depressed second metatarsal head. *(F),* Lateral x-ray study demonstrating the depressed second metatarsal head. *(G and H),* Before and after excision of the second ray (see text).

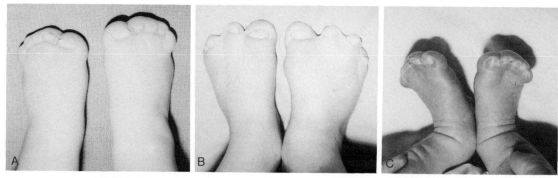

FIGURE 34–7. *(A to C)*, Clinical presentations of bilateral feet in Apert's syndrome.

thickness graft. Some hyperpigmentation does occur but is of little consequence in this hidden site; the plantar and dorsal surfaces look relatively normal (Fig. 34–11).

When I perform this procedure, I prepare the groin area and the leg and foot as one sterile area, block drape the inguinal crease, and hold the towels on with a "sticky" drape material. After the remaining extremity drape is completed, a sterile pneumatic tourniquet is placed high on the thigh. After exsanguination with the elastic bandage, the tourniquet is inflated and an elastic bandage is also placed around the knee to prevent early back-bleeding. The surgery is performed with the surgeon seated at the end of the operating table (so that the surgeon's knees can extend under the table). Loupe (3.5 to 4.5×) magnification is used.

The incision lines are indicated with a skin-marking pen. The dorsal midline of the in-

volved digits is noted, and parallel lines are drawn along the midline for the dorsal flap from the metatarsophalangeal joints to about three-quarters of the distance to the proximal interphalangeal joints. The length-to-width ratio of the flap is about 1.5:1.0. The distal end of the flap is oblique and is therefore slightly flared. On the plantar surface, a matching but shorter one-to-one flap is created, starting in the midline of the digits and extending from the flexion crease approximately half the distance to the proximal interphalangeal joint crease. The distal end of the flap is similarly slanted to match the dorsal end.

From the midline of each distal edge, the incision is zig-zagged to the distal end of the combined digits. If there is a complete syndactyly and the nails are compound, they must be divided, and distal S-shaped flaps must be constructed on the distal toes to create an eponychium (Fig. 34–12).

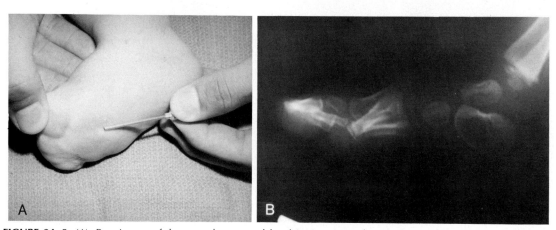

FIGURE 34–8. *(A)*, Prominence of the second metatarsal head in Apert's syndrome (closeup view of Fig. 34–6*E*). *(B)*, X-ray study of a depressed second metatarsal.

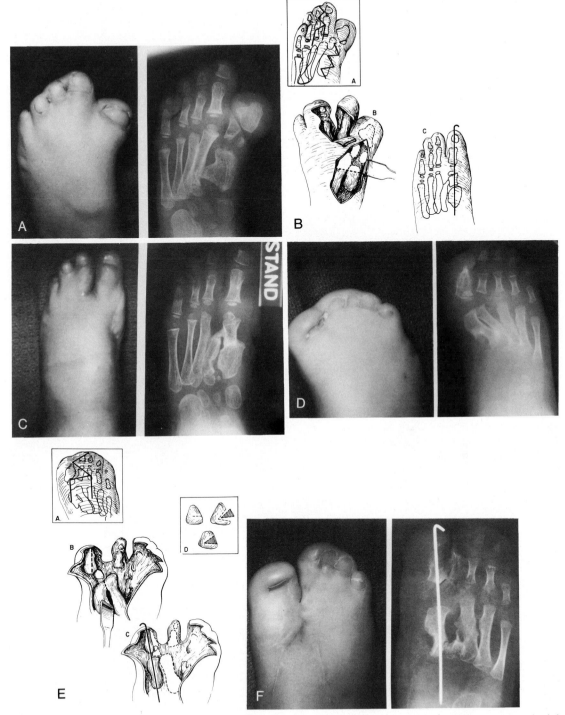

FIGURE 34–9. Dell and Sheppard's approach to Apert's feet.[7] *(A)*, Clinical and x-ray presentations of the anomaly (left foot). *(B)*, Illustration of the surgical plan to hallucize the second ray with deletion of the first. *(C)*, Clinical and x-ray presentations of completed hallucization. *(D)*, Clinical and x-ray appearances of widened spatulate right forefoot. *(E)*, Illustration of planned realignment of the first ray and deletion of the second. *(F)*, Completion of the surgical procedure to narrow the forefoot.

590   *Problems of the Pediatric Foot*

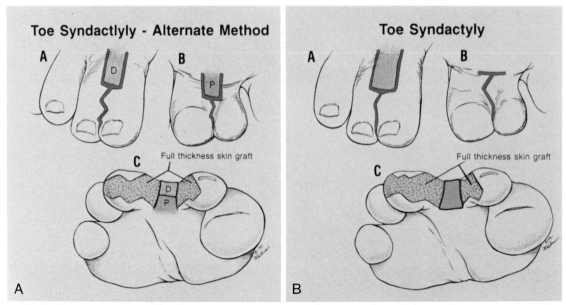

FIGURE 34–10. Toe syndactyly reconstruction techniques. *(A)*, Dorsal (D) and plantar (P) flaps are created with skin grafting of the sides (see text). The distal edges of the flaps are slanted more than shown here. *(B)*, Only the dorsal flap is used for the creation of the commissure.

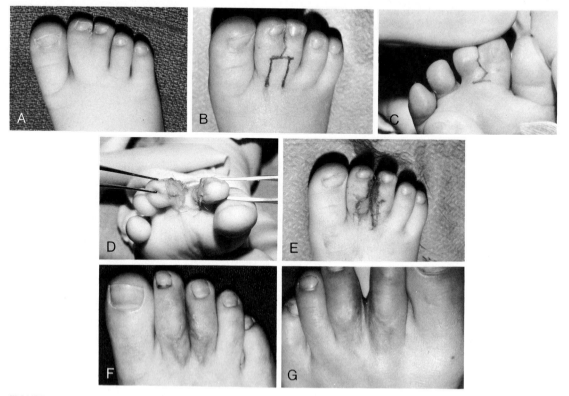

FIGURE 34–11. Reconstruction of the 2–3 web using the technique shown in Figure 34–10*B*. *(A)*, Simple incomplete 2–3 syndactyly. *(B)*, Marking of the dorsal flap. *(C)*, Plantar marking. *(D)*, The completed commissure and grafted sides. *(E)*, The completed web from the dorsum. *(F and G)*, Later appearances of similar reconstructions.

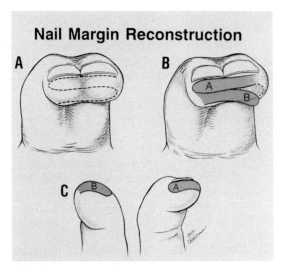

Nail Margin Reconstruction

A   B

C

FIGURE 34–12. Technique of reconstruction of the nail margins.

After marking the dorsal areas as indicated, I make my incision with a No. 15 blade and carry the incision dorsally to the extensor tendon level, cauterizing bleeders with a bipolar cautery as needed and initially leaving all the excessive subcutaneous fat on the flaps rather than on the tendon surface. Excessive fat is then quickly and easily removed from the flap with curved tenotomy scissors. The plantar incisions extend through the subcutaneous tissue to expose the neurovascular bundles.

The nail division is done sharply with a No. 64 Beaver blade through nail plate and sterile and germinal matrices. After this division, the created apical flaps resurface the bare blunt surfaces of the distal phalanges and nails. If there is a synostosis of the distal phalanges, it is divided by a digital osteotome. At this point, a fine, fibrous retinaculum, like natatory ligaments, is encountered between the digits. This is divided, separating the digits and further exposing the neurovascular bundles plantarward. The dissection can be carried proximally to the bifurcations of the digital nerves and arteries. More depth can be created by teasing apart the common nerve, but the bifurcation of the artery is an absolute barrier unless the surgeon decides to sacrifice a digital vessel to one digit. This is rarely necessary. However, it is important, to reach this intersection and divide the true natatory ligaments to "unpack" the toes and allow for a smooth, slanted surface between the toes.

If a hidden polydactyly exists, the excision of this component is carried out at this time. If additional nerves or blood vessels are present, apparently related to this component, they are not necessarily deleted but are referred to one digit or another. If the duplication extends into the metatarsal area, one of the dorsal longitudinal incision lines may have to be extended proximally. Through this extension, the additional component may be deleted. If there is a shared joint between the duplicated phalanges and the contiguous normal phalanx or metatarsal that is unstable after excision, a flap of periosteum from the deleted digit but based on the remaining digit must be used to recreate a collateral ligament, which is sutured across the joint with dissolving suture. I usually use 4–0 or 5–0 Vicryl for this maneuver. (Further discussion of this problem is given in the section on duplication.)

After defatting, the plantar and dorsal flaps are brought together and sutured without tension with a 6–0 dissolvable suture. (I use Vicryl on a P-1 needle.) The skin graft is harvested after the defects are measured and the amount of skin is determined. The total amount of skin required is converted to an ellipse, which can be marked specifically to correspond to each component defect or can be simply used, as needed, first on one side and then on the other, saving as much from the first side as possible as the graft is stretched onto the defect. The graft is defatted as it is harvested. Further defatting is subsequently performed to expose the rete pegs on the graft. I close the groin defect with deep subcutaneous 4–0 dissolving suture and the deep dermis or subcuticular layer with a running 5–0 dissolving suture as well. The wound is steri-stripped and is then covered with a plastic barrier material.

After the commissure and tip have been constructed, the tourniquet is released to check for any significant bleeding before graft application. When the graft is applied, it is important to stretch it onto its base, sewing the margins and quilting the graft by sewing it onto its bed, also with dissolving suture. The zigzags must be followed and the graft must be darted to avoid longitudinal contracture. Long linear reaches and areas of granulation and epithelialization lead to linear contracture. Longitudinal contracture can cause an angular deformity of the digits, either with healing or with subsequent growth. The zig-zag incision lines tend to lessen this possibility.

After completion of the procedure, the incision lines are covered with antibiotic ointment and nonadherent material. I then pack the web loosely with cotton balls soaked in Bunnell's solution (one-third 0.25-percent acetic acid, one-third glycerol, and one-third antibiotic solution). This combination, which I have used for years over skin grafts, tends to absorb serum from under the graft, and the acetic acid creates an acidic pH, which is apparently less conducive to the growth of certain types of bacteria. The glycerol tends to prevent the cotton ball from adhering to the tissues. At the time of dressing change, soaking the cotton balls with sterile saline allows them to be easily removed. A bulky dressing is applied, followed by a plaster or fiberglass shell, which may be carried above the flexed knee in younger, less contoured legs, simply for protection of the surgical site. Two weeks postoperatively, the shell and underlying dressing are removed, and the foot is mobilized. If there has been a significant slough of graft or flap tissues, it is important to carry out a series of dressing changes, followed by regrafting of the denuded area. Allowing this area to granulate and re-epithelialize will lead to reformation of the web or to signficant angular contracture. When regrafting has not been performed, either through neglect or through parental refusal to allow further surgery, the outcomes have been universally unsatisfactory. On the other hand, minor slough areas frequently heal with little consequence.

The 2–3 web may normally be slightly long relative to the 3–4 and 4–5 webs. For short simple syndactylies, however, with the webbing to the proximal interphalangeal joints or not much more than 1 cm in length, the three-flap web plasty may be used (Fig. 34–13).

The three-flap web plasty[17, 31] is designed to make maximum use of the available adjacent

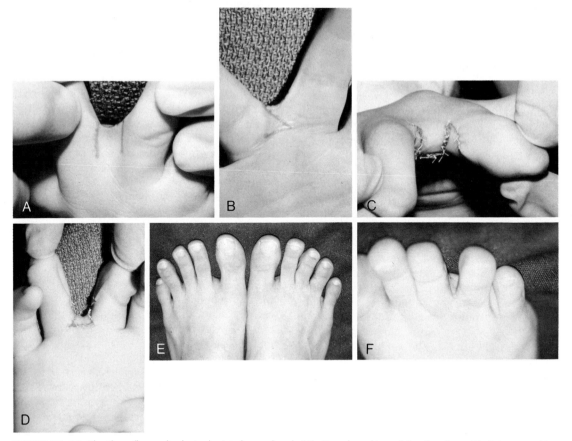

FIGURE 34–13. The three-flap web plasty depicted on a hand. *(A),* Dorsal marking of the first flap. *(B),* Palmar marking of the two triangular flaps. *(C),* The flaps are cut; the dorsal flap is advanced to the palm side and the triangular flaps are rotated into place on each side. *(D),* Palm view. *(E and F),* The 3–4 webs on the feet were reconstructed with this technique.

web skin and to provide a properly slanted commissure between the toes. Its use is limited to short syndactylies, but it is a very helpful technique. The length of the web is marked with a pen and measured. This length is equal to the longitudinal incisions that create the flap and to the distance that the flap can be advanced. The line is drawn along the web, and the two parallel lines are drawn on the dorsum of the midline of the digits, extending from the web proximally for the appropriate amount. From the distal edge of the web, an equal distance is then measured to the plantar skin, and a horizontal line of the same length is drawn. A diagonal line connects the web to the plantar horizontal line.

The incisions are cut and the flaps developed. Excessive fat is removed. The dorsal flap is advanced to the plantar transverse incision line and sutured in place with 6–0 dissolvable suture. The two triangular flaps are rotated to fill the triangular defects on the sides of the digits.

Reconstruction of 4–5 syndactylies is not ordinarily a particular problem, although the risk of creating instability on the tibial side of the metatarsophalangeal joint can be significant and may result in an abduction deformity, which will cause significant shoewear problems. This possibility is particularly relevant in syndactylies that also include a hidden or not-so-hidden duplication (see Fig. 34–5*A* and *B*). When the inner or tibial member of a duplication is of proper size, shape, and angulation, it is often preferable to excise the outer or fibular component so as not to threaten the joint stability at the metatarsophalangeal level. When removal of the inner component is important, it is performed easily if the duplication does not extend proximally to the metatarsal level. When it does, the surgeon must reconstruct the metatarsophalangeal joint collateral ligament with a periosteal flap and pin the joint, protecting it for 4 to 6 weeks to ensure stability.

Although hereditary simple syndactyly is usually expressed as a mirror-image syndactyly on the opposite foot, occasionally different degrees of syndactyly occur on each member. On one side, for example, there may be a simple complete syndactyly, whereas on the other, syndactyly may be simple and incomplete. One side may have a simple syndactyly, and the other, a complex one. The more complex syndactylies are usually sporadic (mu-

tations), but not in all situations. In addition to simple syndactyly and complex syndactylies that involve synostoses and duplications, various other conditions may have associated syndactyly. These include both hypo- and hyperplasia, failure of formation, and duplications. These additional elements are dealt with in conjunction with procedures, such as those described earlier, for the syndactyly component. A special type of syndactyly, known as acrosyndactyly, is associated with congenital constriction band syndrome. This peculiar type of webbing problem is thought to be not a failure of segmentation but a fusing of digits related to an event occurring in late pregnancy. This condition and the congenital constriction band problem itself are discussed further in a later section.

Rehabilitation for surgery related to syndactyly reconstruction is usually unnecessary. After healing of the flaps and grafts, the skin is massaged with standard skin lubricants; otherwise, however, there is little need for special care. Complications in this type of surgery are usually minor and insignificant. The major concerns are infection, graft and flap slough, subsequent angular deformity, and neurovascular compromise. Infection can lead to loss of an entire skin graft, but this complication can usually be managed by clearing of the infection and later regrafting. Meticulous technique, including good hemostasis and proper dressings, with at least local antibiotic coverage, should minimize the occurrence of these events. In cases of previous infection, systemic antibiotics are also given. Angular deformity is usually treated by excision of the offending scar and by adequate regrafting with appropriate darting of linear incisional areas to prevent recontracture. On occasion, a transpositional flap of normal skin may be rotated into the defect to break up the linear scar with grafting of the fresh defect from the donor site. This has been particularly helpful for salvage of recalcitrant cases. Loss of digital nerve function to the web is of little consequence, but it is also relatively insignificant to lose a single digital nerve on the grafted side because the plantar and dorsal aspects of the toe are usually well innervated by the digital nerve on the opposite side. This is also true for circulation to the toe, which comes from both webs. On the other hand, this risk to nerves and vessels might be cited as a reason to avoid reconstruction of adjacent webs. Although this recon-

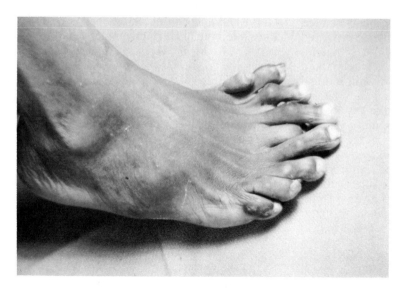

FIGURE 34–14. A "mirror" foot with eight rays.

struction is only occasionally required, the surgeon should not challenge a digit with simultaneous reconstruction of adjacent webs. When reconstruction of adjacent webs is necessary, an interval of 3 months should elapse between reconstructions, and every attempt is made to preserve the digital nerves and vessels on each occasion. Consequently, when both webs are reconstructed, the risk to viability of the toe could be significant. Careful surgery,

under magnification, is necessary to prevent an unfortunate mishap.

Duplication

Duplication, or polydactyly, may involve a single toe, part of a toe, an entire ray, or multiple rays.[4, 6, 33] Polydactyly of the little toe may be duplication of a simple skin tag only, of parts of the toe, or of the entire ray. All of

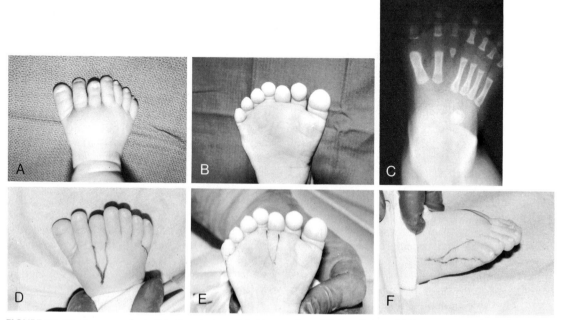

FIGURE 34–15. Seven-ray foot. (A), Dorsal view. (B), Plantar view. (C), Insufficient third ray. (D), Markings for wedge resection of the third ray. (E), Plantar view of the wedge markings. (F), Wedge resection of the seventh ray.

the involved components are surgically excised so as not to leave a remnant that will require further surgery. (I also prefer surgical excision of skin tags, rather than ligation, for the same reason.) Occasionally, I have encountered a "mirror foot" with as many as eight rays (Fig. 34–14).[47] Either the x-ray findings or the clinical appearance often indicates the best choices for deletion. If a toe is "riding high" or is hypoplastic, it is chosen for deletion. The removal of central rays creates a gap, which is rectified by creating metatarsal plantar plate flaps. These flaps are sutured together, usually with absorbable suture. Splaying with growth is not unusual, and reclosure of the gap may be necessary later. Excision of the most fibular ray may also be a good choice to narrow the foot without producing a gap. The peroneus

brevis must be reattached to the base of the new fifth metatarsal (Figs. 34–15 and 34–16).

Central Duplication

The technique for deletion of a central duplication involves a wedge- or pie-shaped dorsal incision that becomes broader distally, toward the base of the toe. On the plantar side, a narrow wedge is taken. A racket incision around the base of the proximal phalanx completes this incisional area. From the dorsum, the extensor mechanism to the toe is delineated, and with protection of the extensors to the adjacent toe, the tendon is divided. The level for excision of the base of the duplicated metatarsal may be determined easily if there is no real articulation proximally, or if the

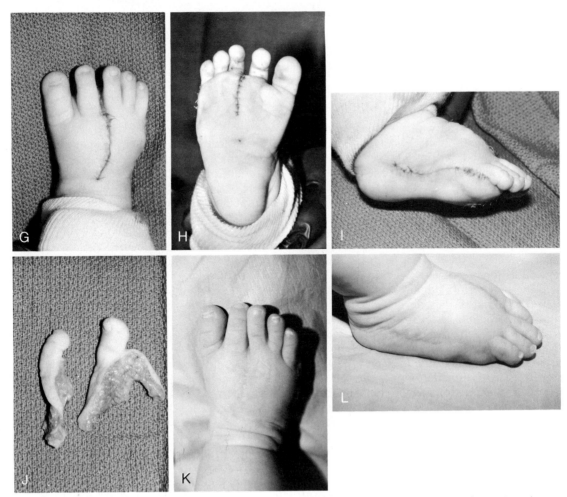

FIGURE 34–15 *(Continued) (G)*, Completed appearance of the reconstruction from the dorsum. *(H)*, Plantar view; the gap has been narrowed. *(I)*, Lateral view; the peroneus brevis has been reattached to a new fifth ray base. *(J)*, Removed segments. *(K)*, The healed foot from the dorsum. *(L)*, Lateral view of the healed foot.

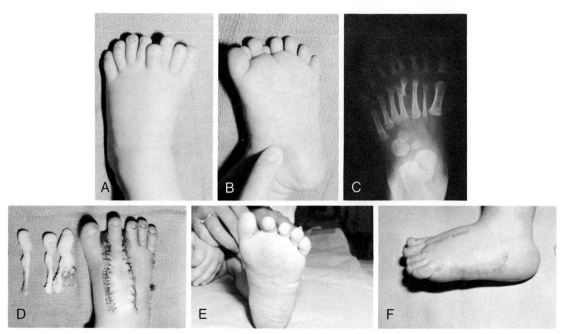

FIGURE 34–16. Eight-ray foot. *(A)*, Dorsal view. *(B)*, Plantar view; note that toes two and four are high riding. *(C)*, X-ray showing eight rays; the second ray is hypoplastic. *(D)*, After resection of rays two, four, and eight. *(E)*, Plantar view of the healed foot. *(F)*, Lateral view.

articulation is shared with an adjacent metatarsal on a cuneiform, disarticulation can simply be performed. At times, a wedge must be taken from the cuneiform in order to narrow it sufficiently to narrow the entire foot. Extending the incision distally, the surgeon divides the intrinsic interosseous attachments to the proximal phalanx of the toe. On the plantar side, the surgeon must dissect the neurovascular bundles of the toe that is to be deleted, as well as those of each of the adjacent toes. This must be performed fairly distally, starting at the proximal phalanx level, to avoid interrupting the digital vessel to the adjacent toe. If the neurovascular dissection is performed at the metatarsal level, the common digital vessel or nerve to the adjacent toes may be interrupted. Therefore, the digital vessels and nerves are located on the proximal phalanx, and the vessels are followed back proximally to the bifurcation. Obviously, the division of vessels and nerves is carried out distal to the bifurcation. The flexor tendons are divided at the metatarsophalangeal joint level. The intermetatarsal ligaments are removed from the metatarsal to be deleted, leaving a fringe of tissue on the remaining metatarsal heads and plantar plates.

After the ray to be excised is delivered, reconstruction is necessary between the metatarsals to eliminate the gap. I usually use heavy materials such as 2–0 or even 0 absorbable suture between the fringes of the plantar plate intermetatarsal ligament in order to close the gap. If the gap does not close well, one may need to do the wedge osteotomy in the cuneiform to achieve the closure. Usually, this is not necessary. The gap may be held together with a threaded 0.062-inch fixation pin between the metatarsal heads during the healing period. This pin is removed after 4 to 6 weeks.

Fifth Toe Duplication

With duplication of the little toe, the surgeon usually attempts to remove the fibular component so as not to destabilize the metatarsophalangeal joint on the tibial side and thus create an abducted toe (Fig. 34–17).[30] If this is not possible because of a markedly deformed or hypoplastic tibial component, it may be necessary to remove the inner duplication and to realign the fifth toe or ray. The collateral ligament may need to be reconstructed using periosteal flaps, and osteotomy of the fifth metatarsal may be needed to bring it in against the fourth metatarsal and eliminate the splay. The specific site for the metatarsal osteotomy is determined by the level of the deformity. If the entire metatarsal is splayed, an osteotomy can be done at the base of the metatarsal, either with a closing wedge or a concentric (dome) cut. I favor the latter because there is minimal shortening with this technique and I can place the distal segment exactly where I want it. I make the cut with a curved concentric saw blade on an oscillating saw handle. The osteotomy site is pinned with a 0.045- or 0.062-inch fixation pin, which is left in place until healing has occurred, at 6 weeks or later. Although long, oblique diaphyseal osteotomies are useful, they seem relatively unnecessary in the younger child, in whom healing seems to occur readily with

osteotomies performed through the proximal metaphysis. If the distal metatarsal tends to flair out significantly, as may occur in some of these duplications, it is more appropriate to carry out an osteotomy distally. For this purpose, I use a distal chevron technique, which is also appropriate for the type of bunionette that also has this type of flair (see Chapter 7).

Hallux Duplication

Duplication of the hallux provides a particular challenge.[20, 24] Even triplication has been seen (Fig. 34–18). Almost all such duplications are associated with a short, wide first metatarsal[18] and varus positioning of the articular facets on the metatarsal (Fig. 34–19). The obligation is to fully delete the most medial

Text continued on page 602

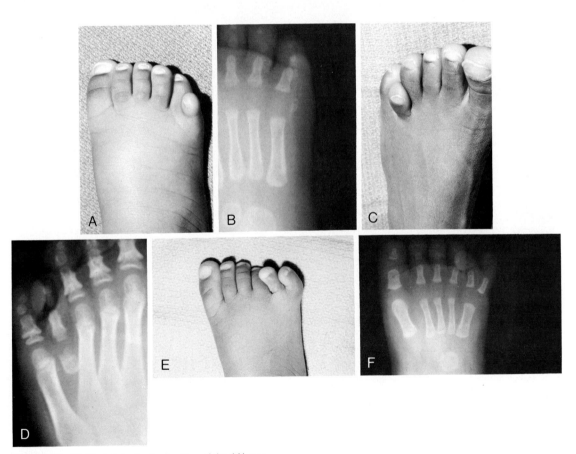

FIGURE 34–17. Variations in duplication of the fifth toe.

(A and B), Incomplete duplication of the distal and middle phalanx without articulation with the fifth ray.

(C and D), A high-riding incomplete duplication lying between the fourth and fifth rays. In addition to excision of the insufficient ray, an osteotomy of the base of the fifth ray was necessary to eliminate the 4–5 splay.

(E and F), Duplication of the toes with a common articulation at the metatarsophalangeal joint. Excision of the fibular facet and reconstruction of the collateral ligament were necessary (see text).

Illustration continued on following page

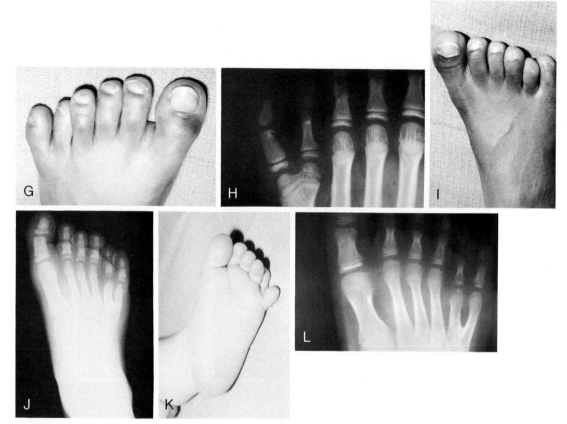

FIGURE 34–17 (Continued)

(G and H), Similar to E and F, the duplication here occurs just proximal to the epiphyseal plate. A capsular and collateral ligament reconstruction for the fibular side of the tibial component was fashioned from the structures on the tibial side of the deleted component. When this tissue is not present, a ligament and periosteal graft may be taken from the fibular side of the deleted component, stripping the tissue down from distal to proximal. After the excision, this flap is reattached to the residual joint.

(I and J), Duplication of the ray begins at the midmetatarsal. Although the inner component is somewhat smaller, excision of the fibular component leaves a nicely contoured lateral border without fifth metatarsal splay.

(K and L), Duplication begins at the proximal third of the metatarsal. The reconstruction is the same as in I and J.

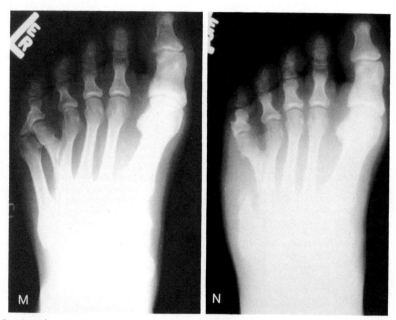

FIGURE 34–17 *(Continued)*

(M and N), In this interesting metatarsal duplication, the problem is the wide, prominent fifth metatarsal head. Although the obvious "interloper" is the fibular branch of the fourth metatarsal, excision of it creates an alignment and potentially a tibial collateral ligament problem for the biphalangeal little toe and the metatarsophalangeal joint and also necessitates an osteotomy at the base of the fifth metatarsal. Excision of the fifth metatarsal, leaving the peroneus brevis attachment at the base and an easy reconstruction of the fibular collateral ligament, was the logical cosmetic and functional solution. Note that this patient's growth plates are closed, and the outcome will not be affected by growth. The procedure could have been done earlier, as well.

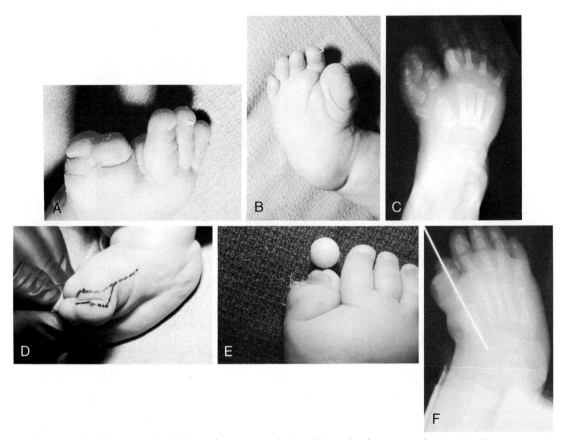

FIGURE 34–18. Triplication of the hallux at the metatarsophalangeal joint level. *(A),* Dorsal view. *(B),* Plantar view. *(C),* X-ray appearance. *(D),* Medial markings. *(E),* Dorsal view of the realigned remaining segment. *(F),* X-ray of the realigned residual toe with Kirschner wire stabilization of the reconstruction.

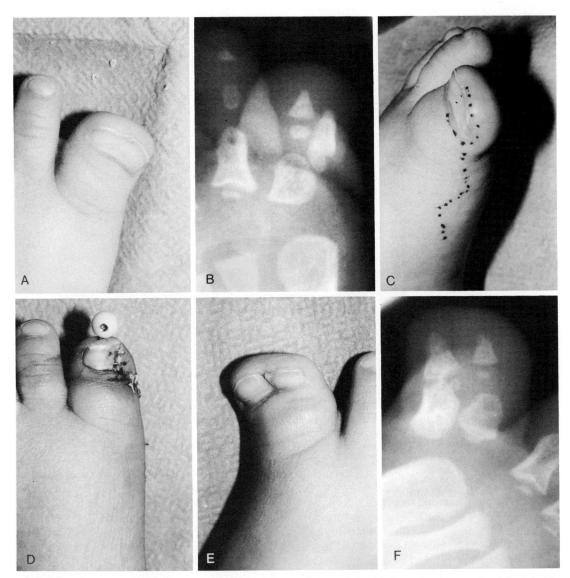

FIGURE 34–19. Bilateral duplications of the hallux. *(A)*, Dorsal view of the left foot. *(B)*, X-ray study of the left side. Duplication is at the interphalangeal joint level. *(C)*, Zig-zag markings for incision to prevent linear contracture from deviating the residual member. *(D)*, An appropriate nail width was determined, and an equal amount of soft tissue was placed on the tibial side to reconstruct the eponychium. *(E)*, Right-sided duplication. *(F)*, X-ray study of the right side demonstrates duplication at the metatarsophalangeal joint, with varus alignment of the toe components.

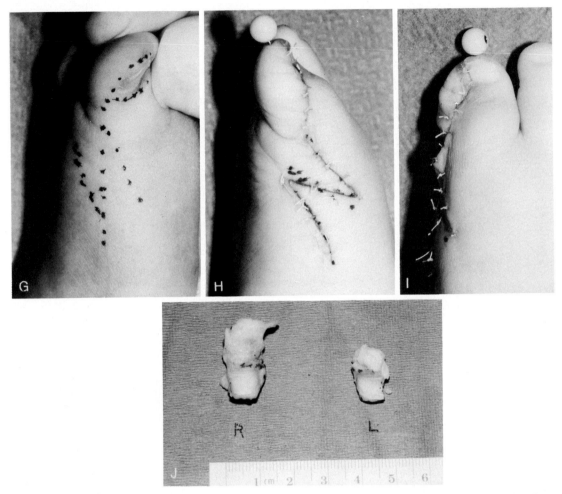

FIGURE 34–19 *(Continued) (G)*, A Z-plasty is marked medially to eliminate skin contracture. *(H)*, The completed Z-plasty. *(I)*, The completed reconstruction. *(J)*, The deleted components.

(tibial) extra ray, or phalanges; to narrow a portion of the metatarsal; and to realign the residual toe on the metatarsal head. This typically requires a medial release or Z-plasty of the skin and lengthening of the abductor hallucis. The medially facing facet on the metatarsal needs to be realigned by a laterally based wedge on the distal first metatarsal head. The surgeon may attempt to reverse the wedge and place it in medially to create an articular surface perpendicular to the long axis of the metatarsal to avoid creating further shortening. However, I have had problems securing the wedge well, and a simple closing wedge seems to suffice. A concentric osteotomy distally is also a consideration here. On occasion,

not only is the great toe in varus secondary to the duplication but all of the toes are angulated medially at the metatarsophalangeal joints. When this occurs, I realign the first ray, carry out capsulotomies on the tibial side of each metatarsophalangeal joint of the lesser toes, and pin the joints in the corrected position for 4 to 6 weeks. By this time, the osteotomy on the first ray has also healed. Overall, this has created a satisfactory result. Although treatment of some hallux duplications can be fairly straightforward (Fig. 34–20), full correction of other duplications requires a thorough knowledge of reconstructive foot surgery (Fig. 34–21).

The major complications of surgery for poly-

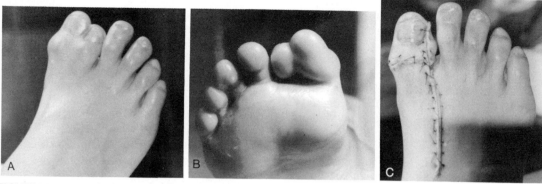

FIGURE 34–20. Simple duplication on the fibular side of the hallux. *(A)*, Dorsal view. *(B)*, Plantar view. *(C)*, Completed reconstruction. (Courtesy of Dr. Richard Herrick, M.D., Opelika, AL.)

dactyly are uncorrected angular deformities or recurrence of angular deformities after surgery or growth. In addition, gaping at sites of central ray deletion may also occur. These can be avoided by appropriate surgery at the time of the deletion of the duplication, or if these deformities occur later, reconstruction can be performed at that time. The reconstructions usually involve appropriate osteotomies or carrying out maneuvers that were originally indicated.

Hyperplasia

The potential causes of hyperplasia (overgrowth or macrodactyly) include Albright's polyostotic fibrous dysplasia, osteoid osteoma,

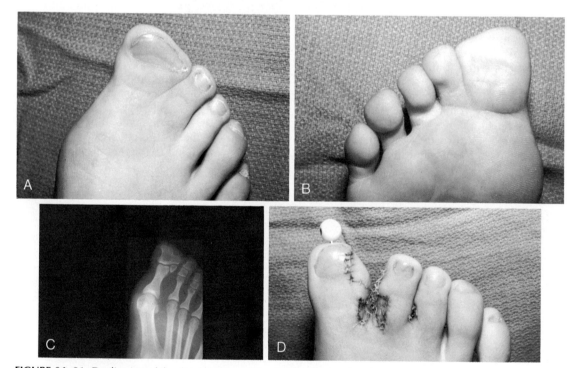

FIGURE 34–21. Duplication of the distal phalanx of the hallux associated with simple syndactyly to the second toe, and an adolescent bunion in a teenage girl. *(A)*, Dorsal view. *(B)*, Plantar view. *(C)*, X-ray study of the duplication and the bunion. *(D)*, Dorsal appearance after excision of the duplication, reconstruction of the syndactyly, and correction of the bunion with the chevron technique.

lymphedema, arteriovenous fistula, lymphangioma, hemangioma and associated Klippel-Trenaunay-Weber syndrome, and von Recklinghausen's neurofibromatosis. True macrodactyly, however, has two clinical forms: the static type, in which the infant is born with the enlarged digit and growth of the digit remains proportional to that of the remaining digits throughout the growth period, and the progressive type, in which there is more rapid growth in the part than in the rest of the foot. The first type appears to be somewhat more common.[1] Typically, the enlargement is noted at birth or within a few months, and males are affected more often than females. The great toe and the second and third toes are more commonly involved than the fourth and fifth toes. Distal portions of the digits are more commonly and more severely involved than the proximal portions. The growth rate is more rapid in the first few years than later.[1, 9, 12]

Typically, with macrodactyly, digital nerves are enlarged, and the enlargement may involve the digit alone or extend proximally to involve the metatarsal. Enlargement may be in length, circumference, or both. Efforts to deal with the problem surgically range from amputation of the toe or ray to maneuvers to retard the overgrowth and reduce the size of the part. Whereas in the hand, the loss of function, particularly stiffness, that follows efforts at reconstruction may militate against these attempts, in the toe, surgery is done primarily for shoe fitting and appearance and may be very satisfactory in some cases. Although deletion of a single involved toe is not deforming, dysfunctional, or devastating to a patient, this condition may involve multiple toes or even

the entire foot. As the situation becomes more encompassing, efforts to find solutions intensify. In the worst scenario, major amputations might well be considered, but another consideration is to provide appropriate accommodative footwear until both the surgeon and the family are prepared for a more drastic deletion procedure. In addition to providing extra-depth footwear, skillful pedorthists can split the last on a shoe and fill in the central portion with more material, thus accommodating the significantly wider foot without the need for and expense of a completely custom-made shoe.

Neurolysis and Debulking

The first surgical maneuvers that can be carried out with a single enlarged digit or even with several enlarged minor digits, include a technique described by Tsuge[45, 46] as an extended neurolysis. In this procedure, the digital nerves are exposed through a plantar zigzag incision. All of the branches of the digital nerve are divided. This maneuver is anticipated to decrease the circumferential growth due to neural stimulation of the digit. Although I have performed this procedure on various occasions, I have not had a control digit to determine whether it has really been effective. It is my impression that this technique has limited value.

Associated with this maneuver, I have carried out a wedge resection at the tip of the toe. An incision is made transversely just plantar to the edge of the nail. The incision is deepened to the distal phalanx. A concave ellipse is completed, with the second incision

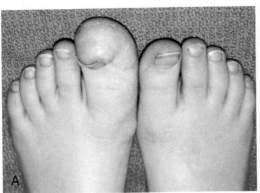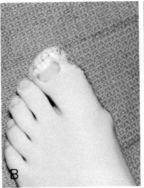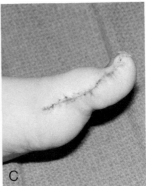

FIGURE 34–23. The Tsuge toe-shortening technique. *(A)*, Enlarged third and fourth toes to be shortened by the Tsuge technique. *(B)*, Bone excision sites. *(C)*, The skin incision. *(D)*, Shifted segments and the residual dorsal hump. *(E)*, Excision of the soft tissue hump 3 months after the initial procedure.

more plantarward. This somewhat radical "smile" wedge excision seems to eliminate the bulk in the toe at its distal-most point and to result in at least some improvement in the dorsal-plantar diameter. Further debulking maneuvers are carried out later, first on one side of the digit and, 3 months later, on the other. In these maneuvers, performed through a midlateral incision, a portion of the tissues dorsal and plantar to the midlateral line is removed, but the adjacent neurovascular bundles, which lie under Cleland's ligaments, are preserved. This type of debulking maneuver has been particularly useful in teenagers with a bone age of older than 13 in girls and 15 in boys, in whom growth might be expected to be complete. It appears to be a more temporizing procedure in the young child (Fig. 34–22).

Although debulking is probably appropriate in patients of any age, after continuing efforts to carry out this procedure and after further growth and development, the digits become increasingly scarred and stiff. This militates against the value of the procedure in the hand; however, if the resultant size and appearance are satisfactory in the foot, the ultimate result is functional.

Enlargement of the part typically continues throughout the growth period, and the excessive growth may occur in either girth, length, or both. Often, the overdevelopment occurs in both parameters. In some cases, however, excessive growth in length is not really a difficult problem. Based on the length of the normal part in the parent of the same gender, I make a decision concerning the interruption of longitudinal growth in the patient's involved part. The standard approach is to perform an epiphysiodesis on all the bones that have reached full length. Therefore, if there does not appear to be any overgrowth in the metatarsal, the growth arrests are carried out only in the phalanges.

Epiphysiodesis

My approach is to make a midlateral incision on both sides of the digit. The growth plate is identified through a limited subperiosteal dissection in the proximal part of the bone. The growth plate is usually easy to recognize because of its whitish appearance compared with the more bony color of the adjacent epiphysis and diaphysis. If there is any question about this, x-ray studies and insertion of a pin can be used to identify the proper site. After I have identified the growth plates on each of the bones, I begin curettage with a small digital curette. An effort is made to remove several millimeters of the growth plate from either side, but no attempt is made to remove all of the cartilaginous material. The epiphyseal plate is V shaped and not specifically perpendicular to the long axis of the bone. It is also not really feasible to perform a classic Phemister bone block technique[34] because the bone is actually too small to carry out this maneuver. The growth arrest has to be carried out on each side of each of the three phalanges. I usually obtain some small plugs of cancellous bone, either from the iliac crest or from the os calcis, by using a semiclosed lateral approach to this area. The dissection to the os calcis is carried out plantar to the peroneal tendons through a short curvilinear incision. The sural nerve and its branches are carefully avoided by using a blunt dissection to the lateral cortex. With a small trephine, very adequate small plugs of cortical and cancellous bone can be obtained. These are used to pack the defects created after curettage. The periosteum is closed as well as possible over the defects. If too vigorous a curettage is carried out, a fracture can occur into the adjacent joint. If there is a suspicion that curettage may have been too vigorous, a longitudinal Kirschner wire can be used to stabilize the digit during the healing period of 4 to 6 weeks. There is no experience, to my knowledge, with efforts to use miniature Blount staples.

In addition, little information is available about the success or failure of the epiphysiodesis technique in the phalanges. However, my observations of procedures that referring physicians, my colleagues, and I have carried out suggest that failure to obtain successful growth arrest is not at all uncommon. Consequently, if the development of a definite bony bridge does not occur within 6 weeks to 3 months, the surgeon should assume that the effort was not successful and will require revision.

Digital Shortening

Techniques for digital shortening, which I have found particularly applicable in the young teenager, are described by Barsky[1] and Tsuge.[45, 46] Although simple amputation to the appropriate length could be carried out, efforts are generally taken to preserve the appearance of the end of the toe. Giannestras recommended removal of the entire proximal phalanx and as much as necessary of the middle phalanx, with surgical syndactylization considered to the adjacent toe.[15]

In Barsky's technique, the distal half of the middle phalanx is removed, and the tip of the remaining shaft is shaped to a pencil point.[1] The articular surface of the distal phalanx is reamed to create a receptacle, which is then fitted over the end of the middle phalanx. Intramedullary Kirschner wires are used to hold the position. An arch-shaped incision is made across the dorsum of the digit at approximately the mid–middle phalanx level and carried down to approximately the midsagittal line. A parallel arch is made somewhat more distally at the distal interphalangeal joint level, and both of these arch-shaped incisions meet a midsagittal incision carried distally. The soft tissue is excised over the dorsum, and the underlying bony work is subsequently carried out. A hump is created with the redundant plantar tissue, which can be excised at a later date. The circulation to the distal pulp and dorsal residual skin is at significant risk with this procedure, but in view of the nature and purpose of this procedure, the risks can probably be accepted if explained well to the patient and family.

The procedure described by Tsuge[45, 46] is somewhat different (Fig. 34–23). The plantar three-quarters of the distal phalanx and the excessive plantar pulp are excised along with an equivalent length of the dorsal half of the middle phalanx. The nail and dorsal portion of the distal phalanx are then recessed onto the residual plantar portion of the middle phalanx. This is carried out through a midlateral incision, which provides easy access to excision of the lower portion of the distal phalanx and the dorsum of the middle phalanx.

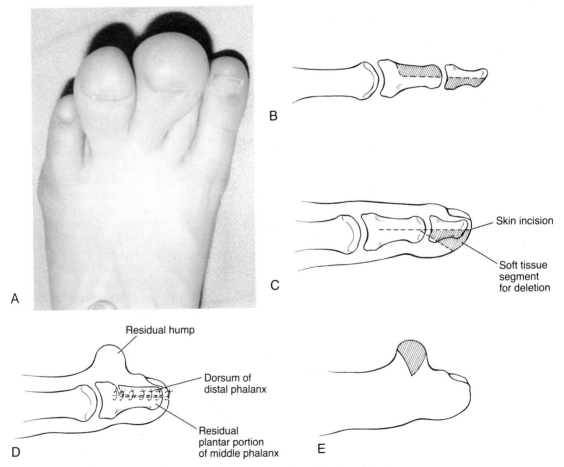

FIGURE 34–23. The Tsuge toe-shortening technique. *(A)*, Enlarged third and fourth toes to be shortened by the Tsuge technique. *(B)*, Bone excision sites. *(C)*, The skin incision. *(D)*, Shifted segments and the residual dorsal hump. *(E)*, Excision of the soft tissue hump 3 months after the initial procedure.

A dorsal hump is created that can be partially removed at this time to allow closure of the sagittal incision line; the remainder of the dorsal hump is removed later. The circulation to the dorsal skin and nail is precarious, and in the several patients in whom I have carried out this procedure, although the skin survived, there was sloughing of the nail, indicative of the marginal blood supply. However, even with the problem with nail growth, the contour of the digit and its overall appearance were superior to that of a simple amputation.

The final procedure to be considered in macrodactyly is actual deletion of the part (Fig. 34–24). Although this procedure must obviously be considered for resolution of an ongoing problem, it is not altogether necessary to perform it or even to recommend it at the time of the initial visit. In my opinion, the seed for this procedure should be planted in the minds of the parents early on: if the procedure then becomes necessary, it will not be totally unexpected (Fig. 34–25). In view of the variability in the presentation of this con-

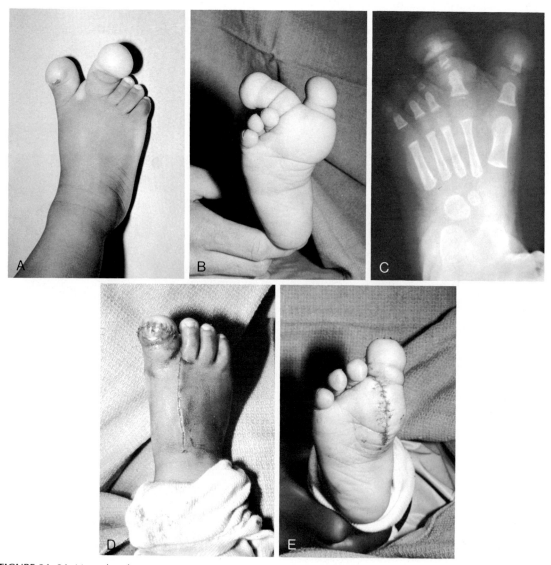

FIGURE 34–24. Macrodactyly reconstructed by ablation. *(A)*, Dorsal view of macrodactyly of the second toe. *(B)*, Plantar view. *(C)*, X-ray study showing the enlarged second toe. *(D and E)*, The entire second ray, except the base, leaving Lisfranc's ligament intact, is excised to allow narrowing of the gap between the great and third toes. This prevents a secondary bunion from forming.

dition, the surgeon should have knowledge of all of these approaches and of perhaps still others[19, 21, 35, 36, 39, 48] and should consider the applicability of each in each circumstance in which this condition is encountered.

Complications of surgery for macrodactyly include continued overgrowth and failure to achieve an adequate reduction, requiring further revision. Scarring and stiffness, which usually appear to be part of the sequelae, are less significant in the toes than in the fingers. As long as protective sensibility is maintained, damage or excision of nerve branches is not of much consequence. Loss of circulation to a part is certainly a possibility with these various maneuvers, and it should be explained to the parents as a possible consequence of efforts to reduce the part. Carrying out the surgery with loupe magnification and attention to the location of the vascular supply will help prevent premature loss of parts.

Hypoplasia

Hypoplasia is rarely an indication for surgical intervention. Usually, an accommodative insert helps fill out the shoe, allowing the wearing of matched pairs. Hypoplasia of a single toe is particularly of no consequence, unless an angular deformity occurs in the adjacent digit. Again, the use of inserts can

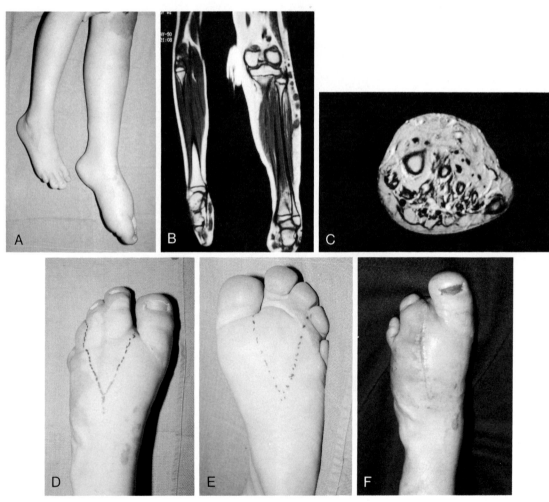

FIGURE 34–25. Macrodactyly of toes three and four on the right foot, with hemihypertrophy on the left. *(A)*, Both lower extremities. *(B)*, Magnetic resonance image demonstrating the enlarged soft tissues and increased vascularity. *(C)*, Cross-sectional magnetic resonance image of the left forefoot. *(D and E)*, Dorsal and plantar markings for deletion of the second and third rays. *(F)*, Dorsal view after ray deletions.

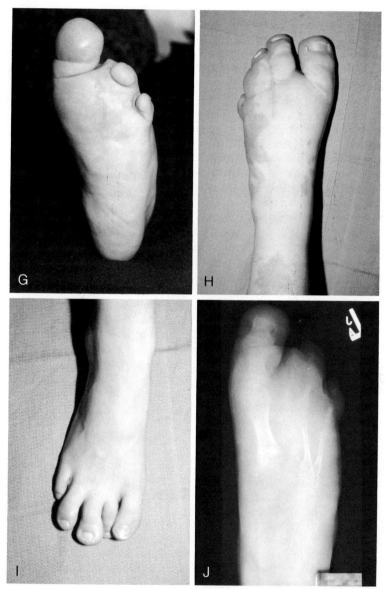

FIGURE 34–25 *(Continued) (G),* Plantar view after ray deletions. The procedure made shoeing significantly easier. *(H and I),* Current views of the left and right feet. Macrodactyly toes have yet to be reconstructed. In this 7-year-old, further reconstructive ablations will have to be considered. *(J),* X-ray study after ray excisions.

protect the adjacent toes from migrating into the area. Typically, hypoplasia is seen in conditions in which there is a failure of formation of parts, rather than as the formation of a completely normal toe or ray that is hypoplastic.

Short metatarsals, on the other hand, may well result in decreased length of the entire ray. This may or may not be of consequence. Shortness of the first metatarsal was first implicated by Morton.[29] He suggested that this condition would lead to uneven weight bearing along the plantar aspect of the foot, resulting in metatarsalgia and increased pronation. He stressed that this would only be an occasional problem. Subsequently, Harris and Beath reported that the short first metatarsal would rarely, if ever, be the cause of significant foot problems.[18] A shortened fourth metatarsal, although often cited as a skeletal variation in calcium and phosphorus abnormalities, is typically unrelated to metabolic disorders. Shortening may be seen in the third metatarsal as well or in both the third and fourth metatarsals. These patients rarely seem to have true problems with weight bearing and are primarily disturbed by the appearance of the shortened toe. If weight bearing is a problem, the use of accommodative total contact inserts should be sufficient to deal with the problem. Lengthening efforts with typical two-dimensional lengthening devices have been a problem. The more recent use of the small Ilizarov-type equipment may be a better approach (see Chapter 31). Other approaches are described in the literature.[13, 23]

Congenital Constriction Band Syndrome

Congenital constriction band syndrome is a rare and poorly understood entity. It apparently occurs sporadically, with an incidence of one in 15,000 births.[32] Although Temtamy and McKusick,[43] as well as Streeter,[40] believe that this is a germ plasm defect, Torpin[44] described constrictions by amniotic bands, a phenomenon occurring late in pregnancy, as the cause of this disorder. The current consensus is that Torpin's interpretation is correct.[27, 37, 38] The phenomenon presents in a variety of ways: constriction rings that may completely or incompletely surround a part; rings with the amputation of distal parts; rings with marked swelling of the distal component; and acrosyn-

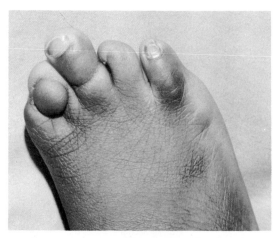

FIGURE 34–26. Congenital constriction band syndrome. Bands, an enlarged distal segment, and a congenital amputation are demonstrated.

dactyly (Fig. 34–26).[8, 11] In acrosyndactyly, the tips of various digits are joined, with typical loss of portions of the distal components and various degrees of residual web formation. At times, the swelling and cyanosis of the distal part dictate immediate release of the band for preservation of the distal part. In the area of the constriction, important structures such as the neurovascular bundles and even tendons may be severely compromised and may or may not be in full continuity. When neurolysis is carried out, it is important to start well proximal and distal to the ring to identify the normal structures.[8]

The standard approach in dealing with the rings is to carry out a series of Z-plasties, involving only half of the circumference of the digit initially and then involving the second half several months later.[11] It is important to excise the band and to interdigitate the 60-degree Z-plasties. An alternate technique is to carry out a W-plasty. Typically, I perform the Z-plasties on the dorsum initially and then perform those on the plantar side later. On occasion, it appears appropriate to involve half of the dorsal side and half of the plantar side each time, but this is technically a little more difficult.

The persistent problem encountered with this condition is distal swelling of the digit, particularly on the dorsal side. My usual approach is to initially carry out the Z-plasties and then to look for a reduction in the swelling over the course of the next year. If the swelling does not recede, I perform a second procedure to debulk the digit by creating a distally based flap, still maintaining interdigitations proximally at the site of the previous band. The flap is raised down to the level of the extensor mechanism. Interestingly, the thickened tissue is not boggy and edematous, but rather a thick, fibrofatty layer of relatively dense tissue. This is thinned down at the time of the surgery, leaving significant[14] redundant skin. The excess is trimmed and reinterdigitated at this second procedure.

Acrosyndactyly

Acrosyndactyly is thought to be a refusion of digits after the webs have been formed. In some instances, it is easy to make this diagnosis, whereas in others, it is difficult to differentiate acrosyndactyly from an extensive complex syndactyly. However, the presence of skin-lined sinuses between the dorsal and plantar surfaces confirms that some form of web probably existed at one time in utero. I have classified this condition into three types, each of which has a specific surgical approach.[17a] In type I, the tips are joined, but the webs are well formed to the proper depth. Unfortunately, in many of these, there has been a distal amputation at the site of the band, and the toes are particularly short. I believe that it is important not only to separate the tips but also to excise the ever-present seed-like nubbins on the tips of these digits, to round them off, and then to carry out a closure with available skin (Fig. 34–27).

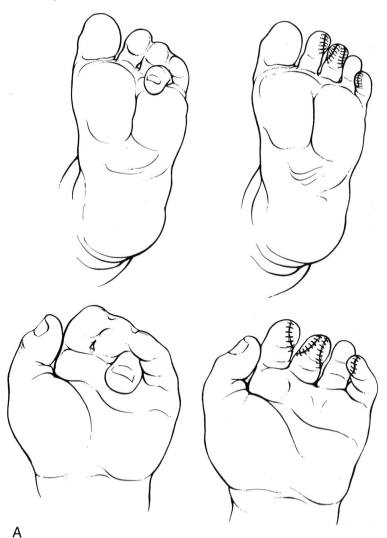

A

FIGURE 34–27. Type I acrosyndactyly (tips joined). *(A)*, Artist's drawing *(feet above, hands below)*. Tips are released, nubbins excised, and fingers or toes closed *(right)*.

Illustration continued on following page

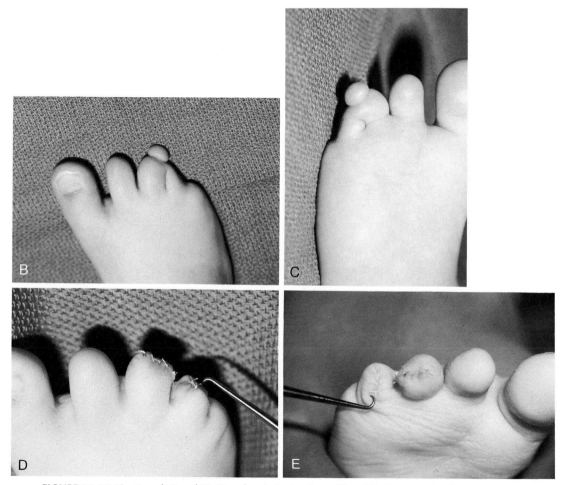

FIGURE 34–27 *(Continued)* *(B* and *C),* Dorsal and plantar views. *(D* and *E),* The completed reconstruction.

In type II, the tips are also joined, but the webs, although present, are significantly longer. These may be shortened by use of the three-flap web plasty,[17, 31] as described earlier, or may require a more formal syndactyly reconstruction with the use of full-thickness skin grafting (Fig. 34–28). In type III, although the tips are joined, little web formation is present other than the skin-lined sinuses between the dorsal and plantar surfaces. In these patients, more formal syndactyly reconstruction, as described earlier, is appropriate. Here, we recon-

struct the border digits first and the remaining web 3 months later. An attempt is made to create four digits if four are involved, but the shape of the residual digits and their spacing are important, and it may be necessary to sacrifice a toe in order to provide the best ultimate appearance (Fig. 34–29).

Angular Deformities

Angular deformities include hallux varus (Fig. 34–30), hallux valgus, hallux valgus in-

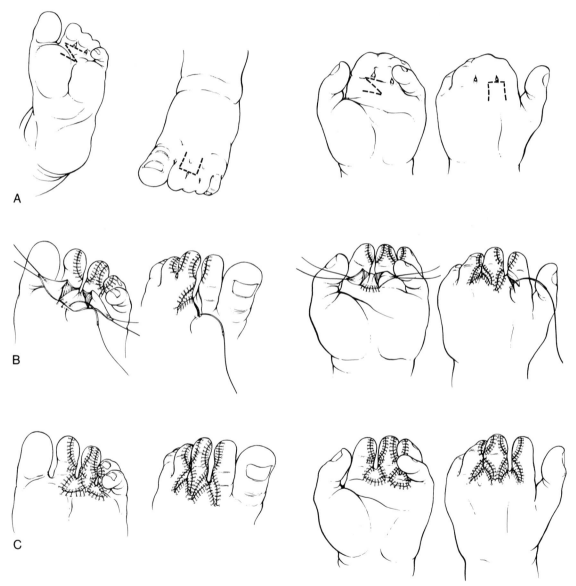

FIGURE 34–28. *(A to C),* Type II acrosyndactyly (tips joined, webs prolonged in feet *(left)* and hands *(right).* Tips are separated and webs are deepened with three-flap web plasties. *(A),* Markings. *(B),* Tips are separated and commissure flaps cut. *(C),* The complete reconstruction.

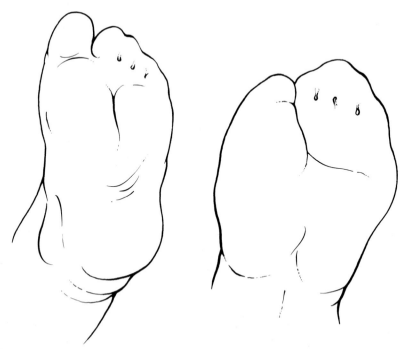

FIGURE 34–29. Type III acrosyndactyly (tips joined, only sinuses between the digits in a foot *(left)* and a hand *(right)*. Reconstruction is carried out with standard syndactyly technique (see text). The web sinuses are excised. Border digits are operated on first.

FIGURE 34–30. Hallux varus deformity secondary to old residual duplication. *(A)*, Dorsal view. *(B)*, X-ray study demonstrating a medially facing metatarsal facet. *(C and D)*, Reconstruction by lateral closing wedge osteotomy of the distal metatarsal metaphysis.

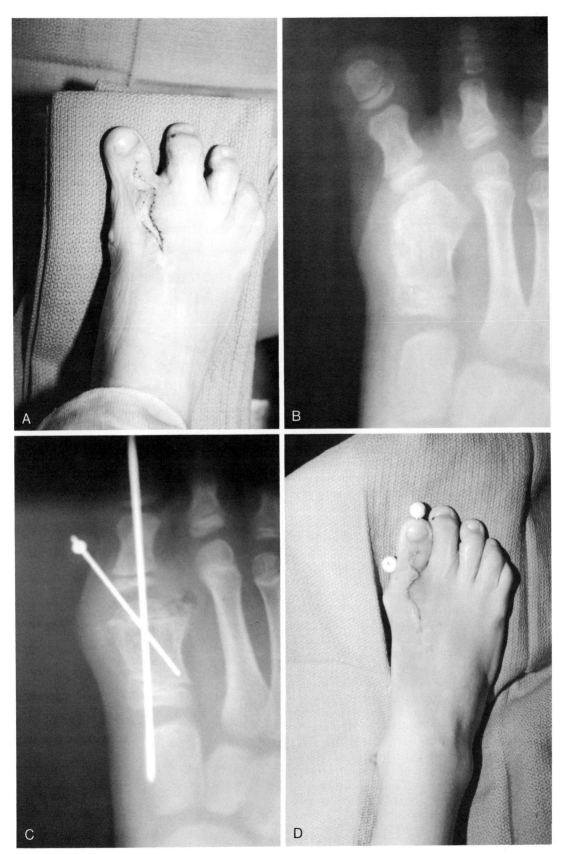

FIGURE 34–30 *See legend on opposite page*

terphalangeus, clinodactyly, hammer toe, clawtoe, and mallet toe, over- and underlapping second and fifth toes, and curly toes. In addition, metatarsus adductus, functional interning, and the skewfoot deformity associated with pronation of the hindfoot and compensatory adduction and varus of the forefoot should be included. Each of these conditions requires significant discussion and involves a variety of surgical techniques. Consequently, they are dealt with in subsequent chapters.

SUMMARY

An approach to congenital anomalies requires a knowledge of the fundamentals of the functional requirements of the foot, including the need for stability and for mobility in certain areas; an appreciation of sociologic factors, including appropriate footwear for a given age group; and an understanding of the psychological considerations related to this portion of the anatomy. Along with an understanding of the physical and emotional needs of the patient, the surgeon must also possess the knowledge and training related to orthopaedic and plastic procedures involving these tissues. A thorough understanding of the anatomy, particularly the neurovascular supply, is important. Finally, a knowledge of potential pedorthic adjuncts helps to bring the issue at hand into perspective, allowing the use of either surgery, nonoperative means, or a combination of both to achieve the desired result.

In the area of surgery for congenital malformations of the feet and toes, more than in perhaps any other area in the foot, a specific operation for a specific problem in a given patient may not yet have been performed or even described. With this in mind, the surgeon must be well grounded in the principles listed previously and must extrapolate them to deal with the given situation. Consequently, a knowledge of fundamental principles, imagination, artistry, technical skill, and a thorough discussion between the surgeon, perhaps the patient, and certainly the parents are needed in order to proceed with ideal reconstructions. Finally, the surgeon must remain open minded and current with technologic advances to provide the best treatment possible for the patient.

References

1. Barsky A: Macrodactyly. J Bone Joint Surg 49A:1255–1266, 1967.
2. Bauer TB, Tondra JM, Trusler HM: Technical modification in repair of syndactylies. Plast Reconstr 17:385–392, 1956.
3. Blanco JS, Herring JA: Congenital Chopart amputation. A functional assessment. Clin Orthop 256:14–21, 1990.
4. Blauth W, Olason AT: Classification of polydactyly of the hands and feet. Arch Orthop Trauma Surg 107:334–344, 1988.
5. Blauth W: The treatment of congenital foot abnormalities. 127:3–14, 1989.
6. Buck-Gramcko D, Behrens P: Classification of polydactyly of the hand and foot. Handchir Mikrochir Plast Chir 21:195–204, 1989.
7. Dell PC, Sheppard JE: Deformities of the great toe in Apert's syndrome. Clin Orthop 157:113–118, 1981.
8. Dobyns JH, Wood VE, Bayne LG, Frykman GK: Congenital hand deformities. *In* Green DP (Ed): Operative Hand Surgery. New York, Churchill Livingstone, 1982, pp 213–450.
9. Edgerton MT, Tuerk DB: Macrodactyly (digital gigantism); it's nature and treatment. *In* Littler JW, Cramer LM, Smith JW (Eds): Symposium On Reconstructive Hand Surgery, Vol 9. St. Louis, CV Mosby, 1974, pp 157–172.
10. Fett-Conte AC, Richieri-Costa A: Acheiropodia: Report on four new Brazilian patients. Am J Med Genet 36:341–344, 1990.
11. Flatt AE: The Care of Congenital Hand Anomalies. St. Louis, CV Mosby, 1977, pp 213–277.
12. Flatt AE: The Care of Congenital Hand Anomalies. St. Louis, CV Mosby, 1977, pp 249–262.
13. Frankel JP, Fleishman JH: Correction of brachymetatarsia with transpositional metatarsal osteotomies. J Foot Surg 30:19–25, 1991.
14. Frantz CH, O'Rahilly R: Congenital skeletal limb deformities. J Bone Joint Surg 43A:1202, 1961.
15. Giannestras NJ: Foot Disorders. Philadelphia, Lea & Febiger, 1967, pp 304–306.
16. Goldner JL: Advances and care of the foot: 1800–1987. Orthopedics 10:1817–1836, 1987.
17. Gould JS: *Syndactyly. In* Carter PR (Ed): Reconstruction of the Child's Hand. Philadelphia, Lea & Febiger, 1991, pp 127–151.
17a. Gould JS, American Society for Surgery of the Hand correspondence letter.
18. Harris RI, Beath T: The short first metatarsal. J Bone Joint Surg 31A:553–565, 1949.
19. Herring JA, Tolo VT: Macrodactyly. J Pediatr Orthop 4:503–506, 1984.
20. Hootnick DR, Packard DS Jr, Levinsohn EM, Factor DA: The anatomy of a human foot with missing toes and reduplication of the hallux. J Anat 174:1–17, 1991.
21. Kalen V, Burwell DS, Omer GE: Macrodactyly of the hand and feet. J Pediatr Orthop 8:311–315, 1988.
22. Lieber MT, Toub AS: Common foot deformities and what they mean for parents. Am J Mat Child Nurs 13:47–50, 1988.
23. Martin DE, Kalish SR: Brachymetatarsia. A new

surgical approach. J Am Podiatr Med Assoc 81:10–17, 1991.

24. Masada K, Tsuyuguchi Y, Kawabata H, Ono K: Treatment of preaxial polydactyly of the foot. Plast Reconstr Surg 79:251–258, 1987.

25. Mason WH, Wymore M, Berger E: Foot deformities in Apert's syndrome. Review of the literature and case reports. J Am Podiatr Med Assoc 80:540–544, 1990.

26. Matev IB: Thumb reconstruction in children through metacarpal lengthening. Plast Reconstr Surg 64:665–669, 1979.

27. Miura T: Congenital constriction band syndrome. J Hand Surg 9A:82–88, 1984.

28. Mondolfi PE: Syndactyly of the toes. Plast Reconstr Surg 71:212–218, 1983.

29. Morton D: The Human Foot. New York, Columbia University Press, 1935.

30. Noagami H: Polydactyly and polysyndactyly of the fifth toe. Clin Orthop 204:261–265, 1986.

31. Ostrowski DM, Feagin CA, Gould JS: A three-flap webplasty for release of short congenital syndactyly and dorsal adduction contracture. J Hand Surg 16A:634–641, 1991.

32. Patterson TJS: Congenital ring constrictions. Br J Plast Surg 14:1, 1961.

33. Phelps DA, Grogan DP: Polydactyly of the foot. J Pediatr Orthop 5:446–451, 1985.

34. Phemister DB: Operative arrestment of longitudinal growth of bones, in the treatment of deformities. J Bone Joint Surg 15:1, 1933.

35. Pho RW, Patterson M, Lee WS: Reconstruction and pathology and macrodactyly. J Hand Surg 13A:78–83, 1988.

36. Rawat SS: A new operative technique for congenital gigantism of the toes. Br J Plast Surg 43:120–121, 1990.

37. Ray M, Hendrick SJ, Raimer SS, Blackwell SJ: Amniotic band syndrome. Int J Dermatol 27:312–314, 1988.

38. Rossillon D, Rombouts JJ, Verellen-Dumoulin C, et al: Congenital ring construction syndrome of the limbs; A report of 19 cases. Br J Plast Surg 41:270–277, 1988.

39. Sabapathy SR, Roberts JO, Regan PJ, Ramaswamy CN: Pedal macrodactyly treated by digital shortening and free nail graft; A report of two cases. Br J Plast Surg 43:116–199, 1990.

40. Streeter GL: Focal deficiencies in fetal tissues and their relation to intra-uterine amputation. *In* Contributions To Embryology Vol. 22, No. 126. Washington, DC, Carnegie Institution of Washington, 1930, pp 1–44.

41. Swanson AB: A classification for congenital limb malformations. J Hand Surg 1:8–22, 1976.

42. Tachdjian MO: The Child's Foot. Philadelphia, WB Saunders, 1985, pp 131–351.

43. Temtamy SA, McKusick VA: Digital and other malformations associated with congenital ring constrictions. Birth Defects 14:547, 1978.

44. Torpin R: Fetal Malformations Caused by Amnion Rupture During Gestation. Springfield, IL, Charles C Thomas, 1968.

45. Tsuge K: Treatment of macrodactyly. Plast Reconstr Surg 39:590–599, 1967.

46. Tsuge K: Treatment of macrodactyly. J Hand Surg 10A:968–969, 1985.

47. Viljoen DL, Kidson SH: Mirror polydactyly: Pathogenesis based on a morphogen gradient theory. Am J Med Genet 35:229–235, 1990.

48. Wood VE: Macrodactyly. J Iowa Med Soc 59:922–928, 1969.

49. Wong HB: Genetic aspects of foot deformities. J Singapore Paediatr Soc 29:13–22, 1987.

35

Angular Deformities of the Lesser Toes

JOHN E. HANDELSMAN

The lesser toes, together with the hallux, play a significant role in normal ambulation. At toe-off, weight is transferred from the metatarsal heads to the extended toes, which plantarflex to provide the spring in comfortable walking. When the toes are dorsally subluxed at the metatarsophalangeal joints, this function is lost. Excessive weight is borne by the metatarsal heads. Skin calluses, digital nerve neurapraxias, and pain may be the outcome. Toe flexion contractures have an equally unsatisfactory effect, often preventing normal weight bearing on the metatarsal heads and resulting in callosities on the tips of the toes, nail abnormalities because of pressure, and dorsal callosities as the acutely flexed toes thrust against the upper portion of the shoes. Toes that deviate sideways and come to underlie or overlie adjacent toes, may be equally nonfunctional.

Angular toe deformities may, therefore, compromise normal weight bearing, result in the development of callosities, and produce pain. Shoe fitting may be difficult, and the toes may be an unacceptable cosmetic blemish, particularly for a teenager. When there is underlying neurologic disease, toe deformity may be relentlessly progressive. Although out of sight, toe deformities may be disabling and warrant correction.

CONGENITAL CURLY TOES

Underlapping Toes

Curly toes are common, frequently familial, and usually affect the lateral three toes, partic-

ularly the third (Fig. 35–1A). The toe is angled, usually toward the tibial side, and somewhat rotated. The toe is almost always flexed, and tightness of the flexor tendons is apparent. Isolated shortness of the long, short or both toe flexor tendons appears to be the primary cause of the condition.

Nonoperative Treatment

Underlapping of the affected toe may be of a minor order, in which the toe straightens with weight bearing. If the appearance is not regarded as unacceptable, no treatment is indicated. However, particularly in infancy, strapping of the affected toe into a dorsiflexed position is an innocuous, easily performed, and effective treatment. A narrow standard adhesive tape is placed so that the affected toe rests on the nonsticky surface and is held dorsiflexed by the tape, which is then wrapped around the two adjoining toes (Fig. 35–1B). The tension is adjusted so that the affected toe is held parallel with its neighbors. If used regularly during sleeping periods and as tolerated during the day, the deformity may be sufficiently corrected. Should this method fail, surgery is a simple and effective alternative and can be performed in the ambulatory setting.

Operative Treatment

Toe Flexor Tendon Tenotomy

A general anesthetic and a tourniquet are preferred. A small transverse incision is made in the proximal flexor crease where the toe

618

FIGURE 35–1. *(A)*, Congenital curly third toe, underlapping the second. *(B)*, Taping of an underlying third toe. Narrow adhesive tape is attached to the adjoining second and fourth toes and is used as an elevating sling underneath the curled down third toe so that it is brought level with its neighbors.

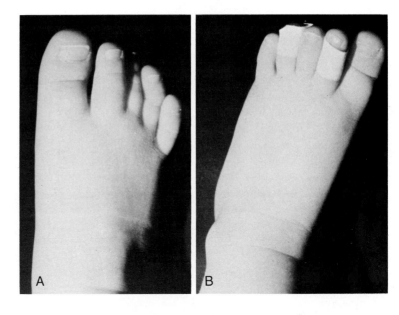

joins the fat pad under of the metatarsal heads (Fig. 35–2A[1]). This is deepened directly to tendon sheath, and small retractors are used medially and laterally to protect soft tissues that contain the neurovascular bundle on each side.

The tendon sheaths are opened, and the flexor digitorum longus tendon is identified over the proximal phalanx and mobilized (Fig. 35–2A[2] and 35–2B). The brevis tendon has split at this point, and its two sections should be sought on each side of the longus tendon. Extension of the toe identifies the tendon that is too short and tight. This is usually the flexor digitorum longus tendon and, if so, the tendon is tenotomized. When only the long flexor tendon is to be released, an oblique cut is satisfactory. If, however, both the long and the short tendons are to be elongated, a Z-lengthening in the long tendon should be performed to assist in retaining continuity and function subsequently. When the short tendon needs to be released, both arms of the split tendon are tenotomized obliquely. No attempt is made to repair the tendons, and subcutaneous tissue and skin are then repaired with fine absorbable sutures. Subcuticular sutures are used for skin whenever practical. Skin closure may be reinforced with adhesive strips, because there is frequently some tension as the toe is straightened.

Postoperatively, the released toe is taped to the dorsum of the foot (Fig. 35–2C) or held in a tape sling in a manner similar to that described for nonoperative treatment. Where several tendons have been released, it is better to apply a short-leg walking cast, incorporating a toe plate to hold the toes moderately dorsiflexed. Splinting is necessary for about 3 weeks.

Flexor function in the toes invariably returns. A potential complication is damage to the plantar digital nerves and vessels.

Overlapping Toes

This condition is usually a familial condition involving the fifth toe, which overlaps the fourth (Fig. 35–3A). Other toes may occasionally be involved. There is contraction of the dorsal and medial capsule of the metatarsophalangeal joint and relative shortness of the extensor tendons. The proximal phalanx is dorsally displaced, adducted, and rotated. The condition is usually bilateral. When other toes are involved, there is frequently congenital shortening of the associated metatarsal. The clinical presentation and management are similar to that for overlapping of the fifth toe.

If the condition is not treated, about half the patients will ultimately have disabling symptoms.[2] Because of difficulty with shoe fitting and callus formation in adulthood, pro-

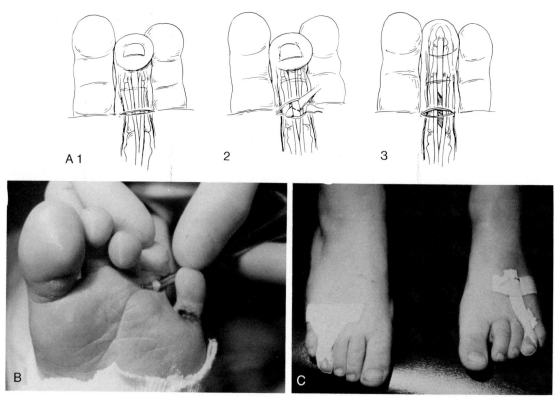

FIGURE 35–2. *(A),* The tight long toe flexor is approached through a transverse incision in the proximal toe crease (1). The long flexor tendon is separated from the split brevis tendon and delivered into the wound (2). The tendon is divided obliquely, permitting straightening of the toe (3). *(B),* The fourth digitorum longus tendon has been delivered into the wound prior to division. The fifth toe has already been corrected surgically. *(C),* Postoperative taping in place after surgical release of the third and fourth toes bilaterally. This taping is left in place for 3 weeks.

cedures such as syndactylization of the fifth to the fourth toes,[5] proximal hemiphalangectomy,[6] and even amputation of the toe have been recommended. Thus, early treatment is strongly advocated.

Nonoperative Treatment

In infancy, stretching of the displaced fifth toe may be helpful, combined with taping the toe into a plantar flexed attitude at night. Stretching should be gentle, but held firmly for a count of three, and be performed twenty times on each toe, at each diaper change. At night the toe is taped, and correction obtained by attaching the tail of the tape under the lateral aspect of the sole. Should this combination of stretching and strapping fail, surgery is advised, preferably before the patient starts walking.

Operative Treatment

Soft Tissue Release for Overlapping Fifth Toe

The procedure consists of Z-lengthening of the fifth toe extensor tendons and a release of the fifth metatarsophalangeal joint capsule, both dorsally and medially.

The key to the procedure is to prevent relapse because of tight dorsal skin. The dorsal tendon and capsule are thus approached through a V-incision, based distally and closed in a Y-fashion, so that skin is advanced. A variation of this procedure that is preferred by the author is Butler's operation described by Cocklin (Fig. 35–3).[2]

Butler's Operation. In this procedure, the approach is modified in that a circumferential incision is made around the base of the fifth toe and a dorsal extension is added to produce

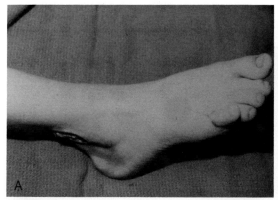
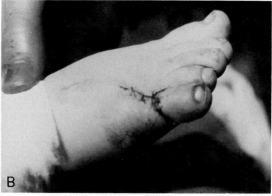
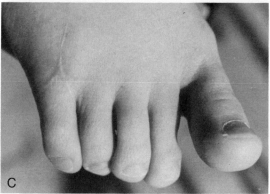

FIGURE 35–3. Cockin's modification of the Butler operation for an overlapping fifth toe. *(A)*, A double racket incision is used. After release of the dorsal and medial capsule of the metatarsophalangeal joint and lengthening of the extensor tendons, the toe is placed in the volar arm of the incision as it is reduced anatomically. *(B)*, Skin closure maintains the correct position of the toe. *(C)*, Two years after surgery, the fifth toe remains corrected.

a racket shape (Fig. 35–3A). This permits adequate exposure of the extensor tendons and the metatarsophalangeal joint and capsule. A second incision on the plantar aspect of the foot is made extending proximally from the circumferential incision, thus producing a second handle to the racket. The extensor tendons are elongated in a Z-fashion, and the capsule of the metatarsophalangeal joint is released dorsally and medially. After release, the toe is pulled into the correct position and comes to lie in the plantar handle. The circumferential incision and dorsal handle are then closed, locking the toe in the reduced position (Figs. 35–3B and C).

In performing the procedure, care must be taken to retract the soft tissue containing the small dorsal neurovascular bundles and to perform the medial portion of the metatarsophalangeal joint capsulotomy with care so that the larger volar neurovascular bundle is not damaged. Even when it does not appear tight, a limited lengthening of the extensor tendons is always necessary to prevent recurrence of the deformity. However, do not overlengthen the extensor tendons or hold the toe too plantar-flexed postoperatively, because overcorrection can occur.

TRUE ANGULAR TOE DEFORMITIES

Sometimes, a toe may deviate because of true angulation within a phalanx and not because of the tethering effect of a short tendon. The lateral toes are more prone to be involved, and the condition is usually bilateral and frequently familial.

Since angular toes usually do not overlap or underlap, the condition is often no more than a cosmetic blemish and may not warrant treatment. However, if the appearance is unacceptable or if there is functional compromise, correction can be obtained by osteotomy of the offending phalanx.

Surgical intervention should be withheld until the toe is sufficiently large. This toe usually deviates in a tibial direction, and the offending phalanx should be approached through a dor-

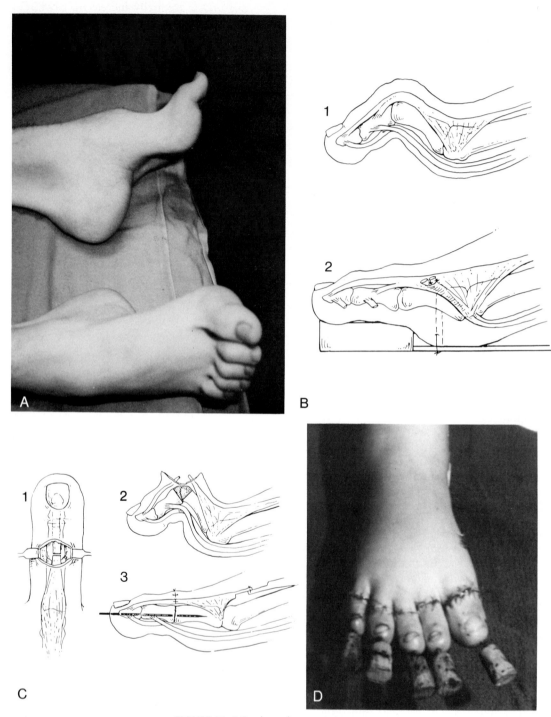

FIGURE 35–4 *See legend on opposite page*

solateral incision. Blunt dissection to the periosteum is used to avoid damaging the neurovascular structures.

The periosteum is incised and cleared over the point of maximum angulation. Care should be taken to avoid stripping the periosteum beyond the proximally situated growth plate. The site is predrilled, and the osteotomy is performed using an osteotome. The osteotome provides better control than a power saw, which may also burn the bone and produce delayed union. If necessary, a small wedge of bone may be removed. After careful closure of periosteum, the toe may be sufficiently stable. If not, a thin smooth Kirschner wire is passed through the tuft of the toe and is inserted to the base of the proximal phalanx. A short-leg walking cast with an adequate toe plate is always used for 6 weeks or until union is adequate. The Kirschner wire can be removed at the third or fourth postoperative week.

CLAWING OF THE TOES

Flexion at the interphalangeal joints and extension at the metatarsophalangeal joints occurs when there is loss of innervation of the intrinsic muscles of the foot. The essential function of the interossei and lumbrical muscles is to flex the metatarsophalangeal joints, because their tendons are volar to the joints, and to extend the interphalangeal joints through their insertions into the extensor expansions. For practical purposes, the long toe flexor tendons flex only at the interphalangeal joints, and the long toe extensors extend only at the metatarsophalangeal joints. Unopposed,

these tendons gradually produce a clawtoe deformity. Ultimately, the deformity becomes fixed and a gradually increasing cavus deformity of the foot frequently follows (Figs. 35–4A and 35–4B[1]). This train of events is obvious when a loss of innervation of the intrinsic muscles of the foot is seen, as in Charcot-Marie-Tooth disease, low myelomeningocele, and occasionally, with cord tethering syndromes. The cause of familial cavus and clawtoe deformities is less clear. However, it is reasonable to assume that a subtle muscle imbalance with intrinsic muscle weakness is a significant factor. All these conditions respond to methods that replace the intrinsic muscle functions.

Nonoperative Treatment

Toe clawing may be present at birth or may become apparent soon thereafter. It will occur gradually at an older age in children with spinal cord tethering syndromes. When the deformity is mobile, stretching of the toes into flexion at the metatarsophalangeal joints and extension at the interphalangeal joints may help to slow the process. Footwear should be broad enough and of sufficient length to prevent any pressure on the toes. When toe deformity becomes fixed and cavus commences, orthotic support under the metatarsal necks may relieve the metatarsal head discomfort and callus formation that occurs in the established case. In all instances, intrinsic muscle foot exercises are important.

Operative Techniques

The aim of surgery is to replace intrinsic muscle function. Two methods are available.

FIGURE 35–4. *(A)*, Fixed clawing of the toes and bilateral cavus deformity in a 14-year-old boy. *(B)*, The Girdlestone operation. Typical clawing, with hyperextension at the metatarsophalangeal joints and flexion at the proximal interphalangeal joints, resulting from relative weakness of the intrinsic muscle (1). The flexor digitorum longus and brevis tendons are detached close to their insertions, are brought to the dorsum of the foot lateral to the proximal phalanx, and are attached to the extensor expansion using a buttonhole technique: Note that the tendons remain on the volar surface of the axis of the metatarsophalangeal joint. A heavy suture is passed close to bone on each side of the proximal phalanx, and through the plantar skin. This suture is tied to a prong of a Lambrinudi plate that supports the toes distally, and proximally it is attached to a short-leg walking cast (2). *(C)*, Proximal interphalangeal joint fusion of the toe. The proximal interphalangeal joint is exposed through an oval dorsal incision, directly over the joint. A small amount of skin that may contain a callus is excised. The extensor expansion is transected transversely (1). The joint is opened, and the head of the proximal phalanx and base of distal phalanx are excised at right angles to the shafts of the bone, as shown in the shaded area (2). After establishing accurate apposition of the stumps of the excised phalanges, the straight attitude of the toe is maintained with a smooth Kirschner wire. The extensor tendon almost always has to be lengthened (3). *(D)*, Interphalangeal joint fusions of all the toes have been performed, and the position is held with Kirschner wires on which corks have been placed. A short-leg plaster of Paris cast was subsequently applied with a suitable toe piece extending beyond the pins and corks.

The first is a transfer of the long toe flexor tendons into the extensor expansion of the toe. This method was first described by Forrester-Brown[3] in 1928 and subsequently developed by G. R. Girdlestone in Oxford, whose name has come to be associated with the operation. The usefulness of this procedure was reported in 112 feet by R. G. Taylor in 1951.[8]

This operation is tedious, and a similar result may be achieved by the simpler technique of fusing the proximal interphalangeal joint of the toe in extension. This type of joint fusion moves the lever arm of the short toe flexor back to the metatarsophalangeal joint, where flexion must now occur. Furthermore, since the flexion range of the terminal phalanx is relatively limited, the effect of the long toe flexor tendon is also transmitted to the metatarsophalangeal joint. For similar reasons, the extensor tendon is able to dorsiflex the toe as a whole and not just the metatarsophalangeal joint. Proximal interphalangeal joint fusion is the preferred procedure.

The Girdlestone Operation

An elongation of the extensor tendons and, when clawing is very fixed, division of the dorsal capsules of the metatarsophalangeal joints, may be necessary before the tendon transfers can be performed.

Each toe is exposed dorsolaterally, the incision extending from the neck of the metatarsal to the distal interphalangeal joint. The extensor expansion is defined, and the soft tissues containing the dorsal neurovascular bundle are protected and retracted laterally. A plane is developed close to the bone at the neck of the middle phalanx, and the flexor digitorum longus tendon is identified, freed, and brought into the wound using a small blunt hook. The tendon is cut at its insertion. A second plane between soft tissues and the neck of the proximal phalanx is similarly developed, the two attachment points of the short tendon to the base of the middle phalanx are identified, and the tendon is detached. Both the long and the short tendons are then brought around the lateral aspect of the proximal phalanx and are sutured into the extensor expansion by the buttonhole method (Fig. 35–4B[2]). To ensure that the deformity remains fully corrected, tension must be maintained in the tendons while they are being sutured. The metatarsophalangeal joint must also be held moderately

flexed and the interphalangeal joints held moderately extended. Indeed, these attitudes must be maintained until plaster of Paris fixation has been secured.

The position of the toes is held by a stay suture that is placed around the proximal phalanx close to the bone and out to the plantar surface of each toe. The suture must lie against the bone to avoid damage to the neurovascular bundles. Each suture is tied to a prong of a Lambrinudi splint that is incorporated into the toe piece of a short-leg cast. The Lambrinudi splint consists of a baseplate with a strong metal wire that extends underneath each toe (Fig. 35–4B[2]). Once the toes have been stabilized, a felt pad is placed over the dressing on the dorsal surface of the toes and the plaster cast is extended over this pad and is gently molded down over the toes.

Postoperatively, the cast is reinforced for weightbearing, and walking may be permitted after a week. The plaster cast and sutures are removed after 6 weeks, and exercises are commenced.

Proximal Interphalangeal Joint Fusion

The operation may be performed on an individual old enough to ensure that the bony epiphyses are sufficiently large for phalangeal fusion to occur. It is advisable to delay surgery until the patient is about 10 years of age.

A tight extensor tendon should first be lengthened in a Z-fashion through a small vertical skin incision over the affected tendon.

The proximal interphalangeal joint is approached through a dorsal elliptical incision, which excises any dorsal bunion formation (Fig. 35–4C[1]). The incision is deepened down to the extensor tendon, and soft tissue is retracted medially and laterally to protect the neurovascular structures. The extensor expansion is then transected transversely and the proximal interphalangeal joint exposed. Articular cartilage of the head of the proximal phalanx and of the base of the distal phalanx is then removed at right angles to the shafts of the bones using a small osteotome or a bone cutter (Fig. 35–4C[2]). The toe is then straightened, and the two flat surfaces of the trimmed phalanges are examined for quality of fit. Bone may have to be trimmed to prevent any residual angulation of the joint. Once a satisfactory position has been achieved, a smooth Kirschner wire is passed in a retrograde fashion through the middle and distal phalanges and out through the pulp of the toe, and then it is passed back across the fusion area while the middle and proximal phalanges are held accurately aligned. The Kirschner wire should engage the proximal phalanx but need not cross the metatarsophalangeal joint unless there is a tendency for extension to occur at that joint. The dorsal expansion is then sutured under moderate tension (Figs. 35–4C[3] and 35–4D). Subcutaneous tissues and skin are then apposed, and a short-leg walking cast is applied with a substantial toe plate extended over suitable padding to maintain correct positioning of the toes. Depending on the age of the patient, the cast and pin immobilization is continued for 6 to 8 weeks. Success of the procedure depends upon a meticulous technique.

Care must be taken to protect the neurovascular structures. Flat surfaces at the distal end of the proximal phalanx and proximal end of the middle phalanx must be obtained to avoid nonunion. Adequate lengthening of the extensor tendon and, where necessary, release of the dorsal capsule of the metatarsophalangeal joint must be obtained and the toe held straight or slightly plantarflexed at that joint. A residual extension deformity at the metatarsophalangeal joint results in a straight toe pointing upward, that is not only unsightly but does not function properly in toe-off during ambulation.

FLEXION CONTRACTURE OF THE TOES

In this condition, there is a flexion contracture at both the metatarsophalangeal and interphalangeal joints so that the toe tips point directly downward. The deformity may be sufficient to prevent weight bearing on the metatarsal heads. Gait is then inefficient, painful callosities may develop under the toe tufts, and nail distortion may also occur. This condition may be a sequel to surgical release of a clubfoot deformity when lengthening of the long toe flexor tendons has not been performed. It most often occurs, however, in neuromuscular diseases that produce an equinus deformity, particularly cerebral palsy. Toe flexion occurs when the equinus deformity is corrected by a lengthening of the tendo calcaneus alone. As the foot is brought into a plantigrade position, long toe flexor tendon

tightness becomes apparent and the toes firmly plantarflex (Fig. 35–5A). These toe flexion contractures do not tend to resolve, and painful plantar callosities, difficulty with shoe fitting, and a compromised gait are the ultimate sequels if the condition is not treated. When tight, concurrent long toe flexor tendon lengthening is thus recommended whenever elongation of the tendo calcaneus is undertaken.

Nonoperative Treatment

When the toes are still flexible, regular stretching of all the toe joints into extension should be performed. If enough extension at the metatarsophalangeal joint can be obtained to bring the metatarsal heads into some prominence, a period of casting with the toes held dorsiflexed may also be helpful. If these methods fail, surgical intervention is indicated.

Operative Techniques

Since the flexor digitorum and flexor hallucis longus tendons are usually tethered in the sole of the foot, both tendons need to be elongated. The long tendons can be lengthened in one of three areas. The first is through an approach under the metatarsophalangeal joint in a manner described earlier in this chapter. This lengthening procedure is indicated if the toe flexion remains equally tight when the foot is plantar flexed, because this indicates tightness in the short toe flexors. On the other hand, if the toe straightens when the foot is plantarflexed, the long toe flexors are tight and should be lengthened. These flexors may be approached either in the sole of the foot or above the medial malleolus between the pulley mechanism and the musculotendinous junction. The author avoids lengthening tendons within the pulley mechanism in order to lessen the possibility of postoperative adhesions.

Lengthening of the long toe flexor tendons in the sole of the foot would only be indicated in a residual clubfoot deformity when this area is already exposed surgically. The tendons of flexor digitorum and flexor hallucis longus are identified between the proximal pulley mechanism and the distal point where they disappear in the region of Henry's knot. Each tendon is then lengthened in a standard Z-fashion and resutured under moderate tension

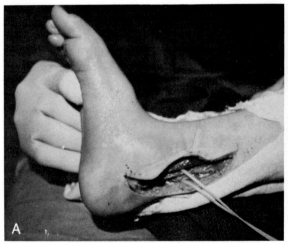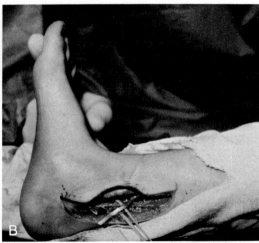

FIGURE 35–5. *(A)*, Equinus deformity in a cerebral palsy patient. The tendo calcaneus has been lengthened through a medial serpentine incision and the foot pushed into dorsiflexion. The toes flex because the flexor digitorum and flexor hallucis longus muscles are tight. *(B)*, The long toe flexor tendons have now been lengthened in a Z-fashion above the medial malleolus, and the toe flexion contracture is corrected.

with the toes and foot slightly overcorrected into dorsiflexion.

It is the author's preference, however, to lengthen toe flexor tendons above the medial malleolus, where they are readily accessible. Lengthening can be easily combined with elongation of the tendo calcaneus. Indeed, when the heel cord is lengthened as part of the management of the equinus deformity of cerebral palsy, tightness of the long toe flexor tendons is always tested, and in the majority of instances, Z-lengthening of these tendons is performed through the same incision during the same procedure.

This procedure is performed under general anesthesia and with a tourniquet. The approach is through a medial serpentine skin incision that extends from behind the medial malleolus up to the distal quarter of the calf. The shape of the incision permits considerable stretching of skin that is frequently tight because of the equinus deformity. Furthermore, should keloid formation occur, contraction is not linear and thus not likely to redeform the foot because of skin tightness. The incision is deepened directly down to the tendo calcaneus, leaving fat both anterior and posterior to the tendon as it is cleared. The neurovascular bundle is located together with the tendons of flexor digitorum longus and tibialis posterior. The wad of fat between the neurovascular bundle and the tendo calcaneus is maintained. The tendo calcaneus is then

lengthened in a Z-fashion. The author prefers a coronal plane lengthening, because this follows the lines of the natural spiral of the tendon. Once it is split, the tendon is detached posteriorly above so that it may be extended beyond the musculotendinous junction, and anteriorly below, close to the calcaneus. In cerebral palsy, the tendon is only partly split so that with dorsiflexion some of the fibers of the tendon remain in continuity. This helps prevent overlengthening.

Once the foot can be dorsiflexed, the toes are tested for tightness. If dorsiflexion is not comfortable and relaxed, Z-lengthening of the long toe flexor tendons is indicated (Figs. 35–5A and B). The neurovascular bundle is then dissected free, with adequate soft tissue protection of the nerve and vessels maintained. The bundle is retracted with a vessel loop away from the nearby tendons. The sheath of the flexor digitorum longus is opened so that the tendon may be mobilized, and this is lengthened in a Z-fashion, extending the lengthening beyond the musculotendinous junction proximally and as far as the pulley mechanism distally. The tendon of the flexor hallucis longus lies deep to the neurovascular bundle, and this is now mobilized. The proximal portion of its pulley mechanism is incised to enable sufficient length of the tendon to be delivered into the wound. The foot is then plantarflexed and inverted, and the hallux is plantarflexed to relax the tendon, which is then brought out into the wound. A Z-lengthening is performed so that the tendon is divided past the musculotendinous junction. It is advisable to immediately secure the distal portion of the tendon with a stay suture, because the tendon may otherwise disappear into the pulley tunnel as the foot is brought into a plantigrade position and the hallux dorsiflexed.

The three lengthened tendons are then repaired so that there is some tension in the tendon when the foot and toes are slightly overcorrected. It is the author's practice to use a 3–0 absorbable suture at each end of the Z-cut and to place an extra one or two sutures in the tendo calcaneus for security. Similar material is used to close the subcutaneous tissues, and a 4–0 suture is used to close the skin in a subcuticular fashion. The wound closure is reinforced with adhesive strips. Before closure, the tourniquet is deflated so that hemostasis can be achieved. If full dorsiflexion creates blanching of the skin flaps, a cast is applied leaving the foot in enough plantar flexion to retain good vascularity in the skin. A week or 10 days later, the cast is changed and the foot placed in the definitive position of moderate dorsiflexion and the toes are held properly extended.

SYNDACTYLY

Syndactyly of the toes occurs in association with other congenital anomalies and syndromes. McKusick[7] described three types, all of which are inherited in an autosomal dominant fashion. Type I is a partial or complete webbing of the second and third toes and is the most common. The fingers may also be involved. Type II describes syndactylization of the fourth and fifth toes. A duplicated fifth toe is frequently included in the common syndactyly web. Type III is syndactyly of the toes with a metatarsal fusion (also see Chapter 34).

Nonoperative Treatment

Syndactyly is usually a cosmetic problem rather than a functional problem, and treatment may be unnecessary. The toes should be observed, however, because differential growth between two syndactylized toes may occur. The longer toe will then be stunted by skin restriction and clawing will result (Fig. 35–6A). In this circumstance or when cosmesis is a major problem, surgical intervention is indicated.

Surgical Release of Syndactyly

A technique similar to that described by Bauer, Tondra and Trusler[1] for the hand is preferred. The foot should be large enough for surgery to be performed comfortably, preferably before walking commences. In the older child, increased clawing of one affected toe requires surgery, which should be done before the age of social awareness at about 5 or 6 years of age.

The principles of surgery are to create interdigitating flaps of dorsal and volar skin that will reasonably mesh when the skin is closed after the tissues are separated. If approximation is fairly close, all gaps will fill by epithelialization, thus avoiding the need for grafting. Zig-zag skin flaps are depicted in Figure 35–6 (1 and 2). The key is a proximally based dorsal flap that must be sufficiently wide and long to create a new web between the toes. Two further lateral flaps are fashioned dorsolaterally and one flap dorsomedially. These should interdigitate with two medial and two lateral volar flaps, as depicted in Figure 35–6B (3). Skin flaps are carefully marked with a methylene blue pen, and when the markings are judged to be correct, the skin is incised. Skin flaps are elevated with fat to maintain vascularity, and soft tissues are then separated between the phalanges of each bone. Care is taken to avoid damaging neurovascular structures, and the medial and lateral soft tissues should be carefully retracted. Any bony union between phalanges is separated at this time. Excessive bone should be trimmed, but great care must be taken not to damage growth plates or articular cartilage.

Closure is achieved by opposing subcutaneous tissue and interdigitating the skin flaps as carefully as possible (Fig. 35–6B[3]). Interrupted subcuticular sutures are useful to oppose flaps without tension. Occasional interrupted simple sutures may be needed. If large gaps are left, skin grafting may be necessary. However, in the author's experience, epithelialization in the child is rapid and leaves a good cosmetic result with pliable skin. The steps required to separate two syndactyly sites in the foot of a 2-year-old girl are shown in Figures 35–6C to J.

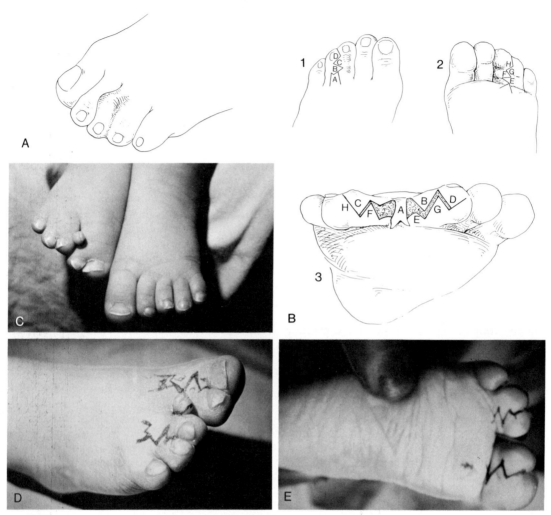

FIGURE 35–6. *(A),* Syndactyly of the third and fourth toes. The third toe is becoming clawed because it is tethered by the shorter fourth toe. *(B),* Physical separation of syndactyly of the toes. Z-cuts are made dorsally (1) and on the volar surface (2) in a manner that will permit flaps to interdigitate once the toes are separated (3). A proximally based flap on the volar surface is used to form the new cleft. Small gaps after the flaps have interdigitated may be left to epithelialize, but occasionally skin grafting may be indicated. *(C),* Syndactyly is present between the first and second, and the third and fourth toes in the right foot of a 2-year-old girl. There is also an accessory digit on the dorsum of the third toe. *(D and E),* Zig-zag incisions are planned and marked on the dorsal and plantar aspects of the conjoined toes.

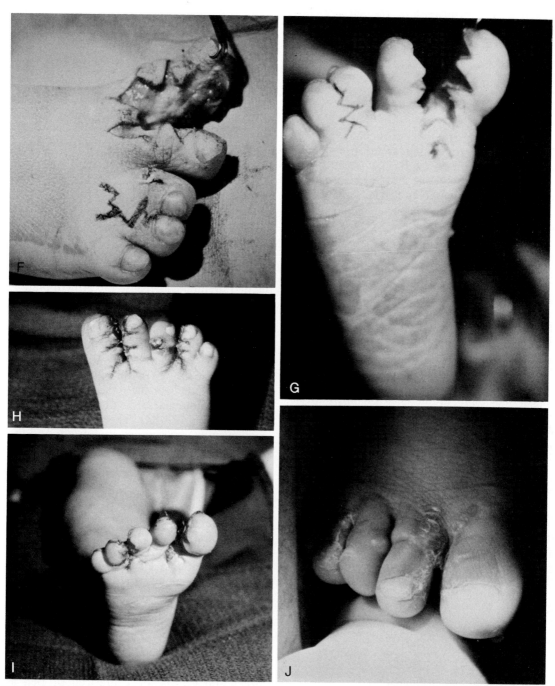

FIGURE 35–6 *(Continued)* *(F and G),* The first and second clefts have been separated. *(H and I),* Satisfactory apposition of skin was achieved at both syndactyly sites without skin grafting. The accessory digit has been excised. *(J),* The result 2 months after separation of both syndactylized areas, and removal of the accessory digit.

When a duplication of the fifth toe is present within the syndactyly web, the smaller toe is removed. The principles of the surgery are otherwise similar to that used for other types of syndactyly. Redundant skin may require trimming.

POLYDACTYLY

Duplication of the toes, particularly of the fifth, may result in an angular deformity. Toe duplication is not rare. It may occur with specific syndromes but is most often isolated and inherited in a dominant fashion. The lesser toes are usually involved, and a similar problem may appear in the hand.

Venn-Watson[9] classified toe duplication morphologically. Duplication may be distal with two separate terminal phalanges articulating with a single Y-shaped middle phalanx. More commonly, two distinct proximal phalanges articulate with a broad or block-shaped metatarsal bone (Fig. 35–7A). The metatarsal bone may be bifid distally and appear in a Y or T configuration. This shape is common with duplication of the fifth toe, and angular deformity of one or both of the double toes is almost inevitable. Sometimes the metatarsal bone may be completely duplicated so that the supernumerary digit appears to be a separate accessory ray (also see Chapter 34).

Nonoperative Treatment

When there is no angulation of the toes and the family is not concerned about the appearance of a foot with an extra digit, surgical excision may not be indicated. However, when there is angulation of a toe, shoe fitting can be extremely difficult because angulation further widens a foot that is already much too broad. Furthermore, there may be pain because of abnormal weight-bearing stresses.

Surgical Treatment of Polydactyly

Surgery should be performed early, before the infant starts walking, and should aim at properly recontouring the foot. The most angulated toe, which is usually the less functional and smaller one, is excised (Figs. 35–7C to E). If the metatarsal head is duplicated, the half

that articulates with the extra toe must be excised and the neck area trimmed to reconstitute a normal contour. When the metatarsal head is Y shaped or T shaped, an osteotomy through the neck of the remaining limb of the metatarsal bone may be necessary in order to realign the retained digit. Sometimes a single broad metatarsal head may have to be trimmed and the remaining proximal phalanx centralized on the metatarsal head. Capsular releases and tendon lengthenings may be necessary. When there is a complete duplication of a ray, the supernumerary metatarsal is removed by performing an osteotomy through the base of the metarsal. It is advisable to leave the metatarsotarsal articulation intact. It may be necessary to perform osteotomies through the bases of some or all of the remaining metatarsals in order to narrow the foot and bring the metatarsal heads together. Caution should be exercised when performing an osteotomy on the first metatarsal because the growth plate is situated proximally and the osteotomy must be performed sufficiently distal to the growth plate to avoid damage.

Excision of an angulated supernumerary digit is performed under general anesthesia and with the use of a tourniquet. A dorsal incision is made over the middle and proximal phalanx and metatarsal head of the toe to be removed (Fig. 35–7C). The extensor tendon mechanism is exposed and mobilized, and the dorsal neurovascular bundle then dissected free down to its bifurcation to the extra digit and the adjoining toe on each side. The branches to the extra digit are tied or cauterized, and they are severed distal to the bifurcation. The extensor tendons are transected as high as possible and allowed to retract. Occasionally, there may be some compromise in tendon function in an adjoining toe, and in this case, they can be anastomosed to the weak adjoining tendons.

A dorsal capsulotomy at the tarsometatarsal joint is then performed, and the toe is flexed to expose the volar structures. The large plantar neurovascular bundles are dissected free, the bifurcation is found on each side, and the nerves and vessels are cauterized or tied as they run to the toe to be removed, distal to the bifurcation. They may then be divided. Where indicated, the flexor tendons may be used to reinforce those of an adjoining toe. More usually, they are pulled into the wound, transected as high as possible, and allowed to retract. The accessory toe is then completely

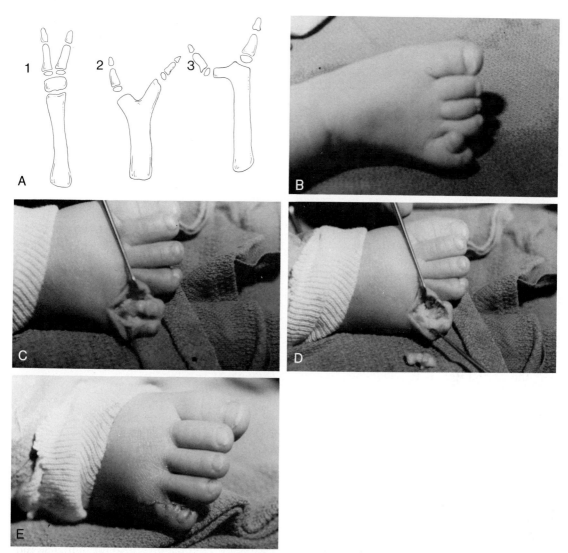

FIGURE 35–7. *(A),* Duplication of a digit. The proximal phalanges may articulate with a broadened metatarsal head (1). Metatarsal heads may be bifid, and have a Y (2) or a T (3) configuration. *(B),* Duplication of the fifth toe. There is partial syndactyly, and the medial toe is angled. *(C),* The medial toe is exposed through a dorsal incision. *(D),* The phalanges are freed and removed. *(E),* The remaining lateral toe is centralized over the metatarsal base, and after removal of excessive skin, closure is achieved.

ablated by incision of remaining soft tissue structures.

At this point, the metatarsal head may need to be refashioned or a bifid head excised. Significant angulation should be corrected by an osteotomy through the metatarsal neck. The adjoining normal toe may need to be suitably repositioned by capsulotomy and tendon sheath realignment. Residual skin must be trimmed so that volar skin is brought into the new cleft as closure is achieved (Fig. 35–7E).

When an accessory metatarsal needs to be excised, the incision is extended dorsally to the base of the metatarsal bone and the shaft of the metatarsal is exposed. The periosteum is left intact but soft tissues are cleared. The bone is divided proximally, close to the talar articulation, using either a small osteotome or a bone cutter. The bone is then enucleated. Basal osteotomies of adjoining metatarsal bones are performed as necessary. Two or three metatarsal bones may be readily approached through a single dorsal incision.

In order to narrow the forefoot and to approximate the remaining metatarsal heads, it is useful to pass a small threaded Kirschner wire through the bases of the metatarsal bones, starting at the fifth metatarsal neck. A power drill should be used to drill the holes. The threaded Kirschner wire is introduced through a small skin incision. The Kirschner wire may skirt the central one or two metatarsal necks because these are at a slightly higher plane than the others when the transverse arch is properly reconstituted. As long as there is a good purchase medially and laterally in the foot, however, and the foot has been held in a narrowed position as the threaded Kirschner wire is applied, it will serve its purpose.

These wounds are closed in layers, and where possible, subcuticular sutures are preferred. Postoperatively, a well-padded cast is applied that is univalved immediately postoperatively but should not initially be spread unless there is an indication to do so. As soon as the swelling subsides, the cast should be closed by adding more plaster. After 4 weeks, the Kirschner wire is removed and a new definitive lightweight walking cast is applied. This cast must hold apposed the metatarsal heads that were previously separated by the accessory ray.

Severe angulation of the lateral digits may occasionally be associated with toe duplication elsewhere (Fig. 35–8A and B). In this patient,

the hallux was duplicated, both feet were extremely broad, and shoes had to be cut out to accommodate the laterally pointing fourth and fifth digits, particularly on the right side. The purpose of surgery was to narrow the foot sufficiently to make normal shoe fitting possible. The duplicated hallux was ignored. Attention was directed solely to the lateral toes, and since it was not possible to reduce the fifth toe into normal alignment because of shortness of the neurovascular structures, it was elected to excise the fifth ray completely, together with the abnormal toe. This was performed bilaterally, through a dorsolateral incision, but the metatarsal base was left intact so that the attachment of the peroneus brevis tendon was left undisturbed, as was the pathway of the peroneus longus tendon. The base of the metatarsal bone was trimmed so that lateral contour of the foot was smooth. The metatarsal bone was excised with its periosteum intact, and care was taken to leave intact the neurovascular structures to the adjoining toe. The flexor and extensor tendons were cut short. On the more affected right side, lateral capsulotomies of the metatarsophalangeal joints were performed on the third and fourth toes, and these were successfully aligned without stress on the neurovascular bundles or tendons. Correction was held with smooth Kirschner wires. A narrowed foot with good function was achieved (Fig. 35–8C).

ANGULAR TOE DEFORMITIES ASSOCIATED WITH CLEFT OR LOBSTER CLAWFOOT

This condition is unusual, occurring in about 1 per 90,000 live births. It is inherited as a mendelian dominant trait but may also occur as a spontaneous mutation.[4] A cleft and other anomalies are common in the hands, and occasionally, cleft palate is also present. The foot exhibits hypoplasia or complete absence of the central rays. It is deeply split, and frequently, the first and fifth metatarsal bones diverge. In time, the remaining fifth toe and hallux incline toward the midline. The deformity increases with age, and the angled digits eventually exhibit a lobster claw appearance (Fig. 35–9A). The condition is a significant cosmetic blemish. The first and fifth metatarsal heads are widely separated, so that the foot is abnormally broad and shoe fitting is extremely

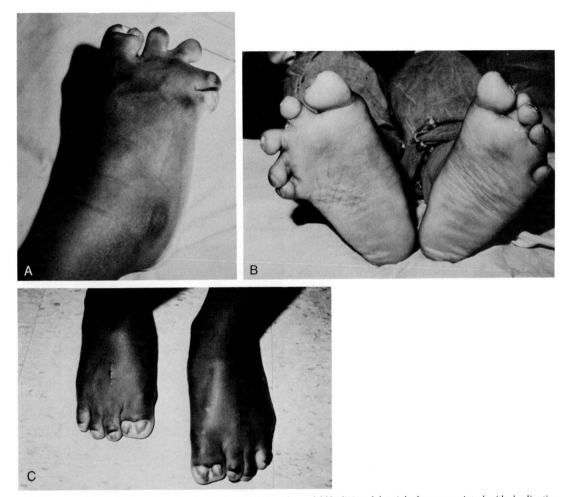

FIGURE 35–8. *(A and B)*, Lateral angulation in the third, fourth, and fifth digits of the right foot, associated with duplication of the hallux. The foot was narrowed by ablating the fifth ray and toe, and repositioning the fourth and third toes by suitable lateral capsulotomies of the metatarsophalangeal joints. *(C)*, The result 4 months later.

difficult. Although toe-off is not normal, most patients adapt remarkably well to their deformity from the functional point of view. Some may develop discomfort and callosities.

The severity of the deformity varies. In milder forms, there may be only a small cleft with absence of one or two toes. Even with the absence of a single digit, however, there is a tendency for the toes to tilt into the space created so that ultimately fixed angular deformities of the toes will occur.

Nonoperative Treatment

Although no improvement of the deformity can be achieved without surgery, patients must clearly understand that particularly when the condition is severe, surgery can only improve the problem at best and cannot replace parts of the foot that are absent. Therefore, surgical goals are limited, and older patients who have adapted to a severe deformity may do well with nothing more than wearing footwear wide enough to accommodate the deformity. In the mild form in which one or two digits are missing, the use of a spacer between existing toes may prevent toe deviation.

In most instances, however, careful surgery performed early can greatly improve appearance, function, and shoe-wearing capabilities. Surgery is indicated as soon as the tissues are large enough to work with comfortably and should be undertaken before walking commences.

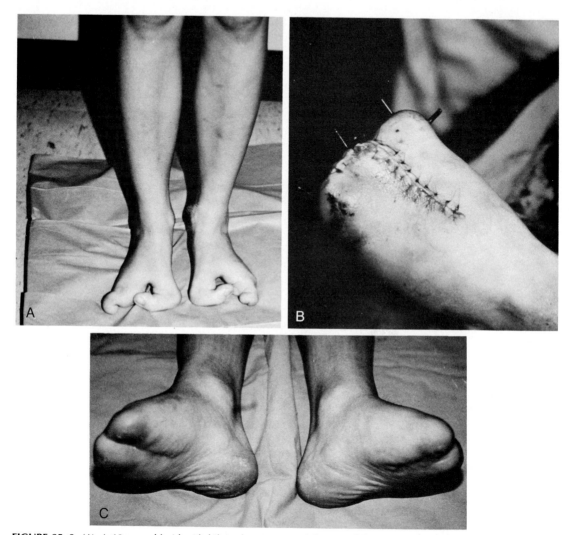

FIGURE 35–9. *(A)*, A 13-year-old girl with bilateral centray ray deficiency (lobster clawfeet) with fixed deviations of the fifth toes and hallux that are apposed. *(B)*, The hallux and fifth toe were ablated, and the broad feed narrowed by performing osteotomies of the bases of the remaining metatarsal bones. The position was held with a threaded Steinmann pin passed through the metatarsal necks and smooth pins running through the metatarsals into the tarsals. *(C)*, Six months later, the patient's feet were toeless but well shaped, and function was good and shoe fitting easy.

Principles of Operative Treatment

The purpose of surgery is to narrow the foot at the metatarsal head level and to maintain or achieve a proper attitude of the toes. The cleft should be opened on each side and re-alignment of residual metatarsals achieved by basal metatarsal osteotomies. When an oste-otomy is performed on the first metatarsal bone, the proximal growth plate must be avoided. The forefoot is narrowed and so held by placing a threaded Kirschner wire or small Steinmann pin across the necks of the meta-tarsal bones. Soft tissues in the cleft are ap-posed, redundant skin is excised, and the cleft is closed. If they are flexible, angulated toes may be held straight with smooth Kirschner wires passed through the toes into their meta-tarsals. If there is resistance to correction, capsulotomies of the metatarsophalangeal and the interphalangeal joints and, possibly, lengthening of tendons may be necessary. In the older patient, it is frequently impossible to correct the toes because of shortening of soft tissues, particularly of the neurovascular bun-dles. In this instance, amputation of the of-fending toes (usually the fifth toe and hallux) (Fig. 35–9*B*) produces a foot that is very functional, well shaped, and able to fit into normal footwear (Fig. 35–9*C*).

If amputation is necessary, a racket incision is made around the base of the proximal pha-lanx of the toe to be removed so that the handle of the racket extends into the incision to open the cleft. The large volar and small dorsal neurovascular bundles are dissected free, and these bundles are either cauterized or tied, and then transected. The extensor tendons are pulled distally, divided proximally, and allowed to retract. The capsule of the metatarsophalangeal joint is then opened dor-sally, and the division of the capsule is ex-tended medially and laterally so that the toe remains tethered to the foot by the volar plate and flexor tendons. The plate is then separated from its proximal attachment to the metatarsal bone. The sheath around the flexor tendons is divided and the tendons pulled distally. Divi-sion of these tendons permits the toe to be removed completely. The larger volar skin flap is then brought up to meet the dorsal skin. The flap is suitably trimmed to allow a com-fortable closure without tension but also with-out redundant soft tissue. Suturing of these flaps must also interdigitate with closure of the cleft.

Postoperatively, a cast is kept in place for 4 weeks. Thereafter, any Kirschner wires or Steinmann pins that were required to stabilize the foot are removed and a definitive, light-weight cast is applied maintaining the nar-rowed and plantigrade attitude. The patient may commence partial weight bearing and progress to full weight bearing by 6 weeks. The cast is removed at about 8 weeks when the basal osteotomies are healed, and rehabil-itation is commenced.

References

1. Bauer TB, Tondra JM, and Trusber HM: Technical modification in repair of syndactylism. Plast Reconstr Surg 17:385, 1956.
2. Cocklin J: Butler's operation for an overriding fifth toe. J Bone Joint Surg 50B:78, 1968.
3. Forrester-Brown MF: Tendon transplantation for claw-ing of the great toe. J Bone Joint Surg 20:57, 1938.
4. Handelsman JE: The lobster claw foot. J Bone Joint Surg 8:449, 1984.
5. Kelikian H, Clayton I, Loseff H: Surgical syndactylia of the toes. Clin Orthop 19:208, 1961.
6. Leonard MH, Rising EH: Syndactylization to maintain correction of overlapping 5th toe. Clin Orthop 43:241, 1965.
7. McKusick VA: Mendelian Inheritance in Man: Cata-logues of Autosomal Dominant, Autosomal Recessive, and X-Linked Phenotypes. 2nd ed. Baltimore, Johns Hopkins University Press, 1968.
8. Taylor RG: The treatment of claw toes by multiple transfers of flexor into extensor tendons. J Bone Joint Surg 33B:539, 1951.
9. Venn-Watson E: Problems in polydactyly of the foot. Orthop Clin North Am 7:909, 1976.

36

The Pathophysiology and Treatment of the Juvenile Bunion

MICHAEL J. COUGHLIN

It is uncommon for a juvenile or preteenager to develop a symptomatic hallux valgus deformity.[46, 51] Inconsistent results have been reported in the literature regarding surgical correction of juvenile bunions, and delaying surgery until skeletal maturity has been reached is frequently recommended. Failure rates of bunion repairs in this age group have been inordinantly high.* Success rates have been variable even in series employing a similar operative technique. Thus, there is considerable confusion over the indications, timing, and operative technique for correction of a juvenile hallux valgus deformity.

In 1960, Piggot[51] reported on a series of adult patients with hallux valgus. While 57 percent recalled the onset of their deformity in adolescent years, only 5 percent recalled the development of a hallux valgus deformity after age 20. In an extensive long-term review of patients with hallux valgus, Hardy and Clapham[25] found that 40 percent of bunion deformities occurred prior to age 20, and Scranton[55] reported that a juvenile bunion is rarely seen prior to age 10. On the other hand, most other series report the average age at the time of surgery to be 13 years, thus implying a rather early onset of this condition.

No report has been published regarding the incidence of juvenile hallux valgus deformity or the frequency of its surgical repair in the United States. In 1981, Helal[27] estimated that 2000 operations were performed on juveniles with hallux valgus deformities each year in Great Britain. Most series report that the majority of juvenile patients with hallux valgus undergoing surgical correction are females,* which may correlate with the onset of pain and discomfort following the adoption of high-fashion footwear in the teenage years. By definition, a juvenile hallux valgus deformity has its onset during the preteenage and early teenage years. Certain adult hallux valgus deformities are significantly more difficult to treat than others and have a higher risk of postoperative recurrence, and many of these, particularly in view of their anatomic characteristics, appear to have developed in the juvenile or adolescent years.[12]

A juvenile hallux valgus deformity differs from a typical adult type hallux valgus deformity in several ways.[46, 49] In the juvenile, degenerative changes at the metatarsophalangeal joint are rarely found and bursal thickening over the medial eminence is uncommon. The epiphyseal growth plates at the base of the proximal phalanx and the base of the first metatarsal are often still open. While the magnitude of the medial eminence and the hallux valgus angle at the metatarsophalangeal joint are typically smaller in the juvenile than in the adult, the magnitude of the 1–2 intermetatarsal angle is often greater. Furthermore, the metatarsocuneiform articulation is often rigid in

---

*See references 8, 24, 28, 37, 46, 56, and 59.

This chapter is an adaptation of material published in Coughlin MJ: Juvenile bunions. *In* Mann RA, Coughlin MJ (Eds): Surgery of the Foot and Ankle, 6th Ed. St. Louis, Mosby–Year Book, 1993, pp 297–339. Reprinted with permission of the publisher.

*See references 9, 13, 27, 32, 37, 49, 56, and 61.

comparison to the typical adult onset hallux valgus deformity.

ETIOLOGY

Various postural and anatomic factors have been noted to contribute to the onset and progression of the juvenile hallux valgus deformity, including ligamentous laxity[2, 56] and pes planus.* Scranton and Zuckerman[56] noted a 41-percent incidence of pes planus in association with a juvenile hallux valgus deformity, and Trott[60] reported an incidence of 25 percent in his series of juvenile bunions. The axis of the first ray is altered with the development of pronation of the foot and assumes an oblique orientation with weight bearing. In some patients with pronation, if the metatarsophalangeal joint is unable to withstand the deforming pressures exerted on the medial capsular soft tissue supporting structures, a hallux valgus deformity may develop.

The length of the first metatarsal has been mentioned as a factor in a bunion formation,[24, 45, 56] with a long first metatarsal presenting an increased risk, but it appears that the relationship between metatarsal length and the later development of a hallux valgus deformity is fortuitous.[12, 41] Constricting footwear[2, 12, 20, 41] has been implicated in association with bunion progression in the juvenile. Two possibilities should be considered: an already wide or splayed foot may be constricted by a narrow shoe causing increased symptoms over the medial eminence, or a constricting shoebox may lead to progression of deformity in a foot otherwise at risk for a hallux valgus abnormality.

Variations in shape and anatomic structure may place specific feet at risk for hallux valgus development in the juvenile population. The presence of midfoot and hindfoot abnormalities must be considered as well as the orientation and shape of both the metatarsocuneiform and metatarsophalangeal joint. The metatarsocuneiform joint is one of the key factors in the development of an increased 1–2 intermetatarsal angle and an increased valgus angulation of the first metatarsophalangeal joint. Understanding the components of the hallux valgus deformity is important in planning surgical correction.

---

*See references 16, 22, 24, 30, 35, 45, 55, 56, and 61.

ANATOMY

First Metatarsophalangeal Joint

The shape of the metatarsal and phalangeal articular surfaces has a significant effect on the intrinsic stability of the first metatarsophalangeal joint: they may resist or predispose the hallux to progressive deformity. A chevron-shaped metatarsophalangeal articular surface (Fig. 36–1A) resists progressive deformity,[41] while a round metatarsal head (Fig. 36–1B and C)[41, 45] is more prone to progression of hallux valgus.

In the radiographic analysis of the first metatarsophalangeal joint, the articular surfaces of the base of the proximal phalanx and the distal first metatarsal are not necessarily oriented at right angles in relationship to the long axis of the phalanx and the metatarsal. A hallux valgus angle of 16 degrees or less is normal.[25, 29, 41] Lateral tilting of the articular surface either at the base of the proximal phalanx or at the distal first metatarsal may be the cause of this static valgus orientation. Piggott[51] claimed that while this valgus condition may become symptomatic, it is not prone to progress to a more severe deformity.

The metatarsophalangeal joint orientation must be carefully inspected in the assessment of a juvenile bunion deformity in order to define the pathologic components as well as to plan the appropriate method of repair. The metatarsal articular orientation (MAO) (proximal articular set angle or metatarsal articular angle) (Fig. 36–2A) defines the orientation of the distal metatarsal articular surface in relationship to the long axis of the first metatarsal. Rarely is this angle 0 degrees; frequently it will measure 10 to 15 degrees of lateral inclination. The phalangeal articular orientation (PAO) (distal articular set angle or phalangeal articular angle) (Fig. 36–2B) defines the orientation of the articular surface at the base of the proximal phalanx in relationship to the long axis of the proximal phalanx. Often slight valgus inclination is present but rarely does it exceed 5 degrees. When this angle is abnormally high, a hallux valgus interphalangeous deformity will occur. Thus, a hallux valgus abnormality may be due to an abnormally large MAO, PAO, or a combination of both. This is considered to be a static structural abnormality: although it may become symptomatic, it is unlikely to progress.[12, 51]

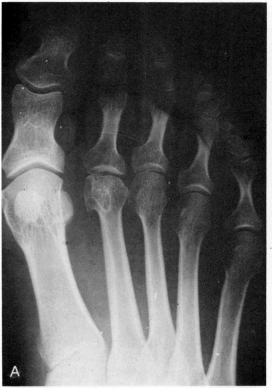

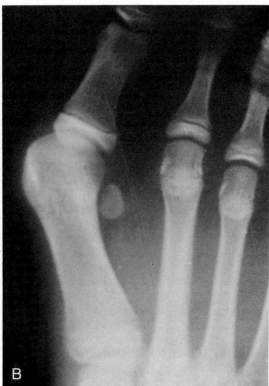

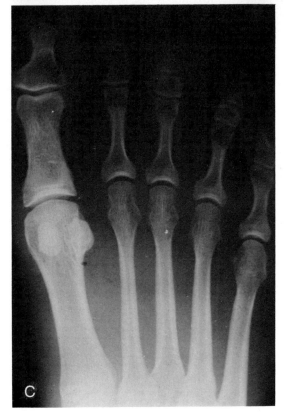

FIGURE 36–1. (A), A chevron-shaped metatarsal head is more stable and resists subluxation. (B), A round metatarsal head is at risk for subluxation. (C), A flat metatarsal head is relatively stable. (From Coughlin MJ, Mann RA: The pathophysiology of the juvenile bunion. Instr Course Lect 36:123, 1987.)

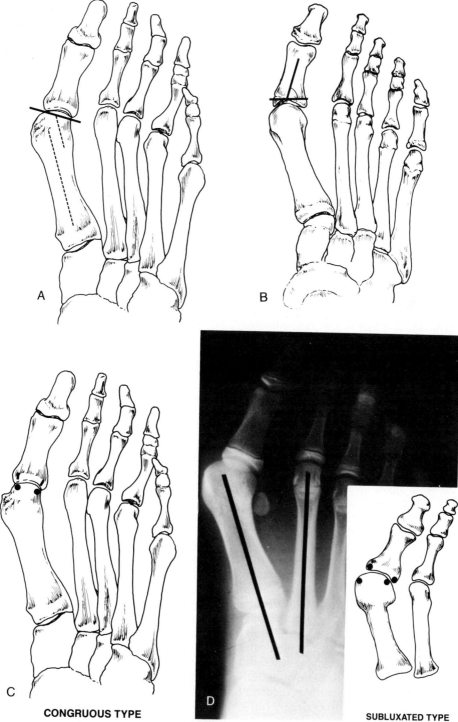

CONGRUOUS TYPE

SUBLUXATED TYPE

FIGURE 36–2. *(A),* The metatarsal articular orientation (MAO) (distal metatarsal articular angle) defines the relationship of the long axis of the first metatarsal to the distal metatarsal articular surface. *(B),* The phalangeal articular orientation (PAO) (proximal phalangeal articular angle) defines the relationship of the long axis of the proximal phalanx to the proximal articular surface. *(C),* A congruent joint has a concentric relationship between the corresponding articular surfaces of the first metatarsal and proximal phalanx. In spite of this, significant hallux valgus may be present. *(D),* Metatarsophalangeal subluxation occurs in a noncongruent joint with widening of the 1–2 intermetatarsal angle. *(A, B,* and *C* from Coughlin MJ, Mann RA: The pathophysiology of the juvenile bunion. Instr Course Lect 36:123, 1987. *D* is courtesy of Michael J. Coughlin, M.D.)

The concept of *joint congruity* forms a basis for understanding the origin of the juvenile bunion deformity as well as assisting in the planning of a surgical correction. With a congruous metatarsophalangeal joint, the corresponding articular surfaces of the base of the proximal phalanx and the first metatarsal head are aligned in a concentric fashion (Fig. 36–2C). If the peripheral extent of the margins of the articular surface of the first metatarsal and base of the proximal phalanx are marked, the corresponding marks on one articular surface will align closely with the marks on the opposing articular surface. A significant amount of valgus at the metatarsophalangeal joint can be present, however, due to angulation in the orientation of either articular surface (MAO or PAO).

With an incongruous metatarsophalangeal joint, the base of the proximal phalanx may subluxate or deviate in a lateral direction in relationship to the articular surface of the first metatarsal head; in other words, the margins of the articular surface no longer correspond. What may originally begin as mild subluxation of the first metatarsophalangeal joint may progress with time, leaving the medial aspect of the metatarsal articular surface uncovered (Fig. 36–2D). Piggott[51] hypothesized that a congruous metatarsophalangeal joint was an intrinsically stable joint and would not progress to a significant hallux valgus deformity. On the other hand, an incongruent metatarsophalangeal joint with slight deviation is likely to progress to metatarsophalangeal joint subluxation.

The valgus orientation of the metatarsophalangeal joint can be attributed to a tilting of the articular surface in relationship to the long axis of the metatarsal (MAO) or proximal phalanx (PAO), to joint subluxation, or to both. It is important to appreciate this distinction. If a symptomatic hallux valgus deformity with a congruent metatarsophalangeal joint requires surgical correction, an intra-articular realignment of the metatarsophalangeal joint may place the metatarsophalangeal joint surfaces at significant risk for either recurrent hallux valgus or postoperative degenerative joint disease.

Metatarsocuneiform Joint

The orientation and flexibility of the metatarsocuneiform joint are probably the most

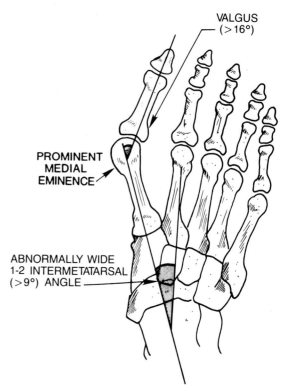

FIGURE 36–3. The 1–2 intermetatarsal angle. (From Coughlin MJ, Mann RA: The pathophysiology of the juvenile bunion. Instr Course Lect 36:123, 1987.)

important factors in the development of a hallux valgus deformity and an increased intermetatarsal angle. A 1–2 intermetatarsal angle (Fig. 36–3) of 9 degrees or less is considered normal.[3, 9, 14, 25, 29, 52] The stability of the first ray depends to a great extent upon the orientation and shape of the metatarsocuneiform joint. A horizontal orientation (Fig. 36–4A) tends to resist an increase in the 1–2 intermetatarsal angle, while an oblique orientation (Fig. 36–4B) is associated with an increased 1–2 intermetatarsal angle. A curved metatarsocuneiform joint articulation (Fig. 36–4C) appears to correlate with increased joint mobility and may allow progressive medial deviation of the first metatarsal with a widening of the 1–2 intermetatarsal angle.[40] A facet (Fig. 36–4D) located at the proximal lateral base of the first metatarsal may create a rigid metatarsocuneiform articulation that resists surgical reduction following distal soft tissue realignment.[35, 40, 41] The distal surface of the first cuneiform articulates with the proximal aspect of the first metatarsal and is oriented in a transverse (coronal) plane. The concave surface of the proximal metatarsal is somewhat elliptical in shape and oriented in a plantar-medial direction.[23, 54]

Ewald in 1912[18] and Berntsen in 1930[6] reported that an obliquely oriented metatarsocuneiform joint resulted in a varus inclination of the first metatarsal and was associated with a hallux valgus deformity. The metatarsocuneiform joint is difficult to visualize on a routine radiograph, and Simon[60] questioned the "apparent orientation" of this joint and wondered if some of the findings were radiographic artifacts. With computer-assisted imaging this perplexing question may eventually be answered. Following numerous metatarsocuneiform resections, Haines and McDougall[23] concluded that when present, a hallux valgus deformity was often associated with an oblique orientation of the first metatarsocuneiform joint. Both they and Truslow[62] hypothesized that an abnormality of the proximal base of the first metatarsal led to metatarsus primus varus. The first metatarsocuneiform joint orientation appears to be the major factor associated with the magnitude of the 1–2 intermetatarsal angle. Mitchell[49] and others[14, 27, 36, 46, 62] have concluded that an increase in the 1–2 intermetatarsal angle is the result of an abnormal orientation of the metatarsocuneiform joint.

The factor most commonly associated with hallux valgus is an increased 1–2 intermetatarsal angle.[8, 20, 25, 59] Whether this is a primary or secondary deformity distinguishes the juvenile and the adult hallux valgus deformities.[12] Inman[30] and Piggott[51] hypothesized that as metatarsophalangeal subluxation occurs, there is a concomitant increase in the 1–2 intermetatarsal angle. Antrobus[3] speculated that following corrective surgery at the first metatarsophalangeal joint (without metatarsal osteotomy) if the 1–2 intermetatarsal angle is reduced to a normal range following a distal soft tissue repair, then it follows that the increased 1–2 intermetatarsal angle is secondary to the distal hallux valgus deformity. DuVries[16] stated that metatarsus primus varus is a secondary change in the adult with hallux valgus resulting from the metatarsophalangeal subluxation; while in the juvenile, the increased 1–2 intermetatarsal angle is responsible for the development of hallux valgus. It has frequently been postulated that in a juvenile, an increased 1–2 intermetatarsal angle is

the primary deformity and the hallux valgus the secondary acquired deformity.* This is an important distinction, for metatarsocuneiform joint flexibility can have a significant influence upon both the development of hallux valgus and the specific type of surgical repair selected and its ultimate success. A rigid, wide 1–2 intermetatarsal angle carries risk of postoperative recurrence if only a distal soft tissue realignment is performed. On the other hand, a hallux valgus deformity with an intermetatarsal angle of similar magnitude that occurred secondarily following the development of metatarsophalangeal joint subluxation has inherent flexibility at the first metatarsocuneiform joint, and an adequate correction with a distal soft tissue realignment can be achieved without metatarsal osteotomy.[41] Thus, the inherent flexibility of the first metatarsocuneiform joint plays an integral part in any surgical correction.[36] Unfortunately, this flexibility often can only be assessed intraoperatively following the release of the soft tissue contractures at the first metatarsophalangeal joint. It is intriguing that Mann and Coughlin[41] reported a 5.2 degree decrease in the 1–2 intermetatarsal angle following a distal soft tissue repair utilizing the modified McBride procedure (without a first metatarsal osteotomy), and Hawkins[26] reported an average correction of the 1–2 intermetatarsal angle of 5.2 degrees following a distal metatarsal osteotomy (Mitchell procedure). These results imply that in many cases there is a degree of flexibility at the metatarsocuneiform articulation that may allow a decrease in the 1–2 intermetatarsal angle with either a distal soft tissue realignment or a distal metatarsal osteotomy.

The 1–2 intermetatarsal angle must be assessed in relationship to the remaining lesser metatarsals. As previously mentioned, the upper range of normal for the 1–2 intermetatarsal angle is 9 degrees. However, it is the orientation of the second metatarsal and the other lesser metatarsals in relationship to the first metatarsal that determines this actual measurement.[52] If the lesser metatarsals are aligned in what is considered a normal orientation, then the 1–2 intermetatarsal angle should give an accurate indication of the magnitude of metatarsus primus varus. Price[52] advocated calculating the angle subtended by the first and

---

*See references 8, 9, 10, 14, 16, 32, 36, 37, 49, 62, and 63.

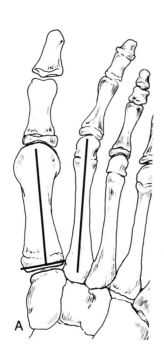

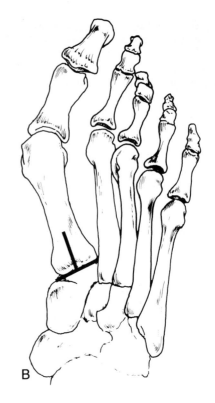

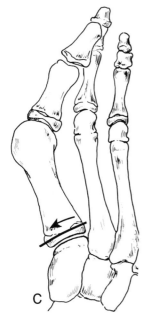

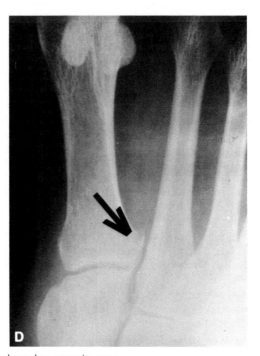

Staight
metatarsocuneiform
joint

Oblique
metatarsocuneiform
joint

Curved
metatarsocuneiform
joint

FIGURE 36–4 *See legend on opposite page*

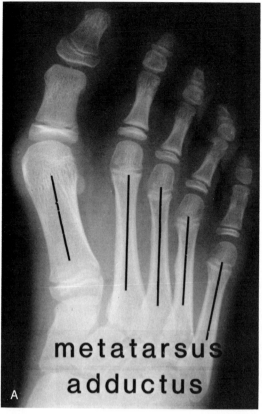

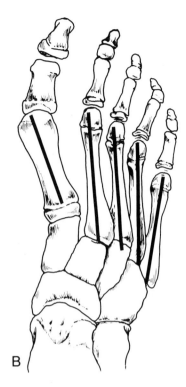

**Juvenile Hallux Valgus with
Metatarsus Adductus**

FIGURE 36–5. *(A)*, A radiograph demonstrating a child with metatarsus adductus and metatarsus primus varus. *(B)*, It is difficult to reduce the metatarsus primus varus when metatarsus adductus is present. *(B from Coughlin MJ, Mann RA: The pathophysiology of the juvenile bunion. Instr Course Lect 36:123, 1987.)*

fifth metatarsals in order to assess the true medial inclination of the first metatarsal. He believed that an angle greater than 29 degrees was abnormal. In the absence of metatarsus quintus valgus (in combination with hallux valgus, a splay foot) or metatarsus adductus, he found this to be a more reliable guide than measuring the 1–2 intermetatarsal angle. This technique has not been widely used in calculating the magnitude of the medial inclination of the first metatarsal.

It is not uncommon for a juvenile hallux valgus deformity to be associated with meta-

tarsus adductus (Fig. 36–5*A* and *B*). With an adducted forefoot, the 1–2 intermetatarsal angle does not give true representation of the amount of varus of the first ray since the point of reference (the second metatarsal) is deviated medially as well.[22, 24] Hallux valgus in association with metatarsus adductus has been reported in the juvenile population[22, 24, 37, 45, 52, 61] and this presents a very difficult condition to treat as there is little room to realign the first metatarsal laterally. Houghton and Dickson[29] hypothesized that there was no significant increase in the medial inclination of

FIGURE 36–4. The metatarsocuneiform joint. *(A)*, A horizontal orientation is typically stable. *(B)*, An oblique orientation is often inflexible, and at surgery, a first metatarsal osteotomy may be necessary to decrease the 1–2 intermetatarsal angle. An opening wedge cuneiform osteotomy also might be used, especially in the presence of a short first ray. *(C)*, A curved metatarsocuneiform joint is often flexible. A decrease in the 1–2 intermetatarsal angle may occur with a distal soft tissue realignment. *(D)*, A facet between the first and second metatarsal may create a first metatarsocuneiform joint that is resistent to correction with a distal soft tissue realignment. *(From Coughlin MJ, Mann RA: The pathophysiology of the juvenile bunion. Instr Course Lect 36:123, 1987.)*

the first metatarsal in patients with hallux valgus and concluded that the magnitude of the 1–2 intermetatarsal angle was due to an increased valgus of the lateral metatarsals. Helal[27] disagreed with this conclusion and reported significant varus of the first metatarsal in 99 percent of the juvenile patients that he treated. The lateral inclination of the second ray does not influence the magnitude of the true varus of the first metatarsal, but lesser metatarsal orientation does indeed influence the magnitude of the 1–2 intermetatarsal angle. Significant adduction of the lesser metatarsals may make repair of a juvenile hallux valgus deformity difficult.

Open Epiphysis

Postponement of surgery until skeletal maturity has been recommended on the basis that progression of a hallux valgus deformity may occur postoperatively due to further epiphyseal growth.* Another consideration is the possibility of epiphyseal injury either at the base of the proximal phalanx or at the proximal aspect of the first metatarsal.

A high rate of postoperative recurrence following surgical correction has been reported in the juvenile. Scranton and Zuckerman[56] reported a 20 percent recurrence rate in juveniles with an open epiphysis, while Bonney and MacNab[8] noted a recurrence rate of 42 percent. Although the presence of an open epiphysis is not a contraindication to an osteotomy, it is important to determine the exact location of the phalangeal or metatarsal epiphyses when an osteotomy is performed in these regions to avoid iatrogenic injury. Surgical repair of a hallux valgus deformity in a juvenile frequently requires an osteotomy in order to obtain an acceptable correction, and it is important to be aware of exactly how much growth can be expected in the foot postoperatively. If an epiphyseal injury does occur, one can then postulate what effect it will have on phalangeal or metatarsal growth. Analysis of the rate of growth in the female foot[7, 17] has determined that full foot growth is usually achieved by age 14. At 12 years of age an average of less than 1 cm of total foot growth remains, and probably less than 50 percent of this will occur at the first metatarsal epiphy-

sis.[12] Thus, an iatrogenic epiphyseal arrest or partial epiphyseal plate closure will probably be inconsequential at this age. However, termination of growth in adolescent males does not occur until an average age of 16 years, and at age 12, there is almost 3 cm total foot growth remaining, with approximately one-half of the longitudinal foot growth occurring at the first metatarsal epiphysis (approximately 1.5 cm). Postponement of surgery may be advisable until skeletal maturity is approached (approximately age 15 or 16).

The proximal first metatarsal epiphyseal orientation may play a role in the increased magnitude of the 1–2 intermetatarsal angle as well as postsurgical recurrence of metatarsus primus varus. Luba and Rosman[37] postulated that medial inclination of the first metatarsal epiphysis, according to Wolff's law, causes tension to develop on the lateral aspect of the epiphysis and compression on the medial aspect of the epiphysis (Fig. 36–6). This theoretically leads to an increased growth rate on the lateral aspect of the epiphysis with subsequent medial inclination of the first metatarsal. An osteotomy performed on the medial aspect of the first ray can potentially alter these forces, decreasing the lateral tension forces

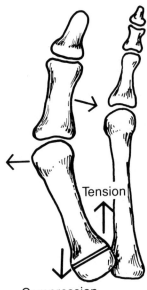

FIGURE 36–6. The orientation of the proximal first metatarsal epiphysis may stimulate lateral epiphyseal growth (by tension forces laterally), leading to an increase in the 1–2 intermetatarsal angle. (From Coughlin MJ, Mann RA: The pathophysiology of the juvenile bunion. Instr Course Lect 36:123, 1987.)

---

*See references 8, 10, 24, 27, 46, 56, and 59.

and thereby affecting the growth rate of the lateral aspect of the epiphysis. An osteotomy performed distal to the metatarsal epiphysis may realign the first ray and diminish lateral epiphyseal growth; it may also run the risk of recurrence if lateral epiphyseal overgrowth occurs. For this reason, a first cuneiform osteotomy may achieve correction proximal to the metatarsocuneiform joint at the site of the abnormality and thus avoid the possibility of damage to an open epiphysis.

A partial lateral epiphyseal arrest in the early teenage years theoretically allows gradual correction of the 1–2 intermetatarsal angle. Ellis[17] and Fox and Smith[19] have suggested selective partial lateral epiphyseal arrest as a means of decreasing metatarsus primus varus. However, its efficacy remains hypothetical, and no controlled long-term evaluation of this technique has been reported.

TREATMENT

Conservative Care

For most juvenile patients with a bunion deformity, conservative care will be adequate to relieve symptoms.[10] A mild hallux valgus deformity that is symptomatic may be periodically evaluated for progression. A medial arch support[45, 46, 55] can be used in patients with a flexible pes planus deformity or a low collagen syndrome with associated pes planus. Roomy footwear that reduces extrinsic pressure on the medial eminence and medial hallux is probably the single most important factor in achieving symptomatic relief of pain, but it is difficult to achieve compliance in this age group.[10] There is no doubt that constricting footwear will exacerbate symptoms in patients with a hallux valgus deformity and that low-heeled shoes with an adequate toe box will relieve discomfort. If a patient continues to have significant pain over the medial eminence with conservative footwear, surgical intervention may be contemplated.* A further indication for surgery is progression of a hallux valgus deformity.[22, 55, 59] While cosmesis is a relative indication,[9, 13, 37, 63] pain should be the major reason for surgical correction. It may, however, be difficult to distinguish between cosmetic concerns and actual discomfort in juvenile patients.

Conservative care is also indicated in patients with moderate and severe deformities, especially if compliance is a problem. Rapid progression of a deformity is uncommon and often a patient can be evaluated over a lengthy period of time. Nonsurgical care is also advised in juveniles with hyperelasticity, a low collagen syndrome, or significant pes planus. Surgery is never done on an emergency basis. Postoperative recurrence is quite common in this age group.

Decision-Making in Juvenile Hallux Valgus

In the evaluation of a juvenile with hallux valgus, it is important to recognize concomitant abnormalities that may have an effect on either the development of a hallux valgus deformity or the results of the intended surgery. When examining a patient, care should be taken to evaluate tightness of the Achilles tendon as well as any spasticity that may be present. Hyperelasticity, pes planus, hindfoot valgus, or other postural abnormalities may influence the overall success rate. Radiographic evaluation must be done to assess the magnitude of the hallux valgus angle and 1–2 intermetatarsal angle as well as joint space congruity.

In the case of a mild hallux valgus deformity (hallux valgus angle of 25 degrees or less), a distal soft tissue realignment may be performed. A modified McBride procedure (without excision of the lateral sesamoid), a chevron osteotomy, or a Mitchell osteotomy are all acceptable methods of repair. When the hallux valgus angle is greater than 25 degrees with concurrent metatarsophalangeal joint subluxation, a distal soft tissue realignment can be combined with a proximal first metatarsal osteotomy to reduce the 1-2 intermetatarsal angle. The location of an osteotomy in the first ray depends upon the patient's age and whether the proximal first metatarsal epiphysis remains open, and if so, how much estimated growth remains. A metatarsal osteotomy can be placed distal to the epiphysis, or an opening wedge first cuneiform osteotomy can be performed if the first ray is not already excessively long.[12]

---

*See references 9, 13, 32, 37, 46, 55, 59, and 63.

Piggott[51] reported a 9-percent incidence of congruous metatarsophalangeal articulations in patients with hallux valgus. While he felt these deformities were less likely to progress, this deformity does occasionally require surgical correction. A first metatarsophalangeal joint realignment is contraindicated since it will create a noncongruous joint and may place the first metatarsophalangeal joint at risk for later degenerative changes or recurrence of deformity (Fig. 36–7A and B). In this situation, an extra-articular repair is indicated. Different procedures may be selected depending upon the magnitude of the deformity. A distal metatarsal osteotomy,[20, 26, 49, 50, 53, 65] a proximal phalangeal osteotomy,[40] a proximal phalangeal osteotomy combined with a proximal metatarsal osteotomy,[12] a metatarsocuneiform arthrodesis,[35, 36] or a cuneiform osteotomy[8, 64] with a phalangeal osteotomy may be contemplated.

In all these situations, an attempt must be made to create an extra-articular realignment of the metatarsophalangeal joint when a congruous joint is present. Osteotomies in the proximal aspect of the proximal phalanx and in the proximal aspect of the first metatarsal must be positioned meticulously in order to avoid epiphyseal injury. When a proximal osteotomy is performed, the choice of an opening, closing, or crescentic osteotomy depends to a great extent on whether one desires to increase, decrease, or maintain first metatarsal length (Fig. 36–8A to C).

Metatarsocuneiform joint flexibility will indicate whether the 1–2 intermetatarsal angle is a fixed or flexible deformity. The preoperative examination may give an indication of metatarsocuneiform flexibility; however, not uncommonly this can be determined only at the time of surgery following a release of the soft

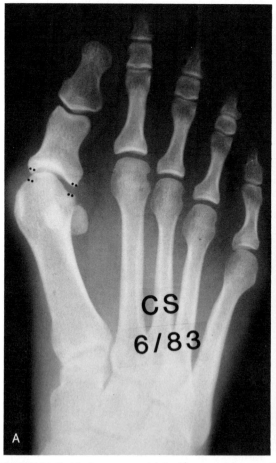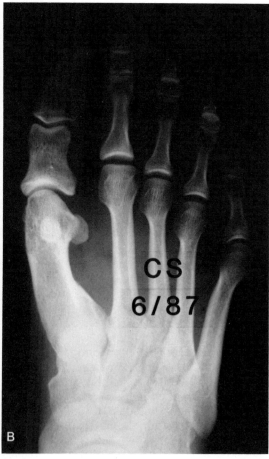

FIGURE 36–7. *(A),* A congruous joint with concentric apposition of the corresponding phalangeal and metatarsal articular surfaces. *(B),* A distal soft tissue realignment was performed on this congruent joint causing incongruity and increasing the chance of either postoperative recurrence or degenerative arthritis of the first metatarsophalangeal joint. (From Coughlin MJ, Mann RA: The pathophysiology of the juvenile bunion. Instr Course Lect 36:123, 1987.)

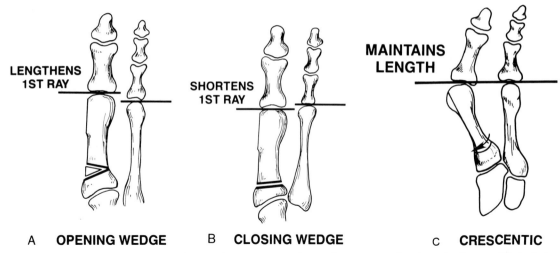

FIGURE 36–8. Proximal first metatarsal osteotomy. *(A)*, An opening wedge osteotomy lengthens the first ray. *(B)*, A closing wedge osteotomy shortens the first ray. *(C)*, A crescentic osteotomy maintains the first ray length. (Modified from Mann RA, Coughlin MJ: Surgery of the Foot and Ankle, 6th Ed. St. Louis, Mosby–Year Book, 1993, p 325.)

tissue contractures at the first metatarsophalangeal joint. The metatarsocuneiform joint is further assessed by preoperative radiographic examination. A fixed obliquity of the metatarsocuneiform joint is often a rigid deformity that resists correction following a distal soft tissue release, while a curvilinear orientation of the metatarsocuneiform joint is often more amenable to spontaneous intraoperative correction of the 1–2 intermetatarsal angle following a distal soft tissue release and realignment. A juvenile bunion is frequently characterized by a metatarsocuneiform joint that has little flexibility. The first metatarsal often has a significant 1–2 intermetatarsal angle that does not diminish following the release of the soft tissue contracture at the first metatarsophalangeal joint. Frequently, an osteotomy of the first metatarsal is necessary to correct the intermetatarsal angle, and when this is not performed, postoperative recurrence is significant.[13, 14, 49, 59] While a distal soft tissue realignment may correct the hallux valgus, a proximal osteotomy (of the metatarsal or cuneiform) is necessary to reduce the 1–2 intermetatarsal angle. At the time of surgery, all elements of the hallux valgus deformity must be corrected to avoid recurrence.[8, 12, 46, 61, 62]

Surgical Repair

Numerous surgical procedures have been described for the repair of a juvenile hallux valgus deformity. A first metatarsal osteotomy is frequently an integral part of the technique because of the need to correct the 1–2 intermetatarsal angle. A distal metatarsal osteotomy, while not necessarily close to the true deformity, may allow adequate correction if the hallux valgus is not severe. As the magnitude of the deformity increases, a more proximally oriented osteotomy is necessary in order to achieve reduction of the increased 1–2 intermetatarsal angle.

Akin Procedure

Indications

The Akin procedure[1, 57, 58] involves a medial eminence resection and a medial capsular reefing combined with a medial closing wedge osteotomy of the proximal phalanx. This operation can be utilized for a hallux valgus interphalangeus deformity in the juvenile. When there is a congruous joint with significant deformity, an extra-articular repair utilizing an Akin osteotomy of the proximal phalanx can be combined with a metatarsal or cuneiform osteotomy. An extra-articular repair may prevent a disturbance of the concentric orientation of the metatarsophalangeal articulation. An isolated phalangeal osteotomy does not address an increased 1–2 intermetatarsal angle. Therefore, if there is a significant metatarsus primus varus deformity, an Akin procedure must be combined with a more proximal osteotomy, or another procedure should be chosen. On occasion, a phalangeal osteotomy can be done without a medial eminence resection and medial capsular reefing if an osteotomy is sufficient to realign the hallux.

Technique

A medial longitudinal incision is centered over the medial eminence beginning at the interphalangeal joint and extending proximally to a point proximal to the medial eminence. Care must be taken to protect the neurovascular bundles on the dorsal and plantar aspect. A U-shaped distally based capsular flap is created, and the capsule is carefully reflected off the medial eminence. The plantar incision is placed along the superior border of the abductor hallucis tendon. The capsular incisions are repaired later. The medial eminence is resected using an oscillating saw often at a point slightly medial to the sagittal sulcus, and any remaining osteophyte is resected with a

rongeur. There is generally little if any osteophyte formation in the juvenile patient.

The phalangeal osteotomy in the juvenile is made in the mid to proximal diaphyseal region. Since the phalangeal epiphysis is located in the proximal metaphyseal region, care must be taken to protect the growth plate. Once the epiphyseal plate is isolated with a small needle the osteotomy can be performed. A subperiosteal dissection is utilized to reflect soft tissue from the phalangeal metaphyseal region. Care is taken to protect the distally based capsular flap. A small, medially based wedge of bone (base approximately 2 mm in width) is resected with an oscillating saw (Fig. 36–9A and B). The lateral cortex is left intact and the osteotomy site is closed and fixed with a smooth 0.062-inch Kirschner wire placed in an oblique fashion. In accomplishing internal fixation, care should be taken to avoid penetration of the interphalangeal and metatarsophalangeal joints as well as the epiphyseal plate. An

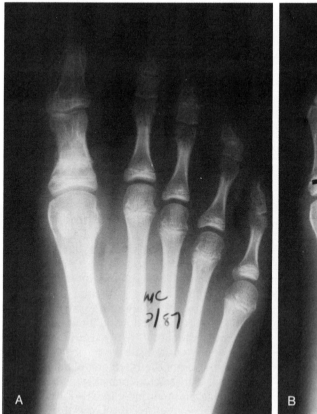
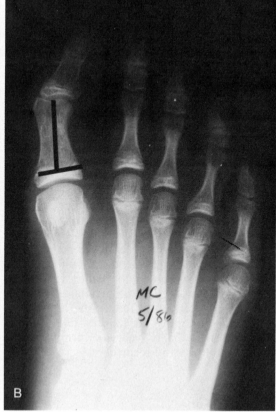

FIGURE 36–9. *(A)*, Preoperative radiograph demonstrating hallux valgus interphalangeus. *(B)*, Following Akin's osteotomy, realignment of the hallux is achieved. (Modified from Mann RA, Coughlin MJ: Surgery of the Foot and Ankle, 6th Ed. St. Louis, Mosby–Year Book, 1993, p 313.)

intraoperative radiograph may aid in visualizing the Kirschner wire in relation to the epiphysis and joints of the hallux. With a phalangeal osteotomy, toe pronation can be corrected by rotating the osteotomy site at the time of surgery. The medial capsule is then sutured to the remaining metatarsophalangeal capsule on the dorsal-proximal and plantar aspect. If insufficient capsule is present on the dorsal-proximal aspect, a small drill-hole may be placed in the metaphyseal cortex and the capsular flap reefed to the bone.

Postoperative Care

Casting is usually not necessary following a phalangeal osteotomy. A gauze compression dressing is applied at surgery and is changed weekly, and the patient is allowed to ambulate in a wooden-soled shoe. Four to six weeks following surgery the fixation pin is removed, and range-of-motion exercises may be initiated at that time.

Complications

Complications are uncommon following the Akin osteotomy. Internal fixation minimizes the occurrence of malunion or nonunion. In his description of this procedure,[1] Akin advised that a lateral metatarsophalangeal capsular release be performed, but this should be avoided as it may devascularize the proximal phalangeal fragment. Furthermore, extensive soft tissue stripping is contraindicated because it can lead to avascular necrosis. Again, when a hallux valgus deformity is associated with a significant intermetatarsal angle, consideration must be given to treatment of the metatarsus primus varus deformity as well.

Distal Metatarsal Osteotomy

The Chevron Procedure

Indications

The chevron procedure was initially described by Austin and Leventen in 1968.[4] Corless,[11] Johnson,[31] and Zimmer[65] have also reported on their experience using this procedure for mild and moderate hallux valgus deformities with an intermetatarsal angle of less than 15 degrees and a hallux valgus angle of less than 30 degrees. The chevron osteotomy achieves an extra-articular repair and thus may be used to correct both a subluxated and a noncongruous metatarsophalangeal joint deformity as well as a hallux valgus deformity with a congruous joint.

Technique

A medial longitudinal incision is centered over the medial eminence starting at the midportion of the proximal phalanx and extending approximately 5 cm. The dissection is carried down to the metatarsophalangeal capsule and dorsal and plantar skin flaps are developed. The dorsal and plantar cutaneous nerves are contained within these flaps and protected by this type of dissection. A U-shaped distally based capsular flap is developed. The plantar limb of this incision is made just superior to the abductor hallucis tendon. The medial eminence is resected with an oscillating saw or an osteotome. This osteotomy is usually performed just medial to or within the sagittal sulcus. Any remaining osteophyte is removed with a rongeur. A drill hole (Fig. 36–10A) is then made in the metatarsal head in a medial to lateral direction to mark the apex of the osteotomy. A drill hole is placed in the very center of the metatarsal head, an equal distance from the articular surface and the dorsal and plantar surfaces. The chevron osteotomy is made with an oscillating saw, using a very fine blade to minimize shortening at the osteotomy site. The osteotomy is made in a medial to lateral direction with the apex of the angle approximately 60 degrees. The proximally based osteotomy is made in the metaphyseal region, providing a large area for bony contact that aids rapid healing (Fig. 36–10B to D). The chevron shape of the osteotomy makes a very stable osteotomy in a dorsal plantar direction.

During the surgical dissection, care should be taken to avoid excessive soft tissue stripping as this may endanger the circulation to the first metatarsal head. Although Austin and Leventen[4] recommend a lateral capsular release and a release of the conjoined adductor tendon, it is preferable to avoid this. While Austin probably achieved greater surgical correction by a lateral release,[4] Meier and Kenzora[47] and Mann[38] noted several cases of partial and total avascular necrosis in the metatarsal head following the chevron procedure in adults (Fig. 36–10E and F). A lateral release

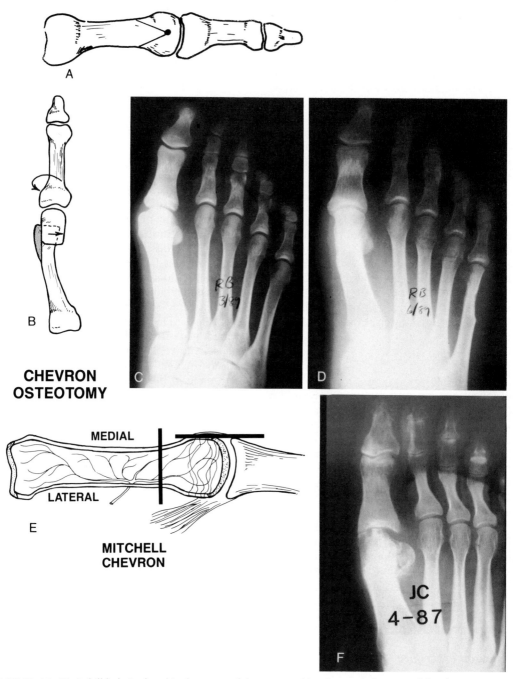

FIGURE 36–10. *(A),* A drill hole is placed in the center of the metatarsal head to mark the apex of the chevron osteotomy. *(B),* The capital fragment is displaced in a lateral direction. *(C),* Preoperative radiograph demonstrating a moderate hallux valgus deformity in a skeletally mature individual. *(D),* Postoperative radiograph following a chevron hallux valgus repair. *(E),* A distal metatarsal osteotomy is performed through a medial incision. If a lateral capsular and adductor tendon release is performed, the possibility of avascular necrosis of the metatarsal head is increased. (The black lines indicate disruption of vascular supply medially following medial capsulorrhaphy, and transversely following the distal metatarsal osteotomy. The rest of the circulation is derived from the lateral capsular structures.) *(E),* Following distal metatarsal osteotomy, avascular necrosis may occur if a lateral release is carried out as well. *(A, B, E,* and *F* from Mann RA, Coughlin MJ: Surgery of the Foot and Ankle, 6th Ed. St. Louis, Mosby–Year Book, 1993, p 315.)

may indeed compromise circulation to the first metatarsal head and for this reason is probably unwise. Following the osteotomy, the metatarsal head is displaced in a lateral direction approximately one-third of the metaphyseal width of the first metatarsal. The osteotomy site is then impacted and fixed with a 0.062 Kirschner wire directed in a proximal dorsal to distal plantar direction. Care is taken not to penetrate the metatarsophalangeal joint. The osteotomy is stable in a dorsal plantar direction, but the possibility of medial displacement and loss of correction makes internal fixation desirable. The U-shaped medial capsular flap is repaired with interrupted absorbable sutures. If there is insufficient proximal medial capsule with which to repair the capsular flap, drill holes may be placed in the medial metaphyseal cortex to aid in the capsular repair.

Postoperative Care

Cast immobilization is usually not necessary. A gauze compression dressing is applied at surgery and is changed weekly. The internal fixation is removed 3 weeks following surgery under local anesthesia. Range-of-motion exercises may then be initiated. The patient is allowed to ambulate in a postoperative shoe and later in an open-toed sandal.

The Mitchell Procedure

Indications

The Mitchell procedure was initially described by Hawkins, Mitchell, and Hedrick in 1945.[26] By using a lateral displacement-angulation osteotomy of the distal metatarsal metaphysis, the increased 1–2 intermetatarsal angle and valgus deviation of the great toe are corrected. The indications for this procedure are mild to moderate hallux valgus deformities with an intermetatarsal angle of less than 16 degrees and a hallux valgus angle of less than 40 degrees. The Mitchell procedure achieves an extra-articular repair and may be used to correct both a subluxated and a noncongruous metatarsophalangeal joint as well as a hallux valgus deformity with a congruous joint.

Technique

A dorsomedial curvilinear incision is extended from the base of the proximal phalanx to the midportion of the first metatarsal, and dissection is carried down to the metatarsophalangeal joint capsule with care taken to protect the neurovascular bundles. The metatarsophalangeal joint capsule is incised longitudinally, exposing the medial eminence, and a sagittal saw is used to remove the medial eminence in line with the medial border of the foot. Retractors are placed and two dorsoplantar drill holes are created for later fixation of the osteotomy site. The most distal drill hole emerges on the plantar aspect of the first metatarsal head just proximal to the articular cartilage of the first metatarsal. The proximal drill hole is placed approximately 1 cm proximal and 0.5 cm lateral to the distal hole. The distal osteotomy cut is only a partial osteotomy and is placed about 3 to 4 mm proximal to the distal drill hole at a right angle to the longitudinal axis of the metatarsal shaft. A second osteotomy cut completely across the metatarsal is made just proximal to the first partial osteotomy cut. These cuts should be only 1 to 2 mm apart on the dorsal surface of the first metatarsal. They diverge in a lateral and plantar direction, which allows the creation of 10 to 15 degrees of plantar inclination at the osteotomy site to minimize postoperative lateral metatarsalgia. The excess bone at the osteotomy site is removed with a rongeur and the first metatarsal head is displaced laterally and engaged on its bony ledge. Heavy nonabsorbable sutures are then passed in a dorsal plantar direction through the proximal hole and in a plantar dorsal direction through the distal hole. With the osteotomy site compressed, the first suture is tied, then the second suture is tied, tightly compressing the osteotomy site. Any excess bone on the medial aspect of the first metatarsal is removed, and the medial capsule is closed in a pants-over-vest fashion.

Initially a bulky compression dressing is placed. A sterile tongue depressor may be used to give rigidity to the dressing. The foot is initially elevated and then approximately 1 week after surgery, the dressing is changed and a slipper toe spica cast is applied with the toe in neutral alignment. Immobilization is continued for 6 to 8 weeks until the osteotomy site is solidly healed.

Results of Distal Metatarsal Osteotomy

Distal osteotomy for treatment of juvenile bunions has had varying results. Mitchell[49] reported a 22-percent and Ball and Sullivan[5] a 44-percent incidence of postoperative metatarsalgia. While satisfactory results were reported in several series,[9, 13, 37, 49] Ball and Sullivan[5] reported a 61-percent recurrence rate with the Mitchell repair. Displacement of the small distal fragment with a Mitchell osteotomy, rotational instability, nonunion, dorsiflexion or plantar flexion malunion, incomplete correction, and avascular necrosis are just some of the complications that have been reported following the Mitchell procedure.[5, 9, 13, 22, 46] Due to the unstable nature of this osteotomy, postoperative displacement and malunion may occur.

Zimmer and coworkers[65] have published the only report on use of the chevron procedure in the juvenile patient. In their series of 20 patients, there was a recurrence rate of 20 percent and no cases of avascular necrosis. There was an average correction in the hallux valgus angle of 8.1 degrees (preoperative 28.6 degrees, postoperative 20.5 degrees) and a correction in the 1–2 intermetatarsal angle of 4.8 degrees (preoperative 12.3 degrees, postoperative 7.5 degrees). They concluded that the indications for the chevron procedure in the juvenile patient were a hallux valgus angle of less than 40 degrees and a 1–2 intermetatarsal angle of less than 15 degrees. The authors found little correlation between the radiographic measurement and the overall results; however, the rather limited hallux valgus correction reported in their article would tend to limit this procedure to patients with a relatively mild deformity. This operation is also indicated when a congruent metatarsophalangeal joint is present; however, if there is a significant 1–2 intermetatarsal angle, a proximal osteotomy may be necessary to achieve a greater correction.

Complications

The most significant, albeit uncommon, complication following a chevron osteotomy is avascular necrosis of the first metatarsal head.[38, 47] Hallux varus, excessive shortening,[40] and postoperative migration or recurrence[50] are seen as well. Postoperative recurrence is more likely when this procedure is utilized for more severe deformities. In a hallux valgus deformity with an angle greater than 40 degrees, or with a 1–2 intermetatarsal angle of greater than 15 degrees, a more aggressive procedure should be contemplated.

The most significant complication following a Mitchell bunionectomy is lateral metatarsalgia. Dorsal angulation or displacement can occur due to the instability of this osteotomy. Ball and Sullivan[5] reported a high incidence of postoperative metatarsalgia, and avascular necrosis is a possibility with any distal osteotomy, although it is less common with the Mitchell procedure. Excessive shortening can develop following a Mitchell procedure, and plantar angulation of the osteotomy site may help to diminish postoperative metatarsalgia. Postoperative recurrence is more common when this procedure is used for severe deformities. The upper limits of this procedure are a hallux valgus angle greater than 40 degrees with a 1–2 intermetatarsal angle greater than 16 degrees. The indications for either a chevron or a Mitchell procedure are similar, although a Mitchell procedure can be used for a slightly more severe deformity because the osteotomy is slightly more proximal than in the chevron technique.

Distal Soft Tissue Realignment

The modified McBride procedure has been recommended for the repair of mild to moderate hallux valgus deformities.[43, 44, 48] As originally described, this procedure included a lateral capsular release, an adductor tendon transfer (with implantation into the lateral metatarsal head), lateral sesamoid excision, medial eminence resection, and medial capsular repair. Later, DuVries[15] modified this procedure and incorporated the adductor tendon into the lateral capsular reefing. Continued modification of this procedure makes the use of the eponym "McBride procedure" inappropriate; a more descriptive term is "distal soft tissue realignment," which highlights the fact that this is an intra-articular repair of the first metatarsophalangeal joint. A proximal first metatarsal or cuneiform osteotomy at times may be utilized in association with a distal soft tissue realignment.

Technique

A 2- to 3-cm dorsal longitudinal incision is centered in the first intermetatarsal web space, and a Weitlaner retractor is used to distract the first and second metatarsals, exposing the adductor hallucis tendon. The tendon is dissected free from the lateral sesamoid, and the distal adductor tendon insertion is left attached to the base of the proximal phalanx and the tendon is released approximately 1.5 cm proximal to the insertion at the level of the musculotendinous junction. This distal tendon stump is marked with a suture and is later sutured to the lateral metatarsal capsule. The adductor hallucis muscle is allowed to retract, the lateral sesamoid is freed of any contracted tissue, and the transverse intermetatarsal ligament is incised. Care must be taken to avoid injury to the flexor hallucis longus tendon and the common digital nerve, which lies directly beneath the transverse intermetatarsal ligament. The lateral sesamoid is rarely removed. The lateral capsule is then perforated with several puncture wounds and the toe angulated in a medial direction causing the lateral capsule to tear. By avoiding an abrupt incision of the lateral capsule and instead tearing the capsule, it is hoped that scar tissue will develop to provide some postoperative stability to the lateral aspect of the metatarsophalangeal joint.

The stump of conjoined tendon that was left attached to the base of the proximal phalanx is later used to reinforce the lateral capsule to minimize the possibility of a hallux varus deformity.

A 4-cm medial longitudinal incision is centered over the medial eminence. The dissection is carried down directly to the capsule and dorsal and plantar skin flaps are raised. Within these skin flaps lie the digital nerves that are protected by retractors. A U-shaped distally based capsular flap is then developed. The plantar extent of the capsular flap lies at the superior border of the abductor hallucis tendon.

The medial eminence is resected using an oscillating saw or osteotome (Fig. 36–11*A* and *B*). The osteotomy is performed in a line parallel with the diaphyseal cortex of the first metatarsal. Occasionally, a sagittal sulcus is present in the juvenile, but this is more common in the adult with hallux valgus deformity. The osteotomy is made without regard to the

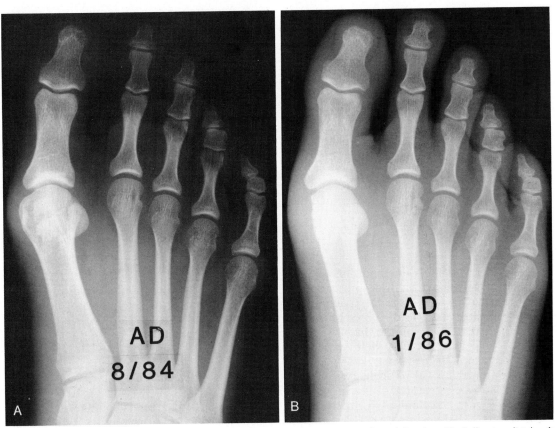

FIGURE 36–11. *(A)*, Preoperative radiograph demonstrating moderate hallux valgus deformity. *(B)*, Following distal soft tissue realignment. (Modified from Mann RA, Coughlin MJ: Surgery of the Foot and Ankle, 6th Ed. St. Louis, Mosby–Year Book, 1993, p 323.)

site of the sagittal sulcus, which varies. Following the osteotomy of the medial eminence, any remaining edge or bony prominence is removed with a rongeur.

Three interrupted 2–0 sutures are then used to approximate the lateral capsule of the first metatarsal with the medial capsule of the second metatarsal. These sutures are placed and later tied following the medial capsule repair. After the sutures are tied, compression is placed on the transverse metatarsal arch in order to approximate the first and second metatarsal heads. The stump of the conjoined adductor tendon is then sutured into the lateral metatarsal capsular cuff to further stabilize the lateral repair.

With the great toe held in appropriate rotation and alignment, several interrupted 2–0 absorbable sutures are used to repair the medial capsule, and several more sutures are placed along the plantar capsular incision. Occasionally, it is difficult to achieve an adequate dorsal-proximal capsular repair due to the absence of proximal capsular tissue. In this situation, drill holes may be placed in the dorsal-medial metaphysis of the first metatarsal through which the dorsal-medial capsular flap is stabilized.

Postoperative Care

A gauze compression dressing is applied at surgery and changed on a weekly basis. Ambulation is allowed in a wooden-soled shoe, and 6 weeks following surgery, a stiff-soled sandal may be substituted. At this point the patient is instructed in the manipulation of the toe in a dorsal-plantar plane. Eight weeks after surgery the dressings are discontinued and the patient may use a roomy shoe.

Results

Mann and Coughlin[41] in reporting on the results of the modified McBride procedure in 100 patients noted an average correction in the 1–2 intermetatarsal angle of 5.2 degrees and an average correction of the hallux valgus angle of 17 degrees. It was their conclusion that if an intermetatarsal angle exceeded 15 degrees or the hallux valgus angle exceeded 40 degrees, then an osteotomy of the first metatarsal base was also indicated. Meier and Kenzora[47] reported on 21 patients who underwent a modified McBride procedure and sug-

gested that if the intermetatarsal angle was less than or equal to 14 degrees and the hallux valgus angle less than or equal to 50 degrees, this procedure would be effective. In the 21 patients operated upon, an overall hallux valgus correction of 20 degrees and an overall average correction in the 1–2 intermetatarsal angle of 4.2 degrees was reported. Both of these series involved hallux valgus in the adult patient.

Scranton and Zuckerman[56] reported a 75-percent failure rate with the modified McBride procedure in juvenile patients. Bonney and MacNab[8] found that following a distal soft tissue realignment without a metatarsal osteotomy, the 1–2 intermetatarsal angle returned to its original preoperative angle or actually increased in 63 percent of the operated cases. Helal and colleagues[28] reported a 46-percent failure rate with this technique and suggested that the correction did not hold up well with the passage of time.

Complications

A frequently reported complication following distal soft tissue realignment is hallux varus. Mann and Coughlin[40] reported postoperative hallux varus in 11 percent of their series of adult patients, although it was a significant deformity in only 4 percent. They recommended that a lateral metatarsophalangeal release be performed without a lateral sesamoidectomy. Following this modification, a 2-percent incidence of hallux varus was reported.[39]

Another significant complication is postoperative recurrence. Both Mann and Coughlin[40, 41] and Meier and Kenzora[47] advocate a distal soft tissue realignment if the 1–2 intermetatarsal angle is less than or equal to 14 degrees. A hallux valgus angle of less than 40 degrees is the upper limit for a distal soft tissue realignment. Because of the high rate of recurrence of a hallux valgus deformity in the juvenile, a proximal metatarsal osteotomy is frequently recommended in conjunction with a distal soft tissue realignment.[12, 22, 59]

Proximal Metatarsal Osteotomy

Proximal metatarsal osteotomies have been used with varying success in the treatment of the juvenile bunion. While Bonney and

MacNab[8] recommend an opening wedge osteotomy for the repair of a juvenile hallux valgus deformity, Scranton and Zuckerman[56] reported a 35-percent failure rate with this procedure. Goldner and Gaines[22] reported that an opening wedge first metatarsal osteotomy leads to tightening of the extensor mechanism and postoperative recurrence. Scranton and Zuckerman[56] recommended a closing wedge osteotomy despite a 25-percent recurrence rate. Wilson[63] reported an 88 percent satisfactory repair with a midmetatarsal oblique osteotomy, while Helal[27] had excellent results with a similar technique.

While an opening or closing wedge osteotomy of the first metatarsal may be performed, it is usually not necessary to either lengthen or shorten the first ray. For this reason, a crescentic osteotomy of the proximal first metatarsal has been advocated.[39, 40] The metaphysis of the first metatarsal is selected as the osteotomy site because it provides a rather broad surface that permits fairly rapid healing and is relatively stable in a plantar direction.

Indications

Due to the frequent recurrence of a hallux valgus deformity in juvenile patients, serious consideration must be given to correction of the increased 1–2 intermetatarsal angle. A proximal first metatarsal osteotomy or an osteotomy at some location along the first ray is frequently necessary to achieve a diminution of the metatarsus primus varus. Frequently the first metatarsocuneiform joint in a juvenile is quite rigid and thus an osteotomy may be indicated with a 1–2 intermetatarsal angle of less than 14 degrees. Following a distal soft tissue realignment or some other distal procedure, a proximal osteotomy should be considered if the 1–2 intermetatarsal angle cannot be reduced.

Technique

A 3-cm dorsal longitudinal incision is centered over the proximal first metatarsal, and the dissection is carried down on either the medial or lateral aspect of the extensor hallucis longus tendon. A subperiosteal dissection is used to expose the proximal first metatarsal shaft. The metatarsocuneiform joint should be identified so that it is not penetrated with the osteotomy. A crescentic osteotomy is then performed 1 cm distal to the metatarsocuneiform joint using a power-driven, curved sawblade.

The osteotomy is made in a dorsal to plantar direction at about a 120-degree angle with the first metatarsal shaft. On occasion, depending upon the thickness of the first metatarsal metaphysis, an osteotome can be utilized to complete the plantar cut. The proximal fragment is held with an elevator and the distal fragment is then rotated in a medial direction approximately 2 to 3 mm in order to decrease the 1–2 intermetatarsal angle. Care must be taken not to overcorrect the osteotomy and create a negative 1–2 intermetatarsal angle. The osteotomy is fixed with a 0.062-inch Kirschner wire, then the distal fragment is drilled with a 3.5-mm drill and the proximal fragment with a 2.5-mm drill. The fixation hole is tapped and a "206" Synthes screw is used to compress and fix the osteotomy site. The distal screw hole is placed 1 cm distal to the osteotomy site and oriented in a proximal direction. By keeping the drill as close to parallel as possible to the distal metatarsal shaft, the plantar aspect of the proximal fragment can be engaged and stabilized (Fig. 36–12*A* and *B*). It should be noted that a proximal osteotomy with internal fixation is performed where the epiphyseal line has completed growth. If the epiphysis is open, a proximal crescentic osteotomy may be performed, but screw fixation is contraindicated. The osteotomy can be placed distal to the epiphyseal plate; however, careful placement of internal fixation is necessary to avoid an epiphyseal injury. Steinmann pins can also be used to stabilize the distal first metatarsal to the second metatarsal and can be removed following successful healing of the osteotomy site.

When a Kirschner wire is used, it is bent at the surface of the first metatarsal shaft and left in place. Dual fixation with both a Kirschner wire and a compression screw provides not only compression but also rotational stability at the osteotomy site. Intraoperative x-ray films may be taken to evaluate the correction of the 1–2 intermetatarsal angle and the location of internal fixation. Often while an anteroposterior radiograph appears to show the fixation penetrating the metatarsocuneiform joint, a lateral film will confirm that the fixation is within the first metatarsal. Should the metatarsocuneiform joint be penetrated, the internal fixation device can be removed postop-

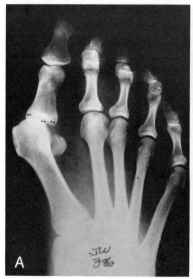
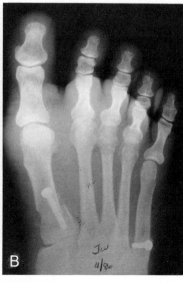

FIGURE 36–12. (A), Preoperative radiograph of a patient with a splay foot deformity and marked subluxation of the first metatarsophalangeal joint. (B), Following proximal first metatarsal osteotomy and distal soft tissue realignment, correction of the first ray is achieved. (A bunionette repair was also performed.) (From Coughlin MJ, Mann RA: The pathophysiology of the juvenile bunion. Instr Course Lect 36:123, 1987.)

eratively following adequate healing at the osteotomy site. Internal fixation is frequently removed under local anesthesia 6 weeks after surgery.

Postoperative Care

A soft gauze dressing is applied at surgery and changed weekly for 8 weeks following surgery. Ambulation in a wooden-soled shoe is permitted initially, and a stiff-soled sandal substituted at 6 weeks. The patient can begin to manipulate the toe in a dorsal-plantar plane 7 to 8 weeks after surgery.

Results

Mann[39] reported the results of a combined proximal metatarsal osteotomy with distal soft tissue realignment in the adult patient. In a series of 50 patients, an average correction of the hallux valgus angle of 22 degrees and an average correction of the 1–2 intermetatarsal angle of 8.9 degrees was noted. These patients had moderate deformity (21 to 39 degrees). An average correction of 30 degrees for the hallux valgus angle and 8.6 degrees for the 1–2 intermetatarsal angle was reported in patients with severe deformity (hallux valgus angle greater than 40 degrees). Mann[39, 41] has emphasized the versatility of this procedure. For relatively mild deformities, where the metatarsophalangal joint is incongruent or subluxated, a distal soft tissue realignment can be performed. In the case of moderate or severe

deformities, following a distal soft tissue realignment, a proximal osteotomy can be also done to achieve a correction of the increased 1–2 intermetatarsal angle.

Complications

The major complication following a distal soft tissue realignment with a proximal first metatarsal osteotomy is overcorrection or hallux varus deformity. The incidence of hallux varus can be reduced by avoiding an excessive medial eminence resection. An intraoperative radiograph is helpful in assuring adequate correction and preventing overcorrection at the osteotomy site. While malunion (plantar or dorsal angulation) is possible, the use of internal fixation lessens the possibility of this complication. It is rare for a delayed or nonunion to occur with a proximal first metatarsal osteotomy.

First Cuneiform Osteotomy

According to Kelikian,[33] Riedl in 1886 was the first to report an opening wedge first cuneiform osteotomy to correct a wide intermetatarsal angle. Young[64] used this technique in 1910 and Bonney and McNab[8] also employed a medial cuneiform osteotomy to realign the metatarsocuneiform joint without disturbing the proximal metatarsal epiphysis. So far, all reports of this technique have been of individual cases.

Indications

The indications for a medial cuneiform opening wedge osteotomy are a juvenile hallux valgus deformity with an open proximal first metatarsal epiphysis with an abnormally wide 1–2 intermetatarsal angle. Marked obliquity of the metatarsocuneiform joint with an abnormally wide 1–2 intermetatarsal angle. Realignment of the metatarsocuneiform joint may reverse the tension and compression on the proximal metatarsal epiphysis and according to the rationale of Luba and Rosman[37] may diminish the growth rate on the lateral aspect of the epiphysis, decreasing the chance of recurrence of a widened 1–2 intermetatarsal angle.

Technique

A medial incision is centered over the first cuneiform. Care is taken to identify the metatarsocuneiform and the cuneiform navicular joints. This is a relatively small bone in both the coronal and sagittal planes. The osteotomy is centered in the first cuneiform, which has an overall length of approximately 2 cm, and is made in a direct medial-lateral plane and carried to a depth of approximately 1.5 cm. The coronal dimension of the first cuneiform is approximately 3 cm in height, and the osteotomy must be completed from the dorsal to the plantar cortex. While some have used the medial eminence as an interposition bone graft, in the juvenile very little medial eminence is resected. Therefore, if a cuneiform osteotomy is performed, it is best to remove the donor bone from the iliac crest, usually in a longitudinal fashion. Due to the height of the first cuneiform, a fairly long graft must be placed in a dorsal-plantar plane. The graft, which is usually less than 1 cm at the base and tapers to a fine point at the apex, is prepared so that all cortical bone is removed. Then the osteotomy site is levered open with a small osteotome or lamina spreader and the bone graft is impacted into place. Any instability at the osteotomy site should be fixed with a Kirschner wire. Frequently, the osteotomy site is under such tension that it is very stable (Fig. 36–13A and B). The wound is closed in a routine fashion.

Postoperative Care

In an unreliable patient a short-leg walking cast may be applied, but in most a compression gauze dressing can be used. Usually if the osteotomy is combined with a distal soft tissue realignment, a compression gauze dressing is helpful in aligning the toe. When an interposition iliac crest graft is used, the osteotomy will often be healed at 6 weeks following surgery.

Results

Unfortunately, there has been no series reported utilizing cuneiform osteotomy in the juvenile patient. Nevertheless, this is a useful technique for treating a juvenile hallux valgus deformity in which the proximal metatarsal epiphysis remains open.

Complications

The main complication is displacement of the osteotomy site, which requires internal fixation. It is important that the osteotomy be wedged open on the medial aspect so that diminution of the 1–2 intermetatarsal angle can be achieved. An intraoperative x-ray study is helpful to ascertain whether adequate correction has been attained.

Metatarsocuneiform Arthrodesis

An arthrodesis of the first metatarsocuneiform joint achieved popularity following Lapidus' description in 1934.[35] Kelikian[33] reported that Albrecht first described this procedure in 1911 and that Kleinberg advocated its use in 1932. The eponym "Lapidus procedure" is another term for arthrodesis of the first metatarsocuneiform joint.

Indications

DuVries[16] recommended the use of a metatarsocuneiform fusion for juvenile hallux valgus, and Giannestras[21] also advocated metatarsocuneiform fusion as a means of reducing and stabilizing the 1–2 intermetatarsal angle in juvenile hallux valgus. Goldner and Gaines[22] used the Lapidus procedure for juvenile bunion and found that while this arthrodesis eliminates motion at the metatarsocuneiform joint, its absence is unnoticed by most patients. They felt that a Lapidus procedure was advantageous when the first cuneiform–metatarsal articulation had an obliquity of greater than 30 degrees and when the first metatarsal was significantly longer than the second metatarsal.

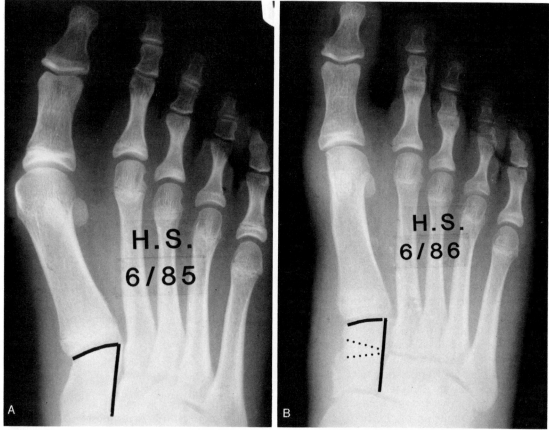

FIGURE 36–13. *(A)*, Preoperative radiograph of juvenile hallux valgus. *(B)*, Postoperative radiograph following distal soft tissue realignment and opening wedge cuneiform osteotomy. (From Coughlin MJ, Mann RA: The pathophysiology of the juvenile bunion. Instr Course Lect 36:123, 1987.)

Technique

A metatarsocuneiform fusion is frequently combined with a distal soft tissue realignment, Akin procedure, or other distal hallux valgus repair. A 3-cm skin incision is centered over the dorsal aspect of the metatarsocuneiform joint. The capsule is incised on the dorsal aspect as well as on the dorsal medial aspect. A subperiosteal stripping is carried out between the base of the first and second metatarsals with care not to damage the dorsalis pedis artery. The lateral tuberosity of the first metatarsal is excised. The medial base of the second metatarsal and the lateral base of the first metatarsal are roughened to promote an arthrodesis. A small wedge of bone is removed on the lateral aspect of the metatarsocuneiform joint, and the articular cartilage of the proximal metatarsal and distal cuneiform are excised. Care must be taken not to remove an

excessive lateral wedge nor to significantly destabilize this joint. Lapidus[36] noted that too large a resection "is not favorable for bony fusion." Lapidus advocated translating the first metatarsal in a slight plantarward direction to decrease pronation. Goldner and Gaines[22] recommended medial translation of the base of the first metatarsal in relationship to the medial cuneiform.

It is also helpful to remove a bone block from the proposed fusion area. If this block is removed in an eccentric fashion so that more bone is removed from the cuneiform and less from the proximal metatarsal, it can be rotated to assist in achieving an arthrodesis. Care must be taken when performing a metatarsocuneiform fusion to avoid damaging an open epiphysis.

Lapidus[35] recommended a chromic catgut suture as a means of stabilizing this fusion, while Goldner[22] advised pin fixation at the fusion site. Giannestras[21] did not utilize internal fixation at the metatarsocuneiform joint, but instead placed a transverse Steinmann pin at the distal aspect of the first and second metatarsals for stabilization.

The arthrodesis may be augmented by an autogenous bone graft. An iliac crest graft can be used to fill in any defects at the metatarsocuneiform joint and can also be used to effect an arthrodesis at the base of the first and second metatarsals. While the medial eminence may be morselized and used in this area, frequently very little medial eminence is resected, which leaves little bone available for grafting.

Postoperative Care

In his initial report Lapidus advocated plaster immobilization;[35] in his later report,[36] he recommended rigid immobilization without casting. DuVries[16] stabilized the metatarsocuneiform joint with a small staple and used a non–weight-bearing cast for 4 weeks and then a walking cast for 6 more weeks.

Today, the compression screw technique used for the basilar osteotomy of the metatarsal is used for this arthrodesis, with a second stabilizing cortical screw placed between the first and second metatarsals.

Results

In 1960, Lapidus[36] published a report on "the author's bunion operation from 1931 to 1959" but actually failed to describe results in any series of patients. In 1976, Goldner and Gaines[22] reported on 25 juvenile patients in whom hallux valgus repairs had been performed. They reported on 40 feet in which correction had been achieved and noted 25 excellent, 10 good, and 5 fair results. They included six case reports in their series, but it is difficult to tell how many of these patients underwent a metatarsocuneiform arthrodesis. The authors were enthusiastic about this technique, but it was difficult to ascertain their success rate with the Lapidus procedure. DuVries in 1965[16] reported that "in over 100 cases . . . results have been uniformly satisfactory." No information on pre- and postoperative hallux valgus or 1–2 intermetatarsal angles was given in this series, making it difficult to ascertain the actual success rate with

this procedure. Mauldin and associates[42] reported on 30 patients who underwent a limited metatarsocuneiform arthrodesis in which fusion was achieved with removal and rotation of a bone block. In this series of adult patients, the average correction of the hallux valgus angle was 18.5 degrees and the average improvement in the 1–2 intermetatarsal angle was 5.9 degrees. Postoperative radiographs demonstrated a successful arthrodesis in only 25 percent. In spite of this, there was little symptomatology at the metatarsocuneiform joint, and the authors inferred that a fibrous union at this joint was comparable to a true arthrodesis. Kwong and Aubuchon[34] reported a high rate of nonunion and a significant malunion rate in attempts to fuse the metatarsocuneiform joint.

Complications

The most frequent complication following an attempted arthrodesis at the metatarsocuneiform joint is nonunion. This is a difficult joint to fuse, especially if it is destabilized. A rotated bone block may be helpful in achieving arthrodesis. Augmentation with autogenous bone graft both in the interval between the first and second metatarsals and at the metatarsocuneiform joint may increase the fusion rate. Rigid internal fixation likewise may be helpful, but it may be difficult to achieve in a juvenile with an open epiphysis. Distal metatarsal fixation between the first and second metatarsals may be helpful when there is an open proximal metatarsal epiphysis. Malunion is another significant complication and can develop if the first metatarsocuneiform joint is destabilized. In situ fusion and correction of the intermetatarsal angle appear to offer a lower rate of complication.

DISCUSSION

A single operation is not suitable for all juvenile patients with a hallux valgus deformity. A pre-existing contracted Achilles tendon or severe hindfoot valgus deformity must be corrected prior to hallux valgus repair.

With a greater 1–2 intermetatarsal angle, a more proximally oriented osteotomy will achieve greater correction than a distal metatarsal osteotomy. With significant obliquity of

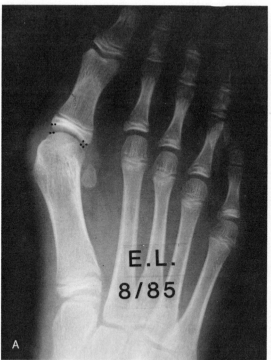

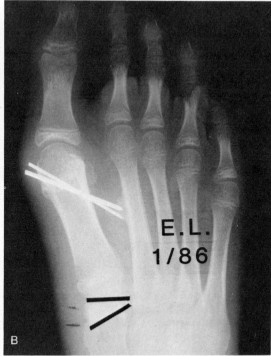

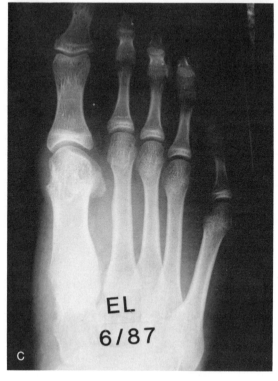

FIGURE 36–14. *(A),* Preoperative juvenile hallux valgus deformity with congruous metatarsophalangeal articulation with increased 1–2 intermetatarsal angle. *(B),* Postoperative radiograph following distal closing wedge osteotomy and opening wedge cuneiform osteotomy. *(C),* Radiograph 18 months postoperatively. (From Coughlin MJ, Mann RA: The pathophysiology of the juvenile bunion. Instr Course Lect 36:123, 1987.)

the metatarsocuneiform joint, or if the epiphysis still has considerable growth remaining, a first cuneiform osteotomy may be the treatment of choice.

Radiographic assessment is necessary in order to quantitate the magnitude of the hallux valgus angle, the 1–2 intermetatarsal angle, and the obliquity of the metatarsocuneiform joint and to ascertain whether the joint is congruous or noncongruous, as this will determine, whether an extra-articular repair or an intra-articular repair is indicated. In a noncongruous joint with significant metatarsophalangeal subluxation, a distal soft tissue realignment is the treatment of choice. When significant subluxation at the metatarsophalangeal joint is combined with a wide 1–2 intermetatarsal angle, a distal soft tissue realignment with either a proximal metatarsal osteotomy or a cuneiform osteotomy is acceptable. A metatarsocuneiform arthrodesis may also be performed in combination with a distal soft tissue realignment if there is increased flexibility at the metatarsocuneiform joint or an oblique orientation of the metatarsocuneiform joint.

The treatment of a hallux valgus deformity with a congruous joint requires periarticular osteotomies. For a hallux valgus interphalangeus deformity, a proximal phalangeal osteotomy such as an Akin procedure may be used, but care must be taken to protect the proximal phalangeal epiphysis. For a congruous joint with a moderate hallux valgus deformity, a chevron distal metatarsal osteotomy is preferable to the Mitchell procedure because of its inherent stability. Helal[28] used the Wilson midshaft osteotomy for similar conditions. For a more severe hallux valgus deformity with a congruous metatarsophalangeal joint, a double osteotomy as recommended by Durman[14] can be done (Fig. 36–14*A to C*). He performed an open wedge proximal phalangeal osteotomy and a closing wedge distal metatarsal osteotomy; however, other variations may be employed. Amarnek and associates[2] recommended a crescentic phalangeal osteotomy combined with a crescentic metatarsal osteotomy. Both Durman and Amarnek reported success with these procedures, but the surgeon must be careful not to disturb an open phalangeal or metatarsal epiphyseal plate in the juvenile patient.

While a chevron osteotomy may be combined with a cuneiform osteotomy, it is difficult to combine a chevron osteotomy with a proximal metatarsal osteotomy because this requires significant soft tissue stripping of the first metatarsal shaft.

The orientation of the lesser metatarsals must be considered, as significant metatarsus adductus is frequently associated with the juvenile bunion[12] and is difficult to treat. Correction of the metatarsus primus varus may require a proximal metatarsal osteotomy. A negative (overcorrected) intermetatarsal angle may be necessary in order to achieve adequate correction.

Postoperative complications are frequent following juvenile hallux valgus surgery. Care must be taken to avoid excessive metatarsal head resection when removing the medial eminence, devascularization of the metatarsal head resulting in avascular necrosis, overcorrection of a first metatarsal osteotomy, or excessive shortening following a first metatarsal osteotomy.

Any procedure selected should correct all the components of the deformity—the hallux valgus deformity, pronation of the hallux, a prominent medial eminence, a widened 1–2 intermetatarsal angle, and obliquity of the metatarsocuneiform joint.

Often, a surgeon utilizes a single operation in repairing adult hallux valgus deformities, but surgical versatility is most important in dealing with juvenile bunions. Different juvenile bunions may require completely different operative approaches.

It is important not to stretch the indications for a hallux valgus procedure. If a more severe deformity is present, a more aggressive procedure should be utilized to correct the deformity. The fact that different success rates are reported for various bunion techniques emphasizes the fact that juvenile bunions are not all alike and are not suited for any one standard hallux valgus repair. The surgeon must vary the surgical technique for a juvenile hallux valgus deformity depending upon the anatomic and pathologic abnormalities present.

References

1. Akin OA: The treatment of hallux valgus: A new operative procedure and its results. Med Sentinel 33:678, 1925.
2. Amarnek D, Jacobs A, Oloff L: Adolescent hallux valgus: Its etiology and surgical management. J Foot Surg 24:54, 1985.

3. Antrobus J: The primary deformity in hallux valgus and metatarsus primus varus. Clin Orthop 184:251, 1984.
4. Austin DW, Leventen EO: A new osteotomy for hallux valgus: A horizontally directed "V" displacement osteotomy of the metatarsal head for hallux valgus and primus varus. Clin Orthop 157:25, 1981.
5. Ball J, Sullivan J: Treatment of the juvenile bunion by Mitchell osteotomy. Orthopaedics 8:1249, 1985.
6. Berntsen A: De l'hallux valgus, conribution à son etiologie et à son traitement. Rev D'Orthop 17:101, 1930.
7. Blais M, Green W, Anderson M: Lengths of the growing foot. J Bone Joint Surg 38A:998, 1956.
8. Bonney G, MacNab I: Hallux valgus and hallux rigidus. A critical survey of operative results. J Bone Joint Surg 34B:366, 1952.
9. Carr C, Boyd B: Correctional osteotomy for metatarsus primus varus and hallux valgus. J Bone Joint Surg 50A:1353, 1968.
10. Cholmeley J: Hallux valgus in adolescents. Proc R Soc Med 5:903, 1958.
11. Corless JR: A modification of the Mitchell procedure. J Bone Joint Surg 58B:138, 1976.
12. Coughlin MJ, Mann RA: The pathophysiology of the juvenile bunion. Instr Course Lect 36:123, 1987.
13. Das De S: Distal metatarsal osteotomy for adolescent hallux valgus. J Pediatr Orthop 4:32, 1984.
14. Durman D: Metatarsus primus varus and hallux valgus. Arch Surg 74:128, 1957.
15. DuVries H: Static deformities. *In* DuVries HL (Ed): Surgery of the Foot, 1st Ed. St. Louis, CV Mosby, 1959.
16. DuVries H: Static deformities of the forefoot. *In* DuVries HL (Ed): Surgery of the Foot, 2nd Ed. St. Louis, CV Mosby, 1965.
17. Ellis V: A method of correcting metatarsus primus varus. J Bone Joint Surg 33B:415, 1951.
18. Ewald P: Die Aetiologie Des Hallux Valgus. Dtsch Z Chir 114:90, 1912.
19. Fox I, Smith S: Juvenile bunion correction by epiphysiodesis of the first metatarsal. J Am Podiatry Assoc 73:448, 1983.
20. Funk FJ, Wells RE: Bunionectomy with distal osteotomy. Clin Orthop 85:71, 1972.
21. Giannestras NJ: The Giannestras modification of the Lapidus operation. *In* Giannestras NJ (Ed): Foot Disorders, Medical and Surgical Management. Philadelphia, Lea & Febiger, 1973.
22. Goldner J, Gaines R: Adult and juvenile hallux valgus: Analysis and treatment. Orthop Clin North Am 7:863, 1976.
23. Haines R, McDougall A: The anatomy of hallux valgus. J Bone Joint Surg 36B:272, 1954.
24. Halebain J, Gaines S: Juvenile hallux valgus. J Foot Surg 22:290, 1983.
25. Hardy R, Clapham J: Observations on hallux valgus. J Bone Joint Surg 33B:376, 1951.
26. Hawkins FB, Mitchell CL, Hedrick DW: Correction of hallux valgus by metatarsal osteotomy. J Bone Joint Surg 27:387, 1945.
27. Helal B: Surgery for adolescent hallux valgus. Clin Orthop 157:50, 1981.
28. Helal B, Gupta S, Gojaseni P: Surgery for adolescent hallux valgus. Acta Orthop Scand 45:271, 1974.
29. Houghton G, Dickson R: Hallux valgus in the younger patient. The structural abnormality. J Bone Joint Surg 61B:176, 1979.
30. Inman V: Hallux valgus: A review of etiologic factors. Orthop Clin North Am 5:59, 1974.
31. Johnson KA, Cofield RH, Morrey BF: Chevron osteotomy for hallux valgus. Clin Orthop 142:44, 1979.
32. Jones A: Hallux valgus in the adolescent. Proc R Soc Med 41:392, 1948.
33. Kelikian H: Hallux Valgus and Allied Deformities of the Forefoot and Metatarsalgia. Philadelphia, WB Saunders, 1965.
34. Kwong P, Aubuchon C: Relief of second metatarsalgia by first metatarsal-cuneiform joint fusion. Presented at the 17th Annual Meeting of the American Orthopaedic Foot and Ankle Society, San Francisco, California, January 21, 1987.
35. Lapidus P: Operative correction of the metatarsus varus primus in hallux valgus. Surg Gynecol Obstet 58:183, 1934.
36. Lapidus P: The author's bunion operation from 1931 to 1959. Clin Orthop 16:119, 1960.
37. Luba R, Rosman M: Bunions in children: Treatment with a modified Mitchell osteotomy. J Pediatr Orthop 4:44, 1984.
38. Mann RA: Avascular necrosis of the metatarsal head following a chevron osteotomy. Foot Ankle 3:125, 1982.
39. Mann RA: Hallux valgus. Instr Course Lect 35:339, 1986.
40. Mann RA, Coughlin MJ: Hallux valgus—etiology, anatomy, treatment, and surgical consideration. Clin Orthop 157:31, 1981.
41. Mann RA, Coughlin MJ: Hallux valgus and complications of hallus valgus. *In* Mann RA (ed): Surgery of the Foot, 5th Ed. St. Louis, CV Mosby, 1986.
42. Mauldin DM, Sanders M, Whitmer W: Correction of hallux valgus with limited metatarsocuneiform arthrodesis. Presented at the 18th Annual Meeting of the American Orthopaedic Foot and Ankle Society, Atlanta, Georgia, February 7, 1988.
43. McBride ED: A conservative operation for bunions. J Bone Joint Surg 10:735, 1928.
44. McBride ED: The conservative operation for "bunions" and results and refinement of technic. JAMA 105:1164, 1935.
45. McHale KA, McKay DW: Bunions in a child: Conservative versus surgical management. J Musculoskel Med 3:56, 1986.
46. Meehan P: Adolescent bunion. Instr Course Lect 31:262, 1982.
47. Meier PJ, Kenzora JE: The risks and benefits of distal first metatarsal osteotomies. Foot Ankle 6:7, 1985.
48. Meyer JM, Hoffmeyer P, Borst F: The treatment of hallux valgus in runners using a modified McBride procedure. Int Orthop 11:197, 1987.
49. Mitchell C, Fleming J, Allen R, et al: Osteotomy-bunionectomy for hallux valgus. J Bone Joint Surg 40A:41, 1958.
50. Peabody DW: Surgical care of hallux valgus. J Bone Joint Surg 13:273, 1931.
51. Piggott H: The natural history of hallux valgus in adolescence and early adult life. J Bone Joint Surg 42B:749, 1960.
52. Price G: Metatarsus primus varus: Including various clinicoradiologic features of the female foot. Clin Orthop 145:217, 1979.

53. Reverdin J: De la deviation en dehors du gros orteil et de son traitement chirurgical. Trans Int Med Cong 2:408, 1881.
54. Sarrafian SK: Anatomy of the Foot and Ankle. Philadelphia, JB Lippincott, 1983.
55. Scranton P: Adolescent bunions: Diagnosis and management. Pediatr Ann 11:518, 1982.
56. Scranton P, Zuckerman J: Bunion surgery in adolescents: Results of surgical treatment. J Pediatr Orthop 4:39, 1984.
57. Seelenfreund M, Fried A: Correction of hallux valgus deformity by basal phalanx osteotomy of the big toe. J Bone Joint Surg 55A:1411, 1973.
58. Silberman FS: Proximal phalangeal osteotomy for the correction of hallux valgus. Clin Orthop 85:98, 1972.
59. Simmonds F, Menelaus M: Hallux valgus in adolescents. J Bone Joint Surg 42B:761, 1960.
60. Simon WV: Der Hallux Valgus und seine chirurgische Behandlung mit besdonderer Berucksichtigung der Ludlof'schen Operation. Beitr Klin Chir 3:467, 1918.
61. Trott A: Hallux valgus in adolescents. Instruct Course Lect 21:262, 1972.
62. Truslow W: Metatarsus primus varus or hallux valgus? J Bone Joint Surg 7:98, 1925.
63. Wilson D: Treatment of hallux valgus and bunions. Br J Hosp Med 24:548, 1963.
64. Young JD: A new operation for adolescent hallux valgus. Univ Penn Med Bull 23:459, 1910.
65. Zimmer TJ, Johnson KA, Klassen RA: Treatment of hallux valgus in adolescents by the chevron osteotomy. Foot Ankle 9:190, 1989.

37

Congenital Hallux Varus

JOHN G. THOMETZ

Hallux varus may lead to disability by making it difficult to wear shoes and causing significant discomfort. The patient may also feel the appearance is unacceptable. Careful preoperative planning is required, as there tends to be a significant tendency for varus to recur postoperatively.

Hallux varus has been divided into a number of subcategories.* The primary type is described as an isolated deformity with no other associated congenital anomalies. In this case, a taut fibrous band extends from the medial aspect of the hallux to the base of the first metatarsal. This has been hypothesized to be the result of arrested development in utero of a medial accessory hallux, which later becomes a fibrous or cartilaginous band that progressively pulls the hallux into varus. The second type of hallux varus is associated with a block metatarsal (a short, broad first metatarsal, generally with medial angulation at the metatarsophalangeal joint). A rare third type of hallux varus has been associated with the delta phalanx. A fourth type of hallux varus is associated with accessory bones in variations of preaxial polydactyly. The last type of hallux varus is associated with extensive skeletal developmental abnormalities such as diastrophic dwarfism.

Soft tissue abnormalities are usually present. In Falliner's experience with eight patients who had congenital hallux varus and polydactyly of the hallux,[4] muscle and tendon anomalies were found in all patients. In four patients, signifi-

cant fibrous bands extended from the rudimentary hallux to the tarsus. In five patients, the abductor hallucis muscle was found to be quite contracted. Therefore, in addition to removal of the supernumerary digit, these contracted muscles must be lengthened or the fibrous bands divided.

Neil and Conacher stated that isolated hallux varus due to a delta phalanx of the hallux is extremely rare.[14] There have been only a few case reports of it in the literature. They disagreed with the conclusion of Watson and Boyes, who stated in their review of congenital anomalies of the hand and feet that the delta phalanx was "routinely a manifestation of polydactylism," although they noted that there was appreciable variation in the degree of the triangular shape of the delta phalanx.[18] Jaeger and Refior observed that these triangular deformities are located not only in the phalanges but also in the metatarsals.[7]

Many of the cases of hallux varus reported in the literature have been associated with preaxial polydactyly of the foot. In two large series of polydactyly of the foot, cases of preaxial polydactyly constituted about 15 percent of the series.[11, 15] Polydactyly of the foot can occur with various genetic syndromes or chromosomal abnormalities.[17] The anomaly most commonly associated with polydactyly of the foot is polydactyly of the hand. Polydactyly has been reported to have a higher incidence in blacks and in Asians.[11, 15] Preaxial polydactyly may occur with a normal metatarsal with distal duplication, proximal duplication, or (most commonly) a block metatarsal[15] (Figs. 37–1 and 37–2).

*See references 1, 2, 5, 9, 11, 15, and 16.

664

FIGURE 37–1. Duplication of both the proximal and distal phalanx with hallux varus.

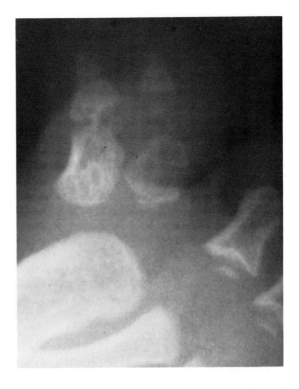

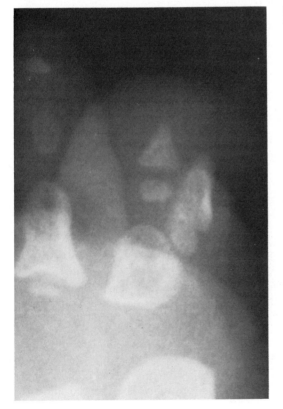

FIGURE 37–2. Duplication of the distal phalanx with hallux varus.

PREOPERATIVE ASSESSMENT

Careful clinical assessment should be made of the size, appearance, and function of both toes when duplication of the hallux is present. The most medial digit is not always the one that should be excised; the less functional and cosmetically unacceptable toe is the one that should be removed. Jahss and Nelson,[8] in a review of patients with an average 21-year follow-up, found that the best results occurred when the lateral hallux was excised. Although it may be difficult, the tendon function to each toe should be evaluated, and reconstruction is performed as needed to avoid leaving the child with a flail toe.

Radiographic assessment is essential to determine the hallux with the smaller, less developed bone, which should be removed (Figs. 37–3 to 37–5).

OPERATIVE TECHNIQUE

Surgery should be done before the child begins walking. Phelps and Grogan[15] believed

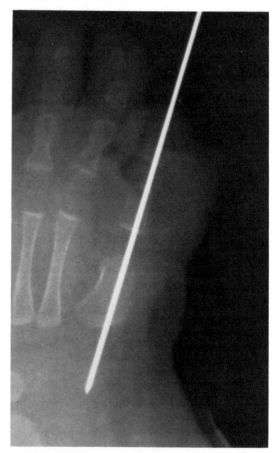

FIGURE 37–4. Excision of the medial hallux with pin stabilization of the lateral hallux.

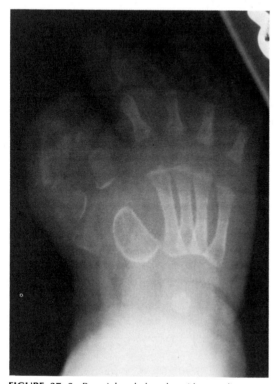

FIGURE 37–3. Preaxial polydactyly with a rudimentary medial hallux.

that surgery should be delayed until the child is about 1 year of age to provide better visualization of the anatomic structures about the foot. The use of magnification may allow surgery to be performed earlier.

If the medial hallux or ray is to be excised, Jahss[8] stresses that the incision on the medial aspect of the toe should be as dorsal as possible to avoid problems with scar contracture. He found that excessive scar formation resulted when a straight medial incision was used. Medially contracted skin may require Z-plasty or X-plasty. In Jahss' series, severe medial scar formation over the years led to hallux varus interphalangeus, requiring rather complex attempts at reconstruction. Care should be taken to protect the medial plantar sensory branch.

The abductor and the adductor hallucis tendon insertions must be identified. It is helpful to delineate the accessory sesamoids as an aid to finding the tendons. The divided adductor

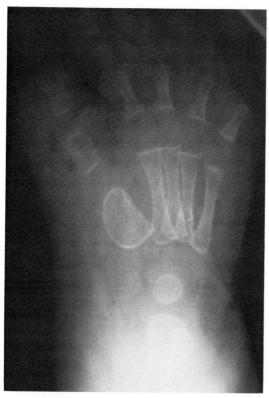

FIGURE 37–5. Postoperative radiograph.

series the results were poor.[13] Another option to be considered is a reverse Akin procedure of the proximal phalanx.[6]

In cases associated with polydactyly, the conjoined nail bed should be divided down its middle cleavage plane. The use of the Bilhaut-Cloquet procedure to treat Wassel class IV duplications of the hallux is poorly documented in the literature and is therefore not recommended. In patients with a duplicated proximal phalanx, the metatarsal head may become excessively prominent after excision of the medial proximal phalanx. Excision of this medial prominence of the metatarsal head will provide a better contour for the foot.

SPECIFIC PROCEDURES

Farmer's Technique

In mild cases of hallux varus, Farmer's technique[5] may be used (Fig. 37–6). Here, a skin flap is transported to the medial aspect of the base of the toe to allow lengthening of the contracted soft tissue on the medial aspect of the foot. The flap may be either plantar based or dorsally based. The flap is obtained from both the lateral aspect of the hallux and the medial aspect of the second toe; it extends roughly across the proximal third of the toes. The flap is then carried proximally. The proximal end of the medial incision is carried medially around the base of the metatarsophalangeal joint. The medial aspect of the metatarsophalangeal joint is then incised to allow the toe to move in a more lateral position. When the flap is transposed medially, tension may develop on the lateral aspect of the flap. To avoid this, a small triangular area is left open and then is filled with a full-thickness skin graft. Syndactylization is performed between the first and second toes at their bases in order to prevent any recurrent tendency toward hallux varus. To prevent the web space from becoming too narrow, a Z-plasty must allow the base of the syndactyly to be a bit wider. A cast is then applied for 3 weeks.

McElvenny's Technique

McElvenny's technique[12] involves release of the medial aspect of the metatarsophalangeal joint of the hallux combined with removal of the accessory digit. The alignment of the hallux

or abductor tendon should be reattached after resection of the appropriate hallux. In severe cases, in addition to lengthening of the abductor, release of the tibial head of the flexor hallucis brevis may be necessary. Transection of the lateral capsule should also be avoided unless absolutely necessary because this may result in an unstable metatarsophalangeal joint. Phelps and Grogan routinely use pin fixation of the metatarsophalangeal joint postoperatively.[15] They also recommend a meticulous capsular repair and reinsertion of this lengthened abductor tendon. In cases in which the accessory lateral first ray is excised, a significant dead space may remain. Therefore, Jahss recommends tightening the intermetatarsal ligament between the first and second metatarsals along with removing the redundant dorsal web space skin.

Additional osseous procedures have been employed occasionally to improve the alignment of the hallux. Metatarsal osteotomies have been employed to correct medial angulation of the metatarsophalangeal joint and thereby straighten the toe. However, in one

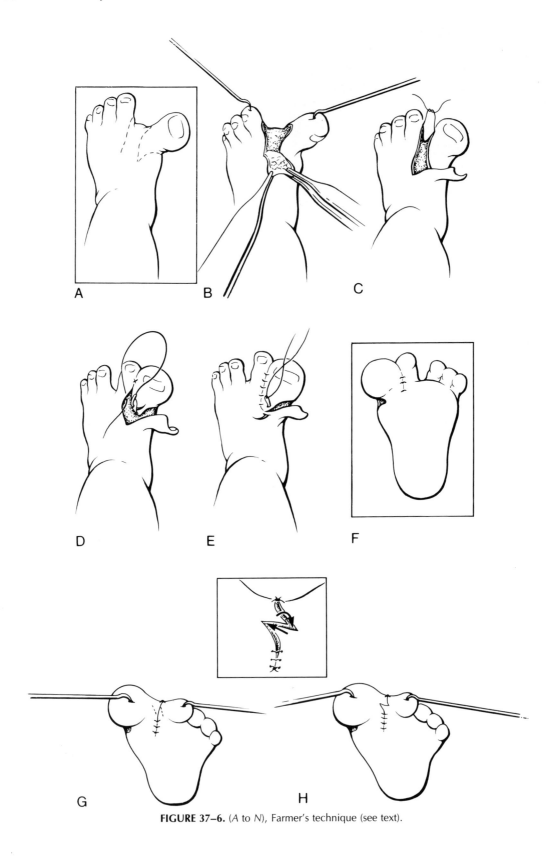

FIGURE 37–6. (*A* to *N*), Farmer's technique (see text).

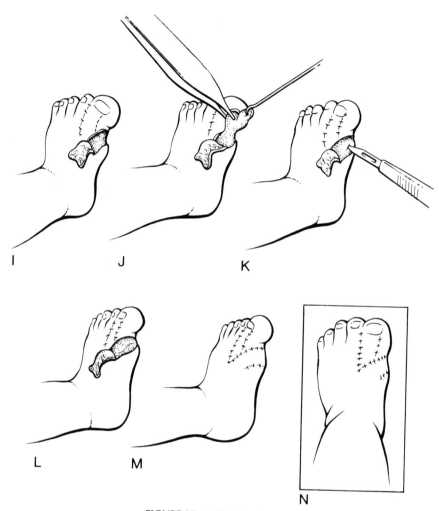

FIGURE 37–6 *(Continued)*

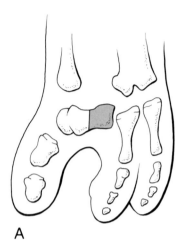 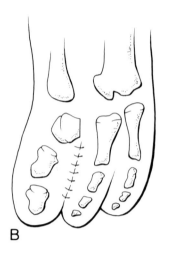

A   B

FIGURE 37–7. (A and B), Kelikian's technique (see text).

is maintained by transferring the extensor hallucis brevis tendon in combination with a distally based lateral capsular flap. Syndactylization is performed between the first and second toes, and a Kirschner wire is used to maintain stability.

Kelikian's Technique

The technique of Kelikian[10] may be useful in more complex anomalies (Fig. 37–7). Kelikian described a case in which the first metatarsal lay at a right angle to the lateral metatarsals, with the axis of the first metatarsal pointing medially. In this patient, the metatarsal shaft and base were resected, and syndactylization was performed between the first and second rays, with a satisfactory result.

Carstam's Technique for Delta Phalanx

An opening wedge osteotomy to correct delta phalanx (Figs. 37–8 and 37–9) can cause the skin to be so contracted that skin grafting may be required following surgical correction with the bone graft. Because of this, Carstam uses a reverse wedge osteotomy to correct the deformity.[1] Through a dorsal incision, a laterally based wedge is first removed and is then inserted into the medial aspect of the osteotomy in the phalanx. This causes less lengthening of the hallux medially and permits easier skin closure. A Kirschner wire is inserted through the distal phalanx, across the proximal phalanx, and into the metatarsal for stabiliza-

tion. I have used this technique in two cases. The short-term result has been satisfactory.

Procedures for Apert's Syndrome

Patients with Apert's syndrome (craniosynostosis with complex syndactyly of the hands and feet) present more complex problems (Fig. 37–10). In patients with mild or moderate

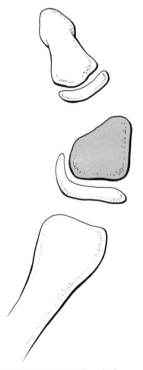

FIGURE 37–8. Delta phalanx.

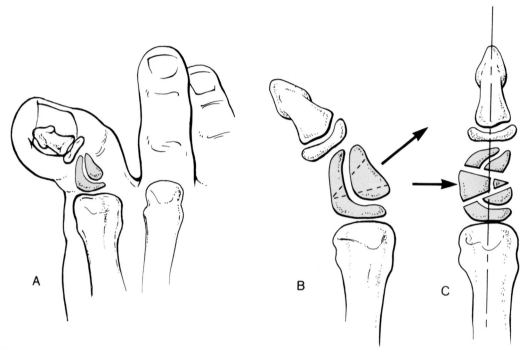

FIGURE 37–9. (*A* to *C*), Carstam's technique to correct delta phalanx (see text). This technique for the hand works equally well for the foot.

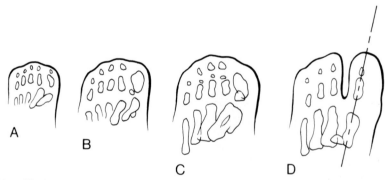

FIGURE 37–10. (*A* to *D*), Apert's syndrome (reconstructive procedures as described by Dell and Sheppard). Deletion of the second ray.

angulation of the proximal phalanx, Dell and Sheppard recommend an osteotomy of the proximal phalanx and narrowing of the foot by resection of the second ray.[3] For a markedly shortened and angulated hallux with appreciable skeletal abnormalities, Dell and Sheppard excise the hallux and perform hallucization of the second toe with the creation of a commissure between the second and third toes.

SALVAGE TECHNIQUES

Metatarsophalangeal arthrodesis[13] is indicated when hallux varus is accompanied by significant pain and arthritis. Amputation is useful when other methods have failed and there is still an appreciable problem with the ability to wear shoes.[13] Lengthening of the shortened first metatarsal may cause an asymptomatic foot to become symptomatic. Therefore, its use for this problem is controversial.

COMPLICATIONS

Complications include recurrence of varus, excessive scar formation, skin necrosis (when

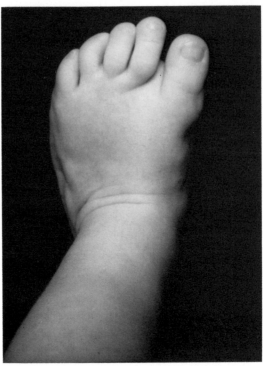

FIGURE 37–12. Clinical appearance of the foot in Figure 37–11 following Z-plasty of the previous incision, release of the medial metatarsophalangeal joint, removal of the triangular wedge of bone from the lateral aspect of the first metatarsal, and placement of the wedge medially.

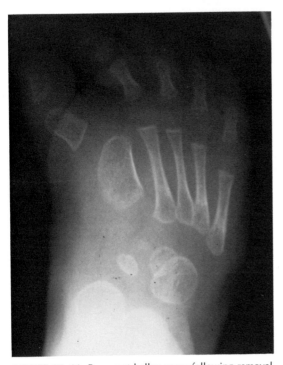

FIGURE 37–11. Recurrent hallux varus following removal of the medial hallux.

flaps have been used), metatarsalgia, and flail toe.

Recurrent varus occurred in 50 percent of Venn-Watson's cases[17] (Figs. 37–11 and 37–12). He recommended pin stabilization, capsular repair, and appropriate tendon balancing to reduce the incidence of recurrence. Placing the incision dorsomedially should help diminish the frequency of extensive scar formation, which may cause the toe to deviate medially. Jahss advises against the use of Z-plasty for undermining skin to create flaps, as this could result in skin sloughs with secondary contractures.[8] Care should be taken to avoid tension on the flaps to prevent skin necrosis.

Metatarsalgia may occur without surgery. It also occurs following surgery, with transfer lesions developing beneath the second and third metatarsal heads, especially in patients with a short first metatarsal. Phelps and Grogan reported on one patient with significant anterior metatarsalgia.[15] Metatarsalgia is usually mild and is often controlled with orthotics. If conservative treatment is unsuccessful, osteotomy of the base of the painful metatarsals plus Kirschner wire fixation usually relieves symptoms.

References

1. Carstam N, Theander G: Surgical treatment of clinodactyly caused by longitudinal bracketed diaphysis (delta phalanx). Scand J Plast Reconstr Surg 9:199, 1975.
2. Christian JC, Cho KS, Franklin EA, Thompson BH: Dominant preaxial brachydactyly with hallux varus and thumb abduction. Am J Hum Genet 24:694, 1972.
3. Dell PC, Sheppard JE: Deformities of the great foot in Apert's syndrome. Clin Orthop 157:113, 1981.
4. Falliner Z: Orthopedics 126(3):239, 1988.
5. Farmer AW: Congenital hallux varus. Am J Surg 95:274, 1958.
6. Gould J, Medical College of Wisconsin, personal communication.
7. Jaeger M, Refior HJ: The congenital triangular deformity of the tubular bones of hand and foot. Clin Orthop 81:139, 1971.
8. Jahss MH, Nelson J: Duplication of the hallux. Foot Ankle 5:26, 1984.
9. Joseph B, Chacko V, Abraham T, Jacob M: Pathomechanics of congenital and acquired hallux varus: A clinical and anatomical study. Foot Ankle 8:137, 1987.
10. Kelikian H, Clayton L, Loseff H: Surgical syndactylia of the toes. Clin Orthop 19:208, 1961.
11. Masada K, Tsuyuguchi Y, Kawabata H, Ono K: Treatment of preaxial polydactyly of the foot. Plast Reconstr Surg 79:251, 1987.
12. McElvenny RT: Hallux varus. Q Bull Northwest Med School 15:277, 1941.
13. Mills JA, Menelaus MB: Hallux varus. J Bone Joint Surg 71B:437, 1989.
14. Neil MJ, Conacher C: Bilateral delta phalanx of the proximal phalanges of the great toes; A report on an affected family. J Bone Joint Surg 66B:77, 1984.
15. Phelps DA, Grogan D: Polydactyly of the foot. J Pediatr Orthop 5:446, 1985.
16. Thomson SA: Hallux varus and metatarsus varus; A five-year study (1954–1958). Clin Orthop 16:109, 1960.
17. Venn-Watson EA: Problems in polydactyly of the foot. Orthop Clin North Am 7:909, 1976.
18. Watson HK, Boyes JH: Congenital angular deformity of the digits. J Bone Joint Surg 49A:333, 1967.

38 Metatarsus Adductus

SEYMOUR ZIMBLER
CLIFFORD L. CRAIG
BENJAMIN A. ALMAN

Metatarsus adductus is a congenital deformity of the foot in which there is increased adduction of the forefoot. The major component of the deformity is medial deviation of the metatarsals at the tarsometatarsal joint. Varying degrees of forefoot inversion and supination can be associated with the adduction. The diagnosis of this disorder is relatively straightforward and usually can be made on physical examination. Radiographs can help to distinguish this disorder from other, more complex, foot deformities. Most patients can be treated nonoperatively with abduction exercises in the flexible deformity and serial casting in the less flexible deformities. Operative therapy is reserved for the deformed foot that is resistant to nonoperative treatment or that has been neglected.

The incidence of the deformity is about three per 1000 children.[18] Other anomalies can be associated with metatarsus adductus. Up to a 10 percent incidence of congenital dysplasia of the hip is found in children with the deformity.[8] Adduction of the forefoot can be associated with other foot abnormalities. One such deformity is skewfoot, in which there is rigid hindfoot valgus (fixed eversion) in addition to the forefoot deformity. It is important to distinguish a skewfoot from metatarsus adductus because the skewfoot usually requires additional treatment. Occasionally, a patient who was treated for a clubfoot deformity will present with a residual adducted forefoot. These feet often have hindfoot deformity and require more than treatment for the metatarsus adductus alone.

ASSESSMENT

The patient with metatarsus adductus presents with some degree of adducted forefoot at birth. The deformity may progress in severity over the first 6 weeks of life as muscular activity increases. Physical examination will reveal a concave medial border of the foot, with a convex lateral border and a prominent fifth metatarsal base. There is often wide separation of the first and second toes (Fig. 38–1).[19] The child who is not yet ambulatory may have some degree of hindfoot valgus. The older child with rigid hindfoot valgus is more likely to have a skewfoot deformity.[12] The evaluation of a child with metatarsus adductus must include a complete physical examination to look for associated abnormalities such as congenital dysplasia of the hip.

The severity of the deformity can be classified using a longitudinal line that bisects the heel. In the normal foot, the line crosses between the second and third toes. If the bisector line crosses the third toe, there is a mild deformity; if it crosses between the third and fourth toes or through the fourth toe, there is a moderate deformity; and if it crosses lateral to the fourth toe, there is a severe deformity. Flexibility of the foot can be classified by the degree of passive abduction of the forefoot against a fixed hindfoot. If the foot can be abducted beyond the heel bisector, the deformity is mild; if the foot can be abducted to the neutral position, the deformity is classified as moderate; and if the foot cannot

674

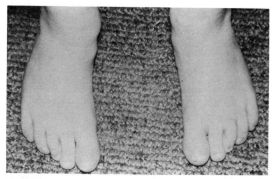

FIGURE 38–1. A 5-year-old with metatarsus adductus. (The condition is more severe in the right foot than in the left.) Dynamically, there is a significant spread of the great toe from the second toe, indicating increased activity of the abductor hallucis.

be abducted to the neutral position, the deformity is considered severe.[5]

Radiographs can help distinguish between metatarsus adductus and skewfoot. On a standing anteroposterior radiograph of a normal foot, a longitudinal line through the talus bisects the base of the first metatarsal. There is a neutral or valgus angle between the shaft of the first metatarsal and the axis of the talus. The foot with metatarsus adductus will have a varus angle between the shaft of the first metatarsal and the axis of the talus. In skewfoot, there is also a valgus hindfoot with a talocalcaneal angle that is greater than 35 degrees on a standing anteroposterior radiograph. Both types of deformity can occur with a lateral shift of the midportion of the foot. The axis of the calcaneus crosses the base of the fourth metatarsal in the normal foot. In the foot with lateral shift of the midportion, this axis crosses medial to the base of the fourth metatarsal (Figs. 38–2 and 38–3).[2]

ETIOLOGY

Several etiologies have been proposed for metatarsus adductus. Intrauterine positioning or molding has been suggested as the cause of the deformity. Several studies have shown abnormal muscle insertions. An abnormal insertion of the anterior tibial tendon has been suggested by some investigators. Anatomic and intraoperative observations suggest a more distal insertion, onto only the first metatarsal, which is wider than normal and winds onto the

plantar surface of the foot.[17] An abnormal insertion of the abductor hallucis tendon has been suggested as a possible contributor to the deformity. Anatomic descriptions by Thompson show an insertion of the abductor hallucis onto only the medial aspect of the proximal phalanx instead of the normal insertion onto the medial sesamoid and the capsule of the metatarsophalangeal joint.[16]

NONOPERATIVE TREATMENT

Most children with metatarsus adductus can be treated nonoperatively. The major decision to be made with these children is whether or not casting is required. Bleck showed, in a series of patients treated without surgery, that results were related directly to a patient's age at the onset of treatment, rather than to the type of treatment.[5] Children who were under 8 months of age with feet that had mild deformity and were flexible did well regardless of the treatment regimen. Bleck suggested that the mild deformities in these young children could be treated without serial casting.[5] In a series of 142 patients (218 feet) who were treated with passive forefoot abduction exercises in feet that could be corrected to neutral (moderate flexibility deformity) and 57 patients who were treated with corrective serial casting for feet that could not be corrected to neutral, there were excellent results in all patients.[19]

The patient with mild deformity can be

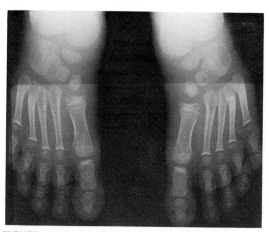

FIGURE 38–2. Standing anteroposterior radiograph of metatarsus adductus. (The left foot has more severe involvement.)

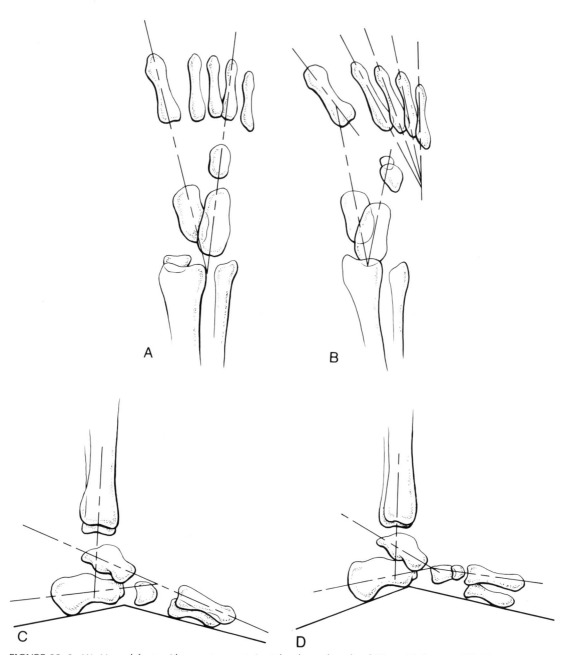

FIGURE 38–3. *(A)*, Normal foot, with an anteroposterior talocalcaneal angle of 20 to 40 degrees. *(B)*, Metatarsus varus (adductus), with adduction of all metatarsals. *(C)*, Normal foot, with a lateral talocalcaneal angle of 30 to 50 degrees. *(D)*, Metatarsus varus (adductus), with increased hindfoot valgus and an increased lateral talocalcaneal angle.

treated with passive abduction exercises at each diaper change. When shoe wear is begun, a straight last or reverse last shoe is advised until a neutral foot position is obtained. For the moderate or severe deformity, serial casting at weekly intervals is used. The casts are applied after manipulation of the forefoot into maximal abduction, with careful molding over the first metatarsal head and the base of the fifth metatarsal. Long-leg plaster casts with the knee in 60 to 90 degrees of flexion, anteroposterior thigh molds, and adhesive material on the skin are used to prevent slippage. Once the forefoot can abduct to neutral, below-knee casts can be used. When the foot can remain at neutral or abduction without support, night splints, shoes, or corrective bivalved night casts can be continued for an additional 4 to 6 months.[19]

OPERATIVE TREATMENT

Operative treatment for metatarsus adductus is reserved for deformities that have been neglected or that have not responded to nonoperative therapy. Additionally, some of the procedures can be used to treat a residual metatarsus adductus within the clubfoot deformity. There are three basic types of procedures: tendon releases or transfers, mobilization of the tarsometatarsal joints, and osteotomies. Each type of procedure has its own specific indications. Tendon releases are used in young patients who have tightness or contractures of a specific tendon, or overactivity despite nonoperative therapy. Mobilization of the tarsometatarsal joints can be used in patients whose bones still have the capacity to remodel. Osteotomies are reserved for older children who have resistant deformities or for patients who have foot deformity associated with other congenital musculoskeletal disorders.

Abductor Hallucis Tendon Release

Abductor hallucis release is indicated in patients who have a palpably tight abductor despite nonoperative therapy. The release is also effective in patients with cerebral palsy who have a spastic abductor. Intraoperative observations by Thompson suggest that there is an anomalous insertion of the abductor hallucis

onto only the medial aspect of the proximal phalanx in metatarsus adductus.[16] In a series of properly selected patients between the ages of 1 and 4 years, this procedure had a success rate of 80 to 90 percent. Hallux valgus is reported as a complication in 12 percent of cases.[10, 11, 16] A spastic abductor hallucis can lead to metatarsus adductus in patients with cerebral palsy. In a small series of patients, the release of the abductor led to correction of the deformity.[4]

Technique.[10, 11] Release of the distal insertion of the abductor can be carried out using a small longitudinal incision over the distal first metatarsal. The abductor tendon is dissected free of the capsule of the metatarsophalangeal joint and is then sharply divided or Z-lengthened. An alternative method is to release the muscle from its origin. A medial curved incision over the proximal abductor is used. The neurovascular bundle is identified. The muscle is released from its calcaneal attachment. The neurovascular bundle is protected as release is continued over the flexor retinaculum, plantar aponeurosis, and spring ligaments. The foot is held in a corrective cast for 6 weeks to allow fibrosis of the capsule and to maintain the muscles in a new position. A fractional lengthening of the abductor hallucis can be carried out more distally in the tendon and is probably a good alternative procedure.

Anterior Tibial Tendon Transfer

The anterior tibial tendon has also been suggested as a causative factor in some patients with metatarsus adductus. Intraoperative observation suggests that the tendon inserts more distally than usual and winds toward the plantar side of the foot.[17] Patients with resistant metatarsus adductus after clubfoot treatment occasionally have a tight anterior tibial tendon. These feet can be corrected by an anterior tibial tendon procedure as long as there is potential for the child's foot to remodel. This exists until age 7.[1] Transfer of the anterior tibial tendon laterally can lead to a pes valgus deformity.[7, 13] A split anterior tibial tendon transfer, rather than complete transfer, has been recommended to correct the metatarsus varus without producing the complication of pes valgus.

Technique (Fig. 38–4).[7] Two incisions are made to mobilize and divide the anterior tibial

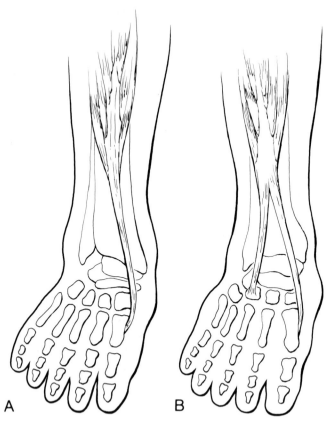

FIGURE 38–4. Split anterior tibial tendon transfer. *(A),* Normal insertion of the anterior tibial tendon. *(B),* Split anterior tibial tendon with insertion of the lateral half into the third cuneiform.

A

B

tendon. Distally, a small, longitudinally oriented incision is made over the insertion of the tendon onto the first cuneiform. Proximally, a second longitudinal incision 3 to 4 cm in length is made over the lateral aspect of the tendon and tibia at the junction of the middle and distal thirds of the tibia. The lateral half of the tendon is removed from its insertion and divided longitudinally from the intact medial half through the distal incision. A tendon passer and whipstitch suture are then used to pass the lateral half of the tendon into the proximal wound through the tibialis anterior sheath. A third incision is made longitudinally over the dorsum of the third cuneiform. A tendon passer is guided subcutaneously, superficial to the transverse retinacular ligament, into the proximal incision. The lateral half of the tendon is passed through the subcutaneous tunnel. A Bunnell-type weave is used to place a stainless steel wire through the distal 2 cm of the tendon. A pull-out stainless steel wire is passed through the most proximal loop. A drill hole is made in the cuneiform, and a straight needle is used to pass the pull-out wire

through the drill hole and out the plantar surface of the foot. The pull-out wire is secured over a felt button under the plantar surface of the foot. The wounds are closed, and the foot is casted in a corrected position for 8 weeks.

We prefer a different type of tendon attachment to bone rather than the pull-out wire, which is cumbersome. Our standard attachment has been a trapdoor within bone as well as adjacent drill holes. The tendon end plus the whipstitch suture is pulled into the trapdoor. The suture ends are passed through the drill holes and tied over bone as a mattress suture. This has always been quite successful. However, several new metallic attachments now allow suture material to be buried securely within the bone. These techniques will eventually eliminate the pull-out wire as well as the trapdoor.

Tarsometatarsal Joint Mobilization

Tarsometatarsal joint mobilization, or capsulotomy, can be used in children between the ages of 3 and 8 who have metatarsus adductus that is the residual deformity of a clubfoot or primary metatarsus adductus that has not responded to nonoperative therapy. The procedure releases the resultant joint contractures but does not address the underlying cause of the deformity. The procedure produced an asymptomatic foot in 92 percent of patients in a series by Kendrick and colleagues.[9] A more recent series shows a higher incidence of a painful foot (50 percent at late follow-up) and poor results with the use of the procedure for feet in patients with associated deformities such as myelomeningocele and ring constriction syndrome.[14] Complications include degenerative arthritis of the tarsometatarsal joints, avascular necrosis of the cuneiforms, and dorsal prominence of the first metatarsal.

Technique (Fig. 38–5).[6, 9] A transverse incision is made from the base of the first metatarsal to the base of the fifth metatarsal over the dorsum of the foot. Skin flaps are developed proximally and distally. Care is taken during the procedure to preserve the extensor tendons and the neurovascular structures. The deep fascia over the first tarsometatarsal joint is incised in a longitudinal fashion. The dorsal, medial, and lateral interosseous ligaments of the first cuneiform–metatarsal joint are identified, and they are sharply divided using a U-shaped incision in the dorsal capsule. This capsulotomy follows the base of the first metatarsal. A mosquito hemostat is then placed in the interval between the first and second metatarsal bases, and the intermetatarsal ligament

is identified. This is sharply divided from distal to proximal. The dorsal capsule of the second cuneiform–metatarsal joint is similarly sharply divided, following the base of the metatarsal. The intermetatarsal ligament between the second and third metatarsals is identified and divided.

Similar releases of the dorsal and intermetatarsal ligaments are carried out on the remainder of the tarsometatarsal joints, but the lateral capsule of the fifth joint is preserved. After release of all the dorsal capsules, the toes are plantarflexed, and under direct vision, with care taken to preserve the articular surfaces, the plantar capsules of the joints are sharply divided. The foot is brought into a corrected position. There will be joint incongruity when the deformity is corrected. The foot is held in the corrected position for a total of 4 months to allow remodeling to correct the incongruity. During the first 3 weeks, the patient is non–weight bearing. One or two longitudinal smooth Steinmann pins can be used to maintain the forefoot in the corrected position rather than using the cast alone for corrective position.

Osteotomy Procedures

In children over the age of 8, the ability of bone to remodel sufficiently for correction by a soft tissue procedure is lost. The treatment for these patients involves osteotomies to correct the deformity. Several types of metatarsal

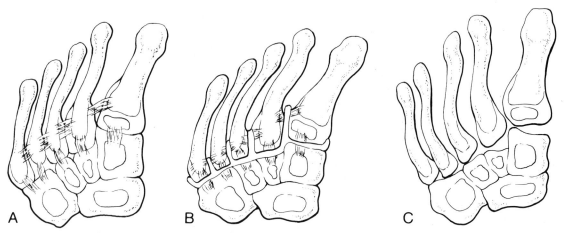

FIGURE 38–5. *(A),* Bone, cartilage, and ligament structures in metatarsus adductus. *(B),* Sites of tarsometatarsal capsulotomies. *(C),* The foot in the corrected position after completion of the capsulotomies.

osteotomies can be performed. The type of osteotomy chosen depends somewhat on the type of bony deformity. In long-standing deformity, the medial structures become shortened, and closing lateral wedge osteotomies will correct both the deformity and the unequal bone lengths. In the younger patient or the patient without significant loss of medial foot bone length, dome osteotomies can be performed. Proximal metatarsal osteotomies are indicated for older children (those at least 5 years of age) or adults with residual metatarsus adductus of any etiology.[3, 15] Multiple metatarsal osteotomies produced asymptomatic feet in 84 percent of patients in a series by Berman and Gartland.[3] Complications included a 10-percent nonunion rate (but all these patients were asymptomatic) and a loss of length of the medial aspect of the foot, either from growth plate damage or malpositioning of the corrected foot.[3]

Technique (Fig. 38–6).[3] Two longitudinal incisions are made over the dorsum of the foot, one between the first and second metatarsals, and the other over the fourth metatarsal. Skin flaps are developed so that the bases of the first and second metatarsals can be approached through the medial incision and the bases of the other metatarsal can be approached through the lateral incision. The bases of the metatarsals are identified. In the child with open epiphyses, these are identified and avoided. The attachment of vessels and capsule to the area of the epiphysis is usually obvious, but a Keith needle or a small drill

point can be used with radiographic or fluoroscopic control to definitively show the position of the first metatarsal and confirm that the proposed osteotomy site is away from this. Subperiosteal dissection is then carried out in the proximal metaphyseal regions of the metatarsals, with care taken to protect the growth plates if they are open. Osteotomies of all proximal metatarsals are performed. A dome osteotomy of the metaphyseal region is performed if there is no shortening of the bone structures of the medial foot. A closing lateral wedge osteotomy is performed if there is shortening of the medial structures. Preoperative radiographs should be used to plan the osteotomies. Smooth Steinmann pins are passed from proximal to distal along the shafts of the first and fifth metatarsals through the osteotomy sites and out the skin on the plantar aspect of the foot. The foot is brought into a corrected position, and the pins are advanced in a retrograde fashion to hold the correction. Intraoperative radiographs are obtained to verify correction. The foot is immobilized in a cast for 6 weeks, at which time the pins are removed. The foot is held in a cast until union is noted radiographically.

Authors' Preferred Approach

Our indications for surgical treatment are (1) any residual deformity resistant to nonoperative treatment, (2) the neglected foot, (3) an abnormal gait due to the deformity, (4) an

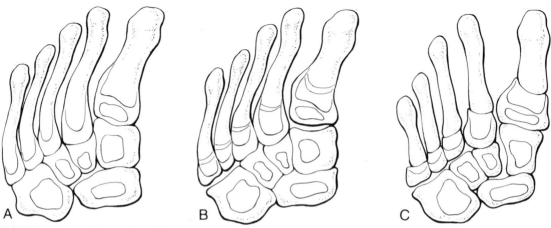

FIGURE 38–6. *(A),* Bone and cartilage structures in metatarsus adductus. *(B),* Sites of proximal metatarsal dome-shaped osteotomies. *(C),* The foot in the corrected position after completion of the osteotomies. An open-up cuneiform osteotomy could be substituted for the proximal first metatarsal osteotomy in a younger child. The domes may also be cut convex distally.

inability to fit into shoes, and (5) a skewfoot deformity. The foot that can be corrected by an isolated tendon procedure is unusual. Occasionally these procedures can be used in addition to a tarsometatarsal release or along with multiple osteotomies in patients with a deforming anterior tibial tendon or abductor hallucis. Multiple tarsometatarsal capsulotomies will correct a deformity in younger children. In older children, a combination of a capsulotomy and osteotomy of each metatarsal base may be required for correction. The capsulotomy alone appears to give the best results in children under the age of 5. Multiple osteotomies and capsulotomies will be needed in older children because the deformity becomes rigid and the bones lose the capability of remodeling. In the skewfoot, the hindfoot valgus must be addressed. This is corrected with an extra-articular subtalar arthrodesis, simultaneously or as a second stage after correction of the forefoot. An opening wedge osteotomy of the anterior calcaneus has been used in cases of severe planovalgus deformity. It is probably applicable to the skewfoot, although we have no experience with this procedure.

We prefer multiple longitudinal incisions to a single transverse incision. These incisions are placed between the first and second metatarsals and over the fourth metatarsal. The capsulotomies are carried out using the technique of Heyman and colleagues.[6] When the foot is brought into the corrected position, there is often a prominent lateral midfoot, which is usually related to the cuboid. A closing wedge cuboid osteotomy can be performed to correct it. When there is residual shortening of the medial aspect of the foot, an opening wedge osteotomy of the first cuneiform can be performed. Bone graft for the opening wedge osteotomy can be obtained from the bone removed from the cuboid, from the iliac crest, or from the proximal tibia. A deforming abductor hallucis or anterior tibial tendon can be addressed at this point. Often the peroneal tendons will be quite loose when the forefoot is corrected. Peroneal reefing can be performed to tighten the slack tendons. The closing wedge osteotomy in the cuboid is held with a staple or Steinmann pins. The corrected foot is held with two Steinmann pins, one placed through the calcaneus into the forefoot and the other placed transversely across the metatarsals from medial to lateral to hold the corrected medial forefoot (Figs. 38–7 and 38–8). The transverse metatarsal pin usually contacts the first and fifth metatarsals to preserve the transverse arch. Patients over the age of 5 are treated with multiple metatarsal osteotomies. An osteotomy of the first cuneiform is preferred over a proximal metatarsal osteotomy, especially in a child with an open growth plate, because the proximal metatarsal osteotomy results in a prominent base of the first metatarsal. The foot is held in a cast until the osteotomies heal. After the foot is removed from the cast, forefoot stretching exercises and peroneal strengthening exercises are begun.

FIGURE 38–7. *(A)*, Standing anteroposterior radiograph of a 5-year-old with metatarsus adductus. The patient underwent tarsometatarsal capsulotomies with closing wedge osteotomy of the cuboid. *(B)*, The foot 3 years after surgical correction. Mild residual adduction is present.

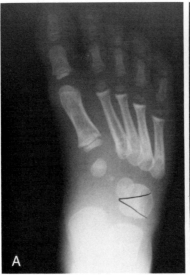
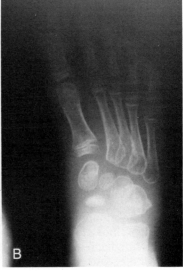

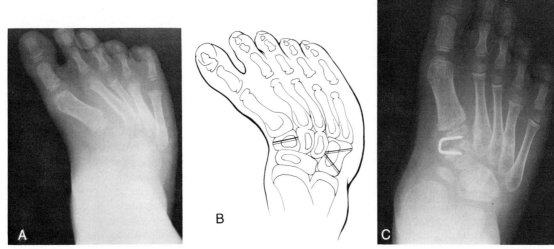

FIGURE 38–8. *(A)*, Severe metatarsus adductus associated with a valgus hindfoot (skewfoot). *(B)*, Sites of closing wedge cuboid osteotomy and opening wedge cuneiform osteotomy. *(C)*, Postoperative radiograph of a first-stage correction of the forefoot in a severe skewfoot deformity. An opening wedge osteotomy has been carried out through the first cuneiform, and a staple is holding it in place. The staple is in cartilage. Correction of the first metatarsal was incomplete. A closing wedge osteotomy of the cuboid was also carried out. The hindfoot will require a subtalar arthrodesis or another procedure at a later stage.

The foot is kept in a night brace or cast until strength returns and the foot remains in the corrected position without support.

Failure in the surgical treatment of metatarsus adductus is related to errors in patient selection. Rotational malalignment of the femur or tibia can give the appearance of an inverted foot. A superficial evaluation of the patient with rotational malalignment can lead to an erroneous diagnosis of metatarsus adductus with a gait abnormality. Surgical correction of the foot in this case will do little to help the patient. Failure to recognize a skewfoot deformity and to treat it appropriately will also lead to failure to correct the major foot deformity. Alternatively, the misdiagnosis of skewfoot will lead to surgical treatment for feet that might be corrected with serial casting.

SUMMARY

Metatarsus adductus can be treated either with abduction exercises or with serial casting in most patients. In the patient who does not respond to nonoperative treatment, surgical therapy is indicated. Soft tissue procedures, such as tarsometatarsal capsulotomies, can be done in the younger child, whose bones have

the capability to remodel. If a specific tendon is a deforming force, release or transfer of the tendon will help to correct the deformity. Closing wedge osteotomy of the cuboid and opening wedge osteotomy of the first cuneiform can be helpful adjuncts to the soft tissue procedures. In the child who is 5 to 8 years old or older, the correction must rely on multiple metatarsal osteotomies. Children with multiple congenital anomalies may have less satisfactory results from soft tissue procedures and may benefit from multiple osteotomies. Treatment of a skewfoot deformity includes management of the hindfoot valgus and should be differentiated from treatment of the simpler metatarsus adductus.

References

1. Beaty JH: Congenital metatarsus adductus. *In* Crenshaw AH (Ed): Campbell's Operative Orthopaedics, 7th Ed. St. Louis, CV Mosby, 1987.
2. Berg EE: A reappraisal of metatarsus adductus and skewfoot. J Bone Joint Surg 68A:1185, 1986.
3. Berman A, Gartland JJ: Metatarsal osteotomy for correction of adduction of the fore part of the foot in children. J Bone Joint Surg 53A:498, 1971.
4. Bleck EE: Spastic abductor hallucis. Dev Med Child Neurol 9:602, 1967.

5. Bleck EE: Metatarsus adductus: Classification and relationships to outcomes of treatment. J Pediatr Orthop 3:2, 1983.
6. Heyman CH, Herdon CH, Strong JM: Mobilization of tarsometatarsal and intermetatarsal joints for the correction of the fore part of the foot in congenital clubfoot or congenital metatarsus varus. J Bone Joint Surg 40A:299, 1958.
7. Huurman WW: Congenital foot deformities. *In* Mann RA (Ed): Surgery of the Foot. St. Louis, CV Mosby, 1986.
8. Jacobs JE: Metatarsus varus and hip dysplasia. Clin Orthop 16:19, 1960.
9. Kendrick RE, Sharma NK, Hassler WL, Herndon CH: Tarsometatarsal mobilization for resistant adduction of the fore part of the foot. J Bone Joint Surg 52A:61, 1970.
10. Lichblau S: Section of the abductor hallucis tendon for correction of metatarsus varus deformity. Clin Orthop 110:227, 1975.
11. Mitchell GP: Abductor hallucis release in congenital metatarsus varus. Int Orthop 3:299, 1980.
12. Peterson HA: Skewfoot (forefoot adduction with heel valgus). J Pediatr Orthop 6:24, 1986.
13. Specht EE: Major congenital deformities and anomalies of the foot. *In* Inmann VT (Ed): DuVries' Surgery of the Foot. St. Louis, CV Mosby, 1973.
14. Stark JG, Johanson JE, Winter RB: The Heyman-Herndon tarsometatarsal capsulotomy for metatarsus adductus: Results in 48 feet. J Pediatr Orthop 7:305, 1987.
15. Steytler JCS, Ven der Walt ID: Correction of resistant adduction of the forefoot in congenital club-foot and congenital metatarsus varus by metatarsal osteotomy. Br J Surg 53:558, 1966.
16. Thompson SA: Hallux varus and metatarsus varus. Clin Orthop 16:109, 1960.
17. Tonnis D: Skewfoot. Orthopade 15:174, 1986.
18. Wynne-Davis R: Family studies and the cause of congenital clubfoot—talipes equinovarus, talipes calcaneovalgus and metatarsus varus. J Bone Joint Surg 46B:445, 1954.
19. Zimbler S, Banks HH, Craig CL: Metatarsus adductus: A treatment plan and evaluation of long term results. *In* Gould JS (Ed): The Foot Book. Baltimore, Williams & Wilkins, 1988.

39
Clubfoot

GEORGE W. SIMONS

As used in this chapter, "clubfoot" excludes the neurovascular forms, including arthrogryposis, as well as the simple positional clubfoot that occurs from intrauterine molding during the last trimester of pregnancy.

There are two prerequisites for understanding the various surgical methods for the treatment of clubfoot: a clear knowledge of the pathoanatomy of the clubfoot and a thorough knowledge of the technique of obtaining and evaluating radiographs. Not only do properly taken radiographs yield information that cannot be perceived clinically (e.g., mild degrees of varus, flat-top talus, calcaneocuboid subluxation), intraoperatively they are essential to the precise realignment of the foot and, thus, the prevention of under- and overcorrection.

PATHOANATOMY

The pathoanatomy of clubfoot is considered from the standpoint of soft tissues, then bone. The discussion of bony changes addresses the structural alterations in the individual bones, which have been well described in the literature, and the changes in positional relationships among the various bones of the fully deformed foot. These changes are less well understood and have given rise to competing theoretical models. Finally, the movements of the joints that are required to reposition the foot into normal alignment and the surgical steps necessary to produce this correction are detailed.*

---

*For a thorough discussion of pathoanatomy, the reader is referred to reference 106.

Soft Tissue Changes

All of the soft tissue structures on the posterior and medial aspects of the foot and ankle are contracted: skin, fascia, neurovascular tissues, tendons, muscles, and ligaments. The severity of contracture depends upon both the degree of contracture present at birth and the success of previous conservative treatment. In addition, the plantar structures may also be contracted, especially if the child has gone without treatment for a prolonged period or if conservative treatment has been inadequate. The structures on the dorsal and lateral sides of the foot are generally stretched beyond their normal length.

It is now generally understood that the most severe contractures exist in the ligaments, and they represent the final barrier to correction.[50, 81, 99] Sequential release of skin, fascia, and tendons without the appropriate capsular and ligamentous release fails to produce radiographically verifiable correction of moderate and severe deformities. It is not until the necessary capsules and ligaments have been released that objective radiographic correction can be achieved.

Bony Deformity

Talus

The talus is the most severely deformed bone in the clubfoot.[50, 86] It is smaller than normal, with decreased height, width, and length. The neck is angulated downward and medially, with a smaller than normal circumference and length. The medial angulation of the talar neck is about 160 degrees as compared with the normal 115 to 135 degrees; i.e., it is 25 to 40 degrees more angulated medially (Fig. 39–1). The talar neck is also angled downward. The talar head is small, and it is directed almost medially and slightly plantarward. The inferior surface of the talus may be devoid of facet development or show some development of the posterior facet.[50, 86]

Whether these changes represent primary deformities, i.e., secondary to a germ plasm defect,[50] or are themselves secondary to external forces outside of the talus (but which act maximally on the talus) is controversial. Certainly, structural changes of the other bones are much less severe and are generally accepted as being secondary.

Calcaneus

The shape and size of the calcaneus are relatively normal. The sustentaculum is poorly developed, and there is no significant angulation of the distal calcaneus.[50, 86]

Navicular

The navicular is smaller than normal, is of relatively normal shape, and may have a well-

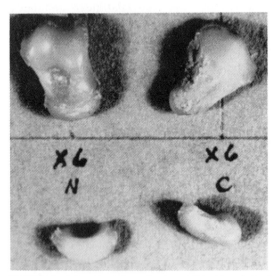

FIGURE 39–1. Late fetal dissection in a child with unilateral clubfoot: normal talus and navicular *(left)*, clubfoot talus and navicular *(right)*. The talar head and neck are much smaller than normal. The talar neck is inclined medially and inferiorly 20 to 45 degrees more than the normal side. (From Irani RN, Sherman MS: The pathological anatomy of idiopathic clubfoot. J Bone Joint Surg 45A:45, 1963.)

developed medial facet where it articulates with the tibia.

Cuboid

The cuboid is essentially normal in size and shape.

Articular (Positional) Relationships

Talus to Ankle Mortise

The talus is rotated forward around a coronal axis in the fully deformed club foot. This is accompanied by a few degrees of forward displacement of the lateral trochlea. In addition, it is generally believed that the talus is not abnormally rotated within the mortise, either around a vertical axis in the sagittal plane or an anteroposterior (AP) axis in the horizontal plane (Fig. 39–2A). However, Adams,[2] Swann and associates,[105] Carroll and others[14] are of the opinion that there is lateral or external rotation of the talus in the ankle mortise occurring around a vertical axis (Fig. 39–2B). Conversely, Goldner believes that the body of the talus is internally rotated around a vertical axis and around an AP axis (Fig. 39–3).[38] The entire talus is inverted around an AP axis and the entire talus is in equinus, having rotated around a medial-lateral axis. The apparent prominence of the body of the talus with reference to the bimalleolar axis of the tibia and fibula makes the talus appear to be lateral to the internally directed head and neck of the talus. Goldner states that his studies have shown that the body of the talus is internally rotated because of the high angle of the tibiofibular axis. This may explain the discrepancy between his concept and that of Carroll: that is, one of terminology and perception rather than a true anatomic difference. Walsham and Hughes also believe that the talar body is inclined medially as well as forward and downward (i.e., presumably rotated inward around the vertical axis).[114]

Talus to Calcaneus

The calcaneus is tilted into varus. It is also rotated around a vertical axis according to McKay[62, 63] and Simons.[93, 95, 97] This rotation involves medial movement of the anterior portion of the calcaneus and lateral movement of

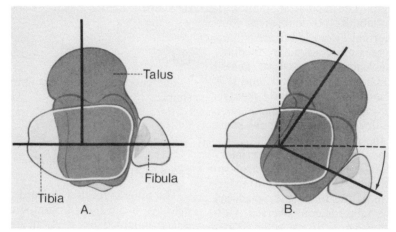

FIGURE 39–2. Concept of talar position in the ankle mortise as proposed by Lloyd-Roberts. *(A),* Normal position of the talus in the ankle mortise. *(B),* External rotation of the talus in the ankle mortise. The talus externally rotates while the tibia remains stationary. The fibula rotates posteriorly with the talus. This concept is also held by Carroll. (Courtesy of George W. Simons, M.D.)

the posterior portion of the calcaneus, so that the axis of rotation passes through the central portion of these two bones, i.e., through the interosseous talocalcaneal ligament (Fig. 39–4). As the posterior calcaneus has rotated laterally, it is tightly bound to the fibula. In addition, the calcaneus is slightly displaced posteriorly beneath the talus.

Talus to Navicular

The navicular is displaced medially and plantarward on the head of the talus and is rotated

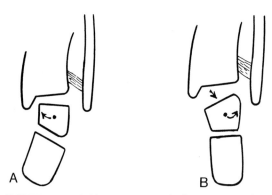

FIGURE 39–3. Goldner's concept of talar position within the mortise and rotation around an AP axis. *(A),* Internal rotation of the talus within the mortise. *(B),* Repositioning of the talus by anterior, medial, and posterior capsulotomy at the ankle joint as described by Goldner. (From Simons GW: Symposium: Current practices in the treatment of idiopathic clubfoot in the child between birth and five years of age. Contemp Orthop 17:63, 157, 1988.)

around an AP axis. The inferior surface of the navicular rotates medially while the superior surface rotates laterally. It also rotates around a vertical axis. This three-plane displacement of the navicular on the head of the talus allows the navicular to be displaced proximally as well. Often a pseudoarticular facet forms with the distal anterior medial tibia. The longer the navicular remains in this medially displaced position, the more the talar head and neck become deformed, so that the talonavicular joint eventually develops in a markedly displaced medial and inferior position.

Calcaneus to Cuboid

The anterior end of the calcaneus appears nondeformed in the fetus,[50, 86] but in infants it may be inclined inward with the lateral portion being more distal. When the calcaneus has this anterior inclination, the cuboid is angled inward to a variable degree (Fig. 39–5). There may also be an element of medial subluxation at the calcaneocuboid joint. In addition, the calcaneus and cuboid are supinated as a unit, so that they lie below the talus and navicular, respectively.

The tarsals and the metatarsals are supinated so that the cuboid and lateral metatarsals lie beneath the cuneiforms and the medial metatarsals. There is also considerable adduction of the metatarsals.

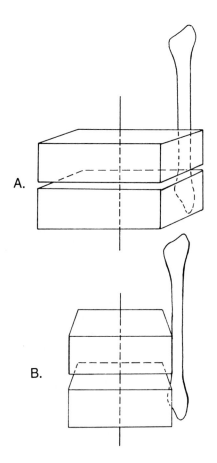

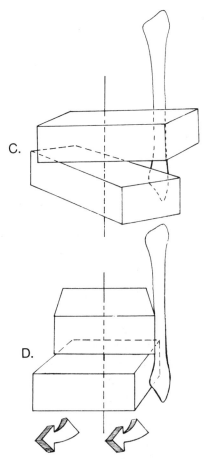

FIGURE 39–4. Concept of calcaneal rotation as proposed by McKay. The boxes simulate the position of the talus *(top)* and the calcaneus *(bottom)* in the uncorrected clubfoot. *(A)*, Note the vertical axis passing upward through the subtalar joint in the regions of the interosseous talocalcaneal ligament. The calcaneus anterior to the axis is medially displaced and the posterior portion is laterally displaced and tightly bound to the inferior aspect of the fibula by the calcaneofibular ligament. *(B)*, The talus, calcaneus, and fibula as viewed posteriorly. The calcaneus is tightly bound to the fibula by the calcaneofibular ligament. *(C and D)*, Lateral and posterior views of the talus and calcaneus following complete subtalar release and including release of the calcaneofibular ligament *(C)*. The calcaneus has been rotated away from the fibula *(D)*. The posterior view shows the rotation of the posterior calcaneus away from the fibula after incision of the calcaneofibular ligament.

Movement of the Joints of the Foot and Ankle

Normal Movements

If a normally standing patient (Fig. 39–6*A*) pronates the feet maximally, the talar head will move medially, will tend to slide off the sustentaculum tali, and may protrude on the medial plantar surface of the foot. The anterior talus rotates internally around a vertical axis that passes through the middle of the talus. Simultaneously, the trochlea of the talus rotates and thereby guides the distal tibia and fibula as the ankle mortise moves as a unit. Thus the fibular malleolus rotates anteriorly and the tibial malleolus rotates posteriorly. At the same time, the knee and upper leg also rotate inwardly (Fig. 39–6*C*).[89]

If the same patient moves feet into maximal

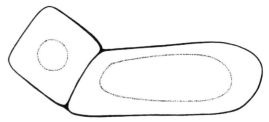

FIGURE 39–5. Calcaneocuboid malalignment, grade 2. The light lines represent the cuboid and calcaneal ossification centers, and the heavy lines outline the unossified cartilage of the calcaneus and the cuboid. Note the angulation of the distal calcaneus and possible slight medial subluxation of the cuboid.

supination, the anterior calcaneus then moves medially so that it comes to lie beneath the talar head and neck. These structures are then supported by the sustentaculum tali. Concurrently, the talar body rotates externally around

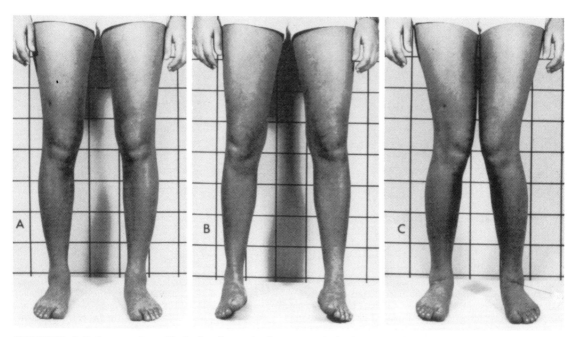

FIGURE 39–6. Patient standing with the feet flat on the floor *(A)*, with the feet inverted *(B)*, and with the feet everted *(C)*. In *A*, the patient's knees point straight ahead. In *B*, when the patient everts the feet, the anterior calcaneus moves inward beneath the talus so that the sustentaculum supports the talar head. The talar head and neck move into external rotation around a vertical axis passing up through the interosseous ligament. The lateral trochlea of the talus rotates posteriorly while the medial trochlea rotates anteriorly. Thus, the talar dome guides the position of the malleoli. As the lateral trochlea rotates posteriorly, the lateral malleolus also moves posteriorly. As the medial trochlea moves anteriorly, the medial malleolus also moves anteriorly. Thus, the whole leg above the ankle rotates externally as shown by the position of the knee. The greater trochanter also moves posteriorly. Figure C demonstrates the opposite movement, i.e., pronation of the feet. In this position the talar head rotates internally and tends to slide off the sustentaculum tali. As this happens, the trochlea guide the malleoli so that the lateral malleolus rotates forward and the medial malleolus rotates backward. Simultaneously the knees rotate medially and the greater trochanter rotates forward. The position of the feet seen in *B* is similar to that with clubfoot except that the foot is not in equinus as the patient is not standing on his toes. The position of the foot in clubfoot deformity is an exaggeration of *B*. In addition, the foot would be in more equinus. (From Campos da Paz A Jr, DeSouza V: Talipes equinovarus: Pathomechanical basis of treatment. Orthop Clin North Am 9:177, 1978.)

the vertical axis, passing upward through its center. Therefore, the trochlea of the talus guides the movements of the malleoli, with the medial malleoli moving anteriorly and the lateral malleoli moving posteriorly. These movements in turn cause external rotation of the entire leg above the ankle joint, as can be seen by the external rotation of the patella (Fig. 39–6B). These positional changes occurring with maximal supination are seen both in normal children and in children with clubfeet, but in the latter, the foot is inverted and supinated beyond the normal range of movement.[89]

Movement of the Clubfoot and the Surgical Steps Required to Reposition the Foot

Moving a clubfoot from the fully deformed position to the fully corrected position requires changes in position that are both three dimensional and complex. One may think of the fully deformed clubfoot as a normal foot that has undergone plantar flexion, inversion of the mid- and hindfoot, and supination and adduction of the forefoot, all of which have been carried beyond their normal limits. Thus, to correct the foot, the opposite movements must be achieved.

The movements required at the individual joints are also complex. Correction at each joint must be satisfactorily achieved to create as nearly normal a foot as possible. The exact surgical steps required to accomplish correction are often poorly understood and controversial.

In the foot that has had conservative treatment, varying degrees of correction will have been achieved at each of the joints. The movements of the bones and joints that must take place to correct the fully deformed foot are as follows.

Ankle Joint

The talus must move into dorsiflexion with a slight degree of posterior movement on the lateral side of the talus. Dorsiflexion should occur to the extent that the talus forms approximately a 70 to 80 degree angle with the tibia as determined by a lateral radiographic projection. To achieve this, the tight tendon structures require lengthening, specifically the Achilles tendon and posterior tibial tendon. Next, a posterior capsulotomy of the ankle is extended medially to the level of the posterior tibial tendon sheath and laterally to the level of the posterior talofibular ligament with release of this ligament. Releasing the posterior capsule alone will not achieve maximal movement.[92]

Subtalar Joint

In moving from the completely deformed position to the completely corrected position, the calcaneus must be rotated beneath the talus like a boat rolling on waves. As the bow of the boat pitches upward (i.e., the anterior calcaneus) it approaches the corrected position. Thus, it moves from the plantarflexed supinated position to a pronated dorsiflexed position, and the anterior calcaneus comes to rest on the lateral side of the talar head. Simultaneously, the posterior portion of the calcaneus descends inferiorly and moves medially away from the fibula, and in doing so the posterior calcaneus pronates, bringing the posterior medial tuberosity of the calcaneus into an inferior position. As the calcaneus goes into the fully corrected position, the anterior end (the bow of the boat) pitches or rises and its posterior end (the stern) plunges while the body turns on itself. When the posterior calcaneus moves into a dorsiflexed position, the opposite movements occur (Fig. 39–7A through F).

The subtalar joint requires complete subtalar release in the fully deformed foot, as has been mentioned. Paramount in this release is the incision of the calcaneofibular ligament, which allows rotary movement of the calcaneus beneath the talus as described by McKay.[63]

Talonavicular Joint

In accomplishing correction of the talonavicular joint, one must consider the movement of the combined talonaviculocubocalcaneal complex. The navicular, cuboid, and calcaneus move as a unit around the talar head like a ball in a socket: the talar head represents the ball and the complex of the other three bones, the socket. However, the socket moves around the head rather than the head in the socket. When the foot is corrected, these bones move laterally and dorsally and rotate so that the hindfoot, midfoot, and forefoot tend to come into abduction, eversion, and pronation (Fig. 39–7A through F). To achieve this, complete

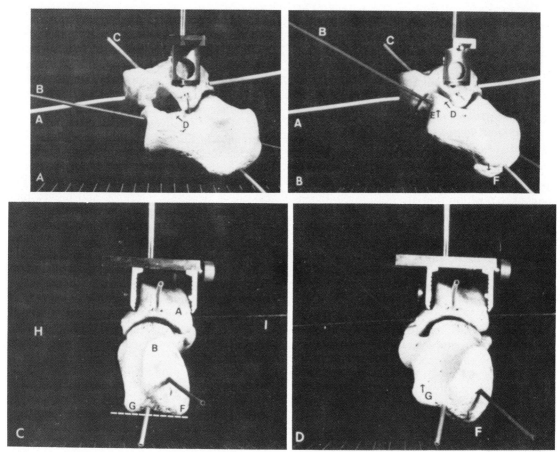

FIGURE 39–7. Movements of the calcaneus under the talus (left foot). Pins have been inserted into the talus and calcaneus to simulate the longitudinal axis of the talus *(A)*, calcaneus *(B)*, and subtalar joint *(C)*. *(A)*, Lateral view with the foot in supination. The anterior end of the calcaneus moves in plantar flexion. The sinus tarsi is open. *(B)*, Lateral view in pronation. The sinus tarsi is closed. The anterior end of the calcaneus is elevated into dorsiflexion and the posterior tuberosity (F) is displaced into plantar flexion. *(C and D)*, Posterior views of the left foot. In C, the calcaneus is in maximal supination. The lateral and medial tubercles of the posterior tuberosity of the calcaneus (G and F) are at the same level. In D, the calcaneus is pronated and the medial tubercle has migrated plantarward. *(E and F)*, Anterior views of the left talus and calcaneus. In E the calcaneus is supinated and in F, pronated. The calcaneus shows the same movements under the talus. In transition from supination to pronation, the anterior end of the calcaneus (E) is elevated into dorsiflexion and the medial tubercle of the posterior tuberosity (F) is displaced into plantar flexion. (From Campos da Paz A Jr, DeSouza V: Talipes equinovarus: Pathomechanical basis of treatment. Orthop Clin North Am 9:172–175, 1978.)

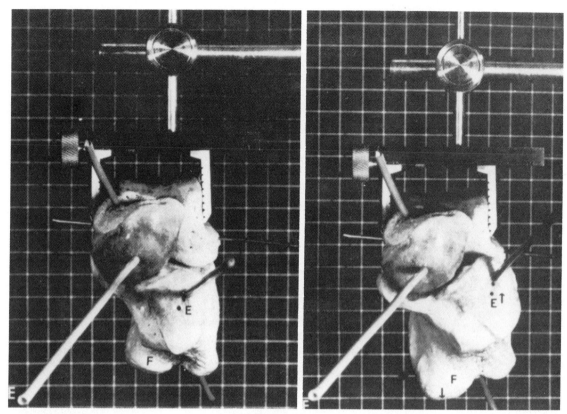

FIGURE 39–7 *Continued.*

circumferential release of the talonavicular joint is required, as well as release of the subtalar complex. This involves releasing the interosseous talocalcaneal ligament, unless very minimal contracture has occurred in this ligament, which is unusual except during the first month or two of life.

Calcaneocuboid Joint

In the infant, there may be considerable medial angulation at the calcaneocuboid joint as well as medial subluxation of the calcaneus on the talus. The anterior portion of the calcaneus may be very underdeveloped on its medial side, while the lateral side apparently continues to grow normally. Thus, the cuboid may lie in a medially angulated position with respect to the end of the calcaneus (see Fig. 39–5). However, the cuboid may also subluxate a variable degree. When the angulation and/or subluxation is significant, the movements that are required for correction are lateral tilt and lateral translation. Restoration of this joint to a position of complete correc-

tion when it is moderately or markedly angulated or subluxated is achieved only by complete capsulotomy of the joint. Opening the medial, dorsal, and volar surfaces while leaving the lateral capsule intact will not achieve satisfactory correction in most cases.

Naviculocuneiform Joint

This joint typically shows very little deformation and therefore requires no capsulotomy.

Tarsometatarsal Joints

These joints are adducted and supinated to varying degrees. They often yield to conservative treatment, although frequently the result is less than full correction. Capsulotomies of these joints must achieve correction of both adduction and supination. Therefore, pronation and abduction are necessary after release.

Once the three bones (calcaneus, cuboid, and navicular) have been released from the talus, a dramatic change can be seen at the level of the ankle joint when the ankle is

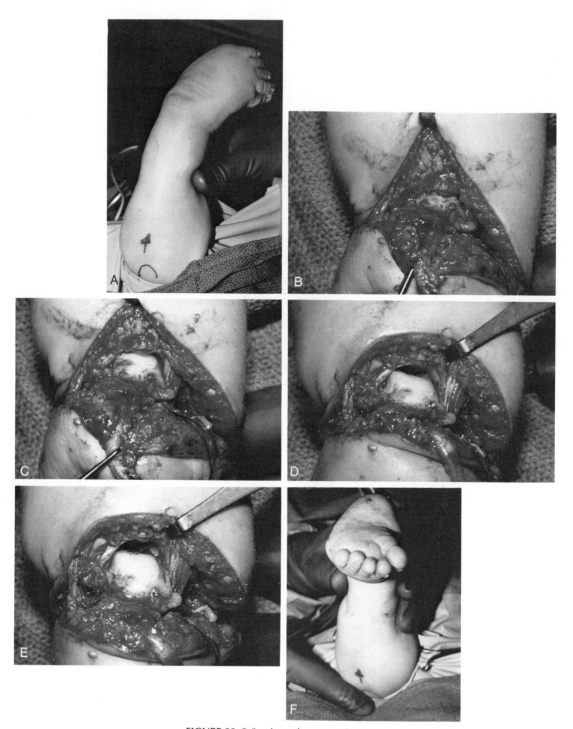

FIGURE 39–8 *See legend on opposite page*

viewed from behind. If the foot is placed into its fully deformed position, attempts to rock it into plantar flexion and dorsiflexion will be seen to occur roughly at a right angle to the plane of motion of the talus. It is not until the foot is externally rotated (approximately 60 to 80 degrees) that the calcaneus and the rest of the foot can be placed in normal alignment with the talus. When they are placed in this externally rotated position and pinned to the talus, attempts at plantar flexion and dorsiflexion of the foot coincide with dorsiflexion and plantar flexion of the talus. The surgery required for this correction is complete release of the subtalar joint (Fig. 39–8*A* through *F*).

CLINICAL ASSESSMENT

The diagnosis of the clubfoot is unmistakable, as the foot is in a position of marked deformity. The degree of stiffness of the foot varies considerably, however. In the postural clubfoot, which develops late in pregnancy, the foot can usually be manipulated to a neutral position, perhaps even further. In the severe neurovascular clubfoot, the deformities may be rigid and yield very minimally to attempts at manual correction. The typical clubfoot has a degree of stiffness between these two extremes.

The involved calf is smaller than the normal calf. The heel is small and in a position of equinus and varus. The skin on the dorsolateral aspect of the foot is frequently thin, and there is little subcutaneous tissue. Once correction of the foot has taken place, this dorsolateral skin becomes wrinkled and never develops the thickness of the normal soft tissues in this area.

There may be deep creases on the plantar surface of the foot, which indicate a poor prognosis. An atavistic (i.e., shortened to a marked degree in comparison with the other rays) first metatarsal is also unpromising. Thus, a "terrible triad" of marked stiffness, deep medial and plantar skin creases, and an atavistic first metatarsal indicates a very poor prognosis in the typical clubfoot.

In the clinical assessment, it is also important to identify the presence of any of the 30 or more syndromes, some very rare, in which clubfeet have been observed.[102] Abnormal fascies, major organ defects, and associated congenital anomalies are frequently present in these syndromes. When a patient with a clubfoot has obviously abnormal facial features or other congenital anomalies, genetic consultation is indicated before surgery. A child who has a syndrome with a poor prognosis is not a candidate for extensive clubfoot surgery.[102]

RADIOGRAPHIC EVALUATION

Advantages and Disadvantages

The use of radiographs in the evaluation and treatment of clubfeet is controversial. The primary reason for skepticism is that at birth the ossification centers of the midfoot and hindfoot are sometimes too small to be used for the measurement of angles and axes. In addition, the ossification center of the cuboid is occasionally absent at birth, while the ossification center of the navicular frequently does not appear until 3 years of age or later. Another reason is that the ossification center of the talus does not lie within the body of the talus but rather in the neck of the talus.[76] Finally, the patient may move the foot at the time the radiograph is taken or the radiograph may be taken in a nonstandardized manner. For these

FIGURE 39–8. (*A*), Uncorrected clubfoot. The anesthetized and prone patient's knee is flexed to 90 degrees. The foot is turned inward markedly and is in equinus. The axis of the ankle is essentially parallel to the knee axis but is externally rotated 60 to 80 degrees; thus, to flex and extend the ankle with the foot markedly deformed at the subtalar joint (due to medial rotation of the anterior calcaneus and lateral rotation of the posterior calcaneus) requires inversion and eversion. To restore the foot to the normal position so that it dorsiflexes and plantarflexes in normal alignment with the leg requires the foot to be externally rotated around the talus about 60 to 80 degrees. (*B* to *E*), A complete subtalar release has been performed through a Cincinnati incision, and the talonavicular and talocalcaneal joints have been pinned. The knee has been extended and the foot is being viewed through the Cincinnati incision. The heel is at the bottom. These four photographs show the ankle joint opening posteriorly, progressively from *B* through *E*. As the dome of the talus comes progressively into view, the talus appears not to rotate around an AP axis or around a vertical axis but rather to rotate solely around a transverse axis. (*F*), The knee is flexed, the patient is prone, and the foot is maximally dorsiflexed (forefoot moved toward the table). When plantarflexed and dorsiflexed, the foot moves in normal alignment with the leg (compare with *A*).

reasons, the x-ray films may be difficult to interpret.

It is the author's contention that although the ossification centers may not be present or may be too small for measurement of their axes at birth, by the time the patient is ready for surgery (i.e., when the foot is at least 8 cm long, generally between 3 and 6 months of age), the ossification centers are sufficiently developed to permit angular measurements. Furthermore, although the talar ossification center is located in the talar neck, its position is constant in all feet, and therefore it qualifies as a valid reference point for measurement.

When deformities are extensive, as in the newborn, radiographs are not of great value. Gross deformities such as varus of the hindfoot, in which the talus and the calcaneus are completely overlapping, do not need to be measured in order to establish that there is varus or rotational deformity between these two bones. Angular measurements may be helpful when the foot has undergone considerable correction by conservative treatment and improvement has reached a plateau. Moreover, when standardized radiographic and measurement techniques are used, most of the remaining objections can be overcome.[88]

Indications

There are four times when radiographs may be helpful. The first is during conservative treatment. At this time the position of the talar axis in relation to the base of the first metatarsal is useful to tell when the talonavicular subluxation has been reduced. When the talar axis passes through the base of the first metatarsal, the navicular has been reduced on the distal aspect of the talus. The next step in the correction of the hindfoot (i.e., correction of varus) cannot take place until the navicular has been "unlocked." Even the experienced surgeon may not be able to ascertain this by careful clinical examination.

When varus of the heel appears to be clinically corrected, an AP film will verify that correction of hindfoot varus has been achieved. This is established by the presence of a normal AP talocalcaneal (APTC) angle (20 to 40 degrees). Finally, when equinus is corrected, a lateral projection should show that the lateral talocalcaneal (TC) angle measures greater than 35 degrees.

The second time radiographs are useful is preoperatively, to determine the persisting deformity and thereby to decide on which primary and ancillary procedures to use.

The third time radiographs are useful is during the intraoperative evaluation. These are the most valuable radiographs that the surgeon can obtain in the treatment of clubfoot. These films verify that complete correction of the foot has been achieved intraoperatively and that overcorrection is not present.

Radiographs are also useful in the postoperative phase. Early and late postoperative films are compared with one another and with the intraoperative films to determine whether correction is being maintained, is relapsing, or is slowly changing into an overcorrected position (which is unusual). When comparing films over a period of several years, it is important to recognize that the APTC angle normally decreases gradually with age.[88, 112]

Standardized Radiographic Method

The radiographic evaluation of the clubfoot involves the use of standardized two-plane radiographic techniques. It is mandatory to follow a standardized method for obtaining and interpreting the radiographs.* This method involves positioning both the patient and the tube and the cassette in a specific way, inspecting and rejecting inadequate films, and (when necessary) making precise measurements of the various angles.

Technique

Films of the patient with clubfeet should be taken in a simulated or true standing position whenever possible. If sitting, the patient should be positioned on a small stool with the knees flexed and the feet flat on the cassette. An AP view should be taken of each foot individually, although both feet may be taken on the same cassette. The tube should be angled approximately 27 degrees from the vertical, so that the beam is directed at the talar head. The foot should not be allowed to plantarflex, invert, evert, or rotate when the radiograph is taken (Fig. 39–9). On the lateral view,

---

*For a complete discussion of the standardized radiographic technique used by the author, the reader is referred to reference 88.

FIGURE 39–9. Technique of obtaining AP x-ray views of the foot. The patient is placed in a simulated standing position with the feet flat on the cassette. The x-ray machine is angulated 30 degrees from the vertical and the beam directed at the talar head. (From Simons GW: A standardized method for the radiographic evaluation of clubfeet. Clin Orthop 135:107, 1978.)

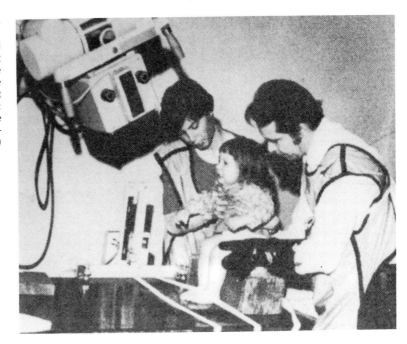

the patient should be placed straddling a cassette, which is preferably positioned in a slotted board on the x-ray table, or alternatively, the cassette may be held vertically by the orthopedic or radiographic technician. The cassette must be vertical, while the child's foot should be placed parallel with the cassette. If there is significant medial deviation of the midfoot or forefoot, then the hindfoot should be moved away from the cassette so that it is parallel with the cassette. The lower leg should not be allowed to rotate or the foot to supinate or plantarflex (Fig. 39–10).

Evaluation

The surgeon should be aware of the specific criteria for rejecting radiographic views that have not been taken according to a standardized technique. Clues to whether or not the

FIGURE 39–10. Technique of obtaining the lateral x-ray view. The patient is placed in a standing position straddling the cassette with the feet placed flat on the cassette. The ankle is maximally dorsiflexed. If the anterior portion of the foot is markedly deviated medially, the back of the foot must be moved laterally so that the hind portion is parallel to the cassette. (From Simons GW: Standardized method for the radiographic evaluation of clubfeet. Clin Orthop 135:107, 1978.)

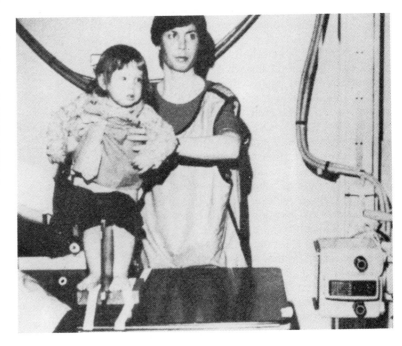

TABLE 39–1. CLUES THAT SUGGEST IMPROPER RADIOGRAPHIC TECHNIQUE

LATERAL VIEW

Extreme Posterior Positioning of Fibula with Respect to Tibia

The hindfoot may have been positioned in some external rotation causing a false increase in the talocalcaneal (TC) angle. Significant medial deviation of the midfoot or forefoot on the AP view suggests this, along with the clinical appearance of the foot.

Loss of Overlapping Appearance of Metatarsals

This suggests that the whole foot was inverted when the film was taken therefore causing a false decrease in the TC angle. Comparing the films with the clinical appearance of the foot may verify this.

Lack of Ankle Dorsiflexion

This suggests that the ankle was not adequately dorsiflexed when the film was taken or that significant equinus exists. Inadequate dorsiflexion will cause a falsely diminished TC angle. Comparing the films with the clinical appearance of the foot may verify this.

ANTEROPOSTERIOR VIEW

Anterior Ends of Talus and Calcaneus at Different Levels

If the anterior ends of these bones are more than 2–3 mm apart the x-ray tube was not positioned at 30° or the foot was malpositioned in plantar flexion. This may result in an error in angular measurement.

Significant Overlapping of Metatarsals

This indicates that the film may have been taken with the whole foot inverted and suggests a falsely diminished TC angle. Compare the film with the clinical appearance of the foot.

Visualization of Shafts of Tibia and Fibula

This suggests that the film was taken without adequate dorsiflexion of the ankle or that significant equinus prevented dorsiflexion. Inadequate dorsiflexion will cause a false decrease in the TC angle. Compare the film with the clinical appearance of the foot.

From Simons GW: A standardized method for the radiographic evaluation of clubfeet. Clin Orthop 135:107–118, 1978.

foot has been positioned properly are as follows (Table 39–1): On the lateral view, improper technique may be indicated by a posterior position of the fibula in relation to the tibia. The radiograph gives the appearance of an AP projection of the tibia and fibula, while the foot gives the appearance of a lateral projection. This incongruity occurs when there is significant mid- or forefoot adduction and the hindfoot is not placed parallel to the cassette but rather is externally rotated (Fig. 39–11). With the medial surface of both the forefoot and hindfoot against the cassette, an external oblique radiographic view will be obtained. If the metatarsals are not overlapping but appear side by side, and the clinical appearance does not correspond, then the foot was held in a position of inversion when the radiograph was taken and a fallaciously small lateral TC angle may be present. If the ankle was not fully dorsiflexed, the film will show the ankle to be less dorsiflexed than the foot appears clinically, and as a result, the lateral TC angle will be falsely diminished (Fig. 39–12A and B). On the AP view, the anterior ends of the talus and calcaneus should be approximately at the same level. If the talus is too far forward, the x-ray beam was too vertical to the cassette, whereas if the calcaneus is too far forward, the beam was too horizontal

(Fig. 39–13). If the foot has been supinated, the metatarsals will appear to overlap and there will be incongruity with the clinical appearance of the foot. If the foot has been

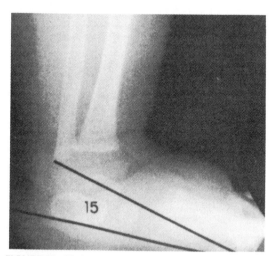

FIGURE 39–11. Apparent posterior rotation of the fibula in the ankle mortise caused by improper technique in taking the radiograph. There was significant medial deviation of the forefoot (metatarsus adductus) and the entire foot was placed parallel to the cassette resulting in an oblique projection. When significant metatarsal adduction exists, the foot must be moved away from the cassette so that the hindfoot is parallel with the cassette. (From Simons GW: A standardized method for the radiographic evaluation of clubfeet. Clin Orthop 135:107, 1978.)

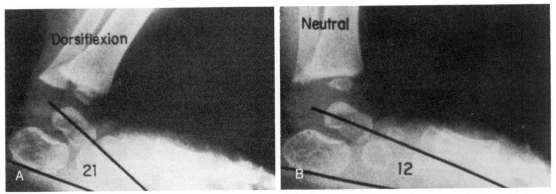

FIGURE 39–12. *(A),* Lateral TC angle (12 degrees) when the foot is placed in a plantargrade position with the ankle in the neutral position. *(B),* With the ankle fully dorsiflexed, the true lateral TC angle of 21 degrees is seen. This shows the importance of positioning the foot in full dorsiflexion. (From Simons GW: A standardized method for the radiographic evaluation of clubfeet. Clin Orthop 135:107, 1978.)

plantarflexed, the tibia and fibula will be seen, which may indicate that there is inadequate dorsiflexion at the ankle (unless there is significant fixed equinus deformity, which prevents dorsiflexion).

Measurement of Radiographic Angles

As indicated earlier, measurement of the radiographic angles on the preoperative films is most useful when small or moderate degrees of deformity persist. With greater deformity, particularly in the newborn, the foot is so distorted that measuring the angles is useless. By 2 or 3 months of age the ossification centers have usually become large enough to be useful for angular measurements. Once the surgical release is completed and the foot is thought to be normally aligned, intraoperative x-ray evaluation is more precise than clinical evaluation.

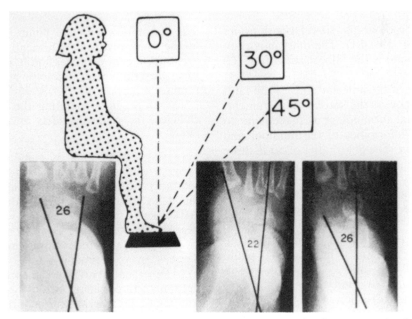

FIGURE 39–13. Method of determining whether the x-ray machine was positioned at the proper angle relative to the foot. The x-ray film on the left shows the calcaneus too far anterior to the talus while that on the right shows the talus too far anterior to the calcaneus. The central film shows the head of the talus and the head of the calcaneus at the same level. This is the proper position and is obtained when the x-ray unit is positioned at 30 degrees from the vertical. (From Simons GW: A standardized method for the radiographic evaluation of clubfeet. Clin Orthop 135:107, 1978.)

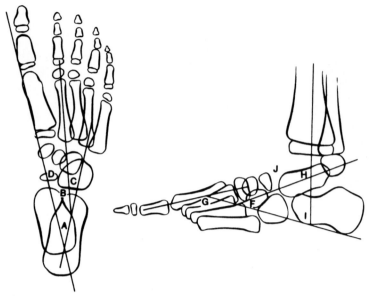

FIGURE 39–14. AP and lateral radiographic measurements with normal values for the child less than 5 years old. On the AP radiograph, A is the (AP) talocalcaneal angle (20–40 degrees); B, the (AP) talocalcaneal divergence (0–+1); C, the position of the ossification center of the cuboid relative to the calcaneus (normal position is grade 0); and D, the navicular in normal (0–+1) position (i.e., the talar axis passes through the base of the first metatarsal).

On the lateral radiograph, F is the lateral (TC) angle (35–50 degrees); G, the calcaneal–first metatarsal angle (0 degrees); H, the tibiotalar angle in dorsiflexion (70–100 degrees) and in plantar flexion (120–180 degrees); I, the tibiocalcaneal angle in dorsiflexion (25–60 degrees); and J, the navicular position relative to the talar head (0–normal). Notice that there is mild dorsal subluxation of the navicular on this film and that the talar axis passes plantar to the first metatarsal (i.e., +1). (From Simons GW: The complete subtalar release in clubfeet. II. Comparison with less extensive procedures. J Bone Joint Surg 67A:1056, 1985.)

On the AP radiograph, six relationships are evaluated (Fig. 39–14*A*). The most important angle to evaluate is the talocalcaneal (APTC) angle.

Divergence of the anterior ends of the talus and the calcaneus is the second measurement.

Conventional terminology is inadequate to describe the deformities of the hindfoot and their correction. The deformities occur in three planes and their surgical correction takes place simultaneously in all three. In the fully deformed hindfoot, the position of the calcaneus cannot be adequately described with singular terms such as "varus" and "valgus" (e.g., the calcaneus is rotated in a horizontal plane around the vertical axis, in a coronal plane around an AP axis, and to a slight degree in the sagittal plane around the medial-lateral axis). Thus, the correction of the talocalcaneal relationship, when described as correction from varus to normal or to valgus, describes only one plane of correction (the coronal plane): it neglects rotational correction in the horizontal plane. Attempts to overcome this deficiency have been made by combining the

axis of rotation with the plane of movement of the bone involved. Although this is more accurate, it is nevertheless quite cumbersome. Ideal descriptive terminology has yet to be found.

Therefore, in considering the radiographic changes, the following facts must be kept in mind.

1. The APTC angle is a measurement of varus or valgus of the hindfoot (coronal plane rotation) and rotation of the calcaneus beneath the talus (horizontal plane rotation). The APTC angle normally measures between 20 degrees and 40 degrees. Fewer than 20 degrees indicates undercorrection and more than 40 degrees, overcorrection.[88]

2. Divergence between the anterior ends of the talus and calcaneus is mostly the result of rotation of the anterior aspect of the calcaneus. Failure of divergence indicates persistence of calcaneal rotation, while excessive divergence indicates overcorrection into valgus (i.e., rotary valgus) (Figs. 39–14*A* and 39–15).[94]

3. Percentage of overlap of the talus and calcaneus is a result of translation of the cal-

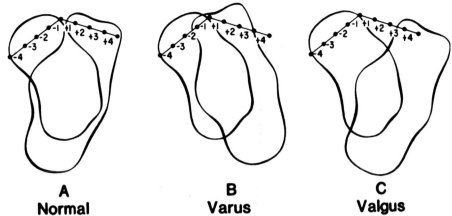

A
Normal

B
Varus

C
Valgus

FIGURE 39–15. Talocalcaneal divergence. Divergence of the anterior ends of the talus and the calcaneus is normal in children who are less than 5 years old; that is, a cleft exists at the anterior ends. Overlap is measured in one quarter increments (−1 to −4); divergence is designated as +1 to +4. (Divergence and overlap are based on the transverse diameter of the talar head at the distal end of the talus at the points where their forward curvature begins.) (From Simons GW: The complete subtalar release in clubfeet. II. Comparison with less extensive procedures. J Bone Joint Surg 67A:1056, 1985.)

caneus beneath the talus and rotation of the calcaneus beneath the talus.

Normally there should be approximately 50 percent overlap in the young child's foot. Less than this indicates translation of the calcaneus beneath the talus.

When these three facts are considered together, a more accurate three-dimensional assessment can be made as the line drawings of

the talus and calcaneus in Figure 39–16 demonstrate.

The third sign to evaluate on the AP views is overlap of the talus and the calcaneus.

The fourth parameter to evaluate is the position of the talar axis relative to the base of the first metatarsal. The talar axis normally passes through the base of the first metatarsal. If it passes lateral to it, this indicates the presence of medial talonavicular subluxation.

TALOCALCANEAL RELATIONSHIPS

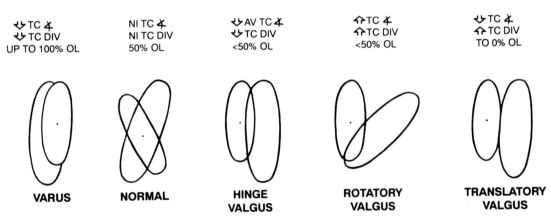

FIGURE 39–16. Line drawings of the talar and calcaneal relationships. The utilization of these three measurements, i.e., APTC angle, APTC divergence and AP overlap, when taken together can be used to diagnose not only varus and valgus but also rotation and translation.

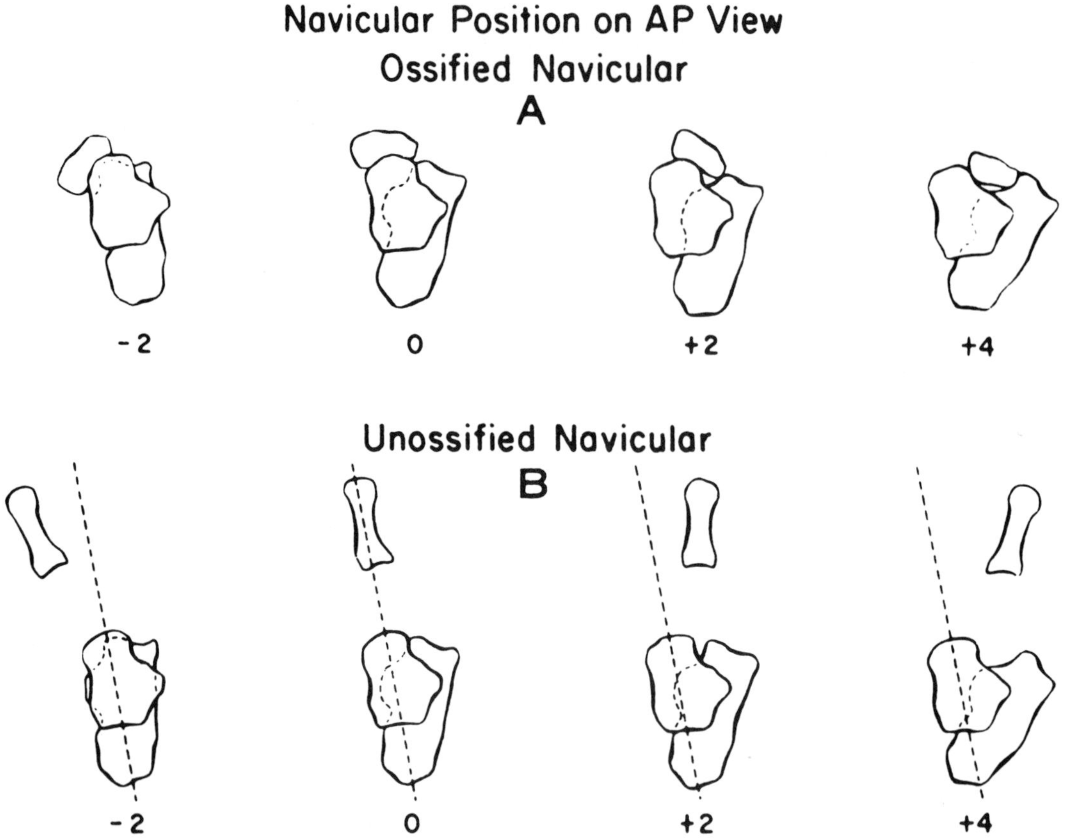

Navicular Position on AP View
Ossified Navicular
A

-2   0   +2   +4

Unossified Navicular
B

-2   0   +2   +4

FIGURE 39–17. Navicular position on the anteroposterior radiograph. *(A)*, Method of determining the navicular position after ossification has occurred. The position of the navicular is graded as 0 if the navicular is positioned centrally on the distal end of the talus. If it is laterally or medially displaced by one-quarter of the diameter of the talar head, a grade of +1 or -1, respectively, is given. If it is laterally or medially displaced by one-half of the diameter of the talar head, a grade of +2 or -2 is given. Similarly, grades of 3 and 4 are given for displacement of three-quarters and complete displacement of the navicular from the talar head, respectively. On the AP radiograph, the central position of the navicular with respect to the talar head is the normal position. Mild and moderate lateral deviation is seen in hypermobile flat feet; this condition is usually asymptomatic and is compatible with good function. Thus a grade of +1 or +2 is satisfactory but is considered overcorrection, while a grade of +3 or +4 represents marked overcorrection and, therefore, a complication. Grades of -1, -2, and -3 are all unsatisfactory and represent a major complication. *(B)*, Method of determining the navicular position before ossification has occurred. When the talar axis passes through the base of the first metatarsal, the navicular is in normal alignment with the talus and the navicular position is then rated 0. When it passes medial or lateral to the base of the first metatarsal by one-half of the width of the base of the first metatarsal, a grade of -1 or +1, respectively, is given. When it passes medially or laterally the full width of the base of the first metatarsal, a grade of -2 or +2, respectively, is given, and so on. Grades of 0, +1, and +2 are considered satisfactory, while ratings greater or less than this are considered to represent a major complication. (From Simons GW: The complete subtalar release in clubfeet. II. Comparison with less extensive procedures. J Bone Joint Surg 67A:1056, 1985.)

If it passes medially, there is lateral subluxation of the navicular (Figs. 39–14*A* and 39–17).[80]

The fifth parameter is the location of the central point of the cuboid ossification center in relationship to the calcaneal axis. Normally, this lies on the long axis of the calcaneus. Varying degrees of medial subluxation may occur from grade 1 to grade 3, with grade 3 being complete medial subluxation of the cuboid off the distal end of the calcaneus and

proximal migration of the cuboid to a level where the central point of the ossification center lies proximal to the distal end of the ossified talus. (See Figure 39–47*A* and related text.)

The sixth parameter is metatarsal alignment. Normally the metatarsals diverge, but in the clubfoot, all metatarsals converge medially. When corrected the metatarsals should no longer converge but should diverge with a relatively straight lateral border of the foot, the fifth metatarsal being more or less parallel with the calcaneus in this projection (Fig. 39–14A). Some surgeons use the calcaneal–fifth metatarsal angle for measuring this parameter. The normal measurement is 0 degrees.

The lateral radiograph allows evaluation of two angles and one axis relationship (Fig. 39–14B). The normal lateral TC angle measures 35 degrees to 50 degrees.[88] Smaller values indicate persistent hindfoot equinus, whereas larger values indicate calcaneus deformity.

The talar axis–first metatarsal basis relationship may be a difficult radiographic parameter to measure because of overlapping metatar-sals. However, normally the talar axis passes through the base of the first metatarsal. If the talar axis points inferiorly to the base of the first metatarsal, either the navicular is subluxated dorsally or the talus is in excessive plantarflexion. If the talar axis passes dorsal to the first metatarsal, the navicular is in an inferiorly subluxated position, which is rare (Figs. 39–14B, 39–18, and 39–19).

The second angle to evaluate on the lateral radiograph is the talar–first metatarsal angle, which indicates the presence of a cavus deformity or rocker-bottom deformity. The normal measurement of this angle is 0 to 20 degrees.[81]

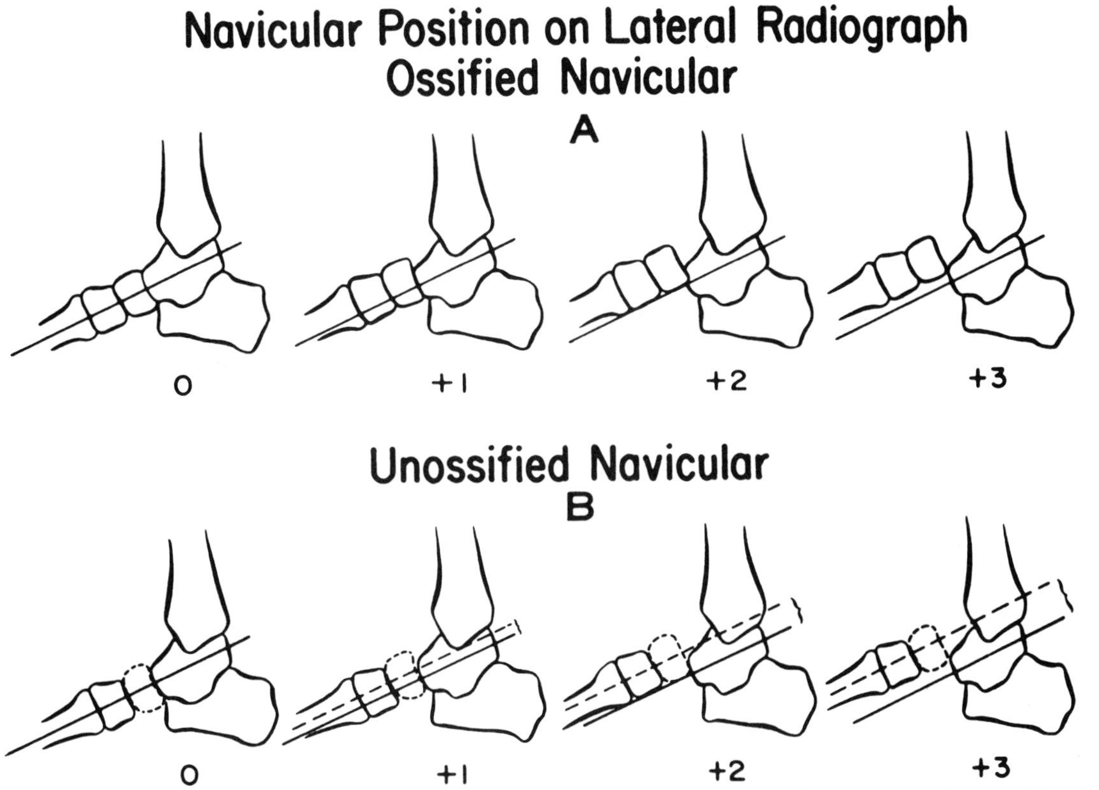

Navicular Position on Lateral Radiograph
Ossified Navicular
A

| 0 | +1 | +2 | +3 |

Unossified Navicular
B

| 0 | +1 | +2 | +3 |

FIGURE 39–18. Navicular position on the lateral radiograph. *(A),* Method of determining the presence or absence of dorsal subluxation of the navicular after ossification has occurred. On the lateral radiograph, the navicular is normally not displaced dorsally with respect to the talus. This normal position of the navicular is graded as 0. Superior displacement of approximately one-third or less of the height of the ossified navicular head is graded +1, superior displacement of between one-third and two-thirds is graded +2, and superior displacement of more than two-thirds is graded +3. A grade of +1 is considered satisfactory (but overcorrected), whereas grades of +2 and +3 are considered unsatisfactory and indicative of a major complication. *(B),* Method of determining the presence or absence of dorsal subluxation of the navicular before ossification has occurred. When a line is drawn through the talar axis and another line is drawn through the first metatarsal axis, the distance between these two parallel lines represents the dorsal subluxation of the navicular. Grades are determined by comparing the distance between the two lines to the height of the talar head; that is, 0 to one-third, +1; one-third to two-thirds, +2; and two-thirds to 1, +3. Occasionally the overlap of the metatarsals makes identification of the first metatarsal impossible. In that case, a line along the superior surface of the most dorsal metatarsal may be used. If it passes above the talar head, the navicular is dorsally subluxated. Normal position is graded 0; +1, satisfactory; and more than +1, unsatisfactory. In the presence of a cavus deformity, this measurement is unreliable. (From Simons GW: The complete subtalar release in clubfeet. II. Comparison with less extensive procedures. J Bone Joint Surg 67A:1056, 1985.)

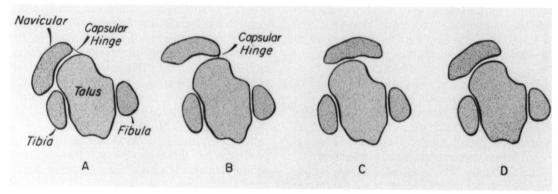

FIGURE 39–19. *(A)*, Medial position of the navicular bone in the uncorrected club foot. *(B)*, The capsule of the talonavicular joint has been excised except for the lateral portion. This permits hinging open of the joint but does not allow lateral translation and correction of the talonavicular subluxation. *(C)*, Excessive lateral translation (overcorrection) following total release. *(D)*, The proper amount of translation. The edge of the navicular should protrude slightly medially and there should be no irregularity of the joint surfaces laterally. (From Simons GW: The complete subtalar release in clubfeet. Orthop Clin North Am 18:667, 1987.)

The most important radiographic projections are the intraoperative PA and lateral views. These define the degree of correction or overcorrection that is present at the time of surgery. In most cases, the surgical results seen radiographically will remain fairly stable following surgery, although the APTC angle tends to decrease with age.[113] The most important single measurement is the APTC angle, which indicates the degree of correction of hindfoot varus and of rotary correction of the calcaneus beneath the talus.

SURGERY

Three major types of surgery are employed for clubfoot: soft tissue, bone, and joint procedures. Soft tissue procedures are generally employed from birth to 4 years of age. The age range between 4 and 8 years represents a gray zone in which either soft tissue or bone procedures may be performed. Between 8 and 12 years of age, bone procedures are indicated, and over 12 years of age, joint procedures are indicated.

The reason for this chronologic grouping is the degree of ossification present in the bones of the mid- and hindfoot at these ages. Since the bones are either nonossified or normally ossifying in the first 4 years of life, osteotomy through the bones will not permit good bone-to-bone apposition for healing, and a fibrous or nonunion can be expected. In addition, joint resection in the child between 4 and 12 years of age requires excision of a large amount of cartilage before the outer surfaces of the ossification centers are adequately exposed for arthrodesis. Thus, osteotomies of the midfoot and hindfoot are usually not performed before 4 years of age and preferably not until 8 years of age, while arthrodesis is not performed before 10 years of age and preferably only after 13 years. (An exception to this principle regarding osteotomies may be severe calcaneocuboid subluxation which is difficult to reduce after a calcaneocuboid capsulotomy.)

Soft Tissue Procedures

The three main types of soft tissue procedures in use today are grouped by the anatomic regions that they involve. These procedures are the posterior release, the posterior medial release, and the posterior, medial, and lateral release. Most of the procedures that have been devised fall into one of these three main categories.

A number of soft tissue operations have been designed or modified by various authors according to the pathologic anatomy that they believe to be present in the foot. In 1969, Goldner described a posterior, medial, and anterior ankle joint release. He believed that the major deformity is due to internal rotation of the talus in the ankle mortise and that this occurs principally around a vertical axis passing through the talocalcaneal joint in the region of the interosseous ligament. He also theorized that an internal rotational deformity occurs around a second axis (i.e., around an AP axis), so that the talus is rotated into a varus position (see Fig. 39–3). Thus there is no true varus of the calcaneus, but the varus position in which it lies is secondary to primary talar varus. To correct these deformities, he operated at the ankle level rather than at the subtalar level, which he left virtually undisturbed. The procedure is essentially a circumferential release at the ankle level, except for the lateral aspect of the ankle capsule, which is left intact.[38, 41, 97, 98]

Turco's posterior medial release (1971), essentially a refinement of Codivilla's procedure described in 1906, became widely used about two decades ago[109, 110] and is probably the most commonly used posterior medial release today.[14] A release of the anterior, medial, and posterior aspects of the subtalar joint including the medial, dorsal, and volar aspects of the talonavicular joint allows these two joints to hinge open like the covers of a book rather than the rotated or translated movements that are now believed to be necessary for the correction of these two joints (Fig. 39–19). Turco held that the principal deformity involves the talonavicular joint, and he was the first to advocate Kirschner wire fixation following surgery at this level.

Over the past decade, several new procedures have been developed. Carroll[14] maintains that the principal deformity is external rotation of the talus in the ankle mortise around a vertical axis (see Fig. 39–2). To correct this, he performs a partial ankle capsulotomy and partial subtalar capsulotomy, then rotates the talus medially and simultaneously rotates the calcaneus in the opposite direction.[14, 97, 98]

McKay believes that the primary deformity of the hindfoot is calcaneal rotation beneath the talus around a vertical axis (see Fig. 39–4). He performs a complete subtalar release and in most instances releases the interosseous ligament, although he occasionally leaves a portion of the lateral capsule intact.[62, 63, 97, 98]

The author's surgical release (complete subtalar release) is based on McKay's concept. While very similar in principle to McKay's technique, it differs in a number of surgical steps. There is invariably a release of the interosseous talocalcaneal ligament, while McKay releases it the majority of the time. He routinely performs a plantar release while the author does so only in selected cases. His treatment of the tendons differs in that he rolls back the tendon sheath before lengthening the tendons; the author retains the posterior tibial tendon sheath to retain its pulley effect in supporting the medial longitudinal arch. The technique of realigning the foot and verifying its position also differs from McKay's. Probably the most important difference between the two methods, however, is not with the procedure itself, but rather with the use of intraoperative radiographs to verify the precise realignment of the foot. McKay does not use intraoperative radiographs, while the author considers them an integral part of the complete subtalar release.[93–95, 97, 98] The reader who wishes to have a more detailed explanation of these procedures should consult the articles cited in references 14, 38, 41, 62, 63, 97, 98, and 105.

Ancillary Procedures

There are several ancillary procedures that many surgeons use as part of their extensive subtalar release in the presence of certain abnormalities. For example, the plantar release may be used for forefoot adduction and cavus. The calcaneocuboid release[54, 55, 93, 107] may be used for calcaneocuboid subluxation, and metatarsal capsulotomies[46, 51] or osteotomies[6, 104] for forefoot adduction.

Limited Soft Tissue Procedures

When the only deformity is hindfoot equinus, a limited version of the extensive procedures may be performed (see Partial Subtalar Release).

Other Soft Tissue Procedures

The most frequently used tendon transfer is an anterior tibial tendon transfer to the lateral side of the foot or to the center of the foot.*

This is used to correct supination following surgery. With few exceptions, posterior tibial tendon transfers are no longer used in nonneurogenic clubfoot surgery because of the risk of marked planovalgus deformity following the transfer.[12, 37, 98, 100, 115, 116]

Transfer of the flexor digitorum longus has been described but is not commonly used, and the author has no experience with it.[76]

---

*See references 13, 19, 32, 34–36, 53, 74, 101, 103.

Bone Procedures

Cervical Osteotomy of the Talus

This has been described by several authors.[47, 48, 70, 82, 121] Although this procedure is conceptually appealing because it realigns the marked abnormally angulated cervical neck of the talus, it has the inherent danger of damage to the blood supply of the talus, although this has apparently not been a significant complication. It is indicated only in the older patient between 8 and 12 years of age.

Talectomy

Originally described by Whitman in 1922[119] for severe residual deformities of the hindfoot, a talectomy is used in the older child after multiple previous procedures. In the author's opinion, this is a destructive operation that removes the "keystone" of the foot.[124] Instability and pain that may occur following talectomy are difficult to treat and may require tibiocalcaneal arthrodesis. In most instances, reconstruction of the foot may be accomplished by other means.

Calcaneal Osteotomy

Numerous calcaneal osteotomies have been devised to correct deformities of the calcaneus.* Dwyer has described both open and closing wedge oblique osteotomies through the posterior calcaneus just anterior to the apophysis for the correction of varus deformity.[7, 26, 27, 28, 59, 118] Horizontal opening wedge osteotomies and translatory osteotomies have been described for valgus of the heel due to overcorrection.[8] V-shaped osteotomies have been reported in which two slanting vertical osteotomy cuts, one anterior and one posterior through the calcaneus, have been used to correct equinus and other calcaneal deformities.[49] Also, a U-shaped osteotomy for equinus of the hindfoot[49] and a T-shaped osteotomy for cavovarus of the hindfoot have been used.[70] The author also occasionally uses anterior lateral vertical closing wedge osteotomies for shortening the lateral column of the foot. Calcaneal osteotomies have also been recommended for cavus deformities.[26, 116]

---

*See references 8, 10, 24, 31, 68, 69, 78, 117.

Naviculectomy

Navicular resection has been described for rare severe cases, but in the author's opinion it is contraindicated. If adequate soft tissue dissection is performed, the navicular can usually be replaced on the distal talus in a more normal relationship. Removal of the navicular shortens an already shortened medial column of the foot.

Cuboid Osteotomy

Closing wedge cuboid osteotomy[21, 75] was first described by Ogston and was performed without concomitant cuneiform-navicular capsulotomy. This procedure is used to shorten the lateral column of the foot, thus lateralizing the adducted metatarsals. However, it does not achieve this goal unless the medial half of the tarsus is allowed to open while the lateral half closes. Consequently, it should not be used unless cuneiform-navicular capsulotomy or cuneiform osteotomy is done at the same time.

Tarsal Osteotomy

Dorsal wedge resection of the anterior lateral calcaneus is effective when used to align the cavovarus deformity of the midfoot, provided the major deformities primarily involve the tarsus rather than the metatarsals. However, it does not significantly improve deformity of the hindfoot.

Metatarsal Osteotomy

Selected or multiple metatarsal osteotomies of all five metatarsals have been used to correct residual forefoot adduction and cavus deformities.[46, 104] This should generally be preceded by plantar release, as occasionally enough correction may be obtained that this will be unnecessary. This procedure may be combined with an extensive soft tissue release, in which case it may be used much earlier than the usual age of 4 to 6 years.

Tibial Osteotomy

Lateral tibial rotation osteotomy has been described for internal tibial torsion and residual medial deviation of the foot following previous surgery. However, it has been well established that internal tibial torsion is not one of the deformities of clubfeet.[107] Furthermore, medial deviation of the foot following surgery is usually secondary to residual deformity within the foot. Consequently, external tibial rotation osteotomy is not an appropriate procedure as it produces a second deformity at a distance from the first.

Medial tibial rotation osteotomy has been described for severe residual deformities of the foot in the older child[57, 65] with an apparent posterior rotation of the fibula. Lloyd-Roberts and associates believed that this condition was due to external rotation of the talus in the mortise of the ankle. Their medial tibial derotation osteotomy was followed by a second-stage procedure to abduct the foot. This concept is not generally accepted today.[57]

Joint Procedures

The main joint procedure is the triple arthrodesis.[60] In addition, various combinations of procedures such as the Dwyer calcaneal osteotomy and metatarsal osteotomies may be employed in this age range. The triple arthrodesis has the distinct advantage that significant deformities can be corrected in multiple planes. However, in doing so, joint surfaces have to be resected, which makes this procedure unsuitable for patients under 10; preferably the patient should be between 12 and 14 years of age. The peripheries of the tarsal bones are mainly cartilaginous in the young child and have a thicker cartilaginous surface to resect to permit bone-to-bone apposition when the foot is fused. Therefore, in the young child, this requires resection of large areas of joint surface, which results in shortening of a foot that is often short to begin with.

Sometimes preferable to a triple arthrodesis are combined procedures, such as the Dwyer operation, to correct hindfoot varus and metatarsal osteotomies to correct the forefoot adduction and/or cavus while leaving the midtarsus uncorrected. By doing hindfoot and forefoot surgery and leaving the midportion of the foot uncorrected, a plantigrade foot can be achieved. However, if significant supination is present preoperatively, this combined procedure is not indicated, because the prominence at the base of the fifth metatarsal on the plantar surface of the foot will persist. The patient will walk on the lateral plantar border of the foot and may experience considerable discomfort and callus formation. Cubocuneiform lateral closing and medial opening wedge osteotomies are the combined procedures of choice. The advantage of performing these combined osteotomies rather than the triple arthrodesis is that if significant joint motion remains it will be at the subtalar and midtarsal levels, which is advantageous, particularly for walking on uneven surfaces. The combined procedure is especially suitable for the patient who has a flat-top talus or markedly limited ankle motion.

Procedures Utilizing External Fixation

Grill and Franke have recently reported the results of their treatment of older children and adults with the Ilizarov distractor.[42] Ten feet in nine children, ages 8 to 15 years, were operated on. Only three of these feet had congenital talipes equinovarus; the other disorders were arthrogrypotic, neurogenic, or post-traumatic in origin. All 10 feet achieved the plantigrade position following treatment with the Ilizarov device, but all showed significant stiffness with very little motion at the midtarsal and subtalar joints. The ankle joint had an average of only 20 degrees of motion. However, all these feet were quite stiff prior to surgery. No muscular or sensory deficits occurred.

The advantages of this procedure in the older patient are that no bone resection is done and consequently no additional shortening results. Skin necrosis, pseudoarthrosis, infection, and vascular injury were avoided. Finally, it is not necessary to wait until the completion of skeletal growth for application of the device.

At this time, this procedure is restricted to the older child. It is unlikely that the Ilizarov distractor will replace the early use of conventional conservative and surgical techniques in younger patients.

INDICATIONS FOR SURGERY

General Indications

The general indications for surgery are a plateau in conservative treatment, the development of complications during or after conservative treatment, and the length of the foot.

The major indication for surgery is the failure of conservative treatment to achieve full correction. It may be difficult to determine exactly when a plateau has been reached. It is the author's opinion that if three or more radiographs demonstrate a lack of progress, a plateau has definitely been reached. Clinical criteria are less accurate; however, over a period of time it will become obvious that correction is not progressing.

Generally, at least 6 weeks of conservative treatment should be tried before surgery is employed. However, it may be ascertained as early 3 or 4 weeks that a plateau has been reached, particularly if the foot is very stiff and multiple manipulations, taping, or serial casting have been tried unsuccessfully. In this situation, holding casts should be used until the foot is 8 cm long.

The second indication for surgical treatment is the appearance of complications of conservative treatment. Some mild, spurious corrections are reversible, such as rocker-bottom deformity. However, other complications, such as the development of flat-top talus, are not reversible. If flat-top talus can be detected early by radiographic means, damage to the talus may be minimized. It is therefore prudent to use radiographic as well as clinical assessment.

The third indication for surgery is a foot length of more than 8 cm. The length of the foot is a better indication than the age of the child, as foot size can vary considerably at a given age, and it is the size of the foot that determines when surgery can be done. A foot that is smaller than 8 cm can easily be operated upon but the small tendons may pull apart following lengthening and repair.

There appears to be no well-defined cut-off point for any of the extensive soft tissue procedures (including complete subtalar release) at this time, although about 4 to 6 years is suggested as an upper age limit. The author has performed the complete subtalar release as late as 9 years of age with satisfactory results, although the patient has been followed for only 3 years.

Specific Indications

Specific indications are the residual deformities that are present when a plateau has been reached. These include equinus, varus, persisting calcaneal rotation (around the vertical axis), talonavicular subluxation, calcaneocuboid subluxation, forefoot adduction, supination, and cavus. In addition, other deformities resulting from spurious correction by conservative treatment or from previous operative procedures may require specific treatment modalities.

Indications for Extensive Soft Tissue Release

1. Persistence of varus deformity of the hindfoot despite conservative treatment. (Talonavicular subluxation may or may not be present. It requires the same treatment as varus.)
2. Significant uncorrected calcaneal rotation following an adequate trial of conservative treatment.
3. Failure of a partial subtalar release to correct hindfoot equinus deformity.

Indications for Limited Soft Tissue Release

1. Equinus is the only indication for a limited soft tissue release. (The author performs a more extensive variation of the commonly used posterior release—the partial subtalar release. See discussion under Author's Preferred Procedures.)

Indications for Ancillary Procedures

1. Calcaneocuboid capsulotomy is required for grade 2 and 3 calcaneocuboid subluxation.
2. Plantar release is required for forefoot adduction, cavus deformity, and calcaneocuboid subluxation.
3. Metatarsal osteotomies are required for forefoot adduction and cavus deformity not completely corrected by plantar release. It is difficult to quantify the degrees of metatarsus adductus and cavus that require surgery. However, when the foot is manually straightened, there should be no significant recoil when it is released. When there is significant recoil or the foot cannot be fully straightened, metatarsal osteotomies are indicated.
4. Calcaneal osteotomy is required for forefoot adduction and calcaneocuboid subluxation in the child over 3 years of age if plantar release is inadequate.

CONTRAINDICATIONS TO SURGERY

The contraindications to complete subtalar release are (1) a flat-top talus, (2) anterior ankle contracture, and (3) two or more previous extensive soft tissue procedures. The first two result in a restricted range of ankle motion, while the third produces excessive fibrosis. Flat-top talus results from forceful dorsiflexion during conservative treatment, while anterior ankle contracture may follow prolonged cast immobilization with the talus in the fully dorsiflexed position. This may occur either during or after conservative treatment or after previous surgery.

When the ankle is dorsiflexed and relatively fixed in this position, complete subtalar release (CSTR) or other extensive soft tissue release requires placement of the calcaneus into a position of deformity with respect to the talus, that is, the front of the foot will be elevated excessively (and fixed in this position) while the heel is too low, so that in walking, the front of the foot cannot be brought down into the toe-off position.

When a restricted range of motion is present preoperatively, it is imperative that lateral dorsiflexion–plantar flexion views be obtained to ascertain the extent of restriction of ankle motion and the location of the restricted range within the arc (Figs. 39–20A and B and 39–21A and B). When there is less than 30 degrees of motion and it is present only or mainly in the dorsiflexion range of the arc, a lateral arthrogram of the ankle will indicate whether this is due to a flat-top talus (Fig. 39–20C) or to an anterior ankle contracture (Fig. 39–21C). This is an important differentiation, because a flat-top talus does not respond well to surgical treatment, while an ankle contracture may be treated by an anterior ankle capsulotomy (performed before the definitive soft tissue release) in the older child (Fig. 39–21A to C). If a CSTR or other extensive soft tissue release is performed in the presence of either a flat-top talus or an anterior ankle contracture, the results will be compromised.

After two extensive soft tissue procedures the possibility of damage to the neurovascular tissues and articular surfaces due to postsurgical fibrosis is significant. Therefore, in this situation, it is best to wait until the child is old enough for bone surgery, usually at about 6 to 8 years of age.

AUTHOR'S PREFERRED PROCEDURES

The author prefers to perform either the partial subtalar release or the CSTR using the Cincinnati approach.[7, 18, 52]

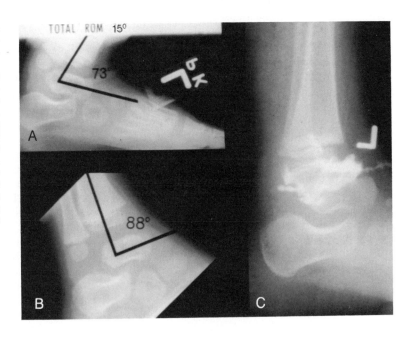

FIGURE 39–20. (A), Tibiotalar angle with the foot in maximal dorsiflexion. (B), Lateral tibiotalar angle with the foot in maximal plantar flexion. Note that the range of motion is decreased to 15 degrees with the motion restricted to the dorsiflexion portion of the arc. The restriction of motion of less than 30 degrees in this portion of the arc indicates either flat-top talus or anterior ankle contracture. (C), Arthrogram of the ankle showing flattening of the talar dome due to flat-top talus. (From Simons GW: The complete subtalar release in clubfeet. Orthop Clin North Am 18:667, 1987.)

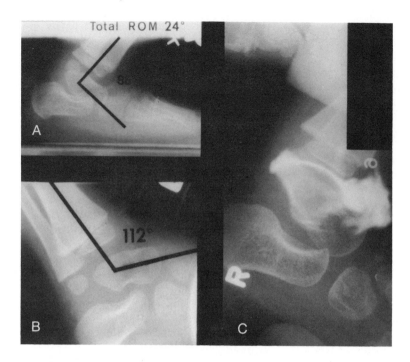

FIGURE 39–21. *(A)*, Dorsiflexion of foot with a tibiotalar angle of 88 degrees. *(B)*, Ankle in plantar flexion with a tibiotalar angle measuring 112 degrees. Therefore, the total range of ankle motion is 24 degrees with the range of motion in the dorsiflexion part of the arc. *(C)*, Ankle arthrogram with an almost normal dome of the talus. This indicates that the ankle does not have a flat-top talus but rather that the restriction of motion at the ankle joint is due to an anterior ankle contracture.

Definitions

The CSTR can be defined as a complete release of the following structures: the entire subtalar joint and talonavicular joint, the interosseous talocalcaneal ligament, the calcaneofibular ligament, the lateral subtalar capsule, and the capsule of the lateral aspect of the talonavicular joint, in addition to all the structures released through the conventional posterior medial release. In essence, the entire foot is released from the talus, then repositioned and pinned to the talus in a more normal relationship.

Partial subtalar release (PSTR) implies the surgical release of fewer structures than the CSTR. This, however, may vary from Achilles tendon and posterior tibial tendon lengthening with posterior capsulotomies of the ankle and subtalar joints to virtually complete subtalar release. The presence of equinus deformity (as the only residual deformity of the hindfoot) after conservative treatment is the only indication for PSTR. (In the uncorrected foot, on the AP view, the talocalcaneal angle should be less than 20 degrees, and there should be very slight or no divergence between the anterior talus and calcaneus, while the lateral view should show a talocalcaneal angle of less than 30 degrees.)

In a study of nine feet in which the only

significant deformity of the hindfoot was equinus, each anatomic structure was released that is normally released with the CSTR. Radiographs were taken after each stage of the release to identify those structures that had to be released in order to provide radiographically verifiable correction of the equinus deformity (Fig. 39–22). Unfortunately, release of the same structures was not required in every case. It was established, however, that certain structures must always be released, while the release of others was of varying importance. The structures that invariably require lengthening or release are the Achilles tendon, the posterior tibial tendon, the calcaneofibular ligament, the posterior ankle capsule, and part of the capsule of the subtalar joint. The incision in the ankle capsule must extend medially to the posterior tibial tendon sheath and laterally to the posterior talofibular ligament. The incision in the subtalar capsule must include the posterior capsule, and it must extend around the medial and lateral sides of the joint at least halfway to the front of the subtalar joint.

Release of the interosseous talocalcaneal ligament is required in some cases, but not all. In the more resistant cases, it is necessary to release the entire lateral subtalar capsule. In the most recalcitrant cases, this incision must be carried across the entire talonavicular joint,

FIGURE 39–22. Progressive improvement in the range of dorsiflexion at the ankle joint (progressive decrease in the lateral tibiotalar angle) as well as in the lateral tibiocalcaneal angle (not drawn). (A), Preoperative lateral view. (B), After lengthening of the Achilles tendon and posterior tibial tendon. (C), After posterior capsulotomies of ankle and subtalar joints. (D), After release of the calcaneal fibular ligament, posterior talofibular ligament extension of the ankle capsulotomy medially to the posterior tibial tendon sheath, and extension of the subtalar capsulotomy medially and laterally to approximately the midpoint of the subtalar joint. It is not until the structures in D have been released that significant improvement in both ankle dorsiflexion (the lateral tibiotalar angle) and subtalar movement (the lateral tibiocalcaneal angle) occurs.

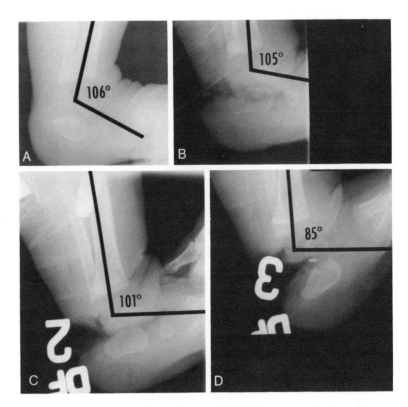

as well as medially, to release the entire medial subtalar joint, the talonavicular joint, and the anterior portion of the subtalar joint. In other words, the most severe cases require complete subtalar release.[92]

Cincinnati Approach

Advantages and Disadvantages

The major advantage of the Cincinnati approach over the conventional straight, oblique, or hockey stick medial incision is that it allows direct, easy access to all the areas of dissection, except for the small dorsal aspect of the talonavicular joint (Fig. 39–23). (Incisions favored by other surgeons are shown in Figures 39–24 and 39–25.)

This area underlies the skin bridge on the dorsum of the foot and can be released easily by dissection through the medial and lateral aspects of the Cincinnati incision. Adequate lengthening of the Achilles tendon can be

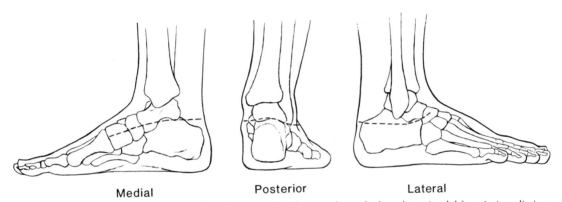

Medial   Posterior   Lateral

FIGURE 39–23. The Cincinnati incision. (From Simons GW: The complete subtalar release in clubfeet. I. A preliminary report. J Bone Joint Surg 67A:1044, 1985.)

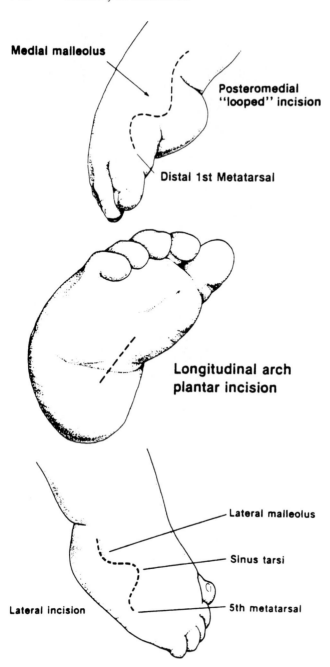

FIGURE 39–24. Incisions preferred by Gould and Goldner. (From Simons GW: Symposium: Current practices in the treatment of idiopathic club foot in the child between birth and five years of age. I. Contemp Orthop 17:63, 1988.)

achieved by subcutaneous dissection medially and laterally beneath the proximal skin flap.

The second advantage of this procedure is that with the patient in the prone position the foot is easily movable, so that one may switch from the medial to the posterior to the lateral wound with ease and with equally good visibility through all portions of the wound. The third advantage is that this procedure provides the best visualization of pathology and assessment of the ankle anatomy and motion of any incision. The fourth advantage is cosmetic: the scar is completely hidden by a shoe. The sole disadvantage of the Cincinnati approach is that there may be a slightly greater incidence of wound edge necrosis in the child over 3 years of age.

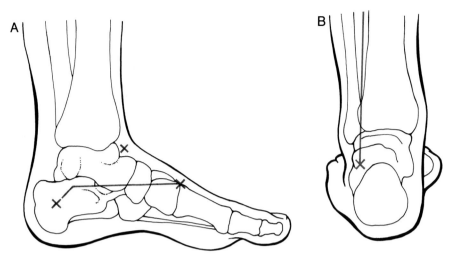

FIGURE 39–25. (*A* and *B*), Incisions preferred by Carroll. (From Simons GW: Symposium: Current practices in the treatment of idiopathic club foot in the child between birth and five years of age. I. Contemp Orthop 17:63, 1988.)

The Technique of the Complete Subtalar Release And Ancillary Procedures

Because of the complexity of the pathologic anatomy, the CSTR should be undertaken only by experienced surgeons who have knowledge of both the anatomy and the pathology involved.

When scheduling surgery, an extra one-half hour should be added so that the surgeon has adequate time at the end of the procedure to reposition the pins and obtain new radiographs if necessary. One of the most frequent mistakes is not allowing enough time for pin replacement and radiographs and therefore to accepting a result that intraoperative x-ray films would show to be unacceptable.

Marking and Exsanguination of the Leg

With the patient in the prone position, the knee is draped out so that it is visible when flexed. The patella and tibial apophyses are marked with an indelible pen for rotational orientation of the foot later in the procedure. The leg and foot are partially exsanguinated with an Ace bandage and the tourniquet inflated. Partial exsanguination makes identification of the neurovascular bundle easier, whereas complete exsanguination may totally occlude the veins, rendering them invisible.

The Incision

The Cincinnati incision may be less extensive on the medial and lateral side of the foot when a PSTR is performed. The incision for the CSTR needs to be extended only to the level of the first metatarsal-tarsal joint medially and to the calcaneocuboid joint laterally.

Superficial Medial Dissection

The superficial dissection is most easily carried out by using small, sharp-pointed tenotomy scissors inserted at a right angle to the wound to spread the underlying fat and subcutaneous tissues. Dissection of the abductor hallucis is performed on the medial side of the foot (Fig. 39–26). The superior edge of the midportion of the abductor hallucis muscle overlying the proximal first metatarsal and cuneiform is identified and reflected plantarward. The superficial portion of the abductor hallucis muscle is reflected inferiorly; a deep portion can be seen to originate from the fascia overlying the first metatarsal. In the proximal portion of this area, it takes its origin from fascia that often has the appearance of a double arcade (Fig. 39–27). The significance of locating this structure is that the medial branch of the plantar nerve, artery, and vein pass beneath the upper arcade. It is not necessary to open this arcade, but simply to be aware of it. However, the deep central origin of the abductor hallucis muscle may be reflected off this upper arcade and the arcade opened for better visualization. The superficial portion of the muscle may be transected, if desired, for better visualization of the neurovascular bun-

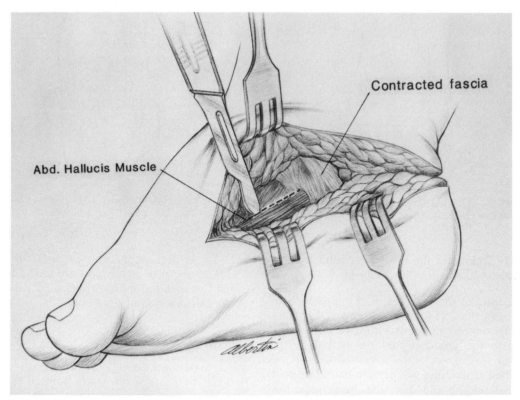

FIGURE 39–26. Dissection of the abductor hallucis from underlying tissues. (From Simons GW: The complete subtalar release in clubfeet. Orthop Clin North Am 18:667, 1987.)

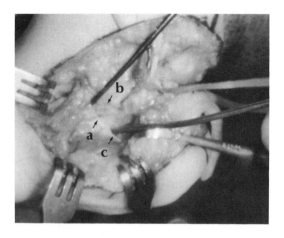

FIGURE 39–27. Double arcade from which the deep portion of the abductor hallux takes origin in the midfoot. The upper probe lies within the upper arcade (a). The neurovascular bundle can be seen passing beneath the upper arcade just below the probe (b). A second probe lies within the second arcade. A portion of the abductor hallucis remains attached to the lower arcade (c). (From Simons GW: The complete subtalar release in clubfeet. Orthop Clin North Am 18:667, 1987.)

dle, particularly the medial plantar nerve, which crosses in this part of the wound.

Frequently, a dense thickening of the fascia passes vertically across the neurovascular bundle in the area overlying the talonavicular joint and is particularly prominent in those feet that have a deep medial skin or plantar crease. This fascial band often appears contracted and may be difficult to release. If this band is very dense and extends deeply into the tissues, it is most easily handled by a scored Frazier dural elevator. The elevator is first inserted beneath one edge of this tissue, and the overlying tissue incised. Then the elevator is inserted beneath the opposite edge. Thus, by moving from one side to the other, one can work safely into the depth of this deep fibrous band without cutting into the neurovascular structures.

The next stage involves the dissection of the neurovascular bundle (Figs. 39–28 and 39–29). This is most easily achieved by first identifying the underlying veins that pass just behind the medial malleolus. By spreading the overlying adipose tissue, the laciniate ligament (crural fascia) overlying the neurovascular sheath comes into view. If one uses this plane of dissection, staying outside of the laciniate ligament, one can easily dissect the soft tissues overlying the ligament as far proximally as necessary, which brings the entire neurovascular bundle in this area into view. The veins in the neurovascular bundle can usually be visualized through the ligament.

When dealing with normal neurovascular structures, the laciniate ligament is incised and reflected from the neurovascular structures proximally and distally as far as the wound will permit (see Figs. 39–28 and 39–29). An umbilical tape can be inserted around the bundle for retraction. In dissecting the neurovascular bundle, it must be remembered that the bundle overlies the flexor hallucis longus tendon, which in turn overlies the subtalar joint on the medial side of the foot. The medial subtalar capsule must be released eventually. Therefore, the neurovascular bundle has to be dissected distal to the level of Henry's knot in order to achieve the freedom of retraction that

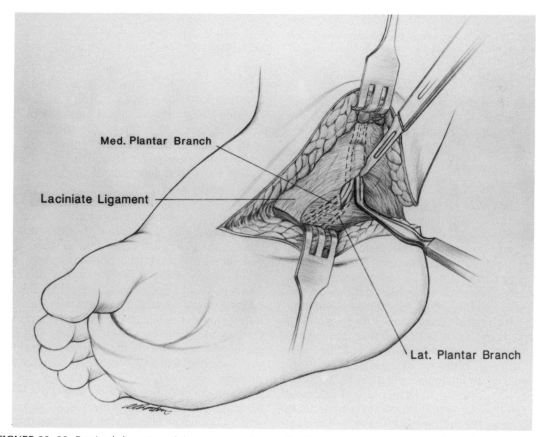

FIGURE 39–28. Proximal dissection of the neurovascular bundle. (From Simons GW: The complete subtalar release in clubfeet. Orthop Clin North Am 18:667, 1987.)

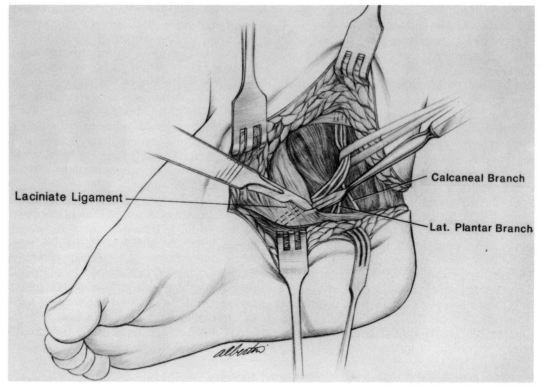

FIGURE 39–29. The laciniate ligament is incised from the level of the malleolus distally to the area where the neurovascular bundle passes into the midfoot. (From Simons GW: The complete subtalar release in clubfeet. Orthop Clin North Am 18:667, 1987.)

will be needed for this portion of the exposure. The calcaneal branch should be preserved, but the other minor branches should be released.

Identification and Treatment of an Anomalous Blood Supply

If the veins are not visible through the laciniate ligament, the tourniquet should be released for 1 to 2 seconds and, if necessary, this procedure should be repeated several times until the veins perfuse. Failure of the veins to perfuse after the tourniquet has been released several times should alert the surgeon to the possibility of an anomalous blood supply, which occurs in perhaps 1 to 2 percent of cases. If the veins fail to perfuse, the neurovascular bundle can be opened and the veins and arteries within it examined. If they are absent, an anomalous circulation exists (however, the posterior tibial nerve and calcaneal branch have been present within the bundle in three cases the author has observed). The next step is to carefully dissect posteriorly to iden-

tify the posterior peroneal artery and veins crossing obliquely over the lower end of the flexor hallucis longus tendon. In the proximal portion of the wound, these vessels will lie directly posteriorly (Fig. 39–30).

One must then determine if there are additional major arteries to the foot. The vessels should be manually occluded or occluded with smooth forceps and the tourniquet released. The location of the capillary refill gives an indication as to which vessels are present. One can see the skin on the dorsum of the foot filling slowly if the dorsalis pedis is present, but one should not expect to see the plantar surface of the foot filling adequately until the deep peroneal is released. If the circulation is coming only from this vessel, blood flow should readily be restored to the plantar surface of the foot but will only slowly return to the dorsum.

When the posterior peroneal vessel has been identified, it should be protected at all costs and additional smaller vessels protected if they are found. The peroneal vessel should be dis-

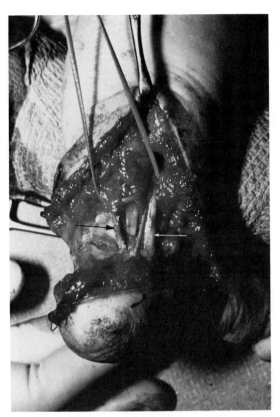

FIGURE 39–30. Anomalous circulation arising from the posterior peroneal artery. The posterior tibial artery is absent. *Top arrow,* anomalous artery; *bottom arrow,* posterior tibial nerve.

sected from surrounding tissues proximally and distally as much as possible, so that the vessel can stretch when the foot is brought out of its equinus position at the end of the procedure.

The flexor digitorum communis tendon is then dissected out of its sheath (Fig. 39–31). A long incision is made in this sheath from as far proximal as the skin incision will allow and distally to the level of Henry's knot in the plantar aspect of the foot. (Henry's knot is the thickening in the tendon sheaths of the flexor digitorum communis and flexor hallucis longus where they cross one another in the medial plantar surface of the foot.)[44] Care should be used in dissection of the sheath at this level as the plantar nerve lies very close to the distal end of the sheath. This tendon is freed from its sheath but not lengthened at this time. The posterior tibial tendon sheath is opened in a similar manner, approximately to the level of the ankle joint, but not distal to it, and then

the posterior tibial tendon is Z-lengthened. The Z-lengthening is carried as far proximally as the wound will permit (Fig. 39–32). The tendon of the flexor hallucis longus is exposed in the posterior medial aspect of the wound from as far proximally as the incision will allow and distally to the point where it passes beneath the medial edge of the talus and the neurovascular bundle. This exposure permits subsequent retraction of the tendon and bundle when the posterior medial capsulotomies of the ankle and subtalar joints are performed.

In addition to the vascular anomalies already mentioned, occasionally there is complete absence of the posterior tibial tendon. There may also be accessory tendons present, three of which insert into the calcaneus and two of which pass into the foot and insert into the flexor digitorum longus or the quadratus plantae. These tendons are as follows: the fibulocalcaneal tendon, the tibiocalcaneal tendon, the accessory soleus-calcaneal tendon, the accessory flexor digitorum longus tendon, and the accessory quadratus plantae tendon.[75] If an accessory tendon restricts correction it should be sectioned or lengthened.

Posterior Dissection

In performing the dissection posteriorly, first the Achilles tendon is lengthened (Fig. 39–32), either in the coronal or in the sagittal plane. The author prefers lengthening in the sagittal plane so that the distal medial attachment of the tendon can be released, thereby allowing a more lateral pull of the remaining distal portion of the tendon once it is repaired. The dissection should be extended as far proximal beneath the skin edge as possible. An Army-Navy retractor is used for greater visualization under the retracted flap, as often a greater length of Achilles tendon is necessary at the completion of the surgery than one anticipates. The Achilles tendon should be lengthened a minimum of 4 cm, and this should be increased proportionately for larger feet. This technique obviates the need for a second incision above the first in order to extend the tendon incision more proximally.

The next step in the dissection is capsulotomy of the posterior ankle joint. As one begins dissection at this level, the deep peroneal artery should be identified. It is usually a very small artery and can be transected, but if it is sizable, it should be dissected free and retained

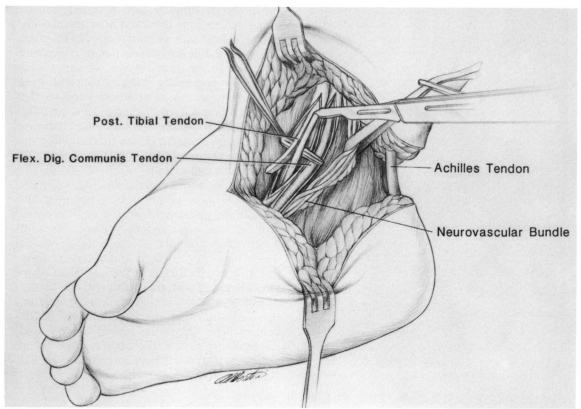

FIGURE 39–31. The flexor digitorum communis tendon lying within its sheath, which has been opened down to and including Henry's knot. However, this tendon is not lengthened at this time. The posterior tibial tendon is lengthened by the Z-lengthening technique. (From Simons GW: The complete subtalar release in clubfeet. Orthop Clin North Am 18:667, 1987.)

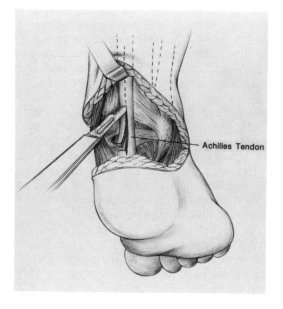

FIGURE 39–32. Achilles tendon lengthening by Z-lengthening technique.

if possible. The level of the capsulotomy is most easily discerned by flexing and extending the ankle while using the tip of an instrument to feel the level of the joint. A transverse incision is then made through the capsule, with care taken not to cut deeply. If one incises too proximally, the posterior physis of the tibia can be injured. Once the joint has been entered, the incision is extended laterally to the level of the peroneal tendons but not into the tendon sheaths. The incision is extended medially by keeping the knife within the joint while incising from within outward. This prevents injudicious incision of joint cartilage. As the dissection progresses medially, the flexor hallucis longus and neurovascular bundle are retracted first posteriorly and then anteriorly. By this means, the incision in the capsule can be extended further forward on the medial side of the foot to the level of the posterior tibial tendon sheath but not through the sheath. If this incision is extended too far distally, the talus will possibly subluxate out of the mortise. Therefore, if this capsular incision is extended distal to the posterior tibial tendon sheath, it should be repaired by one or two interrupted sutures. If the posterior tibial tendon sheath has not been dissected this far distally, it should be opened to the level of the ankle capsulotomy.

The next structure to be released is the posterior capsule of the subtalar joint (Fig. 39–33), which can be identified at the level of the flexor hallucis longus, where the tendon passes beneath the posterior medial edge of the talus. After the capsule is opened, this incision should be carried laterally to the level of the peroneal tendons, but no further. Medially, the incision can be extended to the lateral side of the flexor hallucis longus tendon. However, carrying the incision too far forward on the medial side at this stage of the dissection may injure the tendon or the joint surfaces and therefore is not advised. Next, the posterior talofibular ligament is incised vertically, just medial to the level of the peroneal tendon sheaths (Fig. 39–33). However, this ligament should not be incised too far inferiorly to avoid possible instability of the ankle joint. Once this ligament has been incised, the ankle joint will open further (Fig. 39–34). If the posterior talus is then moved up and down, it is easy to tell if enough of the posterior talofibular ligament has been released. When the ligament is adequately released, the posterior aspect of the joint usually opens relatively widely. If there is anterior ankle capsular contracture or flattening of the dome of the talus, movement of the talus in the ankle mortise will be restricted.

Lateral Dissection

Dissection then continues on the lateral side of the foot. The sural nerve is dissected prox-

FIGURE 39–33. The incision of the posterior talofibular ligament and posterior capsules.

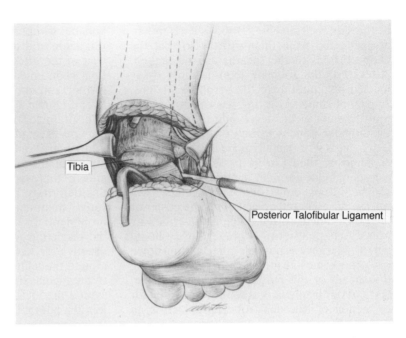

Tibia

Posterior Talofibular Ligament

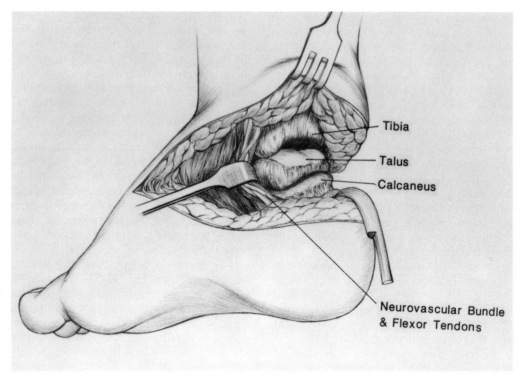

FIGURE 39–34. The hindfoot following posterior capsulotomy of the ankle joint and the posterior subtalar capsulotomy. The posterior talofibular ligament has been incised. The ankle and subtalar joints are open widely and easily seen. (From Simons GW: The complete subtalar release in clubfeet. Orthop Clin North Am 18:667, 1987.)

imally and distally 2 cm, then retracted posteriorly. The peroneal tendons are identified. The incision in the peroneal tendon sheath is made at the level of the subtalar joint, parallel to the skin incision (Fig. 39–35). The tendons are retracted from their sheaths so that the deep portions of the sheaths can be incised. After this, the subtalar joint is most easily located just anterior to the peroneal tendons. A pair of sharp dissecting scissors is inserted into the joint at this level, and the capsule of the subtalar joint is incised distally for about 2 to 3 cm and proximally beneath the tendons. A hemostat then can be passed beneath the calcaneofibular ligament, from posterior to anterior. Cutting down onto this ligament will release this tight tether as it binds the posterior lateral calcaneus to the fibula as described by McKay (Fig. 39–36). However, one should stay as inferiorly as possible when cutting down onto the hemostat in order to avoid opening the sheath of the peroneal tendons. The release of this ligament is absolutely essential for correction of calcaneal rotation, which is an

inherent part of the clubfoot deformity. Once the calcaneofibular ligament has been released, it is necessary to release the remainder of the posterior lateral subtalar capsule. It is then possible to open the subtalar joint further by retraction and to incise the posterolateral aspect of the interosseous ligament. The dissection is continued in the lateral subtalar capsule further anteriorly to allow entrance into the lateral talonavicular joint (Fig. 39–37). If it is difficult to locate the talonavicular joint, retraction is maintained to keep the subtalar joint open as one is incising distally. The lateral aspect of the talar head is prominent in this area if there is talonavicular subluxation. If this deformity has been corrected by conservative treatment, the talar head will not be prominent. In that case, it is imperative that the dissection follow the subtalar joint as far distally as necessary. One should dissect around the talar head and, if necessary, return to the medial side of the talonavicular joint to extend the incision laterally from that area to join the lateral incision. Misdirected dissection

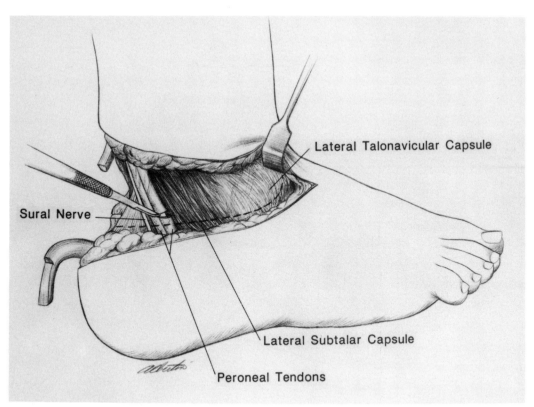

FIGURE 39–35. Incision of peroneal tendon sheaths at the level of the skin incision. (From Simons GW: The complete subtalar release in clubfeet. I. A preliminary report. J Bone Joint Surg 67A:1044, 1985.)

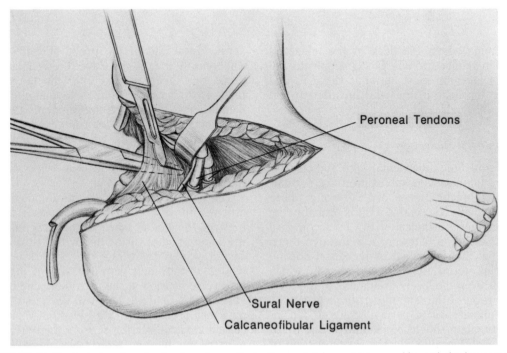

FIGURE 39–36. The technique for releasing the calcaneofibular ligament. A hemostat is passed beneath this ligament from the posterior wound into the lateral wound, and a scalpel is used to cut through the ligament onto the underlying hemostat. (From Simons GW: The complete subtalar release in clubfeet. Orthop Clin North Am 18:667, 1987.)

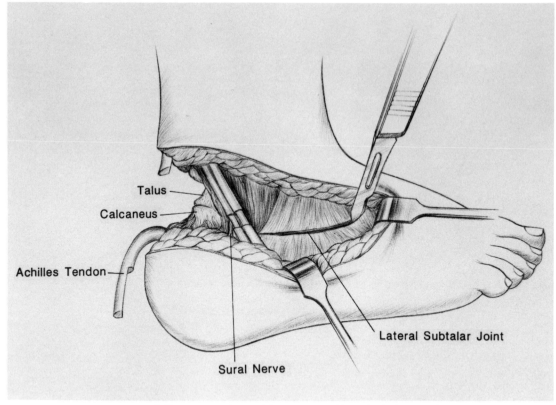

FIGURE 39–37. Release of the anterior and lateral subtalar capsule.

can extend across the neck of the talus and result in damage to the blood supply to the talus. Dissection must be made distal to and around the head of the talus in order to find the talonavicular joint.

Deep Medial Dissection

Locating the talonavicular joint and correcting the talonavicular subluxation are perhaps the most difficult aspects of CSTR, and failure to completely release this joint is probably the most common technical error. To accomplish this dissection, a blunt probe is inserted down the canal that is formed by the distal portion of the posterior tibial tendon sheath, which extends from the level of the ankle to the level of insertion of the tendon on the navicular. A longitudinal incision perpendicular to the inserting tendon should be made over the tip of the probe (Fig. 39–38). The distal portion of the tendon is passed out through this incision

at the distal end of the probe (Fig. 39–39). The reason that a special effort is made to retain this sheath is that after the tendon is replaced, it acts as a pulley to maintain the medial longitudinal arch and prevents the development of a flatfoot deformity. In addition, better excursion may be achieved by maintaining the tendon sheath as a canal. If the sheath is opened, more adhesions may form during the healing process.

The next step is to locate the tibionavicular articulation, a pseudoarticulation that forms between the medial aspect of the navicular and the anteromedial distal tip of the tibia. The easiest way is to retract the posterior tibial tendon distally and with the scalpel make a transverse incision at the proximal edge of the base of this tendon. This will open the tibionavicular articulation (Fig. 39–40). A pair of curved sharp dissecting scissors then are used to carry the incision in the fascia dorsally and volarward for several millimeters. This permits

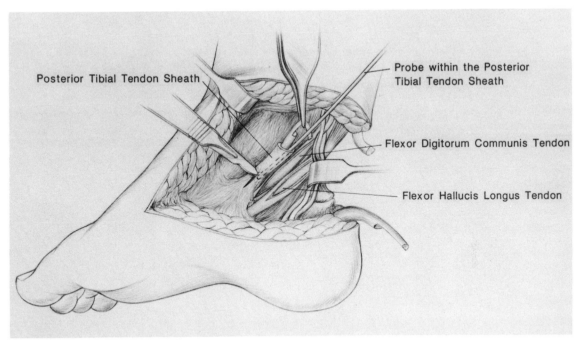

FIGURE 39–38. Incision made at the tip of the blunt probe which has been passed down through the posterior tibial tendon sheath.

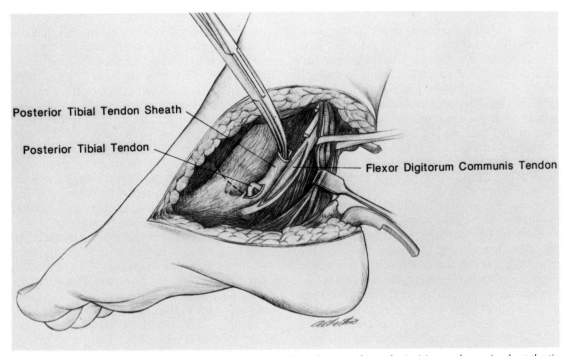

FIGURE 39–39. Passage of the posterior tibial tendon down through its canal into the incision made previously at the tip of the probe. (From Simons GW: The complete subtalar release in clubfeet. Orthop Clin North Am 18:667, 1987.)

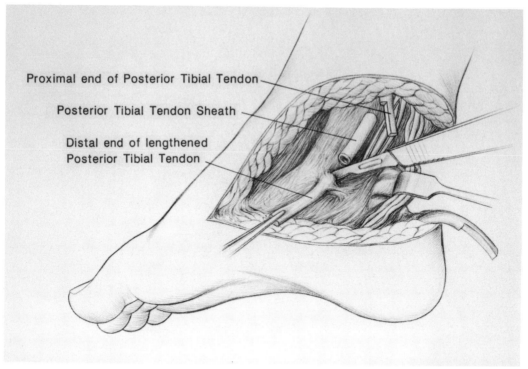

Proximal end of Posterior Tibial Tendon

Posterior Tibial Tendon Sheath

Distal end of lengthened
Posterior Tibial Tendon

FIGURE 39–40. Retraction of the posterior tibial tendon distally and incision at the base of the tendon to identify the tibionavicular articulation.

better visualization into the depth of this pseudoarticulation. If the real (talonavicular) joint is not visible, dissection is carried a little further dorsally and volarward while continued traction is applied to the posterior tibial tendon (Fig. 39–41). By taking a Beaver scalpel* with a right-angle Beaver blade and cutting into the base of the fascia at the depth of the tibionavicular articulation, one is usually able to enter the talonavicular joint without injuring the head of the talus, which lies within the depth of this articulation (Fig. 39–42). Once the talonavicular joint is identified, the anterior capsulotomy can be continued across the dorsum of the talonavicular joint, but care must be taken not to dissect proximally onto the talar neck, where the blood suppy enters the talus. In a similar manner, the dissection can be carried posteriorly around the plantar aspect of the talonavicular joint through the spring ligament complex. The talonavicular joint can be hinged open by pulling the posterior tibial tendon distally, while progressive dissection is made across the dorsum of the

*Rudolph Beaver Co., Waltham, MA.

joint. It is imperative while doing this that the dissecting scissors be kept beneath the tendons and the neurovascular bundle while staying on the capsule. This is made easier by inserting the blunt end of a Senn retractor beneath the tendons and neurovascular bundle as one proceeds across the dorsum of the foot to incise the capsule. At this point, it is possible that the dorsal talonavicular capsular incision on the medial side of the foot can be connected with the incision on the lateral side of the foot. If not, it may help to return to the lateral side of the foot momentarily and carry that incision medially to join the medial incision.

The neurovascular bundle lies superficial to the flexor hallucis longus tendon as it passes distally beneath the malleolus. The neurovascular bundle must be retracted anteriorly far enough to permit the flexor hallucis longus tendon sheath to be incised distally to the level of Henry's knot in the medial plantar aspect of the foot. It is imperative that the neurovascular bundle be retracted carefully at its distal portion, as the plantar nerve can easily be cut during incision of this portion of the sheath. Once this tendon has been released from its

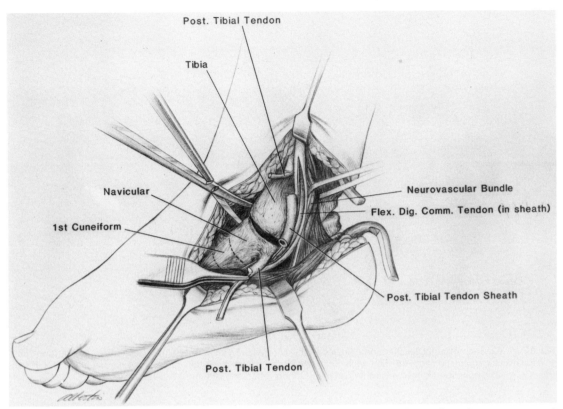

FIGURE 39–41. Dorsal (and volar) dissection of the capsule of the tibionavicular articulation allows the surgeon to reach the talonavicular joint, which lies in the depth of this wound. (From Simons GW: The complete subtalar release in clubfeet. I. A preliminary report. J Bone Joint Surg 67A:1044, 1985.)

sheath, it can be retracted anteriorly, giving the surgeon direct access to the superficial deltoid ligament and the medial subtalar capsule, which must be incised to effect complete release of the subtalar joint on the medial side of the foot (Fig. 39–43). In carrying out the subtalar dissection, one should progress posteriorly to anteriorly. As the anterior one-half to one-third of this joint is approached, locating the joint line can be greatly facilitated by looking into the posterior aspect of the subtalar joint through the posterior wound. On the medial side of the joint, a small cartilaginous column often can be seen projecting from the talus down to the calcaneus (Fig. 39–44); this column is actually a part of the inferior surface of the talar head and neck that overlies the sustentaculum tali. This is the structure that is often mistaken for a bar, as it is difficult to see the joint line across this area. When the joint line cannot be seen, the surgeon should release the interosseous ligament in its entirety and

then incise transversely through this vertical column at its base, not at its dorsum.

Dissection should then extend into the talonavicular joint and across the anterior portion of the subtalar joint, releasing the small anterior aspect of the joint. Once this has been achieved, any remaining portion of the interosseous talocalcaneal ligament can be released fully.

It is imperative that the connection between the medial and lateral aspects of the talonavicular joint be released by completely incising the dorsal capsule. Often one or more strands remain in this area, in which case adequate mobilization of the foot from the talar head cannot be accomplished. A hemostat should be passed across the subtalar joint and upward around the head of the talus from both the medial and lateral sides to make certain that residual strands of interosseous ligament or dorsal capsule of the talonavicular joint have been completely released.

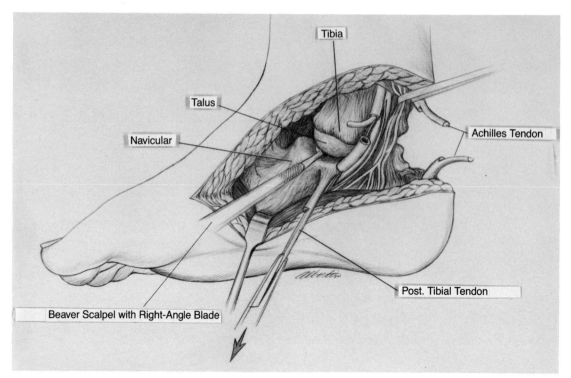

FIGURE 39–42. Technique for locating the entrance to the talonavicular joint. The joint is opened by cutting down into the talonavicular articulation with the right-angle Beaver blade, which is angled toward the distal portion of the foot. (From Simons GW: The complete subtalar release in clubfeet. Orthop Clin North Am 18:667, 1987.)

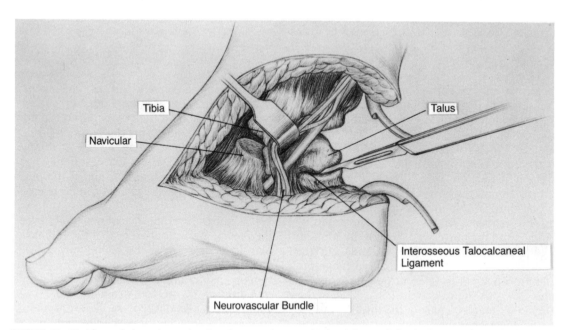

FIGURE 39–43. The technique for performing the posterior two-thirds of the medial subtalar capsulotomy. The flexor hallucis longus (FHL) lies between the neurovascular bundle and the medial capsule of the subtalar joint. The neurovascular bundle must be mobilized distally and retracted anteriorly to permit the incision in the tendon sheath of the FHL to be extended distally across Henry's knot. The medial plantar nerve lies close to the FHL as it approaches Henry's knot and must be identified and retracted carefully. The FHL must be released from its sheath until it permits exposure of the underlying medial subtalar capsule. After the capsulotomy of the posterior medial two-thirds of the subtalar joint has been made, the remaining part of the interosseous talocalcaneal ligament is incised. (From Simons GW: The complete subtalar release in clubfeet. Orthop Clin North Am 18:667, 1987.)

724

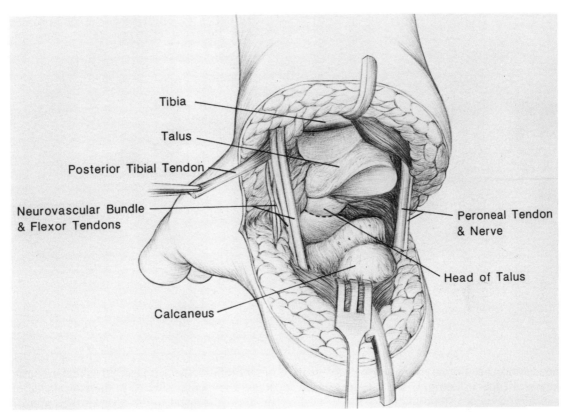

Tibia

Talus

Posterior Tibial Tendon

Neurovascular Bundle
& Flexor Tendons

Peroneal Tendon
& Nerve

Head of Talus

Calcaneus

FIGURE 39–44. An apparent cartilaginous column extending between the talus and calcaneus at the anterior aspect of the medial subtalar joint is actually the inferior surface of the talar head and neck. Visualized from the posterior wound, this may appear to form a vertical cartilaginous bar. The joint lies at the base of this structure and must be opened in order to release the medial subtalar joint. The dotted line indicates the area where the incision should be made. (From Simons GW: The complete subtalar release in clubfeet. Orthop Clin North Am 18:667, 1987.)

When the dissection is complete, the foot should be mobilized from the talus in the following manner. The foot should be plantar-flexed and then maximally inverted; thus, the plantar surface of the tibia will become fully exposed (Fig. 39–45). If the foot cannot be easily dislocated medially, the subtalar or the talonavicular joints have not been released completely. In the foot that has not had previous surgery, failure of medial dislocation of the foot is usually due to residual strands of the dorsal capsule of the talonavicular joint.

Once the foot has been dislocated medially from the talus, one has excellent vision of the plantar surface of the talus and the posterior aspects of the ankle and subtalar joint. If the foot is reduced into its preoperative position and rotated about 60 to 70 degrees externally into its proper, new position in relation to the ankle and leg, one can discern the true nature of the pathology that exists at the ankle level. This can be seen best through a Cincinnati incision.[7, 18, 90] By rotating the foot back into the fully deformed position, it is apparent that true ankle motion in this position involves eversion and inversion of the foot, whereas when the foot is placed into its fully corrected position, ankle flexion and extension occur in the normal plane with respect to the leg. Thus, the true nature of the pathology is demonstrated. Talar flexion and extension occur with minimal rotation within the mortise.

The talonavicular pin is now inserted unless one or more of the ancillary procedures are to be employed. The foot should be replaced beneath the talus before carrying out any ancillary procedure.

Ancillary Procedures

Once a complete subtalar release has been performed, a decision has to be made regarding the need for (1) plantar release, (2) calca-

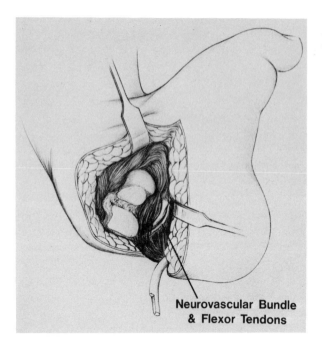

FIGURE 39–45. Medial dislocation of the foot off the talus. The plantar surface of the talus is viewed from the inferior aspect.

Neurovascular Bundle & Flexor Tendons

neocuboid capsulotomy or anterior calcaneal lateral wedge osteotomy, and (3) metatarsal capsulotomies or osteotomies.

Plantar Release

The first question is whether a plantar release is needed. If the plantar structures are tight on the medial side of the foot with significant residual forefoot adduction, if there is significant cavus deformity, or if there is significant subluxation of the calcaneocuboid joint, plantar release should be performed. Furthermore, the foot should be floppy and not tend to spring back strongly to the deformed position with manual correction. If the foot springs backward, then the release should be carried out. Definite contraindications for a plantar release are flatfoot or rocker-bottom deformity preoperatively. Failure to release plantar structures when indicated often results in recurrence of deformity. Yet in one case followed for 8 years in which there was marked residual forefoot adduction at the end of surgery, the deformity corrected gradually over that time span.

The plantar release is accomplished by making a small incision in the subcutaneous tissues just beneath the skin adjacent to the area where the calcaneal nerve and the main branch of the posterior tibial nerve bifurcate. A pair of tenotomy scissors is inserted subcutaneously across the plantar surface to the lateral side of the foot just distal to the level of the anterior calcaneus. This incision is kept superficial to the plantar fascia. The scissors are spread as they are removed. Thus, this dissection extends superficially to the plantar fascia all the way across the foot. A second small incision is made in the axilla of the bifurcation between the calcaneal branch and the lateral branch of the plantar nerve but deep to the plantar fascia, abductor hallucis, and quadratus plantae. This incision is also spread open with the dissecting scissors. Using a heavier pair of scissors such as curved Mayo scissors, one blade is placed into each of these two wounds with the tip pointed proximally toward the calcaneus. With one stroke, the plantar fascia, superficial and deep portions of the abductor hallucis, quadratus plantae, and flexor hallucis brevis are released. If the scissor tips are kept on the anterior edge of the calcaneus, the lateral plantar artery and nerve will not be injured (Fig. 39–46). A gloved finger may be inserted into the depth of the wound to determine whether any tight structures originating from the plantar surface of the calcaneus remain. If so, they should be released also. Unless there is a fixed cavus deformity or forefoot deformity, improvement in the alignment of the foot will be seen.

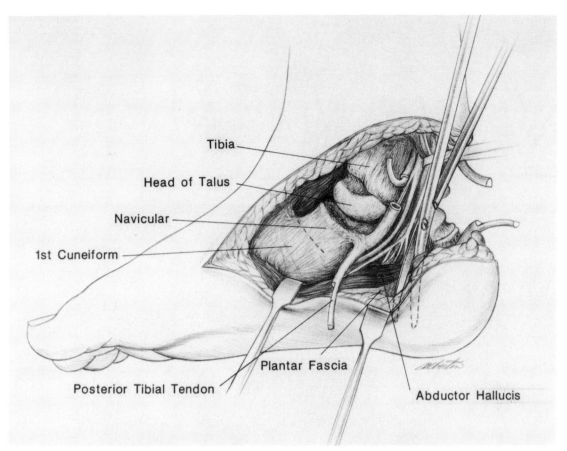

Tibia

Head of Talus

Navicular

1st Cuneiform

Plantar Fascia

Posterior Tibial Tendon

Abductor Hallucis

FIGURE 39–46. Technique of plantar release. (From Simons GW: The complete subtalar release in clubfeet. I. A preliminary report. J Bone Joint Surg 67A:1044, 1985.)

Calcaneocuboid Capsulotomy

In a child under approximately 3 years of age, the author prefers a calcaneocuboid capsulotomy to a calcaneocuboid osteotomy. Calcaneocuboid capsulotomy is indicated for persistent calcaneocuboid subluxation following complete subtalar release. While mild calcaneocuboid subluxation is frequently present, it is only occasionally found in moderate and marked degrees (about 25 percent). Diagnosis of calcaneocuboid subluxation is made on the anteroposterior radiograph, which shows that the central point of the ossifying cuboid bone is medially displaced with respect to the longitudinal axis of the calcaneus (Fig. 39–47A).[107]

The grades of subluxation are as follows:

Grade 0—The central point of the cuboid ossification center normally lies on the longitudinal axis of the calcaneus.

Grade 1—The central point of the cuboid ossification center lies between the longitudinal axis of the calcaneus and a line along the medial border of the calcaneus parallel to the longitudinal axis (the medial tangent).

Grade 2—The central point of the ossification center lies medial to the medial tangent (Fig. 39–47B).*

Grade 3—The ossification center of the cuboid has migrated proximally to the distal ossified portion of the calcaneus (Fig. 39–47B).

Grade 1 subluxation does not appear to cause significant secondary displacement of any other joints and, therefore, does not require correction. Surgical correction is indicated if grade 2 or 3 subluxation is present.

The release of this joint on the dorsal,

---

*As the valgus deformity decreases, the outline of the sustentaculum comes into view and makes the medial border of the calcaneus irregular. The medial line must then be drawn from the point where the distal rounded medial end of the calcaneus straightens out or curves medially. It is drawn through this point parallel to the axis of the calcaneus.

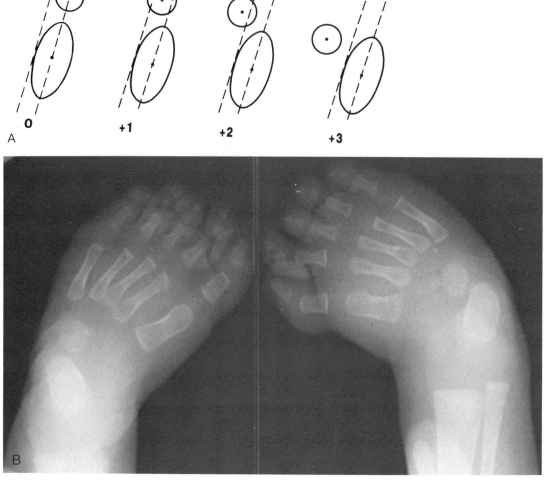

FIGURE 39–47. (A), Radiographic classification of calcaneocuboid subluxation (see text for details). (B), Grade 2 calcaneocuboid subluxation bilaterally.

medial, and volar surfaces while the lateral capsule remains intact has resulted in marked deformity of the calcaneus. Apparently the oblique end of the calcaneus allows the cuboid to rotate on the distal end of the calcaneus, and the calcaneus then moves into a marked degree of valgus (Fig. 39–48A and D). Correction of this deformity requires a circumfer-ential incision of the calcaneocuboid capsule, reduction on the distal end of the calcaneus, and fixation with one or two threaded Kirschner wires (Fig. 39–49). Figure 39–50 illustrates the consequences of (1) no treatment, (2) failure to employ a calcaneocuboid capsulotomy when indicated, (3) partial release, (4) complete release, and (5) translation.

FIGURE 39–48. (A), Preoperative radiograph showing calcaneocuboid subluxation. (B), Following dorsal, volar, and medial capsulotomy of the calcaneocuboid joint leaving the lateral capsule intact. There is excessive external rotation of the calcaneus with the calcaneocuboid subluxation considerably worse. The plantar release had not been performed at this stage but the lateral capsule remained intact. (C), Attempted manipulation and pinning only made the situation worse. The metatarsal adduction was more severe. (D), Following removal of the pins, complete calcaneocuboid capsulotomy, plantar release, replacement of the cuboid on the distal end of the calcaneus, and pinning. Note the satisfactory calcaneocuboid alignment following this procedure.

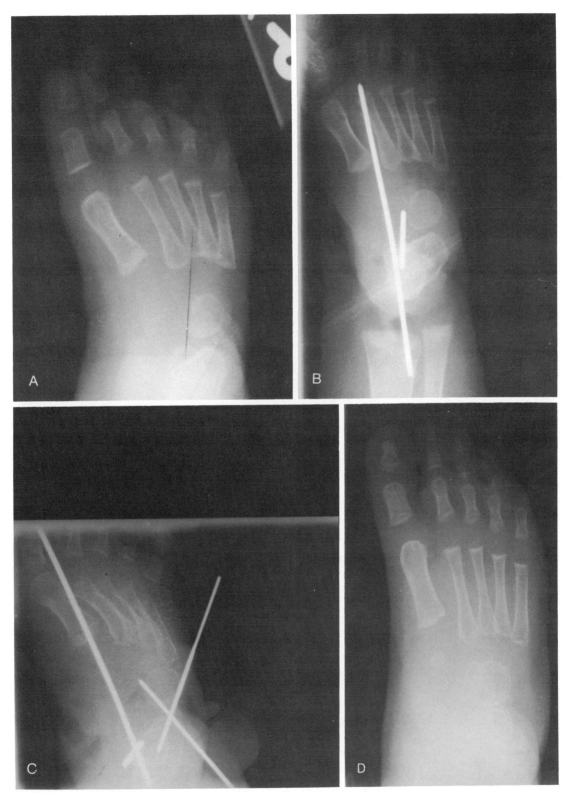

FIGURE 39–48 *See legend on opposite page*

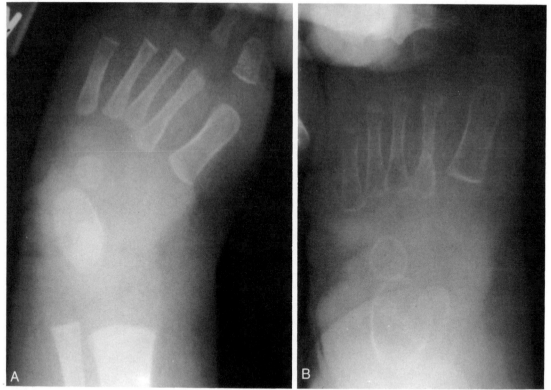

FIGURE 39–49. (A), Marked calcaneocuboid subluxation preoperatively. (B), Postoperative correction of the calcaneocuboid malalignment. Note also that the talar axis passes through the base of the first metatarsal, the APTC angle is normal, and the metatarsal alignment is normal.

In performing this capsulotomy, the approach is made through the anterior portion of the lateral wound. The joint line, which is sometimes difficult to palpate, is located at the apex of the bony prominence in this area. The anterior calcaneus has an inclination at the apex of which the joint line is most easily found. Also, the joint itself is oriented to the lateral surfaces of the calcaneus and cuboid, so that it is directed obliquely posteriorly and medially. Release of this joint requires careful dissection beneath the peroneal tendons and placement of a small Homan retractor between the inferior surface of the calcaneus and the tendons. Once this has been inserted, the lateral and plantar surfaces of the joint capsule

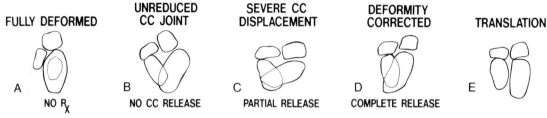

FIGURE 39–50. Drawings of the various anatomic configurations that may be seen in feet with calcaneocuboid subluxation. (A), Untreated foot. (B), The navicular is reduced on the talar head but calcaneocuboid subluxation is still present. The calcaneus has rotated into a valgus position because the navicular, cuboid, and calcaneus act as a single unit of bone when they are entirely released from the talus. (C), Reduction of the navicular on the talus but even greater subluxation of the cuboid and calcaneus following partial release of the calcaneocuboid joint. (D), Complete correction of calcaneocuboid subluxation following complete release of the calcaneocuboid joint. (E), Translation with persisting calcaneocuboid subluxation. (Translation may also exist without calcaneocuboid subluxation.)

can be easily incised. However, when incising into the depth of this joint, one often has to carry the dissection deeper than is initially anticipated. The cuboid should move freely on the calcaneus once the joint is completely released. It is a common mistake to release this joint incompletely. Consequently, the lateral translation that is required for its correction may not be achieved.[107]

Finally, a plantar release should be performed when the calcaneocuboid joint is released if tightness of the medial plantar structures becomes more prominent or persists after the calcaneocuboid joint is reduced.

Calcaneal Osteotomy

In the child over 3 years of age in whom there is significant residual forefoot adduction or cavus following complete subtalar release or in the child over 3 years of age who presents with significant calcaneocuboid subluxation, the author prefers to use a laterally based, vertical closed wedge osteotomy of the anterior aspect of the calcaneus, staying approximately 0.5 to 1 cm proximal to the joint margin (Fig. 39–51). By performing an osteotomy at this level, it is possible to realign the midfoot and forefoot to a significant degree. In conjunction with a plantar release, this will often provide satisfactory repositioning of the forefoot so that no subsequent surgery of the forefoot is necessary. The advantage of calcaneal osteotomy over the Evans[1, 29, 30] and Lichtblau[56] procedures is that the articular surfaces of the calcaneocuboid joint are left intact. The sole disadvantage of this osteotomy is that it crosses the anterior facet joint, which may cause mild incongruity at this level in the older patient. This has not been a major problem in any of

our patients, however, so that this objection seems to be more theoretical than actual.

Metatarsal Capsulotomy or Osteotomy

In the author's experience, the plantar release and calcaneocuboid capsulotomies (or anterolateral calcaneal osteotomies) have reduced the need to perform forefoot correction.

Various techniques can be used to correct the forefoot, ranging from capsulotomy at the first metatarsal cuneiform joint to capsulotomies of all five metatarsal-tarsal joints. We have also done metatarsal osteotomies of the second and third metatarsals as well as osteotomies of all five metatarsals. Selective osteotomies at the bases of the second and third metatarsals were done on the assumption that the second metatarsal was wedged into a mortise at its base and that the osteotomy of the second and third metatarsals would allow mobilization of all five. Mobilization of the second and third metatarsals by osteotomy, however, did not prove completely satisfactory. Complete correction was not achieved in some cases, and in malunion and nonunion occurred in some patients less than 2 years of age. Now we rarely perform capsulotomies or osteotomies to correct the forefoot at the same time that a complete subtalar release is performed.

Repositioning and Pinning of the Foot

Two or three threaded pins are used to fix the midfoot and hindfoot in the corrected position: the talonavicular pin, the calcaneotalar pin, and occasionally a calcaneocuboid pin.

The Calcaneocuboid Pin

If the calcaneocuboid joint has been released, this pin is inserted first. This pin is inserted into the anterior aspect of the calcaneus to exit posteriorly, and it is then passed from posterior to anterior to cross the calcaneocuboid joint and the cuboid and come out the dorsal lateral side of the foot. As it is being inserted, three-point pressure is applied so that the calcaneocuboid joint is maximally corrected. The cuboid may tend to subluxate dorsally or plantarward, and the positions of these bones should be checked radiographically after pin insertion.

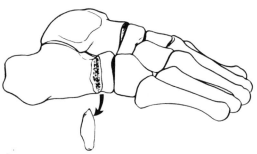

Lateral Calcaneal Osteotomy

FIGURE 39–51. Removal of a lateral wedge from the anterior lateral calcaneus to shorten the lateral column of the foot.

The Talonavicular Pin

Insertion of the talonavicular pin is facilitated by medially dislocating the foot. To accomplish this, the foot is plantarflexed and then everted. With the foot held in this position, a threaded 6-inch Kirschner wire with pointed tips at both ends is inserted into the center of the most distal point of the talar head (Fig. 39–52). Complete exposure of the talar head is paramount for pin placement. While we formerly placed the pin through the posterior aspect of the talus in a forward direction, we now believe it is better to insert this pin through the talar head. Thus exact central placement of the pin in the talar head is achieved and secure fixation of the navicular obtained. Posterior insertion may permit eccentric location of the pin as it exits through the talar head, with poor purchase in the navicular (Fig. 39–53).

Once the pin has been placed through the talar head, it should emerge at or near the posterior lateral ridge of the talus. If it is more than several millimeters from the ridge, it should be withdrawn and reinserted. Drilling through the talus continues until the pin protrudes several inches posteriorly. The drill bit

is removed from the anterior end of the pin and is attached to the posterior end. The pin is then drilled retrograde until the anterior tip is buried just beneath the articular surface of the talar head (Fig. 39–54). This is time consuming, but it is the easiest way to achieve exact positioning for pinning of the talonavicular joint.

Repositioning the Foot on the Talus

Accurate repositioning of the foot is the most important part of the procedure. Unfortunately, it is difficult and requires considerable experience. The foot must be replaced as closely as possible to the normal position. Two millimeters of misplacement is often too much to accept! To achieve this degree of accuracy, the foot is held by the surgeon with the palm of the hand over the plantar surface of the foot, the thumb placed over the medial side of the talonavicular joint, and the index or long finger placed in the lateral wound. Simultaneously, the posterior aspect of the subtalar joint is observed. The important clinical features for repositioning are as follows: (1) The navicular must protrude a short distance medially be-

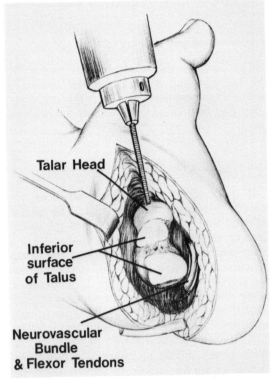

FIGURE 39–52. Insertion of the talonavicular pin into the center of the talar head.

Talar Head

Inferior surface of Talus

Neurovascular Bundle & Flexor Tendons

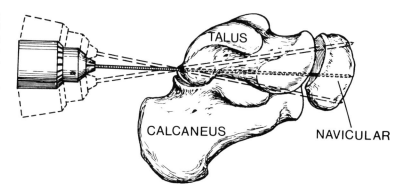

FIGURE 39–53. Improper insertion of the talonavicular pin through the posterior talus. Note that if the pin is not positioned with extreme accuracy, it will pass anteriorly, inferiorly, medially, or laterally, with possible poor fixation of the navicular. Therefore, pin insertion through the talar read is perferable.

TALUS

CALCANEUS

NAVICULAR

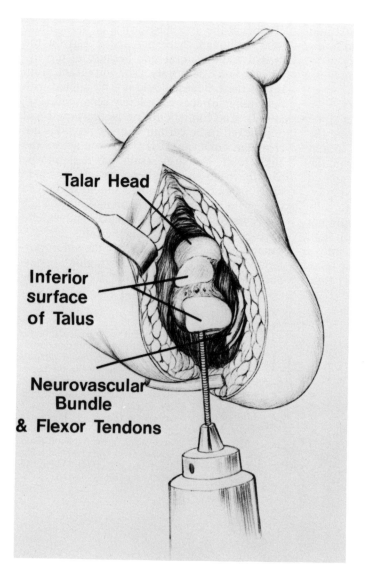

Talar Head

Inferior
surface
of Talus

Neurovascular
Bundle
& Flexor Tendons

FIGURE 39–54. Retrograde drilling for removing the pin backward until the point reaches the subchondral bone of the talar head. At this point the navicular is reduced on the talus and pinning of the joint is carried out by drilling the pin forward.

yond the talar head. It should not be placed flush with the medial aspect of the talar head (Fig. 39–55). (2) The dorsal surface of the navicular should correspond to the level of the dorsal surface of the talar head. (3) The talus must be in longitudinal alignment with the navicular and midfoot (i.e., it should not be markedly plantarflexed or dorsiflexed). (4) The index or long finger in the lateral wound should palpate the talonavicular joint as the pinning takes place, and there should not be a step-off at this joint. (5) The posterior aspect of the subtalar joint should be closed.

The pin is inserted across the talonavicular joint very slowly. If inserted rapidly, the pin may push the navicular away from the talus before penetrating it, leaving a gap between these two bones. In general, the pin should be aimed toward the cleft between the first and second metatarsal on the dorsum of the foot.

Checking the Position of the Foot Clinically

Next, the position of the foot should be checked carefully. This is done by flexing the knee and holding the foot and the leg so that the foot is at a right angle to the leg. From the front, the alignment of the foot is compared with the knee, which was marked previously. The foot should not appear to be internally rotated with respect to the tibia. It should not be in a supinated or a pronated position, and it should not be translated or tilted into a valgus position. The foot should appear to be absolutely plantigrade and have normal rota-

tion, so that it is in 0 to 20 degrees of external rotation with respect to the tibial apophyseal landmark (Fig. 39–56).

The Calcaneotalar Pin

The final pin is placed through the plantar surface of the calcaneus across the subtalar joint and into the talus but not into the ankle joint or the tibia. This pin should be placed while light lateral pressure is applied to the heel to push it away from the fibula. The posterior lateral surfaces of the calcaneus and talus should not have a step-off, and the articular surfaces should be closed as much as possible with the calcaneus in a vertical position; that is, the calcaneus should not be tilted into varus or valgus. This usually allows closure of most of the articular surface of the subtalar joint, although there may be a gap on the medial and/or lateral side because of the significant bony deformity. The important point is that these bones should not be pinned with their joint surfaces completely separated (Fig. 39–57). The foot should be plantarflexed and dorsiflexed to be certain that the pin does not cross the ankle joint. If the pin is across the ankle joint, no harm results but it should be withdrawn so that it does not restrict ankle range of motion. The ankle should be moved through a maximal range of motion at each cast change. Once the navicular and cuboid have been repositioned on the talus and calcaneus, a remarkable change in the anteroposterior (AP) and lateral radiographic appearances will occur with very little, if any, opening

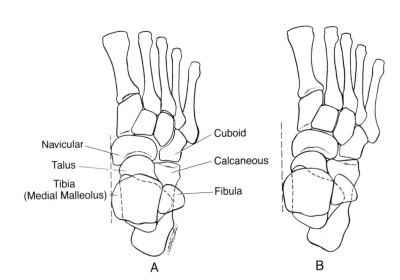

Navicular

Talus

Tibia
(Medial Malleolus)

Cuboid

Calcaneous

Fibula

A   B

FIGURE 39–55. (A), Normal repositioning of the navicular on the talar head, i.e., the medial portion of the navicular should protrude slightly medially while the lateral aspect of the talonavicular joint should be flush, without a step-off. (B), Overcorrection of the navicular on the talar head. This results in lateral talonavicular subluxation and valgus of the hindfoot. (From Simons GW: The complete subtalar release in clubfeet. Orthop Clin North Am 18:667, 1987.)

FIGURE 39–56. The abnormal and normal positions of the foot, which may be seen on careful clinical inspection once pinning has been achieved. (From Simons GW: The complete subtalar release in clubfeet. I. A preliminary report. J Bone Joint Surg 67A:1044, 1985.)

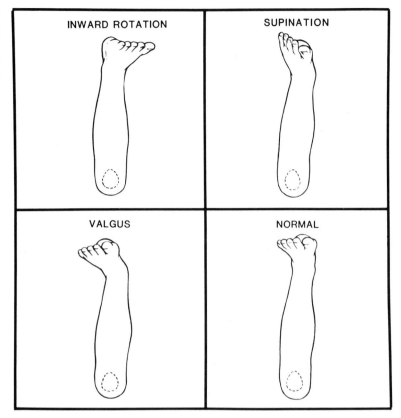

of the subtalar joint. The AP and lateral talocalcaneal angles should be restored to normal.

The Flexor Tendons

Before radiographs are taken, the toe flexor tendons should be examined to determine whether they should be lengthened. If the toes cannot be brought to the neutral position with the foot plantigrade, the tendons should be Z-lengthened. Frequently, the flexor hallucis longus requires lengthening, but the flexor digitorum communis does only occasionally.

Following placement of the pins and lengthening of the toe flexor tendons, the position of the foot should again be examined clinically as previously described before intraoperative radiographs are obtained. If the posterior portion of the talonavicular pin blocks plantar flexion, it should be drilled anteriorly until the tip lies just beneath the cartilage of the posterior talus.

Intraoperative Radiographic Evaluation

Positioning the Foot

It is imperative that the position of the foot be checked radiographically during surgery after pin placement. Failure to do this deprives the patient of one of the most important aspects of the entire procedure: ascertaining that the foot is properly corrected (i.e., neither overcorrected nor undercorrected). When the intraoperative radiographs are taken, posteroanterior and lateral views should be obtained. For the posteroanterior view, the cassette is placed near the end of the table and the foot is simply laid on the cassette, as the patient is already in the prone position. They x-ray beam is angled 25 to 30 degrees from the vertical position. The x-ray unit should be absolutely perpendicular to the foot, not tilted to one side or the other. When this view has been taken in the proper manner, the anterior portion of the talar head will appear at the same transverse level as the anterior portion of the calcaneus. If the calcaneus is too far forward, the film was taken with the x-ray unit too horizontal; when the talar head is in front of the calcaneus, the beam was taken with the x-ray unit too vertical. Occasionally in the very young child whose talar ossification center is small, the x-ray unit must be positioned at a greater angle from the vertical, perhaps as much as 45 degrees (see Fig. 39–13). In addi-

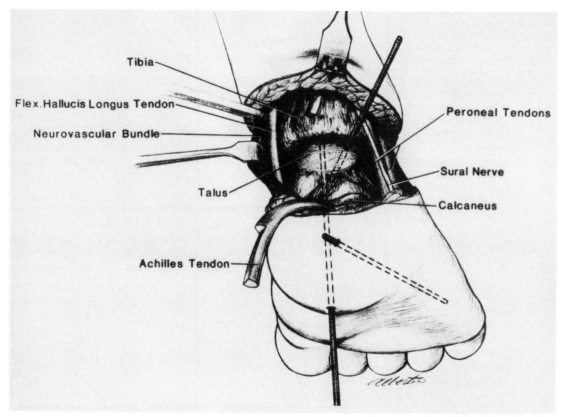

FIGURE 39–57. Posterior view of the ankle with all three pins in place. Note that the subtalar joint is virtually closed except on the medial side. (From Simons GW: The complete subtalar release in clubfeet. I. A preliminary report. J Bone Joint Surg 67A:1044, 1985.)

tion, the foot should be positioned so that it is tilted neither medially nor laterally; thus, a projection is taken at a true right angle to the foot.

The lateral view is a routine cross-table lateral projection with the foot held in maximum dorsiflexion and parallel to the cassette. As much of the metatarsals should be included as possible without exposing the surgeon's fingers.

Interpretation of the Radiographs

The posteroanterior (PA) radiograph provides the same measurements as the AP radiograph and should show the following six features if acceptable correction has been achieved: (1) The posteroanterior talocalcaneal (PATC) angle should be between 20 and 40 degrees (see Fig. 39–14A). (2) There should

not be a very deep cleft at the anterior ends of the talus and calcaneus; that is, the depth of the divergence between these two bones should be minimal (see Fig. 39–16). A deep cleft implies that the anterior calcaneus has been rotated laterally or the whole calcaneus translated too far laterally. (3) About 50 percent of the ossification centers of the talus and calcaneus should overlap in a medial-lateral direction. Less overlap implies that the whole calcaneus has been translated laterally. When minimal overlap exists, the foot may not be stable and the talar head may subluxate medially off the sustentaculum tali (Fig. 39–58B). (4) The talar axis should pass across the base of the first metatarsal. It does not have to pass down the shaft to be in proper alignment, because there may be some residual forefoot adduction or abduction (see Fig. 39–15). (5) The calcaneocuboid joint must be reduced if

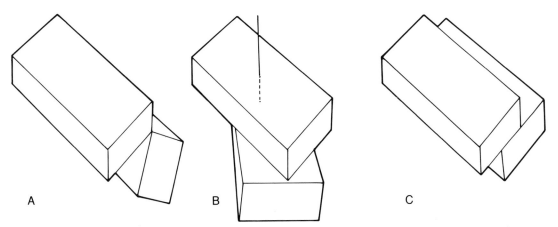

FIGURE 39–58. Three types of valgus that can occur as complications following surgery for clubfoot deformity. *(A)*, Hinge valgus occurs when the anterior, medial, and posterior subtalar joints are released, leaving the lateral subtalar capsule intact. This may occur following Turco's procedure. *(B)*, Rotary valgus can follow complete release of the subtalar joint (with or without release of the interosseus talocalcaneal ligaments). The anterior calcaneus rotates excessively in a lateral direction while the posterior calcaneus remains stationary or rotates inward excessively. *(C)*, Transitory valgus occurs when the entire calcaneus translates laterally after release from the talus.

it shows grade 2 or 3 subluxation (see Fig. 39–17). (6) The metatarsals should not converge but should diverge with a relatively straight lateral border of the entire foot, the fifth metatarsal being more or less parallel with the calcaneus in this projection (see Fig. 39–14A). The normal calcaneal–fifth metatarsal angle is 0 degrees.

On the lateral view, the lateral talocalcaneal angle should measure 30 to 55 degrees (see Fig. 39–14B). The talar axis should bisect the base of the first metatarsal (see Fig. 39–14B and 39–18). It may be hard to evaluate the position of the first metatarsal because of the overlap of the other metatarsals. However, the metatarsals should not be markedly displaced above or below the level of the talar head on the lateral projection. The foot should not appear to have a marked cavus component (see Fig. 39–14B). The lateral talar first metatarsal angle normally measures 0 degrees.[88] Finally, there should be neither superior nor inferior subluxation of the calcaneocuboid joint if the joint has been released.

If these criteria are not met, the pins should be removed and the foot repositioned and repinned. As little as 2 mm of movement in the young child may realign the foot to the fully corrected position. The surgeon should try to limit the pin insertions to a maximum of three. With experience, satisfactory insertion can usually be accomplished on the first attempt. More than three attempts can be made

if necessary but damage to the ossification center may occur, although the author has never seen this. New radiographs are required for re-evaluation after each set of pin placements. About 15 minutes is needed to take, process, and read each set of films.

Wound Closure and Cast Application

Once proper pin placement is verified radiographically, the anterior tip of the talonavicular pin is backed out in an anterior direction until its posterior tip lies within the talus. All pins are then cut off just beneath the surface of the skin. As all pins are threaded, migration has not been a problem and pin tract infection has been virtually nonexistent.

After hemostasis has been obtained, the tendons are repaired with absorbable sutures. The posterior tibial tendon is replaced through its tunnel beneath the medial malleolus. Traction should be placed on both ends of this tendon by the assistant while the surgeon places the suture. This assures proper tension when the sutures are inserted. Once repaired, the tendons should be just minimally tight with no slack. If lengthened, the toe flexor tendons are repaired and replaced in their sheaths. The Achilles tendon, likewise, is repaired under slight tension with the foot in approximately 10 degrees of dorsiflexion. The subcutaneous tissues are closed with interrupted sutures. A tight subcutaneous closure around the heel, particularly on its medial side, is important for skin healing without necrosis. A continuous absorbable suture is placed in the skin. The skin is carefully checked for capillary refill by dorsiflexing the foot maximally and letting it down slowly into a plantarflexed position until capillary return is observed. Steritapes are applied and a small strip of cotton is placed along the dorsum of the foot and front of the leg before cast padding is applied. This protects the foot if it is inadvertently moved into dorsiflexion during cast application. In this way, an internal ridge that may form within the cast or constriction by the cast padding will not cut into the dorsum of the foot, jeopardizing the blood supply and viability of the skin in this area. This pad should be about 1/4 inch thick and 1 to 2 inches wide. If the cast needs to be split, this pad also protects the underlying skin.

After padding, plaster is applied with the foot in 10 degrees of plantar flexion beyond the point where capillary refill was observed and in about 20 degrees external rotation with respect to the knee. Three-point pressure is applied to the foot so that the forefoot can be brought into maximal abduction. The knee is placed at 90 degrees, and the cast includes the proximal thigh.

Postoperative Care

The patient is placed in a crib or bed and the foot is immediately placed in a sling suspended from an overhead bar to hold the heel slightly above the level of the knee. Using this technique, it is rarely necessary to split the cast.

The first cast change at 10 days allows inspection of the wound and manipulation of the ankle joint to break up early adhesions that may be forming within the ankle and to stretch the newly forming capsule. At 3 weeks the cast is changed again, and the pins are removed unless a calcaneal osteotomy has been performed, in which case the pin crossing this joint remains for the duration of casting, a total of 6 weeks. The first two casts are changed under a light general anesthetic on an out-patient basis. The third cast is removed in the clinic, at which time the child is measured for a Seattle night brace,[61] which should be worn for 2 years. The parents are instructed in stretching exercises which should continue for 2 years. Radiographs are taken periodically and compared with the intraoperative radiographs to determine whether there has been recurrence of deformity or gradual late drift into an overcorrected position; both are now unusual in our experience. Follow-up should ideally continue until the patient is an adult.

COMPLICATIONS OF SURGICAL TREATMENT OF CLUB FEET

Numerous complications can occur with surgical treatment of congenital talipes equinovarus (Table 39–2), but fortunately most are rare. The incidence of complications is greater with the more extensive surgical procedures. Furthermore, certain complications are peculiar to specific procedures; for example, hinge valgus occurs as the result of the posterior medial release (PMR) but not the complete subtalar release (CSTR).

Most complications are preventable, provided the causes are known and provided that treatment, especially surgery, is performed by experienced individuals. Many of the mild and moderate deformities resulting from treatment do not require additional treatment or at most only orthotic modifications, while the more significant complications require surgical treatment. Uncorrected deformities that persist following surgical treatment should perhaps not be considered as complications. However, surgery is frequently required to correct these and thus they have been included here as complications.

The complications of surgical treatment have been grouped according to the joint(s) primarily involved: the ankle joint, subtalar joint, proximal tarsal joints, tarsal-metatarsal joints, and the metatarsophalangeal joints. In addition, other complications of bone and soft tissues can occur.

Ankle Joint

Complications involving this joint include (1) equinus; (2) calcaneus; (3) valgus; (4) arrest of the posterior distal tibial physis; and (5) restriction of ankle range of motion.

Equinus

Equinus of the ankle joint may result from inadequate lengthening of the Achilles tendon

TABLE 39-2. CLASSIFICATION OF SURGICAL COMPLICATIONS

COMPLICATIONS INVOLVING JOINTS
Ankle Joint
  Equinus
  Calcaneus
  Valgus
  Growth arrest of the posterior distal epiphyseal plate
  Restricted range of motion of the ankle joint
Subtalar Joint
  Varus
  Valgus
    Hinge valgus
    Rotary valgus
    Translatory valgus
  Uncorrected calcaneal rotation
  Restricted range of motion of the subtalar joint
Proximal Tarsal Joints
  Medial talonavicular subluxation
  Dorsal talonavicular subluxation
  Lateral talonavicular subluxation
  Volar talonavicular subluxation
  Proximal tarsal cavus
  Collapse of the medial longitudinal arch
  Supination
  Calcaneocuboid subluxation
Midtarsal Joints
Tarsometatarsal Joints
  Forefoot adduction
  Forefoot abduction
  Cavus
  Flatfoot
  Growth arrest of the physis of the first metatarsal
Metatarsophalangeal Joints
  Hammer toe
  Hallux varus
  Dorsal bunion

OTHER COMPLICATIONS
Bone and Cartilage Complications
  Transection of the sustentaculum tali
  Transection of the talar head
  Avascular necrosis
    Talus
    Navicular
    Calcaneus
    Cuneiform
    Metatarsals
Soft Tissue Complications
  Spasm of the posterior tibial artery
  Transection of the neurovascular bundle
  Deep wound infection
  Skin necrosis
  Compartment syndrome

A third cause is the failure to perform stretching exercises postoperatively. Probably the most common cause, however, is failure to perform an adequate release. Slipping of a below-knee cast may rapidly lead to a fixed equinus deformity.

It is a popular misconception that the conventional posterior release will correct equinus deformity. The "typical" posterior release involves posterior ankle capsulotomy and posterior subtalar capsulotomy with lengthening of the Achilles tendon and the posterior tibial tendon. A study by the author in which radiographs were performed at each stage of a sequential release of the posterior, medial, and lateral structures determined which structures require incision or lengthening in order to produce complete radiographic correction of the equinus deformity.[92] These structures are the posterior ankle joint, the Achilles tendon, the posterior tibial tendon, the calcaneofibular ligament, and at least the posterior one-half of the subtalar joint. In more severe cases, a release of the interosseus talocalcaneal ligament and even complete subtalar release (including complete talonavicular capsulotomy) were required to obtain a normal talocalcaneal angle on the lateral radiograph (see Fig. 39-20). The variety of structures that may require release indicates the importance of using intraoperative radiographs to verify correction.

Calcaneus Deformity

Two postsurgical causes for this deformity have been identified: overlengthening of the Achilles tendon and anterior ankle contracture. Anterior subluxation of the peroneal tendons is a third possible cause of calcaneovalgus deformity.

Miller and Bernstein observed that the calcaneus may be shortened in its ultimate length due to overlengthening of the Achilles tendon. They theorize that normal tension on the posterior apophysis is necessary for linear growth. These changes are observed on the anteroposterior radiograph as hypoplasia of the posterior aspect of the calcaneus and on the lateral view as an increase in Boehler's angle.[71]

This deformity may be prevented by the repair of the Achilles tendon with the foot in no more than 10 degrees of dorsiflexion and with tension placed on each end of the tendon when it is repaired. Pinning of the subtalar joint with the joint virtually closed except for

or from placing the foot in plantar flexion to relieve skin tension during wound closure. If the foot is left in a cast for an excessive period of time in this position (i.e., more than 2 weeks), the equinus may become permanent.

a slight medial or lateral gap due to deformation of bone surfaces is the proper technique. The joint should not be allowed to open posteriorly.

Wijesinha and Menalaus have reported their experience with calcaneus deformity resulting from surgery.[120] Three patients had calcaneus; one of them also had associated hindfoot valgus while another had supination. All three had some ill-defined neurologic or joint disorder, one of which involved spastic diplegia. The etiology of the calcaneus deformity was thought to be overlengthening of the Achilles tendon with possible contributions by the generalized disorders in each of the patients. The incidence of these deformities was three cases in approximately 500 clubfeet. The indications for surgery were footwear problems and progression of deformity.

The treatment they recommended was as follows:

I. For nonfixed calcaneus deformity of the ankle (without fixed dorsiflexion contracture) due to overlengthening of the Achilles tendon, they recommended shortening of the Achilles tendon.
II. For fixed calcaneus deformity of the ankle:
  A. Anterior capsulotomy of the ankle joint.
  B. Lengthening of the flexor digitorum and flexor hallucis longus tendons and peroneus tertius tendons.
  C. Transfer of the anterior tibial tendon to the heel. Prior to performing a transfer of the anterior tibial tendon to the heel, however, fixed calcaneus deformity of the ankle (talus) must be corrected. The talus must be brought down to about 20 degrees of plantar flexion. The anterior tibial tendon is the strongest tendon available for transfer. This transfer does not result in a drop foot gait because of the residual amount of ankle stiffness.
III. For fixed calcaneus deformity of the heel which was vertically aligned (pistol-grip deformity), calcaneal osteotomy.
IV. For fixed valgus deformity of the heel, calcaneal osteotomy.
V. For supination deformity, excision of a plantar based wedge from the metatarsal first-cuneiform joint with fusion of the joint.

The osteotomy used to simultaneously correct the fixed calcaneus and the fixed valgus deformities was resection of a superiorly based wedge with medial translation and angulation of the posterior calcaneus. The results were less than perfect, although all cases were improved. The patients had plantigrade feet with improved gait. Also the shoe-wear problem was considerably improved.[120]

Our treatment for the child with a calcaneus deformity has been very similar. Achilles tendon shortening alone is not adequate. If the cause is an anterior ankle contracture, the child is treated by simultaneous anterior ankle capsulotomy, lengthening of the tight dorsiflexion tendons, and tightening of the Achilles tendon. Our unpublished results of three patients are similar to those of Wijesinha and Menalaus.[120] We have lengthened but not transferred the anterior tibial tendon and we have not used calcaneal osteotomies, although for the more severe and combined deformities they are probably necessary. This has helped considerably as far as improvement of the calcaneus gait, although it does not usually provide a normal range of plantar flexion nor a completely normal gait.

Valgus

Valgus deformity of the ankle joint results from excessive release of the medial ankle capsule, i.e., the medial aspect of deep deltoid ligament. This complication is more likely to occur with Goldner's procedure where the primary capsular release is at the ankle level. With other extensive soft tissue release procedures, if the posterior medial ankle capsulotomy is carried beyond the level of the posterior tibial tendon sheath, ankle valgus may result. If this is recognized at the time of surgery, the capsule can be resutured to the level of the posterior tibial tendon sheath. If not, the foot will appear to be in valgus postoperatively. Standing AP x-ray views of the ankle will show that the talus is tilting into valgus in the ankle mortise. Treatment of this condition requires a medial displacement horizontal osteotomy of the calcaneus.[8]

Growth Arrest of the Posterior Distal Tibial Epiphyseal Plate

This complication may result from traumatic attempts to open the posterior capsule of the ankle joint. If care is not taken, one can cut into the growth plate, causing premature growth arrest. The joint can be located by palpating with a probe or with a gloved finger while moving the foot into plantar flexion and dorsiflexion. This rare complication requires repeated opening wedge osteotomies or bar resection of the posterior physis.

Restricted Range of Motion of the Ankle Joint

Significantly restricted range of plantar flexion following surgery is due to anterior ankle contracture and possibly anterior subluxation of the peroneal tendons. Ankle motion may be restricted in the typical clubfoot both pre- and postoperatively and may occasionally be severely limited. Nomura's study of patients following various combinations of posterior release and posterior medial release demonstrated a variable but surprising loss of ankle motion, especially in plantar flexion. Some patients had a total range of motion of only 20 to 40 degrees. The group with the greatest range of motion was the posterior release group (45 degrees). There was a corresponding slight increase in forefoot motion.[73]

Although plantar flexion was markedly limited in most groups, this did not interfere with the ability to stand or walk. However, it did interfere with the patients' ability to hop for extended periods.[73]

Moreau and Dick, reporting on ankle motion in the clubfoot following extensive soft tissue release, concluded that clinical measurements of ankle motion were inaccurate and that actual motion measured by maximal dorsiflexion and plantar flexion radiographs showed significant decrease in range of motion. They concluded that a good functional result was noted despite an average range of ankle motion of only 20 degrees, a figure far lower than the 39 degrees reported by Nomura.[72]

In a study by the author, ankle range of motion was evaluated in 50 patients following extensive soft tissue releases. Although the procedures chosen differed from case to case, the method of restoring ankle mobility was essentially the same in all. Specifically, the releases involved the following steps: Z-lengthening of the Achilles tendon and posterior tibial tendon, posterior capsulotomy of the ankle with extension of the capsulotomy medially to the posterior tibial tendon sheath,

posterior talofibular and calcaneofibular ligament release, and posterior subtalar release. Fifty feet were evaluated by determining the pre- and postoperative lateral tibiotalar angles on plantar flexion and dorsiflexion lateral radiographs.[93]

The average preoperative range of motion was 31 degrees and the average postoperative range of motion was 29 degrees. The total change in ankle range of motion was −2 degrees. Thirty percent of the feet had less than 25 degrees of ankle motion preoperatively; 28 percent of the feet had less than 25 degrees of motion postoperatively. The average change in dorsiflexion was +10 degrees, and the average change in plantar flexion was −12 degrees. Eighty-two percent of the feet gained dorsiflexion, while 88 percent lost plantar flexion.[92]

In conclusion, it was observed that the total range of motion was minimally affected by soft tissue release. The arc of motion was changed approximately 10 degrees toward dorsiflexion. One-third of the feet had marked decrease in range of motion preoperatively and one-third had marked decrease in range of motion postoperatively.[92]

Our conclusions differ with those of Nomura and associates[73] in that we have not frequently observed incongruity of the ankle joint. Once the posterior talofibular ligament is released and the ankle capsulotomy is carried to the posterior tibial tendon sheath medially, good range of motion of the ankle joint is usually restored, provided that an anterior ankle contracture or a flat-top talus is not present. In the latter case, restriction of motion is considerable, as it is with anterior ankle contracture. We also disagree with Nomura and associates regarding adhesions and thickening of the posterior capsule. In our view, posterior capsule contracture does not cause restricted plantar flexion (rather it produces restricted dorsiflexion), while *anterior* capsular contracture does. Adhesions of tendons no doubt cause restricted motion, but this is very difficult to evaluate independently of other factors.[73, 92]

Procedures directed primarily at the correction of equinus deformity (e.g., posterior release) are not usually responsible for restricted ankle range of motion. This occurs with more extensive procedures. We do agree that long-term postoperative immobilization and contracture of the anterior capsule restrict ankle motion. Another causative factor may be anterior subluxation of the peroneal tendons, which can result from the improper release of the tendon sheath during the release of the posterior lateral aspect of the subtalar joint.[73, 92]

Finally, it was observed that despite good restoration of motion at the time of the operative procedure, a moderate loss of ankle motion occurs between the second and third week postoperatively. This is possibly associated with maturation of the healing collagenous tissues.[92]

We now feel that the foot should be immobilized for no more than 6 weeks following extensive soft tissue correction, and possibly even less. Early removal of fixation pins and repeated manipulation under anesthesia during the first few weeks of cast applications may improve the range of ankle motion. In addition, McKay's hinged ankle cast following extensive soft tissue procedures may be efficacious.[63] McKay has also described the use of tendon sheath dissection to improve range of motion.[63] We have not used his technique for tendon lengthening but have tried his hinged cast. It is very laborious to apply, and the heel component frequently slips off the foot. The use of a constant passive motion machine may soon be tested at our center.

When the peroneal tendons are found to be anteriorly subluxated at surgery, they should be repositioned and their position maintained by a soft tissue sling.

Subtalar Joint

Four complications of operative treatment can occur at the subtalar joint: (1) varus, (2) valgus—hinge, rotary, and translatory, (3) calcaneal rotation, and (4) restricted range of subtalar motion.

Varus

Varus of the subtalar joint results from uncorrected deformity during surgery, more frequently following the posterior medial release than the CSTR. It may result from the incomplete release of any of the following structures: (1) the medial subtalar capsule (superficial deltoid ligament), (2) the small anterior subtalar capsule, (3) the entire capsule of the talonavicular joint, i.e., the spring ligament and associated ligaments of the medial talo-

navicular joint, as well as the lateral capsule of the talonavicular joint, (4) the interosseous talocalcaneal ligament, (5) the calcaneofibular ligament, and (6) the lateral subtalar capsule.

Varus invariably results when a posterior release is performed when varus and/or talonavicular subluxation are present. A posterior release is inadequate to correct these deformities. Persistent varus deformity can be prevented by CSTR and intraoperative radiographs to confirm complete correction. In the young child, the treatment of choice is an extensive soft tissue release (CSTR). In the child 6 to 8 years of age, a Dwyer procedure[27, 28] may be used to correct hindfoot varus. If the child is over 12 years of age and there are other associated deformities, a triple arthrodesis may be employed.

Valgus

Valgus of the subtalar joint can occur in one of three forms: hinge valgus, rotary valgus, or translatory valgus.

Hinge Valgus. Whereas rotary valgus takes place around a vertical axis, hinge valgus (see Fig. 39–58A) takes place around an AP axis in the horizontal plane. This usually results from the conventional posterior medial releases, in which the subtalar capsule is opened posteriorly, medially, and anteriorly along with the interosseus talocalcaneal ligament (Fig. 39–59). With the lateral subtalar capsule in-

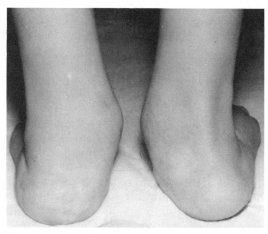

FIGURE 39–59. Bilateral valgus of the hindfoot. Hinge valgus following release of the posterior, medial, and anterior subtalar joints as well as the interosseous ligament by the Turco technique. The lateral subtalar capsule remains intact.

tact, this release allows the calcaneus to hinge open laterally beneath the talus. This deformity may be prevented by the use of the CSTR rather than the conventional posterior medial release in which the lateral subtalar capsule is retained.[98, 100] The treatment for this deformity is horizontal calcaneal osteotomy with medial displacement of the inferior fragment. Busch and co-workers recently reported an 87 percent rate of good and excellent results with this procedure.[8]

Rotary Valgus. Rotary valgus implies that the calcaneus has been rotated excessively beneath the talus around an axis passing vertically upward through the center of the interosseous talocalcaneal ligament. This usually occurs following an extensive soft tissue release of the posterior medial and lateral type (Fig. 39–58*B*).[93, 95] In our experience, this is usually due to placement of the navicular too far

laterally on the head of the talus (with Kirschner wire fixation) during surgery. The navicular is attached to the cuboid, which in turn is attached to the calcaneus. Thus, displacement of the navicular too far laterally results in displacement of all three bones (Fig. 39–60). A second cause is failure to correct marked calcaneocuboid subluxation. Leaving the cuboid in a medially subluxated position when the navicular is properly repositioned on the talar head will laterally displace the calcaneus to an excessive degree (see Calcaneocuboid Subluxation) (see Fig. 39–50*B*). Very rarely, rotary valgus may be due to late drift or gradual shift in position after the release of the interosseous ligament, the talonavicular joint, and the subtalar joint. Late drift seems to be associated with excessive ligamentous laxity. This deformity may be prevented by correction of the position of the navicular and

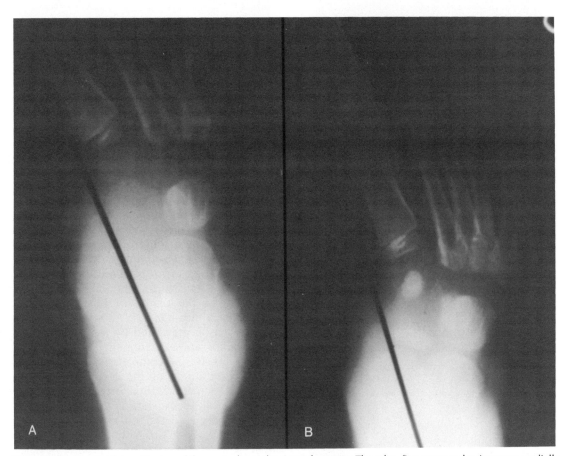

FIGURE 39–60. *(A)*, Malpositioning of the navicular at the time of surgery. The talar–first metatarsal axis passes medially to the base of the first metatarsal. It could be predicted at this point that the patient will have a lateral talonavicular subluxation when ossification occurs. *(B)*, Same patient after ossification of navicular with lateral subluxation of the talonavicular joint, grade 2.

the replacement of Kirschner wire fixation when intraoperative radiographs show the initial position of the navicular to be too lateral. It may also be prevented by correction of calcaneocuboid subluxation when this is present. In addition, if excessive ligamentous laxity can be diagnosed preoperatively, which may be difficult in the young child, this deformity should be corrected only to the lower limits of normal rather than into the mid or upper range of the normal radiographic measurements. Mild rotary valgus requires no treatment. Moderate lateral rotation of the navicular on the head of the talus is seen in many children with flatfeet who are asymptomatic.

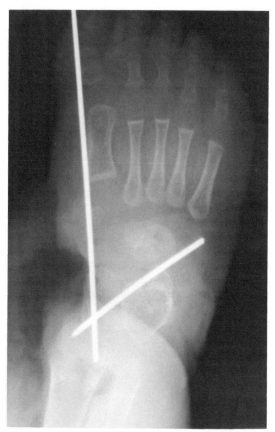

FIGURE 39–62. Translation of the calcaneus beneath the talus.

When this deformity is excessive (Fig. 39–61), the treatment of choice is another CSTR, medial displacement osteotomy of the calcaneus,[8] or in the older child, triple arthrodesis.

Translatory Valgus. This third type of valgus of the hindfoot results from improper pinning of the heel during a complete subtalar release. The entire calcaneus is allowed to translate laterally rather than to rotate around the vertical axis in the region of the interosseous talocalcaneal ligament.

This can be prevented by use of intraoperative radiographs. Treatment is difficult and usually involves a complete subtalar release with repositioning of the calcaneus beneath the talus or a horizontal osteotomy through the entire calcaneus, shifting the posterior portion medially as described by Busch and colleagues (Fig. 39–62).[8] Although we have patients with mild to moderate translatory valgus, they have not yet required osteotomy, and we have had no personal experience with surgery for this complication.[8]

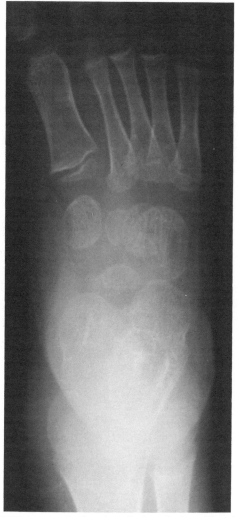

FIGURE 39–61. Grade 4 lateral talonavicular subluxation with the navicular sitting in the cleft between the anterior talus and calcaneus, the latter of which is in marked rotary valgus.

Uncorrected Calcaneal Rotation

The importance of this deformity has recently been described by McKay (Fig. 39–63).[62] Conservative treatment only occasionally corrects this deformity, as the contracted calcaneofibular ligament is resistant to manual stretching. Calcaneal rotation can occasionally be corrected during conservative treatment by pulling medially as well as downward on the posterior superior aspect of the calcaneus, but surgical release of the calcaneofibular ligament is usually required before the calcaneus can be positioned in normal rotary alignment with the talus. CSTR, including calcaneofibular ligament release, complete subtalar capsular release, and even interosseous talocalcaneal ligament release, may be required if conservative treatment fails. Persistence of this deformity results in a significant in-toeing gait with a rotary malalignment between the talus and calcaneus.[62]

Restricted Range of Motion of the Subtalar Joint

There are a number of possible causes of restricted motion at this joint. Restricted range of motion preoperatively is always present to some degree and in some cases may be excessive. It is common following extensive soft tissue procedures, particularly those involving release of the interosseous talocalcaneal ligament. Presumably the incised edges of the interosseous ligament and/or subtalar capsule and ligaments heal with more fibrosis, which renders the ligaments less elastic than prior to surgery, and thus motion is restricted. The second most likely cause is poorly developed subtalar articular facets. Ponseti and coworkers observed that these facets did not develop normally in their patients undergoing conservative treatment and/or Achilles tendon lengthening.[80] It is not yet known whether facet development occurs following operative cor-

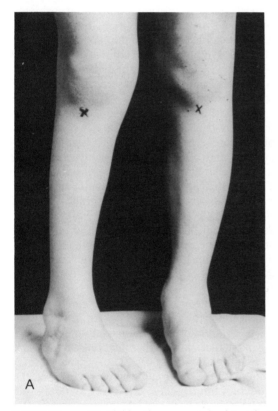

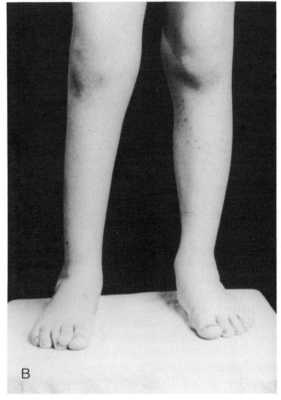

FIGURE 39–63. *(A)*, Child with uncorrected calcaneal rotation of the right foot. *(B)*, Following complete subtalar release and rotation of the anterior calcaneus laterally (around a vertical axis passing through the interosseous talocalcaneal ligament), the foot is now in normal alignment with the leg and knee. (From Simons GW: The complete subtalar release in clubfeet. I. A preliminary report. J Bone Joint Surg 67A:1044, 1985.)

rection of the subtalar deformities by extensive procedures such as CSTR. However, motion at this joint following surgery is rarely, if ever, equal to that in the contralateral normal foot. A third cause of restricted motion is damage to the articular cartilage during surgery, which may result in fibrous ankylosis. Fourth, a small anteromedial cartilaginous or osseous bridge may be present in the region of the sustentaculum tali, and failure to release it at the time of surgery will also result in restricted subtalar motion. Fifth, prolonged pin retention and cast retention following surgery can cause restricted range of motion. Finally, poor cooperation by the parents in the performance of postoperative stretching exercises may be contributory.

Significantly restricted motion can be diminished by removing the pins at 3 weeks and the cast at 6 weeks, by performing stretching exercises, and by postoperative night bracing. The use of a passive range of motion machine for the subtalar joint may improve range of motion, but as yet there are insufficient data to support this view.

Proximal Tarsal Joints

Eight deformities may occur as the result of surgery: (1) medial talonavicular subluxation, (2) dorsal talonavicular subluxation, (3) lateral talonavicular subluxation, (4) volar talonavicular subluxation, (5) proximal tarsal cavus, (6) collapse of the medial longitudinal arch, (7) supination, and (8) calcaneocuboid subluxation.

Medial Talonavicular Subluxation

This is most commonly seen in clubfeet following a conventional posterior medial release or when a posterior release is used for varus of the hindfoot. Frequently, the navicular is not released in the lateral portion of its articulation with the talus; the joint is simply wedged open and gradually closes following surgery. This may be prevented by the use of the complete subtalar release, in which the entire talonavicular joint, as well as the subtalar joint (including the interosseous talocalcaneal ligament) is released, and the navicular is then realigned with the talus.[93, 95] This deformity is usually accompanied by incomplete correction of subtalar varus as well. Medial talonavicular subluxation requires a repeated

extensive soft tissue release (CSTR) in the young child. In the child between 6 and 8 years of age, the varus can be treated by Dwyer osteotomy,[27, 28] while accepting the deformity at the talonavicular joint. This results in a plantigrade straight hindfoot, although there is usually significant restriction of motion in this part of the foot. After the age of 10 to 12 years, triple arthrodesis is indicated.

Dorsal Talonavicular Subluxation

Turco reported the occurrence of dorsal talonavicular subluxation with the one-stage posteromedial release but did not report the incidence of this complication or its functional implications.[110]

Schlafly and associates reported extensively on their experience with this complication in 46 patients with 61 clubfeet.[84] All patients had a one-stage posteromedial release performed by Turco's technique (however, only 88 percent had a talonavicular pin inserted); 43 percent developed dorsal talonavicular subluxation.

The incidence of dorsal talonavicular subluxation in Miller and Bernstein's series was 54 percent (13 of 24 feet). They also used a one-stage posteromedial release using Kirschner wire fixation.[71]

The author reported the incidence of this deformity (Figs. 39–64 and 39–65) in his series of 25 cases treated by CSTR before radiographic and clinical criteria were established for proper realignment of this joint at surgery. The incidence of clinically significant dorsal subluxation of the navicular (grade 2+ and 3+) was 12 percent (3 of 25).[94] Following the development of precise clinical and intraoperative radiographic criteria for accurate positioning of the foot following surgical release, the incidence of this complication decreased to 2 percent.

Turco believes that dorsal talonavicular subluxation may be caused by one of four factors: (1) malpinning of the talonavicular joint with the navicular dorsally subluxated at the time of pinning (Fig. 39–64); (2) excessive plantar flexion of the talar neck and trochlea at the time of pinning (Fig. 39–65); (3) decreased ankle dorsiflexion, which occurs more frequently in the older patient with severe equinus deformity; and (4) manipulation and casting postoperatively.[110, 111]

In their extensive study of patients with

FIGURE 39–64. Dorsal subluxation of the navicular, grade 1. The heel is in marked calcaneus deformity.

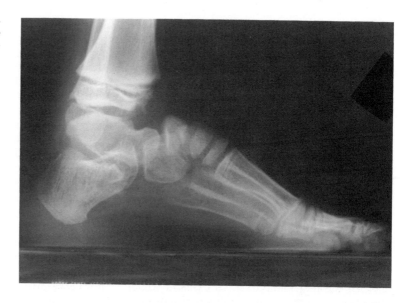

dorsal talonavicular subluxation, Schlafly and colleagues were able to verify only the first of these causes.[84] In our recent study, almost all the cases of dorsal talonavicular subluxation were due to malpinning of the navicular at the time of surgery. A few were due to excessive plantar flexion of the talus at the time of pinning. There were several cases of dorsal talonavicular subluxation that occurred gradually over a 1- to 2-year period following surgery. These patients all had excessive ligamentous laxity, and it is our opinion that this was the causative factor in those rare cases (unpublished data).[95]

Schlafly and associates state that it is easy to malpin the talonavicular joint because it is difficult to decide on the optimal position of the navicular. A small error in placement of the navicular in the younger child will be magnified with growth, and marked deformity of the talar head in the older patient makes placement difficult. Furthermore, they believe that the critical step of pinning the navicular accurately on the head of the talus must be performed without the benefit of radiographic verification, as the navicular has not yet ossified. Therefore, the surgeon may not know for many months whether pinning and fixation were done accurately.[84]

The navicular does not normally ossify until 3 or 4 years of age, and ossification may be delayed considerably longer in children with

FIGURE 39–65. Dorsal subluxation of the navicular. In this case, the talus is in marked plantar flexion as the talonavicular joint was pinned with these two bones in this position. The talus should have been dorsiflexed so that the talar axis passed through the first metatarsal base. Also note the contrast between the position of the calcaneus in this foot, which has complete flattening of the plantar arch, and the position of the calcaneus and the midfoot in Figure 39–64.

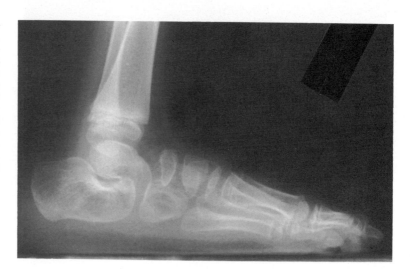

clubfeet. Consequently, the navicular is usually not ossified at the time of the initial surgical procedure. This has led many surgeons to believe that the position of the navicular may be difficult to evaluate by intraoperative radiographic techniques. Until recently, inability to verify the correct positioning at surgery by radiographic means was a major cause of overcorrection of the navicular both dorsally and laterally.

In a retrospective study of our cases, we compared the late postoperative lateral radiographs with those taken intraoperatively. We ascertained that those patients with a normal position of the navicular on the late postoperative lateral radiographs (in which navicular ossification was present) all had a common radiographic finding: the talar axis bisected the base of the first metatarsal. In cases in which the navicular was dorsally subluxated, both the lateral intraoperative and the late lateral postoperative films showed that the talar metatarsal axis passed volar to the base of the first metatarsal. Since then we have been able to use this finding as a radiographic criterion for determining the proper placement of the bones at the time of surgery.

Working from this radiographic criterion (and a similar finding on AP radiographs for lateral talonavicular subluxation), we were able to establish clinical criteria for the normal placement of the bones at the time of surgery. In the vertical plane, the navicular is in proper position when the dorsum is at the same level as the dorsum of the talus. Also, the talus

should not be placed in a plantarflexed position with respect to the navicular when pinning is performed. Since we have used these criteria, the incidence of significant dorsal talonavicular subluxation with CSTR has dropped from 12 percent to less than 2 percent.

An associated finding with dorsal talonavicular subluxation is wedging of the navicular (Fig. 39–66), which Schlafly and colleagues found in 30 percent of their patients treated by one-stage posterior medial release.[84] They were not able to determine whether this had an adverse effect on the prognosis, however. The presence of dorsal talonavicular subluxation did not correlate with the overall clinical results. In particular, there was no functional impairment on short-term follow-up, and even extreme dorsal talonavicular subluxation did not necessarily preclude a satisfactory result in their series. To treat this complication they attempted an open reduction of the dorsal talonavicular subluxation, which failed in one case. Therefore, they recommend that operative reduction not be employed. Likewise, we have attempted one open reduction of a dorsal talonavicular subluxation, which also failed. Our short-term results, too, have shown that functional impairment has not been a problem except for one patient who developed dorsal foot pain about 7 years following posterior medial and lateral release. Our current feeling, although completely speculative, is that a minor degree of dorsal talonavicular subluxation (grade 1) requires no treatment. Possibly grade 2 (dorsal subluxation of 1/3 to 2/3) and grade

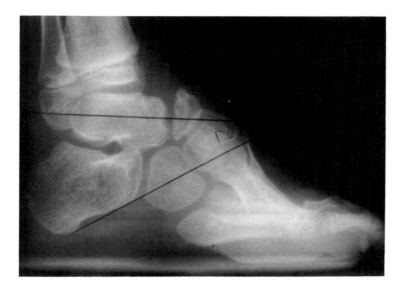

FIGURE 39–66. Cavus at the proximal tarsal level as well as the distal tarsal level. The navicular is subluxated dorsally. This is frequently followed by a compensatory cavus at either the proximal or distal tarsal joints or both to bring the medial ray to the ground for more effective push-off.

3 (complete dislocation) should be treated. Simple open reduction of the talonavicular joint is inadequate. More extensive release and realignment of the entire midfoot and hindfoot are probably necessary (see Fig. 39–66). If cavus deformity has developed, a plantar release may also be necessary. In the patient over 12 years of age, a triple arthrodesis is probably indicated.

Lateral Talonavicular Subluxation

This deformity results from overcorrection of the medial talonavicular subluxation (see Figs. 39–60 and 39–61). In our experience, it is almost invariably due to overcorrection at the time of surgery rather than gradual drift subsequent to surgery. When it occurs as a gradual displacement or late drift, it is usually in the patient who has marked ligamentous laxity. In addition, lateral talonavicular subluxation is most commonly associated with an increased AP talocalcaneal angle, implying that rotary valgus of the calcaneus is also present. The navicular, cuboid, and calcaneus are moved as a unit when this deformity is corrected by CSTR, and therefore overcorrection of the navicular in a lateral direction is accompanied by an excessive lateral rotary or translatory repositioning of the calcaneus (unless the supination of the foot at the talonavicular level remains undercorrected).

Lateral talonavicular subluxation occurring intraoperatively was studied in the same way as dorsal talonavicular subluxation, i.e., the late postoperative radiographs were compared with intraoperative films. On the intraoperative AP view, when the talar axis passed through the base of the first metatarsal, the late postoperative films (with one exception) showed the navicular to be anatomically reduced on the talar head. When the talar axis passed medial to the base of the first metatarsal (see Fig. 39–60A), the navicular, when fully ossified, was laterally subluxated (see Fig. 39–60B), and when the talar axis passed lateral to the base of the first metatarsal, medial subluxation was present on the late postoperative radiograph. The degree of subluxation was quantitated and classified as 1+ to 4+. Grades 1+ and 2+ were thought to be clinically insignificant as these changes are frequently seen in physiologic asymptomatic flatfeet. The incidence of lateral talonavicular subluxation of significant degrees (grades 3 and +4) was 8 percent (see Fig. 39–61).

As in the case of dorsal talonavicular subluxation, clinical criteria for repositioning the navicular at surgery were developed to determine the correct position of the navicular on the talar head in the mediolateral plane. Surprisingly, when the navicular was positioned with its medial side flush with the medial side of the talus, the ultimate position of the navicular was one of lateral subluxation. For proper repositioning, the navicular must be allowed to protrude medially to a slight degree, which varies from 3 to 4 mm in the small child to 1 cm in the older child. Also, there must be no step-off on the lateral aspect of the talonavicular joint. Since the use of the proper clinical and radiographic techniques, the incidence of this deformity has decreased dramatically to less than 2 percent. Therefore, these clinical and radiographic criteria now assume a key role in prevention of this problem with the CSTR.[91]

In our original study, only one case in 51 feet showed significant late drift into a laterally subluxated position.[94] This patient had marked ligamentous laxity, which probably accounted for this late deformity. We now believe there is an additional cause for lateral talonavicular subluxation which accounted for the remaining cases (see Calcaneocuboid Subluxation).

In the report of Schlafly and associates, lateral talonavicular subluxation usually was associated with good results even though it may have been of marked magnitude, whereas medial talonavicular subluxation was usually associated with poor results.[84] The mild degrees of this deformity (grades 1+ and 2+) require no treatment. However, moderate and severe degrees may require a repeated extensive soft tissue procedure, medial displacement osteotomy of the calcaneus,[8] or in the older child, triple arthrodesis.

Volar Talonavicular Subluxation

Magone and coworkers reported this complication following excessive soft tissue release.[66] We believe that this complication occurs as a result of improper pinning at the time of surgery and seldom if ever develops subsequently. This problem can be prevented by applying the clinical criteria described previously for repositioning the navicular on the talus and by verifying the position of the bones during surgery with intraoperative radiographs. Although we have not experienced this complication, we would recommend open reduction with realignment of the talonavicular joint, pinning, and verification of position of reduction with intraoperative radiographs.

Proximal Tarsal Cavus

Cavus may originate from two areas of the tarsus: the proximal tarsal row (i.e., the talonavicular and the calcaneocuboid level) and the distal tarsal row (i.e., the metatarsal-tarsal joints). Most frequently, cavus originates from both the proximal and distal tarsal levels; however, one is usually predominant. In the newborn infant with clubfoot, cavus is not usually one of the major deformities present. It usually develops gradually in the foot that is not corrected by either conservative or surgical measures. It may also be seen with dorsal talonavicular subluxation (see Fig. 39–66). The primary cause for the gradual development of cavus is no doubt muscle imbalance, but the exact etiology is not understood. Early correction of the other major deformities, either by conservative or surgical measures, will prevent this complication. Treatment in the young child is by plantar release; the older child may require dorsal wedge resection of the tarsus, calcaneal osteotomy for associated deformities of the hindfoot, or (in the child over 14 years of age) triple arthrodesis, which is especially indicated if there are other major deformities present.[26, 29, 79, 117, 118]

Collapse of the Medial Longitudinal Arch

This complication is caused by transfer or by releasing the posterior tibial tendon without reattaching it before wound closure. The tendinous support of the arch is thus lost, and it collapses without the heel going into valgus (Fig. 39–67). This commonly occurs following a plantar release or a release of the long plantar ligament. Prevention requires removal of the posterior tibial tendon from its sheath beneath the malleolus during surgical correction, followed by replacement and repair of the tendon under physiologic tension prior to wound closure. Posterior tibial tendon transfer or release is contraindicated in the typical clubfoot, in our opinion. This deformity may also result when plantar release is performed when the patient has flatfoot or rocker-bottom deformity.

Turco observed that most of his patients had flatfeet postoperatively. He routinely performs plantar release and originally released the posterior tibial tendon. He observed that this condition improved with growth and required no treatment.[100, 101] We believe that this condition requires no treatment unless the foot is painful or unless shoe wear is marked, in which case a custom-made orthotic is recomended in children under the age of 12 to 14 years. Triple arthrodesis is the procedure of choice in the child over this age who has significant pain, significant shoe wear, or marked deformity and who does not respond to conservative measures, but this is rarely required. (This complication is discussed further in the section on Flatfeet.)

Supination

This deformity is due to incomplete correction of supination (which occurs mainly at the

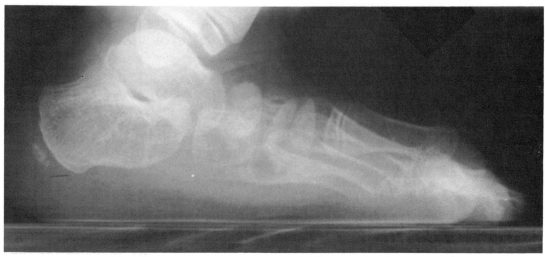

FIGURE 39–67. Loss of the medial longitudinal arch.

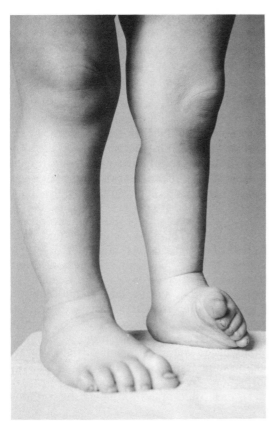

FIGURE 39–68. Marked supination following extensive soft tissue procedure.

talonavicular joint) at the time of surgery (Fig. 39–68). It may also be caused by a muscle imbalance between a normal anterior tibial muscle and a weak peroneus longus muscle. The first cause may be prevented by complete release of the talonavicular joint, by careful repositioning of the foot prior to placement of the talonavicular pin, and following pinning by clinical inspection of the foot with the knee and foot at 90 degree angles. If supination is present, the pin must be removed and supination corrected. If left untreated, this deformity may eventually lead to dorsal bunion formation. Treatment of fixed supination arising at the tarsometatarsal level is by a plantar-based wedge osteotomy of the base of the first metatarsal. Occasionally a plantar-based wedge is also removed from the first cuneiform.[53]

An imbalance between the anterior tibial muscle and the peroneus longus muscle may be due to multiple factors, such as injury to the peroneus longus tendon during surgery.

An anterior tibial tendon lengthening or transfer laterally may be performed if it can be demonstrated that there is muscle imbalance between the peroneus longus and the anterior tibial tendon.

Calcaneocuboid Subluxation

The cause of calcaneocuboid subluxation is not known. It may occur in utero; however, several fetal studies have failed to show angulation at the distal portion of the calcaneus. This deformity has not been seen before early conservative treatment. It is therefore conceivable that the deformity may be due to improper manipulation and cast techniques.

When this deformity is treated by CSTR without calcaneocuboid release, valgus of the hindfoot will result, because the three-bone unit (navicular, cuboid, and calcaneus) will move laterally as a block. Each bone subsequently displaces the other bones further laterally so that when the talonavicular subluxation has been fully corrected, the calcaneus will have rotated abnormally into an excessive degree of valgus deformity.

If this deformity is treated by release of the dorsal, medial, and plantar capsule of the calcaneocuboid joint, leaving the lateral capsule intact, the calcaneocuboid subluxation may become markedly worse and severe valgus of the heel will occur (see Fig. 39–48). The lateral capsule should be released, the cuboid repositioned, and the joint pinned. Grade 2 and 3 deformities require complete release of the calcaneocuboid joint with repositioning of the cuboid on the calcaneus and pinning. In addition to complete subtalar release, plantar release is also helpful. Grade 3 deformity may require additional surgical procedures for complete reduction of the joint. Radiographic verification of correction is important.[96, 107]

Midtarsal Joints

No significant deformities occur at this level in the clubfoot.

Tarsal-Metatarsal Joints

Five deformities can occur at these joints following surgery: (1) forefoot adduction, (2) forefoot abduction, (3) cavus, (4) flatfoot, and (5) arrest of the physis of the first metatarsal.

Forefoot Adduction

This results from undercorrection of the forefoot during surgery. Turco reports that severe metatarsus adductus is often associated with overcorrection of the hindfoot (hinge valgus), resulting in a skew or serpentine foot[110] and/or overcorrection of the navicular into a laterally subluxated position. Forefoot adduction results from inadequate release during the primary operative procedure. Although a plantar release may produce complete correction of mild or moderate degrees of forefoot adduction and may be enhanced by the release of the abductor hallucis or capsulotomy of the first metatarsal-tarsal joint, these steps are usually not adequate to bring about a full correction of the adduction at all five metatarsal-tarsal joints. Treatment of this deformity requires capsulotomies at the base of all five joints if there is a significant degree of metatarsus adductus following the extensive soft tissue release and plantar release.[46, 51, 58, 77] Releasing the capsules of both the dorsal and volar aspects may result in significant instability and dorsal subluxation of these joints later on. Release of just the dorsal capsules and fixation of the bases of the second and fifth metatarsals to the tarsus with Kirschner wires will substantially reduce the tendency for these joints to partially subluxate. In addition, a simple suture can be placed across the additional joints to prevent dorsal subluxation. We have performed metatarsal capsulotomies with the extensive soft tissue release of the midfoot and hindfoot with no adverse effects. This is an extensive procedure to perform on the foot at one time, and most surgeons would prefer to do the metatarsal capsulotomies as a second-stage procedure.

While Wynne-Davies has stated that this deformity corrects gradually with time,[122] we have noticed only gradual correction between the initial surgery and maturation of the foot. Moreover, this gradual correction is generally not complete, and surgery is usually required in the more severe cases. A second-stage metatarsal capsulotomy or osteotomy of all five rays following a first-stage extensive soft tissue release and plantar release may be indicated in the very deformed foot.[6, 104] Another alternative is combined closing wedge osteotomy of the cuboid with opening wedge osteotomy of the medial cuneiform bone or capsulotomy of the naviculocuneiform joint.[75] However,

there may be a tendency for this deformity to gradually improve with time, as long as growth continues.

Forefoot Abduction

This occasionally occurs as a late result following calcaneocuboid joint excision and arthrodesis associated with the posterior medial release procedure as described by Evans[1, 29, 30] or following capsulotomies of the tarsal-metatarsal joints or metatarsal osteotomies. Forefoot abduction typically results when the Evans procedure is performed too early (i.e., at 3 or 4 years of age) because of subsequent tethering of the lateral column of the foot and overgrowth of the medial column. This deformity can be prevented by doing an anterior vertical closing wedge osteotomy of the calcaneus instead of the Evans procedure. In addition, the surgeon should use Kirschner wire fixation of the capsulotomy or osteotomy sites. Abduction may be corrected by an opening wedge osteotomy of the lateral calcaneus or the calcaneocuboid joint (especially if the cause was overcorrection by Evans' procedure) or by metatarsal osteotomies to realign the forefoot.

Cavus

Whenever cavus is found at the tarsal-metatarsal level, it is probably also present to some degree at the proximal row of tarsal joints. This results from failure to perform a plantar release with the extensive soft tissue procedure when significant cavus is present. If it persists following surgery, it can occasionally be corrected by a plantar release through a plantar incision, followed by a walking cast with an anterior heel. In the older foot with fixed bone deformity, persistent cavus may require a dorsal closing wedge osteotomy of the first metatarsal if only the first ray is involved. If all metatarsals are involved, dorsal wedge resection of the midtarsal area can be performed.

Flatfoot

Flatfoot deformity may be caused by the improper release of several structures during an extensive surgical release. As mentioned, if the posterior tibial tendon is released or transferred, it will fail to support the medial arch of the foot and ultimately the plantar arch will be lost. Therefore, it is imperative that the posterior tibial tendon be repaired at the time of surgery and that transfer of this tendon not be undertaken in the child with a clubfoot. Additionally, release of the spring ligaments and talonavicular complex, with pinning of the navicular too far *dorsally* on the talar head, may lead to subluxation of the talar head off the sustentaculum tali and its subsequent protrusion into the medial plantar aspect of the foot. If the navicular is placed to far *laterally* on the talar head, producing lateral talonavicular subluxation, the talar head may also descend off the sustentaculum tali of the calcaneus, because the calcaneus, the cuboid, and navicular represent a unified segment of the foot. If one part of this block is overcorrected, overcorrection in the other parts may result. If the navicular, for example, is placed too far laterally, the calcaneus may likewise be moved too far laterally into a valgus position.

Release of the long plantar ligament of the foot in addition to the complete subtalar release may allow the anterior aspect of the calcaneus to drop inferiorly without the loss of the talocalcaneal relationship. That is, the talar head may not move medially off the sustentaculum tali but may remain in normal relationship to it, while the anterior portion of the calcaneus drops inferiorly in its anterior aspect.

This movement of the talar head off the sustentaculum tali can be prevented by positioning the navicular accurately on the distal part of the talar head with neither superior nor lateral deviation. This placement should be verified radiographically at the time of surgery. If the anterior calcaneus drops plantarward, the treatment is proper pinning of the talonavicular and calcaneotalar joints. This should be done with the calcaneus in the normal position rather than with the anterior aspect plantarflexed.

Growth Arrest of the Physis of the First Metatarsal

Growth arrest can occur as a result of surgical correction of adduction of the first metatarsal.[33] When the physis is inadvertently damaged, two problems can develop: angular deformity with incomplete arrest or (less likely) complete arrest of the proximal physis with a short first toe at the termination of growth. The latter is a crippling deformity and fortunately very rare. Single or repeated opening wedge osteotomies are required for angular

deformity. Physeal bar resection is also theoretically possible for partial physeal injury with angular deformity, but the author has had no experience with this technique at this site. Lengthening the first ray is also a theoretical possibility for treating a short toe.

Metatarsophalangeal Joints

Three deformities may occur at the metatarsophalangeal joints as a result of complications of surgery: (1) hammer toe, (2) hallux varus, and (3) dorsal bunion.

Hammer Toe

This rare deformity occurs when the foot has been corrected by extensive soft tissue procedures and the long toe flexor tendon has not been lengthened (Fig. 39–69). This tendon will frequently stretch to some degree following surgery, but when the toe cannot be passively extended to the neutral position with the foot in the plantigrade position at the time of surgery, the tendon should be lengthened. If the tendon is not lengthened at the time of the primary surgery, it can be lengthened later; however, because the muscular part of the musculotendinous unit extends almost to the level of the malleoli, lengthening must be performed below this level. Thus, extensive surgery on the medial side of the foot is necessary to expose the tendon, making it preferable to lengthen this tendon during the extensive soft tissue procedure, if needed.

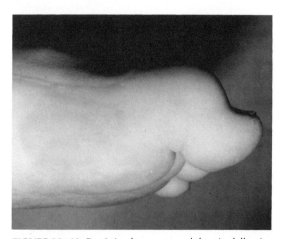

FIGURE 39–69. Persisting hammer toe deformity following extensive soft tissue procedure with failure to elongate the flexor hallucis longus.

Hallux Varus

This is often associated with a flexion deformity in the first ray and is usually due to contracture of the flexor hallucis brevis (Fig. 39–70). Correction requires Z-lengthening of the flexor hallucis brevis just proximal to its insertion. The lateral toes tend to follow the great toe and can often be corrected by lengthening the common flexor tendons.

Dorsal Bunion

This is a rare complication of extensive soft tissue release (Figs. 39–71 and 39–72).[64] Probably one of the best understood but least

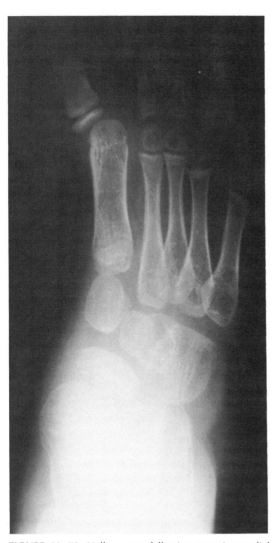

FIGURE 39–70. Hallux varus following posterior medial releases.

common causes is inadvertent transection of the peroneus longus tendon, which can occur during surgery when a calcaneocuboid osteotomy is performed on the lateral side of the foot, during posterior capsulotomies of the ankle and subtalar joints, or during release of the plantar aspect of the calcaneocuboid joint through a medial incision. If this is recognized at the time of surgery, it should be repaired. Following surgery, it is difficult to determine the cause, as the child is usually too young to cooperate with manual muscle testing. In this case, electromyography can be employed or the tendon can be explored through a small incision to determine whether it is in continuity. If the tendon is found to be functioning, another cause must be sought. Other causes for dorsal bunion formation are conditions that significantly decrease the medial longitudinal arch of the foot, causing increased tension within the flexor hallucis brevis. The flexor hallucis brevis then flexes the proximal phalanx, and the metatarsal head is gradually pushed into a superior position. Over time, the metatarsophalangeal joint adapts to the position of hyperflexion and becomes fixed with eventual formation of a dorsal bunion. Various factors that can cause loss of the medial longitudinal arch are pre-existing flatfoot or rocker-bottom deformity resulting from conservative management, plantar release, excessive ligamentous laxity, release or transfer of the posterior tibial tendon, and pin fixation of the talonavicular joint with the forefoot in supination. Usually, more than one factor is causative when dorsal bunion formation takes place (see Fig. 39–72).

In addition, overlengthening of the Achilles tendon will increase the distance between the origin and the insertion of the flexor hallucis longus (FHL). If the FHL remains unlengthened, there will be increased tension within the muscle and it will tend to flex the distal phalanx. Contraction of the flexor hallucis brevis will increase the tendency for dorsal bunion formation.

This condition can be prevented by judicious care during a calcaneocuboid capsulotomy, posterior ankle or subtalar capsulotomy, or anterior calcaneal osteotomy. Also, a plantar release is contraindicated if flatfoot or rocker-bottom deformities are present. Posterior tibial tendon transfer or release is likewise contraindicated.

Dorsal bunion is treated in the young patient by McKay's procedure (i.e., transfer of the

FIGURE 39–71. Dorsal bunion formation following posterior medial release.

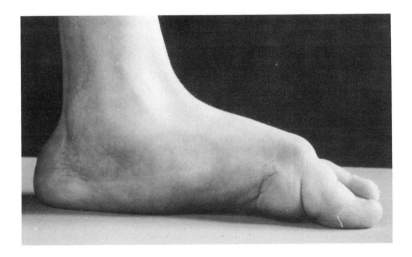

flexor hallucis brevis, the adductor, and the abductor tendons to the dorsum of the first metatarsal).[64] In the older patient, volar wedge osteotomy of the proximal first metatarsal combined with transfer of the flexor hallucis longus to the neck of the first metatarsal may be required in addition to other soft tissue reconstruction.

Bone and Cartilage Complications

Transection of the Sustentaculum Tali

This complication results from spurious dissection of the medial subtalar joint as the surgeon attempts to release the superficial layer of the deltoid ligament. If the neurovascular bundle has not been adequately dissected and the flexor hallucis longus has not been released completely from its sheath to the level of Henry's knot,[44] adequate visualization at this level will be difficult. The joint normally has a slight S-shaped or reversed S-shaped contour. It is occasionally difficult to follow the plane of dissection of the joint line from the medial side. When one is unsure of the plane, it is helpful to return to the posterior aspect of the joint and to spread the subtalar joint open posteriorly with a hemostat and thus locate the level of the dissection. Occasionally, a medial cartilage pillar is seen that seems to join the inferior surface of the talus to the superior surface of the calcaneus. Dissection at this point should be directed to the base of the pillar and then extended anteriorly

(see Fig. 39–44). Occasionally, a small osseous or cartilaginous bar exists in this region, which should be transected.

Although the author has not experienced this complication, if a significant fragment of the sustentaculum is accidentally transected, it may be replaced and pinned with one or two threaded Kirschner wires.

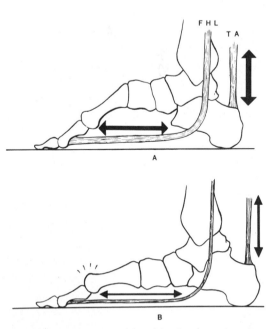

FIGURE 39–72. Causes of dorsal bunion formation. Anything that causes loss of the medial longitudinal arch of the foot puts the flexor hallucis brevis under tension. This flexes the first metatarsophalangeal joint with subsequent dorsal movement of the first metatarsal head and eventual joint fixation in this position.

Transection of the Talar Head

This complication occurs when the inexperienced surgeon tries to open the tibionavicular joint, not realizing that the talar head lies within its depths. Even the experienced surgeon may find identification of the talonavicular joint difficult at times. If dissection is carried too far into the depth of the tibionavicular joint, it is easy to cut into the soft cartilaginous tissue of the talar head or neck. If the surgeon encounters difficulty in locating the talonavicular joint, he or she should return to the medial subtalar joint and complete the dissection of this joint along with the anterior subtalar joint and the interosseous talocalcaneal ligament. In so doing, one is usually able to open the foot medially to a greater extent and to locate the talonavicular joint. The incision can be extended from the subtalar joint into the talonavicular joint rather easily once the talocalcaneal joint is completely freed. Occasionally, a flat talar head may occur from forceful conservative treatment and lead the unsuspecting surgeon to believe that he or she

has amputated the head. Once the subtalar joint has been completely released, if an accidental partial or complete transection has occurred, fixation of the partially transected head with the body should be performed using Kirschner wires in the hope that cartilaginous union will occur. The author has never experienced this complication.

Avascular Necrosis

Talus. This has occurred once in the author's experience (Fig. 39–73).[4, 43] It is due to the inadvertent incision of the blood supply to the talus on the dorsolateral side of the foot. When dissecting the talonavicular joint, either through a posteromedial or a lateral incision, the dissection is accidentally carried dorsally onto the talar neck. Talar neck osteotomy can also produce talar avascular necrosis localized to the head and neck segment.

Talar avascular necrosis was reported in one case of a series of 61 patients treated by single-stage posterior medial release by Schlafly and colleagues.[84] This complication had previously been reported only when a posterior medial

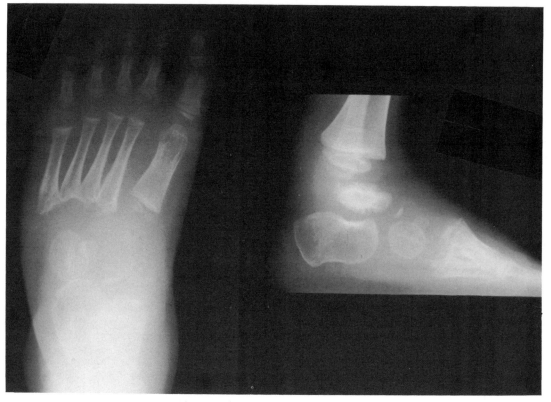

FIGURE 39–73. Talar avascular necrosis, best seen on the lateral radiograph.

release was combined with a lateral release. Schlafly and coworkers did not describe the treatment or final result in their single case.

In a study by Aplington and Riddle, 203 patients with 321 congenital clubfoot deformities had a total of five cases of avascular necrosis of the talus, all of which occurred among a group of 35 patients who had combined medial and lateral releases.[4] It was their belief that this complication resulted from the extensive lateral as well as medial dissection. All cases were noticed as early as 3 months following surgery. These authors believe that subtalar dissection, except at the talonavicular joint, is contraindicated unless absolutely necessary to achieve proper anatomic relationships. The lateral release employed in their 35 patients involved dissection of the sinus tarsi, the calcaneocuboid joint, and frequently the lateral subtalar and talonavicular joints. They did not give a follow-up report on their patients nor did they mention the type of treatment employed.

In performing the CSTR, we routinely release the entire lateral subtalar joint, talonavicular joint, and interosseus talocalcaneal ligament. This involves dissection in the lower lateral aspect of the sinus tarsi. It is the author's belief that the main blood supply to the talus arises from a more superior lateral area of the talar neck. If the dissection is kept distally on the head of the talus and is not allowed to progress up onto the neck, this complication can be avoided. However, once it occurs, there is probably no satisfactory treatment other than a weight-relieving patellar tendon–bearing orthosis. Diagnosis is established by postoperative radiographic evidence of sclerosis and fragmentation within the body of the talus. A search of the literature did not reveal any studies of the long-term effects of this complication or the immediate treatment employed once it is diagnosed.

Navicular. In the series of 61 clubfeet treated by one-stage posterior medial release reported by Schlafly and colleagues,[84] there were two cases of navicular avascular necrosis and seven cases of fragmentation of the navicular. These authors felt that the fragmentation may have been secondary to irregular ossification occurring from multiple ossification centers but that the two cases of avascular necrosis were associated with marked delay in ossification, one of which went on to an excellent result. They therefore do not believe that this complication is associated with functional impairment.

Calcaneus. Magone and coworkers recently reported five cases of this complication following the use of the Cincinnati incision.[66] This entity is very rare, and we have had only one patient with this complication (Fig. 39–74). Calcaneal avascular necrosis, which occurred in both feet, followed bilateral complete subtalar releases. The patient, who had not had previous surgery, postoperatively developed large necrotic areas on both heels that eventually healed by granulation over a period of 3 months. During this time, both calcanei developed changes that appeared to be those of avascular necrosis. Since his surgery 6 months ago, the patient has done well and is fully ambulatory (Fig. 39–75).

Cuneiform. Avascular necrosis of the cuneiform is very rare, and although it has been

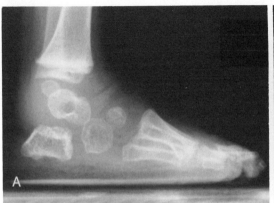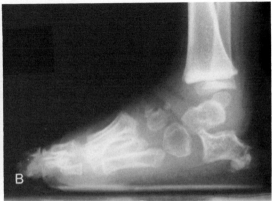

FIGURE 39–74. Bilateral calcaneal avascular necrosis.

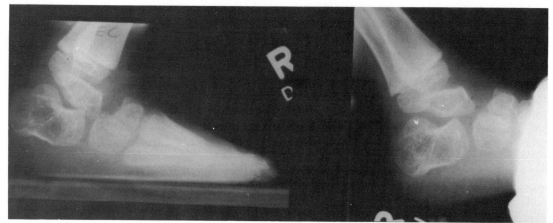

FIGURE 39–75. Persistent absence of the ossification center of the navicular in a 4-year-old boy due to avascular necrosis of the navicular. Flat-top talus and flattening of the talar head can also be seen.

reported, the author has never experienced this complication.

Metatarsal. This deformity is extremely uncommon. Neither it nor its underlying cause (i.e., compartment syndrome) have been pre- viously reported in the literature. In our pa- tient, it followed an extensive soft tissue pro- cedure for a recurrent clubfoot that had been treated by posterior medial release elsewhere. At 3 years following the CSTR, the patient

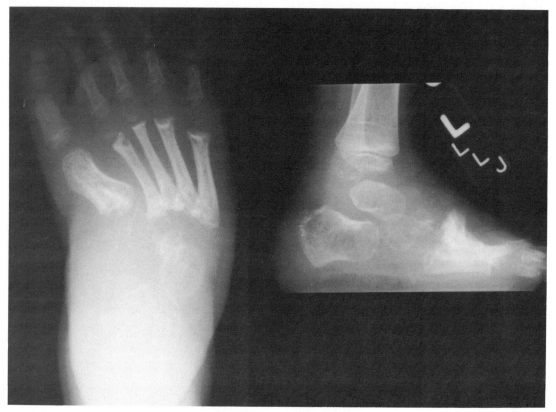

FIGURE 39–76. Metatarsal avascular necrosis following compartment syndrome in a 1-year-old child. Notice the marked plantar flexion of the first metatarsal and the sclerosis of the medial metatarsals.

remains ambulatory but has a significant inward deviation of the foot and a limp. The end results of this complication are unknown at this time (Fig. 39–76).

Soft Tissue Complications

Spasm of the Posterior Tibial Artery

Spasm of the posterior tibial artery may occasionally occur following dissection around the neurovascular bundle. When either transection or spasm of the neurovascular bundle is suspected, the tourniquet should be immediately released and the blood supply to the foot carefully checked. If no definite area of transection can be visualized, bathing the vessels in a papavarine-soaked sponge will relieve the spasm and allow circulation to return to the foot.

Transection of the Neurovascular Bundle

This is a rare but serious complication that may eventuate in a necrotic foot with subsequent need for amputation. The author has transected the posterial tibial artery in two instances: one was in a previously operated foot with extensive fibrosis around the neurovascular bundle, and the second was in a patient with congenital absence of the posterior tibial artery in whom the major blood supply was through the peroneal vessels. In both cases the vessels were repaired and the feet survived. Great care should be used when the posterior tibial artery or nerve is not in its normal location, and the posterior peroneal vessels should be sought posteriorly.

In addition, when dissecting the neurovascular bundle in a previously operated foot that has had an extensive release, it is prudent to begin the dissection superiorly where the neurovascular bundle has not become encased in scar tissue and work from normal to abnormal tissues. The author has found it helpful to dissect the neurovascular bundle en bloc along with the encasing fibrous tissue off the medial surface of the talus to the level of the bifurcation of the vessels in the subtalar region. Once the neurovascular bundle is freed from the talus, dissection of the medial subtalar joint is greatly facilitated.

Deep Wound Infection

This is an extremely uncommon complication. We have had no deep wound infections in our series, although we now routinely use pre- and postoperative antibiotics. If infection occurs, it can cause marked contracture of the wound and deformity of the foot, with restriction of motion of the midfoot and hindfoot. Any subsequent surgery is made especially difficult by the fibrosis and scarring around the neurovascular bundle. Recurrent deformity will occur if the internal fixation pins are removed prematurely, and they should be retained until the likelihood of skin retraction is no longer present.

Skin Necrosis

Skin necrosis is an occasional complication following posterior medial release and complete subtalar release (Fig. 39–77). The incidence of skin necrosis is probably very similar following either procedure, although it may be slightly more common with the Cincinnati incision than with the medial incisions. In most instances, the necrosis involves an area less than 2 cm in diameter and rarely, if ever, requires skin grafting and usually heals with

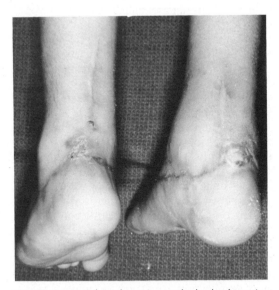

FIGURE 39–77. Bilateral scarring on the heels of a patient who had previous posterior medial release then complete subtalar release using the Cincinnati incision. Healing occurred without grafting. (From Simons GW: The complete subtalar release in clubfeet. Orthop Clin North Am 18:667, 1987.)

granulation tissue and fibrosis with residual scar formation. This has also been Turco's experience.[110] Despite the adverse cosmetic appearance, function is usually not compromised. If extensive, wound healing may require as long as 2 to 3 months (see Fig. 39–76).

Compartment Syndrome

This complication is also extremely rare and to our knowledge has not been reported previously in the literature. The clinical situation was unique in that the child, who had undergone a previous posterior medial release performed elsewhere, was given an epidural block for postoperative pain control, which resulted in peripheral vasodilatation at the completion of surgery. While on the operating table, the foot appeared to have normal circulation, but in the recovery room the fourth and fifth toes became cyanotic. Over the ensuing several days, the patient developed all the characteristic features of compartment syndrome of the foot, including increased pressures within the interosseous muscles of the foot but not of the lower leg.

The foot incision was opened and the grayish muscle tissue quickly filled with blood and regained normal color. Contractility of these muscles did not return promptly, however. Compartment release including each interossei was carried out through the medial wound.

At that time the pins across the talonavicular joint and the calcaneotalar joints were left in place. In retrospect this was a mistake as the fully corrected position of the foot no doubt stretched the neurovascular bundle and caused further ischemia.

The patient's foot survived the ischemic insult. The foot did not become necrotic, although the two toes appeared to. Their entire covering of skin and nails became detached, leaving underlying normal skin and nailbeds. The foot went on to revascularize without evidence of Volkmann's ischemic contracture. Several months following surgery, the avascular metatarsals were first observed. There has been little change in their appearance in the 3 years since surgery. The long-term results of this complication are as yet unknown.

RESULTS

Until recently, little evidence has been available to scientifically validate any of the theories proposed by different surgeons regarding the positional relationships of the bones in untreated clubfoot. Proof of any of these hypotheses, however, would be of considerable importance, as each of the theorists has developed operative techniques based on their pathoanatomic concepts.[14, 38, 62, 105]

The most direct proof was supplied in an article by Herzenberg and coworkers in which a three-dimensional computer model study was performed on two patients, one with a normal foot and one with a clubfoot.[45] This study gave the greatest validity to McKay's theory that the calcaneus rotates around a vertical axis, in that there was approximately 40 degrees of calcaneal rotation at the subtalar joint in the fully deformed clubfoot. In addition, there also seemed to be some support for Carroll's theory of external rotation of the talus in the mortise (around the vertical axis). This study revealed that there was approximately 11 degrees of external rotation of the talus. They also found that the talus rotated internally around an AP axis giving some credence to Goldner's theory of talar inversion. This study must be repeated on a significantly larger number of patients before it can be considered valid.

Recent evidence from different centers allows us to compare the results of the various procedures that have been advocated. The first of these studies compares Goldner's procedure and Turco's procedure. Yngve, Miller, and Herndon performed simultaneous bilateral clubfoot procedures in which Turco's technique was performed on one foot and Goldner's operation on the other. The medial subtalar joint was released in the first and the medial tibiotalar joint was released in the second. Evaluation on the basis of range of motion, six radiographic measurements, and ShuTrac gait measurements revealed essentially no difference between the two groups. However, both groups had a tendency for residual toeing-in, adductus of the forefoot, varus of the heel, and increased lateral plantar pressure.[123]

In another study, Magone and colleagues[66] evaluated three procedures: Turco's, Carroll's, and McKay's. Twenty four feet were operated upon by Turco's procedure with 12.5 percent excellent results, 33.3 percent good results, 16.7 percent fair results, and 37.5 percent poor results. Using Carroll's technique, they operated on 35 feet and found the results to be as follows: 11 percent excellent, 37 percent good,

29 percent fair, and 23 percent poor. Seventeen feet were operated upon using McKay's procedure with 12.5 percent excellent, 50 percent good, 12.5 percent fair, and 25 percent poor results. If one reclassifies these results as satisfactory (excellent or good) or unsatisfactory (fair or poor), Turco's procedure yielded 46 percent satisfactory and 54 percent unsatisfactory results, Carroll's technique showed 48 percent satisfactory and 52 percent unsatisfactory results, and McKay's yielded 62 percent satisfactory and 37 percent unsatisfactory results. While the techniques of Turco and Carroll had nearly comparable results, the outcome with McKay's technique was clearly better. However, because of the smaller number of feet in McKay's group and the short follow-up in all groups, the authors were not prepared to state that McKay's procedure was unequivocably superior (Table 39–3).

In another study involving these same three procedures, an intraoperative control study was carried out by Davidson. Eleven clubfeet were corrected by sequentially performing first the Turco, then the Carroll, and then the McKay release under the same anesthetic. Their conclusion again was that the best results were obtained with McKay's procedure.[23]

In a study by the author published in 1985, a complete subtalar release was compared with procedures that we had performed in the past, such as posterior medial release, and posterior medial and lateral release associated with an anterior subtalar capsule release. Clearly the best results occurred in those who had the complete subtalar release.[95]

TABLE 39–3. EVALUATION OF THREE PROCEDURES*

PROCEDURE		SATISFACTORY	UNSATISFACTORY
Turco	(N = 24)	46%	54%
Carroll	(N = 35)	48%	52%
McKay	(N = 17)	62%	37%

*See reference 66.

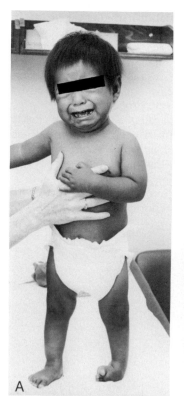
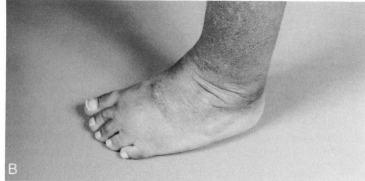
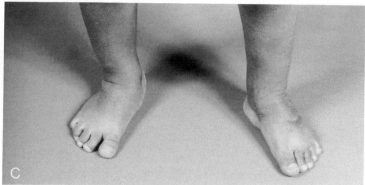

FIGURE 39–78. *(A)*, Three-year-old with a club foot that had never been treated. *(B and C)*, Postoperative results following complete subtalar release, calcaneocuboid release, plantar release, and second and third metatarsal osteotomies. Note that the alignment of the foot appears virtually normal.

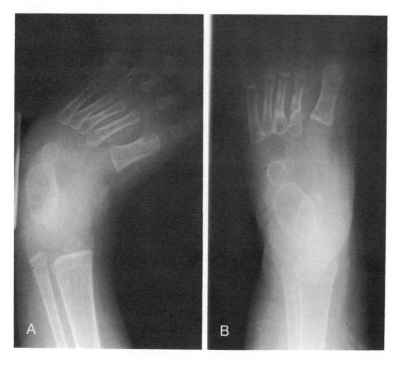

FIGURE 39–79. *(A)*, Preoperative AP view of the same patient shown in Figure 39–78. *(B)*, AP view of the same patient after surgery. All of the following corrections have been achieved: normal anteroposterior TC angle, moderate divergence of the anterior end of the talus and calcaneus, 50 percent overlap of the talar and calcaneal ossification centers, passage of the talar axis through the base of the first metatarsal, normal calcaneocuboid alignment. Mild residual convergence of the metatarsals persists but is acceptable.

More recently Cummings and associates attempted to ascertain whether the circumferential soft tissue release based on McKay's concept of rotation of the calcaneus was improved by this surgery.* They utilized computerized axial tomography to evaluate the bimalleolar axis and concluded that the "medial spin" (rotation) of the calcaneus in clubfeet was in fact improved by the circumferential soft tissue release but was not helped by the posterior medial release. They also concluded that the results of the circumferential soft tissue release could be compromised by previous soft tissue procedures.[20]

Most of the data available at this time clearly support the concept that the complete release at the subtalar level yields the greatest amount of correction and the most anatomically realigned feet.

The results of our early experience with CSTR have been reported previously.[95] Since

---

*Two additional terms have recently been used to describe variations of the posterior medial and lateral release. The term *circumferential release*, as used by Cummings, implies release of the entire subtalar joint without release of the interosseous talocalcaneal ligament.[20] The term *peritalar release,* used by Tachdjian,[106] implies release of all of the ligaments from the talus, including an entire ankle capsulotomy. Actually his procedure does not include an extensive ankle capsulotomy and frequently omits the interosseous talocalcaneal ligament but does include the entire talonavicular capsulotomy and subtalar capsulotomy. Thus, it is a complete subtalar release.

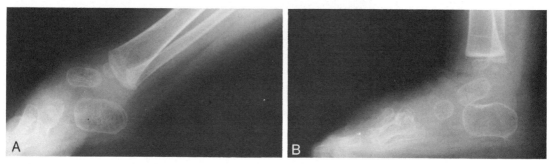

FIGURE 39–80. *(A)*, Lateral preoperative radiograph of the same patient shown in Figure 39–81. *(B)*, Lateral postoperative view demonstrates that the lateral talar axis passes through the base of the first metatarsal and that the lateral TC angle is normal. There is no cavus deformity.

then, further use of the CSTR, the determination of clinical and x-ray criteria for intraoperative radiographic verification of correction, and recognition of the significance of calcaneocuboid subluxation have dramatically decreased the incidence of overcorrection. While recent data have not yet been studied fully, it is clear that significant under- or overcorrection is now infrequent. Satisfactory results are seen in two patients (a 3-year-old and an 8-year old) with a previously unteated clubfoot. Both patients had complete subtalar releases as well as several ancillary procedures (Figs. 39–78 through 39–82).

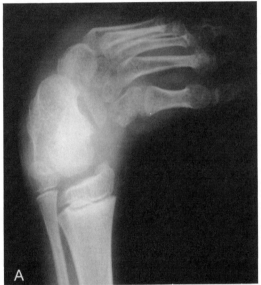

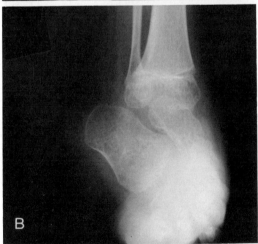

FIGURE 39–81. (A), AP view of the foot and ankle demonstrate severe clubfoot deformity in 8-year-old untreated male. (B), Lateral radiograph of the same foot.

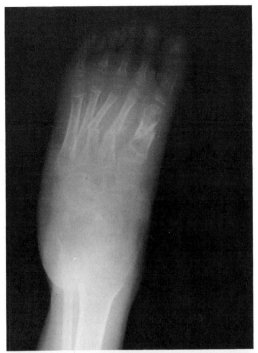

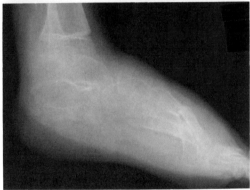

FIGURE 39–82. Same patient as in Figure 39–81. Postoperative radiographs following complete subtalar release, plantar release, lateral calcaneal closing wedge osteotomy, and metatarsal osteotomies of all five metatarsals.

References

1. Abrams RC: Relapsed club foot. The early results of an evaluation of Dillwin Evans' operation. J Bone Joint Surg 51A:270, 1969.
2. Adams W: Club Foot: Its Causes, Pathology and Treatment. London, J. & A. Churchill, 1866.
3. Addison A, Fixsen JA, Lloyd-Roberts GC: A review of the Dillwyn Evans type collateral operation in severe club feet. J Bone Joint Surg 65B:12, 1983.
4. Aplington JP, Riddle CD: Avascular necrosis of the body of the talus after combined medial and lateral release of congenital club foot. South Med J 69:1037, 1976.

5. Barenfeld PA, Weseley MS, Munter M: Dwyer calcaneal osteotomy. Clin Orthop 53:147, 1967.

5a. Barnett A, personal communication.

6. Berman A, Gartland JJ: Metatarsal osteotomy for the correction of adduction of the fore part of the foot in children. J Bone Joint Surg 53A:498, 1971.

7. Brougham DI, Nicol RO: Use of the Cincinnati incision in congenital talipes equinovarus. J Pediatr Orthop 8:696, 1988.

8. Busch M, Diaz L, Tachdjian M: Surgical treatment of severe hindfoot valgus by medial displacement osteotomy of the os calcis. Presented at the 54th Annual Meeting of AAOS. San Francisco, CA, 1987.

9. Campos da Paz A Jr, De Souza V: Talipes equinovarus: Pathomechanical basis of treatment. Orthop Clin North Am 9:171, 1978.

10. Carlioz H: Les osteotomies calcanennes et tibiales dans le traitement du pied bot varus. *In* Le Pied Bot Varus Equin Congenital. Cahiers d'Enseignement de la S.O.F.C.O.T. Paris, Expansion Scientifique Francaise, 1976.

11. Carmack JC, Hallock H: Tibiotarsal arthrodesis after astragalectomy. A report of eight cases. J Bone Joint Surg 29:476, 1947.

12. Caroyan A, Bourges M, Touge M: Dual transfer of the posterior tibial and flexor digitorum longus tendon for drop foot. J Bone Joint Surg 49A:144, 1967.

13. Carpenter EB, Huff SH: Selective tendon transfers for recurrent club foot. South Med J 46:220, 1953.

14. Carroll NC, McMurtry R, Leete SF: The pathoanatomy of congenital club foot. Orthop Clin North Am 9:225, 1978.

15. Codivilla S: Sulla cura del piede equino varo congenito. Nuovo metodo di cura cruenta. Arch Chir Ortop 23:245, 1906.

16. Coleman SS: Complex foot deformities in children. Philadelphia, Lea & Febiger, 1983.

17. Collburn RC: Flat-top talus in recurrent club foot. J Bone Joint Surg 44A:1018, 1962.

18. Crawford AH, Marxsen JL, Osterfeld DL: The Cincinnati incision: A comprehensive approach for surgical procedures for the foot and ankle in childhood. J Bone Joint Surg 64A:1355, 1982.

19. Critchley JE, Taylor RG: Transfer of the tibialis anterior tendon for relapsed club foot. J Bone Joint Surg 34B:49, 1952.

20. Cummings R, Desce M, Bradshaw J, et al: The circumferential club foot release—Does it accomplish what it is intended to? POSNA Annual Meeting, Toronto, Canada, May 18, 1987.

21. Curtis FE, Muro F: Decancellation of the os calcis, astragalus, and cuboid in correction of congenital talipes equinovarus. J Bone Joint Surg 16:110, 1934.

22. Dangelmajor RC: A review of 200 club feet. Bull Hosp Spec Surg 4:73, 1961.

23. Davidson R: Intraoperative controlled comparison of the Turco, Carroll and McKay releases of idiopathic club foot. POSNA Annual Meeting, Hilton Head, SC, May, 1989.

24. Dekel S, Weissman SL: Osteotomy of the calcaneus and concomitant plantar stripping in children with talipes cavo-varus. J Bone Joint Surg 55A:802, 1973.

25. Dunn HK, Samuelson KM: Flat-top talus. A long-term report of twenty club feet. J Bone Joint Surg 56A:57, 1974.

26. Dwyer FC: A new approach to the treatment of pes cavus. Societe Internationale de Chirurgie Orthopedique. Sixieme Congres International de Chieurgie Orthopedique. Brussels, MA Bailleux, 1955, p 551.

27. Dwyer FC: The treatment of relapsed club foot by the insertion of a wedge into the calcaneum. J Bone Joint Surg 45B:67, 1963.

28. Dwyer FC: Treatment of the relapsed club foot. Proc R Soc Med 61:783, 1968.

29. Evans D: Treatment of cavo-varus foot and club foot. J Bone Joint Surg 39B:789, 1957.

30. Evans D: Relapsed club foot. J Bone Joint Surg 43B:722, 1961.

31. Fisher RL, Shaffer SR: An evaluation of calcaneal osteotomy in congenital club foot and other disorders. Clin Orthop 70:141, 1970.

32. Frassi GA: Lateral transplant of the tibialis anterior in the treatment of congenital club foot and its recurrences. Arch Orthop 76:93, 1963.

33. Gamble J, Decker S, Abrams R: Short first ray as a complication of multiple metatarsal osteotomy. Clin Orthop 164:241, 1982.

34. Garceau GJ: Anterior tibial transposition in recurrent congenital club foot. J Bone Joint Surg 22:932, 1940.

35. Garceau GJ: Anterior tibial tendon transfer for recurrent clubfoot. Clin Orthop 84:61, 1972.

36. Garceau GJ, Palmer RM: Transfer of the anterior tibial tendon for recurrent club foot. A long-term follow-up. J Bone Joint Surg 49A:207, 1967.

37. Gartland JJ: Posterior tibial transplant in the surgical treatment of recurrent club foot. A preliminary report. J Bone Joint Surg 46A:1217, 1964.

38. Goldner JL: Congenital talipes equinovarus—fifteen years of surgical treatment. Curr Pract Orthop Surg 4:61, 1969.

39. Gordon SL, Dunn EJ: Peroneal nerve palsy as a complication of club foot treatment. Clin Orthop 101:229, 1974.

40. Gould J: Personal communication.

41. Gould J: Foot Book. Baltimore, Williams & Wilkins, 1988.

42. Grill F, Franke J: The Ilizarov distractor for the correction of relapsed or neglected club foot. J Bone Joint Surg 69B:593, 1987.

43. Haliburton RA, Sullivan CR, Kelly PJ, et al: Extra-osseous and intra-osseous blood supply of the talus. J Bone Joint Surg 40A:1115, 1958.

44. Henry AK: Extensile Exposure, 2nd Ed. London, ES Livingston, 1966.

45. Herzenberg J, Carroll N, Christofferson M, et al: Club foot analysis with three dimensional computer modeling. Presented at the Annual Meeting of the American Foot and Ankle Society. San Francisco, CA, Jan. 22, 1987.

46. Heyman CH, Herndon CH, Strong JM: Mobilization of the tarsometatarsal and intermetatarsal joints for the correction of resistant adduction of the forepart of the foot in congenital club foot or congenital metatarsus varus. J Bone Joint Surg 40A:299, 1958.

47. Hjelmstedt A, Sahlstedt B: Talo-calcaneal osteotomy and soft tissue procedures in the treatment of club feet. I. Indications, principles and technique. Acta Orthop Scand 51:335, 1980.

48. Hjelmstedt A, Sahlstedt B: Talo-calcaneal osteotomy and soft tissue procedures in the treatment of club feet. II. Results in 36 surgically treated feet. Acta Orthop Scand 51:349, 1980.

49. Ilizarov GA: Calcaneal osteotomies. Quoted by D.

Paley, course on advanced Ilizarov techniques. Baltimore, MD, June 26, 1989.

50. Irani RN, Sherman MS: The pathological anatomy of idiopathic clubfoot. J Bone Joint Surg 45A:45, 1963.

51. Kendrick RE, Sharma NK, Hassler WL, et al: Tarsometatarsal mobilization for resistant adduction of the forepart of the foot. A follow-up study. J Bone Joint Surg 52A:61, 1970.

52. Kuo K, Kramer G, Lee Z-L, et al: Posterior medial release for idiopathic talipes equinovarus using Cincinnati exposure. Presented at the Annual Meeting of the Pediatric Orthopedic Society of North America. Hilton Head, SC, May 19, 1989.

53. Langenskiold A, Ritsala V: Supination deformity of the forefoot. Acta Orthop Scand 48:325, 1977.

54. LeNoir JL: Congenital idiopathic talipes. Springfield, IL, Charles C Thomas, 1966.

55. LeNoir JL: A perspective focus on the indicated surgical treatment of resistant club foot in the infant. South Med J 69:837, 1976.

56. Lichtblau S: A medial and lateral release operation for club foot. A preliminary report. J Bone Joint Surg 55A:1377, 1973.

57. Lloyd-Roberts GC, Swann M, Catterall A: Medial rotational osteotomy for severe residual deformity in club foot. A preliminary report on a new method of treatment. J Bone Joint Surg 56B:37, 1974.

58. Lowe LW, Hannon MA: Residual adduction of the forefoot in treated congenital club foot. J Bone Joint Surg 55B:809, 1973.

59. Lundberg BJ: Early Dwyer operation in talipes equinovarus. Clin Orthop 154:223, 1981.

60. McCauley J: Triple arthrodesis for talipes equinovarus deformities. Clin Orthop 34:25, 1964.

61. McCollum RG: A functional brace for congenital club foot. A preliminary report. Clin Orthop 89:197, 1972.

62. McKay DW: New concept of and approach to club foot treatment. I. Principles and morbid anatomy. J Pediatr Orthop 2:347, 1982.

63. McKay DW: New concept of and approach to club foot treatment. II. Correction of the club foot. J Pediatr Orthop 3:10, 1983.

64. McKay DW: Dorsal bunion in children. J Bone Joint Surg 65A:975, 1983.

65. Magnusson R: Rotation osteotomy—a method employed in a case of congenital club foot. J Bone Joint Surg 28:262, 1946.

66. Magone J, Torch M, Clark R: Comparative review of surgical treatment of idiopathic club foot. Presented at the POSNA Annual Meeting. Toronto, Ontario, May 18, 1987.

67. Malan MM: The key role of the calcaneocuboid joint in surgical correction of resistant congenital club feet. Presented at the Eighth Combined Meeting of the Orthopedic Associations of the English-Speaking World. Washington, DC, May 7, 1987.

68. Masse P, Taussig G, Bazin G: External wedge-shaped osteotomy of the calcaneus in the treatment of talipes equinovarus. Rev Chir Orthop 60 (Suppl 2):135, 1974.

69. Masse P, Taussig G, Jacob P: Osteotomy of the calcaneus in the treatment of congenital varus equinus club foot. Rev Chir Orthop 66:51, 1980.

70. Matsuno S, personal communication.

71. Miller JH, Bernstein S: The roentgenographic ap-

pearance of the "corrected club foot." Foot Ankle 6:177, 1986.

72. Moreau M, Dick D: Ankle motion in the surgically corrected club foot. Presented at the POSNA Annual Meeting. Toronto, Canada, 1987.

73. Nomura S, Kondo M, Maekawa M, et al: Limited plantar flexion of the ankle in the surgically treated congenital club foot. Fukuoka Acta Med 73:476, 1982.

74. Nyga W: Results of relocating the anterior tibial muscle in treating congenital club foot. Beitr Orthop Trauma 26:44, 1979.

75. Ogston A: A new principle of curing club foot in severe cases in children a few years old. Br Med J 1:1524, 1902.

76. Ono K, Hiroshima K, Tada K, et al: Anterior transfer of the toe flexors for equinovarus deformity of the foot. Int Orthop 4:225, 1980.

77. Otremski I, Salama R, Khermosh O, et al: Residual adduction of the forefoot. J Bone Joint Surg 69B:832, 1987.

78. Pandey S, Jha SS, Pandey AK: "T" osteotomy of the calcaneum. Int Orthop 4:219, 1980.

79. Paulos L, Coleman SS, Samuelson KM: Pes cavovarus. Review of a surgical approach using selective soft tissue procedures. J Bone Joint Surg 62A:942, 1980.

80. Ponseti I, El-Khoury G, Eppiolito E, et al: A radiographic study of skeletal deformities in treated club feet. Clin Orthop 160:30, 1981.

81. Reimann I: Congenital idiopathic club foot. Thesis. Copenhagen, Munsgaard, 1967.

82. Roberts JM, personal communication, 1982.

83. Sarrafian S: Anatomy of the Foot and Ankle. Philadelphia, JB Lippincott, 1983.

84. Schlafly B, Butler J, Siff S, et al: The appearance of the tarsal navicular after posteromedial release for club foot. Foot Ankle 5:222, 1985.

85. Scott WA, Hosking SW, Catterall A: Observations on the surgical anatomy of club feet. J Bone Joint Surg 66B:31, 1984.

86. Settle GW: The anatomy of congenital talipes equinovarus: Sixteen dissected specimens. J Bone Joint Surg 45A:1341, 1963.

87. Shapiro F, Glimcher JJ: Gross and histological abnormalities of the talus in congenital club foot. J Bone Joint Surg 61A:522, 1979.

88. Simons GW: A standardized method for the radiographic evaluation of clubfeet. Clin Orthop 135:107, 1978.

89. Simons GW: Movements of the normal limb. Presented at the Pediatric Orthopedic International Seminar. Chicago, IL, May, 1979.

90. Simons GW: Cincinnati approach for complete subtalar release of club feet. Presented at the Annual Meeting of the Pediatric Orthopedic Study Group, April 22, 1982.

91. Simons GW: Lateral talonavicular subluxation—A complication of extensive soft tissue release for club feet. Orthop Trans 8:448, 1984.

92. Simons GW: Ankle range of motion in club feet. Presented at the Annual Meeting of the Pediatric Orthopedic Society of North America. San Antonio, TX, 1985. Orthop Trans 9:502, 1985.

93. Simons GW: The complete subtalar release in clubfeet. I. A preliminary report. J Bone Joint Surg 67A:1044, 1985.

94. Simons GW: The complete subtalar release in clubfeet. II. Comparison with less extensive procedures. J Bone Joint Surg 67A:1056, 1985.
95. Simons GW: The complete subtalar release in club feet. Orthop Clin North Am 18:667, 1987.
96. Simons GW: Calcaneal capsulotomy for calcaneocuboid subluxation in clubfeet. Presented at the Annual Meeting of the European Pediatric Society. Budapest, March 20, 1987. J Pediatr Orthop 8:98, 1988.
97. Simons GW: Symposium: Current practices in the treatment of idiopathic clubfoot in the child between birth and five years of age. I. Contemp Orthop 17:63, 1988.
98. Simons GW: Symposium: Current practices in the treatment of idiopathic clubfoot in the child between birth and five years of age. II. Contemp Orthop 17:61, 1988.
99. Simons GW, Sarrafian S: The microsurgical dissection of a stillborn fetal club foot. Clin Orthop 173:275, 1983.
100. Singer M: Tibialis posterior transfer in congenital club foot. J Bone Joint Surg 43B:717, 1961.
101. Singer M, Fripp AT: Tibialis anterior transfer in congenital club foot. J Bone Joint Surg 40B:252, 1958.
102. Smith D: Recognizable patterns of Human Malformation, 2nd Ed. Philadelphia, WB Saunders, 1976.
103. Spotorno A: Stabilization of congenital equinovarus following surgical and non-surgical therapy by means of transplantation of anterior tibial onto fifth metatarsal. Arch Orthop 63:98, 1950.
104. Steyler JCA, Van Der Walt ID: Correction of resistant adduction of the forefoot in congenital club foot and congenital metatarsus varus by metatarsal osteotomy. Br J Surg 53:558, 1966.
105. Swann M, Lloyd-Roberts GC, Catterall A: The anatomy of uncorrected club feet. A study of rotation deformity. J Bone Joint Surg 51B:263, 1969.
106. Tachdjian M: Pediatric Orthopedics. Philadelphia, WB Saunders, 1990.
107. Thometz J, Simons G: Deformity of the calcaneocuboid joint in patients who have talipes equinovarus. J Bone Joint Surg 75A:190–195, 1993.
108. Thompson GH, Richardson AB, Westin GW: Surgical management of resistant congenital talipes equinovarus deformities. J Bone Joint Surg 64A:652, 1982.

109. Turco VJ: Surgical correction of the resistant club foot. One-stage posteromedial release with internal fixation: A preliminary report. J Bone Joint Surg 53A:477, 1971.
110. Turco VJ: Resistant congenital club foot—one stage posteromedial release with internal fixation. A follow-up report of a fifteen-year experience. J Bone Joint Surg 61A:805, 1979.
111. Turco VJ: Club foot. *In* Current problems in orthopaedics. New York, Churchill Livingstone, 1981.
112. Turner JW, Cooper RR: Anterior transfer of the tibialis posterior through the interosseous membrane. Clin Orthop 83:241, 1972.
113. Vanderwilde R, Staheli L, Chew D, et al: Measurements on radiographs of the foot in normal infants and children. J Bone Joint Surg 70A:407, 1988.
114. Walsham WJ, Hughes WK: Treatment of talipes equinus. *In* The deformities of the human foot. London, Bailliere, Tindall & Cox, 1895, p 294.
115. Watkins M, Jones JB, Ryder CT, et al: Transplantation of the posterior tibial tendon. J Bone Joint Surg 36A:1181, 1964.
116. Watts AW: Anterior transplantation of tibialis posterior tendon. Aust N Z J Surg 34:284, 1965.
117. Weseley MS, Barenfeld PA: Calcaneal osteotomy for the treatment of cavus deformity. Bull Hosp Joint Dis 31:93, 1970.
118. Weseley MS, Barenfeld PA: Mechanism of the Dwyer calcaneal osteotomy. Clin Orthop 70:137, 1970.
119. Whitman A: Astragalectomy and backward displacement of the foot. An investigation of its practical results. J Bone Joint Surg 4:266, 1922.
120. Wijesinha S, Menalaus M: Operation for calcaneus deformity after surgery for club feet. J Bone Joint Surg 71B:234, 1989.
121. Wilkins K, DeHaan J: Talar osteotomy in the treatment of resistant equinovarus deformities. Presented at the Annual Meeting of the Pediatric Orthopedic Society of North America, May 5, 1986.
122. Wynne-Davies R: Talipes equinovarus. A review of eighty-four cases after completion of treatment. J Bone Joint Surg 46B:464, 1964.
123. Yngve V, Miller P, Herndon W: Modified Turco vs. modified Goldner release for idiopathic club foot. Toronto, Canada, May 18, 1987.
124. Young AB: Club foot treated by astragalectomy. 50-year follow-up of a case. Lancet 1:670, 1962.

40

Vertical Talus

ROBERT S. ADELAAR

Vertical talus, or convex pes valgus, was first described by Henken in 1914.[1] Lamy and Weissman gave the first comprehensive review in the literature in 1939 and suggested the term *congenital vertical talus*.[2, 3] Many investigators have contributed to our knowledge of this disorder over the last few decades,[4] including Goldner,[10] Coleman and colleagues,[5, 6] Drennan and Sharrard,[7] Herndon and Heyman,[8] and Patterson and colleagues.[9] The treatment philosophy used at the Richmond Children's Hospital has been a modification of the surgical approach used by Goldner from Duke University Medical Center. In a previous study, the Goldner-type release was found to be superior to other approaches and to conservative cast treatment for the true vertical talus.[10]

CLINICAL FEATURES

The clinical features of this condition (Fig. 40–1) are usually constant, regardless of the associated disorders. Many associated disorders have been described in conjunction with vertical talus,[10–13] such as malformation of the neural arch, arthrogryposis, congenital dislocation of the hip, microcephaly, and mongolism.

The severity of the bone and soft tissue changes described in this disease is often related to the age at diagnosis and initiation of treatment. The hindfoot is in equinus and eventually goes into eversion because of the action of the peroneal and extensor tendon groups. The sole of the foot is convex (see Fig. 40–1), with the talus being the lowest bony prominence that can be palpated. The talus is rigid to any manual reduction. The forefoot is held in dorsiflexion and abduction. A dorsal lateral crease is often found near the junction of the talus and navicular (see Fig. 40–1); this space is usually filled with the anterolateral extensor tendon groups.

Range of motion is difficult to evaluate after secondary changes have occurred. In the early vertical talus (before 3 months of age), the talus and subtalar joints are rigidly locked and there is some instability of the talotibial articulation secondary to the narrow posterior talus position in the mortise. Dorsiflexion occurs at the junction between the talus and navicular and is blocked when the navicular rides onto the talus. It is important to recognize that vascular anomalies have been reported, particularly hypoplasia of the posterior tibial artery.[14] This is important for the surgical approach and care of the posterior tibial vessels. There has also been a high association with other congenital conditions, as stated previously, and the examination should be complete to rule out other associated disorders.

RADIOLOGIC FEATURES

The main diagnostic feature on a lateral radiograph is a plantarflexed talus with a talonavicular dislocation (Fig. 40–2). It is important to have dorsiflexion and plantar flexion views to demonstrate that the talus remains in the plantarflexed position in order to differentiate it from a flexible plantarflexed talus or an oblique talus (Fig. 40–3). The oblique talus will demonstrate correction on dorsiflexion stress (Fig. 40–4). The navicular, which does not ossify until the later half of the second year, is normally usually aligned with the remainder of the forefoot. The metatarsal axis will approximate the area where the navicular is to be found on the lateral radiograph (see Fig. 40–2). The anteroposterior radiograph demonstrates talar medial deviation, with an

767

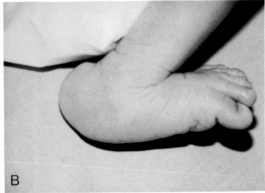
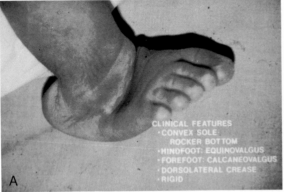

FIGURE 40–1. (*A* and *B*), The clinical features in complex pes valgus in a 1-month-old with Larsen's syndrome. (From Adelaar RS, Williams RN, Gould JS: Congenital pes valgus: Results of early comprehensive release and a review of congenital vertical talus at Richmond Crippled Children's Hospital and the University of Alabama in Birmingham. Foot Ankle 1:62, 1980. © American Orthopaedic Foot and Ankle Society 1980.)

increased angle between the talus and the os calcis (see Fig. 40–2). Another radiographic feature that indicates severity of the condition and is a poor prognostic sign is a diastasis or dislocation of the calcaneocuboid joint (Fig. 40–5).

ETIOLOGY

The etiology of this disorder is not known, but many clues have been found in stillbirth dissections and genetic studies. Approximately 2 percent of all babies are born with flatfeet, and a much smaller percentage of these babies have vertical talus.[12] More than 90 percent of

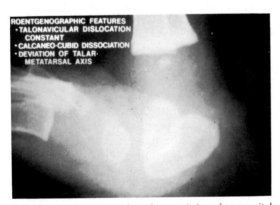

FIGURE 40–2. Radiographic characteristics of congenital vertical talus. (From Adelaar RS, Williams RN, Gould JS: Congenital pes valgus: Results of early comprehensive release and a review of congenital vertical talus at Richmond Crippled Children's Hospital and the University of Alabama in Birmingham. Foot Ankle 1:62, 1980. © American Orthopaedic Foot and Ankle Society 1980.)

children with Down's syndrome have plantar-flexed tali, and 10 percent of children with myelomeningocele have rigid vertical tali.[15] Two main theories have stood the test of time: (1) the condition is caused by an abnormality in tarsal evolution combined with intrauterine molding, and (2) the condition results from a neuromuscular disorder.

Böhm thought that the cause of vertical talus was an intrauterine molding problem resulting from an alteration in a normal tarsal derotation between the second and fourth months of gestation.[16] In the first stage of tarsal evolution, between 6 and 8 weeks of gestation, the foot and tibia are in the same plane in equinus. In the second stage, between 8 and 10 weeks, the foot is in equinus but supination in the forefoot starts. In the third stage, between 10 and 12 weeks, the equinus improves and the forefoot begins to abduct and supinate. In the last stage, between 12 and 14 weeks, the foot approaches neutral and starts to pronate.[13] Therefore, an alteration in the evolution after the forefoot is abducted and supinated could be responsible for the vertical talus.

The neuromuscular theory postulates a relative overactivity of the anterolateral muscle groups as well as the peroneals, with subsequent fibrosis of the anterior structures and contraction of the anterior ankle and talonavicular capsule. The plantar intrinsic muscles have been found to be deficient in certain children, but usually these are children with myelomeningocele or other paralytic abnormalities.[15, 17] Therefore, increased activity or fibrosis of the anterior muscle groups and

FIGURE 40–3. Like the normal foot, the oblique talus aligns with the metatarsal axis in forced plantar flexion. The vertical talus still remains dissociated from the metatarsal axis in plantar flexion. (From Adelaar RS, Williams RN, Gould JS: Congenital pes valgus: Results of early comprehensive release and a review of congenital vertical talus at Richmond Crippled Children's Hospital and the University of Alabama in Birmingham. Foot Ankle 1:62, 1980. © American Orthopaedic Foot and Ankle Society 1980.)

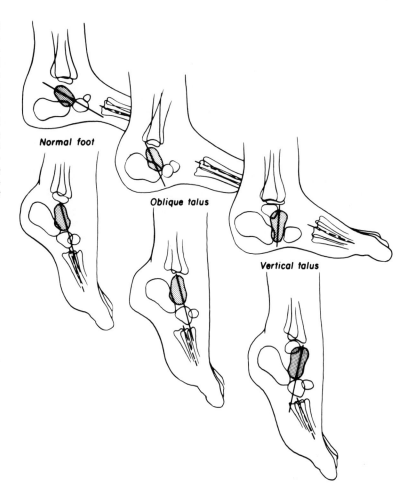

Normal foot

Oblique talus

Vertical talus

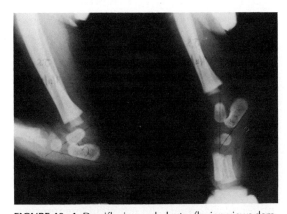

FIGURE 40–4. Dorsiflexion and plantar flexion views demonstrating that the talus is flexible and reduces with alignment of the talar-metatarsal axis. (From Adelaar RS, Williams RN, Gould JS: Congenital pes valgus: Results of early comprehensive release and a review of congenital vertical talus at Richmond Crippled Children's Hospital and the University of Alabama in Birmingham. Foot Ankle 1:62, 1980. © American Orthopaedic Foot and Ankle Society 1980.)

peroneals, combined with a relatively weak plantar intrinsic muscle and possibly an insufficient tibialis posterior, would produce a midtarsal talonavicular dislocation. The Achilles tendon is thought to be overactive to compensate for the weak plantar flexion group and therefore causes the hindfoot to be in equinus.

The genetic correlations are sporadic, but the condition has been found in identical twins and isolated family members.[12] The strongest genetic correlation is a report of five generations of defects in the upper and lower extremity carried by a single autosomal dominant gene in a condition called digitotalar dysmorphism.[18] In our study group, there was a set of identical twins with bilateral vertical talus.[10]

PATHOLOGY

The soft tissue pathology and bone pathology have been well described by stillbirth dis-

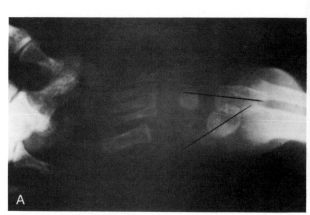
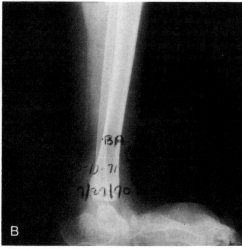

FIGURE 40–5. Radiographs revealing an increased angle between the talus and os calcis (*A*) and calcaneocuboid diastasis (*B*). (From Adelaar RS, Williams RN, Gould JS: Congenital pes valgus: Results of early comprehensive release and a review of congenital vertical talus at Richmond Crippled Children's Hospital and the University of Alabama in Birmingham. Foot Ankle 1:62, 1980. © American Orthopaedic Foot and Ankle Society 1980.)

sections.[4–6, 9, 12, 16, 19–24] It is important to differentiate adaptive changes in older specimens from early changes. The os calcis has been shown to demonstrate several architectural abnormalities in the fetal specimens, such as absence of the anterior facet, hypoplasia of the middle facet, and abnormal slanting of the posterior facet. The slanting of the posterior facet, which is the main support keeping the talus upright, is a significant problem when the talus is being reduced during surgery.[9, 21] The talus is directed plantar and medial, with evidence of hypoplasia of the head and neck. The navicular, which does not ossify until the later part of the second year, is in normal alignment with the metatarsal axis. The navicular is normal in its development and undergoes adaptive changes secondary to prolonged talonavicular dislocation. The navicular is noted to have developed posterior erosion from the superior surface of the talus when it is held in its dislocated position.[17] The calcaneocuboid joint often dislocates after prolonged dorsiflexion (see Fig. 40–5). The greater the separation in the calcaneocuboid joint, the worse the prognosis for reduction without a separate lateral approach to the calcaneocuboid.[7]

The heel cord, posterior ankle, and subtalar capsule are contracted from the equinus position. The talonavicular capsule, interosseous talocalcaneal ligament, spring ligament, and calcaneocuboid ligament are all abnormal from adaptive changes. The posterior tibial and peroneus tendon groups are anteriorly subluxed and contribute an abnormal bending movement to the forefoot. The anterior muscle groups and corresponding retinacular ligaments have been found to be histologically abnormal, with increased fibrous content. Hypoplasia of the plantar intrinsic muscle has also been reported.[7, 21, 22, 24]

NONSURGICAL TREATMENT

No treatment other than surgery can be used for complete reduction of a true vertical talus. Cast treatment is not an effective form of total treatment; rather, it is used for maintaining flexibility of soft tissue until the patient can be safely operated on. If cast treatment is effective, a diagnosis of oblique talus rather than vertical talus should be considered. Therefore, casting and taping are used until the patient is in good medical condition to undergo surgery.

Early manipulative reduction attempts in some of our patients with vertical tali who had other congenital problems for which they required early surgery did not yield any improvement in the disorder.

SURGICAL TREATMENT

Many types of surgical procedures have been described, depending on what the surgeon believes to be the primary etiologic factor and depending on the patient's age at the time of treatment. In patients younger than 1 year of age, lengthening of the anterior tibial tendon, the extensor group, and the peroneals has been advocated with or without a talonavicular capsulectomy.[7] Tendon transfers have been used by those who believe in the neuromuscular etiology with plantar insufficiency.[24] The anterior tibial tendon is transferred to the neck of the talus after reduction is obtained, and the peroneus brevis is transferred to the tibialis posterior if it is believed to be insufficient.

A series of bony procedures have been advocated, particularly for children who have not been surgically treated until they are older than 3 years of age. I believe that this is a failure of diagnosis and that these procedures should be used only for salvage situations. A subtalar arthrodesis is advocated in a primary reduction for the child older than 3 because the talus cannot be reduced and maintained on the abnormal facets of the os calcis. Lamy and Weissman advocated a partial or total talectomy in the older patient and obtained good results.[3] We believe that this has no place in the modern treatment of this disorder because talectomy has a poor cosmetic outcome and results in an unstable foot. Because the medial border of the foot is thought to be elongated, navicular excision has been used to gain reduction in the older child, as advocated by Eyre-Brook,[20] Robbins,[25] Stone,[26] and Clark and colleagues.[19] In the series of Clark and colleagues, the navicular excision was combined with a medial inferior talar release.

Author's Recommended Early Treatment

Casting and taping are used for stretching and maintaining flexibility of the anterior talotibial and talonavicular capsules, as well as of the anterior and lateral muscle groups. Surgery is performed as soon as the patient is a safe risk considering the high association with other disorders. Three months of age is our earliest and preferred time to operate. The operation is a comprehensive release that has been adapted from the procedure of Goldner[10] (Fig. 40–6). The objective of the procedure is to perform a soft tissue release without devascularizing the talus and to achieve a stable reduction of the talus. It is our philosophy that the primary bone pathology is between the talus and os calcis, with the rest of the bone changes being adaptive to long-term dislocation. The goal is to reduce the talus on the os calcis and to maintain this reduction by pin fixation because the os calcis articular facets are maldeveloped. We believe that the navicular and forefoot changes are adaptive and will be reversed by early correction. It is important to note that this procedure should be performed early in life and with loupe magnification in order to avoid injury to vital vascular structures. Meticulous care of the cartilage should be used.

With a posterolateral approach (see Fig. 40–6C), the incision is made long enough so that the Achilles tendon, peroneus brevis, and peroneus longus can be lengthened. In addition, from the lateral side, the contracted posterior ankle capsule and subtalar capsule are released. The deltoid ligament is not taken down. The lateral incision can also be extended to include an open reduction of the calcaneocuboid joint if subluxation occurs (see Fig. 40–5).

In the second step of this two-incision approach, a medial incision is made, centered at the midpoint of the talus (see Fig. 40–6D). Subcutaneous tissue is elevated carefully, the neurovascular bundle is identified, and a loop refractor is placed around the neurovascular bundle. The posterior tibial nerve and artery are not separated unless they are in the way of the dissection. It should be noted that the posterior tibial nerve divides into four branches near the area of the abductor hallucis longus. The posterior tibial tendon is identified, and the surgeon should remember that there may be anterior subluxation over the medial malleolus. The anterior talonavicular capsule is released, and flaps are made that can be used after reduction to support the talonavicular joint (see Fig. 40–6D). The spring ligament is identified; usually, this does not need to be released because it has been stretched, but it may need plication at the conclusion of the procedure. The medial subtalar joint is then released, including the interosseous ligament between the talus and the tibia (see Fig. 40–6E).

At this point, the talus should be able to be moved toward a more dorsiflexed position. The anterior tibiotalar capsule is released under loupe magnification to avoid injuring any vessels penetrating into the neck area of the talus. The central portion of the deltoid is not released, but in order to gain reduction, it may be necessary to release the anterior and posterior superficial portions. If the talus is noted to be mobilized with difficulty, release of the

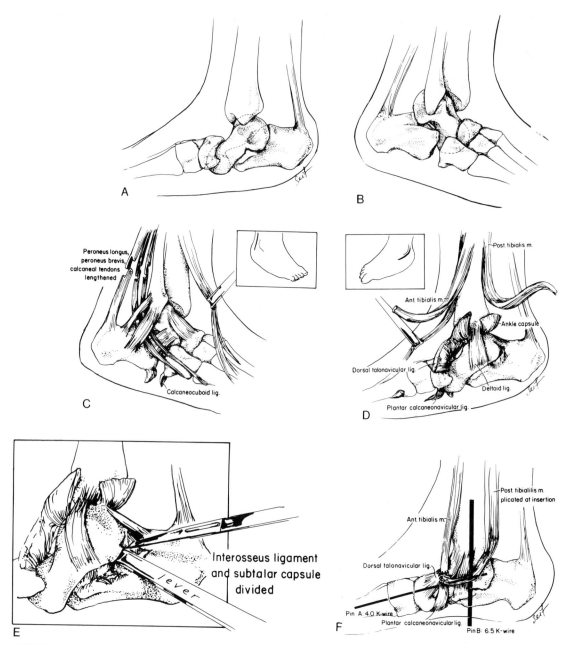

FIGURE 40–6. Comprehensive surgical correction. (*A*), Medial profile. (*B*), Lateral profile. (*C*), Posterolateral approach with lengthening of the peroneal tendons and Achilles tendon. (*D*), Medial approach with peritalar and subtalar release. (*E*), The posterior tibial tendon is advanced, and the anterior tibial tendon is placed into the reduced talus. (*F*), Stabilization with Kirschner wires. (From Adelaar RS, Williams RN, Gould JS: Congenital pes valgus: Results of early comprehensive release and a review of congenital vertical talus at Richmond Crippled Children's Hospital and the University of Alabama in Birmingham. Foot Ankle 1:62, 1980. © American Orthopaedic Foot and Ankle Society 1980.)

calcaneocuboid joint may also be needed in order to completely free the talus from the midtarsal joint. The talus is positioned on the os calcis, with note taken of the hypotrophic facets, particularly the posterior facets, and 0.062-inch Kirschner wires are used to stabilize the os calcis, talus, and ankle in a neutral position (Fig. 40–7). Radiographs are now

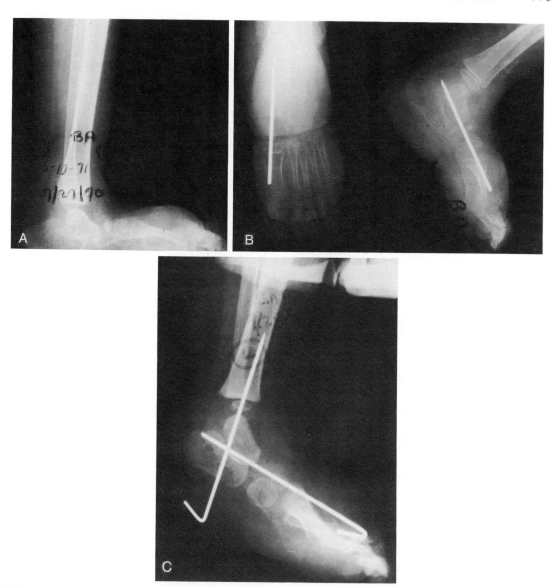

FIGURE 40–7. (*A* to *C*), Radiographs of the vertical talus, which aligns with the metatarsal axis after release. Kirschner wire fixation is used for 6 weeks. (From Adelaar RS, Williams RN, Gould JS: Congenital pes valgus: Results of early comprehensive release and a review of congenital vertical talus at Richmond Crippled Children's Hospital and the University of Alabama in Birmingham. Foot Ankle 1:62, 1980. © American Orthopaedic Foot and Ankle Society 1980.)

obtained to determine the initial reduction of the hindfoot. It is important to determine that the talus is positioned upright on the posterior articular facet and held in a horizontal position supported by the middle and anterior facets. If the facets are not able to support the talus, a subtalar extra- or intra-articular arthrodesis should be considered. Another 0.062-inch

Kirschner wire is passed from the navicular in retrograde fashion into the forefoot, and the navicular is positioned on the head of the talus. The calcaneocuboid joint is also reduced, inspecting it from the lateral side. Pin fixation can be used on the calcaneocuboid joint but is usually not needed.

The capsules that have been fashioned over

the talonavicular and anterior tibial tendon are then sutured after reduction of the forefoot. The anterior tibial tendon is transferred to the neck of the talus to maintain it in a horizontal position (Fig. 40–6*F*). A separate incision is made on the anterior surface, with care taken to preserve the anterior tibial vessel, which may be the only vessel present. The extensor tendons may need lengthening, particularly in an older child. It is important that the peroneal tendons then be positioned behind the malleoli, particularly if they are subluxed, and new retinacular flaps should be made. With this comprehensive release, we have not had any problem with the young child in reducing the elongated medial forefoot. There has been no need in our series of young people to excise the navicular, which we believe is normal in this condition.[22] It is important, in our opinion, to preserve the navicular, which is the keystone of the medial longitudinal arch. Preoperative assessment of the posterior tibial artery, which is achieved with Doppler imaging, should be performed if there is any question of hypoplasia of this vessel.[4] Great care must be taken not to compromise the anterior tibial circulation.

In the postoperative period, the patient is maintained in a long-leg cast, with the pins external to the skin and with the knee flexed 20 degrees for 6 weeks. The cast is applied at the time of surgery and is not changed until 6 to 8 weeks after surgery. Absorbable suture is used so that there is no need to inspect the wound. The pins are removed at 6 weeks, and a new, short-leg, non–weight-bearing cast is applied. At 3 months, the patient is placed in a short-leg weight-bearing cast. Four months postoperatively the cast is removed, and the foot is placed in a straight-laced high-top shoe with a semirigid leather arch. The shoe is attached to a short-leg brace. This is worn for another 3 to 6 months, followed by containment with only a high-top straight-laced shoe until 2 years of age. Care should be taken to perform radiography repeatedly to check for recurrent subluxation.

Surgical Treatment of the Older Child

In the child older than 3 years of age, soft tissue reconstruction usually does not give a concentric reduction because of the secondary deformity that has occurred from the prolonged dislocated position of the talonavicular joint and the talocalcaneal joint. For this age group, we recommend an intra- or extra-artic-

ular arthrodesis because in most cases the talus cannot be supported on the hypoplastic articular facets of the calcaneus. In the older child, a calcaneocuboid release is almost always required to obtain reduction of that joint. In addition, if the talonavicular cannot reduce after the talus is placed in a horizontal position, a navicular excision is sometimes necessary. We try to avoid talectomy except in cases in which arthrogryposis may be the primary disorder. A tendon transfer to the neck of the talus is always required in an older child, in addition to a complete release of the extensor tendons. Peroneal recentralization underneath the fibula with retinacular reconstruction is also necessary. A triple arthrodesis can always be carried out to salvage the severe longstanding deformity. A large portion of the inferior talus will require excision for subtalar fusion, and a navicular excision with fusion of the talus to the first and second cuneiforms may be required.

The postoperative care in the older child usually consists of cast application with pin fixation for 6 weeks, followed by continued non–weight bearing in a cast for a total of 3 months. A firm orthotic and longitudinal arch are often necessary, in addition to night bracing with a short-leg brace or a splint, for approximately 6 months after the cast has been removed.

Complications

The main complication in our series of cases has been the failure to obtain an anatomic reduction at the time of the initial surgery between the talonavicular and talocalcaneal joints.[10] It is mandatory to fix these joints because of their inherent lack of formation and tendency to redislocate. Minor degrees of skin slough are often encountered, but this condition usually does not lead to any long-term or deep-seated infections. Avascular necrosis is also a potential problem with the navicular and talus. In our series, one case of avascular necrosis of the talus occurred in one of the older children, no evidence of collapse was noted. It should be stated that magnetic resonance imaging was not used to evaluate the postoperative circulation in that series; therefore, we cannot state that the vascularity of the talus and navicular was intact. The problem with calcaneocuboid subluxation is usually a failure to recognize that the calcaneocuboid will subluxate or dislocate in long-standing cases.

Conclusions

Vertical talus is a difficult problem that requires early surgical treatment. The use of loupe magnification and care for the soft tissue and cartilage surfaces are absolute requirements. The surgeon should be aware that hypoplasia of the posterior tibial artery has been noted, which mandates careful preoperative assessment and Doppler imaging if there is any question of vascular compromise.[14]

A comprehensive surgical approach using at least two incisions, performed as early as the child is medically able to undergo the procedure and anesthesia, is the preferred treatment. It is important to approach the three-dimensional aspects of the deformity in one comprehensive procedure. The patient must leave the operating room with a full reduction of the talocalcaneal and talonavicular joints. Transfer of the anterior tibial tendon to the neck of the talus is important for maintenance of long-term reduction. The peroneus brevis is occasionally transferred to the tibialis posterior with insufficiency. It is important to recognize that the peroneal tendons can be subluxed in this condition, and they should be re-established in an anatomic location. The calcaneocuboid joint should be evaluated preoperatively to determine whether a separate approach needs to be used in this area.

For the older child, a subtalar arthrodesis may be carried out; a navicular excision is rarely used, and a talectomy should never be performed. Early recognition and treatment will, it is hoped, avoid the need for subtalar arthrodesis and bone excision procedures. A triple arthrodesis is the final salvage procedure in this disorder.

References

1. Henken R: Contribution a l'etude des formes osseuses du pied plat valgus congenital. These de Lyon, 1914.
2. Nove-Josserand: Formes anatomiques de pied plat. Rev Orthop 10:117, 1923.
3. Lamy L, Weissman L: Congenital convex pes valgus. J Bone Joint Surg 21:79, 1939.
4. Osmand-Clark H: Congenital vertical talus. J Bone Joint Surg 38B:334, 1956.
5. Coleman S, Stelling FH, Jarrett J: Congenital vertical talus: Pathogenesis and treatment. J Bone Joint Surg 48A:1422, 1966.
6. Coleman S, Stelling FH, Jarrett J: Pathomechanics and treatment of congenital vertical talus. Clin Orthop 70:62, 1970.
7. Drennan JE, Sharrard WJW: The pathologic anatomy of convex pes valgus. J Bone Joint Surg 53B:455, 1971.
8. Herndon CH, Heyman CH: Problems in recognition and treatment of congenital convex pes valgus. J Bone Joint Surg 45A:413, 1963.
9. Patterson WR, Fitz DA, Smith WS: The pathologic anatomy of congenital convex pes valgus. J Bone Joint Surg 50A:464, 1968.
10. Adelaar RS, Williams RN, Gould JS: Congenital convex pes valgus. Foot Ankle 1:62, 1980.
11. Lloyd-Roberts GC, Spence AJ: Congenital vertical talus. J Bone Joint Surg 40B:33, 1958.
12. Giannestras NJ: Congenital rigid flatfoot (congenital convex pes valgus). *In* Giannestras NJ (Ed): Foot Disorders: Medical and Surgical Management, 2nd Ed. Philadelphia, Lea & Febiger, 1973, p 184.
13. Tachdjian MO: Congenital convex pes valgus. *In* Pediatric Orthopedics. Philadelphia, WB Saunders, 1972, p 1359.
14. Ben Menachim Y, Butler JE: Arteriography of the foot in congenital deformities. J Bone Joint Surg 56A:1625, 1974.
15. Sharrard WJW, Grosfield J: The management of deformity and paralysis of foot in myelomeningocele. J Bone Joint Surg 50B:456, 1968.
16. Böhm M: Der Fotal Fuss: Beitrag zur Entschung des pes planus, des pes valgus und des pes plano-valgus. Z Orthop 57, 1932.
17. Specht EE: Congenital paralytic vertical talus. J Bone Joint Surg 57A:842, 1975.
18. Beighton PH, Sallis JG: Digito-talar dysmorphysm. J Bone Joint Surg 57A:842, 1975.
19. Clark MW, D'Ambrosia RD, Ferguson AB Jr: Congenital vertical talus. J Bone Joint Surg 59A:816, 1977.
20. Eyre-Brook A: Congenital vertical talus. J Bone Joint Surg 49B:618, 1967.
21. Searfoss R, Bendana A, King G, Miller G: Vertical talus of unusual etiology. J Bone Joint Surg 57A:409, 1975.
22. Silk FF, Wainwright D: The recognition and treatment of congenital flatfoot in infancy. J Bone Joint Surg 49B:623, 1967.
23. Storen H: Congenital convex pes valgus with vertical talus. Acta Orthop Scand Suppl 94:1–104, 1967.
24. Duckworth T, Smith TWD: The treatment of paralytic convex pes valgus. J Bone Joint Surg 54B:305, 1974.
25. Robbins H: Naviculectomy for congenital vertical talus. Presented at the Annual Meeting of the American Orthopedic Foot Society. Dallas, TX, 1974.
26. Stone KH: Congenital vertical talus: A new operation. Proc R Soc Med 56:12, 1963.

41 Cavus Foot

DAVID M. DRVARIC

The cavus foot is a perplexing abnormality characterized by a fixed equinus of the forefoot on the hindfoot. Nicholas Andry, in L'Orthopedie (1741), first described the condition as "bolt feet." Since this description, the literature abounds with theories on the etiology and development of the deformity and methods of treatment. The cavus foot is most often a sign of underlying neurologic disorder. Evaluation of the patient and the foot require detailed orthopaedic, neurologic, and radiographic examinations. Treatment is individualized according to the nature of the underlying abnormality, the age of the patient, and the site and degree of structural change.

DEFINITION

The term *pes cavus* refers to a fixed equinus of the forefoot on the hindfoot, resulting in a pathologic elevation of the longitudinal arch. Pes cavus may occur as an isolated deformity (simple pes cavus); however, it is most often seen in association with other deformities. *Pes cavovarus* refers to a fixed forefoot equinus deformity, with either a fixed or flexible varus hindfoot deformity. *Pes calcaneocavus* is characterized by the calcaneus position of the hindfoot and the fixed equinus position of the forefoot, while in *pes equinocavus* the ankle, hindfoot, and forefoot are in equinus.

ETIOLOGY

The etiology of the cavus deformity can be divided into five major categories: neuromus-

cular, congenital, idiopathic, traumatic, and miscellaneous (Table 41–1).

The cavus deformity is most often a sign of underlying neurologic disease.[14, 40] The disorders that can lead to pes cavus are varied and may affect any level of the neuromuscular unit. Charcot-Marie-Tooth disease or peroneal-ulnar muscular atrophy is a hereditary peripheral neuropathy that is the most common cause of pes cavus.[*] Duchenne's muscular dystrophy, which is primarily a muscle disease, often demonstrates cavus deformities of the feet, particularly in the latter stages of the disease.[26] Lesions of the anterior horn cell produced by conditions such as poliomyelitis[†] and myelomeningocele,[13, 14, 40, 50] long tract abnormalities such as Friedreich's ataxia,[14, 40, 58, 90, 101] and central nervous system abnormalities such as cerebral palsy,[11, 33] although rare, can also produce cavus deformity.

Some cases of cavus foot deformity are congenital. These are usually the residua of clubfoot deformities.[‡] Arthrogryposis multiplex congenita has classically been included in this category[90]; however, more current theories regarding the etiology of arthrogryposis allow us to consider this condition among the neuromuscular etiologies.

Isolated congenital cavus foot deformities have also been described.[7, 107] This type may not be recognized immediately owing to the soft tissues covering the neonatal and infantile foot; however, the deformity will become evident with time. Barenfeld and colleagues[7] be-

---

*See references 4, 14, 17, 32, 47, 62, 81, 82, and 90.
†See references 8, 14, 15, 20, 23, 68, and 97.
‡See references 1, 12, 20, 24, 29–31, 34, and 92.

TABLE 41–1. ETIOLOGY OF PES CAVUS

CLASSIFICATION	REFERENCES
Neuromuscular	
Charcot-Marie-Tooth disease	Alexander et al,[4] Brewerton et al,[14] Brody et al,[17] Dyck et al,[32] Gilroy,[37] Heron,[40] Jacobs et al,[47] Levitt et al,[55] Mann et al,[60] Sabir et al,[81, 82] Shapiro et al[90]
Spinal dysraphism	Brewerton et al,[14] Duckworth,[27] Hayes et al,[39] Heron,[40] James et al,[50] Mayer,[62] Sharrard et al[91]
Poliomyelitis	Bradley et al,[13] Brewerton et al,[14] Brewster et al,[15] Drennan,[26] Heron,[40] Lipscomb[56]
Diastematomyelia	Heron,[40] James et al,[50] Winter et al[111]
Friedreich's ataxia	Brewerton et al,[14] Heron,[40] Makin,[58] Shapiro et al,[90] Tyrer et al[101]
Syringomyelia	Pashiro et al,[70] Williams[109]
Cerebral palsy	Bleck,[11] Brewerton et al,[14] Eilert,[33] Gilroy[37]
Trauma	Bigos et al,[10] Rivera-Dominguez et al[79]
Miscellaneous	Brewerton et al,[14] Dyck et al,[32] Heron,[40] Rapin et al,[77] Rivera-Dominguez et al,[79] Shapiro et al,[90] Tyrer et al[101]
Congenital	
Isolated deformity	Barenfeld et al,[7] Brockway,[16] Gilroy,[37] Mayer,[62] Wein et al,[105] Weseley et al[107]
Residual deformity of clubfoot	Abrams,[1] Bost et al,[12] Cole,[20] Dekel et al,[24] Dwyer,[29–31] Fisher et al,[34] Jahss,[48] Mayer,[62] Samilson,[85] Sherman et al[92]
Idiopathic	Brewerton et al,[14] Ibrahim,[46] Lovell et al,[57] Mayer,[62] Tachdjian[99]
Traumatic	
Malunion of fracture	Ibrahim,[46] Lovell et al[57]
Compartment syndrome	Horne,[43] Karlstrom et al,[54] Matsen et al,[61] Owen et al[69]
Miscellaneous	
Dermatologic	Lovell et al,[57] Port et al[75]
Endocrine	Carney et al,[18] Rasmusson,[78] Saltzman et al,[83] Schwankhaus et al[88]
Iatrogenic	

lieve that several factors play a role in the development of this type of cavus, which is most likely related to intrauterine posture.

Idiopathic cavus foot deformity is not common. Brewerton and colleagues reported a combined retrospective and prospective study from the Pes Cavus Clinic at the Royal National Orthopaedic Hospital.[14] Their preliminary retrospective review of 577 patients placed 81 percent of the patients in the idiopathic category. Of the first 77 patients investigated after the institution of the Pes Cavus Clinic, 66 percent were shown to have an underlying neurologic abnormality. Based on these figures, only one-third of the patients with a cavus foot have an idiopathic deformity.

Traumatic etiologies for cavus deformity are becoming more widely recognized. In addition to malunion of tarsal and metatarsal fractures, more remote fractures and injuries may also cause this deformity. Karlstrom and colleagues reported 23 cases of cavus deformity of the foot following tibial shaft fracture.[54] They believed that this deformity was secondary to "fibrous contracture of the muscles in the deep posterior compartment caused by vascular damage, swelling in the deep posterior com-

partment, or severe muscle laceration." It is now well recognized that this is a late manifestation of a deep posterior compartment syndrome.[61, 69] Other documented traumatic etiologies include ankle fractures[43] and peroneus longus tendon laceration.[25]

There are many other known causes of cavus deformity[46, 57, 99] other than those discussed here. Ledderhose's disease, or plantar fibromatosis, rarely is identified as the cause but must be considered, particularly in patients with other sites of fibromatosis. Iatrogenic overlengthening of the tendo Achillis may lead to a calcaneocavus deformity. Dermatologic abnormalities,[75] multiple endocrine neoplasia,[18, 83] and other endocrinopathies[78, 88] are also seen in association with cavus deformity of the feet.

PATHOGENESIS

The exact pathogenesis and mechanics of cavus foot deformity remain unclear, as no one theory can account for all clinically identified types of the deformity. Proposed theories can be categorized as either intrinsic muscle imbalance, extrinsic muscle imbalance, a combination of intrinsic and extrinsic imbalance, and nonmuscular causes.

Intrinsic Muscle Imbalance

The earliest of the intrinsic muscle imbalance theories was described by Duchenne in 1867. He postulated a primary weakness, or paralysis, of the intrinsic musculature of the foot, which would produce clawing analogous to that seen in the hand; however, it is now recognized that the interossei of the foot are anatomically different from those in the hand.[59] Coonrad and colleagues,[23] and later Garceau and Brahms,[36] convincingly demonstrated that functioning interossei are required in order to develop the cavus deformity.

Extrinsic Muscle Imbalance

Extrinsic muscle imbalance has also been postulated as a cause of cavus foot. The most widely espoused theory maintains that the first metatarsal is plantarflexed, and the entire forefoot is pronated by the peroneus longus muscle acting against a relatively weak anterior tibial muscle. The long toe extensors further exaggerate the deformity by hyperextending the proximal phalanges of the toes, forcing the metatarsals into plantar flexion by the so-called windlass mechanism.[19, 21, 99]

Mann and Missirian performed a detailed investigation into the etiology of cavus foot deformity in patients with Charcot-Marie-Tooth disease.[60] Their theory maintains that the primary abnormality produces a weakness of the anterior tibial muscle, peroneus brevis muscle, and the intrinsic musculature. Consequently, the unopposed actions of the peroneus longus muscle, the posterior tibial muscle, and the long toe flexors are responsible for, respectively, the plantar flexion of the first metatarsal and pronation of the forefoot, the hindfoot varus, and the forefoot adduction.

Other theories of primary extrinsic muscle imbalance have been put forth. Scheer and Crego[87] noted the development of severe calcaneocavus deformity with paralysis of the gastrocnemius-soleus complex. Bentzon noted that in selected patients with cavus deformity, excluding those with Charcot-Marie-Tooth disease and poliomyelitis, transplantation of the peroneus longus tendon to the peroneus brevis tendon reduced the plantar flexion of the first metatarsal and the subsequent cavus.[9] Finally, Karlholm and Nilsonne proposed that transfer of the posterior tibial tendon alone would avoid recurrence of the deformity.[53]

Nonmuscular Causes

Nonmuscular causes of cavus deformity have also been postulated. Intrinsic bony abnormality, improper shoewear, and gravity have all been implicated in the development of this deformity. Primary contracture of the plantar fascia has been proposed by many authors, including Rugh,[80] Jahss,[48] and Dwyer,[29] as the mechanism to which the deformity can best be attributed.

Combined Muscle Imbalances

Each of the foregoing proposed mechanisms has some theoretical merit. However, because of the synergism in the foot, a combination of imbalances in both the intrinsic and extrinsic muscle groups, as proposed by Chuinard and Baskin, is most likely to be responsible for the development of this deformity.[19] Their theory states that a right triangle of muscle forces is responsible for ankle-foot function and balance—the gastrocnemius-soleus group, the plantar muscles, and the tibialis anterior. Weakness or contracture in any one of these three groups causes an imbalance in these forces, with resultant cavus deformity (Fig. 41–1).

EVALUATION

The patient presenting for evaluation of a cavus foot usually will not complain of the deformity per se, but rather of symptoms such as pain, clumsiness, or abnormal shoe wear. The pain may be generalized to the entire leg or foot, or it may be specifically related to callosities that have developed either beneath the metatarsal heads or at the base of the fifth metatarsal. Clumsiness, or an abnormality of gait, is often seen in the older child with a progressive neurologic condition. Patients with a fixed rigid deformity may complain of abnormal shoe wear, and patients with an asym-

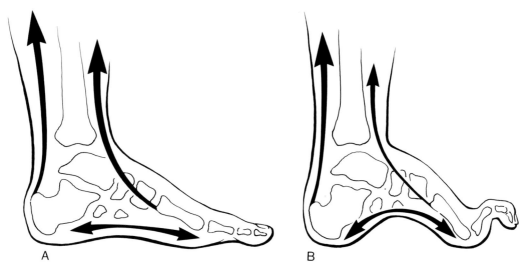

FIGURE 41–1. *(A)*, The normally balanced foot. The balanced forces of the gastrocnemius-soleus, the plantar musculature, and the anterior tibial muscle approximate a right triangle. *(B)*, In the foot with pes cavus, imbalance in any of these forces can result in deformity. (Redrawn from Chuinard EG, Baskin M: Claw-foot deformity. Treatment by transfer of the long extensors into the metatarsals and fusion of the interphalangeal joints. J Bone Joint Surg 55A:360, 1973.)

metrical deformity (Fig. 41–2) may have difficulty in obtaining comfortable shoes as well.

An extensive diagnostic evaluation to determine the underlying etiology is mandatory in the patient with a cavus foot. A thorough history, including family history, is necessary to rule out any heritable disorders that are associated with cavus feet. A complete physical examination must include close examination of the skin to determine whether there are any manifestations of a spinal dysraphism such as a sinus, dimple, or hairy patch. Palpation of the thyroid is necessary to establish the presence of a nodule, which might indicate

medullary thyroid carcinoma associated with multiple endocrine neoplasia type 2b. Cardiovascular evaluation is performed to rule out cardiac involvement, which is typical of inherited neurologic conditions, such as Friedreich's ataxia, to screen for some of the less common etiologies of cavus deformity. Orthopaedic evaluation includes a detailed motor and sensory evaluation of both the upper and lower extremities as well as a comprehensive physical evaluation of the spine.

Consultation with a neurologist is warranted in all patients with cavus feet, as a comprehensive electrodiagnostic evaluation, including

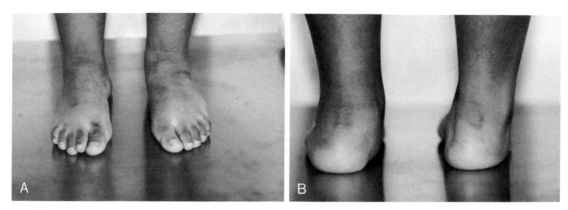

FIGURE 41–2. Standing anteroposterior *(A)* and posteroanterior *(B)* clinical photographs of an 8-year-old girl presenting for an evaluation of "funny feet." She had difficulty wearing shoes for several years. Note the exaggeration of the longitudinal arch on the right, the supination of the forefoot in stance, and the varus attitude of the heel.

electromyography or nerve conduction velocity determinations, is usually necessary.

Clinical evaluation of the patient's gait may reveal abnormalities that may be diagnostic. An ataxic gait, a wide-based steppage gait, the so-called pegleg gait, and spastic gait patterns are easily recognized. The underlying etiology, or at least the predominant pattern of weakness, is often readily appreciated. Formal gait analysis with dynamic electromyography may be beneficial in patients in whom tendon transfers are contemplated.[74]

Evaluation of the footprint in individuals with cavus feet is important. Many techniques are available, including the use of pedobarographs, to evaluate not only the structure of the foot but to assess the local pressures beneath the foot.[3, 51, 72] In comparison with the normal footprint, the cavus foot will usually show a deepening of the concavity of the medial border of the foot, and a prominence laterally in the region of the base of the fifth metatarsal. As the deformity progresses, the footprint eventually becomes divided into two; ultimately, the toe prints will disappear in the most severe cases associated with secondary clawtoe deformity (Fig. 41–3).

Japas has classified the cavus foot into anterior, posterior, and combined forms.[51] He emphasized that the components of the foot are interdependent and must therefore be evaluated individually, because treatment will be based on the position of the apex of the deformity and on the relative flexibility of the foot.

The forefoot of the cavus foot must demonstrate fixed plantar flexion of the first ray. Pronation of the entire forefoot—following the first ray—is also evident. The flexibility of the lateral four rays should be assessed in the non–weight-bearing position; if flexible, they should easily reduce passively onto the midfoot. If the entire forefoot is fixed in equinus, this corresponds to the "global" form of cavus described by Japas, whereas if only the first ray is fixed in plantar flexion, this is simple "cavus deformity of the first ray."

The midfoot is often the apex of the deformity, particularly in the global form of the condition. The relationship and mobility of the midfoot to both the forefoot and hindfoot should be assessed. Any limitation of motion, or pain localizing to this region, should be noted.

The position of the hindfoot is variable. It may be in equinus, calcaneus, varus, or valgus position and may be either flexible or fixed. In the most common presentation, the hindfoot is initially situated in varus but is reducible passively; however, with time the varus position of the hindfoot becomes fixed. The lack of triceps surae in individuals with myelomeningocele or poliomyelitis predisposes them to development of a calcaneus hindfoot; these individuals often have a pistol-grip heel and significant functional disability. Heel strike in varus leads to recurrent lateral ankle ligament sprains and potential instability.

The plantar surface of the foot should be

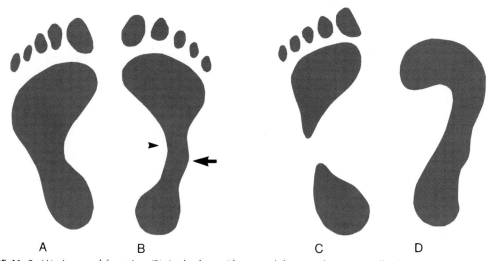

FIGURE 41–3. *(A)*, A normal footprint. *(B)*, In the foot with cavus deformity, there is initially deepening of the concavity of the medial column *(arrowhead)* with prominence of the base of the fifth metatarsal *(arrow)*. *(C)*, The footprint eventually becomes divided into two parts. *(D)*, Ultimately, with severe clawing of the toes, the toeprints disappear.

examined closely. As a rule, the plantar structures, particularly the plantar fascia, are tight. There will often be callosities underneath the metatarsal heads and, after the hindfoot varus deformity has become fixed, beneath the base of the fifth metatarsal.

Clawing of the toes is seen in association with cavus deformity. The clawtoe deformity is characterized by hyperextension of the metatarsophalangeal joints and flexion of the interphalangeal joints. This is not a universal finding, but if present, it must be recognized and assessed so that correction of this deformity may be incorporated into the treatment plan. Occasionally, in the most severe stage, the toes do not touch the ground and are functionless. Again, passive manipulation to assess the ability of the toe deformity to correct should be carried out. Elevating the first metatarsal is often adequate to alleviate the toe deformity.

The overall appearance of the foot and the relationship of the forefoot to the hindfoot must be assessed in the weight-bearing position. As described by Paulos and colleagues, the forefoot is fixed by the plantarflexed first ray in pronation.[72] Therefore, the hindfoot must be forced into varus or supination with weight bearing if the foot is to be plantigrade. This is called the "tripod effect" (Fig. 41–4). With growth, adaptive bony changes usually occur, resulting in a fixed cavovarus deformity.

The flexibility of the hindfoot, as it relates to the forefoot, is critical in the evaluation. Given a fixed forefoot deformity and a supple hindfoot, only forefoot correction is necessary to relieve the secondary hindfoot deformation; however, if the hindfoot deformity is fixed, addressing only the forefoot will result in incomplete correction. Coleman and Chesnut have described the standing lateral block test to evaluate hindfoot flexibility.[22] This test is performed as follows: the heel and lateral border of the foot are placed on a block approximately 1 inch in thickness. In the full weightbearing position, this allows the first metatarsal to hang free, thus eliminating the tripod effect. If the hindfoot is flexible, the heel will assume the normal valgus position. Radiographs, clinical photographs, or both can be used to document this correction (Fig. 41–5).

Radiographic evaluation should include standing or simulated weight-bearing anteroposterior and lateral radiographs of the foot. The initial evaluation should also include standing posteroanterior and lateral radiographs of the spine to rule out spinal dysraphism and diastematomyelia as possible etiologies of the deformity (Fig. 41–6). Further

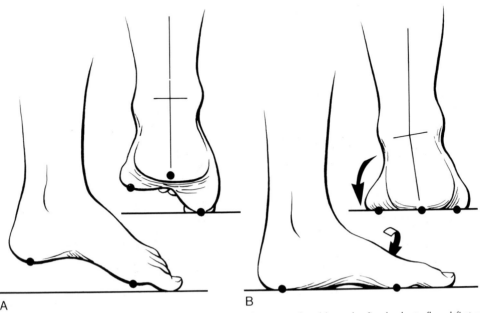

A   B

FIGURE 41–4. The tripod effect. *(A)*, The pronation of the forefoot is attributable to the fixed, plantarflexed first ray. *(B)*, With weight bearing, a flexible hindfoot is forced into supination. (Redrawn from Paulos L, Coleman SS, Samuelson KM: Pes cavovarus. Review of a surgical approach using selective soft-tissue procedures. J Bone Joint Surg 62A:943, 1980.)

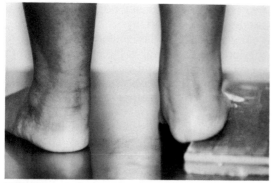

FIGURE 41–5. The lateral standing block test. The patient stands with the heel and the lateral border of the foot on the block, which is of sufficient height to eliminate the effect of the first metatarsal on the hindfoot. If the hindfoot is flexible, as shown here, the normal relationships should be established.

imaging studies of the spine, such as myelography, computed tomography, and magnetic resonance imaging, should be performed if an intraspinal anomaly is suggested on the basis of the clinical examination, electrodiagnostic studies, and plain radiographs.

The anteroposterior radiograph of the foot usually demonstrates the supination of the forefoot as shown by the "stacking" of the metatarsals. Hindfoot varus is indicated by the parallelism of the talus on the calcaneus (Fig. 41–7). The lateral radiograph, again, demonstrates the stacking of the metatarsals and opening of the subtalar joint. The degree of cavus is best measured in the lateral projection. Hibbs described an angle formed by a line drawn through the center of the longitudinal axis of the first metatarsal and a line parallel to the longitudinal axis of the calcaneus, or the lateral calcaneal–first metatarsal angle (Fig. 41–8A).[41] In normal feet, this angle usually measures 140 to 160 degrees. Meary described an angle formed by the longitudinal axes of the lateral talus and the first metatarsal[64]; further work by Vanderwilde and associates has shown this angle to vary according to age,[102] but it is usually between 0 and 20 degrees (Fig. 8B). The relative position of the calcaneus can also be assessed on the lateral radiograph. A calcaneocavus deformity has an increased (greater than 130 degrees) tibiocalcaneal angle, an increased tuber angle of 50 to 70 degrees, compared with a normal angle of 22 to 45 degrees, or an increase in the calcaneus angle of inclination or calcaneal pitch, which is normally 11 to 38 degrees (Fig. 41–8C).[87, 95]

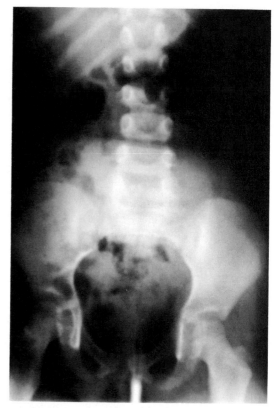

FIGURE 41–6. A standing posteroanterior radiograph of the lumbar spine demonstrates a spina bifida occulta at the level of S1. No associated intraspinal anomalies were identified with magnetic resonance imaging. This radiograph is of the same patient shown in Figures 41–2 and 41–5.

TREATMENT

Nonoperative Treatment

Management of the cavus foot is usually surgical; however, an initial period of obser-

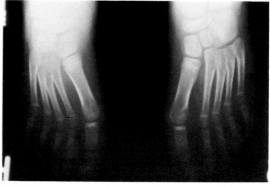

FIGURE 41–7. A standing anteroposterior radiograph of both feet demonstrates the stacking or cascade phenomenon of the metatarsals on the involved *(right)* side.

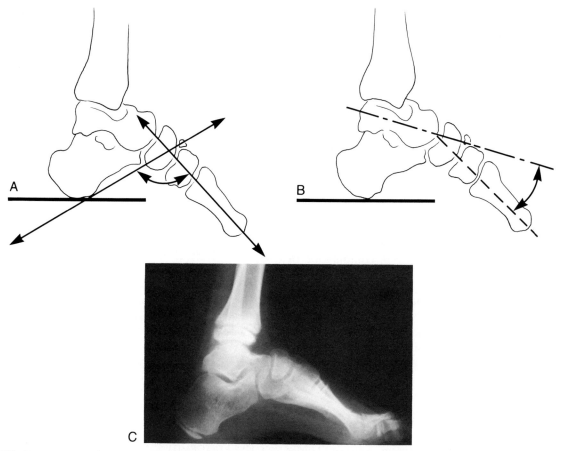

FIGURE 41–8. (A), The Hibbs angle is formed between a line drawn through the longitudinal axis of the first metatarsal and a line parallel to the longitudinal axis of the calcaneus. (B), Meary described an angle formed between a line drawn through the longitudinal axis of the talus and a line drawn through the longitudinal axis of the first metatarsal. (Redrawn from Tachjdian MO: Pes cavus and claw toes. *In* The Child's Foot. Philadelphia, WB Saunders, 1985, p 518.) (C), The calcaneus angle of inclination has a normal range of 11 to 38 degrees. In this case, the angle is greatly increased, which is indicative of calcaneus deformity.

vation and nonoperative management is beneficial. During this period it may be determined whether or not the underlying disease process is progressive. Stretching exercises, particularly those directed at the plantar fascia and often the Achilles tendon, should be carried out several times a day. Symptomatic relief can be provided temporarily by the use of a metatarsal bar, which should be positioned on the sole of the shoe, approximately 1 cm behind the metatarsal heads. The use of custom-molded inserts and padding the tongue of the shoe to relieve local pressure on the plantar surface or dorsum of the foot have also been recommended to provide symptomatic relief. It must be kept in mind, however, that these measures do not correct the deformity, or alter

the natural history of the underlying conditions.

In congenital cavus foot, as described initially by Barenfeld and colleagues,[7] and later by Weseley and colleagues,[107] a course of manipulation and serial casting showed excellent long-term results. Nonoperative management is recommended in these cases because only one patient in the reported series did not respond to this regimen.

Operative Treatment

In cases in which a specific intraspinal abnormality has been identified and is amenable to neurosurgical treatment, this should be carried out before further consideration of treatment alternatives. Often, with correction of the underlying neurologic abnormality, progression of the deficit can be arrested.[50] However, reversal of the deficit should not be expected. The remaining deformity, and often muscle imbalances, must be addressed.

Operative treatment of the cavus foot deformity is indicated when the deformity is progressive, severe, or fixed and when attempted conservative treatment has failed. The goal of all surgery is to provide a painless, plantigrade foot that can fit into a shoe without undue difficulty.

There are many surgical treatment options, including soft tissue releases, tendon transfers, procedures on bone, and any combination of these. The exact procedure or combination of procedures performed is based on the age of the patient, the flexibility of the foot, the apex of the deformity, and the nature of the underlying disease process (Table 41–2). None of the various surgical options, however, are comprehensive; each option is directed at the correction of a specific component of the cavus deformity.

Soft Tissue Release

In all cases requiring surgical correction, soft tissue release is of primary importance. This is primarily directed at the tight plantar fascia and the contracted plantar musculature. Whether this procedure can be used alone or in combination with other procedures depends upon the flexibility of the foot. Paulos and colleagues reasoned that given a supple hindfoot, as demonstrated by the standing lateral block test, release of the plantar structures alone should be adequate to allow correction of the deformity. They recommend the use of the so-called radical plantar release.[72] This procedure is fashioned after the plantar stripping procedure developed originally by Steindler[96] and later modified by Bost and colleagues.[12]

The procedure is performed under tourniquet control with the patient in the supine position. A curvilinear incision superior to the sole of the foot is preferred. This incision extends from the distal portion of the first metatarsal proximally to the middle of the calcaneus (Fig. 41–9A). The tendon of the abductor hallucis muscle is identified distally and released. The muscle is then reflected

TABLE 41–2. OPERATIVE TREATMENT OF PES CAVUS

FLEXIBLE FOREFOOT AND FLEXIBLE HINDFOOT
Radical plantar release[72]
   Steindler's stripping[96]
   Lucas' release[92]
   Tachdjian's midline release[99]
   Proximal medial longitudinal release[104]
Dorsal closing wedge osteotomy of the first
   metatarsal
   First metatarsal–cuneiform-joint fusion[63]
Tendon transfers
   Jones' transfer for the first metatarsal[52]
   Chuinard and Baskin's transfer for the lateral
     metatarsals[19]
   Girdlestone-Taylor flexor-to-extensor transfer[100]
   Frank and Johnson's extensor shift[35]

RIGID FOREFOOT AND SUPPLE HINDFOOT
Steindler's stripping[96]
Akron midtarsal dome osteotomy[106]
   Dorsal tarsal wedge osteotomy[20]
   Multiple metatarsal osteotomies[98, 103]
   First metatarsal–cuneiform-navicular fusion[63]
   Tarsometatarsal truncated wedge arthrodesis of
     Jahss[49]
   Tarsal V-osteotomy of Japas[51]

RIGID FOREFOOT AND VARUS HINDFOOT
Steindler's stripping[96]
Akron midtarsal dome osteotomy[106]
Dwyer's lateral wedge resection of the
   calcaneus[31]—staged procedure

FIXED DEFORMITY
Cavovarus
   Steindler's stripping[20]
   Tendo Achillis lengthening, if necessary
   Triple arthrodesis[2]
     "Beak" triple arthrodesis[93]
     Lambrinudi's triple arthrodesis
   Tendon transfers[44]
Calcaneocavus
   Steindler's stripping[20]
   Samilson's crescentic osteotomy of the
     calcaneus[84]
   Tendon transfers

plantarward, back to the medial tuberosity of the calcaneus. The posterior tibial neurovascular bundle and its divisions should be identified and protected. The sheaths of the flexor digitorum longus and the flexor hallucis longus are released at the master knot of Henry. The origin of the flexor hallucis brevis is then released. At this point the posterior tibial tendon, the origins of the plantar intrinsic musculature, the ligamentous interconnections of the plantar aspect of the foot, the deltoid

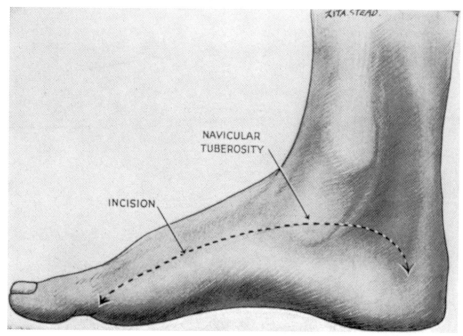

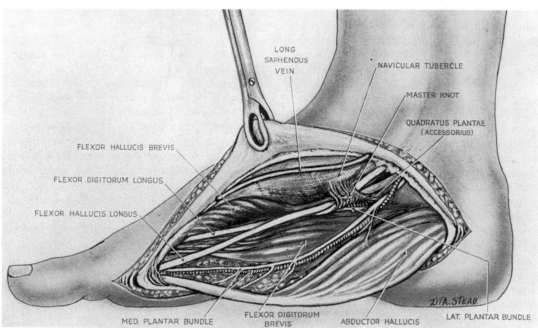

FIGURE 41–9. *(A),* The medial incision of Henry is used for the radical plantar release. *(B),* The abductor hallucis has been released and reflected, allowing visualization of the medial and lateral plantar nerves, the flexor digitorum communis and flexor digitorum longus, and the master knot of Henry.

Illustration continued on following page

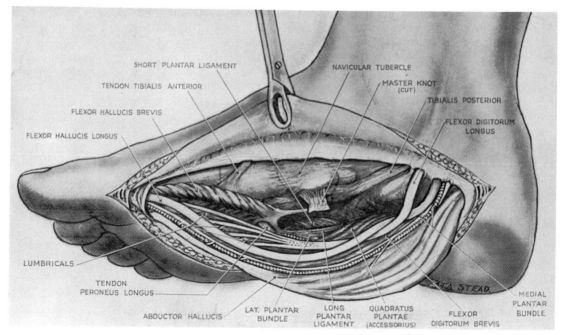

FIGURE 41–9 *Continued (C),* After division of the master knot, the deeper structures and the important supporting ligaments of the plantar surface are exposed for sectioning. (From Henry AK: Exposure of plantar structures. *In* Extensile Exposure, 2nd Ed. New York, Churchill Livingstone, 1970, pp 305–307.)

ligament, and the anterior tibial tendon are exposed (Fig. 41–9*B*). Release of the plantar musculature from its origin, the long and short plantar ligaments, and the spring and bifurcate ligaments is performed sharply, with care taken not to damage the soft cartilaginous elements (Fig. 41–9*C*). Often, opening the talonavicular joint widely allows all or part of the bifurcate ligament to be released; if incomplete division of this ligament complex prevents complete reduction, a second incision laterally may be used to improve visualization of the calcaneonaviculocuboid junction. A complete plantar fasciectomy is recommended; this procedure requires dissection of the plantar fascia from medial to lateral, both dorsal to and plantar to the fascia itself, so that it can be excised in toto, without undue risk to the neurovascular structures and muscles.[45]

When preoperative evaluation has demonstrated a rigid hindfoot, release of the talonavicular joint, medial ankle, and subtalar joint, as well as release of the dorsal, medial, and plantar capsule of the calcaneocuboid joint, can be carried out through this same incision. Recession, lengthening, or release, for transfer of the anterior or posterior tibial tendon, is also easily accomplished through this ap-

proach. Bony procedures, such as dorsal closing wedge osteotomy of the first and second metatarsals, can also be performed through this utilitarian incision.

Alternatives to this extensive dissection and release do exist and have their proponents. The "classic" release was described by Steindler.[96] Tachdjian prefers a single midline incision on the sole of the foot, as he believes the preceding dissection, and that of Steindler, are prone to allow recurrence of the deformity secondary to scar contracture.[99] Sherman and Westin described their experience with the Lucas plantar release procedure performed through a lateral incision, which is thought not to be under tension and not to be prone to contracture.[92] More recently, Ward and Clippinger described a proximal medial longitudinal arch incision beginning in the posterior aspect of the medial longitudinal arch anterior to the middle of the heel pad and curving obliquely to the middle of the medial longitudinal arch for plantar fascia release or partial resection.[104] This approach permits dissection superficial to the neurovascular structures, particularly the calcaneal branch of the posterior tibial nerve.

Postoperative care is critical. All surgical

sites must be drained to prevent accumulation of hematoma, and the use of a bulky compressive dressing, reinforced with plaster splints, is recommended. Elevation is necessary; the use of a Böhler-Braun frame facilitates continuous elevation. After approximately 5 days, the edema usually has diminished, the dressings can be removed, and the patient is placed into a plaster cast in the corrected position. No significant force should be applied to gain correction; if necessary, serial cast changes can be performed, with care taken to flatten the medial longitudinal arch, pronate the hindfoot and midfoot, and supinate the forefoot. Paulos and colleagues[72] and Sherman and Westin[92] emphasize the necessity of gradual correction of the deformity by serial cast changes. Once the foot has been brought into the corrected position, as demonstrated radiographically, this position should be maintained for 6 weeks. Further procedures, such as tendon transfers, may be performed at this time.

Tendon Transfers

Tendon transfers are useful when a dynamic imbalance creates the deformity. These transfers are best used in nonprogressive conditions and only when accurate muscle testing and grading can be performed. Muscle testing should be performed prior to any procedures on the foot. Furthermore, transfers should be used only when there is a full passive range of motion of the affected joints, and only when the fixed cavus deformity has been corrected. It must be remembered that a transfer may lose one full grade of power after the transfer; therefore, only tendons of grade 4 power or better should be transferred. All other principles of tendon transfer must be followed as well: the transfer should be into bone; a nonadherent gliding surface for the transfer must be available; when needed, an adequate pulley must be maintained or constructed; and all bony stabilization procedures should have been completed.

Tendon transfers are divided into forefoot and hindfoot procedures. Those procedures performed most commonly on the forefoot are to correct flexible clawtoe deformity. Hibbs described an en masse transfer of the extensor tendons of the lesser toes into the third cuneiform[41]; however, this fails to dynamically elevate the metatarsal heads and should not be performed. The flexor-to-extensor transfer

devised by Girdlestone and reported on by Taylor[100] and by Barbari and Brevig[6] is recommended in the young patient with deformity that can be corrected passively. In these series, excellent results have been reported by the patients; however, stiffness, persistent pain, and rotational malalignment have also been reported.[76, 99]

Those transfers that can act as dynamic elevators of the metatarsals are the extensor shift procedures described by Frank and Johnson,[35] Jones,[52] and Chuinard and Baskin.[19] Each of these procedures involves a transfer of the long extensor tendons to the neck of the metatarsals. Fusion of the interphalangeal joints, which should accompany these transfers, allows the long toe flexors to flex the metatarsophalangeal joints without producing a hammertoe deformity. I prefer the technique of Jones[52] for the great toe and that of Chuinard and Baskin[19] for the lesser toes; as noted by Shanahan and colleagues,[89] these procedures successfully delay the need for bony correction and minimize growth disturbance.

The procedures are performed under tourniquet control. A plantar release should always be performed. A longitudinal incision is made on the dorsolateral aspect of the first ray, extending from the middle of the proximal phalanx proximally to the middle of the shaft of the first metatarsal. The extensor hallucis tendon is identified and sectioned at its insertion, and the tendon is dissected free as far proximally as possible. The extensor hallucis brevis attachment is preserved. The head of the first metatarsal is then exposed extraperiosteally. A drill hole is made transversely across the metatarsal head through incisions in the periosteum. The extensor hallucis tendon is then passed through this tunnel from medial to lateral. With the ankle in neutral and the forefoot in maximal dorsiflexion so as to raise the dropped metatarsal into proper position, the distal end of the tendon is sutured to the proximal portion of the tendon above its entrance into the bone. The tension is set by pulling the tendon out to about 60 percent of its excursion from no tension to full tension. The tension applied should hold the metatarsal in an elevated position equal to the other. If it does not, the transfer is tightened. Longitudinal incisions are then made between the second and third metatarsals and between the fourth and fifth metatarsals. The long toe extensor of each of the toes is identified and transected from the base of the proximal phalanx. The neck of each metatarsal is exposed extraperiosteally, and a transverse tunnel is made through bone with a drill. Each extensor tendon is transferred to its corresponding metatarsal under equal tension. The distal portion of each tendon is sutured to its proximal portion just above the entrance into bone, similar to the first metatarsal.

The interphalangeal joint of the great toe is fused by denuding its articular cartilage and longitudinal pinning with a Kirschner wire. When the growth plate of the distal phalanx is open, the bone of the epiphyseal body is exposed and lightly burred and the rounded subchondral bone of the proximial phalanx fits into the shallow cup distally.

Fixed clawtoe deformities require fusion. Longitudinal incisions are made on the dorsum of each toe. The proximal interphalangeal joint is exposed and denuded of all articular cartilage. A single smooth intramedullary Kirschner wire is used to stabilize each of the fusions. When the proximal phalanx remains dorsiflexed on the metatarsal head, a dorsal capsulotomy of the metatarsophalangeal joint is performed to provide correct alignment.

The tourniquet is deflated and hemostasis is secured. A bulky compression dressing is applied with plaster splint reinforcement to maintain the corrected position of the forefoot and toes. When the swelling has diminished, a short-leg non–weight-bearing cast is applied. A toe plate must be incorporated into the cast to maintain the position of the toes. This cast is worn for 6 weeks, at which time the Kirschner wires are removed and a new short-leg walking cast is applied.

Many tendon transfer procedures have been described for balancing the hindfoot. Each of these transfers has its own indications based on the observed deformity, the functional disability present, and the tendons available for transfer. Tendon transfers alone, however, should not be expected to provide lasting correction.[47, 55] Anterior transfer of the posterior tibial tendon through the interosseous membrane to the third cuneiform is effective in balancing paralysis of the peroneals, tibialis anterior, and toe extensors.[44, 46] In those instances in which there is partial or complete paralysis of the gastrocnemius-soleus complex and preservation of strong tibialis anterior and common toe extensor function, transfer of the tibialis anterior to the calcaneus, as described by Peabody,[73] should be considered.

Selective Neurectomy

The importance of failing to eliminate or balance the muscular forces acting to deform the foot was stressed by Coonrad and colleagues[23] and by Garceau and Brahms.[36] It was noted that in the otherwise flail foot, the plantar muscles alone may remain functional, resulting in a cavovarus deformity of the foot. A selective denervation of the motor portions of the medial and lateral plantar nerves, myotenotomy of the short toe flexors, and plantarfasciectomy is recommended. I have had no personal experience with the procedure; however, it appears from the published results that this procedure is indicated only in children with deformity secondary to poliomyelitis. The long-term results in congenital clubfeet, arthrogryposis, spina bifida, and "idiopathic" pes cavus have been poor.[99]

Bone Procedures

The child or adult with rigid, fixed structural changes requires a bony procedure to correct the deformity. This procedure may be either osteotomy or arthrodesis. The selection of the appropriate procedure should be based on the clinical and radiographic identification of the apex of the deformity.

Flexible Forefoot and Flexible Hindfoot

In the child with a flexible pes cavus and supple hindfoot, as demonstrated by the lateral standing block test, the use of metatarsal osteotomy has proved to be effective. The procedure is performed simultaneously and through the same incision as the radical plantar release described earlier. The base of the first metatarsal is identified, care is taken to identify the physis (which is proximal in the first metatarsal), and a dorsal closing wedge osteotomy is performed. The osteotomy of the plantar cortex of the metatarsal should not be completed; rather, it should be fenestrated to allow a "greenstick" closure of the osteotomy (Fig. 41–10). Steinmann pin fixation is not necessary to maintain the position, as the forefoot will be dorsiflexed to maintain the correction from the plantar release. A smooth Steinmann pin or Kirschner wire traversing the osteotomy, the physis, and the first metatarsal–cuneiform joint may be used, if preferred by the surgeon, with little risk of producing a growth arrest. Occasionally, in the child, osteotomy of the

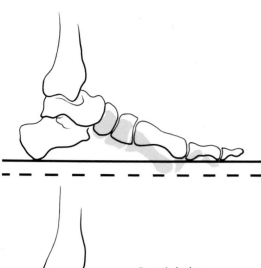

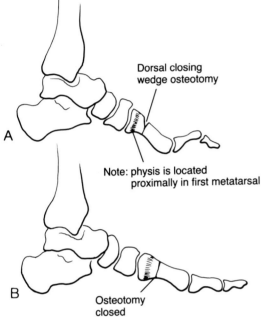

Dorsal closing
wedge osteotomy

A

Note: physis is located
proximally in first metatarsal

B

Osteotomy
closed

FIGURE 41–10. Dorsal closing wedge osteotomy of the first metatarsal. This procedure can be performed at the same time as the radical plantar release through the same incision. Fenestration of the plantar cortex without disruption of the periosteum allows the osteotomy to be closed without the need for Steinmann pin fixation.

second metatarsal may be necessary if osteotomy of the first metatarsal alone does not provide satisfactory correction of the forefoot, or if a transfer lesion is developing beneath the second metatarsal head. This osteotomy should be performed in a similar manner. Postoperatively, a long-leg splint is used until all drains are removed and the swelling has diminished. A long-leg cast is then applied, with care taken to mold the forefoot into dorsiflexion through the osteotomy site, ensuring closure of the osteotomy. Six weeks in the long-leg cast, non–weight bearing, followed by

4 weeks in a short-leg weight-bearing cast, should be adequate.

Rigid Forefoot and Supple Hindfoot

Swanson and colleagues[98] and Wang and Shaffer[103] have advocated the use of multiple metatarsal osteotomies for correction of the rigid cavus foot. This procedure should be used only when the deformity is limited to the forefoot; however, in my experience, it has not been necessary to perform multiple osteotomies for correction of the forefoot equinus.

McElvenny and Caldwell proposed an alternative to first metatarsal osteotomy for use in both the supple cavus foot and the rigid deformity associated with adults.[63] Their procedure, which consists of elevation and supination of the first metatarsal with fusion of the first metatarsal–cuneiform joint and, occasionally, of the navicular-cuneiform joint, recognizes the importance of the depressed first ray in the development of the deformity. As with all procedures on the immature proximal first metatarsal, care must be taken to avoid disturbing the physis, which can lead to significant shortening and deformity.

Many midfoot osteotomies have been described to correct the cavus deformity. These osteotomies are indicated for anterior pes cavus deformities with their apex in the midfoot. The deformity should not be isolated to the first metatarsal and should not be associated with rigid varus of the calcaneus.

In 1935, Saunders was the first to describe an anterior tarsal wedge resection through the midtarsal joints.[86] This procedure was preferred by Cole,[20] as it corrected the deformity at its apex, preserved motion, was cosmetically acceptable, and provided excellent function; however, because of the shortening that must accompany this procedure, it should not be used on the immature foot. Furthermore, vascular compromise is a significant complication of this procedure. Brockway recommended resection of the navicular-cuneiform joint and body of the cuboid to preserve lateral mobility of the foot.[16] However, it was noted that this procedure had limited utility in severe deformities, as the amount of bone available for resection was inadequate. More recently, Jahss described the tarsometatarsal truncated wedge arthrodesis.[49] This osteotomy can correct the forefoot equinus, but usually that is not at the apex of the deformity.

Japas described a V-shaped osteotomy performed between the midtarsal and tarsometatarsal joints, with its apex proximal and at the highest point of the cavus.[51] The limbs of the osteotomy extend through the cuboid and first cuneiform. He reported satisfactory results in 70 percent of cases in his preliminary report; however, this procedure allows only limited correction of associated forefoot adduction or abduction, and rotation.

The midtarsal dome osteotomy of Weiner[106, 108] is preferred. This procedure, performed through the three cuneiform bones, the cuboid, and the base of the fifth metatarsal, allows correction of multiplanar deformities (Fig. 41–11). It allows correction of cavus deformity at the midfoot without shortening the foot or loss of significant motion. As emphasized by Wilcox and Weiner,[108] this is a "salvage" procedure for the foot with a severe rigid cavus or midfoot cavovarus deformity. Further follow-up has demonstrated that this procedure should be performed only in children over 8 years of age.[106] Good and excellent results are reported in 82 percent of their cases, with the highest rate of success in the child nearing, or at, skeletal maturity.

Rigid Hindfoot

Calcaneal osteotomy was introduced by Dwyer.[30, 31] He believed that the varus deformity of the heel was the primary deformity and that by correction of the hindfoot, the deforming forces of the gastrocnemius-soleus muscle group and the plantar fascial structures would gradually be overcome, thus correcting the forefoot deformity. Other authors have demonstrated convincingly that the use of this osteotomy is indicated only in correcting heel varus and that other procedures are necessary to correct cavus or forefoot deformity.[24, 34, 94] An axial, or Harris, view of the calcaneus should be obtained to confirm deformity in the calcaneus before consideration of this osteotomy. The lateral closing wedge osteotomy originally described is preferred.[31]

For the patient with calcaneocavus deformity, the oblique transverse calcaneal osteotomy described by Mitchell[66] or the crescentic osteotomy of the calcaneus described by Samilson,[84] in combination with plantar release, is effective in reducing the calcaneal pitch in fully established deformity. Bradley and Coleman[13] and Coleman[21] have recommended the use of calcaneal osteotomy as part of a staged surgical

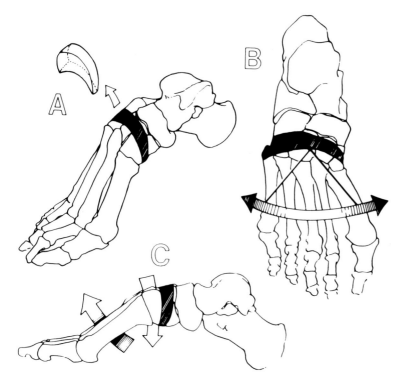

FIGURE 41–11. The Akron midtarsal dome osteotomy. This osteotomy is centered at the apex of the deformity in the midfoot and potentially allows correction in three planes. *(A)*, Correction of the rotary component of deformity. *(B)*, Correction of the adduction deformity. *(C)*, Correction of dorsoplantar deformity. (From Wilcox PG, Weiner DS: The Akron midtarsal dome osteotomy in the treatment of rigid pes cavus: A preliminary review. J Pediatr Orthop 5:335, 1985.)

correction of calcaneocavus deformity in children between 5 and 12 years of age. Others have also emphasized the necessity for tendon transfers following correction of the bony deformity in all calcaneocavus feet.[56, 68]

I prefer the crescentic osteotomy of Samilson.[84] The procedure is performed under tourniquet control. A lateral incision is made posterior to the subtalar joint. The peroneal tendons should be identified anteriorly and protected. Dissection is then carried down to the lateral aspect of the calcaneus. An extensive plantar release is performed according to the technique of Steindler.[96] With retractors placed on the superior and plantar aspects of the tuber of the calcaneus, the line of the osteotomy is marked with multiple drill holes; the osteotomy is completed with an osteotome. The periosteum on the medial aspect of the calcaneus usually needs to be freed by careful dissection with either a Cottle, or other blunt, dissector. A large threaded Steinmann pin is placed through the skin into the posterior fragment of the calcaneus. The posterior segment is then allowed to displace posteriorly and superiorly along the line of the osteotomy (Fig. 41–12). After adequate correction has been confirmed radiographically, the osteotomy is secured by transfixion with a Steinmann pin. Postoperatively, the leg should be maintained in a long-leg non–weight-bearing cast for 6 weeks. At that time the pin should be removed, and a short-leg walking cast is applied for an additional 6 weeks.

Triple Arthrodesis

Triple arthrodesis results in fusion of the subtalar, calcaneocuboid, and talonavicular joints. It should be performed in the adolescent (after age 11) with severe cavovarus deformity or for deformity secondary to a progressive neuromuscular deformity.[2, 38, 47, 55, 71, 112] Many different techniques have been proposed for effecting this arthrodesis, and there are proponents for each of the various techniques,[2, 28, 87, 93] but the ultimate goal of all these procedures is to provide a painless, balanced, plantigrade foot (Fig. 41–13).

My preferred technique of performing triple arthrodesis is described by Adelaar and colleagues[2] and is very similar to the Ryerson arthrodesis shown in Figure 41–13B. The patient is positioned supine, with a roll beneath the ipsilateral hip. A tourniquet is used throughout the procedure. A straight-line incision is used; this incision bisects a line drawn between the distal fibula and the base of the fifth metatarsal. The incision is limited by the peroneus brevis and longus tendons laterally and by the peroneus tertius tendon (if present) or the lateral border of the extensor digitorum communis medially. With an osteotome, an osteoperiosteal flap is elevated. This flap consists of a portion of the periosteum of the anterior calcaneus and the origin of the extensor brevis. The anterior process of the calcaneus is identified and removed with an osteotome parallel to the sole of the foot. The

FIGURE 41–12. The crescentic osteotomy of the calcaneus. (A), The curvilinear osteotomy is performed posterior to the subtalar joint. (B), The tuberosity fragment is displaced posteriorly and superiorly to decrease the calcaneal pitch. This osteotomy is always accompanied by a plantar release. (From Hsu JD, Mann DC, Imbus CE: Pes cavus. *In* Jahss MH [Ed]: Disorders of the Foot. Philadelphia, WB Saunders, 1991, p 888.)

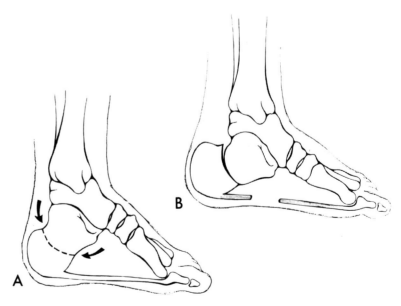

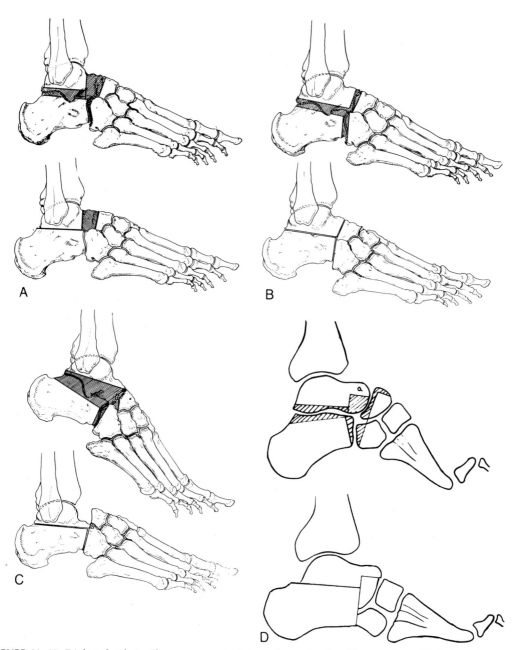

FIGURE 41–13. Triple arthrodesis. There are many techniques for performing this procedure. *(A)*, Hoke arthrodesis. *(B)*, Ryerson arthrodesis. *(C)*, Lambrinudi's arthrodesis. (From Patterson RL, Parrish FF, Hathaway EN: Stabilizing operations on the foot. A study of the indications, techniques used and end results. J Bone Joint Surg 32A:10, 1950.) *(D)*, "Beak" triple arthrodesis. a, residual "beak" of talus. (From Siffert RS, Forester RI, Nachaime B: "Beak" triple arthrodesis for correction of severe cavus deformity. Clin Orthop 45:103, 1966.)

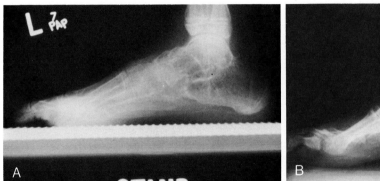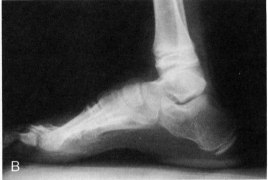

FIGURE 41–14. *(A)*, Standing lateral radiograph of a foot that has undergone plantar release and triple arthrodesis for symptomatic cavovarus deformity. *(B)*, The preoperative radiograph is shown for comparison.

calcaneocuboid joint is widely exposed, and the articular surfaces of this joint are excised perpendicular to the sole of the foot. The subtalar joint is widely exposed and denuded of all articular cartilage. The tendon of the flexor hallucis longus, if unintentionally exposed by completing the medial subtalar capsulotomy while removing the articular cartilage of the subtalar joint, determines the absolute limit of the medial dissection; dissection beyond this risks vascular injury.

Wedges of bone may now be removed, if necessary, to correct osseous deformity. A Hatt spoon, which resembles a shallow melon scoop, is useful to open the talonavicular joint. The articular surface of the talus is removed with a minimal amount of bone, perpendicular to the sole of the foot, as is the articular surface of the navicular. All exposed bony surfaces should be fish scaled with a small, sharp osteotome to maximize the surface area available for fusion. The foot should then be aligned carefully with the ankle mortise, and the foot is displaced posteriorly.

Some surgeons prefer not to use pins or staples for fixation of the arthrodesis; however, I prefer to use a longitudinal pin, inserted through the heel pad, across both the subtalar and ankle joints, with a second pin transfixing the talonavicular joint to maintain the foot in the correct alignment. The previously raised osteoperiosteal flap should be replaced to obliterate the dead space. Subcutaneous tissues are then loosely reapproximated with interrupted sutures, and the skin is closed with interrupted vertical mattress sutures.

Postoperatively, the leg is placed into a long-leg splint and kept elevated. After the edema has diminished, the foot is remanipulated and placed into a long-leg cast if pin fixation is not used. If pins have been used, the incisions and pin tracts should be examined, and new dressings are applied before the long-leg cast is applied. The patient must avoid weight bearing for 6 weeks, when the pins are removed, and then a short-leg weight-bearing cast is applied. This cast is worn for a minimum of 6 weeks, or until clinical and radiographic union of the arthrodesis has occurred (Fig. 41–14).

Overall, triple arthrodesis leads to a satisfactory functional result, providing a stable plantigrade foot. Complications do occur, however, and must be recognized.[5, 67, 71, 110, 112] The most frequent complication is pseudarthrosis, which most commonly occurs at the talonavicular joint. Pseudarthroses are reported in 9 to 23 percent of the feet having stabilization. Wilson and colleagues attributed this problem to lack of internal fixation, poor bony apposition, or early weight bearing.[110] Residual or recurrent deformity, requiring further operation, is noted in a high percentage of feet. Wukich and Bowen reported that 45 percent of the feet in their study had residual deformity and a further 15 percent were overcorrected into planovalgus deformities.[112] A large number of the feet requiring further surgery are in patients in whom an initial triple arthrodesis was performed at a young age. Patterson and colleagues were the first to note the strong association between failure of the arthrodesis and age; 47 percent of the procedures failed when performed in patients younger than 9 years of age, whereas 9 percent of those performed in patients between ages 9 and 12 failed.[71] Hill and colleagues, on the other hand, believe that triple arthrodesis may be performed at any time after the appearance of the ossific nucleus of the navicular, without increasing the risk of pseudarthrosis or shortening of the foot.[42] I strongly disagree with their conclusion and would not perform triple arthrodesis before age 11. Degenerative joint changes have been noted in the ankle, as well as in the midfoot. Radiographic changes have been noted in up to 62 percent of the feet at long-term follow-up.[112] Medhat and Krantz believe that these changes, which they have demonstrated in patients with Charcot-Marie-Tooth disease, are actually a neuroarthropathy.[65] Pain has been a problem in the minority of cases and, when present, was associated with either a pseudarthrosis or severe joint degeneration. Instability has also been noted on objective examination; however, this has not been a subjective problem.

SUMMARY

The cavus foot is a deformity characterized by equinus of the forefoot and a high longitudinal arch. Patients usually present for evaluation of an awkward gait, foot pain, or difficulty wearing shoes. Evaluation of these patients reveals an underlying neuromuscular abnormality as the cause of their foot deformity in the majority of cases.[14] Treatment is ultimately surgical, either to treat the cause or the deformity per se. No single surgical procedure is universally applicable to the treatment of this deformity, and a combination of soft tissue and bony procedures is often necessary to correct the many components of the cavus foot.

References

1. Abrams RC: Relapsed club foot. The early results of an evaluation of Dillwyn Evans' operation. J Bone Joint Surg 51A:270, 1969.
2. Adelaar RS, Dannelly EA, Meunier PA, et al: A long term study of triple arthrodesis in children. Orthop Clin North Am 7:895, 1976.
3. Alcalay J, Lederman N, Kornbrot B: The diagnosis of pes planus and pes cavus in soldiers by the foot-ground pressure pattern. Milit Med 150:215, 1985.
4. Alexander IJ, Johnson KA: Assessment and management of pes cavus in Charcot-Marie-Tooth disease. Clin Orthop 246:273, 1989.
5. Angus PD, Cowell HR: Triple arthrodesis. A critical long-term review. J Bone Joint Surg 68B:260, 1986.

6. Barbari SG, Brevig K: Correction of clawtoes by the Girdlestone-Taylor flexor-extensor transfer procedure. Foot Ankle 5:67, 1984.
7. Barenfeld PA, Weseley MS, Shea JM: The congenital cavus foot. Clin Orthop 79:119, 1971.
8. Barwell R: Pes planus and pes cavus: An anatomical and clinical study. Edinburgh Med J 3:113, 1898.
9. Bentzon PGK: Pes cavus and the m. peroneus longus. Acta Orthop Scand 4:50, 1938.
10. Bigos SJ, Coleman SS: Foot deformity secondary to gluteal injection in infancy. J Pediatr Orthop 4:560, 1984.
11. Bleck EE: Spastic hemiplegia. *In* Bleck EE: Orthopaedic Management in Cerebral Palsy. Philadelphia, MacKeith Press, 1987.
12. Bost FC, Schottstaedt ER, Larsen LJ: Plantar operation to release the soft tissues in recurrent or recalcitrant talipes equinovarus. J Bone Joint Surg 42A:151, 1960.
13. Bradley GW, Coleman SS: Treatment of the calcaneocavus foot deformity. J Bone Joint Surg 63A:1159, 1981.
14. Brewerton DA, Sandifer PH, Sweetnam DR: "Idiopathic" pes cavus. An investigation into its aetiology. Br Med J 2:659, 1963.
15. Brewster AH, Larson CB: Cavus feet. J Bone Joint Surg 22:361, 1940.
16. Brockway A: Surgical correction of talipes cavus deformities. J Bone Joint Surg 22:81, 1940.
17. Brody IA, Wilkins RH: Charcot-Marie-Tooth disease. Arch Neurol 17:552, 1967.
18. Carney JA, Bianco AJ Jr, Sizemore GW, Hayles AB: Multiple endocrine neoplasia with skeletal manifestations. J Bone Joint Surg 63A:405, 1981.
19. Chuinard EG, Baskin M: Claw-foot deformity. Treatment by transfer of the long extensors into the metatarsals and fusion of the interphalangeal joints. J Bone Joint Surg 55A:351, 1973.
20. Cole WH: The treatment of claw-foot. J Bone Joint Surg 22:895, 1940.
21. Coleman SS: The cavovarus foot. *In* Coleman SS: Complex Foot Deformities in Children. Philadelphia, Lea & Febiger, 1983.
22. Coleman SS, Chesnut WJ: A simple test for hindfoot flexibility in the cavovarus foot. Clin Orthop 123:60, 1977.
23. Coonrad RW, Irwin CE, Gucker T, Wray JB: The importance of plantar muscles in paralytic varus feet. The results of treatment by neurectomy and myotenotomy. J Bone Joint Surg 38A:563, 1956.
24. Dekel S, Weissman SL: Osteotomy of the calcaneus and concomitant plantar stripping in children with talipes cavovarus. J Bone Joint Surg 55B:802, 1973.
25. DeLuca PA, Banta JV: Pes cavovarus as a late consequence of peroneus longus tendon laceration. J Pediatr Orthop 5:582, 1985.
26. Drennan JC: Progressive muscular dystrophy. *In* Drennan JC: Orthopaedic Management of Neuromuscular Disorders. Philadelphia, JB Lippincott, 1983.
27. Duckworth T: Management of the feet in spinal dysraphism and myelodysplasia. *In* Jahss MD (Ed): Disorders of the Foot. Philadelphia, WB Saunders, 1982.
28. Duncan J, Lovell WW: Hoke triple arthrodesis. J Bone Joint Surg 60A:795, 1978.
29. Dwyer FC: The present status of the problem of pes cavus. Clin Orthop 106:254, 1975.

30. Dwyer FC: The treatment of relapsed club foot by the insertion of a wedge into the calcaneum. J Bone Joint Surg 45B:67, 1963.

31. Dwyer FC: Osteotomy of the calcaneum for pes cavus. J Bone Joint Surg 41B:80, 1959.

32. Dyck PJ, Lambert EH: Lower motor and primary sensory neuron diseases with peroneal muscular atrophy. I. Neurologic genetic and electrophysiologic findings in hereditary polyneuropathies. Arch Neurol 18:603, 1968.

33. Eilert RE: Cavus foot in cerebral palsy. Foot Ankle 4:185, 1984.

34. Fisher RL, Shaffer SR: An evaluation of calcaneal osteotomy in congenital club foot and other disorders. Clin Orthop 70:141, 1970.

35. Frank GR, Johnson WM: The extensor shift procedure in the correction of clawtoe deformities in children. South Med J 59:889, 1966.

36. Garceau GJ, Brahms MA: A preliminary study of selective plantar-muscle denervation for pes cavus. J Bone Joint Surg 38A:553, 1956.

37. Gilroy E: Pes cavus: A clinical study with special reference to its etiology. Edinburgh Med J 36:749, 1929.

38. Gould N: Surgery in advanced Charcot-Marie-Tooth disease. Foot Ankle 4:267, 1984.

39. Hayes JT, Gross HP, Dow S: Surgery for paralytic defects secondary to myelomeningocele and myelodysplasia. J Bone Joint Surg 46A:1577, 1964.

40. Heron JR: Neurological syndromes associated with pes cavus. Proc R Soc Med 62:270, 1969.

41. Hibbs RA: An operation for "claw foot." JAMA 73:1583, 1919.

42. Hill NA, Wilson HJ, Chevres F, Sweterlitsch PR: Triple arthrodesis in the young child. Clin Orthop 70:187, 1970.

43. Horne G: Pes cavus following ankle fracture. A case report. Clin Orthop 184:249, 1984.

44. Hsu JD, Hoffer MM: Posterior tibial tendon transfer anteriorly through the interosseous membrane. Clin Orthop 131:202, 1978.

45. Hughes WK: Talipes cavus. Br Med J 2:902, 1940.

46. Ibrahim K: Pes cavus. *In* Evarts C (Ed): Surgery of the Musculoskeletal System. New York, Churchill Livingstone, 1983.

47. Jacobs JE, Carr CR: Progressive muscular atrophy of the peroneal type (Charcot-Marie-Tooth disease). Orthopaedic management and end-result study. J Bone Joint Surg 32A:27, 1950.

48. Jahss MH: Evaluation of the cavus foot for orthopaedic treatment. Clin Orthop 181:52, 1983.

49. Jahss MH: Tarso-metatarsal truncated-wedge arthrodesis for pes cavus and equinovarus deformity of the fore part of the foot. J Bone Joint Surg 62A:713, 1980.

50. James CCM, Lassman LP: Spinal dysraphism. The diagnosis and treatment of progressive lesions in spina bifida occulta. J Bone Joint Surg 44B:828, 1962.

51. Japas LM: Surgical treatment of pes cavus by tarsal V-osteotomy. Preliminary report. J Bone Joint Surg 50A:927, 1968.

52. Jones R III: The soldier's foot and the treatment of common deformities of the foot. Part II. Claw-foot. Br Med J 1:749, 1916.

53. Karlholm S, Nilsonne U: Operative treatment of the foot deformity in Charcot-Marie-Tooth disease. Acta Orthop Scand 39:101, 1968.

54. Karlstrom G, Lonnerholm T, Olerud S: Cavus deformity of the foot after fracture of the tibial shaft. J Bone Joint Surg 57A:893, 1975.

55. Levitt RL, Canale ST, Cooke AJ Jr, Gartland JJ: The role of foot surgery in progressive neuromuscular disorders in children. J Bone Joint Surg 55A:1396, 1973.

56. Lipscomb PR: Osteotomy of calcaneus, triple arthrodesis, and tendon transfer for severe paralytic calcaneocavus deformity. Report of a case. J Bone Joint Surg 51A:548, 1969.

57. Lovell WW, Price CT, Meehan PL: The foot. *In* Lovell WW, Winter RB (Eds): Pediatric Orthopaedics. Philadelphia, JB Lippincott, 1986.

58. Makin M: The surgical management of Friedreich's ataxia. J Bone Joint Surg 35A:425, 1953.

59. Mann R, Inman VT: Phasic activity of intrinsic muscles of the foot. J Bone Joint Surg 46A:469, 1964.

60. Mann RA, Missirian J: Pathophysiology of Charcot-Marie-Tooth disease. Clin Orthop 234:221, 1988.

61. Matsen FA, Clawson DK: The deep posterior compartmental syndrome of the leg. J Bone Joint Surg 57A:34, 1975.

62. Mayer PJ: Pes cavus: A diagnostic and therapeutic challenge. Orthop Rev 7:105, 1978.

63. McElvenny RT, Caldwell GD: A new operation for correction of cavus foot. Fusion of first metatarsocuneiform-navicular joints. Clin Orthop 11:85, 1958.

64. Meary R: Le pied creux essentiel. Symposium. Rev Chir Orthop 53:389, 1967.

65. Medhat MA, Krantz H: Neuropathic ankle joint in Charcot-Marie-Tooth disease after triple arthrodesis of the foot. Orthop Rev 17:873, 1988.

66. Mitchell GP: Posterior displacement osteotomy of the calcaneus. J Bone Joint Surg 59B:233, 1977.

67. Monson R, Gibson DA: Long-term follow-up of triple arthrodesis. Can J Surg 21:249, 1978.

68. Mortens J, Pilcher MF: Tendon transplantation in the prevention of foot deformities after poliomyelitis in children. J Bone Joint Surg 38B:633, 1956.

69. Owen R, Tsimboukis B: Ischaemia complicating closed tibial and fibular shafts fractures. J Bone Joint Surg 49B:268, 1967.

70. Pashiro K, Fukazawa T, Moriwaka F, et al: Syringomyelic syndrome: Clinical features in 31 cases confirmed by CT myelography or magnetic resonance imaging. J Neurol 235:26, 1987.

71. Patterson RL Jr, Parrish FF, Hathaway EN: Stabilizing operations on the foot. A study of the indications, techniques used and end results. J Bone Joint Surg 32A:1, 1950.

72. Paulos L, Coleman SS, Samuelson KM: Pes cavovarus. Review of a surgical approach using selective soft-tissue procedures. J Bone Joint Surg 62A:942, 1980.

73. Peabody CW: Tendon transposition. J Bone Joint Surg 20:193, 1938.

74. Perry J, Hoffer MM: Preoperative and postoperative dynamic electromyography as an aid in planning tendon transfers in children with cerebral palsy. J Bone Joint Surg 50A:531, 1977.

75. Port M, Courniotes J, Podwal M: Zosteriform, lentiginous, naevus with ipsilateral rigid cavus foot. Br J Dermatol 98:693, 1978.

76. Pyper JB: The flexor-extensor transplant operation for claw toes. J Bone Joint Surg 40B:528, 1958.

77. Rapin I, Suzuki K, Valsamis MP: Adult (chronic)

GM2 gangliosidosis. Atypical spinal cerebellar degeneration in a Jewish sibship. Arch Neurol 33:120, 1976.

78. Rasmusson B: Bone abnormalities in patients with medullary carcinoma of the thyroid. Acta Radiol [Oncol] 19:461, 1980.

79. Rivera-Dominguez M, Dibenedetto M, Frisbie JH, Rossier AB: Pes cavus and claw toes deformity in patients with spinal cord injury and multiple sclerosis. Paraplegia 16:375, 1979.

80. Rugh JT: An operation for the correction of plantar and adduction contraction of the foot arch. J Bone Joint Surg 6:664, 1924.

81. Sabir M, Lyttle D: Pathogenesis of pes cavus in Charcot-Marie-Tooth disease. Clin Orthop 175:173, 1983.

82. Sabir M, Lyttle D: Pathogenesis of Charcot-Marie-Tooth disease. Gait analysis and electrophysiologic, genetic, histopathologic and enzyme studies in a kinship. Clin Orthop 184:223, 1984.

83. Saltzman CL, Herzenberg JE, Phillips WA, Hensinger RN: Thick lips, bumpy tongue, and slipped capital femoral epiphysis—a deadly combination. J Pediatr Orthop 8:219, 1988.

84. Samilson RL: Calcaneocavus feet. A plan of management in children. Orthop Rev 10:121, 1981.

85. Samilson RL, Dillin WP: Cavus, cavovarus and calcaneocavus. An update. Clin Orthop 177:125, 1983.

86. Saunders JT: The etiology and treatment of clubfoot. Arch Surg 30:179, 1935.

87. Scheer GE, Crego CH Jr: A two-stage stabilization procedure for correction for calcaneocavus. J Bone Joint Surg 38A:1247, 1956.

88. Schwankhaus JD, Currie J, Jaffe MJ, et al: Neurologic findings in men with isolated hypogonadotropic hypogonadism. Neurology 39:223, 1989.

89. Shanahan MD, Douglas DL, Sharrard WJ, et al: The long-term results of the surgical management of paralytic pes cavus by soft tissue release and tendon transfer. Z Kinderchir 40(Suppl 1):37, 1985.

90. Shapiro F, Bresnan MJ: Current concepts review. Orthopaedic management of childhood neuromuscular disease. Part II: Peripheral neuropathies, Friedreich's ataxia and arthrogryposis multiplex congenita. J Bone Joint Surg 64A:949, 1982.

91. Sharrard WJW, Grosfield I: The management of deformity and paralysis of the foot in myelomeningocele. J Bone Joint Surg 50B:456, 1968.

92. Sherman FC, Westin GW: Plantar release in the correction of deformities of the foot in childhood. J Bone Joint Surg 61A:1382, 1981.

93. Siffert RS, Forester RI, Nachaime B: "Beak" triple arthrodesis for correction of severe cavus deformity. Clin Orthop 45:101, 1966.

94. Stauffer RN, Nelson GE, Bianco AJ Jr: Calcaneal osteotomy in the treatment of the cavovarus foot. Mayo Clin Proc 45:624, 1970.

95. Steel MW III, Johnson KA, DeWitz MA, Ilstrup, DM: Radiographic measurements of the normal adult foot. Foot Ankle 1:151, 1980.

96. Steindler A: Stripping of the os calcis. J Orthop Surg 2:8, 1920.

97. Steindler A: The treatment of pes cavus (hollow claw foot). Arch Surg 2:335, 1921.

98. Swanson AB, Browne HS, Coleman JD: The cavus foot-concept of production and treatment by metatarsal osteotomy. J Bone Joint Surg 48A:1019, 1966.

99. Tachdjian MO: Pes cavus and claw toes. *In* The Child's Foot. Philadelphia, WB Saunders, 1985.

100. Taylor RG: The treatment of claw toes by multiple transfers of flexor into extensor tendons. J Bone Joint Surg 33B:539, 1951.

101. Tyrer JH, Sutherland JPM: The primary spinocerebellar atrophies and their associated defects, with a study of the foot deformity. Brain 84:289, 1961.

102. Vanderwilde R, Staheli LT, Chew DE, Malagon V: Measurements on radiographs of the foot in normal infants and children. J Bone Joint Surg 70A:407, 1988.

103. Wang G-J, Shaffer LW: Osteotomy of the metatarsals for pes cavus. South Med J 70:77, 1977.

104. Ward WG, Clippinger FW: Proximal medial longitudinal arch incision for plantar fascia release. Foot Ankle 8:152, 1987.

105. Wein BK, Cowell HR: Genetic considerations of foot anomalies in office practice. Foot Ankle 2:185, 1982.

106. Weiner BK, Weiner DS, Weiner SD: The Akron midtarsal dome osteotomy: An update review of the first 100 cases. Presented at Section on Orthopaedics, American Academy of Pediatrics. Chicago, 1989.

107. Weseley MS, Barenfeld PA, Shea JM, Eisenstein AL: The congenital cavus foot. A follow-up report. Bull Hosp Jt Dis Orthop Inst 42:217, 1982.

108. Wilcox PG, Weiner DS: The Akron midtarsal dome osteotomy in the treatment of rigid pes cavovarus: A preliminary review. J Pediatr Orthop 5:333, 1985.

109. Williams B: Orthopaedic features in the presentation of syringomyelia. J Bone Joint Surg 61B:314, 1979.

110. Wilson FC, Fay GF, Lamotte P, Williams JC: Triple arthrodesis. A study of the factors affecting fusion after three hundred and one procedures. J Bone Joint Surg 47A:340, 1965.

111. Winter RB, Haven JJ, Moe JH, Lagaard SM: Diastematomyelia and congenital spine deformities. J Bone Joint Surg 56A:27, 1974.

112. Wukich DK, Bowen JR: A long-term study of triple arthrodesis for correction of pes cavovarus in Charcot-Marie-Tooth disease. J Pediatr Orthop 9:433, 1989.

42

Neuromuscular Foot Deformities in Children

HELEN M. HORSTMANN

Foot problems in the patient with neuromuscular disease are complicated by many factors. Of special importance are the following factors:

- The coordination of activity from the central nervous system
- The presence or absence of spasticity
- The presence or lack of sensation
- The motor power of each muscle
- The extent of overall involvement (e.g., hemiparesis)
- The progressive (e.g., dystrophies) or non-progressive (e.g., cerebral palsy) nature of the problem
- Other debilitating factors, such as mental retardation

The goal in writing this chapter is to emphasize the complexity of these issues and to present an approach for remedying the deformities while anticipating further problems. Furthermore, this chapter will also serve as a ready reference in planning surgical correction of the deformities as well as the muscle imbalance. Not every possible surgical procedure is discussed; rather, this discussion concentrates on those that seem most pertinent to the present state of knowledge. Not every neuromuscular foot problem is discussed, owing to space constraints. For example, the cavus foot is discussed in Chapter 41; therefore, it will not be covered here. From the types of neuromuscular foot problems presented in this chapter, the reader should be able to extrapolate to those not specifically covered.

CEREBRAL PALSY

Many children with cerebral palsy develop significant foot problems. Cerebral palsy is a nonprogressive encephalopathy. There are many causes, including intraventricular hemorrhage, which is associated with prematurity and anoxia, especially in the neonatal period. Prenatal causes include infections, maternal drug ingestion, and fetal alcohol syndrome. Perinatal causes include problems that occur during birth, such as birth trauma and anoxia associated with placental separation, among other causes. The incidence of athetosis due to erythroblastosis fetalis has markedly decreased.[48] Postnatal causes are associated with meningitis and encephalitis, head injury, and suffocation, as occurs in near-drowning. The etiology may be unknown in as much as 25 percent of the cerebral palsy patient population.[8]

Although cerebral palsy is nonprogressive, it produces a constantly changing picture in a growing child. On the whole, cerebral palsy children are born with normal-looking feet and lower extremities. As they grow, they develop contractures and additional fixed deformities.

Types of Foot Deformity

There are four basic hindfoot deformities in children with cerebral palsy: equinus, varus, valgus, and calcaneus posturing of the foot. In addition, there can be midfoot and forefoot problems, especially valgus of the midfoot. Cavus with midfoot deformity is rare in the child with cerebral palsy. Other causes, such as a tethered cord or a progressive neuromuscular problem, should be sought when cavus is noted. Forefoot adduction is not particularly common in cerebral palsy. Hallux valgus is often associated with a valgus hindfoot and midfoot. A dorsal bunion is not uncommon. Significant toe flexion problems are seen only occasionally in cerebral palsy. Each of these problems is discussed, along with its conservative and surgical management.

Diagnosis

The descriptive diagnosis of the extent of involvement with cerebral palsy is helpful in understanding the child's foot problems. First, one needs to assess the type of motor involvement. Does the child have spasticity, hypotonia, or athetosis? If spasticity is the major problem, lengthening or transferring the offending muscle can help to balance the foot deformity. If athetosis or dystonia is the primary problem, surgical correction is less predictable, and bony stabilization with release of muscles could be the proper solution. If hypotonia is the major problem, bracing stabilization or, less frequently, bony stabilization may be helpful.

It is also important to determine the extent of the motor involvement. The quadriplegic child with involvement of both upper and lower extremities or total body involvement has, by definition, little chance of walking or weight bearing. The quadriplegic child frequently has equinus deformity with associated varus or valgus in the midfoot and hindfoot. The diplegic child has more involvement of the lower than of the upper extremities. Because of balance in the trunk and functional use of the upper extremities, this child usually has the ability to walk. The diplegic child will more often exhibit the equinus and valgus components of foot deformities (Fig. 42–1). The hemiplegic child has spastic involvement of an upper and lower extremity on one side (Fig. 42–2A and B). This child will walk, although usually slightly later than his or her peers. The foot deformity most frequently associated with hemiplegia is an equinovarus deformity, which is often noted in conjunction with a tight hamstring. Heel cord tightness usually develops between the ages of 18 months and 4 years and is generally the first

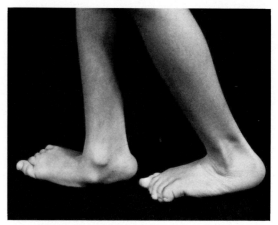

FIGURE 42–1. Diplegic child with valgus feet.

problem noted. The hamstring tightness tends to develop later, between the ages of 2½ and 4½ years.

Although this discussion focuses on the foot deformity in cerebral palsy, one cannot ignore the position of the rest of the extremity[36, 37, 49] and the important relationship with the associated joints.

Gait Evaluation

Analysis of the gait is an intrinsic part of the examination and determining the proper treatment for a child with cerebral palsy (Fig. 42–3). If the child is ambulatory, this requires watching the child walk down a long hallway. Formal gait analysis is becoming increasingly popular and more readily available. With the advent of the home video recorder, motion analysis is a possibility for many more orthopaedic surgeons. This becomes an excellent source of documentation and gives the orthopaedic surgeon a chance for more comprehensive analysis of the child's foot problems. The use of simultaneous electromyographic (EMG) recording requires a more elaborate laboratory and allows a more thorough and more scientific approach to surgical management of the child. No computers, however, can substitute for clinical awareness and clinical judgment. Not too surprisingly, gait analysis of the same child by different observers using the same gait analysis database will yield a variety of opinions regarding the optimal surgical course. It is not an exact science.

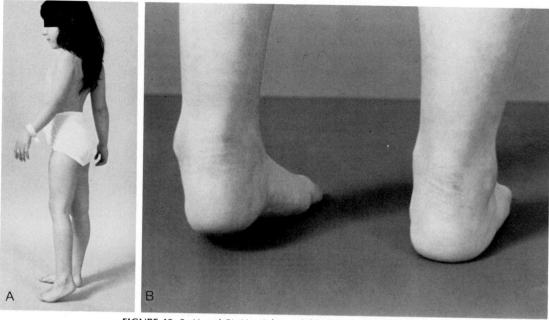

FIGURE 42–2. *(A* and *B),* Hemiplegic child with an equinovarus foot.

FIGURE 42–3. Hemiplegic child with equinovarus deformity in gait analysis with electromyographic monitors and motion analysis surface spotters.

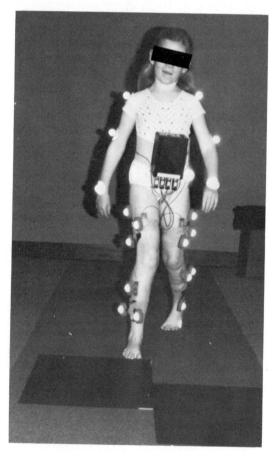

Gait analysis is most helpful when muscles are to be transferred. Spastic muscles tend to have a prolonged firing time. Sometimes they fire continuously throughout the stance and swing phases of gait. Their antagonists may be weak or may not fire at all, and this could be the cause of the problem. The purpose of tendon transfers is to balance a dynamic deformity. Half of a muscle or the whole muscle may be transferred to achieve this. A clinical examination needs to be done primarily to identify the offending muscle.

Muscle grows in response to the stimulus of motion and tension on the muscle. Lengthening a muscle through the tendon area removes some of that tension and changes the arc of motion from a nonfunctional arc to a more functional arc. The actual excursion of the muscle is not changed, however, by lengthening the tendon (Fig. 42–4).[51] As a result of

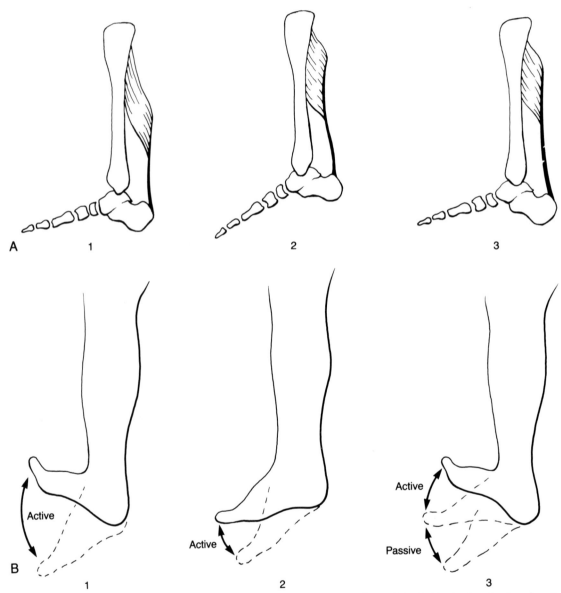

FIGURE 42–4. *(A* and *B)*, Muscle excursion. 1, Normal. 2, Short excursion with spasticity. 3, Tendon lengthening changes the total range of motion by increasing the passive range and displacing the arc of active motion. (Modified from Rang M: Cerebral palsy. *In* Morrissy RT [Ed]: Lovell and Winter's Pediatric Orthopaedics, 3rd Ed. Philadelphia, JB Lippincott, 1990, p 476.)

years of spastic activity, the contracted muscle of a patient with cerebral palsy usually has a shortened muscle body.

Timing of Treatment

A child with cerebral palsy initially will be noted to have developmental delays. Perhaps even before the diagnosis of cerebral palsy is made, occupational and physical therapy intervention is recommended. As soon as the deformity seems to be developing in the feet, bracing becomes appropriate to avoid fixation of this deformity and to allow the therapist to work with the child with the child's feet and limbs in normal positions. In time, this may be insufficient to control the problem, and surgery should be undertaken. Although 4 years of age is frequently recommended as the ideal time for surgery,[8, 36] this is not written in stone, only on paper.

The timing of treatment for cerebral palsy foot problems should be related to the progress of the individual child. Bracing should be initiated as soon as deformities become apparent. Surgery should be performed when a postural deformity develops and causes functional limitations, before the deformity starts to become fixed. This can be as early as 2½ years of age.

> TREATMENT GUIDELINES
> *Begin therapy* when developmental delay is noted (6 to 12 months)
> *Begin bracing* when deformity is flexible (1 to 2 years)
> *Do surgery* before deformity becomes fixed (2 ½ to 6 years)

Equinus Deformity

Equinus results when the gastrocnemius-soleus complex is tight. This can either be associated with fixed contracture or be due to a dynamic tightness associated with functional motion, such as standing or walking. The tibialis anterior is relatively weak compared with the gastrocnemius-soleus complex and therefore can be become elongated as a result of prolonged position in equinus. In the evaluation, the child should be observed carefully to determine whether the knee is flexed and, if so, whether this raises the foot off the ground.

The most conservative management of the equinus deformity consists of stretching the heel cord. This can be done, either actively or passively, with an exercise program, depending on the ability of the child to cooperate and the level of the child's independence. Stretching helps only in the mildest cases of heel cord tightness.

Bracing Management. If the foot can be brought to a neutral position, it can be braced. At present, the preferred brace is the molded ankle-foot orthosis. This allows good control of the position of the midfoot and forefoot, as well as containment of the hindfoot. The brace can be articulated to allow dorsiflexion during ambulation.

The old standard was a Phelps brace (Fig. 42–5A and B), which consists of a single upright bar and allowed motion from neutral position through dorsiflexion. This brace has the advantage of allowing stretch on the heel cord. The shoes that were used for this were traditionally the straight-last shoe. This put the midfoot and forefoot in abnormal positions and was a particular problem with valgus feet, as it allowed further valgus deformity. In addition, it was cosmetically unacceptable.

If the knee tends to go into flexion owing to a weak quadriceps or tight hamstring, an articulating brace is not appropriate, as it does nothing to control the quadriceps. Frequently, a floor reaction brace can help if the knee flexion is coupled with an ankle deformity. This gives a backward push on the tibial tubercle and helps reduce a crouched stance phase during gait (Fig. 42–6A to D).

Brodke and colleagues have compared the use of ankle-foot orthoses with a double-upright brace.[10] In normal children, double-upright metal and leather orthotics were compared with molded plastic orthoses. Their results showed increased knee extension during the stance phase with the use of the molded ankle-foot orthosis and a decrease in the speed of walking and less flexion through the knee joint in the stance phase with the use of a metal and leather brace. The molded plastic ankle-foot orthosis with shoes weighed only 63 percent as much as the metal and leather brace with the shoes.[10] The study further underlines the advantages of molded ankle-foot orthoses.

Surgical Management. There is much discussion regarding the appropriate way to lengthen a heel cord. The Silfverskiöld test was devised to distinguish gastrocnemius tightness from soleus tightness. In this test, the foot is dorsiflexed first with the knee extended

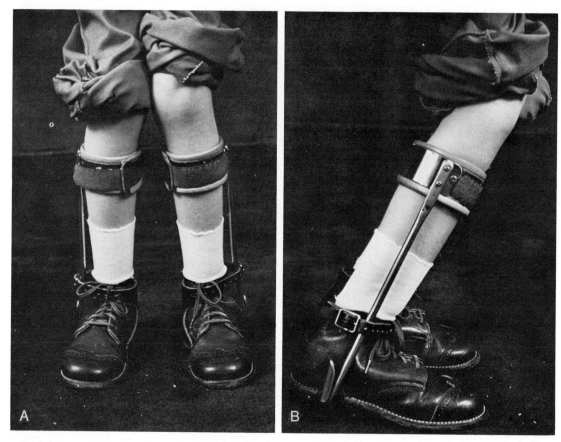

FIGURE 42–5. (A and B), Braces. The Phelps brace allows dorsiflexion and blocks plantar flexion but looks ugly. Ask any child.

and then with the knee flexed. In most cases, the foot can be more easily dorsiflexed with the knee flexed. This is partially due to the relaxation of the gastrocnemius, which originates at the femur and crosses the knee joint.[43] Many children with spasticity have increased dorsiflexion when the knee is flexed, suggesting that the gastrocnemius is spastic or contracted. Perry and Hoffer,[32] however, have shown that positive Silfverskiöld test results do not differentiate the source of the tightness. When EMG studies show that both the gastrocnemius and soleus are spastic during gait, they recommend an Achilles tendon lengthening. If only gastrocnemius spasticity is noted on the EMG, only a gastrocnemius recession should be performed.[32]

One major concern when lengthening a heel cord is the high incidence of calcaneus deformity (Fig. 42–7).[41] A review of gastrocnemius recessions (Silverskiöld operations) showed no such deformity.[44] Calcaneus deformities occurred in eight of 162 heel cord lengthening procedures (5 percent) in Banks and Green's series.[4] Dillin and Samilson considered this problem extensively and noted a high incidence of calcaneus deformity associated not only with heel cord lengthenings but also with posterior tibial tendon transfers.[14] Calcaneus deformity may be much more common than suggested in the older literature; indeed, it may reach as high as 30 percent.[42]

Calcaneus deformities may be related more to the initial indications for surgery than to the exact technique. Hamstring tightness develops later than heel cord tightness! Children lacking quadriceps strength and control seem to have more of a tendency to develop calcaneus deformities. In these children, equinus management should be conservative, and surgical lengthening should be reserved for a markedly fixed contracture.

The gastrocnemius causes deceleration of ankle dorsiflexion during the stance phase of

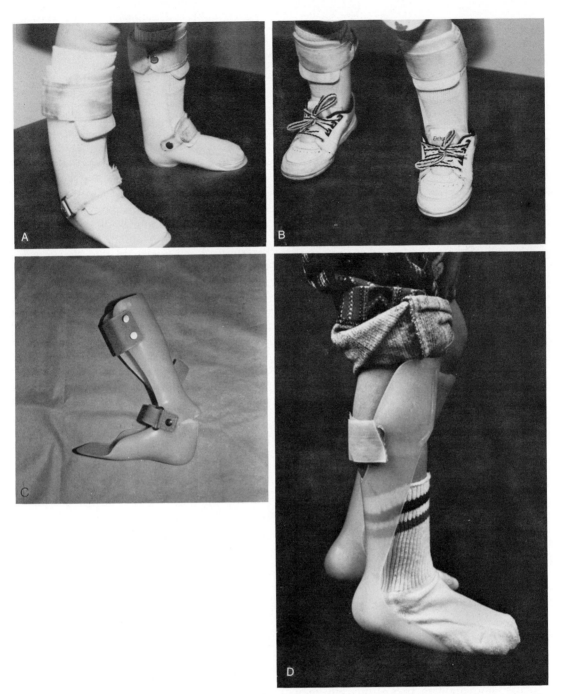

FIGURE 42–6. Molded ankle-foot orthoses. (A), With solid ankle and toe plate extended to the edge of toes to keep toes in extension. (B), Worn in sneakers. (C), With articulating ankle to allow active motion. (D), Floor reaction brace with proximal tibial support to stabilize weak quadriceps and triceps surae.

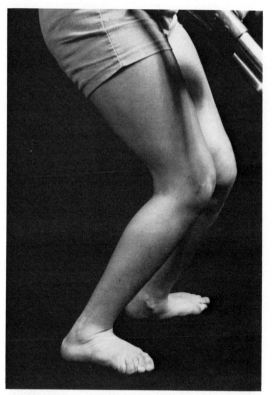

FIGURE 42–7. Iatrogenic calcaneus deformity associated with heel cord lengthening, weak quadriceps, and tight hamstrings.

Vulpius technique, or with the Baker technique, in which a tongue-in-groove inverted-U incision is made through the aponeurosis.

A sliding Hoke Achilles tendon lengthening can be done either with a longitudinal open incision or percutaneously (Fig. 42–8). The percutaneous method can be safely accomplished if it is performed with great care.

I first started using the percutaneous technique after one of my colleague's patients came to me for follow-up with a perfect result. I was embarrassed to note the size of my incisions for an open technique compared with the nearly invisible ones for the percutaneous technique. It is first imperative to draw the proposed cuts in the heel cord on the skin of the ankle. This helps in remembering the direction in which the tendon has already been cut. Then, starting from about 1 cm above the insertion of the heel cord into the os calcis, the blade (a Beaver No. 64) is introduced, initially in a longitudinal direction. Before the blade is turned, the tendon is carefully palpated to be sure that the knife is longitudinally bisecting the tendon at this level. The blade is then turned medially to bisect the heel cord from the midline medially. This process is repeated in the opposite direction about 4 cm more proximally and is again repeated in the initial direction 4 cm more proximal to the

walking and thereby helps to stabilize the knee. In any child with hamstring tightness or quadriceps weakness, the stabilization created by the triceps surae is extremely important, and its strength must be preserved. Therefore, heel cord lengthenings are probably done in too cavalier a fashion. Garbarino and Clancy devised a geometric method of calculating the appropriate amount of Achilles tendon lengthening.[15] The heel cord should be lengthened by one-half the height of the heel off the ground in a standing or passively dorsiflexed position. The use of this calculated method has allowed them to have no instances of overlengthening or residual equinus during an average follow-up of 3.1 years.

Gastrocnemius-lengthening procedures are presently enjoying less popularity, but they still have their place when the gastrocnemius shows excessive spasticity and appears to be the sole offender. In this case, a Strayer procedure can be undertaken. The gastrocnemius can be lengthened as an inverted V, as in the

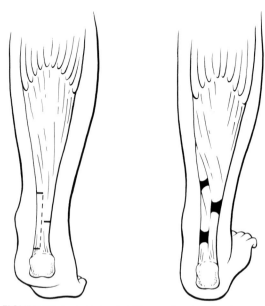

FIGURE 42–8. A Hoke Achilles tendon lengthening procedure.

second cut. The foot is then forcibly dorsi-flexed to about 10 degrees above neutral. A snapping sensation should be felt when the heel cord releases. If this does not occur, further dorsiflexion should not be forced, or a fracture might result! A few fibers in the mid-line may be in continuity. These midline con-tiguous fibers should be incised with special care to be sure that the heel cord is not transected. Although there is some rotation of the heel cord anatomically (proximal medial to distal lateral), this straightforward method of doing a lengthening is simple and effective.

After the heel cord lengthening, the foot should comfortably rest at a neutral position and should be held in a short-leg cast in neutral position with a toe plate. Walking is allowed as soon as the child is comfortable. Sometimes this is the day of surgery, but it may be as long as a week. On an average, most children seem to walk about 3 to 4 days after the surgery. The casts are removed at 6 weeks, and at that time an ankle-foot orthosis can be used if there is any anterior tibial tendon weakness or ten-dency for a suboptimal position.

Varus Foot Deformity

A varus deformity results when there is muscle imbalance causing inversion of the foot (Fig. 42–9). This could be due to a spastic or contracted tibialis posterior or anterior or to weak peroneal muscles that do not counteract the relative strength or tightness of the invert-ers. A varus deformity of the foot tends to be initially rather dynamic. As children get older, it becomes more fixed.

Diagnosis. It is important to analyze the cause of the problem. Initially, this should be done clinically by watching the child walk and feeling the tightness of the tendon. It is helpful to try to palpate the involved muscle as the child walks a step or two and the varus defor-mity is created. Explain this evaluation to the parents so that they do not misinterpret these actions. The offending muscles may be con-tracted, and there may be a fixed bony defor-mity to the hindfoot, midfoot, or both. Varus foot deformity is most frequently seen in a hemiplegic patient.

Surgical Management. A myriad of proce-dures are possible for correction of varus deformity, including muscular lengthening, tendon transfers, and tenotomy.[3, 18, 21, 22, 40]

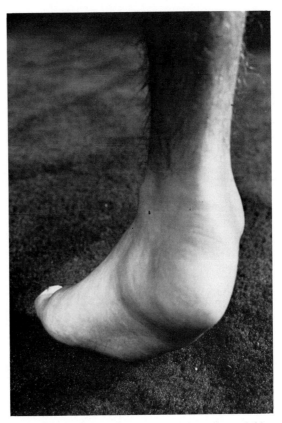

FIGURE 42–9. Equinovarus foot in a hemiplegic child.

Complete tenotomy of the posterior tibial ten-don can sometimes result in midfoot collapse into valgus. If there is weak dorsiflexion in the face of a marked varus deformity, it is helpful to transfer the posterior tibial tendon through the interosseous membrane to augment dorsi-flexion. This should be done after dynamic EMG studies have confirmed that the posterior tibialis is active during swing phase.

Currently, the split posterior tibial tendon transfer is a popular procedure.[17, 27, 28] This operation was devised by Kaufer. It is espe-cially appealing because of its ability to balance the unbalanced foot.

Split Posterior Tibial Tendon Transfer. Be-fore the posterior tibial tendon transfer is undertaken surgically, it is essential that ade-quate assessment be performed with gait anal-ysis and EMG. If the posterior tibial muscle is continuously spastic, it can be of use in bal-ancing the foot. In this procedure (Fig. 42–10*A*), an incision approximately 2 to 3 cm long is made over the insertion of the posterior tibial tendon onto the navicular and medial cuneiform. The more posterior part of it is split and detached from its insertion as far distally as possible. A nonabsorbable suture is then placed through it in a modified Kessler technique.[29] The tendon is divided from its more anterior half by splitting it manually as proximally as can be seen prior to its entrance into the tendon sheath behind the medial malleolus. With a long hemostat (Fig. 42–10B), this suture is retracted into the tendon sheath proximally and is then used to tent the skin in

a more proximal area, about 4 cm above the ankle. An incision is made over that area, and the posterior tibial tendon is pulled through the incision. The tendon is then split longitudinally further up to the musculocutaneous junction. The suture and tendon are then passed back through the incision, using a hemostat and sliding the tendon across the posterior part of the tibia and fibula. It is delivered behind the lateral malleolus at approximately the same level, about 4 to 5 cm above the tip of the malleolus.

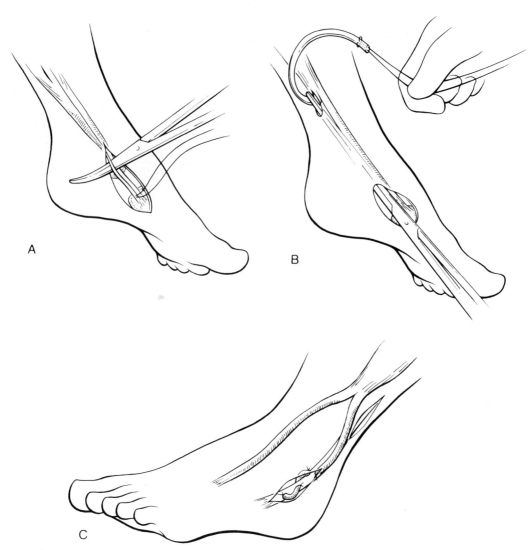

FIGURE 42–10. Split posterior tibial tendon transfer. *(A)*, Medial view of the foot. The posterior half of the distal posterior tibial tendon is split longitudinally, then detached from the bone distally. *(B)*, It is passed proximally through the sheath of the posterior tibial tendon. *(C)*, Lateral side of the foot. The split tendon is passed through the sheath of the peroneus brevis and woven into it.

Another small incision is made at this area, which is just large enough to receive the smallest self-retaining retractor. The length of tendon available is determined by pulling the tendon over the skin paralleling the peroneal tendons. The suture and split posterior tibial tendon are passed subcutaneously through the sheath of the peroneus brevis. A 2.5-cm incision is made over the peroneus brevis. The posterior tibial tendon half is woven into it in the manner of Pulvertaft.[35] The tension on the weave should be such that the length of the tendon is midway between its resting length and maximum passive length. Two nonabsorbable sutures anchor this weave. Any other tight tendons, such as the tendo Achillis, can be lengthened simultaneously. Following wound closure, a short-leg walking cast is applied in neutral position with a toe plate to extend the toes. The cast is removed at 6 weeks. A molded ankle-foot orthosis is then used for 6 to 12 months.

Bone Correction of a Varus Hindfoot. Bone correction of varus hindfoot can be done through a lateral closing wedge through the os calcis (Fig. 42–11).[21, 45] The angle of the wedge to be removed should be estimated by the amount of varus noted through the hindfoot.

Balancing of deforming forces can result in total correction of varus. If, after the preceding measures are undertaken, the foot is still deformed, triple arthrodesis can give satisfactory results.[23, 24] Only rarely should a triple arthrodesis be needed. To perform a triple arthrodesis, an oblique incision is made over the sinus tarsi. A laterally based closing wedge through the subtalar area is done to correct the varus. The talonavicular and calcaneocuboid joints are denuded with appropriate lateral closed wedging to correct midfoot varus. Staples or pins can be used to maintain correction. Casting is used for 10 to 12 weeks. Weight bearing is avoided for the first 6 weeks.

Valgus Deformities

Valgus foot deformities occur principally in spastic diplegic children with cerebral palsy rather than in those with hemiplegia; they are also common among quadriplegic children. The principal causes are peroneal spasticity, posterior tibial inactivity, and ligamentous laxity. Sometimes it is a combination of all of these.[7, 32] Ligamentous laxity will be seen especially in children who tend to be hypotonic.

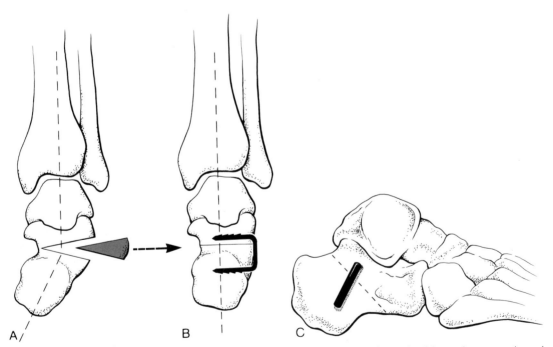

FIGURE 42–11. Lateral closing wedge osteotomy through the os calcis. *(A and B)*, The angle of the wedge removed equals the degree of correction. *(C)*, The line of the osteotomy viewed laterally.

Electromyographic Activity. Analysis of EMG activity in normal subjects shows that the peroneus longus and peroneus brevis begin firing between heel strike and toe strike—that is, through the foot stance of the gait cycle.[53] EMG activity generally ends slightly before toe-off.

Perry and Hoffer studied EMG activity in spastic feet of patients with cerebral palsy.[32] In valgus feet, they noted two patterns of peroneal activity: (1) activity during stance phase only and (2) continual activity during gait. When the peroneus brevis fires during the stance phase only, they transferred it to the tibialis posterior. If the peroneal muscles fired continuously through the gait cycle, they lengthened them. Bennet and colleagues noted valgus deformity due to inactive tibialis posterior.[7] In the face of a weak or nonfunctioning tibialis posterior, transfer of the active peroneus to the tibialis posterior adds balance to the foot.

Adler and colleagues challenged reliance on EMG data for making surgical decisions.[1] They found dynamic EMG studies to be helpful in surgical decision making and anticipating results in only 70 percent of cases. Clinical acumen continues to be an important tool in making surgical decisions. Furthermore, foot switch data from gait laboratories has not been helpful in surgical planning.[56]

Skinner and Lester's dynamic EMG analysis of valgus hindfoot deformities identified three types of abnormal EMG activity: (1) hyperactive peroneals with a strong tibialis posterior, (2) hyperactive peroneal muscles with a weak tibialis posterior, and (3) hyperactive long toe extensors.[46]

X-Ray Assessment. In considering surgery for valgus foot deformities, it is essential to have x-ray delineation of the problem. Both foot and ankle x-ray studies should be obtained. Both should be done in either a standing position or a simulated standing position to show the deformity. It is important to work with the technician to be sure that he or she does not position the foot so as to correct the foot deformity before obtaining the x-ray study. If the child is unable to stand, a simulated standing position should be used, with the foot in the deformed position. The standing mortise ankle x-ray study will help determine whether the valgus deformity is due to the ankle. A Harris view of the heel can help quantitate the amount of overall valgus of the

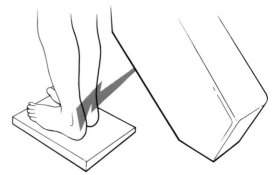

FIGURE 42–12. A standing Harris view of the heel helps to quantitate varus or valgus of the hindfoot. The beam is angled parallel to the line of the osteotomy, and the plate is horizontal.

os calcis (Fig. 42–12). If there is ankle valgus, a subtalar arthrodesis may be insufficient to correct the problem and may place additional strain on the valgus ankle. Ross and Lyne note that four of their bad results from Grice subtalar arthrodeses in 17 feet of patients with spastic cerebral palsy were associated with ankle valgus.[39] Paluska and Blount note that ankle and hindfoot valgus seemed to be independent factors.[31] Nevertheless, early recognition of the ankle component of valgus allows correction of that problem where necessary.

The anteroposterior foot x-ray studies show the talocalcaneal angle. Normally this angle should be between 15 and 25 degrees. Divergence of more than 25 degrees indicates valgus, and that of less than 15 degrees indicates varus (Fig. 42–13). To measure this accurately, the technician has to underexpose the forefoot somewhat in order not to overexpose the hindfoot.

Conservative Treatment. Conservative treatment of a valgus deformity can be tried in the early years, when the deformity begins to develop. Wenger and colleagues indicated that arch supports and molded heel inserts (UCBL from the University of California Biomechanics Laboratory) in corrective shoes are not helpful in affecting the overall outcome of a flexible flatfoot in otherwise normal children.[54] However, in a previous study, Bleck and Berzins demonstrated that use of UCBL shoe inserts can make a difference in control of the hindfoot valgus.[9] When in doubt, x-ray studies can often be enlightening in determining whether a foot is being held in a corrected position inside a shoe. More often than not, the corrective powers of these inserts are less

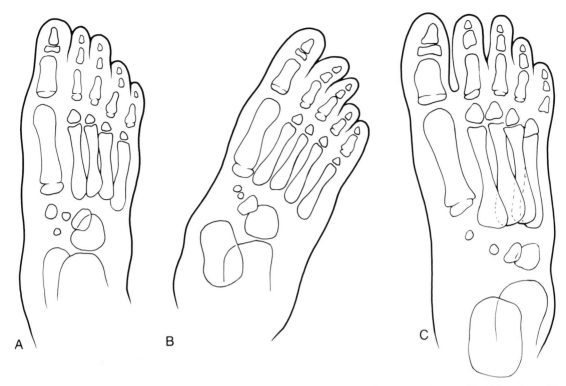

FIGURE 42–13. Talocalcaneal angles. *(A)*, Normal talocalcaneal divergence of 15 to 25 degrees. *(B)*, Valgus foot. *(C)*, Varus foot.

than their ability to obscure definition of the deformity. Perhaps a good sneaker with a firm heel allows the best control of this problem. Fortunately, in most centers, the so-called orthopaedic shoe and its brace have been replaced with a more cosmetic and better-controlling plastic molded foot orthosis. In time, many valgus feet progress to sufficient deformity that surgical intervention is actively sought by the patient or the parents.

Surgical Management. Foot deformities in cerebral palsy can be ameliorated by surgery. These deformities do not resolve spontaneously, and ignoring them can create fixed bony deformities, which are more difficult to correct than the dynamic deformities. Every effort should be made to render the spastic foot plantigrade prior to skeletal maturity.

In surgical management, soft tissue procedures include peroneus tendon lengthening; bone procedures include subtalar arthrodesis, subtalar stabilization, os calcis osteotomy, and triple arthrodesis.

Peroneus Brevis and Longus Lengthening. When the peroneus brevis is tight, contracted, and spastic, as demonstrated by EMG analysis and physical examination, peroneus brevis and longus lengthening is warranted. An incision approximately 1.5 cm long is made longitudinally over the peroneal tendons at about the distal two-thirds of the lower leg. This should be in the area of the peroneus brevis and longus tendon-muscle interface. The tendons can be lengthened while muscle fibers are kept in continuity. The incision is closed subcuticularly, and the extremity is maintained in a short-leg walking cast for 6 weeks. Most often, this procedure is done in conjunction with other procedures, such as heel cord lengthening or even a bone procedure, such as subtalar arthrodesis. By using a similar technique to lengthen the peroneus brevis in 30 feet of patients with cerebral palsy, partial correction was obtained in two-thirds and complete correction in one-third of feet in the study by Nather and colleagues.[30] In their technique, they advise complete division of the peroneus brevis rather than Z-plasty lengthening of it.

Subtalar Arthrodesis (Grice Procedure). Although many articles have discussed the results of subtalar arthrodesis, perhaps we can learn the most from Ross and Lyne's review of procedures performed at two different centers.[39] Almost two-thirds of their results were poor, and among patients with cerebral palsy, 71 percent of 17 patients had poor results. A large number of these poor results were due to ankle valgus. One cannot be sure whether or not this was a preoperative or postoperative problem. Certainly, ankle x-ray studies preoperatively would clarify this. The other problem was delayed union or slippage of the bone graft. The shape of the initial graft could probably allow most of these problems to be eliminated. The Dennyson and Fulford method of stabilization of the bone with a screw has been adopted in most centers with more satisfactory results.[13] In Barrasso's technique, a lateral incision is made obliquely over the sinus tarsi.[5] The extensor digitorum brevis is retracted distally. The sinus tarsi is cleared of fat. The periosteum is retracted and excised. A small trough is made in the lateral talus and os calcis in the area of the sinus tarsi in order to accept the graft. A round[20, 34] or square double-cortex graft that measures 2 mm more than the sinus tarsus site (approximately 2 ×

2 cm) is removed from the iliac crest and introduced into the sinus tarsi. Screw fixation from the dorsum of the head of the talus to the os calcis is then performed. A partially threaded cancellous screw allows fixation into the os calcis. Screw placement is confirmed by x-ray evaluation. The threaded portion of the screw should be distal to the subtalar joint into the os calcis (Fig. 42–14). A short-leg cast is applied. Weight bearing is usually delayed for 6 weeks. The foot is held in a cast for 8 weeks, followed by a molded ankle-foot orthosis for 1 year.

Ross and Lyne also showed the early presence of reactive exostoses at the talonavicular joint and the tibiotalar joint in their follow-up.[39] Talar exostoses were secondary to impingement of the talus on the anterior tibia. The long-term result of fusing the subtalar joint could be marked ankle and midfoot arthritic changes.

Two alternative procedures may alleviate this problem. Bartolozzi and colleagues introduced the concept of true subtalar arthroereisis to maintain the subtalar joint by insertion of a silicone spacer into the sinus tarsi area.[6] It may be necessary to repeat this procedure several

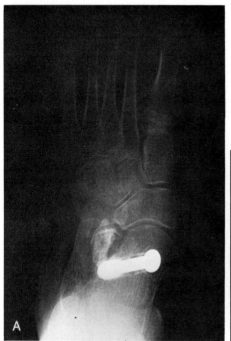
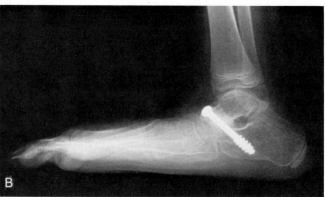

FIGURE 42–14. Postoperative x-ray study of a valgus foot corrected with a subtalar arthrodesis with bone grafting and screw fixation. (A), Anteroposterior. (B), Lateral.

times during the growth process, as the silicone implant may become dislodged or may be of insufficient size to maintain the foot in a neutral position. Some patients complain of the prominence of the silicone in the sinus tarsi area. Arthroereisis can be used as an interim procedure prior to a more definitive subtalar arthrodesis at a later age. This arthroereisis can be done in patients as young as 3 years of age. Caution should be used, however, because silicone can cause a foreign body reaction and a local synovitis.[47]

Subtalar Stabilization Using Staples (Crawford's Procedure). Extra-articular subtalar stabilization without arthrodesis can also be effected by using a laterally placed staple across the subtalar joint.[11] Using an oblique incision, the subtalar joint is opened. The foot is placed into a neutral position. A small trough is made in the os calcis to allow placement of the staple vertical to the weight-bearing surface of the foot. A U-shaped tendon staple is used. The ossific centers of the talus and os calcis must be wide enough to hold the staple. Following closure, the child is placed into a short-leg cast for 6 weeks. This procedure can be done in children as young as 3 years of age. Heel cord lengthening can be done at the same setting, but prior to the subtalar arthrodesis so as not to put additional stress on the corrected foot position once the staple is placed (Fig. 42–15).

Loosening of the staple is the major problem seen with this procedure. This can result in loss of correction and may necessitate more solid fixation. Parents should be warned that this stabilization is less solid than bone grafting, but it potentially gives better long-term results. Time will tell.

Os Calcis Osteotomy. If the valgus deformity is primarily in the hindfoot, an os calcis osteotomy is useful to correct this. A calcaneal osteotomy can be used, even in a child as young as 3 years of age.[52] A transverse or an oblique osteotomy is made from the lateral side of the os calcis from the slope on the lateral tibia from just posterior to the os calcis at about a 45-degree oblique angle anteriorly toward the plantar surface. The heel is then slid over approximately 25 percent of its width so that it is under the weight-bearing axis of the tibia. In a very young child, no fixation is needed. A short-leg cast is applied. I have used this technique and found it helpful in the young child with a worrisome degree of hindfoot valgus (Fig. 42–16).

Generally, in the older group, a Dwyer wedge osteotomy (Fig. 42–17) is preferable. Because it does not interfere with the subtalar joint, it is more physiologic than an arthrodesis. An opening wedge is made from the lateral side. The incision is oblique over the os calcis. An idea of the size of wedge needed can be ascertained by obtaining a Harris view of the foot with the x-ray plate perpendicular to the proposed osteotomy cut and determining how much wedging will bring the heel into a neutral position.[86] A lateral standing foot x-ray study will determine if there is any deformity in this plane. The wedge is packed open with bone graft. Skin closure can be a problem if the wedge is too large. If the wedge is too small, there may be insufficient correction of the deformity.

Staples or smooth Steinmann pins can be used to hold the corrected os calcis after the appropriate wedges are inserted. This is followed by 8 weeks of casting, with no weight bearing during the first 4 weeks.

Triple Arthrodesis. If the child's foot has not been corrected as the child nears maturity, triple arthrodesis can be used.[23, 24] The valgus foot can be corrected by laterally opening the sinus tarsus and denuding the joints (talocalcaneal, talonavicular, and calcaneocuboid). An autogenous iliac bone graft of approximately 2 × 3 cm is wedged into the triple joint (Fig. 42–18).[55]

Ankle Valgus

Ankle valgus must be corrected through the ankle itself. If there is still growth left in the growth plate, medial stapling of the growth plate can allow more lateral growth to occur. The staples can then be removed when the valgus is corrected. Alternatively, a supramalleolar osteotomy can be performed, with resection of the necessary wedge medially. This should be done through a medial longitudinal incision, which could be relatively small (4 cm). Use the image intensifier to ensure correction in the metaphyseal area and to determine that there is no impingement on the physis. The size of the wedge to be removed depends on the extent of valgus deformity of the ankle. A simple way to preoperatively plan for this is to trace the ankle mortise x-ray study and to determine the size of the wedge needed to correct the ankle so that the foot is parallel

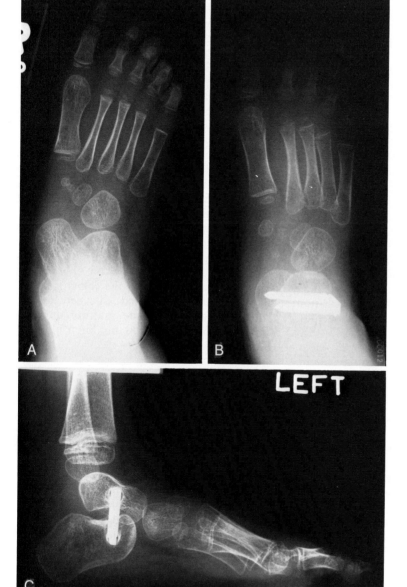

FIGURE 42–15. X-ray study of a valgus foot corrected with Crawford's staple procedure. *(A)*, Preoperative anteroposterior view. *(B)*, Postoperative anteroposterior view. *(C)*, Lateral view. The halo around the staple indicates slight subtalar motion despite excellent clinical correction.

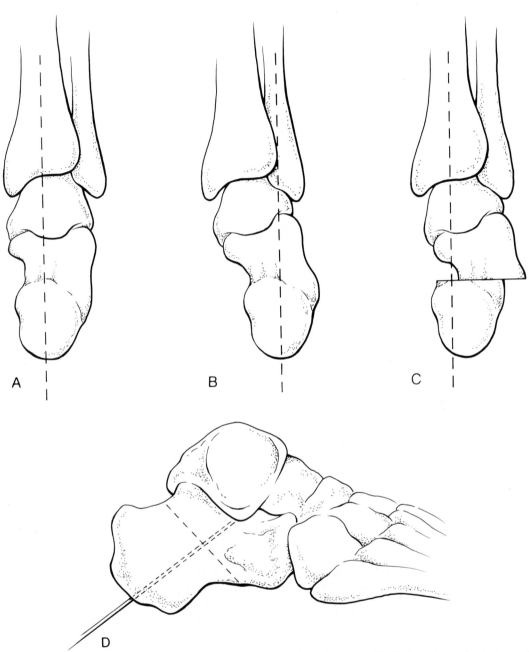

FIGURE 42–16. *(A),* Normal hindfoot alignment. *(B),* Hindfoot valgus alignment. *(C),* Sliding calcaneal osteotomy. *(D),* Line of the osteotomy viewed laterally.

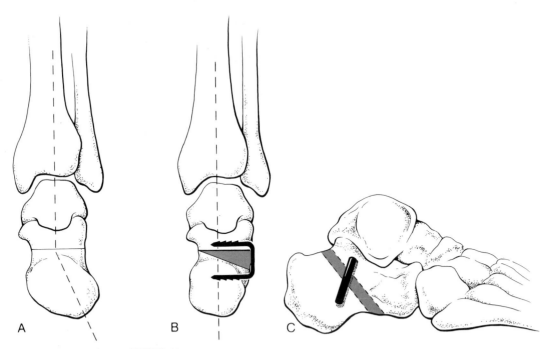

FIGURE 42–17. (*A* to *C*), A Dwyer wedge osteotomy (see text).

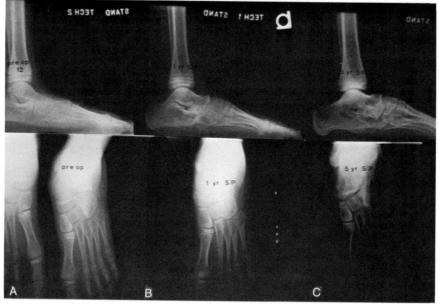

FIGURE 42–18. Triple arthrodesis for valgus foot deformity. (*A*), Preoperative x-ray study. (*B*), One year after operation. (*C*), Five years after operation.

to the ground. Because of the flaring of the metaphysis as it approaches the ankle, a simple closing wedge of the tibia may result in ankle deformity. See Wiltse's method of correction, as discussed in detail under Myelomeningocele (see Fig. 42–31). The osteotomy can be held with several staples. An osteotomy of the fibula may also be necessary at the same time. To correct the valgus deformity, the fibula should be osteotomized about 3 cm above the tibial wedge so as to minimize the instability to the ankle joint.

Hallux Valgus

Hallux valgus is not uncommon in the spastic child (Fig. 42–19). It is seen most frequently in conjunction with a valgus midfoot deformity. It also becomes painful as the child ages. In conjunction with a valgus midfoot deformity, hallux valgus can be seen in quite young children. Correction of the hallux valgus

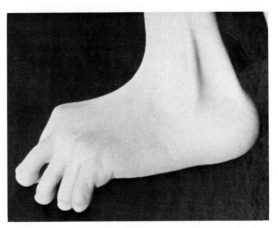

FIGURE 42–20. Dorsal bunion.

should follow correction of hindfoot and midfoot valgus. In a foot that is only moderately spastic, the hallux valgus can be corrected by traditional means, preferably delayed until after skeletal maturity has been reached, and consisting of a modified McBride procedure and proximal first metatarsal osteotomy.

The most definitive procedure for a very spastic foot is a metatarsophalangeal arthrodesis with removal of the exostosis at the first metatarsal head.[38] This is particularly warranted if there is degenerative arthritis of the joint. Make a lateral incision over the metatarsophalangeal joint, and open the capsule longitudinally. Cut off the distal end of the first metatarsal as well as the proximal end of the proximal phalanx. The ideal metatarsophalangeal angle is 25 degrees of dorsiflexion and 15 degrees of valgus. Alternatively, a peg-and-dowel configuration can be used to abut the metatarsal and proximal phalanx.[2, 25] Fixation is held with a Steinmann pin, an AO cancellous screw, or both.

Frequently the proximal phalanx of the great toe is also in a valgus position. An Akin medially based closing wedge osteotomy through the proximal phalanx can correct this. This osteotomy can be fixed with a pin.[16]

Dorsal Bunion

Dorsal bunions are also not uncommon, particularly in the severely involved spastic quadriplegic patient (Fig. 42–20). They are a problem because they cause pain with shoe wear. They are seen in conjunction with spas-

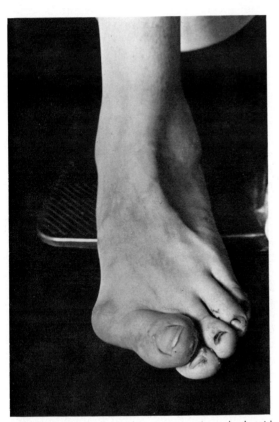

FIGURE 42–19. Hallux valgus in a spastic and athetoid child.

ticity of the anterior tibial tendon as well as the flexor digitorum longus and brevis and flexor hallucis brevis. Surgical treatment of a dorsal bunion must address the causes of the foot deformity. A plantar-based wedge can be removed from the first metatarsal. The anterior tibial tendon is sometimes a dynamic cause of this deformity and can be transferred to the second metatarsal or lengthened if this is the case. The hallucis longus tendon can be lengthened if it is tight. Occasionally the flexor hallucis brevis is also tight and needs to be tenotomized. The osteotomy at the base of the first metatarsal can be held with screw fixation.

The flexor hallucis longus can also be transferred through the neck of the first metatarsal with or without a plantar-based proximal first metatarsal osteotomy.[28a]

MYELOMENINGOCELE

About one child in 1000 is born with myelomeningocele. Previously, most of these children did not survive, but in more recent years, with the advent of shunting and closure of the myelomeningocele defect as well as the use of antibiotics, more children have survived. In Lorber's group of intensively treated patients, 41 percent survived.[89]

The inheritance appears to be multifactorial, with the pathologic change occurring in the early period of gestation. The theories regarding spinal dysraphism can basically be simplified to a failure of closure or rupture of the lumen of the neural tube before the spinal subarachnoid space develops.[98]

The child with myelomeningocele typically has a sensory deficit. He or she will have various muscles innervated to a variable degree. The paralysis can be flaccid or there may be reflex spasticity distal to the cord lesion.[112] The presence of spasticity makes the correction of deformities less predictable. Function is determined not only by neurologic levels but also by the presence or absence of spasticity.[91]

Many factors create foot deformities in myelomeningocele, but the chief cause is muscle imbalance. The deformity cannot be absolutely correlated with the innervation level of paralysis in myelomeningocele. In Lindseth's series,[88] at all levels of paralysis, no deformity was observed in 37 percent of feet, 45 percent had equinovarus deformity, 16 percent had calcaneovalgus deformity, and 2 percent had a

vertical talus deformity. Valgus foot deformities were seen frequently when paralysis was at the L5 level, and the equinovarus deformities were evident throughout all paralysis levels, being increased when paralysis originated at the thoracic level as well as at L4.

In evaluating foot deformities in myelomeningocele, Sharrard and Grosfield found 18 percent to be without deformity, either flail or normal, and a preponderance of varus feet (about 40 percent), with valgus occurring in only 8 percent and equinus in 22 percent.[106] Varus deformity was the preponderant deformity in the series of Hayes and colleagues.[79]

Along with the common foot deformities and valgus ankles, rotational deformities are commonly noted in the myelodysplastic child. Not infrequently, internal tibial torsion is noted.[69]

Increased plantar pressures are common in children with myelomeningocele. These children have smaller feet and weigh more than the average child of the same height, causing increased plantar pressure. In addition, with the foot deformities commonly seen in myelomeningocele, this increased weight is commonly distributed unevenly, causing high-pressure points. These increased plantar pressures can be noted even after the foot deformities are relatively well corrected clinically (Fig. 42–21).[109]

Goals

What type of goals apply to the child with myelomeningocele foot deformity? The foot needs to be plantigrade so that the body weight can be distributed evenly in the standing position. He or she must be able to fit into shoes that are available, so that special shoes are not needed. Shoes are part of our social environment. The handicapped child is already frequently ostracized by society. The child's shoes should be socially acceptable as well as readily obtainable. A plantigrade, albeit insensate, foot will minimize the likelihood of the development of foot ulceration. In many patients with myelomeningocele, the foot deformities eventually cause ulceration, which can preclude walking.

Ambulatory status is determined by a number of factors, including neurologic level, spasticity, hydrocephalus, spinal deformities, upper limb function, contractures, brain damage,

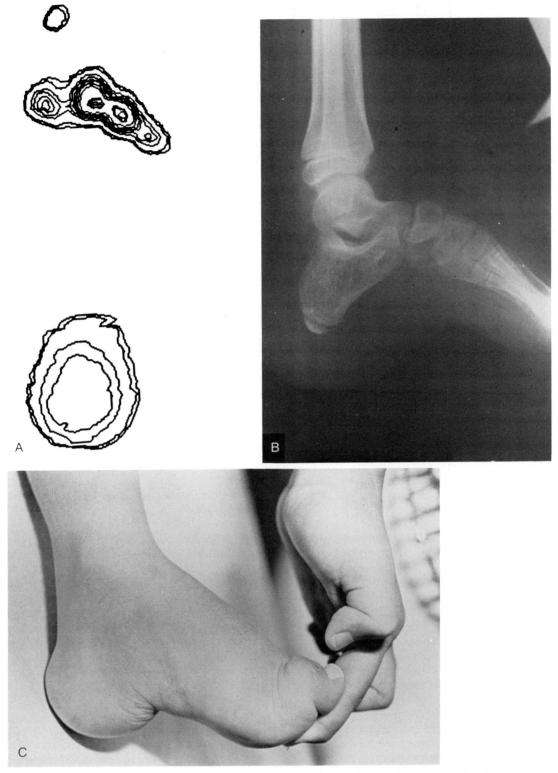

FIGURE 42–21. (A), Uneven foot pressures in a cavus foot deformity in a foot pressure study of children with myelomeningocele. (B), Cavus foot x-ray study shows pressure concentration at the metatarsal heads and os calcis. (C), Cavus foot.

and environmental factors.[82] Community ambulatory status was achieved by 9 years of age
in Hoffer's series.[82] Many children who peaked
as household and nonfunctional ambulators
decreased their ambulatory level as they
reached their teenage years. Some improved
their level of ambulation. Findlay and colleagues found a positive correlation between
the activity at age 7 and the adolescent ambulation level.[72] In general, it has been demonstrated that the presence of a strong quadriceps, particularly in the absence of spasticity,
allows a better quality of life and improved
ability to walk.[93]

Orthotic Management

Orthotics and bracing control for the myelomeningocele patient vary from the very conventional and traditional to those developed
through modern technology. We must first ask
what the function of the brace is. It should be
used not to correct the foot deformity but
rather to hold corrected deformities in a nondeformed position. A molded ankle-foot orthosis with a solid ankle helps to keep the
knee in position, particularly in the presence
of a weak heel cord. If calcaneus deformity is
a problem, the molded ankle-foot orthosis can
be extended throughout the length of the foot
in order to provide a long lever arm to prevent
rollover on the toe.[73] The traditional shoe with
metal upright could be made with a stop at the
ankle to control ankle motion, but when
molded plastic ankle-foot orthoses are available, they should be used (Fig. 42–22). These
orthoses allow cosmetically acceptable shoewear that is more in keeping with that of the
child's peers. The absence of a strong quadriceps necessitates increasing the amount of
bracing to include the knee. This can be done
in leather or by plastic mold with a knee joint
to make a knee-ankle-foot orthosis.

Use of a reciprocal brace has allowed many
children to improve their level of ambulation.
It has made at least household ambulators of
children who were previously not believed to
have any ambulatory potential at all (Fig. 42–
23).

The hip guidance orthosis has been popularized in England and is being used with increasing frequency in North America. It helps to
maintain the momentum of reciprocal walking.
Children with high-level lumbar lesions and

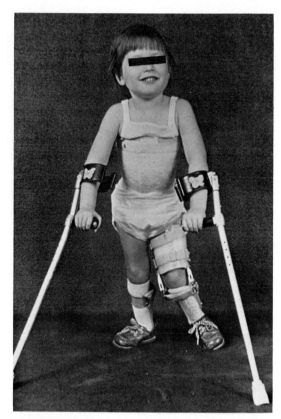

FIGURE 42–22. Child with myelomeningocele in a molded
ankle-foot orthosis and a knee-ankle-foot orthosis.

thoracic lesions have been able to maximize
their walking potential using this despite the
high-level lesion and lower level of function.

A swivel walker has been used not only to
provide mobility but also to continue with the
benefits afforded by gravity in association with
standing. Thus, many children who formerly
would not have been considered potential
weight bearers will now have this capacity for
a much longer period in their lives. The necessity of a plantigrade weight-bearing surface is
thus becoming even more significant as the
expectations for those with myelomeningocele
increase.[102]

Surgical Principles

Before surgery is considered in children with
myelomeningocele and foot deformities, a
thorough evaluation must be made. All deformities should be assessed. If possible, EMG

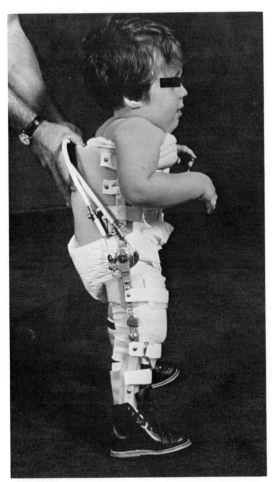

FIGURE 42–23. Child with high-level myelomeningocele in a reciprocal brace.

studies should be obtained to determine the electric activity of the muscles as well as to assess spasticity. Bony defects should be corrected surgically, rather than by casting.

Casts applied with pressure can frequently result in ulcerations, especially in the insensate foot (Fig. 42–24). Although ulcers frequently develop on the weight-bearing surface, they are also known to occur frequently over the dorsum of the foot and the front of the ankle.[106] Pressure and tension on the skin can cause sloughing of skin. In surgery, the skin should be closed without tension, with cast changes at weekly intervals to avoid pressure on the skin. At times, the skin may need to be mobilized with a rotation flap or with silicone tissue expander prior to corrective surgery.

As much surgery as possible should be done

simultaneously to avoid frequent hospitalizations for a child. The goal should be to obtain early weight bearing to correspond with the developmental activity of a normal, nonhandicapped child. Higher sensory or motor levels demand simpler procedures, such as percutaneous tenotomies.

Equinus Deformity

Equinus deformity occurs when the ankle plantar flexors are innervated without the balance of the ankle dorsiflexors (L4, L5), tibialis anterior (L4), and tibialis posterior (L4, L5) (Fig. 42–25).

To provide balance for the fixed equinus foot, Menelaus recommends a tenotomy of the heel cord shortly after birth.[94] This can be performed in the nursery in a child with an insensate foot. The tenotomy would be followed by well-padded casting to gently maneuver the foot into a more neutral position. Braces should be used to maintain the ankle in a neutral position. Many well-respected authorities have adopted this approach with great success.

Tendo Achillis Transfer to the Cuboid. If there is reluctance to sacrifice the active plantar flexors, Ogilvie and Sharrard have proposed a two-stage transfer of the lateral half of the tendo Achillis to the cuboid.[96] This is performed by first elongating the triceps surae with a Z-plasty in the coronal plane. This is followed by transfer of the lateral half of the heel cord to the cuboid. Both stages are done as open procedures with a rather long posterior longitudinal incision. Initially the heel cord is lengthened in the coronal plane as an open

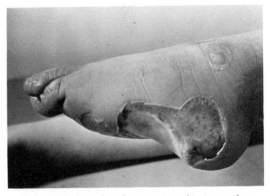

FIGURE 42–24. Ulcer from casting of insensate foot.

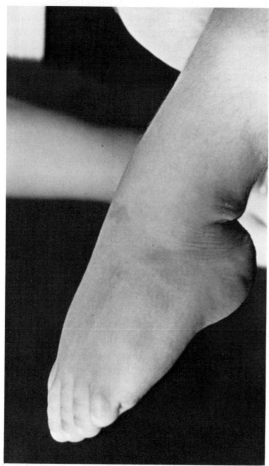

FIGURE 42–25. Equinus foot deformity.

procedure. After 4 to 6 weeks, the lateral half of the heel cord is transferred by detaching it longitudinally from the medial half. The lateral half is then passed subcutaneously with a forceps or tendon passer to the lateral side of the hindfoot. The tendon is then passed through a vertical tunnel in the cuboid, where it is sutured through with a Bunnell pull-out wire. The foot is then immobilized for another 4 weeks.

De Clippelle has suggested a similar one-stage procedure.[66] A small piece of the os calcis is used in this procedure in order to have sufficient length for the transfer and to anchor the tendon within the cuboid.

Calcaneus Deformity

Calcaneus deformity occurs when dorsiflexion is unopposed. The incidence of this defor-

mity, as a component of all foot deformities, is about one-fourth that of equinus.[79] Because foot pressure is then distributed solely on the heel, it can be more troublesome than other deformities. When calcaneus deformity occurs, it is important to assess the extent of the problem, as this will offer the appropriate surgical remedy. EMG studies and gait analysis help to determine the phasicity of muscle activity in the ambulatory child. In the nonambulatory child, these studies can denote the activity of the muscle with attempted voluntary contraction. If the tibialis anterior is active, this muscle can be transferred posteriorly.[64] Transfer of a muscle does not change the phasicity of the muscle during gait.[64] Janda and colleagues corrected the deformity with posterior transfer of the tibialis anteriorly in low-level myelodysplasia.[85] However, they note the formation of new deformities with time. Bliss and Menelaus followed long-term results of tibialis anterior transfers to the os calcis and noted that equinus deformities developed in more than half of the patients.[60] They related this to those who had spasticity of the tibialis anterior. They also noted that those operated on after 5 years of age did better, and most of them had no further surgery. Banta and colleagues,[58] using a modified Peabody technique,[80] noted that this transfer functioned as an Achilles tendon transfer. In this technique, the heel cord is divided at the musculotendinous junction and then tenodesed into the anterior margin of the tibia by suture through a drill hole through the tibia from the posterior aspect.

Anterior Tibial Tendon Transfer to the Os Calcis. The basic technique used to transfer the anterior tibial tendon to the os calcis has been described by Peabody.[75, 99, 117] To use this muscle, the tibialis anterior needs good or excellent strength. Ideally, it should be done before there is fixed bony deformity, but if the bony deformity is present, it should be corrected at the same time.[117] Assessment of the activity of the tibialis anterior is most complete with use of dynamic EMG studies as well as clinical examination.

A small longitudinal incision is made over the insertion of the tibialis anterior. The tendon is freed from its insertion on the first cuneiform and first metatarsal, and an anterior longitudinal incision is then made over the middle third of the tibia. The sheath of the tibialis anterior is opened parallel to the tibial crest. In a modified Kessler technique, a 2–0 nonabsorbable suture is placed into the end of the tendon and is used to pass the tendon.[29] The tendon is then pulled back through its sheath into the anterior tibial wound. The belly of the muscle in the anterior compartment is mobilized to the midleg. Care must be exercised in avoiding the anterior tibial artery, which is lateral to the muscle and just anterior to the interosseous membrane in the proximal half of the leg. The neurovascular bundle enters at the middle third of the muscle and also must be avoided. The interosseous membrane is then incised through the middle third of the leg at its tibial attachment. The suture is then passed through the window in the interosseous membrane, anterior to the soleus muscle and to the tendo Achillis. A longitudinal incision is made posterolaterally from the os calcis for about 7 cm proximally. A tunnel in the bone should be made using a large drill bit. The anterior tibial tendon is interwoven through the tendo Achillis and is further anchored into the os calcis with a Bunnell pull-out wire with the foot in equinus (Fig. 42–26A and B).

Reinforcement for the transferred anterior tibial tendon can be done by tenodesing the heel cord to the tibia. To do this, the Achilles tendon is divided at the musculotendinous junction. A drill hole is then made in the tibia posteriorly at the level of the proximal end of the heel cord. A nonabsorbable 0 suture is then passed through the drill hole to anchor the Achilles tendon to the tibia.

If there are other deforming forces, they must be corrected at the same time. If there is valgus, the peroneus brevis and tertius can be transferred to the os calcis.[77] In the older child with a valgus deformity in association with calcaneus deformity, an extra-articular subtalar arthrodesis can be performed using autogenous bone graft. Although Handelsman uses fibular graft, the graft could be taken from the iliac crest.[13] In teenage years, if there is a pistol-grip deformity of the os calcis, a Steindler plantar fasciotomy is done in combination with lengthening of the long toe extensors and a Steindler plantar fascial release. The bony correction can be obtained with a posteromedially based wedge of the subtalar joint.[77] Preoperative standing foot x-ray studies are used to plan the size of the wedge to be resected.[86]

After wound closure, the leg is held in a

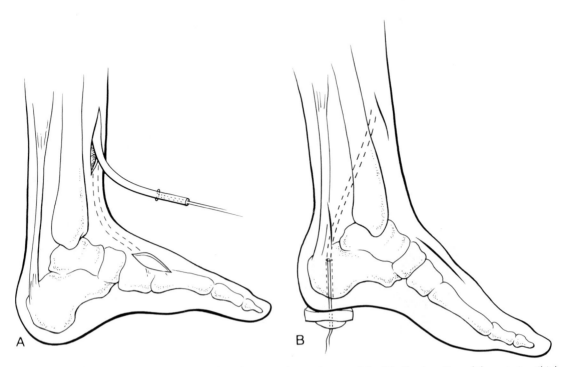

FIGURE 42–26. Transfer of the anterior tibial tendon posterior to the os calcis. *(A)*, The insertion of the anterior tibial tendon is released distally, and the tendon is passed subcutaneously and proximally. *(B)*, The tendon is passed posteriorly through the interosseous membrane, then a hole is drilled in the os calcis and the tendon is secured with a pull-out suture.

long-leg cast with the knee in some flexion and the foot in 15 degrees of equinus. The cast is bivalved, and physical therapy with active motion of the ankle joint is begun at 3 weeks. Walking may begin 6 weeks after surgery. A brace such as a solid ankle molded ankle-foot orthosis is used to avoid forced dorsiflexion.

Valgus Foot and Vertical Talus Deformities

In a vertical talus, the heel is in equinus and the navicular will not reduce on the distal talar head. In a paralytic foot, the peroneals and extensors dorsiflex the forefoot. If the heel is locked in equinus, this should be confirmed with a lateral x-ray study of the foot in plantar flexion (Fig. 42–27). In a vertical talus deformity, plantar flexion does not result in navicular or forefoot reduction onto the talar head. Open reduction of a vertical talus at around age 12 to 18 months can result in good correction.

A Cincinnati horseshoe incision around the hindfoot, at the level of the subtalar joint medially and laterally and proximal to the os calcis posteriorly, allows sufficient exposure.[65]

Extensive releases are necessary, especially through the talonavicular joint, to realign the bone. One or both of the peroneals can be transferred to the posterior tibialis to provide medial balance. The anterior tibialis should be transferred to the talar neck. The tendo Achillis should be lengthened. Steinmann pins maintain bony alignment for the first 6 weeks. The foot initially should be held in a bulky firm dressing to avoid tension on the sutures. At 1 week, the foot should be put into a well-padded cast. The cast can be changed and pins removed at 6 weeks, and the foot is then recast in a weight-bearing cast for 10 to 12 weeks. Alignment is better assured by use of a molded ankle-foot orthosis for at least another year.

Valgus foot deformity is frequently seen, either with equinus or calcaneus deformity. To correct the valgus component of the more supple valgus foot, a Grice procedure has been effective.[59, 95, 101, 103, 104] In conjunction with this, the deforming muscles need to be corrected by either a tendon transfer or tenotomy. One of the key tenets of correction was aptly stated by Wil Westin who said, "Thou shalt not varus."[119] Indeed, one-fourth of the poor results among the Grice procedures he reported on were due to excessive varus. This results in

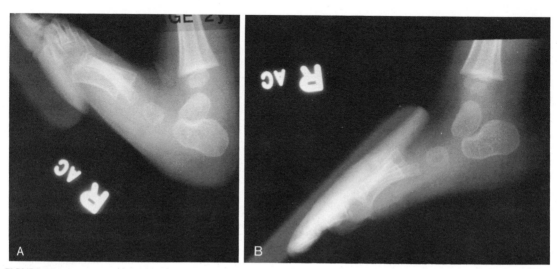

FIGURE 42–27. X-ray studies of vertical talus. *(A)*, Dorsiflexion. *(B)*, Plantar flexion does not result in navicular or forefoot reduction onto the talar head.

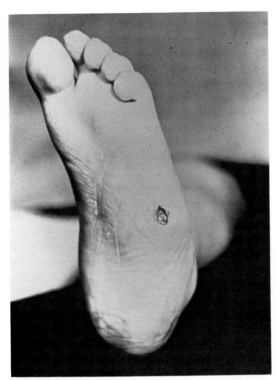

FIGURE 42–28. Foot ulceration at a prominent fifth metatarsal base.

an unsatisfactory weight-bearing pattern and can cause foot ulceration, particularly in the insensate foot (Fig. 42–28). A bone graft is used for the subtalar arthrodesis. If this is taken from the tibia rather than the ilium, an iatrogenic fracture can result. Screw fixation from the talus to the os calcis can be used to stabilize the foot until the bony graft fuses. The leg should be placed in a non–weight-bearing short-leg cast for 6 to 8 weeks. A Dwyer calcaneal osteotomy is not as satisfactory for stabilization of the valgus foot. Because of the laxity noted in the subtalar joint on weight bearing, this joint can open up medially and continue to cause valgus even after a calcaneal osteotomy.

Triple Arthrodesis. Early reports on triple arthrodesis in children with myelomeningocele showed a high incidence of nonunion and the need for revision.[79] Nevertheless, at times it is the only course to create a plantigrade foot. Subsequent studies, using the Williams and Menelaus technique,[121] gave improved results.[97] The Williams and Menelaus technique works nicely to correct a valgus foot deformity.

In this technique, a wedge of bone, usually about 2 cm wide and 4 cm long, is inserted into a prepared bed of slightly smaller size, joining the calcaneocuboid and talonavicular joints (Fig. 42–29). The subtalar joint is also denuded, and cancellous bone is packed into this area to stabilize the subtalar joint as well as the talonavicular and calcaneocuboid joints, allowing correction of the valgus deformity. At the same time, any tight tendons, such as the peroneus brevis and longus, need to be lengthened or tenotomized to eliminate deforming forces.

Ankle Valgus

Ankle valgus is the normal morphologic position at birth. The tibial plafond goes from a valgus tilt of 10 degrees at birth to 0 degrees at age 10.[61] In the normal child, the fibular physis progresses distally. At birth it is located 2 to 3 mm proximal to the dome of the talus, and after 8 years of age it is 2 to 3 mm distal to the dome (Fig. 42–30).[68] Progressive fibular growth occurs relative to the talar dome. In children with myelomeningocele, however, ankle valgus is a significant problem, and progressive shortening of the fibula is common. In Dias' study of 120 ankles of children with myelomeningocele, those under 8 years of age averaged 7.5 mm of shortening of the fibula, and those over 8 years of age averaged 14 mm of shortening of the fibula. Thus, ankle valgus is a very frequent problem in children with

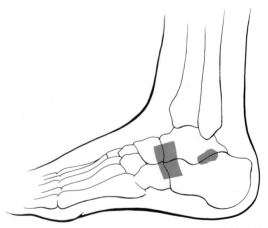

FIGURE 42–29. Menelaus' technique for triple arthrodesis (see text).

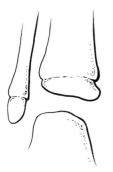 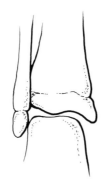 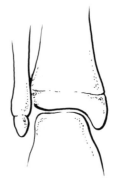

FIGURE 42–30. Normal growth of the fibular physis distally in relation to the dome of the talus at 3, 6, and 12 years of age. (Modified from Dias L: Valgus deformity of the ankle joint: Pathogenesis of fibular shortening. J Pediatr Orthop 5:176, 1985.)

myelomeningocele.[67, 68, 84] Hollingsworth also noted the phenomenon of a triangular physis associated with valgus ankles in a high percentage of these children.[84]

It is important to differentiate between ankle valgus and foot valgus and to address the problem at the level of the deformity.[90] On occasion, a valgus ankle can be seen in combination with tibial torsion. There are two major ways of correcting a valgus ankle. One is a temporary epiphyseodesis, using the stapling technique,[63] and the other is a supramalleolar osteotomy.[105, 122]

Stapling Epiphyseodesis. If there are at least 2 years of growth left in the growth plate, the stapling technique can be used. Be aware that children with myelomeningocele tend to mature physically faster than their chronologic peers. Estimate the growth remaining by obtaining wrist x-ray studies for bone age determination.[76] A medial longitudinal incision is made over the physis. The level of this should be determined prior to incision by fluoroscopy. About six small staples should be used. (They should be arranged to cover an arc of 120 degrees, from just anterior to the posterior tibial tendon, extending around farther anteriorly.) The staples should measure approximately 2 × 1.5 cm. It is important to confirm the position of these staples radiographically and be sure that they do not cross into the ankle joint and that they are parallel to the physis. After closure of the wound, the patient is placed in a short-leg walking cast for 2 weeks. It is important to follow the correction carefully as the child grows. The staples should be removed when the ankle achieves varus angulation of 10 degrees. The patient should be warned that at times the staples can cause skin irritation, especially because of their superficial placement. Occasionally one or more

of the staples needs to be removed prematurely because of this.

Corrective Supramalleolar Osteotomy. If stapling cannot be done because of insufficient growth potential in the distal tibia, a supramalleolar osteotomy is preferable. Preoperative planning for a supramalleolar osteotomy is imperative. A tracing should be made of the ankle and its valgus deformity, and the proposed osteotomy wedge should be cut out and superimposed on the paper. This will allow an estimation of the exact dimensions of the triangle to be removed and precise correction of the ankle deformity. The supramalleolar osteotomy allows correction not only of the valgus ankle deformity but also of any rotational deformities.

A simple closing wedge osteotomy based medially results in relative medial displacement of the foot owing to the increased diameter of the bone distally. The Wiltse technique, using an anterior longitudinal incision, can be done safely by making multiple drill holes through the tibia from an anterior position and connecting these by using an osteotome or power saw.[122] A small triangular wedge should be made with the apex anterior and posterior in the midshaft of the tibia. The medial border of the tibia is then placed in the apex of the triangle, allowing correction of the valgus deformity of the ankle (Fig. 42–31). A lateral oblique osteotomy is made in the fibula, slightly higher than the tibial osteotomy. The ankle is then displaced medially into the wedge of the tibia to correct the valgus deformity of the ankle. Slight overcorrection of the valgus of about 5 degrees will be satisfactory. This can be stabilized using Steinmann pins or screw fixation. After closure of the wound, a long-leg cast should be applied until healing is achieved approximately 8 weeks later.

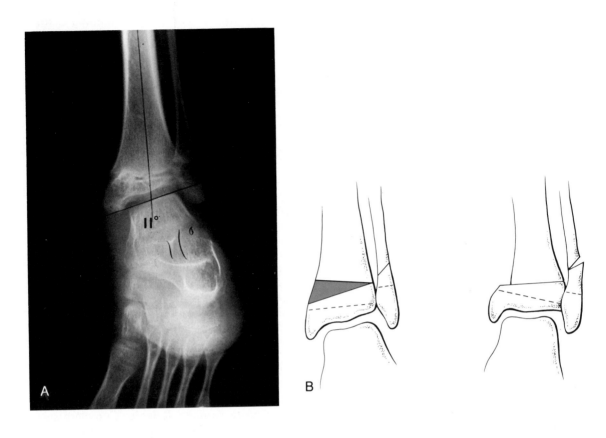

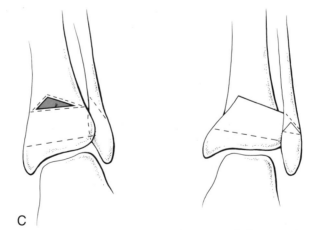

FIGURE 42–31. *(A)*, Valgus ankle (measuring 11 degrees). *(B)*, Medially based closing wedge osteotomy for valgus deformity of the ankle causes ankle deformity. *(C)*, The Wiltse technique uses medial shift and proximal wedging. (Modified from Wiltse LL: Valgus deformity of the ankle. A sequel to acquired or congenital abnormalities of the fibula. J Bone Joint Surg 54A:595, 1972.)

Rotational Problems

A small amount of internal rotation of the lower extremities can be corrected by semitendinosus transfer laterally to the biceps.[69] However, if internal tibial torsion exceeds 10 degrees, a supramalleolar osteotomy may be necessary to correct this rotational problem. If there is no valgus component to the ankle deformity, a supramalleolar tibial osteotomy can be achieved quite simply. A small medial incision is made, about 2 to 3 cm long, proximal to the physis. Use image intensification to verify the position. The osteotomy should be well away (2 cm) from the physeal line to avoid growth disturbance (Fig. 42–32). With care to avoid the posterior tibial nerve and vessels, multiple drill holes are made from the medial cortex of the tibia until these are nearly connected. An osteotome is used to complete the osteotomy. A slightly oblique osteotomy is made about 1 to 2 cm proximal to this through the fibula. Two Kirschner wires are placed parallel to one another both proximally and distally through the tibia. Derotation is then completed by separating the Kirschner wires the desired number of degrees. In the child, the periosteum is thick, and minimal internal fixation is necessary to hold this rotation. One or two smooth Kirschner wires can be passed through the osteotomy sites to secure them. These can be left percutaneously and pulled out about 10 days after surgery. A long-leg cast is worn until healing, which usu-

ally occurs in about 6 weeks. If the patient is not a functional ambulator, rotational deformities are usually not sufficient to warrant surgical intervention.

Equinovarus Deformity

Equinovarus deformities account for a high percentage of foot deformities in the myelomeningocele child.[79, 106] Equinovarus deformities are particularly evident when there is weakness or paralysis of the peroneal muscles. They are also frequently seen in a clubfoot configuration with dysplastic bones. A complete subtalar release, using a Cincinnati incision,[65] can be used to correct the more moderate deformity. The release should be done at an early age, usually before 1 year of age. A complete subtalar release gives more satisfactory results than posteromedial release and can circumvent the need for talectomy if it is done as a primary procedure.[109a] If necessary, a talectomy can be done later, at 2 to 3 years of age.[108, 109, 116] Forefoot adduction can continue to be a problem and may require additional capsular release at the tarsometatarsal level and release of the abductor hallucis.[81]

Complete Subtalar Release. Complete subtalar release can be done using a Cincinnati incision to allow full circumferential correction. The technique is similar to that used to correct a clubfoot. However, the unopposed posterior tibial and Achilles tendons can be

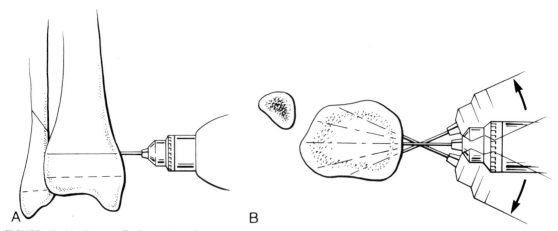

FIGURE 42–32. Supramalleolar rotational osteotomy. *(A),* Anterior view. The drill is used to make multiple cortical perforations in the plane of the osteotomy. *(Broken lines* indicate the epiphyseal growth plate.) (B), Transverse view at the level of the osteotomy. The osteotomy is finished with an osteotome.

tenotomized.[114] The deep deltoid ligament needs to be preserved in order to maintain the stability of the ankle joint. After talonavicular and calcaneocuboid releases, smooth pin fixation of the talonavicular and calcaneocuboid joints maintains correction without tension on the skin. On occasion, a calcaneotalar pin may be necessary for further postoperative stabilization. For the first postoperative week, a bulky long-leg dressing should be used. Thereafter, a long-leg cast can be applied for up to 12 weeks. The cast is changed at 6 weeks and the pins are removed. Simons has had good results with only 3 weeks of pin fixation and 6 weeks of total casting.[109a]

Cavus deformity can require release of the plantar fascia. This should be done under direct visualization from a medial approach. The tibialis anterior can be released and transferred to the midline subcutaneously. A small, separate dorsal incision is made in order to sew this into the second cuneiform bone. This can be sutured into the dorsal ligaments in a young child. This position can be held with Kirschner wires. In order to avoid vascular compromise to the skin, for the first week the foot is held in a bulky soft dressing without tension on the skin and with some equinus and some varus. In a week the foot can be placed into a more neutral position without compromising the skin circulation.

Talectomy. If the equinovarus deformity cannot be satisfactorily corrected with a complete subtalar release, talectomy may occasionally be necessary.[70, 92, 108, 109] Although talectomies can improve a poor correction, ground reaction forces on the plantar surface of the foot show that biomechanically plantigrade feet are seldom achieved with talectomies (Fig. 42–33).[109]

Meticulous attention to talectomy technique[115] is essential. A lateral incision is made over the sinus tarsi. Dissection is carried out in the interval between the extensor digitorum longus and the peroneus tertius. The foot is inverted and plantarflexed to make the talus more prominent. A towel clip is placed around the neck of the talus to secure it as a sharp, deep dissection is made through its ligaments. The talus should be removed intact to avoid leaving fragments of cartilage in the joint. It is important to obtain an x-ray study intraoperatively to be sure that there are no retained fragments of talus. The foot is displaced

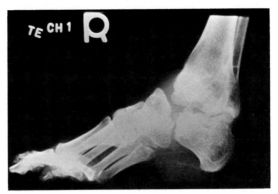

FIGURE 42–33. X-ray study of a foot after talectomy.

posteriorly into the mortise so that the tibial plafond sits on the middle articular facet of the os calcis. The deltoid and lateral collateral ligaments are resected in order to allow satisfactory positioning. If the heel cord is still tight after this, it may be lengthened. The foot should be aligned in relation to the bimalleolar axis of the ankle. Two Steinmann pins are introduced through the os calcis into the tibia to hold this position and are left in place for 6 weeks. A long-leg cast is applied after surgery.[116] Any residual adduction deformity of the forefoot can be corrected with ligamentous releases at the same time. If a talectomy is performed, it is preferable that it be done before the age of 5, while the ankle mortise still has some residual adaptive properties. Casting should be continued for 10 to 12 weeks after surgery. The pins are removed at 6 weeks. Further splinting, using the molded ankle-foot orthosis, is recommended until skeletal maturity.

Triple Arthrodesis. Triple arthrodesis for the deformed foot in spina bifida patients received a bad name following the report of the high failure rate of Hayes and colleagues.[79] Olney and Menelaus, who reported on triple arthrodesis, used this for both varus and valgus deformities, with more satisfactory results.[97] They did not note the high rate of ankle degeneration noted by Duncan and Lovell.[71] In a varus deformity, a lateral incision is made over the sinus tarsi, and lateral wedges are removed from the os calcis and talus to bring the foot into a plantigrade position. The triple arthrodesis has an advantage over the talectomy of allowing additional height in the foot, thereby making shoe fitting easier.[83]

Toe Clawing

In a small number of patients with myelomeningocele, toe clawing can be a problem.[107] It is important to analyze the cause of the problem with gait or motion analysis involving EMG studies and then to correct it. Frequently, the flexor hallucis longus is the offender. This can be tenodesed to the proximal phalanx of the great toe. The cause of the problem must be clearly delineated. EMG analysis is helpful.

Summary

In summary, several principles must be applied to the correction of paralytic foot deformities in patients with myelomeningocele. The deformed foot in such cases is usually at least partially insensate. Plaster cannot be applied with pressure to correct the foot deformities, as this can result in skin slough. Most deformities should be corrected at a young age, while the bones are less calcified and therefore still moldable. Unopposed tendons should be tenotomized in many cases to avoid further deformities. Tendons of active muscles can be transferred to balance the foot. Bony stabilization should be considered a last resort for correction of foot deformities in patients with myelomeningocele.

MUSCULAR DYSTROPHIES

Duchenne's muscular dystrophy is relatively common, occurring in one of 3000 live births. The child with Duchenne's muscular dystrophy initially reaches normal motor milestones but within a few years begins to show evidence of weakness. Initially, the child may begin walking on the toes. This is followed by clumsiness and difficulty in climbing stairs (Fig. 42–34). Frequently there are associated pains, particularly in the calf. As the weakness progresses, the child frequently begins to develop fixed foot deformity. Between the ages of 7 and 10 years, the child's function begins a downward slide.[123, 124]

Generally, the proximal musculature is affected most severely. Initially, the pelvic girdle muscles are involved, and later, the shoulder girdle muscles are involved, with development of progressive scoliosis. Surgery on the lower

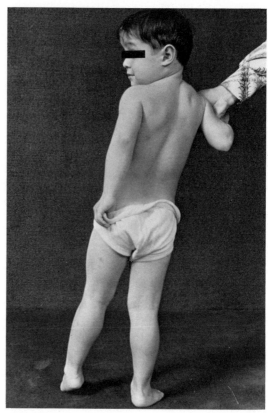

FIGURE 42–34. Child with Duchenne's muscular dystrophy presenting with an initial complaint of flatfeet and incidental clumsiness.

extremities is geared toward maintaining independent ambulation as long as possible.

Equinus Foot Deformity

Equinus deformity is the most common foot deformity in Duchenne's muscular dystrophy. The heel cord will begin to tighten early in the course of Duchenne's muscular dystrophy.[124, 126, 130] At this point, stretching of the heel cord is appropriate, and a molded ankle-foot orthosis may be considered. When the child's foot is no longer plantigrade on standing, consideration should be given to heel cord lengthening. Surgery is generally indicated just as the child is about to discontinue walking. Percutaneous heel cord lengthening, as described previously in this chapter, is especially helpful to these children. Surgery should be followed by 6 weeks of casting in a weight-bearing cast (Fig. 42–35).

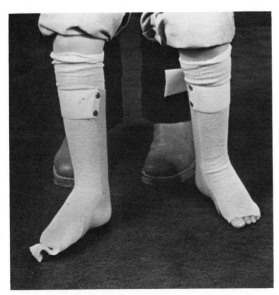

FIGURE 42–35. Bracing after heel cord lengthening.

Varus Foot Deformity

The second most common problem in Duchenne's muscular dystrophy is a varus deformity (Fig. 42–36). The posterior tibial muscle is relatively strong and should be transferred anteriorly to compensate for the weakness of the gastrocnemius-soleus complex.

Technique for Posterior Tibial Muscle Transfer Anteriorly. A small incision is made medially over the insertion of the tibialis posterior at the level of the navicular. The tibialis posterior is released in this area, and 2–0 nonabsorbable suture is threaded through it. This suture should be put into the tendon in a modified Kessler fashion so that it is firmly anchored in the tendon. Using a large hemostat or a tendon passer, the suture should be passed upward in the sheath of the tibialis posterior. The tendon passer should be poked to the side of the skin, and a small incision should be made to pull the tibialis posterior through the skin. This should be at about the level of the distal two-thirds of the tibia. Using a curved Kelly hemostat or a regular hemostat, the suture should then be passed behind the tibia and through the interosseous membrane. An incision measuring about 4 cm in length should be made through the area of the tibialis anterior, at the level of the tendon. A window should be made in the interosseous membrane, and the tibialis posterior should be pulled

through anteriorly. The tibialis posterior should then be passed under the extensor retinaculum with a tendon passer. A 2–0 wire with a pull-out component should be threaded through the tendon. A drill is used to make a hole in the middle of the foot, at the level to which the tendon will reach (approximately in the third cuneiform). The tendon should then be passed through the hole in the third cuneiform, and the wire should be passed through the skin to attach to a button on the plantar surface of the foot. Following transfer of these muscles, it is important to maintain the foot in a molded ankle-foot orthosis to prevent further deformity.

When the child is nonambulatory, the foot deformity may continue to develop. It is still appropriate at this time to consider operative procedures for several reasons. The first is to keep the foot in a plantigrade position to allow the patient to bear weight on the feet for standing as well as for stand and pivot transfers. The second is to prevent skin breakdown. Third, it will allow the patient to continue wearing shoes.[127]

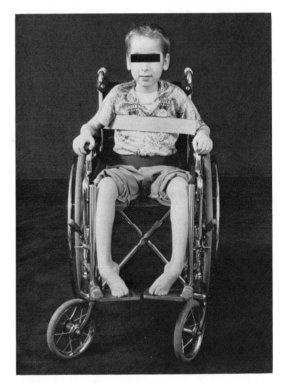

FIGURE 42–36. Equinovarus deformity in a wheelchair-bound child. Surgical correction allows resumption of standing and pivot transfer.

Summary of Foot Problems

Foot deformities will be progressive with the disease process. A plantigrade foot helps to maximize function. Foot bracing helps to maintain foot position and minimizes the need for surgery. Surgery should balance deforming forces or stabilize bones.

SUMMARY

Care of neuromuscular foot problems must be ongoing, taking into account the expected changes due to growth and progression of the disease process. Important factors of relative body involvement, presence of spasticity, absence of sensation, and intellectual status all have an impact on the maintenance of a plantigrade, nondeformed foot. The technology of gait laboratories, bracing advances, and better mobility systems has enhanced our ability to understand the neuromuscular foot. As they have for poliomyelitis, further research advances in prevention will ultimately solve the neuromuscular foot problem by elimination of the disease.

References

Cerebral Palsy

1. Adler N, Bleck EE, Rinsky LA: Gait electromyograms and surgical decisions for paralytic deformities of the foot. Dev Med Child Neurol 31:287, 1989.
2. Alexander I: First metatarsal phalangeal arthrodeses. Presented at the Summer Institute, American Academy of Orthopaedic Surgeons. Chicago, September 1989.
3. Baker LD, Hill LM: Foot alignment in the cerebral palsy patient. J Bone Joint Surg 46A:1, 1964.
4. Banks HH, Green WT: The correction of equinus deformity in cerebral palsy. J Bone Joint Surg 40A:1359, 1958.
5. Barrasso JA, Wile PB, Gage JR: Extraarticular subtalar arthrodesis with internal fixation. J Pediatr Orthop 4:555, 1984.
6. Bartolozzi A, Gregg JG, Trevlun D: Arthroereisis (Silastic implant) in the management of the decompensated flat foot in children. Presented at American Orthopaedic Foot and Ankle Society, 17th Annual Meeting. San Francisco, January 1987.
7. Bennet GC, Rang M, Jones D: Varus and valgus deformities of the foot in cerebral palsy. Dev Med Child Neurol 24:499, 1982.
8. Bleck EE: Orthopedic management of cerebral palsy. Clin Dev Med 99/100:1, 1987.
9. Bleck EE, Berzins UJ: Conservative management of pes valgus with plantar flexed talus, flexible. Clin Orthop 122:85, 1977.
10. Brodke DS, Skinner SR, Lamoreux LL, et al: Effects of ankle-foot orthoses on the gait of children. J Pediatr Orthop 9:702, 1989.
11. Crawford AH, Kucharzyk DO, Roy DR, Bilbo J: Subtalar stabilization of the planovalgus foot by staple arthroereisis in young children who have neuromuscular problems. J Bone Joint Surg 72A:840, 1990.
12. Crawford AH, Marxen JL, Osterfeld DL: The Cincinnati incision: A comprehensive approach for surgical procedures of the foot and ankle in childhood. J Bone Joint Surg 64A:1355, 1982.
13. Dennyson NG, Fulford GE: Subtalar arthrodesis by cancellous grafts and metallic internal fixation. J Bone Joint Surg 58A:507, 1976.
14. Dillin L, Samilson RL: Calcaneus deformity in cerebral palsy. Foot Ankle 4:167, 1983.
15. Gabarino J, Clancy M: A geometric method of calculating tendo achillis lengthening. J Pediatr Orthop 5:573, 1985.
16. Goldner JL: Hallux valgus and hallux flexus associated with cerebral palsy: Analysis and treatment. Clin Orthop 157:98, 1981.
17. Griffin P, Shiavi R: Split posterior tibial-tendon transfer in spastic cerebral palsy. J Bone Joint Surg 65A:748, 1983.
18. Gritzka TL, Staheli LT, Duncan WR: Posterior tibial tendon transfer through the interosseous membrane to correct equinovarus deformity in cerebral palsy: An initial experience. Clin Orthop 89:201, 1972.
19. Gunsolus P, Welsh C, Houser C: Equilibrium reactions in the feet of children with spastic cerebral palsy and of normal children. Dev Med Child Neurol 17:580, 1975.
20. Guttmann G: Modification of the Grice-Green subtalar arthrodesis in children. J Pediatr Orthop 1:219, 1981.
21. Hehne HJ, Baumann JU: Die Calcaneus-Osteotomie nach Dwyer bei der Varusfehlstellung des Rückfusses. [The Dwyer calcaneal osteotomy in varus deformities of the hindfoot.] Z Orthop 117:202, 1979.
22. Hoffer MM, Barakat G, Koffman M: 10-year follow-up of split anterior tibial tendon transfer in cerebral palsied patients with spastic equinovarus deformity. J Pediatr Orthop 5:432, 1985.
23. Horstmann HM, Eilert RE: Triple arthrodesis in cerebral palsy. Orthop Trans 1:109, 1977.
24. Ireland ML, Hoffer M: Triple arthrodesis for children with spastic cerebral palsy. Dev Med Child Neurol 27:623, 1985.
25. Johnson KA: Arthrodesis of the foot and ankle. In Johnson KA: Surgery of the Foot and Ankle. New York, Raven Press, 1989, p 197.
26. Johnston CE, Herring JA: Cerebral palsy. In Helal B, Wilson D (Eds): The Foot, Vol 1. Edinburgh, Churchill Livingstone, 1988, p 286.
27. Kaufer H: Split tendon transfers. Orthop Trans 1:191, 1977.
28. Kling TF, Jr, Kaufer H, Hensinger R: Split posterior tibial-tendon transfers in children with cerebral spastic paralysis and equinovarus deformity. J Bone Joint Surg 67A:186, 1985.
28a. Kuo KN, Fedder DP, Millar EA: Reverse Jones procedure for dorsal bunion following clubfoot surgery. Presented at Annual Meeting, American Academy of Orthopaedic Surgeons. Anaheim, CA, March 1991.

29. Leddy JP: Flexor tendons—acute injuries. *In* Green DP (Ed): Operative Hand Surgery. New York, Churchill Livingstone, 1982.

30. Nather A, Balasubramaniam P, Bose K: A comparative study of different methods of tendon lengthening: An experimental study in rabbits. J Pediatr Orthop 6:456, 1986.

31. Paluska DJ, Blount WP: Ankle valgus after the Grice subtalar stabilization. The late evaluation of a personal series with a modified technique. Clin Orthop 59:137, 1968.

32. Perry J, Hoffer MM: Preoperative and postoperative dynamic electromyography as an aid in planning tendon transfers in children with cerebral palsy. J Bone Joint Surg 59A:531, 1977.

33. Perry J, Hoffer MM, Giovan P, et al: Gait analysis of the triceps surae in cerebral palsy. A preoperative and postoperative clinical and electromyographic study. J Bone Joint Surg 56A:511, 1974.

34. Pirani S, Tredwell SJ, Beauchamp RD: Extraarticular subtalar arthrodesis: The dowel method. J Pediatr Orthop 10:274, 1990.

35. Pulvertaft RG: Tendon grafts for flexor tendon injuries in the fingers and thumb. A study of technique and results. J Bone Joint Surg 38B:175, 1956.

36. Rang M: Cerebral palsy. *In* Morrissy RT (Ed): Lovell and Winter's Pediatric Orthopedics, 3rd Ed. Philadelphia, JB Lippincott, 1990, p 465.

37. Reimers J: Contracture of the hamstrings in spastic cerebral palsy: Study of three methods of operative correction. J Bone Joint Surg 56B:102, 1974.

38. Renshaw TS, Sirkin RB, Drennan JC: The management of hallux valgus in cerebral palsy. Dev Med Child Neurol 21:202–208, 1979.

39. Ross PM, Lyne ED: The Grice procedure: Indications and evaluation of long-term results. Clin Orthop 153:194, 1980.

40. Ruda R, Frost HM: Cerebral palsy: Spastic varus and forefoot adductus, treated by intramuscular posterior tibial tendon lengthening. Clin Orthop 79:61, 1971.

41. Schwartz JR, Carr W, Bassett FH, Conrad RW: Lessons learned in the treatment of equinus deformity in ambulatory cerebral palsy. Orthop Trans 1:84, 1977.

42. Segal LS, Sienko T, Mazur J, Mauterer M: Calcaneal gait in spastic diplegia after heel cord lengthening: A study with gait analysis. J Pediatr Orthop 9:697, 1989.

43. Silfverskiöld N: Reduction of the uncrossed two-joint muscles of the leg to one-joint muscles in spastic conditions. Acta Chir Scand 56:315, 1924.

44. Silver CM, Simon FD: Gastrocnemius recession (Silfverskiöld operation) spastic equinus deformity in cerebral palsy. J Bone Joint Surg 41A:1021, 1959.

45. Silver CM, Simon SD, Spindell E, et al: Calcaneal osteotomy for valgus and varus deformities of the foot in cerebral palsy. A preliminary report on twenty-seven operations. J Bone Joint Surg 49A:232, 1967.

46. Skinner SR, Lester DK: Dynamic EMG findings in valgus hindfoot deformity in spastic cerebral palsy. Orthop Trans 9:91, 1985.

47. Smith DJ, Sazy JA, Crissman JD, et al: Immunogenic potential of carpal implants. J Surg Res 48:13, 1990.

48. Stanley F: Perinatal risk factors in the cerebral palsies. *In* Stanley F, Alberman E (Eds): The Epidemiology of Cerebral Palsy. Clin Dev Med 87:98, 1984.

49. Sutherland DH, Schottstaedt EE, Larsen LJ, et al: Clinical and EMG study of seven spastic children with internal rotation gait. J Bone Joint Surg 51A:1070, 1969.

50. Tardieu C, Lespargot A, Tabaryu C, Bret MD: For how long must the soleus muscle be stretched each day to prevent contracture? Dev Med Child Neurol 30:3, 1988.

51. Tardieu G, Tardieu C, Colbeau-Justin P, Lespargot A: Muscle hypoextensibility in children with cerebral palsy. II. Therapeutic implications. Arch Phys Med Rehabil 63:97, 1982.

52. Treishmann H, Millis M, Hall J, Watts H: A sliding calcaneal osteotomy for treatment of hindfoot deformity. Orthop Trans 4:305, 1980.

53. Walmsley RP: Electromyographic study of the phasic activity of peroneus longus and brevis. Arch Phys Med Rehabil 58:65, 1977.

54. Wenger DR, Mauldin D, Speck G, et al: Corrective shoes and inserts as treatment for flexible flatfoot in infants and children. J Bone Joint Surg 71A:800, 1989.

55. Williams PF, Menelaus M: Triple arthrodesis by inlay grafting. A method suitable for undeformed or valgus foot. J Bone Joint Surg 59B:333, 1977.

56. Wills CA, Hoffer MM, Perry J: A comparison of foot-switch and EMG analysis of varus deformities of the feet of children with cerebral palsy. Dev Med Child Neurol 30:227, 1988.

57. Wolf SL, Binder-MacLeod SA: Electromyographic biofeedback applications to the hemiplegic patient. Changes in lower extremity neuromuscular and functional status. Phys Ther 63:1404, 1983.

Myelomeningocele

58. Banta JV, Sutherland DH, Wyatt M: Anterior tibial transfer to the os calcis with achilles tenodesis for calcaneal deformity in myelomeningocele. J Pediatr Orthop 1:125, 1981.

59. Banta JV, Nichols O: Autogenous fibular subtalar arthrodesis in myelodysplasia. J Bone Joint Surg 55A:1317, 1973.

60. Bliss DG, Menelaus MB: The results of transfer of the tibialis anterior to the heel in patients who have myelomeningocele. J Bone Joint Surg 68A:1258, 1986.

61. Böhm M: Das menschliche Bein. Stuttgart, Ferdinand Enke, 1935, p 42.

62. Bunch WH: Myelomeningocele. *In* Lovell WW, Winter RB (Eds): Pediatric Orthopaedics, 2nd Ed. Philadelphia, JB Lippincott, 1986, pp 397–435.

63. Burkus JK, Moore DW, Raycroft JF: Valgus deformity of the ankle in myelodysplastic patients. Correction by stapling of the medial part of the distal tibial physis. J Bone Joint Surg 65A:1157, 1983.

64. Close JR, Todd JM: The phasic activity of the muscles of the lower extremity and the effect of tendon transfers on joint surgery. J Bone Joint Surg 41A:189, 1959.

65. Crawford AH, Marxen JL, Osterfeld DL: The Cincinnati incision: A comprehensive approach for surgical procedures of the foot and ankle in childhood. J Bone Joint Surg 64A:1355, 1982.

66. de Clippelle H: Hemitransplantation du tendon d'Achille chez une myopathique. Acta Orthop Belg 39:734, 1973.

67. Dias L: Ankle valgus in children with myelomeningocele. Dev Med Child Neurol 20:627, 1978.

68. Dias L: Valgus deformity of the ankle joint: Pathogenesis of fibular shortening. J Pediatr Orthop 5:176, 1985.

69. Dias LS, Jasty MJ, Collins P: Rotational deformities of the lower limb in myelomeningocele. Evaluation and treatment. J Bone Joint Surg 66A:215, 1984.

70. Dias LS, Stern LS: Talectomy in the treatment of resistant talipes equinovarus deformity in myelomeningocele and arthrogryposis. J Pediatr Orthop 7:39, 1987.

71. Duncan JW, Lovell WW: Triple arthrodesis. J Bone Joint Surg 60A:795, 1978.

72. Findley TW, Agre JC, Habeck R, et al: Ambulation in the adolescent with myelomeningocele. I: Early childhood predictors. Arch Phys Med Rehabil 68:518, 1987.

73. Fulford GE, Cairns TP: The problems associated with flail feet in children and their treatment with orthoses. J Bone Joint Surg 60B:93, 1978.

74. Golski A, Menelaus MB: The treatment of intoed gait in spina bifida patients by lateral transfer of the medial hamstrings. Aust N Z J Surg 46:157, 1976.

75. Georgiadis GM, Aronson DO: Posterior transfer of the anterior tibial tendon in children who have a myelomeningocele. J Bone Joint Surg 72A:392, 1990.

76. Greulich WW, Pyle SI: Radiographic Atlas of Skeletal Development of the Hand and Wrist, 2nd Ed. Palo Alto, Stanford University Press, 1959.

77. Handelsman J: Management of paralytic calcaneus deformity of the foot. J Bone Joint Surg 55B:438, 1973.

78. Hay M, Walker G: Plantar pressures in healthy children and in children with myelomeningocele. J Bone Joint Surg 55B:828, 1973.

79. Hayes JT, Gross HP, Dow S: Surgery for paralytic defects secondary to myelomeningocele and myelodysplasia. J Bone Joint Surg 46A:1577, 1964.

80. Herndon CH, Strong JM, Heyman CH: Transposition of the tibialis anterior in the treatment of paralytic talipes calcaneus. J Bone Joint Surg 38A:751, 1956.

81. Heyman CH, Herndon CH, Strong JM: Mobilization of the tarsometatarsal and intermetatarsal joints for the correction of resistant adduction of the fore part of the foot in congenital club-foot or congenital metatarsus varus. J Bone Joint Surg 40A:299, 1958.

82. Hoffer MM, Feiwell E, Perry J: Functional ambulation in patients with myelomeningocele. J Bone Joint Surg 55A:137, 1973.

83. Hoke M: An operation for stabilizing paralytic feet. Am J Orthop Surg 3:474, 1921.

84. Hollingsworth RP: An x-ray study of valgus ankles in spina bifida children with valgus flatfoot. Proc R Soc Med 68:481, 1975.

85. Janda JPS, Skinner SR, Barto PS: Posterior transfer of tibialis anterior in low-level myelodysplasia. Dev Med Child Neurol 26:100, 1984.

86. Krackow KA, Hales D, Jones L: Preoperative planning for performing a Dwyer calcaneal osteotomy. J Pediatr Orthop 5:214, 1989.

87. Lang-Stevenson AI, Sharrard WJW, Betts RP, Duckworth J: Neuropathic ulcers of the foot. J Bone Joint Surg 67B:438, 1985.

88. Lindseth RE: Treatment of the lower extremity in children paralyzed by myelomeningocele (birth to 18 months). Instr Course Lect 25:76, 1976.

89. Lorber J: Results of treatment of myelomeningocele. Dev Med Child Neurol 13:229, 1971.

90. Malhotra D, Puri R, Owen R: Valgus deformity of the ankle in children with spina bifida aperta. J Bone Joint Surg 66B:381, 1984.

91. Mazur JM, Stillwell A, Menelaus M: The significance of spasticity in the upper and lower limbs in myelomeningocele. J Bone Joint Surg 68B:213, 1986.

92. Menelaus MB: Talectomy for equinovarus deformity in arthrogryposis and spina bifida. J Bone Joint Surg 53B:468, 1971.

93. Menelaus MB: Orthopaedic management of children with myelomeningocele. A plea for realistic goals. Dev Med Child Neurol 18(Suppl 37):3, 1976.

94. Menelaus MB: The Orthopaedic Management of Spina Bifida Cystica. Edinburgh, E & S Livingstone, 1971.

95. Moreland JR, Westin GW: Further experience with Grice subtalar arthrodesis. Clin Orthop 207:113, 1986.

96. Ogilvie C, Sharrard WJW: Hemitransplantation of the tendo calcaneus in children with spinal neurological disorders. J Bone Joint Surg 68B:767, 1986.

97. Olney RW, Menelaus MB: Triple arthrodesis of the foot in spina bifida patients. J Bone Joint Surg 70B:234, 1988.

98. Patten BM: Embryologic stages in the establishing of myeloschisis with spina bifida. Am J Anat 93:365, 1953.

99. Peabody CW: Tendon transposition. An end result study. J Bone Joint Surg 20:193, 1938.

100. Peabody CW: Tendon transposition in the paralytic foot. Instr Course Lect 6:178, 1949.

101. Pollock JH, Carrell B: Subtalar extra-articular arthrodesis in the treatment of paralytic valgus deformities. A review of 112 procedures in 100 patients. J Bone Joint Surg 46A:533, 1964.

102. Rose GK, Sankarankutty M, Stallard J: A clinical review of the orthotic treatment of myelomeningocele patients. J Bone Joint Surg 65B:242, 1983.

103. Ross PM, Lyne ED: The Grice procedure: Indications and evaluation of long-term results. Clin Orthop 153:194, 1980.

104. Scott SM, Janes PC, Stevens PM: Grice subtalar arthrodesis followed to skeletal maturity. J Pediatr Orthop 8:176, 1988.

105. Sharrard WJW, Webb J: Supra-malleolar wedge osteotomy of the tibia in children with myelomeningocele. J Bone Joint Surg 56B:458, 1974.

106. Sharrard WJW, Grosfield I: The management of deformity and paralysis of the foot in myelomeningocele. J Bone Joint Surg 50B:456, 1968.

107. Sharrard WJW, Smith TWD: Tenodesis of flexor hallucis longus for paralytic clawing of the hallux in childhood. J Bone Joint Surg 58B:224, 1976.

108. Sherk HH, Ames MD: Talectomy in the treatment of the myelomeningocele patient. Clin Orthop 110:218, 1975.

109. Sherk HH, Marchinski LJ, Clancy M, Melchionni J: Ground reaction forces on the plantar surface of the foot after talectomy in the myelomeningocele. J Pediatr Orthop 9:269, 1989.

109a. Simons GW, personal communication, 1990.

110. Simon SR, Mann RA, Hagy JL, Larsen LJ: Role of

the posterior calf muscles in normal gait. J Bone Joint Surg 60A:466, 1978.

111. Smith TWD, Duckworth T: The management of deformities of the foot in children with spina bifida. Dev Med Child Neurol 18(Suppl 37):104, 1974.

112. Stark GD, Baker GCW: The neurologic involvement of the lower limbs in myelomeningocele. Dev Med Child Neurol 9:1732, 1967.

113. Stillwell A, Menelaus MB: Walking ability in mature patients with spina bifida. J Pediatr Orthop 3:184, 1983.

114. Szalay E: Orthopaedic management of the lower extremities in spina bifida. Instr Course Lect 36:275, 1987.

115. Thompson TC: Astragalectomy and the treatment of calcaneovalgus. J Bone Joint Surg 21:627, 1939.

116. Trumble T, Banta JV, Raycroft JF, Curtis BH: Talectomy for equinovarus deformity in myelodysplasia. J Bone Joint Surg 67A:21, 1985.

117. Turner JW, Cooper RR: Anterior transfer of the tibialis posterior through the interosseus membrane. Clin Orthop 83:241, 1972.

118. Walker G: The early management of varus feet in myelomeningocele. J Bone Joint Surg 53B:462, 1971.

119. Westin GW, quoted in Polloch JH, Carrell B: Subtalar extraarticular arthrodesis in the treatment of paralytic valgus deformities. J Bone Joint Surg 46A:533, 1967.

120. Westin GW, Dingeman RD, Gausewitz SH: The results of tenodesis of the tendo achillis to the fibula for paralytic pes calcaneus. J Bone Joint Surg 70A:320, 1988.

121. Williams PF, Menelaus M: Triple arthrodesis by inlay grafting. A method suitable for undeformed or valgus foot. J Bone Joint Surg 59B:333, 1977.

122. Wiltse LL: Valgus deformity of the ankle. A sequel to acquired or congenital abnormalities of the fibula. J Bone Joint Surg 54A:595, 1972.

Muscular Dystrophies

123. Brooke MH: A Clinician's View of Neuromuscular Diseases. Baltimore, Williams & Wilkins, 1977, p 95.

124. Drennan JC: Neuromuscular disorders. *In* Morrisey RT (Ed): Lovell and Winter's Pediatric Orthopaedics, 3rd Ed. Philadelphia, JB Lippincott, 1990, p 385.

125. Hsu JD, Hoffer MM: Posterior tibial tendon transfer anteriorly through the interosseous membrane: A modification of the technique. Clin Orthop 131:202, 1978.

126. Hsu JD: Management of foot deformity in Duchenne's pseudohypertrophic muscular dystrophy. Orthop Clin North Am 7:979, 1976.

127. Hsu JD, Jackson R: Treatment of symptomatic foot and ankle deformities in the nonambulatory neuromuscular patient. Foot Ankle 5:238, 1985.

128. Melkonian GJ, Cristofaro RL, Perry J, Hsu JD: Dynamic gait electromyography study in Duchenne muscular dystrophy (DMD) patients. Foot Ankle 1:78, 1980.

129. Roy L, Gibson D: Pseudohypertrophic muscular dystrophy and its surgical management: Review of 30 patients. Can J Surg 1:13, 1970.

130. Sutherland DH, Olshen R, Casper L, et al: The pathomechanics of gait in Duchenne muscular dystrophy. Dev Med Child Neurol 23:3, 1981.

43

Flexible Flatfoot

G. PAUL DeROSA

It may seem odd to have a chapter on a condition that rarely requires surgery in a textbook on operative foot surgery, but it is important to be all inclusive as well as to rethink the pathomechanics of flatfeet.

This condition is frequently referred to as pronated foot, relaxed flatfoot, and congenital planovalgus. Basically, the term *flatfoot* is generic, and it is used to describe any condition of the foot in which the longitudinal arch is abnormally low or absent. Perhaps because it is so common, we frequently fail to make the correct diagnosis in the majority of affected children.

In reviewing the medical literature, much has been written about this relatively common problem. These writings include theories of etiology and numerous treatment modalities. There is no agreement on either the theory of the etiology or common treatment practices. Absent from the orthopaedic literature are long-term studies of patients who have had no treatment or of others who have had only conservative care. If anything can be gleaned from the literature with certainty, it is the impression that the large majority of these feet are asymptomatic and will remain so throughout the patient's life. Those who advocate surgical intervention must emphasize the need to limit treatment to patients with substantial symptoms or with severe deformity. Without a clear knowledge of the natural history of the condition, healthy skepticism should be used when reading information about short-term results of operative intervention.

I know of few other subjects that incite as much parental anxiety as do flatfeet, especially when this is coupled with knowledge of an older relative who may be experiencing symptoms in similarly appearing feet.

Certainly, varying degrees of flexible flatfeet are common in young children. For the most part, it can be stated that as long as a young child has feet with normal musculature and normal flexibility, then the feet are normal. It is important to remember that the calcaneovalgus position of the foot (that in which the dorsum of the foot can be placed against the anterior aspect of the tibia) is the most common position of the foot in the newborn. The medial longitudinal arch does not develop until after 2 years of age; therefore, when the normal child starts to stand (at any time from 9 months to 18 months), the feet will appear flat.[27] In addition, there is a prominent pad of fat present in the foot on the medial side anterior to the heel. This effectively can obliterate the longitudinal arch. Ozonoff[43] has stated that by age 10, only 4 percent of children will appear to be flatfooted. Very few of these feet will develop disability or symptoms of pain, or sufficient abnormal shoe wear to warrant a surgical operation. In Crego and Ford's[8] long-term study, they estimated that only one child in 40 with *symptomatic* flatfeet required a surgical procedure; the rest could be treated conservatively.

CLINICAL FEATURES

The term *flexible flatfoot* describes a foot in which the medial longitudinal arch has diminished height and the hindfoot assumes a valgus (pronated) position on weight bearing (Fig. 43–1). In addition, the forefoot is abducted.

834

FIGURE 43–1. *(A* and *B),* Ten-year-old child with mild flatfoot deformity. Note heel valgus.

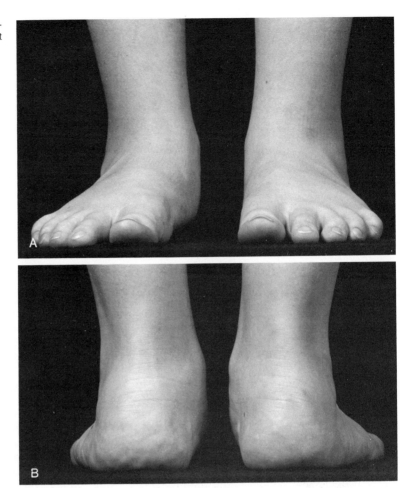

This, combined with the valgus orientation of the heel, results in depression of the longitudinal arch. When weight bearing is relieved, the foot assumes a normal contour and a normal-appearing arch. The depression in the longitudinal arch may result from plantar deviation of any one or all three of the components that make up the arch, namely the talocalcaneal, talonavicular, and naviculocuneiform joints (Fig. 43–2). On weight bearing,

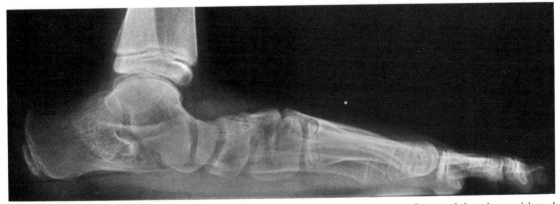

FIGURE 43–2. Standing lateral x-ray study of severe flatfoot deformity, marked plantar flexion of the talus, and lateral rotation of the os calcis. Depression at the talonavicular joint is well seen.

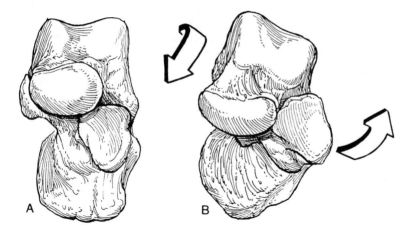

FIGURE 43–3. (A), Normal support of talus by the os calcis. (B), the os calcis fails to support the talus, allowing it to rotate and plantarflex medially.

the os calcis rotates under the talus. The anterior end of the os calcis moves laterally and dorsally, allowing the head of the talus to move medially and plantarward. Because of ligamentous laxity, the plantar calcaneonavicular ligament (spring) does not support the head of the talus, allowing the talus to plantarflex (Fig. 43–3). The navicular abducts (moves laterally) with the anterior end of the os calcis, and the forefoot follows the navicular. In general, patients with relaxed flatfoot have familial ligamentous laxity.

Coleman believes that the term pronated foot is neither accurate nor appropriate for this condition. He bases his conclusion on the fact that the heel is in valgus on weight bearing and that the lateral side of the forefoot cannot be in contact with the floor unless the forefoot supinates to some degree in relationship to the hindfoot. The end result of this complex mo-

tion within the foot is a transfer of the weight-bearing line medial to the normal position (Fig. 43–4). A foot that on weight bearing assumes this valgus posture with medial displacement of the load of body weight produces excessive stresses on the foot. Tachdjian[54] postulates that a child with planovalgoid feet may actively toe in in order to shift the body weight laterally. This, he believes, is a protective mechanism for the child's foot. Normally, weight is borne over the lateral border of the foot and on the first and fifth metatarsal heads. Prolonged weight bearing of the foot in the everted position may result in heel cord contracture. Therefore, heel cord tightness must be carefully assessed when evaluating the planovalgoid foot. The heel must be placed in neutral and the knee extended to obtain a true assessment of ankle dorsiflexion and relative tightness of the Achilles tendon.

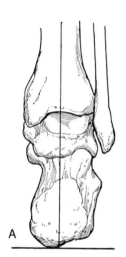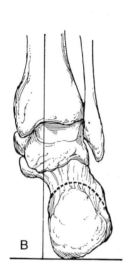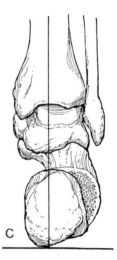

FIGURE 43–4. (A), The normal weight-bearing line coming through the tibiotalar joint to the subtalar joint and through the os calcis. (B), The usual weight-bearing line shifting medially because of heel valgus. (C), The effect of medial shift of the os calcis after an osteotomy has been accomplished.

RADIOGRAPHIC FEATURES

For accurate assessment, radiographs should be taken in the weight-bearing position. On the anterior posterior film, the hindfoot is in valgus, as evidenced by an increase in the talocalcaneal angle. If the long axis of the talus diverges more than 35 degrees from the long axis of the os calcis, excessive heel valgus is considered to be present. In addition, the midtalar line usually passes far medial to the first metatarsal bone. The navicular bone is usually displaced laterally from its position opposite the head of the talus (Fig. 43–5*A*).

On the lateral projection, hindfoot valgus is again noted, with the talus being much more vertical than normal (Fig. 43–5*B*). Meary[36] has described the relationship of the midtalar line to the midmetatarsal line. In a normal foot, this is usually less than −10 degrees. The sag may occur at any one of the joints between these joints or at more than one joint (Fig. 43–6).

PHYSICAL EXAMINATION

When assessing a patient with flexible flatfeet, one must be certain to gather the history including a family history and physical examination. The examination should include inspection for signs of generalized ligamentous laxity at the hands, wrists, elbows, and knees. The spine should be carefully examined for any stigmata of dysraphism, and the reflexes should be examined in both the upper and the lower extremities. The child should be asked to walk first in normal fashion so that alignment of spine, hips, knees, and ankles can be assessed, and then the child should be asked to walk on tiptoe to determine whether or not the longitudinal arch is reconstituted. The child should then walk on the heels to observe the relative flexibility of the Achilles tendon; on outer borders of feet to determine whether or not the arch is again reconstituted and to assess the strength of the anterior tibialis musculature; and then on the inner borders of feet to observe at the mechanics and mobility of the subtalar and midtarsal joints. The child should also be asked to run in order to identify any abnormalities of the lower extremities. The static examination of the foot should then be accomplished. In the weight-bearing position, Jack's test[26] should be employed; that is, dor-siflexion of the great toe should elevate the longitudinal arch in a flexible flatfoot.[23, 47, 48] This is due to the windlass action of the plantar fascia as well as the relative strength of the flexor hallucis longus tendon. (The plantar fascia extends from the plantar medial surface of the os calcis to the base of the proximal phalanges of the toes. As the metatarso-pha-langeal joints are hyperextended, the firm fascia draws the heel toward the forefoot. In a flexible relaxed flatfoot, this action causes an elevation of the longitudinal arch.) If there is significant contracture of the gastrocnemius-soleus group, the patient may not be able to perform Jack's toe-rising test.[26]

ETIOLOGY

As with congenital talipes equinovarus, there is no consensus among numerous authors who have written on the etiology of flatfeet. Because the structures of the foot involve bones, ligaments, and muscle tendon units, various theories of flatfoot revolve around the isolated structures. It is convenient to classify all complex foot deformities into two broad etiologic categories: that is, neurologic and developmental. It is in the neurologic type that the basic underlying cause is paralysis, in which muscle function is compromised. In the second category, the muscle function of the foot and ankle is normal and there is no defined cause of the flatness of the foot. Paralytic feet demand joint stabilization and muscle balance if muscles are available to be transferred. There is no direct approach to flexible flatfoot, as we will see later in this chapter. In reviewing the literature, it is obvious that great men have given considerable thought to the structure and function of the foot and ankle. Many of the surgical procedures that were performed historically had their genesis in the anatomic dissections of previous authors. Harris and Beath[19] believed that the function of the foot and its ultimate shape during weight bearing depended on the design and configuration of the tarsal bones in their relative positions. They believed that a "strong foot" was one in which the tarsal bones articulated so accurately that there was little motion between the bones on weight bearing. In their theory of flatfeet, the valgus position of the os calcis and the secondary shortened Achilles tendon resulted in medial displacement of the head of the talus.

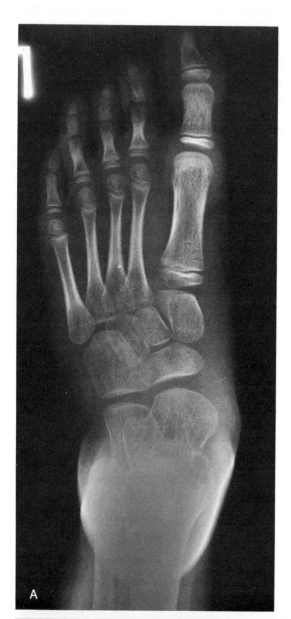

FIGURE 43–5. *(A),* Standing anteroposterior view of a flexible flatfoot, showing the medial deviation and plantar flexion of the talus, with lateral placement of the navicular bone. *(B),* Lateral projection of the same patient in *A* showing markedly plantarflexed talus and flattening of the medial border of the foot.

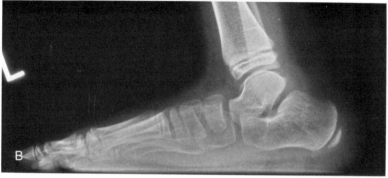

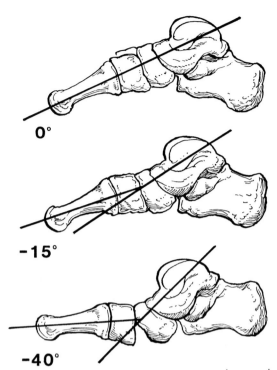

0°

−15°

−40°

FIGURE 43–6. Meary's lines at the top represent the normal relationship; the middle figure, a mild flatfoot; and the lower figure, severe sag of the medial longitudinal arch.

This apparent lateral rotation of the os calcis then allows for the flattening of the longitudinal arch, which could only be maintained by muscle and ligamentous support. Again, in the strong foot, muscles are used to maintain balance, to adjust the foot to the ground, and to propel the body forward. In the weak foot, the muscles are called on to maintain the normal shape of the foot at rest. Gleich,[15] Lord,[33] and Chambers[7] believed that the valgus position of the os calcis and the subsequent loss of support for the talus were important in the cause of the flatfoot, that excessive forefoot abduction resulted in the flattening of the longitudinal arch, and that the stretching of the ligaments was the result and not the primary cause of the problem.

THE MUSCLES

The theory that the muscles control the arch of the foot first arose from the work of Duchenne,[11] who reportedly stimulated the peroneus longus muscle of flatfooted children and was able to develop an arch on the medial side. Jones,[28] Haraldsson,[17, 18] and Niederecker[41, 42] in independent publications supported the concept that the musculature was the most important factor in maintaining a longitudinal arch. Sir Arthur Keith,[29] in his study of the history of the human foot, agreed that the supporting musculature was the most important factor in maintaining the longitudinal arch, and believed that the ligamentous structures of the foot came into play only after muscles had failed. Morton,[39] in his book entitled *The Human Foot*, believed that appreciable muscle exertion is needed only when the center of gravity moved beyond the margins of structural stability. Jones[28] estimated that the tibialis posterior and peroneus longus and brevis bore only 15 to 20 percent of the tension stress on the foot, and he further concluded that both passive elasticity of ligaments and active contractility of muscles controlled the normal longitudinal arch, with the plantar aponeurosis and plantar tarsal ligaments holding together the anterior and posterior pillars of the arch. Hicks[21–23] brought us the concept that the plantar aponeurosis functions as a truss, a triangular structure composed of two rods and a tie. In the foot, the tie is the plantar aponeurosis. Anteriorly, there are five rods radiating from a common posterior rod (i.e., the metatarsal bones and the os calcis). The plantar fascia and aponeurosis resist the deforming effect of body weight. The height of the triangle, or truss, increases when the tie, or the base, shortens. The shortening of the plantar aponeurosis is brought about by the windlass mechanism. The plantar ligament of the metatarsophalangeal joint is an extension of the plantar aponeurosis. When the metatarsophalangeal joint is extended, it thereby tightens the plantar aponeurosis, pulling the os calcis toward the metatarsal heads. Elevation of the arch can thereby be accomplished passively, without muscle force. This was spoken of earlier as Jack's test of extension of the great toe. In a normal foot, it results in elevation of the longitudinal arch, inversion of the hindfoot, lateral rotation of the leg at the ankle, and concomitant tightening of the plantar aponeurosis. Basmajian,[2, 3] using electromyographic studies, showed that there was little or no muscular activity in the intrinsic or extrinsic muscles of the normal foot when a person stands at rest. He tested the flexor hallucis longus, the tibialis anterior, the tibialis posterior, the peroneus longus, the abductor hallucis, and the flexor digitorum brevis muscles. These muscles showed no electrical activity in reaction to loads that actually surpassed those normally applied to a static plantigrade foot. The author believes at this point in time that no consensus as to the etiology of the flatfoot exists and that the definitive paper is yet to be written.

MECHANICS

Numerous authors[21-23, 25, 29] have demonstrated that the joint complex that makes up the hindfoot behaves as a hinge. Unlike the tibiotalar joint, the peritalar and midtarsal joints are placed as oblique hinges. Inman[25] has demonstrated that with eversion of the heel as well as in pronation of the forefoot, all the articulations in the midfoot become unlocked and maximum motion in the talonavicular and calcaneocuboid joints occurs. If the heel is inverted and the forefoot is held firmly fixed, something happens to convert the entire foot into a rigid structure. This implies that the everted foot (heel valgus) is mechanically less stable than the inverted foot.

In the pes planus "planovalgoid" deformity, the patient shifts body weight medially, presumably placing excessive stresses on the ligaments that support the longitudinal arch. The normal pattern of weight-bearing, i.e., the os calcis, lateral border of the foot, combined with the first and fifth metatarsal bones, is now altered so that more pressure and weight is placed over the inner part of the foot. Because of heel valgus position, the talar head loses its support medially and therefore plantarflexes (see Fig. 43–3). The heel valgus causes the Achilles tendon to be functionally shorter and puts it at a mechanical advantage to become an evertor of the hindfoot. If one is to stop the cycle of medial weight bearing, heel valgus, and short Achilles tendon, one must address the problems by restitution of joint stability or ligamentous reconstruction rather than on muscle-balancing procedures or tendon transfers.

TREATMENT

Conservative Treatment

Because many of the affected children have no symptoms whatsoever, conservative treat-ment is difficult to propose. Wenger and colleagues[55] have recently concluded that the time-honored treatment of shoe modification and inserts have no effect whatsoever when applied in random fashion in a prospective manner. Since the natural history is not known, should we treat the condition at all? Penneau and associates[44] radiographically evaluated 10 children with flexible flatfeet. Films were taken with the children barefoot, with a Thomas heel, with an over-the-counter scaphoid insert, and with specially molded plastic foot orthotic devices. The authors noted no significant change in the radiographic appearance of the feet with the shoe modifications. If the physical examination reveals that the patient has a tight heel cord, then heel cord–stretching exercises are indicated. If the complaint is that the child is ruining his shoes and that the condition is financially disabling for the family, then certainly modified UCBL (University of California Biomechanics Laboratory) heel inserts may be used to prolong shoe life for the patient with a severe deformity (Fig. 43–7).[4, 5, 20]

The family must realize that one is treating symptoms and not the deformity per se. No shoe modifications or inserts have been shown to change the ultimate shape of the foot whatsoever.

Certainly, there is no indication that muscle strengthening exercises, such as picking up marbles with toes, have any benefit whatsoever in the treatment of this condition.

Surgical Treatment

Operative intervention to correct the deformity of flatfoot is only indicated when the discomfort in the foot persists despite conservative measures and prevents the patient from taking part in normal activities or when the deformity is so marked that it causes rapid abnormal wear of the shoes. Ideally, surgical correction should result in a foot with a normal longitudinal arch that is free of pain and has as near-normal range of motion and function as possible. In the review of the literature, numerous operative procedures have been described for correction of flexible flatfeet (Table 43–1). In general, they can be divided into four main groups: (1) soft tissue procedures alone, such as ligament tightenings or releases or muscle tendon transfers; (2) arthrodesis of

FIGURE 43–7. A well-worn modified UCBL (University of California Biomechanics Laboratory) heel insert, used by the patient in Figure 43–1*A* and *B*.

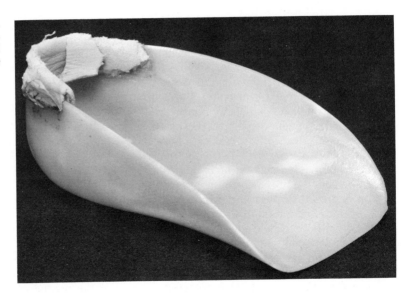

tarsal joints; (3) osteotomy of tarsal bones, with or without bone grafting; and (4) combinations of bone and joint operations with soft tissue procedures.

Soft Tissue Procedures: Tendon Transfers and Ligament-Tightening Procedures

There are several procedures in the literature in which tendon transfers have been proposed to provide dynamic force to elevate the apex of the medial longitudinal arch. Transfer of the anterior tibial tendon to the dorsum of the navicular (without arthrodesis of the tarsal joints) was first performed by Muller,[40] modified by Legg,[32] and popularized by Young.[57]

An intriguing operation proposed by Jones[27] is the transfer of the medial half of the Achilles tendon to the neck of the first metatarsal.

Surgical Technique of the Jones Achilles Transfer

The procedure uses a sagittally split medial half of the Achilles tendon; the upper end of

---

TABLE 43–1 OPERATIVE PROCEDURES FOR FLATFOOT

SOFT TISSUE PROCEDURES
Muller—Anterior tibial tendon transfer to navicular bone
Jones—Medial half Achilles tendon transfer to first metatarsal neck
Phelps—Imbrication of medial soft tissues
Schoolfield—Proximal advancement of deltoid ligament

TARSAL ARTHRODESIS
Hoke—Naviculocuneiform fusion
Miller—Naviculocuneiform-metatarsal fusion and tightening of medial sling
Durham—Naviculocuneiform fusion with ligamentous periosteal flap
Lovell (Scottish Rite)—Osteotomy of cuneiform and proximal-based ligamentous periosteal flap

SUBTALAR ARTHRODESIS
Grice—Bone block in sinus tarsi
Batchelor-Grice—Fibular graft across talocalcaneal joint and subtalar fusion
Dennyson, Fulford—Screw across talocalcaneal joint and subtalar fusion

TRIPLE ARTHRODESIS

CALCANEAL OSTEOTOMIES
Gleich—Medial displacement of os calcis
Evans—Opening wedge anterior lateral osteotomy

ARTHROEREISIS

MEDIAL NAVICULAR RESECTION
Kidner—Accessory navicular resection and tibialis posterior tendon rerouting

the medial half including its fascial prolongation over the muscle belly is divided from muscle but is left attached to the calcaneus at its lower end (Fig. 43–8). A small second incision is made over the medial aspect of the neck of the first metatarsal bone, and a hole is drilled through it. A subcutaneous tunnel from the inferomedial aspect of the os calcis to the second incision is created, and the separated end of the medial strip of the calcaneal tendon is passed through this tunnel. Here, the rolled up fascial prolongation of the tendon is passed through the drill hole in the neck of the first metatarsal and sutured to itself, with the arch held in a corrected position. Wounds are closed, and a padded below-the-knee plaster cast is applied. Six weeks after the operation, a walking plaster is applied, and at 3 months, the child is left unprotected.

Jones[27] presented three cases and had good results in all three. I have no experience with this procedure, but it remains intriguing if one could rely solely on soft tissues for correction.

Other Soft Tissue Procedures

Other soft tissue procedures include tightening of soft tissues on the medial aspect of the foot by division and shortening, as advocated by Phelps.[45] Schoolfield[49] transferred the deltoid ligament proximally, because he believed that the flatfoot was caused by insufficiency of the deltoid ligament. In my personal experience, most plication and shortening operations do not stand the test of time and deform as body weight stresses the repair.

Arthrodesis of Tarsal Bones

In 1931, Hoke[24] introduced naviculocuneiform fusion for correction of flatfoot. This operation did not stand the test of time.[50] Miller[38] described an operation in which the articulations between the navicular bone and the medial cuneiform bone and between the medial cuneiform bone and first metatarsal bone were fused in a corrected position. Simultaneously, the plantar calcaneal navicular ligament and tibialis posterior tendon were transferred distally, thus tightening the sling that supports the medial longitudinal arch and holds the head of the talus in a normal relationship with the anterior end of the os calcis. Durham[6, 13] is credited with an operation that differs from Miller's in only two respects. First,

the cuneiform–first metatarsal joint is not fused, and second, a ligamentous periosteal flap is raised from the medial and plantar aspect of the navicular bone and the medial cuneiform bone, with its base left attached distally on the first metatarsal base. After navicular-cuneiform fusion, the flap is pulled taut and attached to the sustentaculum tali in an attempt to reinforce the spring ligament, i.e., the plantar calcaneal navicular ligament.

Lovell[34] described what is known as the Scottish Rite procedure. It combines elements of the Miller and the Durham procedures.

The Scottish Rite Procedure
(Fig. 43–9*A* to *G*)

A dorsally based opening wedge osteotomy of the medial cuneiform is performed to elevate the longitudinal arch. The naviculocuneiform joint is fused, but the cuneiform–first metatarsal joint is not violated. A proximally based osteoperiosteal flap is raised (Fig. 43–9*D*) and advanced distally and sewn into the first metatarsal–cuneiform area. If this procedure is performed properly, it should accomplish the following: (1) elevate the depressed plantar flexed position of the talus; (2) tighten the soft tissue of the plantar medial aspect of the foot, thereby elevating the longitudinal arch; (3) increase the supination of the first metatarsocuneiform joint by tightening the anterior tibialis tendon and placing the posterior tibialis tendon more distally; (4) increase the "lever arm" (by fusion of the navicular-cuneiform joint) on which the posterior tibial and anterior tibial tendons can work; (5) shorten the medial column of the foot; (6) correct the abnormal talocalcaneal angle; and (7) correct the talonavicular subluxation. (Figs. 43–10 and 43–11).

Although this procedure yields satisfactory results, it is being supplanted by technically easier osteotomies of the os calcis or formal subtalar fusions for more rigidly deformed feet.

Subtalar Arthrodesis

The patients who require surgical correction of flexible flatfoot usually have significant disability with rapid abnormal wear of shoes secondary to the valgus malalignment of the talocalcaneal and talonavicular joints. In our experience, it is the significant valgus of the

Text continued on page 847

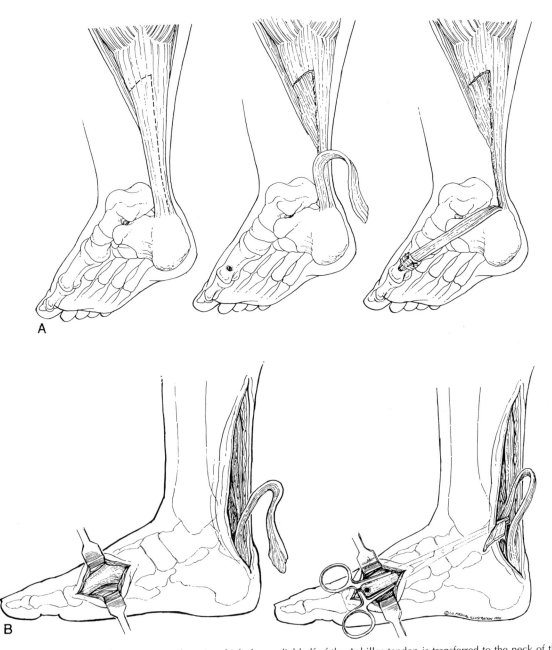

FIGURE 43–8. *(A)*, The Jones procedure, in which the medial half of the Achilles tendon is transferred to the neck of the first metatarsal; the completed transfer is seen on the right.

(B), Medial half of the Achilles tendon left attached distally and transferred through a subcutaneous tunnel to the neck of the first metatarsal. © I.U. Medical Illustration 1990.

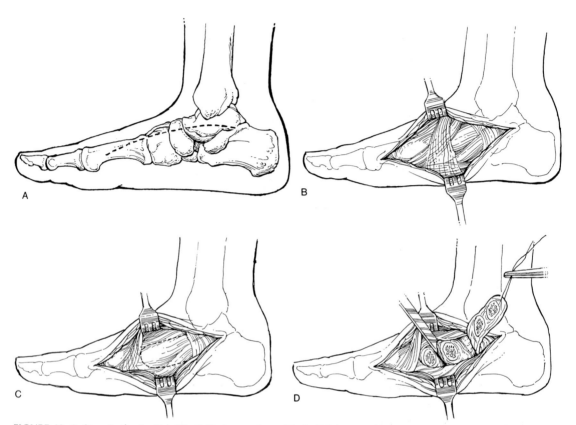

FIGURE 43–9. Steps in the Scottish Rite flatfoot procedure. *(A)*, A slightly curved incision is made over the medial aspect of the foot, beginning immediately posterior to the medial malleolus, extending anteriorly to the navicular tubercle, and ending at the middle of the midshaft of the first metatarsal.

(B), The subcutaneous tissue is divided in line with the skin incision. The wound margins are undermined, elevated, and gently retracted. The abductor hallucis muscle is detached and elevated from the medial and plantar surfaces of the medial cuneiform bone, the navicular bone, and the spring ligament.

(C), The tibialis posterior tendon is identified. The neurovascular bundle is retracted into the sole. An osteoperiosteal flap is developed, with the flap beginning at the attachment of the anterior tibialis tendon and continuing to the medial cuneiform–first metatarsal area. This flap, which should be approximately 1/2 inch in width, extends from the anterior tibialis tendon posteriorly to the attachment of the tibialis posterior on the navicular bone.

(D), The flap is continued proximally, being distally based on the medial aspect of the talus, with a small amount of bone being removed from the navicular. The capsule at the naviculocuneiform joint is incised, and the joint cartilage is removed. The tubercle, or prominence of the navicular bone, should be excised with an osteotome and saved as a bone graft, to be used to elongate and elevate the arch.

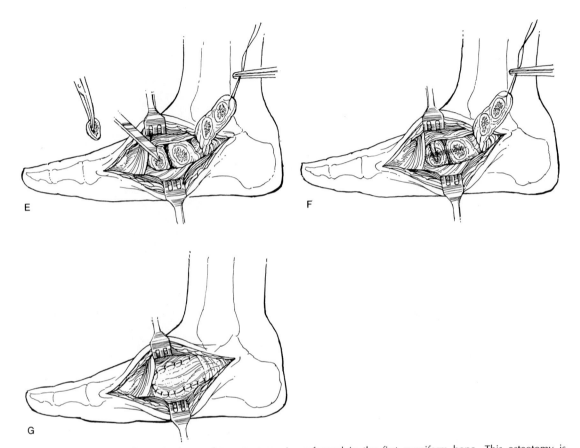

FIGURE 43–9 *Continued (E),* An incomplete osteotomy is performed in the first cuneiform bone. This osteotomy is performed from the dorsal aspect of the cuneiform bone toward the plantar cortex, the latter being left intact so that it can be wedged open to receive the bone graft taken from the navicular bone.

(F), The osteotomy of the cuneiform bone as well as the naviculocuneiform joint is then transfixed with Kirschner's wires or a cancellous bone screw in the "corrected" position.

(G), The previously prepared osteoperiosteal flap is then passed distally under the anterior tibialis tendon, with the foot in slight supination. This flap is sutured to the plantar aspect of the foot. The spring ligament and the posterior tibial tendon plantar expansion are then advanced and tightened with sutures into the osteoperiosteal flap. Heel cord lengthening may be accomplished. The wound is closed, and the extremity placed in a short-leg cast in slight varus and slight equinus. Non–weight-bearing is continued for 6 weeks, followed by the application of a short-leg weight-bearing cast for an additional 6 weeks.

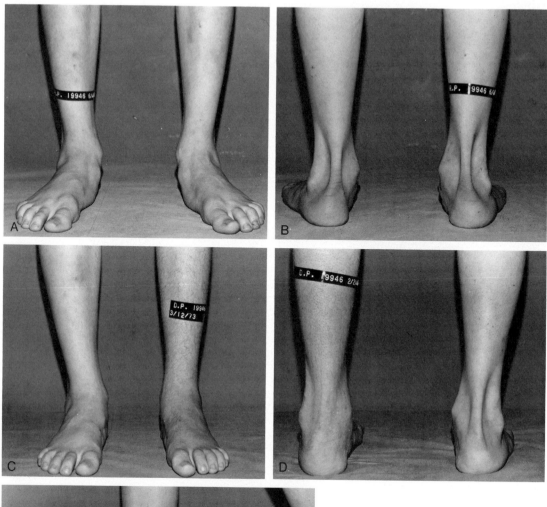

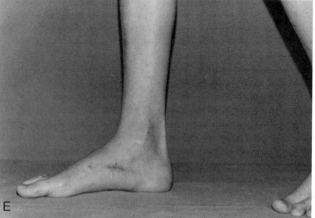

FIGURE 43–10. *(A to E)*, Standing photographs of a 14-year-old boy with moderate to severe flatfeet treated with the Scottish Rite procedure. Postoperatively, one can see the correction of the heel valgus, mild elevation of the longitudinal arch, and the resultant scar on the medial aspect of the foot. His symptoms were markedly improved, and shoe wear was immeasurably improved. (Courtesy of Peter Meehan of the Atlanta Scottish Rite Hospital.)

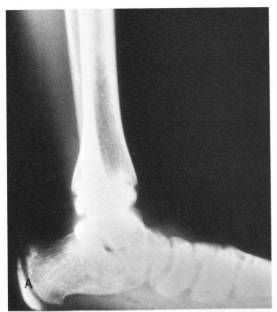

FIGURE 43–11. Radiographs of the patient in Figure 43–10. *(A)*, Preoperative standing lateral x-ray study of the left foot. *(B)*, Postoperative standing lateral x-ray study of the left foot. Notice the change in the position of the talus and fusion of the naviculocuneiform joint

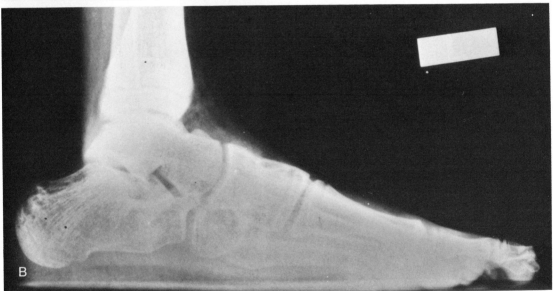

hindfoot that causes problems. Restoration of the hindfoot to a near-neutral position can be accomplished by several methods. The first is by fusion. The criticism is that fusion eliminates motion, but in our experience of over 15 years, the relief of the symptoms has been long lasting, and the author[10] favors a formal subtalar arthrodesis. This combines a transtalar fibular dowel graft (Batchelor technique) with cancellous graft in the subtalar joint and sinus tarsi (Fig. 43–12). Dennyson and Fulford[9] have described a technique of subtalar arthrodesis incorporating metallic internal fixation instead of the fibular graft.

In 1952, Grice[16] described his hindfoot stabilization procedure for children with paralytic flatfeet. The procedure has been widely used for nonparalytic feet as well as in feet of children afflicted with spastic cerebral palsy.[51] Although others have reported excellent results, the author has given up the procedure and uses the formal subtalar fusion described earlier. The criticism of the subtalar fusion has been the fear that it may result in stunted

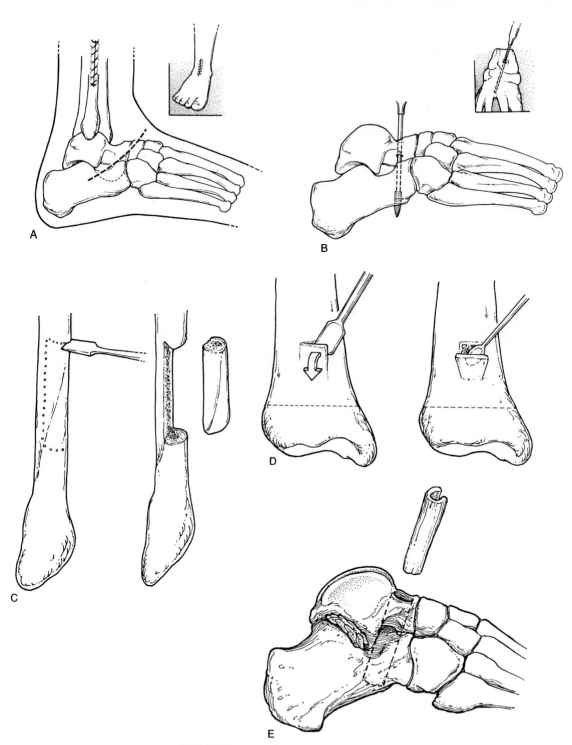

FIGURE 43–12 *See legend on opposite page*

hindfoot growth, which has not been documented in the author's 18 years of personal observation.

It is the author's experience that triple arthrodesis has not been necessary for the symptomatic flatfoot caused by excessive ligamentous laxity associated with generalized conditions such as Marfan's and Down syndromes. The author has been able to manage these syndromes with formal subtalar arthrodesis, as described earlier, usually without lengthening of the Achilles tendon (Fig. 43–13).

If subsequent changes in the calcaneocuboid and talonavicular joints cause pain, then a limited fusion can be accomplished at a later date. If the patient has severe deformity and is near skeletal maturity, triple arthrodesis may be indicated. If a triple arthrodesis is chosen, then I feel the inlay technique of Williams and Menelaus[56] is beneficial, because it does not excessively shorten the foot. The author is aware that many people believe that the restricted motion in the subtalar joint may lead to premature degenerative changes. However, the restriction of motion has not caused symptoms in the author's patients, some of whom have been followed up for a total of 18 years.

Osteotomies of the Os Calcis to Correct Hindfoot Deformity

Osteotomies of the os calcis are intriguing procedures, designed to shift the distal part of the os calcis medially, in an attempt to put the weight-bearing line into a more normal position between the metatarsal bones anteriorly.[52] Medial displacement osteotomy, as described by Koutsogiannis,[31] is a simple calcaneal osteotomy whose principle is not new. The first description was presented by Gleich.[15]

Surgical Technique of the Gleich Procedure

The osteotomy is performed through an incision made over the lateral aspect of the body of the os calcis parallel and immediately posterior to the peroneal tendons; it extends proximally from the lateral margin of the Achilles tendon to the plantar aspect of the heel. The sural nerve should be protected throughout the procedure. The os calcis is exposed on its dorsal, lateral, and plantar surfaces. The periosteum is incised and elevated in line with the skin incision. Once the osteotomy is performed, a laminar spreader is placed in the osteotomy site so that the medial periosteum can be divided under direct vision. The posterior fragment of the os calcis is displaced medially until its medial margin is aligned with the sustentaculum tali. This usually necessitates a displacement of either one-third to one-half the width of the os calcis. The fragments are then transfixed by Steinmann pins (Fig. 43–14). The wound is closed, and a well-padded above-the-knee cast is applied with the ankle in the neutral·position and the knee at

---

FIGURE 43–12. *(A),* Skin incisions used for subtalar arthrodesis. The sinus tarsi is exposed through a slightly curved incision. The contents of the sinus tarsi are sharply elevated from the os calcis, being left attached proximally to the talus, to be repositioned later as a fibrofatty flap. The extensor digitorum brevis is identified and dissected distally in order to expose the calcaneocuboid joint. The dissection is continued medially to expose the talonavicular joint, which is opened. The subtalar joint is mobilized in order to position the os calcis properly under the talus. By so doing, the talonavicular joint is reduced.

(B), The sulcus on the neck of the talus just distal to the tibiotalar joint is cleared of soft tissue, and an awl or burr is used to make a hole in the neck of the talus through the subtalar joint into the os calcis. This is enlarged with No. 3 and 5 curettes, so that it can accept a fibular graft.

(C), The fibular graft is harvested through a longitudinal incision over the fibula in its distal one-third (see *A*). The length of the graft is determined by an intraoperative lateral x-ray study taken with the burr or awl in place, so that length could be measured appropriately. The fibula is subperiosteally stripped, and by using drill holes and an osteotome or a motorized saw, a segment of fibula two-thirds the size of the circumference is removed.

(D), An anterior incision is then made just lateral to the anterior tibial tendon above the ankle joint, as seen in *A,* carried down to periosteum, which is elevated, staying several centimeters above the growth plate. A trap door is made with a chisel, and cancellous graft is obtained using a curette.

(E), The posterior facet and anterior facet of the subtalar joint are curetted of cartilage in preparation for fusion. The fibular graft is then driven through the neck of the talus into the os calcis under direct vision, and the cancellous graft from the distal tibial metaphysis is packed into the subtalar joint around the fibular graft and in the sinus tarsi. The previously prepared flap of fibrofatty tissue from the sinus tarsi is replaced, and the wound loosely closed. A bulky dressing with a posterior plaster splint is applied until swelling subsides; then a short-leg weight-bearing plaster cast is applied for the next 8 to 12 weeks.

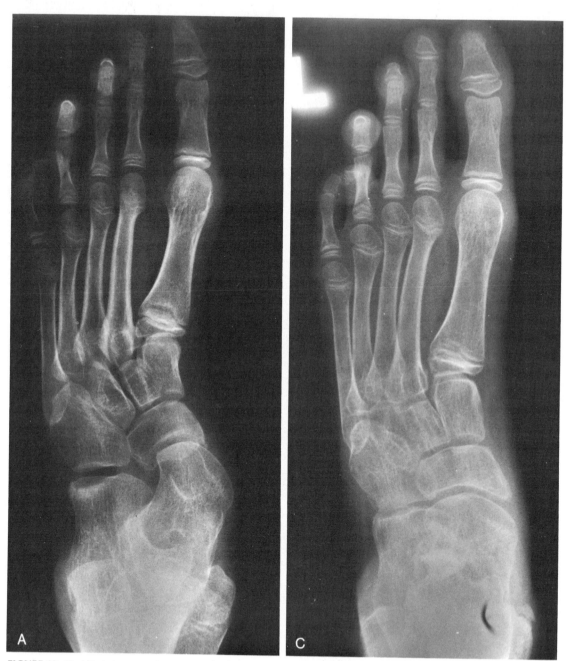

FIGURE 43–13. *(A),* Anteroposterior x-ray study of a young adolescent with severe ligamentous laxity and flatfeet secondary to Marfan's syndrome.

   (C), Weight-bearing anteroposterior roentgenogram taken several years after formal subtalar arthrodesis, revealing correction of the flatfoot deformity.

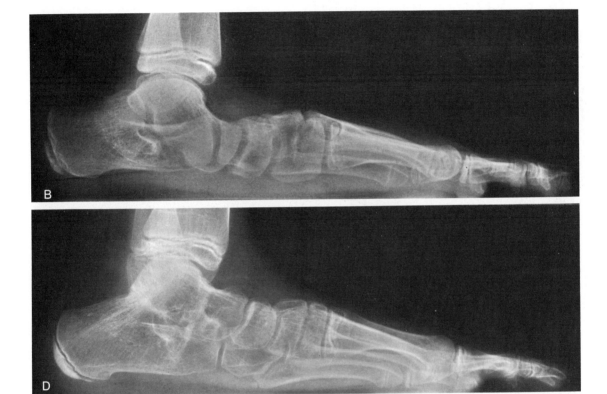

FIGURE 43–13 *Continued*
   (B), Weight-bearing lateral roentgenogram of the same patient.
   (D), Weight-bearing postoperative roentgenogram of the same patient. The "ghost" of the fibular graft is still identified, and the posterior facet has obvious fusion. The present talocalcaneal relationship should be compared with the preoperative relationship.

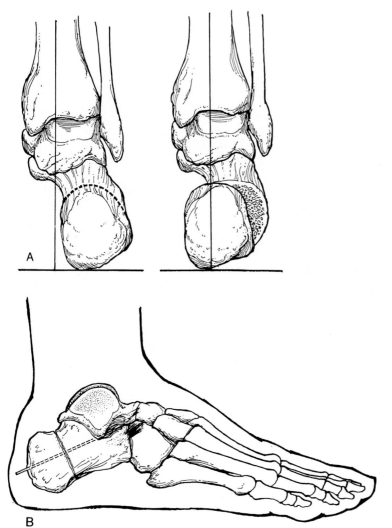

FIGURE 43–14. *(A)*, The weight-bearing line passing medial to the tuberosity of the os calcis. The proposed dotted line of osteotomy of the os calcis prior to medial displacement, which has been accomplished in *B*.

(B), Once medial displacement has been accomplished, it can be held with Steinmann pins while consolidation begins. See text.

45 degrees of flexion. Four weeks after the operation, the pins are removed and a below-knee walking plaster cast is applied for an additional 2 weeks or more.

Koutsogiannis[31] reported the results of this operation in patients whose mean age was 12 years. Function was markedly improved in 17 of 19 patients. The two failures were attributed to a taut Achilles tendon or inadequate medial displacement of the posterior calcaneal fragment. The author concurs that the medial displacement osteotomy is an excellent way to correct a hindfoot valgus in severe symptomatic flatfeet.

The Evans Procedure

Evans[14] strongly believed that the calcaneovalgus foot deformity could be treated by elongation of the lateral column of the foot. First, he stated that varus and valgus are opposite deformities and, second, that the difference between the two in terms of tarsal structure lay in the relative lengths of the two columns of the foot. A long lateral column is associated with varus deformity of the tarsus, including heel varus and also possibly equinus, whereas a short lateral column is associated with valgus deformity of the tarsus, including heel valgus and also calcaneus deformity. He, therefore, performed a reverse of his initial clubfoot operation; that is, an elongation of the lateral column of the foot, preserving the calcaneocuboid joint (Fig. 43–15). He performed an osteotomy at the anterior end of the calcaneus about 1.5 cm proximal to the calcaneocuboid joint in a plane parallel with that joint. The two parts of the os calcis are then forced apart to lengthen the lateral column, and the gap is filled with cortical cancellous bone, which is usually taken from the tibia.

Surgical Technique of the Evans Procedure

At the time of procedure, an incision is made at the surface of the calcaneus parallel with and just above the peroneal tendons, avoiding the sural nerve. The anterior half of the bone is exposed, and the calcaneocuboid joint is identified. The anterior end of the calcaneus is then divided through its narrow part in front of the peroneal tubercle by an osteotome, the line of division being parallel

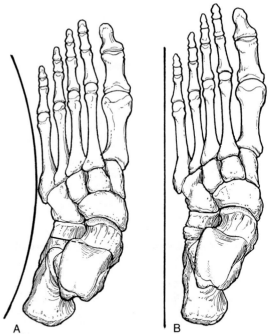

FIGURE 43–15. "Reverse" Evans' procedure for flatfeet. *(A)*, The preoperative position. The bold line across the anterior aspect of the os calcis is the proposed osteotomy site. After osteotomy, a cortical bone graft is inserted. *(B)*, The lateral column is elongated, so that the border of the foot laterally is now straight, whereas previously it was concave.

with and about 1.5 cm proximal to the calcaneocuboid joint. The cut surfaces of the calcaneus are then pried apart by means of a spreader, and a cortical graft taken from the tibia is inserted between the blades of the spreader to maintain separation of the two pieces of the os calcis. The wound is then closed, and the foot is immobilized comfortably in plaster, in a position of slight equinovarus. The plaster is retained for approximately 4 months to allow consolidation of the new os calcis, but weight bearing was allowed as early as 4 weeks (Fig. 43–16).

Evans[1, 46] described the operation for all types of valgus deformities. Nine cases were for rigid flatfeet, and 18 cases were idiopathic valgus, including one case associated with Marfan's syndrome. Evans cautioned that in cases of severe idiopathic valgus, it is necessary to distinguish between simple mild valgus, which is a variant of normal, and severe valgus, which is clearly abnormal. He further stated that overcorrection may occur, and it is all too easy to produce an equinovarus deformity.

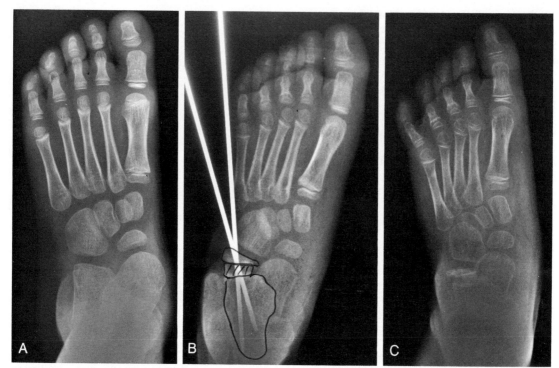

FIGURE 43–16. *(A)*, Preoperative standing anteroposterior radiograph of a child with flexible flatfoot. Notice the lateral position of the navicular bone relative to the talus.

(B), Intraoperative anteroposterior film. The cortical graft is in position, indicated by the cross-hatched section. The elongated os calcis is transfixed with two Steinmann pins. Notice that the navicular bone has translated medially on the talus into a correct position.

(C), X-ray study taken 1 year postoperatively in the same patient. The alignment of the talonavicular joint as well as that of the talocalcaneal joints has been well maintained. The allograft is still visualized in this photo. (X-ray study courtesy of Thomas F. Kling, Jr., M.D.)

Arthroereisis

A discussion is required of a procedure that is described generically as arthroereisis,[53] coming from the Greek words "arthro," or joint, and "reises," or to prop up. This procedure was first described many years ago. A bony plug was inserted beneath the lateral process of the talus in an attempt to prop open the subtalar articulation and thus to reduce valgus of the hindfoot. Recently, arthroereisis has been advocated by some podiatrists, who use a silicone or polyethylene plug, which blocks hindfoot eversion. Although some short-term results have been promising, I am skeptical of the procedure for several reasons. First, from our experience with silicone implants in rheumatoid arthritis patients, we know that it can produce a significant synovitis. Second, it is very easy to overcorrect the foot, especially in young children (3 to 8 years of age). The flexible hindfoot in these children allows over-

correction and, unfortunately, a varus position of the os calcis. This is not a problem in older children, since the tissues are stiffer and, therefore, less mobile. Finally, the author has had to remove three sets of these devices because of persistent pain over the sinus tarsi in immature feet.

ACCESSORY TARSAL NAVICULAR WITH OR WITHOUT FLATFOOT

The accessory tarsal navicular, frequently referred to in the literature as prehallux or os tibiale externum, is present as a separate bone in up to 10 percent of humans (Fig. 43–17). It is a separate center of ossification for the tuberosity of the navicular bone in the fetus. The tibialis posterior tendon is attached to it, passing across the medial aspect of the navicular bone instead of underneath it. In theory, the dynamic support of the longitudinal arch normally afforded by the posterior tibial muscle is weakened. The result may be valgus and planus deformity of the foot, formation of an

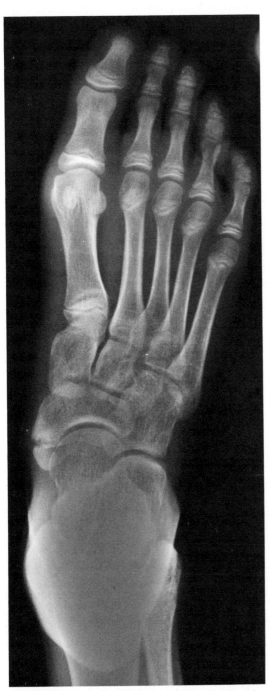

FIGURE 43–17. Weight-bearing anteroposterior view of an adolescent girl with a painful accessory tarsal navicular. This patient was treated with the modified Kidner procedure of excision of the accessory tarsal navicular and advancement of the tibialis posterior tendon.

inflamed adventitial bursa, and perhaps, tenosynovitis of the tibialis posterior tendon. Most cases respond to conservative measures, but if they do not, Kidner's[30] technique of excision of the accessory tarsonavicular with rerouting of the tibialis posterior tendon has produced excellent results.

Surgical Technique of Kidner's Procedure

A dorsally curved incision is made based over the tibialis posterior tendon as it attaches to the accessory navicular. The subcutaneous tissue and deep fascia are divided. Retraction is accomplished to expose the tibialis posterior tendon as it attaches to the tuberosity of the navicular and into the plantar surfaces of the medial cuneiform and base of second, third, and fourth metatarsal bones. The accessory navicular bone can frequently be shelled out of the tendon, but certainly, all other attachements of the tibialis posterior to the bone should be left intact. The accessory tarsal navicular bone is excised, as well as the medial surface of the navicular bone, so that it is flush with the medial borders of the cuneiform bone and the talus. The tibialis posterior tendon is transferred plantarward onto the plantar surface of the navicular, where it is anchored under tension to the periosteum and plantar ligaments using two or three nonabsorbable heavy sutures. These may be anchored to bone, if desired. Hemostasis is achieved. The wound is closed, and a below-the-knee walking cast is applied. The cast is removed in approximately 3 to 4 weeks, and a longitudinal arch support is used for an additional 3 to 4 months.

The usual results of this procedure are excellent if the intent is to remove the medial bulge and to rid the child of symptoms of the pressure and tenosynovitis. If there is an excessive amount of flatfoot deformity present, it will not be corrected by the Kidner procedure alone.

In summary, surgical treatment of flatfeet is rarely indicated and probably should not be performed in patients under the skeletal age of 10 years. Careful physical examination must be performed in all patients to rule out intrinsic bony deformities of the foot, such as coalitions. In addition, careful evaluation of the gastrocnemius-soleus complex must be performed in the search for a heel cord contracture. If it is not possible to passively stretch the contracture, then judicious heel cord lengthening may be performed. Pure soft tissue procedures probably will not stand the test of time for correcting *symptomatic* flatfoot deformity. When the most severe part of the problem is severe hindfoot valgus, medial displacement osteotomy may be indicated. An alternative may be subtalar arthrodesis. When the navicular bone appears to be significantly displaced laterally on the head of the talus and the medial column of the foot appears to be elongated, the reverse Evans procedure of lateral column elongation may be recommended. In severe pes planus, such as that due to excessive ligamentous laxity and in conditions such as Down or Marfan's syndrome, formal subtalar arthrodesis has given good results in our hands. An alternative would be a triple arthrodesis in the nearly skeletally mature foot in whom one fears development of secondary degenerative changes in the talonavicular joint complex.

References

1. Armstrong G: Evans elongation of lateral column of the foot for valgus deformity. J Bone Joint Surg 57B:530, 1975.
2. Basmajian JV, Bentzon JW: An electromyographic study of certain muscles of the leg and foot in the standing position. Surg Gynecol Obstet 98:662, 1954.
3. Basmajian JV, Stecko G: The role of muscles in arch support of the foot. J Bone Joint Surg 45A:1184, 1963.
4. Bleck EE: The shoeing of children: Sham or science? Dev Med Child Neurol 13:188, 1971.
5. Bleck EE, Berzins UJ: Conservative management of pes valgus with plantar flexed talus flexible. Clin Orthop 122:85, 1977.
6. Caldwell GD: Surgical correction of relaxed flatfoot by the Durham flatfoot plasty. Clin Orthop 2:221, 1953.
7. Chambers EFS: An operation for the correction of flexible flatfeet of adolescents. West J Surg 54:77, 1946.
8. Crego CH, Ford LT: An end-result study of various operative procedures for correcting flat feet in children. J Bone Joint Surg 34A:183, 1952.
9. Dennyson WG, Fulford GE: Subtalar arthrodesis by cancellous grafts and metallic internal fixation. J Bone Joint Surg 58B:507, 1976.
10. DeRosa GP, Mesko JW: Modified Batchelor-Brown Subtalar Arthrodesis for Pes Planus. Unpublished data.
11. Duchenne GB: Physiology of Motion. Philadelphia, WB Saunders, 1959, p 337.
12. DuCroquet C, Launay D: Arthrodese du pied. Presse Medicale, June 30, 1909.
13. Durham HA, cited by Caldwell GD: Surgical correction of relaxed flatfoot by the Durham flatfoot plasty. Clin Orthop 2:221, 1953.
14. Evans D: Calcaneo-valgus deformity. J Bone Joint Surg 57B:270, 1975.
15. Gleich A: Beitrag Zur Operativen Plattfussbehandlung. Arch Klin Chir 46:358, 1893.
16. Grice DS: An extra-articular arthrodesis of the subastragalar joint for correction of paralytic flat feet in children. J Bone Joint Surg 34A:927, 1952.
17. Haraldsson S: Operative treatment of pes planovalgus staticus juvenilis. Acta Orthop Scand 32:492, 1962.
18. Haraldsson S: Pes plano-valgus staticus juvenilis and its operative treatment. Acta Orthop Scand 35:234, 1965.
19. Harris RI, Beath T: Hypermobile flatfoot with short tendon Achilles. J Bone Joint Surg 30A:116, 1948.
20. Helfet A: A new way of treating flatfeet in children. Lancet 1:262, 1956.
21. Hicks JH: The function of the plantar aponeurosis. J Anat 85:414, 1951.
22. Hicks JH: The mechanics of the foot. I. The joints. J Anat 87:343, 1943.
23. Hicks JH: The mechanics of the foot. II. The plantar aponeurosis and the arch. J Anat 88:25, 1954.
24. Hoke M: An operation for the correction of extremely relaxed flatfeet. J Bone Joint Surg 13:773, 1931.
25. Inman VT: The human foot. Manitoba Med Rev 46:513, 1966.
26. Jack EA: Naviculo-cuneiform fusion in the treatment of flat foot. J Bone Joint Surg 35B:75, 1953.
27. Jones BS: Flatfoot—a preliminary report of an operation for severe cases. J Bone Joint Surg 57B:279, 1975.
28. Jones RL: The human foot. An experimental study of its mechanics and the role of its muscles and ligaments in support of the arch. Am J Anat 68:1, 1941.
29. Keith A: The history of the human foot and its bearing on orthopaedic practice. J Bone Joint Surg 11:10, 1929.
30. Kidner FC: The prehallux (accessory scaphoid) and its relation to flatfoot. J Bone Joint Surg 11:831, 1929.
31. Koutsogiannis, E: Treatment of mobile flat foot by displacement osteotomy of the calcaneus. J Bone Joint Surg 53B:96, 1971.
32. Legg AT: The treatment of congenital flatfoot by tendon transplantation. Am J Orthop Surg 10:584, 1913.
33. Lord JP: Correction of extreme flatfoot. Value of osteotomy of os calcis (Gleich operation). JAMA 81:1502, 1923.
34. Lovell WW, Price CT, Meehan PL: The foot. *In* Winter RB, Lovell WW (Eds): Pediatric Orthopaedics. Philadelphia, JB Lippincott, 1978.
35. Lowman CL: An operative method for correction of certain forms of flatfoot. JAMA 81:1500, 1923.
36. Meary R: On the measurement of the angle between the talus and the first metatarsal. Symposium: LePied Creux Essentiel. Rev Chir Orthop 53:389, 1967.
37. Miller GR: The operative treatment of hypermobile flatfeet in the young child. Clin Orthop 122:95, 1977.
38. Miller OL: A plastic flat foot operation. J Bone Joint Surg 9:84, 1927.
39. Morton DJ: The Human Foot. New York, Columbia University Press, 1935, p 119.
40. Muller E: Ueber die Resultate der Ernst Muller'schen Plattfussoperation. Beitr Klin Chir, LXXV: 424, 1913.
41. Niederecker K: Operationsverfahren zur Behandlung des Plattfusses. Chir 182–183, 1932.

42. Niederecker, K: Der Plattfuss. Stuttgart, F. Enke, 1959.
43. Ozonoff, M.B.: Pediatric Orthopaedic Radiology. Philadelphia, WB Saunders, 1979, p 300.
44. Penneau K, Lutter LD, Winter RB: Pes planus: Radiographic changes with foot orthoses and shoes. Foot Ankle 2:299, 1982.
45. Phelps AM: The etiology, pathology, and treatment of flat-foot. Post-Graduate 7:104, 1892.
46. Phillips GE: A review of elongation of os calcis for flat feet. J Bone Joint Surg 65B:15, 1983.
47. Rose GK: Correction of the pronated foot. J Bone Joint Surg 40B:674, 1958.
48. Rose GK: Correction of the pronated foot. J Bone Joint Surg 44B:642, 1962.
49. Schoolfield BL: An operation for the cure of flatfoot. Ann Surg 110:437, 1939.
50. Seymour N: The late results of naviculo-cuneiform fusion. J Bone Joint Surg 49B:558, 1967.
51. Seymour N, Evans DK: A modification of the Grice subtalar arthrodesis. J Bone Joint Surg 50B:372, 1968.
52. Silver CM, Simon SD, Spindell E, Litchman HM, and Scala M: Calcaneal osteotomy for valgus and varus deformities of the feet in cerebral palsy. J Bone Joint Surg 49:232, 1967.
53. Smith SD, Millar EA: Arthrorisis by means of a subtalar polyethylene peg implant for correction of hindfoot pronation in children. Clin Orthop 181:15, 1983.
54. Tachdjian MO: Pediatric Orthopaedics. Philadelphia, WB Saunders, 1972, p 1397.
55. Wenger DR, Mauldin D, Speck G, et al: Corrective shoes and inserts as treatment for flexible flatfoot in infants and children. J Bone Joint Surg 71A:800, 1989.
56. Williams PF, Menelaus MB: Triple arthrodesis by inlay grafting—a method suitable for the undeformed or valgus foot. J Bone Joint Surg 59B:333, 1977.
57. Young CS: Operative treatment of pes planus. Surg Gynecol Obstet 68:1099, 1939.
58. Zadek I: Transverse wedge arthrodesis for the relief of pain in rigid flatfoot. J Bone Joint Surg 17:453, 1935.

44

Peroneal Spastic Flatfoot

GEORGE H. THOMPSON
DANIEL R. COOPERMAN

Peroneal spastic flatfoot is a relatively common foot disorder characterized by a painful, rigid valgus deformity of the midfoot and hindfoot and peroneal muscle spasm but without true spasticity.[8, 25, 78, 79, 98, 126, 138, 141] Because of the confusion regarding spasticity, Mitchell has preferred the term spasmodic flatfoot.[95, 96] Although there is an extensive differential diagnosis, the descriptive term, peroneal spastic flatfoot, is usually synonymous with tarsal coalition, a congenital synostosis or failure of segmentation between two or more tarsal bones.

DIFFERENTIAL DIAGNOSIS

Any disorder affecting the normal gliding and rotatory motion of the subtalar (talocalcaneal) joint may produce the clinical appearance of a peroneal spastic flatfoot. The loss of subtalar motion can occur from direct subtalar joint involvement or from abnormalities in the transverse tarsal joint—talonavicular and calcaneocuboid joints. Thus, congenital malformations, arthritis or inflammatory disorders,[53, 64] infections,[64, 92] neoplasms,[66] traumas,[22, 49] and iatrogenic conditions[48, 52] involving the midfoot and/or hindfoot can limit motion, cause pain, and potentially produce a peroneal spastic flatfoot. The differential diagnosis of this condition is presented in Table 44–1. Since treatment varies according to the exact etiology, it is important that a precise diagnosis be established prior to initiating treatment. A careful history, musculoskeletal examination, and appropriate radiographs usually result in the correct diagnosis. Since the majority of individuals with a peroneal spastic flatfoot have a tarsal coalition, the remainder of this chapter is devoted to this disorder.

TARSAL COALITIONS

Tarsal coalitions can be fibrous (syndesmosis), cartilaginous (synchondrosis), or osseous (synostosis). Historically, they have been found in skeletal remains from archeologic studies in the Mayan civilization and in pre-Columbian Indian civilizations in Ohio.[52, 55] Anatomic reports of tarsal coalitions began with Buffon in 1750.[11] The calcaneonavicular coalition was described by Cruveilhier[26] in 1829, the talocalcaneal coalition by Zuckerkandl[156] in 1877, and the talonavicular coalition by Anderson[1] in 1880. Holl[59] proposed a possible relationship between flatfoot and intertarsal bars in 1880; Jones[67] provided the first clinical description of a peroneal spastic flatfoot in 1897; and Kirmisson[71] was the first to radiographically demonstrate tarsal coalitions in 1898. Since then, the correlation between tarsal coalitions and a peroneal spastic flatfoot has been well established.

Etiology and Inheritance

Pfitzner was the first to study the etiology of coalitions and believed they were secondary to incorporation of sesamoid bones or accessory ossicles into the major adjacent tarsal bones.[111] Many investigators supported this theory.[4, 6, 39,

TABLE 44–1. DIFFERENTIAL DIAGNOSIS OF PERONEAL SPASTIC FLATFOOT

ARTHRITIS AND INFLAMMATORY DISORDERS
Rheumatoid arthritis
Ankylosing spondylitis
Gout
Osteoarthritis
Post-traumatic

INFECTION
Septic arthritis
Osteomyelitis

CONGENITAL DISORDERS
Tarsal coalition
Sustentaculum tali malformation
Osteochondrodystrophies
Rigid flatfoot
Relaxed or flexible flatfoot

NEOPLASTIC DISORDERS
Pituitary (acromegaly)
Fibrosarcoma
Bone cyst
Osteoid Osteoma

TRAUMATIC DISORDERS
Osteochondral fracture
Osteochondritis dissecans
Overuse syndromes

IATROGENIC DISORDERS
Overcorrected clubfoot
Grice procedure
Gallie subtalar arthrodesis
Postoperative subtalar arthrodesis

Adapted from Mosier KM, Asher M: Tarsal coalitions and peroneal spastic flat foot. J Bone Joint Surg 66A:976–984, 1984.

[56, 129] Others, however, disagreed.[35, 39, 50, 54, 64] The work of Trolle[143] in 1948, Harris[50] in 1955, and O'Rahilly and associates[105] in 1960 demonstrated that cartilaginous tarsal coalitions occurred in fetal feet as the result of a congenital failure of differentiation or segmentation of the primitive mesenchyme. This is currently the accepted etiologic theory. It is also supported by the association of tarsal coalitions with other congenital musculoskeletal abnormalities, such as carpal coalitions, symphalangism, Apert's syndrome, Nievergelt-Pearlman syndrome, arthrogryposis multiplex congenita, phocomelia, talipes equinovarus (clubfoot), and hand-foot-uterus syndrome.* Tarsal coa-

*See references 3, 13–15, 18, 30, 32, 33, 40, 44, 47, 52, 80, 94, 99, 104, 106–108, 112, and 139.

litions are also seen in monozygous twins[41, 52] and in relatives of involved individuals.

Many genetic studies have indicated that tarsal coalitions are inherited as a unifactorial autosomal dominant trait with nearly full penetrance.* Leonard, in 1974, reviewed 98 first-degree relatives of 31 patients with tarsal coalitions and found that 39 percent had radiographically demonstrable tarsal coalitions.[81] However, none were symptomatic. Studies have also indicated that inherited coalitions may be either unilateral or bilateral.[9, 152] Approximately 60 percent of calcaneonavicular and 50 percent of talocalcaneal coalitions are bilateral.[23]

Incidence

The actual incidence of tarsal coalitions is unknown because many involved individuals are asymptomatic. The reported incidence in the general population varies widely between 0.4 and 6 percent.[53, 55, 111, 136, 144, 154] Harris and Beath, in 1948, reported a 2-percent incidence of peroneal spastic flatfoot on routine physical examination of 3600 Canadian Army recruits.[53] Vaughan and Segal, in 1953, found 21 tarsal coalitions in 2000 Army personnel (1.1 percent) with painful feet.[144] Rankin and Baker in 1974 reported 24 cases of tarsal coalition in 60,000 basic Army trainees (0.4 percent) aged 17 to 22 years.[113] Levine and Scoles, in 1989, found seven tarsal coalitions in 3000 skeletons (0.2 percent) in the Hamann-Todd collection at the Cleveland Museum of National History.[83] There were six talocalcaneal coalitions and only one calcaneonavicular coalition. Based on the current literature, the incidence of tarsal coalitions, both symptomatic and asymptomatic, is approximately 1 percent.

Classification

Almost any tarsal bone can be involved in a coalition. A modification of the classification by Tachdjian[141] is presented in Table 44–2. Of all possible combinations the middle facet talocalcaneal and the calcaneonavicular coalitions are by far the most common.[23, 24, 98, 136] The middle facet talocalcaneal coalition is slightly

*See references 6–9, 25, 31, 40, 41, 81, 118, 149, and 152.

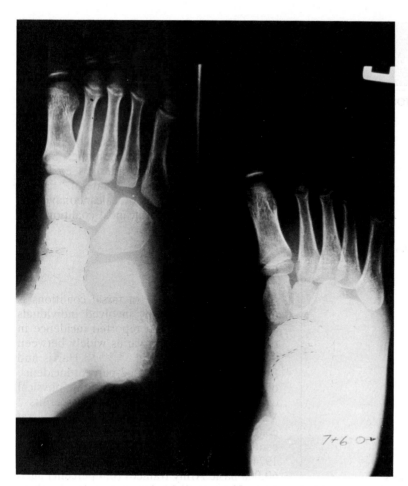

FIGURE 44–1. A partially ossified talonavicular coalition of the right foot in a 7-year-old male. His foot was asymptomatic, and the radiographic diagnosis was made following evaluation for minor trauma.

more prevalent than the calcaneonavicular coalition. Other coalitions that have been described include anterior and posterior facet talocalcaneal,[6, 23, 107, 140] talonavicular,* naviculocuneiform,[45, 84, 93] calcaneocuboid,[20, 85, 145, 147] and cubonavicular.[28, 113, 124, 148] However, these are not as apt to produce symptoms that result in a peroneal spastic flatfoot. Approximately 100 cases of talonavicular coalition have been reported, and only occasionally are they associated with a peroneal spastic flatfoot (Fig. 44–1). Coalitions involving multiple tarsal bones or those occurring at unusual sites are generally associated with other congenital abnormalities, especially symphalangism. Also, more than one coalition can occur in the same foot.[47, 69, 151]

Pathomechanics

The biomechanics of the normal foot and ankle have been studied extensively.* Because of the complex kinetic relationship between the subtalar and the transverse tarsal joints (talonavicular and calcaneocuboid joints), it appears that when motion is lost or altered in one joint, increased stress and shear forces are applied to the remaining joints in a compensatory manner. This results in altered mechanics, ligament stress, and possibly, pain. Cartilage degeneration and osteoarthritis may subsequently develop depending on the degree of deformity.

The pathomechanics of the peroneal spastic flatfoot were succinctly summarized by Mosier and Asher[98] in 1984. During walking, the nor-

---

*See references 1, 9, 15, 20, 38, 39, 58, 60, 76, 77, 101, 106, 113, 119, 122, 136, 150, and 155.

*See references 19, 34, 37, 62, 82, 86, 87, 89, 109, and 153.

TABLE 44–2. CLASSIFICATION OF TARSAL COALITIONS

TALOCALCANEAL
 1. Medial
   a. Complete
   b. Incomplete
   c. Rudimentary
 2. Posterior
 3. Anterior
 	
 CALCANEONAVICULAR
 TALONAVICULAR
 CALCANEOCUBOID
 NAVICULOCUNEIFORM
 CUBONAVICULAR
 MULTIPLE
 MASSIVE
   More than two of the above

Adapted from Tachdjian MO: Tarsal coalitions. *In* Tachdjian MO: The Child's Foot. Philadelphia, W.B. Saunders, 1985, pp 261–294.

mal subtalar joint has both a gliding and rotatory or transverse motion.[19, 106, 107, 153] During dorsiflexion of the foot the calcaneus glides forward on the talus to an appreciable degree until limited by the capsular ligaments. Toward the end of dorsiflexion, an upward gliding motion occurs at the transverse tarsal joint, which allows the wide proximal portion of the navicular bone to move very slightly cephalad on the talar head. Outland and Murphy[107] performed fluoroscopic studies of a foot with a subtalar fusion, which is analogous to a tarsal coalition, and demonstrated that the normal gliding motion at the transverse tarsal joint is lost and it becomes a hinged joint. With the foot in full dorsiflexion, the transverse tarsal joint widens inferiorly and narrows superiorly. When this occurs, the proximal edge of the superior portion of the navicular impinges on and overrides the anterior aspect of the head of the talus. This overriding causes elevation of the talonavicular ligament and periosteum on the dorsal or superior aspect of the head and neck of the talus. The osseous repair of this periosteal avulsion over a period of months or years leads to radiographic "beaking" of the talus. This beak has frequently been interpreted as a sign of degenerative osteoarthritis, but this interpretation is usually incorrect. Resnick has recognized three osseous outgrowths that may appear on the dorsal surface of the talus—ridges, osteophytes, and beaks.[116] Hypertrophy of the normal talar ridge, which is 7 to 14 mm proximal to the talonavicular joint, may occur secondary to excessive stress or motion on the insertion of the capsules and ligaments. This is occasionally seen in athletes with otherwise normal feet. Osteophytes represent degenerative osteoarthritis and arise on the margin of the cartilaginous surfaces. Beaks occur at the talar ridge and are secondary to abnormal motion, but these are larger than the hypertrophied talar ridges and extend distally, terminating near or at the articular margin of the talonavicular joint (Fig. 44–2). The radiographic differentiation among these outgrowths usually is not difficult.

The transverse motion of the normal subtalar joint involves rotation of the calcaneus beneath the talus because there is little or no rotation within the ankle joint. Subtalar rotation occurs on an axis defined as a line deviated 42 degrees from the walking surface, and 16 degrees medial to a line extending from the center of the calcaneus to a point between the heads of the first and second metatarsal bones.[89] This axis allows the translation of the normal rotation of the lower extremity during the walking cycle into the foot.[82, 87] At foot strike, there is a moderate degree of eversion in the subtalar joint and internal rotation of the tibia. This is followed by progressive subtalar joint inversion and external rotation of the tibia until the time of toe-off. The magnitude of subtalar motion in the normal foot is approximately 8 degrees. This internal rotation of the subtalar joint helps to compensate for an average horizontal external rotation of the tibia of 10 to 11 degrees during the last three-quarters of the stance phase.[19, 82, 89] When the rotatory subtalar motion becomes restricted, especially with the hindfoot in an everted, valgus position, the compensatory internal rotation of the subtalar joint is lost, resulting in increased mobility in the transverse tarsal joint. This ultimately results in (1) loss of the medial longitudinal arc; (2) strain on the talonavicular ligament and capsule due to the hinged transverse tarsal joint motion; (3) adaptive shortening of the peroneal tendons; (4) impingement of the talus on the lateral aspect of the calcaneal sulcus, leading to flattening and broadening of the lateral talar process; and (5) narrowing of the posterior talocalcaneal articulation. Talocalcaneal coalitions usually restrict subtalar motion more and are associated with greater valgus deformity than other coalitions.[53, 64] The more severe the valgus deformity or the malalignment of the midfoot and hindfoot, the greater the symptoms.[10, 98]

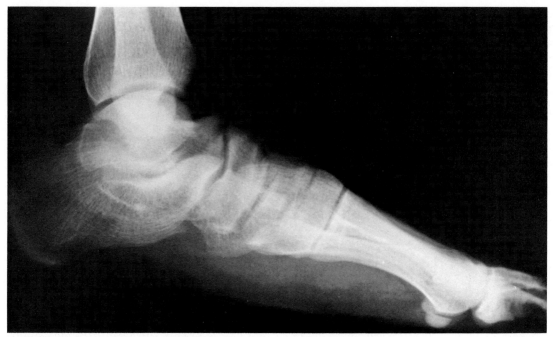

FIGURE 44–2. Lateral weight-bearing radiograph of a 15-year-old male 2 years following resection of a calcaneonavicular coalition of the left foot. The dorsal beak on the neck of the talus is large and persistent, and extends distally over the talonavicular joint. The foot is asymptomatic.

Conversely, the more normal the alignment of the hindfoot, the fewer the symptoms.[23] Pain in a tarsal coalition, therefore, may be attributed to abnormal alignment and mechanics, which result in ligament strain, peroneal muscle spasm, sinus tarsi irritation, subtalar joint irritation,[74] degenerative osteoarthritis, or a combination of all of these conditions.

Clinical Characteristics

The majority of patients with symptomatic tarsal coalitions present with a peroneal spastic flatfoot during late childhood or adolescence. Symptoms usually begin after a minor injury or vigorous activity, such as sports. Although mild limitation of subtalar motion and a valgus deformity are probably present in early childhood, the onset of symptoms appears to vary with the age at which the cartilaginous or fibrous coalition begins to ossify and further decreases subtalar motion.[20, 136, 141] The delay in onset of symptoms may also be secondary to increased stress concentration from greater body weight, increased physical activities such as sports, and abnormal subtalar motion. It has been demonstrated that talonavicular co-

alitions ossify between 3 to 5 years of age, the calcaneonavicular coalition between 8 and 12 years, and the middle facet talocalcaneal coalitions between 12 and 16 years.[23, 64, 65] The pain is usually felt in the tarsal area, laterally near the sinus tarsi, or throughout the hindfoot. Occasionally, the pain radiates laterally along the lateral malleolus and distal fibula. With a talocalcaneal coalition, the pain is frequently felt over the talonavicular joint.[25] Symptoms are frequently aggravated by activities, such as sports, hiking, or walking on uneven ground.

Clinical examination typically reveals a pes planus appearance of the foot with midfoot pronation and heel valgus. In the sitting position, the unsupported, uninvolved foot assumes an equinus position with mild hindfoot varus and forefoot supination, whereas the involved foot demonstrates equinus but with maintenance of heel valgus, flattening of the medial longitudinal arch, and forefoot pronation. Subtalar motion is typically diminished or absent in middle facet talocalcaneal coalitions, and attempts at varus stress may produce pain in the shortened peroneal muscles and reflex peroneal muscle spasm. In calcaneonavicular coalitions, the subtalar and midtarsal joint motion is typically only moderately limited and the hindfoot valgus deformity less severe.[140] A varus deformity, although rare, can occur and usually is attributed to spasm of the tibialis anterior muscle.[20, 128]

During walking, the pes planus and peroneal muscle spasms are visible and the gait is usually antalgic. Occasionally, there may also be a spasm at the tibialis anterior muscle. Limited subtalar motion denies the normal transverse rotation, and this may lead to ankle ligament laxity secondary to repeated sprains due to the horizontal stresses between the foot and tibia being absorbed by the ankle.[17, 132] This ankle ligament laxity and abnormal stress may ultimately give a false impression of subtalar motion and result in an adaptive ball-and-socket ankle joint in a child.[72, 75, 109, 135, 142] Ankle sprains in tarsal coalitions are common, and a fracture of a calcaneonavicular coalition following a sprain has been reported.[117]

The presence of peroneal muscle spasm can be confirmed by a procaine block of the peroneal nerve at the fibular head.[52] Relief of pain and muscle spasm usually is diagnostic. Occasionally, when the symptoms have improved but not completely relieved, injection of the sinus tarsi may be beneficial.

Radiographic Characteristics

The diagnosis of a tarsal coalition is arrived at through the use of radiography. Standard or routine radiographic views combined with special views are usually diagnostic, but occasionally other procedures, such as computed tomography, conventional tomography, technetium bone scans, and magnetic resonance imaging, may be required.

Routine Radiographs

The radiographic evaluation of a patient with a peroneal spastic flatfoot and suspected tarsal coalitions proceeds in a systematic manner and begins with anteroposterior, lateral weight-bearing, and oblique radiographs of both feet. However, these routine radiographs may not demonstrate a tarsal coalition, especially one involving the subtalar or talocalcaneal joint.[29, 57, 90, 110, 137] Bone overlap, oblique orientation, and coalitions of fibrous or cartilaginous origin can make visualization difficult.

Talocalcaneal Coalition. The talocalcaneal joint has two compartments: a posterior and an anterior compartment. Each compartment is separated by the interosseous or talocalcaneal ligament. The posterior compartment contains the posterior facet, whereas the anterior has either a single, large middle facet or a separate anterior and middle facet.[20, 65, 127, 146] Any of the three facets may be involved in a coalition. The medial talocalcaneal coalition may be a complete coalition of the facet; an incomplete coalition, with a mass projecting from the medial aspect of the talus coalesced with a mass projecting from the sustentaculum tali; or a rudimentary coalition, in which only one element at the coalition is present such as an osseous mass projecting upward from the sustentaculum tali or downward from the medial aspect of the talus, in which motion of the subtalar joint is blocked.[139, 141] The complete and incomplete types of coalition are more easily diagnosed radiographically, whereas the rudimentary forms can be quite difficult. Because of the various planes, shapes, and divergences of the facets of the subtalar joint, the lateral radiograph does not allow adequate visualization of its various components (Fig. 44–3A and B). As a consequence, other views or radiographic procedures are necessary for adequate evaluation. The radiographic characteristics suggestive of a talocalcaneal coalition include (1) talar beaking; (2) broadening or rounding of the lateral process of the talus; (3) narrowing of the posterior talocalcaneal joint space; (4) a concave undersurface of the talar neck; (5) a "ball-and-socket" ankle joint; and (6) failure to visualize the middle talocalcaneal facet.[5, 20, 23, 29]

Korvin,[73] in 1934, was the first to describe the penetrated axial view of the calcaneus with varying beam angles, but this was later popularized by Harris and Beath.[53] This view, which is also known as the ski jump view, is necessary to demonstrate the middle facet talocalcaneal coalition. The anterior facet is best visualized in the oblique lateral dorsoplanar view and the posterior facet by the lateral oblique axial view described by Isherwood.[63] When routine radiographic studies, including the penetrated axial view, are normal, it is important to specifically study the anterior facet because this may be the site of an unsuspected coalition.[5, 20, 22, 23]

The proper angle for the penetrated axial view of Harris and Beath can be determined from the standing lateral view by drawing a line through the posterior and middle facet and measuring the angle it forms with the

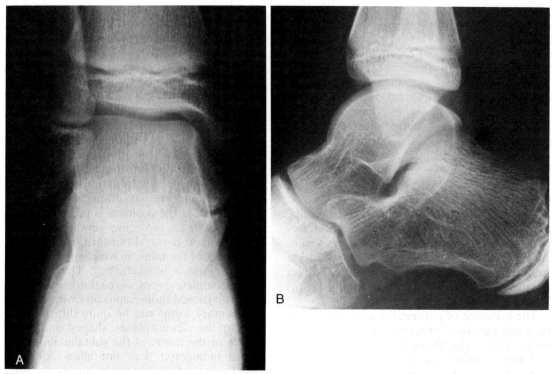

FIGURE 44–3. *(A),* Anteroposterior radiograph of the right ankle of a 13-year-old male with vague hindfoot and ankle pain. Observe the prominent medial portion of the talus and calcaneus and the irregular dish-shaped articulation indicative of the incomplete form of a talocalcaneal coalition. *(B),* The lateral radiograph is essentially normal. The appearance of the subtalar joint shows no evidence to suggest a coalition.

horizontal surface on which the foot is placed. Normally, this angle is approximately 40 to 45 degrees (Fig. 44–4*A* to *C*). In the normal view, the middle and posterior facet joints are in parallel planes. If the two joints are not parallel and the plane of the middle facet joint intersects the plane of the posterior facet, then a cartilaginous talocalcaneal coalition should be suspected even if the joint spaces appear normal.[23, 24] If the coalition is completely ossified, the facet is obliterated, but if the coalition is fibrous or cartilaginous, the joint may be narrowed or irregular. If the correct angle is not determined or used, the coalition may not be seen or the appearance of coalition may be simulated in a noncoalesced subtalar joint.[125, 137] As a consequence, conventional tomography or computed tomography may be necessary to evaluate further the anterior and posterior compartments of the subtalar joint. Arthrography of the subtalar joint has also been recommended in the study of nonosseous talocalcaneal coalitions.[68, 114]

Calcaneonavicular Coalition. The calcaneo-navicular coalition is best visualized on the 45-degree oblique view, as described by Slomann in 1921.[129, 130] Normally, this coalition is approximately 1 cm in width and can vary from fully ossified (Fig. 44–5*A* to *C*) to fibrous or cartilaginous (Fig. 44–6*A* to *C*). In the fibrous or cartilagimous type, the coalition may appear as a sclerotic, irregular line similar to a pseudoarthrosis. Radiographic signs suggestive of a calcaneonavicular coalition include: (1) closer than normal proximity of the calcaneus and navicular; (2) loss of the dense cortical rim at the junction of the calcaneus and navicular; (3) hypoplasia of the head of the talus; and (4) talar beaking.[16, 20, 65, 115, 121] Oestreich and colleagues recently reported on the "anteater nose" sign in calcaneonavicular coalition.[102] This is seen on the standing lateral radiograph and represents the anterior protrusion of the calcaneus.

Conventional Tomography

Lateral tomograms, as described by Conway and Cowell[20] in 1969, can be very beneficial in

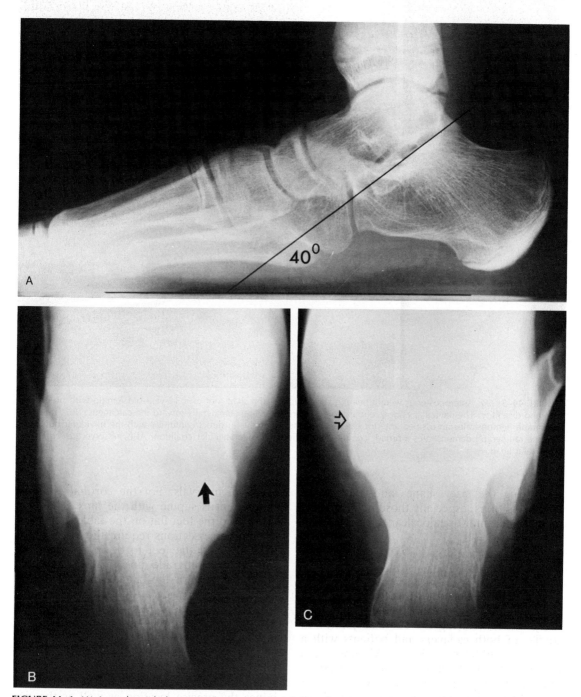

FIGURE 44–4. *(A),* Lateral weight-bearing radiograph of the left foot of a symptomatic 13-year-old male. Note that the line drawn through the posterior facet joint measures 40 degrees with respect to the weight-bearing surface. *(B),* Penetrated axial view of the left hindfoot at 40 degrees demonstrates a middle facet talocalcaneal coalition *(dark arrow). (C),* The penetrated axial view of the right hindfoot at the same degree of angulation shows an open, normal-appearing middle talocalcaneal facet joint *(open arrow).*

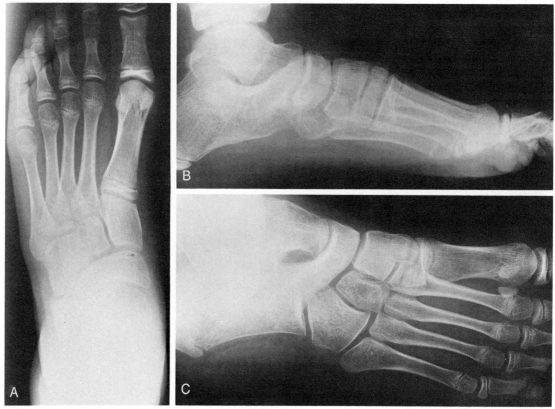

FIGURE 44–5. *(A)*, Anteroposterior weight-bearing radiograph of the right foot of a 12-year-old female with progressive pain and disability. The navicular bone is elongated transversely and tapers laterally toward the calcaneus. *(B)*, The lateral radiograph demonstrates an ossified anterior extension of the calcaneus in direct continuity with the navicular bone. *(C)*, Oblique radiograph demonstrates a broad, completely ossified calcaneonavicular coalition. Also, observe the hypoplasia of the talar head.

identifying the size, shape, and location of tarsal coalitions, especially those involving the middle and anterior talocalcaneal facets (Fig. 44–7*A* to *D*).

Computed Tomography

This technique is currently the procedure of choice in the evaluation of coalitions, especially those involving the subtalar joint.* In studies of both cadavers and patients with a suspected subtalar coalition, Martinez and coworkers[91] and Herzenberg and associates[57] found that computed tomography was superior to routine radiographs and conventional tomography. The scans are obtained in both the coronal and axial or transverse directions at 3-

to 5-mm intervals. For the coronal sections, the patient is supine with the hips and knees flexed and the feet flat on the table. The axial or transverse sections require the knees to be extended and the feet to be in a vertical or simulated plantigrade position. The coronal views are best for the talocalcaneal coalitions because they provide a unique cross-sectional view of the subtalar joint anatomy (Fig. 44–8*A* and *B*). Figure 44–9 shows calcaneonavicular coalitions on radiography (Fig. 44–9*A*) and on computed tomography (Fig. 44–9*B*, *C*). Computed tomography (1) allows simultaneous visualization of both feet; (2) determines the precise location as well as the size of the coalition; (3) distinguishes between osseous and nonosseous coalitions; (4) assesses for other abnormalities such as degenerative arthritis or other coalitions; and (5) is noninvasive.

---

*See references 5, 27, 29, 57, 90, 102, 110, 120, 131, 133, 134, and 137.

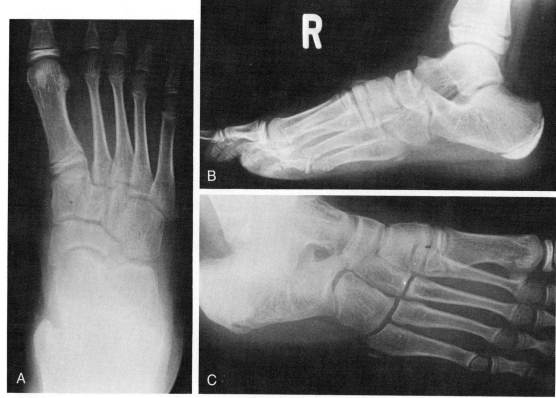

FIGURE 44–6. *(A),* Anteroposterior radiograph of the symptomatic right foot of an 8-year-old female. The extended anteromedial portion of the calcaneus abuts a flattened portion of the tapered, lateral aspect of the navicular. There is a radiolucent line at the coalition indicating fibrous or cartilaginous tissue and incomplete ossification. *(B),* In the lateral radiograph, the extension of the anteromedial portion of the head of the calcaneus is more apparent, producing the so-called "anteater's nose." There is also beaking on the dorsal aspect of the talus. *(C),* The oblique radiograph demonstrates the incompletely ossified calcaneonavicular coalition.

Technetium Bone Scans

Goldman and associates have recommended the use of technetium bone scans as a screening procedure for identifying or confirming symptomatic talocalcaneal coalitions.[42] They showed that the combination of two areas of uptake, superior aspect of the talus and the subtalar area, was indicative of a middle-facet coalition. Deutsch and colleagues also found technetium bone scans useful in localizing middle facet talocalcaneal coalitions prior to computed tomography.[29] Currently, the major indication for bone scans is in the evaluation of a peroneal spastic flatfoot in which a tarsal coalition has not been demonstrated by plain radiographs or computed tomography. They may be beneficial in localizing the site of occult pathology.

Magnetic Resonance Imaging

This procedure has not been widely used in the assessment of tarsal coalition. However, as with technetium bone scans, it may be useful in the evaluation of a peroneal spastic flatfoot that is not secondary to a coalition (see Table 44–1).

Treatment

The treatment of symptomatic tarsal coalitions varies according to the type of coalition, the age of the patient, the extent of the coalition, the presence or absence of degenerative osteoarthritis, and the degree of disability caused by pain and muscle spasm. The treatment may be nonoperative as well as operative. Patients who are affected by the condition

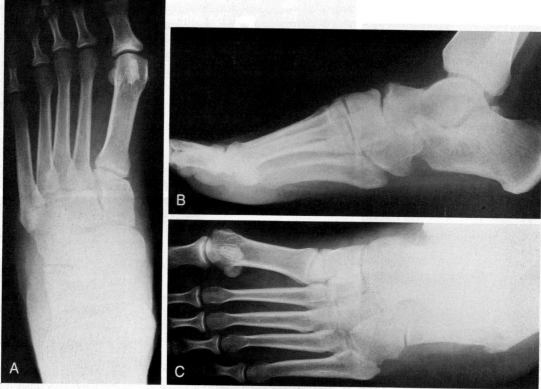

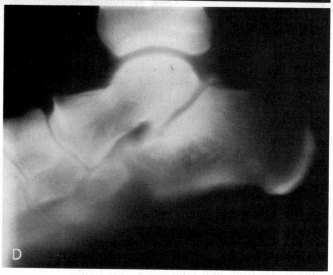

FIGURE 44–7. *(A),* Anteroposterior weight-bearing radiograph of the left foot of a 35-year-old woman. The foot is mildly symptomatic, and the patient has a history of recurrent ankle sprains. The navicular is ovoid and hypertrophied, and there is an absence of the normal talonavicular articulation. Radiographs of the right foot were normal. *(B),* The lateral radiograph demonstrates a complete talonavicular coalition. *(C),* Oblique radiograph shows the enlarged talonavicular coalition. *(D),* Lateral tomogram shows the elongated talonavicular complex with a "beak" on the navicular secondary to osseous hypertrophy at the site of capsular attachment (Courtesy of Donald B. Goodfellow, M.D., Case Western Reserve University.)

but who have few or no symptoms usually do not require treatment. The middle facet talocalcaneal and calcaneonavicular coalitions constitute the majority of cases that require treatment.

Nonoperative Treatment

Nonoperative management is usually the first consideration for symptomatic tarsal coa-litions. This may consist of shoe inserts (arch supports), orthotics (ankle-foot orthoses, Plastizote shoe inserts, University of California Biomechanical Laboratories [UCBL] inserts), shoe modifications (Thomas heel, Whitman plate), and short-leg walking casts. All of these techniques are designed to provide better support to the foot; to decrease stress on the tarsals; to decrease the hindfoot valgus, if

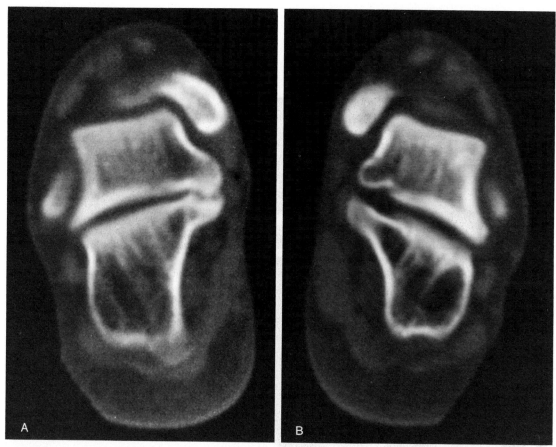

FIGURE 44–8. *(A),* Computed tomography in the coronal plane showing the incomplete right middle facet talocalcaneal coalition of the patient in Figure 44–3*A* and *B. (B),* Tomography of the normal left talocalcaneal joint at the same level.

possible; to reduce irritation and inflammation of the mobile joints; and to reduce associated muscle spasms.[98, 138] Cowell, however, disagreed with conservative treatment of symptomatic calcaneonavicular coalitions because surgery yields a more normal, flexible, and asymptomatic foot.[23]

Indications. All patients usually warrant an initial trial of nonoperative management. If the patient has moderate to severe discomfort, a short-leg walking cast, with the hindfoot molded into slight varus, for 3 to 6 weeks is the best method of treatment.[98] This is followed by a supportive shoe with an insert such as an arch support or a custom-molded Plastizote orthosis. Injection of corticosteroids into the subtalar or midtarsal joint is not recommended.[141] Approximately one-third of the patients treated nonoperatively have relief of their symptoms.[65] Unfortunately, most have recurrence and progression of symptoms. Non-operative treatment is considered to have failed if the patient has persistent or recurrent symptoms after two applications of casts.[25, 98]

Operative Treatment

The currently available methods of surgical treatment include (1) resection of the coalition and interposition grafting; (2) triple arthrodesis; (3) isolated subtalar or talocalcaneal arthrodesis; and (4) os calcis or calcaneal osteotomy to correct the valgus hindfoot.

Indications. The indication for surgical treatment of symptomatic tarsal coalitions is persistence of symptoms following a trial of conservative management. There are specific indications for each of the various surgical procedures.

Resection of Talocalcaneal Coalition

Many recent reports have demonstrated satisfactory results following middle facet talocal-

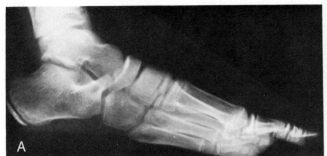

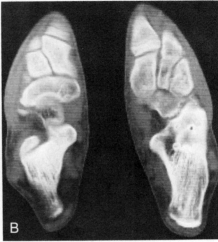

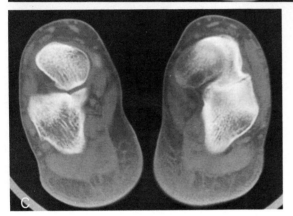

FIGURE 44–9. (A), Lateral radiograph of a mildly symptomatic left foot of a 10-year-old male. There is an extension of the anterior aspect of the calcaneus, producing the so-called "anteater nose" indicative of a calcaneonavicular coalition. This radiograph was interpreted as normal. (B), Computed tomography in the coronal plane demonstrates a broad, incompletely ossified left calcaneonavicular coalition. (C), Computed tomography in the coronal plane also demonstrates the coalition.

caneal coalition resection and interposition grafting.* Hark, in 1960, reported three successful resections in older children but advised triple arthrodesis for older patients.[46] Jayakumar and Colwell[65] had improvement of symptoms in two of four patients and Swiontkowski and associates[140] in four of five following resection. Danielsson reported no pain, good function, good subtalar joint motion, and no regeneration at the coalition in three patients at 1 to 14 years following resection.[27] In 1987, Scranton[123] and Olney and Asher[103] reported good or satisfactory results following resection in 13 of 13 and 8 of 10 feet, respectively. The mean follow-up period in both studies was slightly less than 4 years. The most common problem leading to unsatisfactory results in the study by Olney and Asher was failure to recognize incomplete resection of the coalition.

*See references 27, 38, 46, 64, 65, 97, 107, 123, and 140.

Scranton recommended resection when (1) there was failure of nonoperative treatment; (2) the coalition was less than one-half the surface area of the talocalcaneal joint; and (3) there was no degenerative osteoarthritis of the talonavicular joint. Although beaking of the talus is not considered evidence of degenerative osteoarthritis, Olney and Asher had no patients with excellent results who had this radiographic sign.

The argument against resection is that the subtalar joint is a major weight-bearing joint and that resection increases stress on the anterior and posterior facets and results in delayed degenerative osteoarthritis.[20, 23, 25, 51, 65] The long-term results following resection of this coalition still are not known.

The surgical technique for resection of a middle facet talocalcaneal coalition has been described both by Scranton[123] and by Olney and Asher[103] (Fig. 44–10A and B). A 6-cm incision is made longitudinally over the susten-

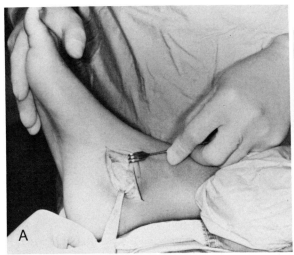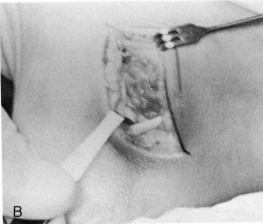

FIGURE 44–10. *(A),* Intraoperative photograph demonstrating a cartilaginous coalition at the right middle talocalcaneal facet. *(B),* The coalition was resected and adipose tissue interposed.

taculum tali. The abductor hallucis muscle is reflected plantarward from its retinacular and calcaneal origins. The flexor digitorum longus muscle and neurovascular bundle are identified, mobilized, and protected. The middle facet of the talocalcaneal joint is located between these two structures. It also lies just superior to the flexor hallucis longus tendon, which passes beneath the sustentaculum tali. The periosteum of the coalition is incised and reflected. The subtalar joint anterior and posterior to the coalition is identified. The coalition is then resected with osteotomes, rongeurs, curettes, or a power burr. Care must be taken to preserve the substance of the sustentaculum tali to provide support for the medial aspect of the subtalar joint. Scranton[123] recommends the resection be only 4 mm in height, whereas Olney and Asher[103] resect between 5 and 7 mm of bone. It is important that the coalition be completely excised and that no subtalar impingement remain. After adequate resection, the remaining articular cartilage, if any, of the middle facet is visible and the motion between the talus and calcaneus is markedly increased and without crepitation. The raw bone surfaces are then sealed with bone wax. Fat obtained locally or from the buttocks is packed into the defect and held there by closing, as much as possible, the overlying periosteum. The flexor retinaculum and the origin of the abductor hallucis are repaired with absorbable sutures. The subcutaneous tissue and skin are closed in a standard fashion.

Postoperatively, the patient is placed in a short-leg plaster of Paris or fiberglass cast for approximately 3 weeks. Initially the patient is maintained on crutches but is allowed to progress to partial weight bearing as tolerated. Following cast removal, the patient is placed on an active range-of-motion exercise program and continued on partial weight bearing with crutches for an additional 3 weeks. Full weight bearing is then allowed and strengthening exercises instituted. The patient is allowed to gradually return to full activities.

Resection of Calcaneonavicular Coalition

Resection is usually the procedure of choice for this condition. The long-term results following calcaneonavicular coalition resection in young patients have demonstrated alleviation of symptoms and improved function of the affected extremity.* However, in older patients, complete ossification at the coalition, the presence of other coalitions, and significant degenerative osteoarthritis in the remaining mobile joints, especially the talonavicular joint, may be contraindications to resection.[2, 25, 43, 61, 95]

Calcaneonavicular bar resection was initially suggested by Badgly in 1927[4] and Bentzon in 1930.[6] Although a portion of the extensor digitorum brevis muscle was interposed by Bentzon through the resection site, his patients

---

*See references 2, 17, 21, 23, 25, 38, 43, 46, 61, 69, 70, 95, 97, and 140.

did not benefit significantly because they were older and had considerable degenerative osteoarthritis. Andreasen[2] reported on the late results of the procedure described by Bentzon and found satisfactory results in 22 of 30 feet (73 percent) at 10 to 22 years postoperatively. However, based on the radiographic evidence of degenerative osteoarthritis and recurrence, either partial or total, of the coalition in 67 percent of his patients, he recommended triple arthrodesis. Mitchell and Gibson,[95] who performed the resection without interposition of soft tissue but cauterized the raw cancellous bone surfaces, had satisfactory results in 41 feet (68 percent) despite a 67 percent incidence of total or partial recurrence of the coalition. Cowell[21, 23, 25] has demonstrated the importance of patient selection, assessment for other unsuspected coalitions, restoration of subtalar motion at the time of surgery, and interposition of soft tissue (extensor digitorum brevis muscle) in achieving satisfactory long-term results. Currently, patients for whom resection is indicated include (1) adolescents, usually less than 16 years of age; (2) persons with symptoms of recent origin; and (3) persons with no degenerative osteoarthritis.[25, 43] Cowell reported that 23 of 26 feet (88 percent) undergoing calcaneonavicular coalition resection had no symptoms and satisfactory motion at a mean follow-up of 5 years.[25] Swiontowski and coworkers reported that 35 of 39 feet (90 percent) were improved following resection at a mean follow-up of 4.6 years.[140] Two of their patients underwent concomitant resection of the associated talar beak, and no degenerative arthritis of the talonavicular joint was found. Chambers and associates, in 1982, reviewed function and gait in 19 patients at a mean follow-up of 8 years following reconstructive surgery for calcaneonavicular coalition.[17] The amount of postoperative subtalar motion correlated with the eventual clinical result with respect to gait and function of the subtalar joint under conditions of stress. Inglis and associates,[61] in 1986, found excellent or good results in 11 of 16 feet (69 percent) at 20 years or more following surgery. Gonzalez and Kumar,[43] in 1990, had similar results in 58 of 75 feet (77 percent) between 2 and 23 years following resection. They discovered partial reformation of the coalition in 17 patients (22 percent) and believed that talar beaking did not affect the final result and was not a contraindication to resection.

The surgical technique for resection of the calcaneonavicular coalition has been described by Cowell (Fig. 44–11*A* to *C*).[23] It consists of an oblique incision (Ollier approach) over the sinus tarsi similar to that for a triple arthrodesis. The extensor digitorum brevis muscle is detached from its origin over the sinus tarsi and retracted distally. The tendons of the peroneus longus and brevis muscles are identified and retracted plantarward. The fat is removed from the sinus tarsi, which usually allows easy visualization of the calcaneonavicular coalition extending from the medial portion of the calcaneal head to the lateral portion of the navicular bone. If the bar is cartilaginous, it will appear as a raised white block. Using a small osteotome, the coalition is excised. Bone or cartilage should be removed from the navicular bone up to the undersurface of the talar head. A rectangle of at least 1.0 cm should be removed. All cartilaginous portions of the coalition should be removed, since the coalition has the potential to reform. Care must be taken not to damage the talonavicular ligament because it will predispose the navicular bone to being displaced superiorly on the talus. With the rongeur, the lateral margin of the navicular bone and medial portion of the head of the talus can be reshaped in a more normal anatomic fashion. Absorbable sutures are then passed through the fascia of the extensor digitorum brevis muscle. Using two Keith needles passed through the defect, the sutures are brought out the medial plantar surface of the foot and the muscle is pulled through the resection site. This obliterates the dead space, limits hematoma formation, and prevents reformation of the coalition. The absorbable sutures are then tied over a padded button on the plantar surface of the foot. Tachdjian prefers to use gluteal fat rather than muscle to fill the defect.[141] The subcutaneous tissues and skin are closed in a standard manner.

Postoperatively, a short-leg non–weight-bearing cast is applied with the foot in a neutral position, and the cast is worn for 7 to 10 days. It is removed and early subtalar motion is allowed. No weight bearing is allowed until the passive subtalar motion is comparable to that obtained intraoperatively following excision of the coalition. Usually full weight bearing can be allowed 4 to 6 weeks after surgery.

Resection of Other Coalitions

Resection of symptomatic coalitions other than the middle facet talocalcaneal and calca-

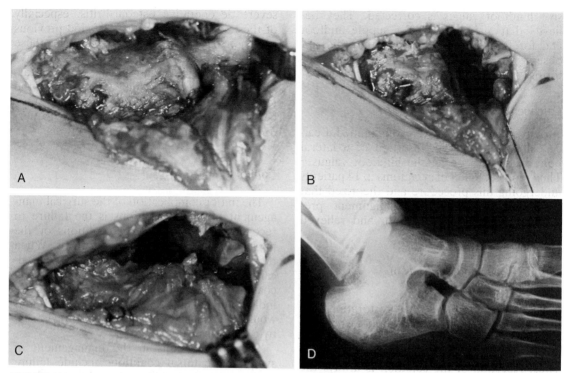

FIGURE 44–11. *(A)*, Intraoperative photograph showing a calcaneonavicular coalition. The anteromedial portion of the head of the calcaneus is extended and coalesced with the lateral portion of the navicular. *(B)*, Photograph following wide resection of the coalition. *(C)*, The origin of the extensor digitorum brevis muscle has been transferred through the coalition. *(D)*, Intraoperative oblique radiograph following resection. Approximately 1 cm of the coalition has been removed to prevent impingement and to allow space for the transferred extensor digitorum brevis muscle.

neonavicular coalitions has been performed. Successful resections for talonavicular,[38] cubonavicular,[24] and anterior and posterior facet talocalcaneal[123, 140] coalitions have been reported.

Triple Arthrodesis

Triple arthrodesis was the previous standard procedure for symptomatic tarsal coalitions, especially the talocalcaneal coalitions. However, its major indications today are extensive talocalcaneal coalition, multiple coalitions, and symptomatic coalitions with extensive degenerative osteoarthritis.[23, 36, 98, 100, 141] It is not commonly indicated. If possible, triple arthrodesis should be postponed until the foot has reached its full growth. However, if disabling symptoms are present during childhood and associated with a severe valgus deformity, it may need to be performed earlier. The procedure does provide good lateral stability and correction of severe foot deformity, and relieves pain caused by degenerative osteoar-

thritis. However, there will be significant stresses applied across the ankle joint. If it is performed early in childhood, it may result in a ball-and-socket ankle joint.

Talocalcaneal Arthrodesis

Isolated subtalar or talocalcaneal arthrodesis has recently been reported to be useful in treating a variety of isolated pathologic subtalar disorders in adults. Mann and Baumgarten have reported the results of subtalar fusions for post-traumatic arthritis, acquired adult flatfoot secondary to posterior tibial tendon rupture, rheumatoid arthritis, and talocalcaneal coalitions.[88] All of the four patients with talocalcaneal coalitions had satisfactory results at a mean follow-up of 3.5 years. The authors believed these patients had better results, both subjectively and objectively, than those patients treated with a subtalar fusion for other reasons. They concluded that subtalar fusion is a satisfactory method of treatment for talocalcaneal coalitions, provided that the excessive hindfoot valgus is corrected. They believed that maintenance of a supple midfoot and forefoot is important, and they did not observe progression of degenerative osteoarthritis.

Calcaneal Osteotomy

Cain and Hyman have recommended a calcaneal osteotomy with insertion of a lateral bone wedge to correct the hindfoot valgus.[12] They reported relief of symptoms in 14 patients undergoing this procedure and theorized that correcting the hindfoot malalignment prevented oblique ligament strain and relieved pain.

Authors' Preferred Methods of Treatment

The authors believe that restoration and preservation of subtalar motion, whenever possible, is the primary goal in symptomatic tarsal coalitions requiring operative treatment. Thus, resection of the coalition is always the preferred method of treatment. Although we are always concerned by the presence of talar beaking, we agree with the other authors that this beak is periarticular rather than articular and is indicative of increased stress across the transverse tarsal joint and does not predict the presence or absence of degenerative osteoarthritis or the ultimate outcome following coalition resection. The published series of both middle facet talocalcaneal and calcaneonavicular coalition resections indicate that a significant majority of patients will have satisfactory long-term results. The age of the patient does not appear to be as important as the presence or absence of degenerative arthritis in the mobile joints. Older adolescents or young adults are acceptable candidates for resection, provided there is not degenerative arthritis in the other tarsal joints. The material interposed in either coalition is probably not critical in the achievement of long-term results. We prefer the method of Cowell for the calcaneonavicular coalitions but interpose fat for the talocalcaneal coalitions. We do not recommend simultaneous excision of large talar beaks because it does not appear to enhance results.

Our indications for triple arthrodesis include extensive coalitions involving multiple tarsal joints; radiographic evidence of moderate to severe degenerative osteoarthritis, especially of the talonavicular joint; and failed previous resection. However, in our experience, these factors are uncommon. When a definite preoperative decision regarding the extent of arthritis cannot be made, then exploration of the joint, in particular the talonavicular joint, may be helpful in deciding whether or not to perform a resection and a triple arthrodesis.

Complications

The major complication of the surgical management of tarsal coalitions is the failure to recognize either additional coalitions or the presence of degenerative osteoarthritis. When these conditions are present, an isolated calcaneonavicular or middle facet talocalcaneal coalition resection will most likely fail. An individual having one of these conditions would be managed better as stated previously, by a triple arthrodesis.

Therefore, pitfalls in the management of symptomatic tarsal coalitions include failure (1) to recognize additional coalitions; (2) to discover the presence of degenerative osteoarthritis, especially of the talonavicular joint; and (3) to adhere to the operative criteria and postoperative management.

References

1. Anderson RJ: The presence of an astragalo-scaphoid bone in man. J Anat Physiol 14:452–455, 1879–1880.
2. Andreasen E: Calcaneo-navicular coalition. Late results of resection. Acta Orthop Scand 39:424–432, 1968.
3. Austin FH: Symphalangism and related fusions of tarsal bones. Radiology 56:882–885, 1951.
4. Badgley CE: Coalition of the calcaneus and the navicular. Arch Surg 15:75–88, 1927.
5. Beckley DE, Anderson PW, Pedegana LR: The radiology of the subtalar joint with special reference to talo-calcaneal coalition. Clin Radiol 26:333–341, 1975.
6. Bentzon PGK: Bilateral congenital deformity of the astragalocalcanean joint. Bony coalescence between os trigonum and the calcaneus? Acta Orthop Scand 1:359–364, 1930.
7. Bersante FA, Samilson RL: Massive familial tarsal synostosis. J Bone Joint Surg 39A:1187–1190, 1957.
8. Blockey NJ: Peroneal spastic flat foot. J Bone Joint Surg. 37B:191–202, 1955.
9. Boyd HB: Congenital talonavicular synostosis. J Bone Joint Surg 26:682–686, 1944.
10. Braddock GTF: A prolonged follow-up of peroneal spastic flat foot. J Bone Joint Surg 43B:734–737, 1961.

11. Buffon G, Conte DE: Histoire naturelle, generrale et particulare. Avec la description du cabinet du roi. Tome 3:47, 1750.

12. Cain TJ, Hyman S: Peroneal spastic flat foot. Its treatment by osteotomy of the os calcis. J Bone Joint Surg 60B:527–529, 1978.

13. Callahan RH: Talipes equinovarus associated with an absent posterior tibial tendon and a tarsal coalition: A case report. Clin Orthop 146:231–233, 1980.

14. Calvert JP: A case of symphalangism with associated carpal and tarsal fusions. Hand 6:291–294, 1974.

15. Challis J: Hereditary transmission of talonavicular coalition in association with anomaly of the little finger. J Bone Joint Surg 56A:1273–1276, 1974.

16. Chambers CH: Congenital anomalies of the tarsal navicular with particular reference to calcaneonavicular coalition. Br J Radiol 23:580–584, 1950.

17. Chambers RB, Cook TM, Cowell HR: Surgical reconstruction for calcaneonavicular coalition. Evaluation of function and gait. J Bone Joint Surg 64A:829–836, 1982.

18. Christian JC, Franken EA Jr, Lindeman JP, et al: A dominant syndrome of metacarpal and metatarsal asymmetry with carpal and tarsal fusions, syndactyly, articular dysplasia and platyspondyly. Clin Genet 8:75–80, 1975.

19. Close JR, Inman VT, Poor PM, Tood FN: The function of the subtalar joint. Clin Orthop 50:159–179, 1967.

20. Conway JJ, Cowell HR: Tarsal coalition: clinical significance and roentgenographic demonstration. Radiology 92:799–811, 1969.

21. Cowell HR: Extensor brevis arthroplasty. J Bone and Joint Surg 52A:820, 1970.

22. Cowell HR: Talocalcaneal coalition and new causes of peroneal spastic flatfoot. Clin Orthop 85:16–22, 1972.

23. Cowell HR: Diagnosis and management of peroneal spastic flatfoot. Instruc Course Lect 24:94–103, 1975.

24. Cowell HR: Tarsal coalition–review and update. Instruc Course Lect 31:264–271, 1982.

25. Cowell HR, Elener V: Rigid painful flatfoot secondary to tarsal coalition. Clin Orthop 177:54–60, 1983.

26. Cruveilhier J: Anatomie pathologique du corps humain. Tome I, 1829–1835.

27. Danielsson LG: Talocalcaneal coalition treated with resection. J Pediatr Orthop 7:513–517, 1987.

28. Del Sel JM, Grand NE: Cubonavicular synostosis. A rare tarsal anomaly. J Bone Joint Surg 41B:149, 1959.

29. Deutsch AL, Resnick D, Campbell G: Computed tomography and bone scintigraphy in the evaluation of tarsal coalitions. Radiology 144:137–140, 1982.

30. Diamond LS: A possible new syndrome in clinodactyly, voluntary shoulder dislocation and massive tarsal coalition. Birth Defects 10:527–530, 1974.

31. Diamond LS: Inherited talocalcaneal coalition. Birth Defects 10:531–534, 1974.

32. Drinkwater H: Phalangeal anarthrosis (synostosis, ankylosis) transmitted through fourteen generations. Proc Roy Soc Med 10 (Part 3):60–68, 1917.

33. Dubois HJ: Nievergelt-Pearlman syndrome. Synostosis in feet and hands with dysplasia of elbows. Report of a case. J Bone Joint Surg 52B:325–329, 1970.

34. Duckworth T: The hindfoot and its relation to rotational deformities of the forefoot. Clin Orthop 177:39–48, 1983.

35. Dwight T: A clinical atlas. Variations of the Bone of the Hands and Feet. Philadelphia, J.B. Lippincott, 1907.

36. Ehrlich MG: Tarsal coalition. *In* Jahss MH (Ed): Disorders of the Foot. Philadelphia, W. B. Saunders, 1982, pp 521–538.

37. Elftman H: The transverse tarsal joint and its control. Clin Orthop 16:41–46, 1960.

38. Elkus RA: Tarsal coalitions in the young athlete. Am J Sports Med 14:477–480, 1986.

39. Gaynor SS: Congenital astragalocalcaneal fusion. J Bone Joint Surg 18:479–482, 1936.

40. Geelhoed GW, Neel JV, Davidson RT: Symphalangism and tarsal coalition: A hereditary syndrome. A report on two families. J Bone Joint Surg 51B:278–289, 1969.

41. Glessner JR Jr, Davis GL: Bilateral calcaneonavicular coalition occurring in twin boys. A case report. Clin Orthop 47:173–176, 1966.

42. Goldman AB, Pavlov H, Schneider R: Radionuclide bone scanning in subtalar coalitions: Differential considerations. Am J Radiol 138:427–432, 1982.

43. Gonzalez P, Kumar SJ: Calcaneonavicular coalition treated by resection and interposition of the extensor digitorum brevis muscle. J Bone Joint Surg 72A:71–77, 1990.

44. Grant AD, Rose D, Lehman W: Talocalcaneal coalition in arthrogryposis multiplex congenita. Bull Hosp Joint Dis 42:236–241, 1982.

45. Gregersen HN: Naviculocuneiform coalition. J Bone Joint Surg 59A:128–130, 1977.

46. Hark FW: Congenital anomalies of the tarsal bones. Clin Orthop 16:21–25, 1960.

47. Harle TS, Stevenson JR: Hereditary symphalangism associated with carpal and tarsal fusions. Radiology 89:91–94, 1967.

48. Harold AJ: Rigid valgus foot from fibrous contractures of the peronei. J Bone Joint Surg 47B:743–745, 1965.

49. Harper MC: Traumatic peroneal spastic flat foot. Orthopaedics 5:466–471, 1981.

50. Harris BJ: Anomalous structures in the developing human foot. [Abstract.] Anat Rec 121:399, 1955.

51. Harris RI: Rigid valgus foot due to talocalcaneal bridge. J Bone Joint Surg 37A:169–183, 1955.

52. Harris RI: Follow-up notes on articles previously published in the journal. Retrospect—peroneal spastic flat foot (rigid valgus foot). J Bone Joint Surg 47A:1657–1667, 1965.

53. Harris RI, Beath T: Etiology of peroneal spastic flat foot (rigid valgus foot). J Bone Joint Surg 30B:624–634, 1948.

54. Heikel HVA: Coalitio calcaneo-navicularis and calcaneus secundarius. A clinical and radiographic study of twenty-three patients. Acta Orthop Scand 32:72–84, 1962.

55. Heiple KG, Lovejoy CO: The antiquity of tarsal coalition. Bilateral deformity in a pre-Columbian indian skeleton. J Bone and Joint Surg 51A:979–983, 1969.

56. Herschel H, VonRonnen JR: The occurrence of calcaneonavicular synostosis in pes valgus contractus. J Bone Joint Surg 32A:280–282, 1950.

57. Herzenberg JE, Goldner JL, Martinez S, Silverman PM: Computed tomography of talocalcaneal tarsal coalition. A clinical and anatomical study. Foot Ankle 6:273–288, 1986.

58. Hodgson FG: Talonavicular synostosis. South Med J 39:940–941, 1946.

59. Holl M: Beitrage zur Chirurgischen Osteologie des Fusses. Arch Klin Chir 25:211, 1880.

60. Illievitz AB: Congenital malformation of the feet. Report of a case of congenital fusion of the scaphoid with the astragalus and complete absence of one toe. Am J Surg 4:550–552, 1928.

61. Inglis G, Buxton RA, MacNicol MF: Symptomatic calcaneonavicular bars. The results 20 years after surgical excision. J Bone Joint Surg 68B:128–131, 1986.

62. Inman VT, Mann RA: Biomechanics of the foot and ankle. *In* Mann RA (Ed): DuVries' Surgery of the Foot. 4th Ed. St. Louis, C.V. Mosby, 1978, pp 3–21.

63. Isherwood I: A radiological approach to the subtalar joint. J Bone Joint Surg 43B:566–574, 1961.

64. Jack EA: Bone anomalies of the tarus in relation to "peroneal spastic flat foot." J Bone Joint Surg 36B:530–542, 1954.

65. Jayakumar S, Cowell HR: Rigid flatfoot. Clin Orthop 122:77–84, 1977.

66. Johnson JC: Peroneal spastic flatfoot syndrome. South Med J 69:807–809, 1976.

67. Jones R: Peroneal spasm and its treatment. [Abstract.] Liverpool Med Chir J 17:442, 1897.

68. Kaye JJ, Ghelman B, Schneider R: Talocalcaneonavicular joint arthrography for sustentacular-talar joint coalitions. Radiology 115:730–731, 1975.

69. Kendrick JI: Treatment of calcaneonavicular bar. J Am Med Assoc 172:1242–1244, 1960.

70. Kendrick JI: Tarsal coalition. Clin Orthop 85:62–63, 1972.

71. Kirmisson E: Double pied bot varus par malformatiaon osseuse primitive associe'a des ankyloses congenitales des doigts et des orteils chez quatre membranes d'une meme famille. Rev d'orthop 9:392–398, 1898.

72. Kolbel R, Hermann HJ: Ball and socket ankle joint and tarsal synostosis. Z Orthop 113:952–956, 1975.

73. Korvin H: Coalitio talocalcanea. Ztschr Orthop Chir 60:105–110, 1934.

74. Kyne PJ, Mankin HJ: Changes in intra-articular pressure with subtalar joint motion with special reference to the etiology of peroneal spastic flat foot. Bull Hosp Jt Dis Orthop Inst 26:181–186, 1965.

75. Lamb D: The ball-and-socket ankle joint. J Bone Joint Surg 40B:240–243, 1958.

76. Lapidus PW: Congenital fusion of the bones of the foot; with report of a case of congenital astragaloscaphoid fusion. J Bone Joint Surg 14:888–894, 1932.

77. Lapidus PW: Bilateral congenital talonavicular fusion. Report of a case. J Bone Joint Surg 20:775–777, 1938.

78. Lapidus PW: Spastic flat foot. J Bone Joint Surg 28:126–136, 1946.

79. Lapidus PW: Flatfoot revisited. Contemp Orthop 3:1002–1013, 1981.

80. Lissoos I, Sousi J: Tarsal synostosis with partial adactylia. Med Proc 11:224–228, 1965.

81. Leonard MA: The inheritance of tarsal coalition and its relationship to spastic flat foot. J Bone Joint Surg 56B:520–526, 1974.

82. Levens AS, Inman VT, Blosser JA: Transverse rotation of the segments of the lower extremity in locomotion. J Bone Joint Surg 30A:859–872, 1948.

83. Levine WN, Scoles PV: Unpublished data, 1989.

84. Lusby HLJ: Naviculo-cuneiform synostosis. J Bone Joint Surg 41B:150, 1959.

85. Mahaffey HW: Bilateral congenital calcaneocuboid synostosis. Case report. J Bone Joint Surg 27:164–167, 1945.

86. Manley MT: Biomechanics of the foot. *In* Helfet AJ, Lee DMG (Eds): Disorders of the Foot. Philadelphia, J.B. Lippincott, 1980, pp 21–30.

87. Mann RA: Biomechanics of the Foot. Instruct Course Lect 31:167–180, 1982.

88. Mann RA, Baumgarten M: Subtalar fusion for isolated subtalar disorders. Preliminary report. Clin Orthop 226:260–265, 1988.

89. Manter JT: Movements of the subtalar and transverse tarsal joints. Anat Rec 80:397–410, 1941.

90. Marchisello PJ: The use of computerized axial tomography for the evaluation of talocalcaneal coalition. A case report. J Bone Joint Surg 69A:609–611, 1987.

91. Martinez S, Herzenberg JE, Apple JS: Computed tomography of the hindfoot. Orthop Clin North Am 16:481–496, 1985.

92. Merryweather R: Spastic valgus of the foot. Proc Roy Soc Med 48:103–106, 1955.

93. Miki T, Yamamuro T, Iida H, et al: Naviculocuneiform coalition. A report of two cases. Clin Orthop 196:256–259, 1985.

94. Miller EM: Congenital ankylosis of joints of hands and feet. J Bone Joint Surg 4:560–569, 1922.

95. Mitchell GP, Gibson JMC: Excision of calcaneonavicular bar for painful spasmodic flat foot. J Bone Joint Surg 49B:281–287, 1967.

96. Mitchell G: Spasmodic flatfoot. Clin Orthop 70:73–78, 1970.

97. Morgan RC Jr, Crawford AH: Surgical management of tarsal coalitions in adolescent athletes. Foot Ankle 7:183–196, 1986.

98. Mosier KM, Asher M: Tarsal coalitions and peroneal spastic flat foot. J Bone Joint Surg 66A:976–984, 1984.

99. Murakami Y: Nievergest-Perlman syndrome with impairment of hearing. Report of three cases in a family. J Bone Joint Surg 57B:367–372, 1975.

100. Musgrave RE, Goulder JL: Results of triple arthrodesis for rigid flat feet. South Med J 49:32–39, 1956.

101. O'Donoghue DH, Sell LS: Congenital talonavicular synostosis. J Bone Joint Surg 25:925–927, 1943.

102. Oestreich AE, Mize WA, Crawford AH, Morgan RC Jr: The "Anteater nose:" A direct sign of calcaneonavicular coalition in the lateral radiograph. J Pediatr Orthop 7:709–711, 1987.

103. Olney BW, Asher MA: Excision of symptomatic coalition of the middle facet of the talocalcaneal joint. J Bone Joint Surg 69A:539–544, 1987.

104. O'Rahilly R: A survey of carpal and tarsal anomalies. J Bone Joint Surg 35A:626–642, 1953.

105. O'Rahilly R, Gardner E, Gray DJ: The skeletal development of the foot. Clin Orthop 16:7–14, 1960.

106. Outland T, Murphy ID: Relation of tarsal anomalies to spastic and rigid flatfeet. Clin Orthop 1:217–224, 1953.

107. Outland T, Murphy ID: The pathomechanics of peroneal spatic flat foot. Clin Orthop 16:64–73, 1960.

108. Pearlman HS, Warren RF: Familial tarsal and carpal synostosis with radial-head subluxation (Nievergelt's syndrome). J Bone Joint Surg 46A:585–592, 1964.

109. Perry J: Anatomy and biomechanics of the hindfoot. Clin Orthop 177:9–15, 1983.

110. Pineda C, Resnick D, Greenway G: Diagnosis of tarsal coalition with computed tomography. Clin Orthop 208:282–288, 1986.

111. Pfitzner, W: Die Variationen im Aufbar des Fussekelts Bertrage zur Kenntniss des Menschlichen Extremitatenskelets. VIII Morphol. Arbeit. 6:245, 1896.

112. Pozanski AD, Stern AM, Gall JC Jr: Radiographic findings in the hand-foot-uterus syndrome (HFUS). Radiology 95:129–134, 1970.

113. Rankin EA, Baker GI: Rigid flatfoot in the young adult. Clin Orthop 104:244–248, 1974.

114. Resnick D: Radiology of the talocalcaneal articulation. Radiology 111:581–586, 1974.

115. Resnick D: Additional congenital or heritable anomalies and syndromes. Diagnosis of bone and joint disorders with emphasis on articular abnormalities. *In* Resnick D, Niwayama G (Eds): Diagnosis of Bone and Joint Disorders. Vol. 4. Philadelphia, W. B. Saunders, 1981, pp 2559–2565.

116. Resnick D: Talar ridges, osteophytes, and beaks. A radiographic commentary. Radiology 151:329–332, 1984.

117. Richards RR, Evans JG, McGory PF: Fracture of a calcaneonavicular bar: A complication of tarsal coalition. A case report. Clin Orthop 185:220–221, 1984.

118. Rothberg AS, Feldman JW, Schuster OF: Congenital fusion of astragalus and scaphoid: Bilateral; inherited. NY State J Med 35:29–31, 1935.

119. Sanghi JK, Roby HR: Bilateral peroneal spastic flat feet associated with congenital fusion of the navicular and talus. A case report. J Bone Joint Surg 43A:1237–1240, 1961.

120. Sarno RC, Carter BL, Bankoff MF, Semine MC: Computed tomography in tarsal coalition. J Comput Assist Tomog 8:1155–1160, 1984.

121. Sartorius DJ, Resnick DL: Tarsal coalition. Arthritis Rheum 28:331–338, 1985.

122. Schreiber RR: Talonavicular synostosis. J Bone Joint Surg 45A:170–172, 1963.

123. Scranton PE Jr: Treatment of symptomatic talocalcaneal coalition. J Bone Joint Surg 69A:533–539, 1987.

124. Sells J, Grand N: Cubo-navicular synostosis. J Bone Joint Surg 41B:149, 1959.

125. Shaffer HA Jr, Harrison RB: Tarsal pseudo-coalition—positional artifact. J Can Assoc Radiol 31:236–240, 1980.

126. Shands AR, Wentz IJ: Congenital anomalies, accessory bones, and osteochondritis in the feet of 850 children. Surg Clin North Am 33:1643–1666, 1953.

127. Shereff MJ, Johnston KA: Radiographic anatomy of hindfoot. Clin Orthop 177:16–22, 1983.

128. Simmons EH: Tibialis spastic varus foot with tarsal coalition. J Bone Joint Surg 47B:533–536, 1965.

129. Slomann W: On coalitio calcaneo-navicularis. J Orthop Surg 3:586–602, 1921.

130. Slomann HC: On the demonstration and analysis of calcaneo-navicular coalition by roentgen examination. Acta Radiol 5:304–308, 1926.

131. Smith RW, Staple TW: Computerized tomography (CT) scanning technique for the hindfoot. Clin Orthop 177:34–38, 1983.

132. Snyder RB, Lipscomb HB, Johnston RK: The relationship of tarsal coalitions to ankle sprains in athletes. Am J Sports Med 9:313–317, 1981.

133. Solomon MA, Gilula LA, Oloff LM, et al: CT scanning of the foot and ankle: 1. Normal anatomy. Am J Roentgen 146:1192–1203, 1986.

134. Solomon MA, Gilula LA, Oloff LM, Oloff J: CT scanning of the foot and ankle: 2. Clinical applications and review of the literature. AJR 146:1204–1214, 1986.

135. Steinhauser J: Further ball-type ankle-joints observed in cases of congenital tarsosynostoses. Z Orthop 112:433–438, 1974.

136. Stormont DM, Peterson HA: The relative incidence of tarsal coalition. Clin Orthop 181:28–36, 1983.

137. Stoskopf CA, Hernandez RJ, Kelikian A, et al: Evaluation of tarsal coalition by computed tomography. J Pediatr Orthop 4:365–369, 1984.

138. Sullivan JA: Tarsal coalition. *In* Morrissy RT (Ed): Lovell and Winter's Pediatric Orthopaedics. 3rd Ed. Philadelphia, J.B. Lippincott, 1990, pp 963–969.

139. Sutro CJ: Anomalous talocalcaneal articulation. Cause for limited subtalar movements. Am J Surg 74:64–65, 1947.

140. Swiontkowski MF, Scranton PE, Hansen S: Tarsal coalitions: Long-term results of surgical treatment. J Pediatr Orthop 3:287–292, 1983.

141. Tachdjian MO: Tarsal coalition. *In* Tachdjian MO (Ed): The Child's Foot. Philadelphia, W. B. Saunders, 1985, pp 261–294.

142. Takakura Y, Tamai S, Masuhara K: Genesis of the ball-and-socket ankle. J Bone Joint Surg 68B:834–837, 1986.

143. Trolle D: Accessory bones of the foot: A radiological, histo-embryological, comparative-anatomical, and genetic study. Translated by Aagesen E. Copenhagen, Mundsgaard, 1948.

144. Vaughan WH, Segal G: Tarsal coalition with special reference to roentgenographic interpretation. Radiology 60:855–863, 1953.

145. Veneruso LC: Unilateral congenital calcaneocuboid synostosis with complete absence of a metatarsal and toe. J Bone Joint Surg 27:718–721, 1945.

146. Viladot A, Lorenzo JC, Salazar J, Rodriguez A: The subtalar joint: embryology and morphology. Foot Ankle 5:54–66, 1984.

147. Wagoner GW: A case of bilateral congenital fusion of the calcanei and cuboids. J Bone Joint Surg 10:220–223, 1928.

148. Waugh W: Partial cubo-navicular coalition as a cause of peroneal spastic flat foot. J Bone Joint Surg 39B:520–523, 1957.

149. Webster FS, Roberts WM: Tarsal anomalies and peroneal spastic flat foot. J Am Med Assoc 146:1099–1104, 1951.

150. Weitzner I: Congenital talonavicular synostosis associated with hereditary multiple ankylosis arthropathies. Am J Roentgen 56:185–188, 1946.

151. Wheeler R, Guerva A, Bleck EE: Tarsal coalitions: Review of the literature and case report of bilateral dual calcaneonavicular and talocalcaneal coalitions. Clin Orthop 156:175–177, 1981.

152. Wray JB, Herndon CN: Hereditary transmission of congenital coalition of the calcaneus to the navicular. J Bone Joint Surg 45A:365–372, 1963.

153. Wright DG, Desai SM, Henderson WH: Action of the subtalar and ankle-joint complex during the stance phase of walking. J Bone Joint Surg 46A:361–382, 1964.

154. Wynne-Davies R: Heritable disorders in orthopaedics. Orthop Clin North Am 9:3, 1978.

155. Zeide MS, Wiessel SW, Terry RL: Talonavicular coalition. Clin Orthop 126:225–227, 1977.

156. Zuckerkandl E: Uber Eine Fall von Synastose Zwischen Talus und Calcaneus. Allg Wein Med Zeit 22:293–294, 1877.

45

Pediatric Ankle Fractures and Foot Fractures

JOHN G. THOMETZ

ANKLE FRACTURES

The proper management of physeal injuries of the ankle is important to the orthopaedic surgeon because these injuries are common and have a high rate of complications. The ultimate prognosis for the ankle depends on many factors, including the severity of the trauma, the age of the patient, the degree of displacement of the fracture, the anatomy of the fracture, and the type of treatment. Other factors that have been implicated include a disrupted vascular supply to the fracture, the adequacy and type of reduction, and the type of internal fixation used. Complications include angular deformity, leg length discrepancy, joint incongruity, and combinations of the three. These complications have been recognized for many years. Owen, in 1891,[44] presented a case of a fracture that passed "across the junction cartilage of the tibia" and checked "the due growth of the tibia," leading to marked inversion of the foot. Elmslie, in 1919,[21] described a "scar" across the "epiphyseal line" and theorized that it would lead to a progressive varus deformity.

Physeal injuries of the ankle are common. In a radiographic review of physeal injuries, Rogers[49] found that injuries to the physes of the distal tibia and fibula accounted for 25 percent of their series of physeal injuries; the physis of the distal tibia is the second most common location for injuries to the growth plate (second only to the distal radius). These fractures generally occur between the ages of 10 and 15 years.[56] It has been recognized since the time of Poland[46] in 1898 that pediatric ankle fractures are different from adult ankle injuries in that the physis is the area of weakness. Injuries to the ligaments are extremely rare in children.[48]

Anatomy

The horizontal portion of the distal tibial epiphysis begins to ossify during the first several months after birth.[43] The medial malleolus begins to ossify around the age of 6 years. An accessory epiphysis of the medial malleolus may be seen but should not be mistaken for a fracture. This accessory epiphysis can be seen in up to 15 percent of cases.[26, 47] Radiographic views of the opposite ankle may be helpful in confirming this appearance, along with stress views. At 2 years of age, widening of the distal tibial epiphysis develops just medial to the midline. This creates an indentation in the metaphysis and creates an irregular contour to the growth plate. Owing to this anatomic development, fractures through the distal tibial physis with displacement are extremely rare unless there is an associated fracture of the metaphysis or fibular shaft. The epiphysis fuses with the metaphysis at the age of 15 in females and 16 in males.[43] The physis closes centrally at first and then medially. Finally, the lateral aspect of the physis closes. This process occurs over a period of about 18 months (Fig. 45–1). During this time, an anterolateral fragment of the distal tibial epiphysis may be displaced traumatically; this is the so-called Tillaux frac-

FIGURE 45–1. Progression of fusion at the physis of the distal tibia.

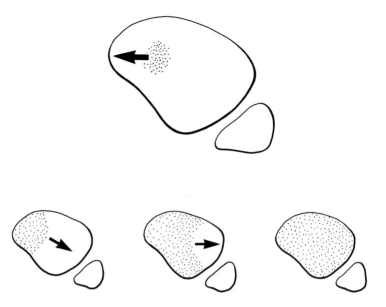

ture.[54] (Ashhurst and Bromer[2] analyzed Tillaux's description of the fracture and concluded that the fracture of Tillaux is actually a fracture of the anterior tibial tubercle.) This pattern of physeal closure, which results in areas of relative strength and weakness, accounts for the fracture pattern of the triplane fracture in the sagittal, coronal, and axial planes.

Classification Systems

One difficulty in reviewing the results of pediatric ankle fractures is that multiple classification systems have been devised to evaluate the fracture patterns. These systems can be broadly divided into two groups: pathomechanic and anatomic. In 1922, Ashhurst and Bromer,[2] in a classic paper, presented the four major causes of pediatric physeal injuries: external rotation, abduction, adduction, and axial compression. In 1932, Bishop[4] modified the classification system and subdivided it into further groups. In 1950, Lauge-Hansen[34] proposed a new classification system based on his experimental observations in which the classification of the fracture could be determined by the position of the foot at the time of trauma and the direction of the abnormal forces. The Lauge-Hansen[34] system was modified for use in the description of pediatric injuries by Gerner-Schmidt[23] and Dias and Tachdjian.[18] No

method of classifying pediatric ankle fractures appears entirely satisfactory; Rang[48] has objected to the pathomechanic classification system, saying it is "conjectural" and difficult for people to agree about the direction of force at the time of injury. The Dias and Tachdjian modification appears to be gaining more popularity and general acceptance; therefore, for the most part, it will be used here as an aid in describing principles of treatment.

Pathomechanic Classification

In 1978, Dias and Tachdjian[18] reviewed 71 cases of ankle fracture and classified them into the following groups.

Supination-Inversion. An inversion force is applied to the supinated foot with two grades of severity: stage 1, displacement of the distal fibular epiphysis (usually quite minimal), and stage 2, an associated Salter-Harris type III or IV fracture of the tibial epiphysis (Fig. 45–2). These injuries have gained a reputation for having a high incidence of subsequent physeal injury, which has often been attributed to a compression injury of the medial growth plate. It also has been noted that this fracture tends to occur in younger children, therefore leaving a greater potential for a serious residual deformity. Supination-inversion injuries account for roughly 15 percent of cases.

Supination–Plantar Flexion. Plantar flexion force is applied to the supinated foot, resulting

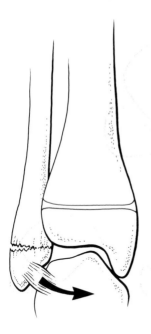
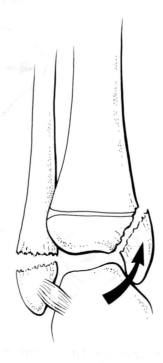

FIGURE 45–2. Supination-inversion, stages I and II.

FIGURE 45–3. Supination–plantar flexion.

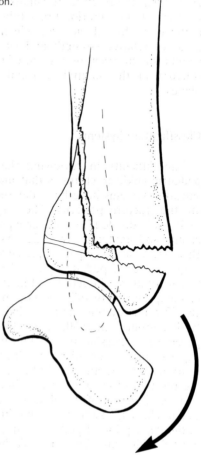

FIGURE 45–4. Supination–external rotation.

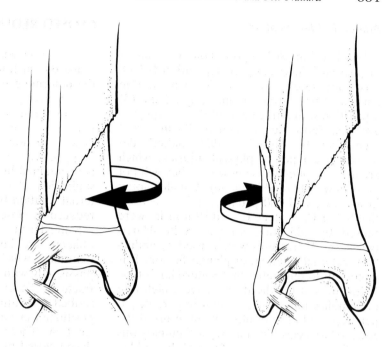

in a Salter-Harris type II fracture of the distal tibial epiphysis with a posterior metaphyseal fragment and posterior displacement of the fracture (Fig. 45–3). Usually a fracture of the

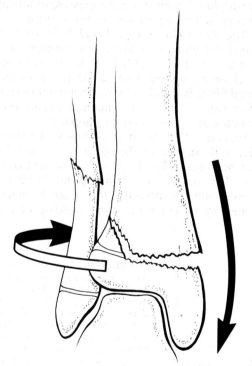

FIGURE 45–5. Pronation–eversion–external rotation.

fibula does not occur. This injury is seen in about 12 percent of cases.

Supination–External Rotation. Supination–external rotation fractures, which represent approximately 25 percent of cases, result when the supinated foot is subjected to an external rotation force. There are two stages: the stage 1 fracture results in a Salter-Harris type II fracture of the distal tibial epiphysis, which starts laterally at the physis and runs proximally and medially. The stage 2 fracture results when the external rotation force continues and produces a spiral fracture of the fibula that begins medially and runs superiorly and posteriorly (Fig. 45–4). Displacement is generally in a posterior direction.

Pronation–Eversion–External Rotation. Finally, the pronation–eversion–external rotation fracture results when the pronated foot is everted and externally rotated. This is the most common mechanism, occurring in about 40 percent of cases. In this fracture, the tibial and fibular fractures occur simultaneously, resulting in a Salter-Harris type II fracture of the distal tibial epiphysis with the metaphyseal fragment on the lateral side and a transverse fibular fracture 4 to 7 cm above the tip of the lateral malleolus (Fig. 45–5). (Excluded from the classification system are the so-called Tillaux fracture and the triplane fracture, which are discussed later.)

Anatomic Classification

Foucher,[22] in 1863, reported on three classes of physeal injury: (1) pure separation (which was quite rare), (2) separation with a thin lamella of bone from the metaphysis, and (3) separation with a fragment off the metaphysis. This was further elaborated by Poland[46] and then again by Aitkin[1] in 1936. Salter[50] described five types of physeal injuries, which are in such common use now that they will not be reviewed here (Fig. 45–6). Canale[8] noted in his review of 100 pediatric ankle fractures that Salter-Harris type III and IV injuries were caused by adduction injuries; Salter-Harris type I and II fractures were caused by abduction, external rotation, or plantar flexion. It is important to remember that Salter-Harris type II fractures of the distal tibia have a high rate of complications. Since several important papers reported their results only in terms of the Salter-Harris classification, we will employ this classification as necessary. Ogden[42] has added a type VI injury to the peripheral physis, which may result in peripheral bridge formation. The type VII injury involves only the medial malleolus (not the physis or weight-bearing areas).

MacNealy and colleagues[37] reviewed fracture patterns in the distal tibial epiphysis of 194 cases of these injuries and studied the incidence of the various types of Salter-Harris fractures. The most common fracture in their series was the Salter-Harris type II (46 percent). Salter-Harris type III fractures constituted 25 percent; Salter-Harris type IV, 10 percent; triplane, 10 percent; and Salter-Harris type I, 6 percent. They also analyzed the fractures as to the mechanism of injury, and the breakdown was as follows: external rotation, 41 percent (Salter-Harris type II, 17 percent; Tillaux, 14 percent; triplane, 10 percent); adduction, 22 percent; plantar flexion, 17 percent; abduction, 14 percent; and miscellaneous, 6 percent.

CLOSED REDUCTION

With knowledge of the mechanism of injury, a closed reduction can be achieved by reversing the deforming forces. For example, the supination-inversion injury is reduced by traction and eversion of the foot. With supination–plantar flexion injuries, the foot is plantar-flexed, traction is applied, and anterior force is applied to the distal fragment. The reduction is maintained by dorsiflexion of the foot. The supination–plantar flexion and supination–external rotation fractures can almost always be reduced by closed techniques.

Salter-Harris type I fractures of the distal tibia are rare, but they may result in a rotatory deformity, which can occur through the distal physis only with no metaphyseal or epiphyseal fractures. Several case reports[6, 7, 41] have described this injury, in which the foot can be positioned at 60 degrees or more of external rotation. These fractures usually can be reduced closed by internal rotation of the foot. To avoid injury to the physis, the reduction should always be done under general anesthesia. The knee and the ankle should be flexed to relax the gastrocnemius-soleus. The reduction should be performed gently. As Carothers and Crenshaw[9] noted, "Accurate reposition of the displaced epiphysis at the expense of forced or repeated manipulations is not justified."

The Salter-Harris type I and II injuries of the distal fibula should be immobilized in a cast for 3 to 4 weeks. Ogden[42] described a case of chronic epiphyseolysis of the physis of the distal fibula in a child who was not immobilized after injury and who remained persistently symptomatic until a cast was applied.

Fractures that result in a displaced Salter-Harris II fracture of the distal tibia generally can be handled by closed reduction and casting. The mechanism of injury should be reversed, and the corrective forces can be maintained by proper three-point molding of the

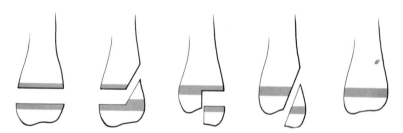

FIGURE 45–6. The Salter-Harris classification of epiphyseal injuries *(left to right)*: type I, through the growth plate; type II, through the plate with the metaphyseal fragment; type III, through the plate with the epiphyseal fragment into the joint; type IV, through the metaphysis and epiphysis; type V, crush injury of the growth plate.

plaster. In the displaced Salter-Harris type II fracture, it is possible for the anterior tibial tendon and neurovascular bundle to become trapped between fragments during reduction.[24] The dorsalis pedis pulse should be checked before and after reduction. A long-leg bent-knee cast should be applied for 6 to 8 weeks. If there is significant swelling at the time of initial cast application, the cast should be changed in a week, after the swelling has subsided, to prevent loss of reduction. The parents should be made aware of the high incidence of physeal injuries in these Salter-Harris type II injuries of the distal tibia.[31, 51] The rotational alignment of the foot after reduction should be with the uninjured side in order to prevent torsional problems. Some residual displacement, particularly in the anteroposterior direction, can be tolerated, but appreciable varus or valgus in the older child will not remodel. If this varus or valgus angulation persists after closed reduction, then an open reduction should be performed.

In a certain number of patients (particularly those with the pronation–eversion–external rotation injury), an interposed piece of periosteum can prevent completion of the closed reduction. There is some controversy as to what to do when this periosteum is interposed. Weber and Sussenbach[58] believed that if the patient was an adolescent, an open reduction should be carried out because the interposed fragment would cause valgus at the fracture site that would not be able to remodel. In the younger child, when the interposed flap is small and there is significant growth remaining, it is more likely that the valgus will resolve with time. However, Dias[19] presented a case of a 10-year-old child with interposed soft tissue that created an initial valgus deformity at the ankle of 12 degrees, which progressed over several months to 17 degrees, requiring a supramalleolar osteotomy. Karrholm and colleagues[28] believed strongly that the interposed periosteum would not lead to further problems over time and would remodel. The preferred approach in the younger child may be controversial, but it is perhaps best to perform an open reduction when there is significant valgus present as the child approaches adolescence. If the fracture is thought to be unstable after removal of the periosteal fragment, it should be stabilized with the use of a lag screw across the metaphysis.

Some controversy surrounds the appropriate management of the Salter-Harris type III and IV fractures of the medial malleolus. If physeal damage results from a Salter-Harris type III or IV fracture of the medial malleolus, a progressive varus deformity can result. Mc-Farland[39] found that varus was a common complication of this injury, and Aitkin[1] believed that this occurred in about 40 percent of all injuries of this type. Because the supination-inversion injury has such a high incidence of physeal injuries, one should particularly strive for an excellent reduction of this fracture. It is generally agreed that fractures with displacement of greater than 2 mm should be reduced. In 1978, Spiegel and colleagues[51] reviewed 237 cases, and 35 patients had a slightly displaced or nondisplaced Salter-Harris type III or IV fracture, with only one case of asymmetrical closure of the growth plate. They concluded that up to 2 mm of displacement was acceptable. Dias also agreed with this approach. However, the data of Kling and colleagues[31] raise the question of whether even 2 mm of displacement is too much. In their series, three children who had 2 mm or less of displacement developed a physeal arrest. These patients had also an associated persistent rotational malalignment of the medial epiphyseal fragment. Kling and colleagues noted that closed treatment resulted in a high incidence of physeal arrest. Their statistical analysis showed that an anatomic reduction of the physis markedly decreased the probability of partial physeal growth arrest. Although some of these physeal injuries may conceivably be due to a compression injury (Salter-Harris type V), in light of the documented reports of growth arrest developing in children left with less than 2 mm of displacement, I believe that it is safest to accept only an anatomic reduction for the Salter-Harris type III and IV fractures as a result of a supination-inversion injury. (The triplane and Tillaux fractures are discussed later.)

Surgical Management

Operative Technique

For open reduction, the patient should be supine, and a tourniquet is utilized. A gently curved incision is made over the medial malleolus, with the anterior border centered over the fracture site. Care should be taken to avoid the long saphenous vein and the two adjacent

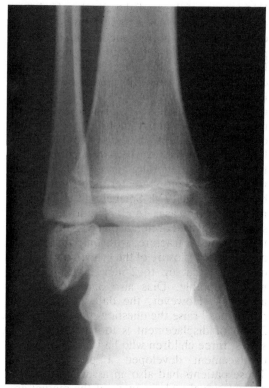

FIGURE 45–7. Preoperative view of an undisplaced supination-inversion injury.

branches of the saphenous nerve. Injury to the saphenous nerve may result in a painful neuroma. After the capsule is opened, the joint should be irrigated to remove any loose osteo-cartilaginous fragments, and a curette may be needed to gently remove a clot from the fracture fragments to allow an anatomic reduction. The exposure should be sufficient to visualize the fracture within the epiphysis and its extension through the physis (Salter-Harris type III) or metaphysis (Salter-Harris type IV). Some authors have recommended removing the metaphyseal fragment to better visualize the reduction; I have been concerned that the removal of this fragment in itself may cause injury to the physis, so I have never removed it.

Once the fracture is reduced, there are several methods of internal fixation. Some authors still recommend using smooth Kirschner wires extending up the medial malleolus, across the physis, and into the metaphysis. Kling and others have noted that bar formation can result even from the placement of smooth pins across the physis. Therefore, this method is to be avoided unless absolutely necessary. Others believe that the use of two smooth pins that either diverge or converge (within the epiphysis) would stabilize the fragment sufficiently. It is my belief that these fractures are best managed by screw fixation in order to apply compressive forces across the fracture site[52]; the fragment is less likely to migrate with screw fixation than if smooth pins are used. After anatomic reduction of the fracture has been achieved, the drill is directed under fluoroscopic control across the fracture site, staying within the epiphysis. Fluoroscopy is used to prevent damage to the physis and to avoid entering the joint. A cancellous screw is generally used to achieve compression and maintain the reduction. The screw should not be excessively tightened or distortion of the reduction may occur. At the time of screw removal, I have had the experience of one case in which the screw fractured within the epiphysis at the junction of the threads and shaft (Figs. 45–7 to 45–9). I have recently used a cortical screw (and washer) in a case in which the fracture fragment was overdrilled to allow

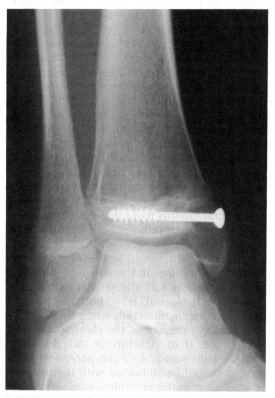

FIGURE 45–8. Reduction and stabilization of the injury in Figure 45–7.

FIGURE 45–9. After attempted screw removal (see Fig. 45–8).

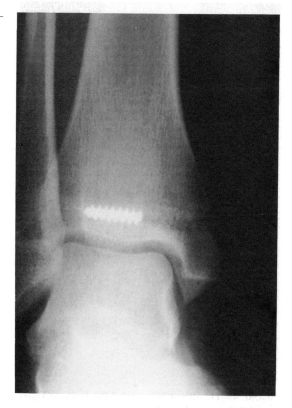

FIGURE 45–10. Displaced supination-inversion injury.

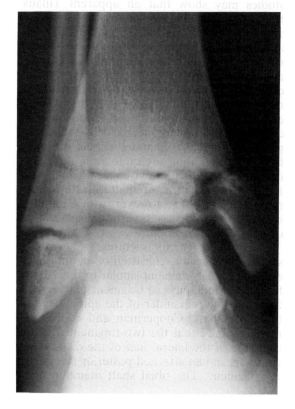

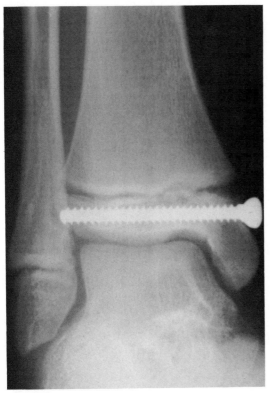

FIGURE 45–11. After stabilization of the injury in Figure 45–10 with a cortical screw.

for compression across the fracture site (Figs. 45–10 and 45–11). The limb is then placed in a long-leg nonwalking cast for 1 month, followed by a short-leg walking cast for 3 weeks.

The patient with a physeal injury should be followed up for at least 2 years in order to check for physeal arrest, as in some cases physeal injury has not been detected until 18 months after injury or later.[31]

Triplane Fracture

Rang[48] summarizes the difficulty in interpreting triplane fracture patterns from radiographs with the statement that "everyone agrees the fracture lines run in three planes, but beyond this, there is uncertainty." Von Laer[56] stated that this fracture "strains the spatial imagination of the surgeon." Discussions of this fracture in the literature have been contradictory. In 1970, Marmor[38] presented the first case report of this fracture, which was given the descriptive term *triplane* in 1972.[37] Cooperman and colleagues,[13] with the aid of computed tomography (CT), be-

lieved that most fractures were composed of two fragments rather than the three parts described by Marmor. On the other hand, Dias and Giegerich[17] documented that the majority of their patients had three fragments (Fig. 45–12). Whether the patient develops a two- or three-part fracture depends on the maturity of the distal physis. Only when the physis is open can a three-part triplane fracture occur. However, if the medial portion of the physis is closed, a two-fragment fracture will result. The triplane fracture is thought to result from an external rotation force on the ankle.[17] Therefore, closed reduction is achieved by internal rotation of the foot followed by application of a long-leg cast. Although originally described as an extremely rare injury, it may be more common than previously thought. Landin and Danielsson[32] found that the triplane and Tillaux's fractures were the third and fourth most common types of pediatric ankle fractures in their series. Transitional fractures (triplane and Tillaux's fractures) generally occur between 10 and 15 years of age. In patients younger than 10 years of age, usually only medial malleolar fractures occur.[56]

Tomography and CT are very helpful in assessing the alignment of the fracture fragments (Fig. 45–13).[10, 27] Occasionally, these studies may show that an apparent Tillaux fracture is actually a triplane fracture. The CT scan may reveal more displacement than that apparent from the plain films. These special studies are key in differentiating between two- and three-part fractures, which is an important distinction because the three-part fracture is more likely to require surgery. If there is any question of the status of the reduction in a child who has undergone a closed reduction, postreduction CT scanning should be performed. Tomograms are quite accurate, but it may be more difficult to visualize mentally and to reconstruct the fracture pattern with tomography than with CT; however, with CT it may be more difficult to assess vertical displacement of the fracture fragments.

The three-fragment fractures,[38, 45, 55] as described by Marmor, consisted of an anterolateral epiphyseal fragment similar to the Tillaux fracture, a metaphyseal fragment that was attached to the remainder of the epiphysis, and the tibial shaft. Cooperman and colleagues' review[13] noted that the two-fragment fracture consisted of the lateral half of the distal tibial epiphysis and an attached posterior metaphyseal fragment. The tibial shaft maintained its

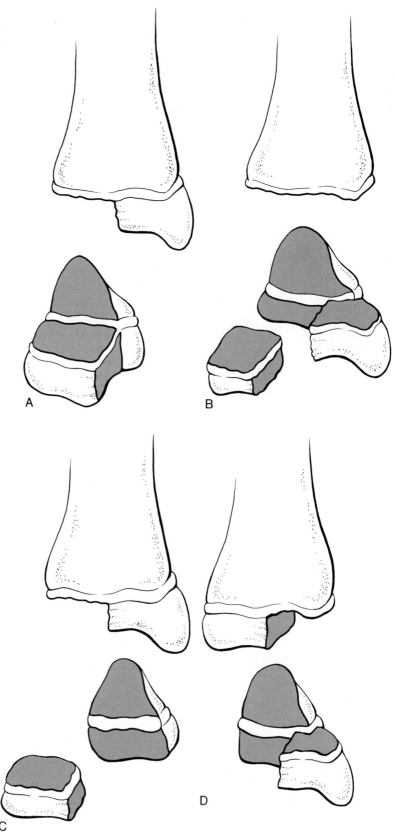

FIGURE 45–12. Various patterns of triplane fractures. *(A)*, Two-part triplane fracture. *(B)*, Classic three-part triplane fracture. *(C)*, Variant three-part pattern. *(D)*, Medial triplane fracture.

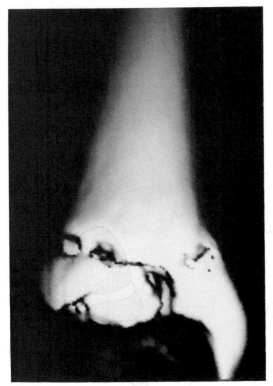

FIGURE 45–13. Three-dimensional reconstruction after computed tomograpy for triplane fracture.

attachment to the medial half of the distal tibial epiphysis. It is unusual to see an associated fibular fracture with the triplane injury.[45]

Von Laer's[56] analysis concluded that the type of fracture that developed depended on the maturity of the epiphyseal plate. The location of the fracture line in the epiphysis correlated with the patient's age; in the more immature patients, with an open medial physis, the fracture line occurs more medially (Fig. 45–14). Occasionally the fracture line may run within the malleolus itself, not involving the weight-bearing surface of the tibia. When the medial portion of the physis is closed, the fracture line runs more laterally through the epiphysis.

Other types of the triplane fracture have been revealed by drawing CT studies. Cone[12] described a variant of the classic three-part fracture that consisted of (1) a free anterolateral epiphyseal fragment, (2) the posterior metaphysis and posterior epiphysis, and (3) the tibial shaft and anteromedial portion of the epiphysis. Denton and Fischer's two-part triplane variant[16] consisted of the tibial shaft and anterolateral epiphyses, and a posterior metaphyseal spike combined with the antero-medial and posterior epiphysis.

Because patients with the two-fragment fracture are generally so close to skeletal maturity, the risk for significant shortening or angulation is small, and the main priority for achieving an anatomic reduction is to prevent the development of degenerative changes within the ankle joint. Cooperman believed that up to 2 mm of displacement could be tolerated; if there is more displacement than this, closed reduction is usually successful. When there is an associated fracture of the fibula, often the two-part fracture cannot be reduced until the fibula is reduced. Von Laer stated that it is unusual for this fracture to have more than 2 mm of displacement. Therefore, open reduction is rarely needed.

Operative Technique for the Classic Triplane Fracture. In order to achieve a satisfactory reduction of the three-fragment triplane fracture, the posteromedial fragment, when displaced, must be reduced first. The reduction is achieved by internal rotation of the foot. Assuming the reduction of the posteromedial fragment is successful, the reduction should be maintained with a cancellous screw. The surgical approach then is anterolateral. The incision begins 1 inch above the ankle joint and curves slightly laterally as it proceeds approximately 1 inch distal to the ankle joint. The extensor tendons along with the neurovascular bundle are protected on the medial border of the incision. After the joint is opened, the anterolateral fragment is reduced under direct visualization anatomically. A cancellous screw is used to maintain the reduction; the screw should not cross the physis.

If the posteromedial fragment is not reduced by closed methods, a medial incision over the distal metaphysis is necessary to reduce this fragment, after which the fracture is held reduced with a screw. Then the anterolateral fragment is reduced and internally fixed. The patient is then placed in a long-leg bent-knee cast for 1 month without weight bearing.

Tillaux's Fracture

Tillaux's fracture actually was initially described by Cooper,[2, 25] and the first large series was that of Kleiger and Mankin.[30] The mechanism of injury is thought by most authors to be an external rotation force to the foot. This causes the anterior inferior tibiofibular liga-

FIGURE 45–14. (A to D), Possible variations in the position of the epiphyseal fracture lines as seen on an anteroposterior radiograph.

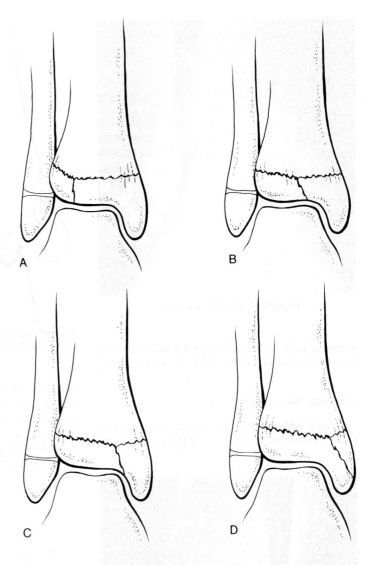

ment to avulse the anterolateral portion of the distal tibial epiphysis, and the fracture is usually displaced either laterally or anterolaterally. The fracture usually occurs in patients who are close to skeletal maturity, in whom the central portion of the physis is closed. Therefore, the risk of clinically significant problems from physeal injury is extremely low, and the chief concern is the maintenance of articular congruity. The radiographs should be examined carefully, as occasionally an apparent Tillaux fracture is actually a triplane fracture. The Tillaux fracture may be missed if it overlaps the fibula.[35] The amount of displacement can easily be underestimated. Internal rotation of the foot usually achieves a satisfactory reduction, although a periosteal flap may

block reduction.[20] After reduction, a long-leg cast is applied with the foot in internal rotation.

Some authors believe that the reduction is satisfactory when there is up to 2 mm of residual displacement. However, the occasional fracture is displaced in an anteroinferior direction, and in this case 2 mm of displacement may lead to osteoarthritis; therefore, anatomic reduction is desirable. Another concern regarding the displaced fracture is diastasis of the anterior tibiofibular joint, which has been documented with this injury.

Although fixation has been described with both smooth pins and a cancellous screw, screw fixation would seem to be most secure. Because this patient is so close to skeletal maturity, it makes little difference whether the

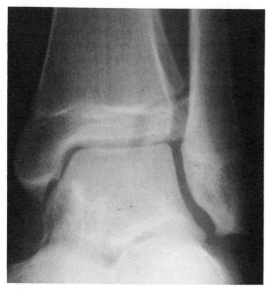

FIGURE 45–15. Tillaux fracture.

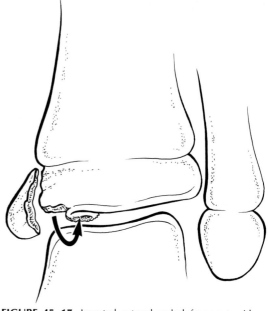

FIGURE 45–17. Inverted osteochondral fragment with a Salter type III fracture.

screw is kept within the epiphysis or crosses the residual physis (Figs. 45–15 and 45–16).

Miscellaneous Injuries

Several other rare injuries may require surgical treatment. Recently, Beaty and Linton[3]

described a child with a Salter-Harris type III fracture of the ankle that had an associated osteochondral fragment that was inverted in the joint and hinged on its cartilage (Fig. 45–17). In this case, the small fragment was excised. Danielsson[15] had a series of five children

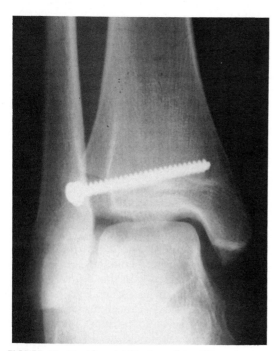

FIGURE 45–16. After stabilization of the Tillaux fracture (see Fig. 45–15).

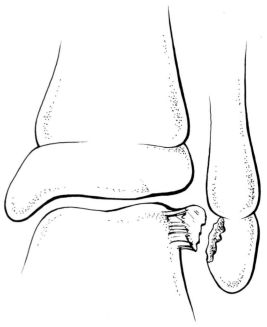

FIGURE 45–18. Bony fragment attached to the anterior talofibular ligament.

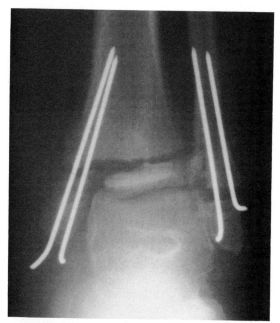

FIGURE 45–19. Radiograph of severe open ankle fracture-dislocation complicated by sepsis, which required multiple débridements before infection was controlled.

who had recurrent symptoms after ankle injuries. They had an osseous fragment that was attached to the anterior talofibular ligament, which was believed to be the cause of their pain. Excision of this fragment resulted in relief of symptoms (Fig. 45–18). Very rarely, the intra-articular tip of the medial or lateral malleolus may become significantly displaced and may not respond to closed reduction; open reduction may then be necessary. Inversion injuries to the ankle may disrupt the tibiofibular ligaments and lead to a tibiofibular synostosis, which becomes symptomatic with activity.[40]

Complications

Physeal injury may lead to progressive angular deformity, leg length discrepancy, or combinations of both (Figs. 45–19 and 45–20). Growth arrest is a well-known complication, and the resultant deformity has been described for over 100 years. As noted earlier, the supination-inversion injury is particularly prone to this complication; growth arrest can occur even after anatomic reduction. Although there are rare reports of spontaneous disruption of a small bony bar,[11] more frequently a small bony

bridge tends to enlarge with time. The distal tibial physis is a common location for the development of a partial growth arrest; in Bright's[5] series of 225 patients surgically treated for a bony bar, the distal tibial physis constituted 26 percent of cases.

Once a growth arrest is evident, proper radiographic assessment is essential to determine the proper treatment.[10, 53] Hypocycloidal tomography, with cuts taken at 3 mm in both the anteroposterior and lateral directions, is critical. CT scans may be useful, but in my experience they are more difficult to interpret. With hypocycloidal tomography, one can construct a map of the physis and determine the cross-sectional area of the bony bridge relative to the cross-sectional area of the entire physis. Bar excision should not be performed if the bar constitutes 50 percent or more of the area of the physis, as it is very unlikely that it will be successful in this case. If significant angular deformity is present, the patient should be positioned in such a fashion so that the tomograms can be taken perpendicular to the plane of the physis; if not, the extent of the bridge may be overestimated.

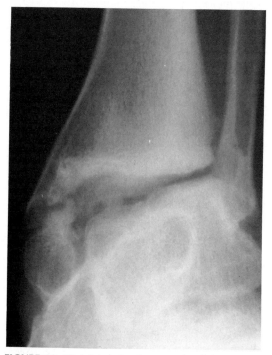

FIGURE 45–20. Joint destruction, angular deformity, and shortening resulting from the conditions in Figure 45–19. The patient had significant pain, and an arthrodesis was performed.

Three types of growth arrest have been identified: peripheral, central, and combined. Tomography will identify the type of lesion and the location. Knowledge of the location is needed to plan the proper approach. The child should have at least 2 years of growth remaining if a bar excision is planned. To summarize, the appropriate therapy for a partial growth arrest of the distal tibia depends on the patient's age and on the location, type, and size of the bridge.

As noted by Cass and Peterson,[10] the options for treatment of growth arrest in this location are varied. One may perform a closure of the remaining open physis of the distal tibia in conjunction with epiphyseodesis of the ipsilateral fibula and contralateral distal tibial and fibular physes. A common method in the past was to perform repeated opening wedge osteotomies to correct recurring deformity,[29] but this method is less desirable today. Osteotomies may be required in conjunction with other procedures when a significant angular deformity is present (especially if the angulation is 20 degrees or greater). If the patient is near maturity, no treatment may be required. Bar resection has been shown[33] to allow resumption of normal growth from the distal tibial physis along with the correction of minor angular deformities.

Angular deformities may also be due to malunion rather than to growth arrest. Minor degrees of deformity in the younger child may resolve spontaneously; in the older child, supramalleolar osteotomy may be necessary. Leg length discrepancies following physeal injury are not infrequent, but the ultimate discrepancy is usually less than 2 cm. If the discrepancy is predicted to be within the range of 2 to 4 cm, an epiphyseodesis of the contralateral proximal tibia and fibular physis can be performed. For discrepancies greater than this, leg lengthening should be considered.

FOOT FRACTURES

Anatomy

There are numerous anatomic variants of the foot that may mimic fractures. As many as 20 percent of children have accessory bones, some of which become symptomatic after trauma[72, 73] (Fig. 45–21). The most common accessory tarsal bones, in order of frequency,

are as follows: os trigonum, 13 percent; os tibiale externum, 10 percent; os fibula, 10 percent; os intermetatarseum, 9 percent; os sustentaculi, 5 percent; and os vesalianum. Occasionally, these may be confused with fractures or surgical lesions; thus, comparison views are helpful.

Talar Fractures

In order to understand the principles of treatment and complication of fractures of the talus, one must appreciate the anatomy of its blood supply (Fig. 45–22). The posterior tibial artery gives a branch to the artery of the tarsal canal, which, in turn, gives branches to the body of the talus, with the largest branches entering the middle of the body. The artery of the tarsal canal then develops an anastomosis with the artery of the tarsal sinus. The dorsalis pedis artery sends branches to the superior surface of the neck. The dorsalis pedis artery gives off a lateral tarsal branch, which communicates with a branch of the perforating peroneal artery to form the artery of the tarsal sinus. This also provides branches to the body of the talus. Small branches from the peroneal artery supply the posterior tubercle area of the talus. The surface of the talus is primarily cartilaginous, and if these vascular branches are significantly compromised, then the bone is at high risk for development of avascular necrosis.[62]

Pediatric talar neck fractures are rare.[61, 79, 80] Hawkins[66] developed a classification system that has been used for talar fractures in adults; it has been adopted by Canale[60] and others and is now generally accepted for evaluation of the pediatric fractures. Type 1 is a minimally displaced fracture through the talar neck. Type 2 is a talar neck fracture with subluxation or dislocation at the subtalar joint. Type 3 combines talar neck fractures with subluxation or dislocation at both the subtalar and ankle joints. Canale has described a type 4 talar neck fracture, which is identical to type 3 but with the addition of dislocation of the talar head from the navicular. The higher the type, the greater the rate of the avascular necrosis. However, Letts and Gibeault[69] noted that there can be an appreciable incidence of avascular necrosis even in the nondisplaced fractures.

For treatment of these fractures, closed reduction and the application of a cast are usually

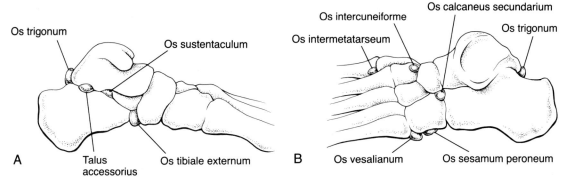

FIGURE 45–21. Medial *(A)* and lateral *(B)* views of the supernumerary tarsal bones.

sufficient. A closed reduction usually can be achieved by plantarflexing and everting the forefoot. A long-leg bent-knee cast is applied with the foot immobilized in plantar flexion and some eversion. One must carefully evaluate the reduction radiographically in order to assess the presence of a varus deformity. In Canale's technique,[60] the foot is maximally plantarflexed and is pronated 15 degrees, and the radiographic beam is directed cephalad at a 75-degree angle from the horizontal (Fig. 45–23). Canale considers a reduction acceptable if there is less than 5 mm of displacement and less than 5 degrees of angulation. In the pediatric population, however, 5 mm may be too much to accept.

If closed reduction is unacceptable, the recommended surgical approach is through a dorsal incision medial to the extensor hallucis longus. The medial aspect of the neck is exposed just enough to achieve reduction, the neurovascular bundle is retracted laterally, and a screw is inserted in order to maintain the reduction. The child needs to be followed long enough to see whether avascular necrosis appears. Hawkins' line is a subchondral lucency beneath the dome of the talus that develops several months after injury and generally indicates that avascular necrosis will not develop. However, it occasionally will not be seen in the child who has been immobilized for only a short period of time. A bone scan can be helpful in questionable cases. Treatment of avascular necrosis is by prolonged non–weight bearing or weight bearing through a patellar tendon–bearing brace.[61]

Fractures of the dome or body of the talus are intra-articular fractures and, as such, need to be reduced anatomically. Rang[74] has recommended multiple Kirschner wire fixation for

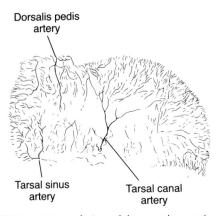

FIGURE 45–22. Lateral view of the vascular supply of the middle third of the talus.

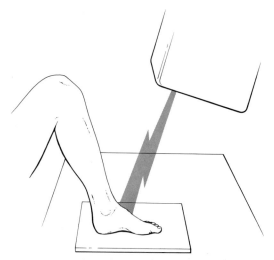

FIGURE 45–23. The technique of Canale to determine the position of fracture at the talar neck (see text).

maintaining a reduction of fractures of the body of the talus. Achievement of anatomic reduction may occasionally require an osteotomy of the medial malleolus, although usually an anteromedial approach provides sufficient exposure to achieve reduction. If an osteotomy of the medial malleolus is performed, care must be taken not to injure the physis.

Another fracture that usually requires surgical treatment is the fracture of the lateral process of the talus. Rang[74] recommends excision of the lateral process, whereas Weber and Sussenbach[82] recommend open reduction and internal fixation in the older child, as this is an intra-articular injury.

Fractures of the posterior process of the talus may be confused with an os trigonum. Weber and Sussenbach[82] recommend open reduction and internal fixation. However, this probably should be undertaken only if the fragment is displaced and involves a significant portion of the articular surface of the dome of the talus.

Calcaneal Fractures

It is generally believed that the need for operative intervention for calcaneal fractures in children is extremely rare. Several studies in the literature evaluate the long-term prognosis. Schmidt and Weiner[78] reviewed 59 fractures and found that, in contrast to the adult population,[64] only 37 percent were intra-articular and 63 percent were extra-articular. The intra-articular fractures are usually either the tongue type or joint depression type (Fig. 45–24). Rasmussen and Schantz[75] found that 34 percent of their patients sustained intra-articular injuries. The predominance of extra-artic-

ular fractures was attributed to the resiliency of the cartilage and soft tissue. Stress fractures of the calcaneus can occur even in the very young child.[59, 63, 72]

Wiley and Profitt[84] found that involvement of the posterior subtalar joint was common in their series, occurring in 28 of 32 fractures of the os calcis in children. Essentially every study has reported severely deformed cases with the use of conservative treatment for calcaneal fractures. A long-term study by Schantz and Rasmussen[77] found that occasionally children can have residual heel tenderness and an increase in width of the calcaneus, often with marked restriction in the range of motion of the subtalar joint. They also noted slight subtalar arthrosis developing in significant tongue fractures. Nonetheless, these problems were thought to be fairly insignificant, for operative intervention was not recommended. Some pediatric patients have shown remodeling of fractures of the calcaneus with an improvement in Böhler's angle over time.[65] Weber and Sussenbach,[82] on the other hand, were of the opinion that intra-articular fractures required open reduction and internal fixation.

My recommendation for patients in the younger age group is conservative treatment, whereas in patients within several years of skeletal maturity who have significant intra-articular injury, the calcaneal fracture can be treated operatively, in a manner similar to that used in the adult population. CT scans are helpful in assessing the more difficult cases.

Tarsometatarsal Injuries

These injuries are rare and are easily missed. Experimentally, it has been shown that the

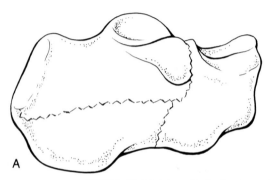 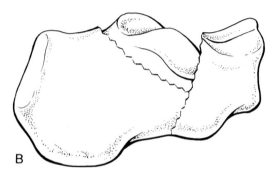

FIGURE 45–24. Intra-articular fractures. *(A),* Tongue type. *(B),* Joint depression type.

FIGURE 45–25. Common mechanism of injury to the base of the metatarsal.

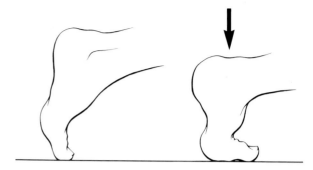

mechanism of injury is forceful plantar flexion of the forefoot combined with rotation; Wilson[85] maintained that a crushing injury alone would not produce dislocation. Gross,[65] however, believed that plantar displacement of the metatarsals could rarely be produced by a falling object. Wiley and Profitt[84] described several mechanisms of injury: landing in the tiptoe position after a jump from a height; a marked compressive load to the heel while the patient is in the kneeling position; and a fall backward while the forefoot is fixed to the ground (Fig. 45–25).

The metatarsal bases are all in the same plane with exception of the second metatarsal, whose base lies more proximally. Therefore, the base of the second metatarsal tends to stabilize the tarsometatarsal joints. If a fracture is present at the base of the second metatarsal, a significant tarsometatarsal joint injury has occurred.

In Wiley's series, all patients were treated with closed reduction, and four of seven had Kirschner wire fixation for 4 weeks. However, in several fractures, they did accept less than a complete reduction and made no attempt to anatomically reduce intra-articular fractures. Several patients were symptomatic at follow-up. In weight-bearing joints, therefore, it seems advisable to perform an open reduction if the dislocation cannot be completely reduced by closed manipulation or if there is significant intra-articular incongruity. Residual dorsal subluxation will produce a painful prominence on the dorsum of the foot.[81] If open reduction is undertaken, one must take care not to injure the physis at the base of the first metatarsal. Such an injury at an early age may lead to a markedly shortened first ray or angular deformity.

The swelling of the foot that occurs with this injury is severe. In the nondisplaced or very minimally displaced fracture, a splint should be applied, the foot elevated, and a short-leg cast applied after several days. Reduction must be performed shortly after injury, or swelling will make reduction difficult. If the closed reduction appears unstable, percutaneous Kirschner wire fixation should be added. The base of the second metatarsal should be fixed, and in more unstable cases, the base of the first and fifth metatarsals should be stabilized also.

Metatarsal Fractures

Fractures of the metatarsal shaft and neck can generally be treated closed (Fig. 45–26). Minimally displaced fractures require about 1 month in a short-leg walking cast. If the fractures are significantly displaced, Chinese finger traps can be helpful in achieving reduction, followed by application of a short-leg cast. The cast should be well molded over the plantar and dorsal aspects of the foot. When the reduction is not stable, a small incision should be made over the fracture site, and the fracture

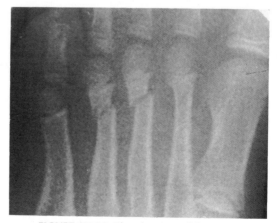

FIGURE 45–26. Closed metatarsal fractures.

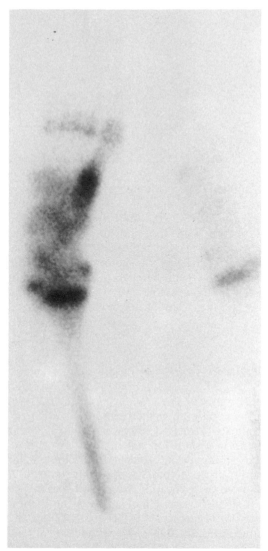

FIGURE 45–27. Bone scan of an open fracture may be helpful in determining the presence of osteomyelitis or septic arthritis.

is reduced and then fixed with a Kirschner wire, which should be inserted antegrade through the distal fragment, exiting on the plantar surface of the foot. The pin is then advanced in a retrograde fashion to stabilize the fracture. Compartment syndromes can occur with this fracture and may require release of all compartments in the foot.

Avulsion fractures of the base of the fifth metatarsal should be differentiated from a fracture through the proximal diaphysis of the fifth metatarsal (the Jones fracture). The Jones fracture has a high incidence of nonunion, even

in the pediatric population. For the athlete, surgical intervention has been recommended for this fracture, with a cancellous bone screw directed proximally to distally across the fracture site from an insertion point on the base of the fifth metatarsal.[68] Ideally, this should decrease the incidence of delayed union or nonunion and allow an earlier return to the patient's athletic activity.

Stress fractures frequently occur in the metatarsals. Treatment is the application of a short-leg cast for several weeks until the child is comfortable.

Fractures of the Phalanges

In minimally displaced fractures, the fractured toe is taped to an adjacent toe with gauze placed between the toes. Evaluation for rotational malalignment should be routinely performed. Only rarely are these fractures so displaced or unstable that percutaneous Kirschner wire fixation is required.

Open Fractures

Treatment of open fractures should follow the same principles that apply in the adult, with the most important aspect being thorough débridement. Puncture wounds of the foot are associated with a high incidence of *Pseudomonas* infections.[67] With *Pseudomonas*, the initial appearance of the wound may appear relatively benign and may mask underlying bone or joint involvement. A bone scan may be helpful in differentiating underlying osteomyelitis from septic arthritis (Fig. 45–27). Puncture wounds should be treated early with decompression and then packed open. Lawn mower injuries cause some of the most severe open injuries of the feet[76] and frequently require microsurgical techniques to repair associated neurovascular injuries.

References

Ankle Fractures

1. Aitken AP: The end results of the fractured distal tibial epiphysis. J Bone Joint Surg 18:685, 1936.
2. Ashhurst APC, Bromer RS: Classification and mechanism of fractures of the leg bones involving the ankle. Arch Surg 4:51, 1922.

3. Beaty JH, Linton RC: Medial malleolar fracture in a child. J Bone Joint Surg 79A:1254, 1988.

4. Bishop PA: Fractures and epiphyseal separation fractures of the ankle. Am J Roentgenol 67:28, 1932.

5. Bright RS: Operative correction of partial epiphyseal plate closure by osseous-bridge resection and silicone rubber implant. J Bone Joint Surg 56A:655, 1974.

6. Broock GJ, Greer RB: Traumatic rotational displacements of the distal tibial growth plate. J Bone Joint Surg 52A:1666, 1970.

7. Cameron HU: A radiologic sign of lateral subluxation of the distal tibial epiphyses. J Trauma 15:1030, 1975.

8. Canale ST: Campbell's Operative Orthopedics. St. Louis, CV Mosby, 1987.

9. Carothers CO, Crenshaw AH: Clinical significance of a classification of epiphyseal injuries at the ankle. Am J Surg 89:879, 1955.

10. Cass JR, Peterson HA: Salter-Harris type IV injuries of the distal tibial epiphyseal growth plate, with emphasis on those involving the medial malleolus. J Bone Joint Surg 65A:1059, 1983.

11. Chadwick CJ: Spontaneous resolution of varus deformity of the ankle following adduction injury of the distal tibial epiphysis. J Bone Joint Surg 64A:774, 1982.

12. Cone RO II: Triplane fracture of the distal tibial epiphysis: Radiographic and CT studies. Radiology 153:763, 1984.

13. Cooperman DR, Spiegel PG, Laros GS: Tibial fractures involving the ankle in children. The so-called triplane epiphyseal fracture. J Bone Joint Surg 60A:1040, 1978.

14. Crenshaw AH: Injuries of the distal tibial epiphysis. Clin Orthop 41:98, 1965.

15. Danielsson LG: Avulsion fracture of the lateral malleolus in children. Br J Accident Surg 12:165, 1980.

16. Denton JR, Fischer SJ: The medial triplane fracture. Report of an unusual injury. J Trauma 21:991, 1981.

17. Dias LS, Giegerich CR: Fractures of the distal tibial epiphysis in adolescence. J Bone Joint Surg 65A:438, 1983.

18. Dias LS, Tachdjian MO: Physeal injuries of the ankle in children. Clin Orthop 136:230, 1978.

19. Dias LS: Fractures in Children. Philadelphia, JB Lippincott, 1984.

20. Dingeman RD, Shaver GB, Jr: Operative treatment of displaced Salter-Harris III distal tibial fractures. Clin Orthop 135:101, 1978.

21. Elmslie RC: The relationship of fracture of the lower epiphysis of the tibia to arrest growth of the bone. J Orthop Surg 1:215, 1919.

22. Foucher: De la divulsion des epiphyses. Cong Med France 1:63, 1863.

23. Gerner-Schmidt M: Ankelbrud Hos Born. Thesis. Kobenhavn, Nyt Nordisk Forlag, 1963.

24. Grace DL: Irreducible fracture separations of the distal tibial epiphysis. J Bone Joint Surg 65B:160, 1983.

25. Gross R: Ankle fractures in children. Bull NY Acad Med 8:739, 1987.

26. Hoed DD: A separate centre of ossification for the tip of the internal malleolus. Br J Radiol 30:67, 1925.

27. Karrholm J, Hansson LI, Laurin S: Computed tomography of intraarticular supination-eversion fractures of the ankle in adolescents. J Pediatr Orthop 1:181, 1981.

28. Karrholm LI, Hansson LI, Laurin S: Pronation injuries of the ankle in children. Acta Orthop Scand 54:1, 1983.

29. Kelikian H: Disorders of the Ankle. Philadelphia, WB Saunders, 1985.

30. Kleiger B, Mankin HJ: Fracture of the lateral portion of the distal tibial epiphysis. J Bone Joint Surg 46A:25, 1964.

31. Kling TF, Bright RW, Hensinger RM: Distal tibial physeal fractures in children that may require open reduction. J Bone Joint Surg 66A:647, 1984.

32. Landin LA, Danielsson LG: Children's ankle fractures. Acta Orthop 54:634, 1983.

33. Langenskiold A: An operation for partial closure of an epiphysial plate in children, and its experimental basis. J Bone Joint Surg 57B:325, 1975.

34. Lauge-Hansen N: Fractures of the ankle. II: Combined experimental-surgical and experimental-roentgenologic investigations. Arch Surg 60:957, 1950.

35. Letts RM: Hidden adolescent ankle fracture. J Pediatr Orthop 2:161, 1982.

35a. Lovell ES: An unusual rotatory injury of the ankle. J Bone Joint Surg 50A:163, 1968.

36. Lynn MD: The triplane distal tibial epiphyseal fracture. Clin Orthop 86:187, 1972.

37. MacNealy GA, Rogers LF, Hernandez R, Poznanski AK: Injuries of the distal tibial epiphysis: Systematic radiographic evaluation. Am J Radiol 138:68, 1982.

38. Marmor L: An unusual fracture of the tibial epiphysis. Clin Orthop 73:132, 1970.

39. McFarland B: Traumatic arrest of epiphyseal growth at the lower end of the tibia. Br J Surg 19:78, 1931.

40. McMaster JH, Scranton PF, Jr: Tibiofibular synostosis a cause of ankle disability. Clin Orthop 3:172, 1975.

41. Nevelos AB, Colton CL: Rotational displacement of the lower tibial epiphysis due to trauma. J Bone Joint Surg 59B:331, 1977.

42. Ogden JA: Skeletal Injury in the Child. Philadelphia, Lea & Febiger, 1982.

43. O'Rahilly R, Gardner E, Gray DJ: The skeletal development of the foot. Clin Orthop 16:7, 1960.

44. Owen E: Cases of injury to the epiphysis: Arrested development of tibia. Lancet 2:767, 1891.

45. Peiro A, Aracil J, Martos F, Mut T: Triplane distal tibial epiphyseal fractures. Clin Orthop 160:196, 1981.

46. Poland J: Pathological anatomy; separation of the lower epiphysis of the tibia; separation of the lower epiphysis of the fibula. *In* Traumatic Separation of Epiphyses. London, Smith, Elder & Col, 1898, pp 70, 817.

47. Powell HDW: Extra centre of ossification for the medial malleolus in children. J Bone Joint Surg 43B:107, 1961.

48. Rang M: Children's Fractures. Philadelphia, JB Lippincott, 1973.

49. Rogers LF: The radiography of epiphyseal injuries. Radiology 96:289, 1970.

50. Salter RB: Injuries of the ankle in children. Orthop Clin North Am 5:147, 1974.

51. Spiegel PG, Cooperman DR, Laros GS: Epiphyseal fractures of the distal ends of the tibia and fibula. A retrospective study of 237 cases in children. J Bone Joint Surg 60A:1046, 1978.

52. Stampfel O, Zoch G, Scholz R, Ferlic P: Ergeonisse der operativen Behandlung von Verletzungen der distalen Tibia Epiphyse. Arch Orthop Unfallchir 84:211, 1976.

53. Tachdjian M: The Child's Foot. Philadelphia, WB Saunders, 1985.

54. Tillaux PJ (reported by Gosselin): Rapport des recherches clinique et experiments sur les fractures malleolaires. Bull Acad Med 1:817, 1872.

55. Torg JS, Ruggiero RA: Comminuted epiphyseal fracture of the distal tibia. Clin Orthop 110:215, 1975.
56. Von Laer L: Classification, diagnosis, and treatment of transitional fractures of the distal part of the tibia. J Bone Joint Surg 67A:687, 1985.
57. Weber BG, Brunner C, Freuler F: Die Frakturenbehandlung bei Kindern und Jugendlichen. Berlin, Springer Verlag, 1978.
58. Weber BG, Sussenbach F: Malleolar fractures. *In* Weber BG, et al (Eds): Treatment of Fractures in Children and Adolescents. Berlin, Springer Verlag, 1980.

Foot Fractures

59. Buchanan J, Greer RB, III: Stress fractures in the calcaneus of a child. Clin Orthop 135:119, 1978.
60. Canale ST, Kelly FB, Jr: Fractures of the neck of the talus. Long term evaluation of 71 cases. J Bone Joint Surg 60A:143, 1978.
61. Canale ST: Campbell's Operative Orthopedics. St. Louis, CV Mosby, 1987.
62. Coltart WD: Aviator's astragalus. J Bone Joint Surg 34B:545, 1952.
63. Devas MB: Stress fractures in children. J Bone Joint Surg 45B:528, 1963.
64. Essex-Lopresti P: The mechanism, reduction, technique and results in fractures of the os calcis. Br J Surg 39:395, 1952.
65. Gross RH: Fractures in Children. Philadelphia, JB Lippincott, 1984.
66. Hawkins LG: Fractures of the neck of the talus. J Bone Joint Surg 52A:991, 1970.
67. Johanson PH: Pseudomonas infections of the foot following puncture wounds. JAMA 204:262, 1968.
68. Kavanaugh JH, Brower TD, Mann RV: The Jones fracture revisited. J Bone Joint Surg 60A:776, 1978.
69. Letts RM, Gibeault D: Fractures of the neck of the talus in children. Foot Ankle 1:74, 1980.
70. Matteri R, Frymoyer J: Fracture of the calcaneus in young children. J Bone Joint Surg 55A:1091, 1973.
71. Mulfinger GL, Trueta J: The blood supply of the talus. J Bone Joint Surg 52B:160, 1970.
72. Ogden JA: Skeletal Injury in the Child. Philadelphia, Lea & Febiger, 1982.
73. O'Rahilly R, Gardner E, Gray DJ: The skeletal development of the foot. Clin Orthop 16:7, 1960.
74. Rang M: Children's Fractures. Philadelphia, JB Lippincott, 1973.
75. Rasmussen F, Schantz K: Radiologic aspects of calcaneal fractures in childhood adolescence. Acta Orthop Scand 57:501, 1987.
76. Ross PM, Schwentker EP, Bryan H: Mutilating lawn mower injuries in children. JAMA 236:480, 1976.
77. Schantz K, Rasmussen F: Good prognosis after calcaneal fracture in childhood. Acta Orthop Scand 59(5):560, 1988.
78. Schmidt TL, Weiner DS: Calcaneal fractures in children. An evaluation of the nature of the injury in 56 children. Clin Orthop 171:150, 1982.
79. Spak I: Fractures of the talus in children. Acta Chir Scand 107:553, 1954.
80. Stephens NA: Fracture dislocations of the talus in childhood: A report of two cases. Br J Surg 43:600, 1956.
81. Trillat A, Lerat JL, Leclerc P, Schuster P: Tarsometatarsal fracture-dislocations. Rev Chir Orthop 62(Suppl):685, 1976.
82. Weber BG, Sussenbach F: Malleolar fractures. *In* Weber BG et al (Eds): Treatment of Fractures in Children and Adolescents. Berlin, Springer Verlag, 1980.
83. Wiley JJ: Tarsometatarsal joint injuries in children. J Pediatr Orthop 1:255, 1981.
84. Wiley JJ, Profitt A: Fractures of the os calcis in children. Clin Orthop Sep(188):131, 1984.
85. Wilson DW: Injuries of the tarso-metatarsal joints. J Bone Joint Surg 54B:677, 1972.

PART **V** *FOOT AND ANKLE*

INJURIES IN SPORTS

Editor
KEVIN P. BLACK

46 *Ankle Injuries in Sports*

LELAND C. McCLUSKEY
KEVIN P. BLACK

The most frequent injury in athletes is injury to the ankle joint. Garrick reported that 45 percent of basketball injuries and 31 percent of soccer injuries involved the ankle ligaments.[41] Acute ankle sprains have been found to represent 21 percent of all sports-related injuries in Finland[81] and 16 percent of all such injuries in Norway.[60]

The lateral ligaments of the ankle are the most commonly sprained structures of the ankle joint; however, the tibiofibular syndesmosis and the medial ligament (i.e., the deltoid ligament) can be torn as well.[16] Although injuries to the ligaments of the ankle are the most frequent of all injuries occurring in sports, the typical ankle sprain is all too often disregarded and undertreated. Tremendous controversy exists regarding methods of evaluation and optimal treatment. Fortunately, most injuries respond to conservative treatment, and surgical intervention is required only when a nonsurgical approach fails.

In addition to ligamentous injuries, this chapter describes osteochondral lesions of the talus, synovial impingement lesions, impingement exostoses, and fractures of the posterior process of the talus. Potential complications following surgical or nonsurgical treatment of ankle injuries and appropriate treatment and salvage protocols complete this discussion of ankle injuries in sports.

ANATOMY AND BIOMECHANICS

The ankle is a modified hinge joint, with the talus articulating into the mortise formed by the tibia and fibula. Motion resulting in upward and downward movement of the foot occurs about a single axis that is oriented obliquely to the long axis of the leg, passes between the medial and lateral malleoli, and is directed 20 to 25 degrees laterally, posteriorly, and distally (Fig. 46–1).[50]

The distal tibia consists of the concave plafond and the medial malleolus. The lateral malleolus, which is located at the distal end of the fibula, is positioned approximately 1.0 cm distal and posterior to the medial malleolus. It has a medial facet for articulation with the talus and a posterior sulcus for passage of the peroneal tendons. The malleoli provide a medial and lateral buttress to the talus that serves

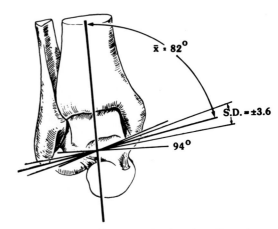

FIGURE 46–1. Ankle joint axis of motion. (From Inman VT: The Joints of the Ankle. Baltimore, Williams & Wilkins, 1976. © 1976, The Williams & Wilkins Company, Baltimore.)

901

as an important link between the ankle and foot.

The posterior process of the talus is composed of medial and lateral tubercles, between which exists a groove containing the flexor hallucis longus tendon (Fig. 46–2). Just posterior to the lateral tubercle of the posterior talar process is the os trigonum, a separate ossification center that is present in 50 percent of adolescents and persists into adulthood as an unfused accessory bone in about 6.5 percent of people (Fig. 46–3).[23] The lateral process of the talus forms both the lateral third of the talar articulation with the posterior calcaneal facet and the superolateral articulation with the distal fibula.

Three major groups of ligaments provide stability to the ankle joint: the lateral ligaments, the tibiofibular syndesmosis, and the medial ligaments. The lateral ligaments consist of the anterior talofibular, calcaneofibular, and posterior talofibular ligaments (Fig. 46–4). The anterior talofibular ligament is an intra-articular thickening of the anterolateral capsule that extends from the anterior border of the distal fibula to the distal anterolateral neck of the talus. It is approximately 2.0 mm thick, 10.0 mm wide, and 20.0 mm long. The calcaneofibular ligament is an extracapsular cord-like

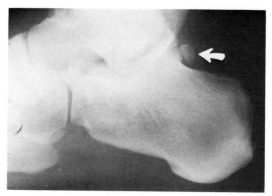

FIGURE 46–3. Os trigonum.

structure running from the inferior aspect of the lateral malleolus distally and posteriorly to a small tubercle on the lateral aspect of the calcaneus. It forms the medial wall of the peroneal tendon sheath and spans both the ankle and the talocalcaneal joints. The ligament averages 3.0 mm in thickness, 5.0 mm in width, and 20.0 mm in length. The posterior talofibular ligament, the strongest of the lateral ligaments, runs horizontally from the distal fossa of the fibula to the lateral tubercle on the posterior process of the talus. It averages 8.0 mm in depth and 30.0 mm in length.[56] Although not truly a structure of the ankle joint, the lateral talocalcaneal ligament blends with the fibers of the anterior talofibular ligament proximally and attaches to the calcaneus adjacent to the calcaneofibular ligament.

The distal tibiofibular articulation is supported by four strong ligaments (i.e., the anteroinferior tibiofibular, posteroinferior tibiofibular, transverse tibiofibular, and interosseous ligaments) and the interosseous membrane (Fig. 46–5). The anteroinferior and posteroinferior tibiofibular ligaments run from superior to inferior in corresponding locations on the anterior and posterior aspects of the syndesmosis. The strong transverse tibiofibular ligament runs from the posterior articular tip of the distal tibia to the fibula and is almost continuous with the inferior margin of the posteroinferior tibiofibular ligament. The distal portion of the interosseous membrane is called the interosseous ligament; it is the strongest of the tibiofibular ligaments.

The major medial ligament is the deltoid, a strong, triangular ligament containing superficial and deep fibers (Fig. 46–6). The fibers of the superficial deltoid are directed more in the

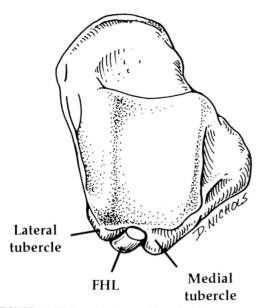

Lateral tubercle

FHL

Medial tubercle

FIGURE 46–2. Superior view of the talus demonstrating the medial and lateral tubercles of the posterior process. The flexor hallucis longus (FHL) tendon lies between the tubercles.

FIGURE 46–4. Lateral view of the ankle demonstrating the lateral ligaments.

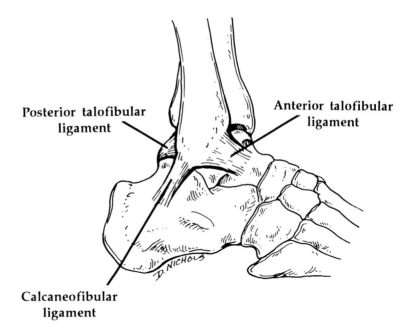

Posterior talofibular ligament

Anterior talofibular ligament

Calcaneofibular ligament

sagittal plane, whereas the fibers of the deep deltoid are nearly horizontal. The superficial fibers run in a continuous sheath from the medial malleolus and consist of the anterior tibiotalar, tibionavicular, tibiocalcaneal, and posterior tibiotalar segments. The most important part of the deltoid ligament is the deep deltoid, which originates on the undersurface of the medial malleolus near its tip and runs a horizontal course intra-articularly to the medial surface of the talus. The tendons of the tibialis posterior and flexor digitorum longus cross superficially over the deltoid ligament.

The biomechanical properties of ligaments and their orientation give valuable information when reconstructive techniques are consid-

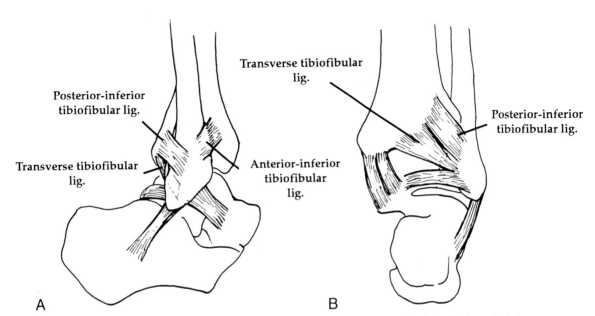

Posterior-inferior tibiofibular lig.

Transverse tibiofibular lig.

Transverse tibiofibular lig.

Anterior-inferior tibiofibular lig.

Posterior-inferior tibiofibular lig.

A   B

FIGURE 46–5. Lateral (*A*) and posterior (*B*) views of the ankle showing the distal tibiofibular articulation.

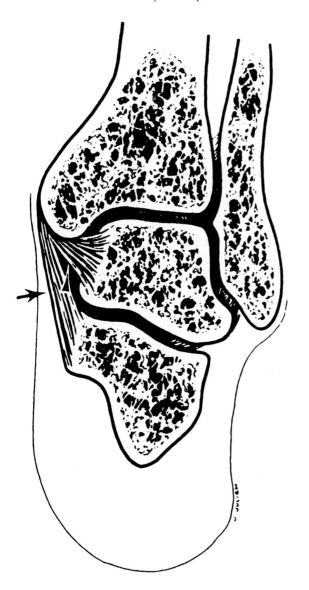

FIGURE 46–6. Coronal section of the hindfoot demonstrating the superficial (*arrow*) and deep (*arrowhead*) components of the deltoid ligament. (From Goergen TG, Danzig LA, Resnick D, Owen CA: Roentgenographic evaluation of the tibiotalar joint. J Bone Joint Surg 59A:874–877, 1977.)

ered. Various combinations of damage to ligaments and osteochondral structures can occur depending on the biomechanical and physiologic conditions present at the time of injury. Storemont and colleagues demonstrated that under physiologic loading (weight bearing), the articular surface of the ankle accounts for 100 percent of the stability to inversion and 30 percent of the stability to internal rotation.[87] Other physiologic conditions important for prevention and rehabilitation include peroneal tendon strength, heel cord tightness, and proprioceptive function.[37, 63] Seemingly similar injuries can result in markedly different injury patterns and severities.

LATERAL LIGAMENT SPRAINS

Mechanism of Injury

Injury to the lateral ligaments occurs from inversion or varus tilt only when the ankle is incompletely loaded (such as at initial ground contact), and it may occur from internal rotation.[87] The anterior talofibular and calcaneofibular ligaments act synergistically: the former approaches vertical orientation to the ground with full plantar flexion, whereas the latter approaches vertical orientation with slight dorsiflexion. Attarian and colleagues showed in cadaveric studies that although the anterior talofibular ligament is the weakest lateral ligament (as demonstrated by its low maximum load and energy to yield point), it has a high strain to failure, which allows for more increase in length before failure and permits physiologic plantar flexion and internal rotation.[6]

Classification of Ligamentous Injuries

O'Donoghue, in 1970, defined sprain as "an injury to a ligament resulting from over-stress that causes some degree of damage to the ligamentous fibers or their attachments."[71] He classified sprains as first, second, or third degree (Fig. 46–7). First-degree sprains consisted of interstitial damage to the ligament without any detectable increase in laxity. Second-degree sprains involved more extensive ligament damage, and although laxity was present, the ligament remained grossly intact. With third-degree sprains, there was a complete tear of the ligament with complete loss of stability.

However, there is some discrepancy in the literature concerning the grading system. Grade III sprains are considered by some authors to be the rare case in which all three lateral ligaments are completely torn, as in a dislocated ankle, but most authors associate grade III injuries with complete disruption of the anterior talofibular ligament and the calcaneofibular ligament.[26]

We prefer to grade acute sprains as mild, moderate, or severe. At 48 hours after injury, individuals with mild sprains have minimal swelling and good range of motion and are able to bear weight comfortably without the need for crutches. Patients with moderate sprains have more swelling, have a limited range of motion of about 0 to 30 degrees of flexion, and typically require the use of crutches or a cane to bear weight on the affected side. Most sprains fall into this category. With severe sprains, the ankle joint is markedly swollen, ecchymosis is present laterally, there is minimal range of motion without pain, and the patient is unable to bear weight on the involved extremity. For the purposes of this chapter, what the literature commonly refers to as a grade I, II, or III ankle sprain roughly corresponds with what we refer to as a mild, moderate, or severe sprain, respectively.

Diagnosis

The symptomatic ankle sprain should be addressed with a thorough history taking, physical examination, and radiographic evaluation to ensure accurate diagnosis and appropriate treatment.

The history often is helpful to the examiner in determining the mechanism of injury. Demonstration by the patient of the precipitating events (with the uninjured ankle) can usually reproduce the mechanism. A thorough history may elucidate prior injuries to the ankle or other pertinent medical problems, such as diabetes or inflammatory disease. In addition, the patient's present and expected activity levels need to be defined.

The physical examination typically reveals a diffusely swollen, plantarflexed, ecchymotic, tender ankle. Patients with severe sprains usually are unable to bear weight on the involved side. The examination should include observations of the patient's general physical condition and any generalized joint laxity. The presence of cavus feet (or, conversely, of hyperpronated feet) should be noted. Cavus feet, which are associated with a rigid varus hindfoot position, predispose the patient to recurrent ankle sprains. Tarsal coalition should be suspected, especially in adolescents with recurrent sprains. Physical examination typically demonstrates a rigid pes planus deformity with peroneal muscle spasm. Calcaneonavicular bars are best seen on oblique radiographs of the foot, whereas talocalcaneal bars are seen on axial (Harris) radiographs and are seen more accurately on semicoronal computed tomographic (CT) scans.

A complete neurovascular check should also be performed. Cases of coexisting superficial and deep peroneal nerve and sural nerve injuries have been reported; they are usually not diagnosed initially.[65] The peroneal tendons can be subluxated, dislocated, or ruptured, especially in dorsiflexion injuries. Compartment syndromes have been reported with peroneal muscle rupture.[5] Careful palpation also should be performed to rule out fractures.

Tenderness is usually found anterolaterally at the ankle and is often noted along the calcaneofibular ligament as well. Funder and colleagues reported that the calcaneofibular ligament was torn in 72 percent of cases exhibiting tenderness over the ligament during examination.[40] However, Broström and others

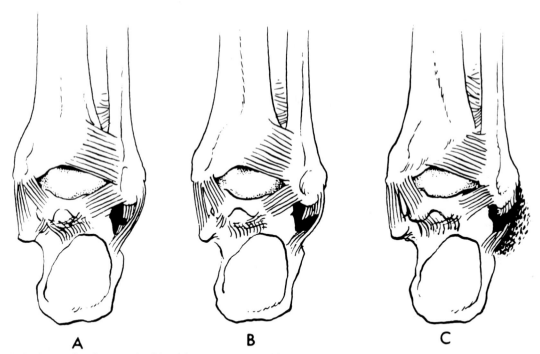

FIGURE 46–7. Classification of mild, moderate, or severe ankle sprains as first (*A*), second (*B*), or third degree (*C*). (From O'Donoghue DH: Treatment of Injuries to Athletes. Philadelphia, WB Saunders, 1970.)

have not found a correlation between areas of tenderness and sites of ligament rupture in ankle sprains.[16] The medial side of the ankle frequently is tender and swollen in association with lateral injuries. Storemont and colleagues demonstrated that the deltoid ligament functions as a primary restraint to internal rotation of the ankle and is probably injured in many "routine" ankle sprains.[87] The syndesmosis often is tender as well and should be examined radiographically with external rotation stress views if necessary.[49]

The extent of ligament damage and instability is assessed primarily by anterior drawer and inversion stress testing. These tests are often not tolerated well by the acutely injured patient, and some authors recommend local, regional, or general anesthesia if sedation is not sufficient.[40] In some patients, only a rotatory instability, in which the talus rotates anteriorly and medially out of the ankle mortise, can be appreciated.[64]

The anterior drawer test is conducted with the patient's knee flexed to relax calf muscles and with the ankle plantarflexed, in a neutral position, and dorsiflexed. According to Seligson and colleagues, the position of the ankle and muscle relaxation do not affect the results

of the anterior drawer test.[82] To perform the test, one hand stabilizes the tibia while the opposite hand directs an anterior force to the heel (Fig. 46–8). Because quantification is difficult, stress radiographs may be used to document the displacement, which is measured from the posterior lip of the tibia to the nearest part of the talus. Comparison must be made with the contralateral ankle in exactly the same position. Normal values for anterior displacement have been reported to range from 2.0 to 9.0 mm, but generally more than 8.0 mm is considered diagnostic of an anterior talofibular ligament tear.[56]

Grace found up to 14.0 mm of anterior displacement in cadaveric ankles with sectioned anterior talofibular ligaments (compared with a maximum of 6.0 mm in control groups) and no significant increase with additional sectioning of the calcaneofibular ligament.[44] However, with the ankle tested in dorsiflexion, Bulucu and colleagues demonstrated a 31-percent increase in displacement when both ligaments were sectioned, compared with when the anterior talofibular ligament was sectioned alone.[22] A 42-percent increase in displacement was reported when the posterior talofibular ligament was also sec-

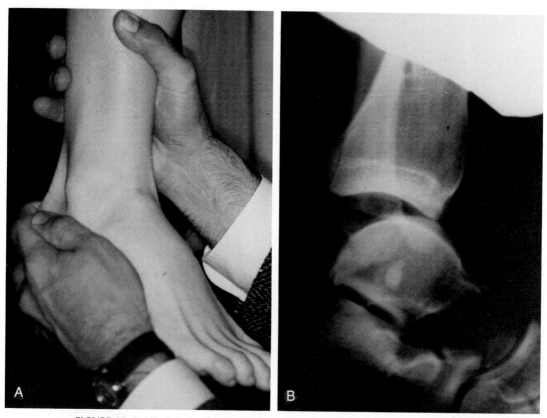

FIGURE 46–8. (*A*), Anterior drawer test (see text). (*B*), Radiograph shows displacement.

tioned. Thus, the anterior drawer test primarily evaluates the anterior talofibular ligament, but the calcaneofibular and posterior talofibular ligaments do provide some stability against displacement during the examination, especially when the ankle is dorsiflexed.

We perform the anterior drawer test with the patient's ankle in neutral and plantar flexion and consider anterior displacement of greater than 5.0 mm compared with that in the contralateral ankle to represent significant disruption of the anterior talofibular ligament. We use this test for patients with chronic symptoms of instability.

The inversion stress test (or talar tilt test) is performed to assess the integrity of the calcaneofibular ligament in particular and that of the anterior talofibular ligament as well. The test is performed with the ankle in a neutral or only slightly plantarflexed position to place more tension on the calcaneofibular ligament. The tibia is stabilized with one hand while the other hand applies varus stress at the level of the calcaneocuboid joint (Fig. 46–9). The an-

gle produced between the tibial plafond and the talar dome can be measured radiographically.

Rubin and Witten reported up to 23 degrees of talar tilt and up to 19 degrees of asymmetry in normal ankles.[79] However, Chrisman and Snook analyzed this study and noted that ankles in 95 percent of normal subjects had less than 10 degrees of asymmetry compared with the contralateral ankle.[28] A study by Cox and Hewes comprising 404 ankles demonstrated normal talar tilt of less than 5 degrees in 98 percent of midshipmen tested.[30] The talar tilt test provides the best noninvasive evaluation of the integrity of the calcaneofibular ligament[30]; however, it has not been shown to predictably differentiate single- from double-ligament tears. We use the test to evaluate patients with chronic symptoms of instability and consider a talar tilt of greater than 10 degrees compared with the contralateral ankle to represent significant mechanical instability.

Several studies have emphasized the unreliability of stress radiographs, especially in non-

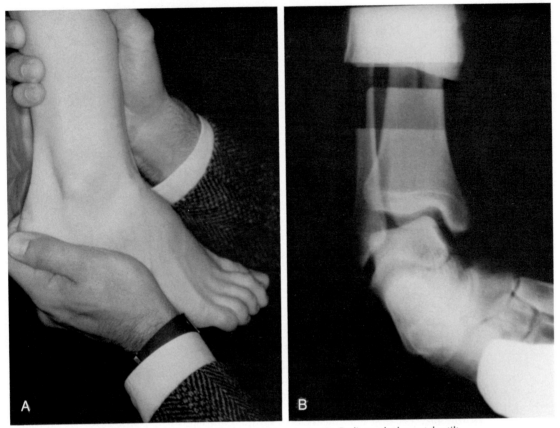

FIGURE 46–9. (*A*), Talar tilt stress test (see text). (*B*), Radiograph shows talar tilt.

anesthetized patients, and recommend ankle arthrography or peroneal tenography.[11, 20, 72] Based on the results of arthrography performed in more than 300 sprained ankles, Broström and colleagues diagnosed anterior talofibular ligament rupture when contrast material escaped the capsule at the tip of the fibula.[20] Dye entering the peroneal tendon sheath suggested calcaneofibular ligament tear, although this was noted in 10 percent of normal ankles. In addition, dye leaked into the flexor hallucis longus and flexor digitorum longus sheaths in 25 percent of cases with a calcaneofibular ligament rupture observed at surgery and into the posterior talocalcaneal joint in 16 to 20 percent of normal ankles. Several studies also have demonstrated a high false-negative rate when arthrograms are used to detect calcaneofibular tears.[39, 86] Arthrograms appear more helpful in evaluating the deltoid or syndesmotic ligaments but must be obtained within 5 to 7 days after injury.

Black and colleagues, in 1978, first described

tenography of the peroneal sheath for the evaluation of calcaneofibular ligament injuries.[11] Bleichrodt and coworkers reported an 88-percent sensitivity and an 87-percent specificity when the test was used to demonstrate surgically proven partial or complete ruptures of the calcaneofibular ligament.[12]

However, these more invasive studies should be performed only if treatment depends on their results. For example, if single- or double-ligament tears will be treated exactly the same, neither arthrography nor tenography is indicated. We treat acute lateral ligament sprains nonoperatively and therefore do not attempt to document the severity of ligament damage with stress radiography or arthrography.

The differential diagnosis of lateral ligament sprain should include peroneal tendon pathology (subluxation, dislocation, or rupture); superficial peroneal or sural nerve injury; injury to the syndesmosis; subtalar joint spasm; fracture of the lateral malleolus, fifth metatarsal base, os trigonum, or lateral process of the talus; and several intra-articular lesions (e.g., osteochondral fractures and impingement lesions). These lesions can accompany an ankle sprain and must always be considered.

Indications for Nonsurgical Treatment

Once the clinical diagnosis has been made, a treatment plan can be implemented. Most authors agree that grade I and II sprains should be treated nonoperatively, with an emphasis on early mobilization and proprioceptive exercises.[51, 52, 77] For acute grade III injuries, several authors have recommended surgical repair,[3, 14, 77, 80] whereas others reserve surgery for high-level athletes[19, 59] and still others recommend initial nonoperative treatment for all acute first-time grade III injuries.[36, 66, 85, 89]

The series of classic articles by Broström and colleagues on ankle ligament injuries included a prospective comparison of grade III injuries treated by primary repair, casting, and strapping.[16-21] Instability symptoms were minimal for all groups; however, they were present to some degree in 20 percent of patients treated with strapping but in only 3 percent of those treated surgically. Broström and colleagues noted that results after late reconstruction were comparable with those after early repair. They concluded that strapping shortened disability time the most and that nonoperative treatment was indicated for the majority of injuries. An exception to the latter is in young athletes, in whom mechanically stable ankles were most important.

Other investigators have found no differences in mechanical stability at follow-up between the primary repair, casting, and strapping treatment groups.[36, 59, 66, 85] In a prospective study, Freeman randomly assigned patients with grade III tears to primary repair, casting, or immediate-mobilization treatment groups.[36] He also found a much shorter period of disability in the group treated with early mobilization. "Functional" instability occurred in 40 percent of patients in each of the three groups. Surgery provided the most "mechanically" stable ankles, as determined by stress radiography, but 1 year after injury, symptoms were present in more of the surgically treated group (75 percent) than of the casting (42 percent) or early-mobilization (47 percent) groups. Freeman suggested that "giving way," or functional instability, is usually due to motor in-

coordination and loss of proprioception, and he proposed a treatment protocol involving coordination exercises that would reduce the symptoms of giving way. Other authors have duplicated these findings.[42]

Of nine prospective, randomized studies documenting late functional instability, three reported better results with nonsurgical treatment,[33, 66, 89] three reported better results with surgical treatment,[19, 59, 77] and three found no difference between the two treatment groups.[36, 57, 70] Therefore, operative treatment does not absolutely minimize late functional instability.

Nonsurgical protocols vary from 8 weeks of casting to immediate protected range-of-motion exercises. Many nonrandomized, retrospective studies support these different treatment options. Kannus and Renström reviewed 12 prospective, randomized studies on the treatment of grade III ruptures and concluded that functional treatment with a short period of protection, followed by early range-of-motion exercises and neuromuscular training, is the method of choice, even as initial treatment in competitive athletes.[52]

We believe that the literature on acute grade III tears of the lateral ligaments clearly supports nonsurgical treatment with early functional mobilization. We implement a nonoperative rehabilitation protocol immediately for mild, moderate, and severe sprains. This treatment choice provides the patient with the best opportunity for early return to work or sport and early recovery of range of motion, without resulting in more mechanical or functional instability than is seen after casting alone or surgery. If necessary, delayed surgical reconstruction can be performed effectively on patients in whom nonoperative therapy is unsuccessful.[26]

Nonsurgical Rehabilitation

It is important to distinguish between nonsurgical treatment and no treatment; with the latter, the physician merely applies an elastic bandage and instructs the patient to return to activities when he or she is "better." Proper rehabilitation of the sprained ankle progresses through four stages: stage I is acute symptom management; stage II is range-of-motion exercises and early strengthening; stage III is aggressive strengthening and proprioception training; and stage IV is a progressive return to functional activities. These stages are not distinct, separate phases but instead represent a rehabilitation program continuum in which there is significant overlap.

The goal of stage I rehabilitation is to minimize pain, swelling, and stiffness. Some authors prefer initial casting for various periods, depending on the severity of injury. Kelikian and Kelikian recommended casting for 5 weeks if rupture of the anterior talofibular ligament alone is suspected and for 3 additional weeks if rupture of the calcaneofibular ligament is also suspected.[56]

Smith and Reischl recommended casting with the ankle in 10 to 15 degrees of dorsiflexion to reduce the torn ends of the anterior talofibular ligament.[84] However, this technique concerns us because of the increased tension placed on the calcaneofibular ligament with the ankle in this position. In addition, immobilization has been shown to weaken the boneligament junction of the medial collateral ligament of the knee.[93] Although no similar scientific studies have been performed on the ankle, there are no data indicating that immobilization in any position promotes ankle ligament healing.

Proponents of initial casting cite increased patient comfort, compliance, and ability to bear weight. However, because of our concerns regarding muscle atrophy and stiffness and because of the potentially deleterious effects of immobilization, we prefer to avoid casting if at all possible. Most patients with acute ankle sprains are comfortable enough with a pneumatic compression splint. This allows them to begin at least partial weight bearing immediately and to initiate range-of-motion exercises at the same time. We "aggressively" rest the ankle with elevation and ice and encourage dorsiflexion and plantar flexion range-of-motion exercises as tolerated. We reserve cast immobilization for individuals with severe pain and swelling that prohibits them from placing their ankles through any range of motion. In such cases, the cast is removed after approximately 1 week, and the pneumatic splint is applied.

Stage II rehabilitation starts as soon as the patient's comfort allows. Strengthening begins with gentle isometrics and proceeds with progressive isotonic and isokinetic progressive resistance exercises. Stage III rehabilitation, which includes proprioceptive exercises, is begun when the patient's strength allows. Stage IV, which includes running and activities involving agility, is started when normal strength has returned. Heel cord stretching should be emphasized throughout rehabilitation to prevent recurrent ankle sprains,[63] and the tilt board and balance disk are helpful in restoring proprioception (Fig. 46–10).

The pneumatic splint is used for a variable period, depending on the severity of the injury, the sport involved, and the level of athletic involvement. The average recreational athlete does not have the luxury of being taped before each game or practice and usually does quite well with any of the commercially available protective splints on returning to activity (Fig. 46–11). Use of the splint is discontinued when the individual feels comfortable and confident. The exception to this is the person who has had several previous sprains; for this patient, we recommend continued protection whenever the patient participates in sports requiring agility. Most professional and intercollegiate athletes prefer taping to splint use, despite the fact that even an excellent "tape job" can stretch within 20 to 30 minutes.

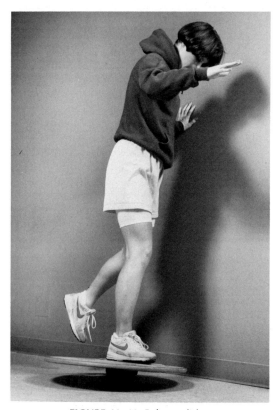

FIGURE 46–10. Balance disk.

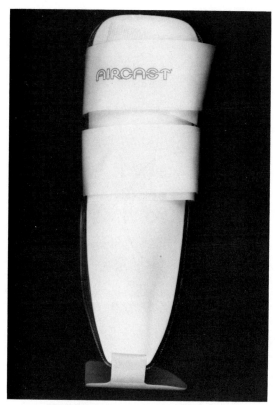

FIGURE 46–11. Functional ankle splint.

Late functional instability, or giving way, is often secondary to the patient's loss of proprioception and decreased muscle coordination and strength. There is no good correlation between functional instability and demonstrable mechanical instability.[37] Thus, even in cases of true mechanical instability and recurrent sprains, an aggressive rehabilitation program should be implemented before surgery is considered. We have seen many patients with chronic functional instability who have improved dramatically as a result of appropriate rehabilitation.

Indications for Surgery

We treat all first-time inversion ankle sprains, regardless of severity, with an aggressive rehabilitation program and reserve surgery for individuals in whom nonoperative treatment has failed. However, surgery may be considered in the acute setting in those rare cases in which associated ankle pathology warrants surgical intervention (e.g., in cases of displaced fractures, displaced osteochondral lesions of the talus, and peroneal tendon ruptures or dislocations).

Clearly, however, these injuries occur infrequently, and the majority of patients on whom we operate are those with chronic functional instability and documented mechanical instability (by stress radiography) who have not benefited from our rehabilitation program. Patients who have a varus hindfoot are predisposed to ankle sprains and to failure of both nonoperative and operative treatment. To correct hindfoot position in these patients, reconstruction of the lateral ligaments should be accompanied by calcaneal osteotomy.

Surgical Procedures

High success rates have been reported with various surgical procedures for repair or reconstruction of the lateral ligaments.[18, 28, 32, 43, 90] Our preferred approach for both acute repair and reconstruction is the Broström-Gould procedure.[18, 43] This technique is essentially an anatomic repair and does not sacrifice any normal structures.

Other common reconstructive procedures (e.g., the Chrisman-Snook, Evans, and Watson-Jones procedures) use the peroneus brevis tendon in different ways to stabilize the lateral aspect of the ankle. Excellent results have been reported for each procedure.[28, 32, 90] We use the Chrisman-Snook modification of the Elmslie procedure to treat those rare patients who have irreparable ligaments or generalized laxity of all ligaments. The Chrisman-Snook procedure is also preferred for patients with associated severe subtalar instability or peroneal tendon subluxation.

Broström-Gould Procedure (Fig. 46–12)

A linear incision is made along the anterior border of the distal fibula, beginning about 5.0 cm proximal to the fibular tip and, after curving posteriorly, stopping at the peroneal tendon sheath. Care is taken to protect the superficial peroneal nerve, which is anterior to the incision, and the sural nerve, which is posterior to the peroneal tendon area. Dissection is then carried down to the capsule anteriorly, and the extensor retinaculum is identified distally. The retinaculum is dissected off the capsule such that it can be used to reinforce

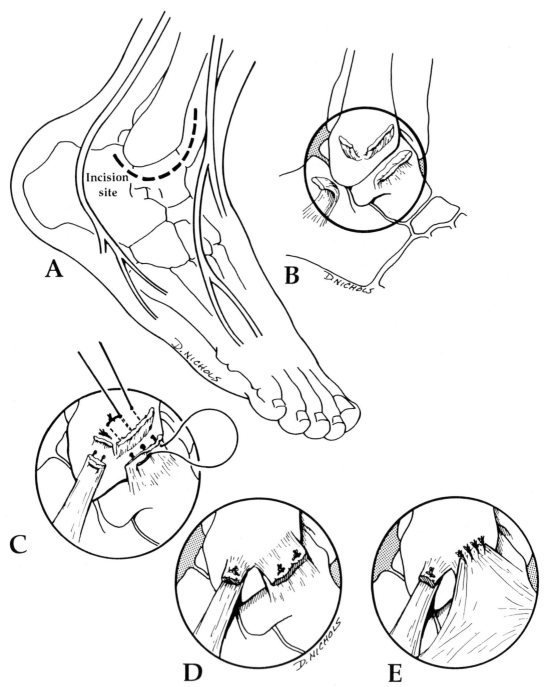

FIGURE 46–12. Broström-Gould procedure. (*A*), Anterolateral curved incision. (*B*), Arthrotomy leaving a 3.0-mm cuff at the fibula. The proximal stump of the ligament is elevated. (*C*), The distal stump of the ligament is sutured into the fibula. (*D*), The proximal stump of the ligament is sutured over the distal stump in a pants-over-vest fashion. (*E*), The lateral extensor retinaculum is sutured over the repair into the fibula.

the repair later in the procedure, as described by N. Gould and colleagues.[43] The capsule is then incised anteriorly and extended to the distal extent of the incision at the peroneal tendon area. A 3.0-mm cuff of capsule is left attached to the fibula.

The anterior talofibular ligament (an intra-articular ligament) can be identified from within this capsule as a well-defined thickening of the capsule. The calcaneofibular ligament (an extracapsular ligament) is next identified at the tip of the fibula, running distally deep to the peroneal tendons until its attachment on the calcaneus. It usually is torn in acute cases and attenuated in chronic cases. Before the ligaments are repaired, the joint is inspected for osteochondral lesions and other evidence of pathology.

In acute cases, the ankle is anatomically reduced and the ligaments are directly repaired with 2–0 nonabsorbable sutures. In chronic injuries, the 3.0-mm stump, which is left attached to the fibula, is elevated, and the remaining distal ligament substance is pulled up and attached directly to the fibula. The proximal stump is then sutured to the distal stump in a pants-over-vest fashion. Drill holes through the fibula or a suture-anchoring device, such as the Mitek, can be helpful in directly attaching the distal ligament substance to the fibula.

The calcaneofibular ligament is repaired first because it is the most difficult to visualize, and then the anterior talofibular ligament is reconstructed. The talocalcaneal ligament can be used to add stability.[43] Stability and range of motion of the ankle are then tested. Next, the lateral extensor retinaculum is pulled over the repair and sutured to the fibula with a 3–0 Vicryl suture. This reinforces the repair and, in addition to the calcaneofibular ligament reconstruction, helps correct any subtalar instability that might be present. The wound is then irrigated, subcutaneous tissue is closed with a 2–0 Vicryl suture, and a running subcuticular suture is used in the skin.

Postoperatively, the patient's lower leg is initially placed in a splint for 3 to 5 days and is then placed in a short-leg walking cast for approximately 4 weeks. After the cast has been removed, the patient is started on range-of-motion, strengthening, and proprioceptive exercises. Full activity is usually resumed within about 12 weeks.

Chrisman-Snook (Modified Elmslie) Procedure (Fig. 46–13)

A curved incision is made along the posterolateral aspect of the ankle directly over the peroneus brevis tendon, beginning 7.5 cm proximal to the tip of the fibula and ending at the base of the fifth metatarsal. Care is taken to avoid injuring the sural nerve. The peroneal sheath is opened, and the peroneus brevis is split lengthwise from its insertion at the metatarsal to the musculotendinous junction. Half of the tendon is detached from the muscle and pulled distally. The skin and subcutaneous tissue are reflected anteriorly to identify the anterior capsule, which is incised, and the joint is inspected.

A drill hole is then made about 2.0 cm proximal to the fibula tip, from anterior to posterior and slightly distal, with care taken not to break through the articular surface. A 6.0-mm drill is usually adequate. With a Hewson suture passer, the tendon is passed, under moderate tension, from anterior to posterior and is fixed to periosteum on the lateral malleolus. Overtightening is avoided to ensure that full range of motion of the ankle is maintained. The talar remnants of the anterior talofibular ligament can be sutured to the tendon at this time.

The peroneal tendons are returned into the fibular groove, and the lateral aspect of the calcaneus is exposed at the insertion of the calcaneofibular ligament. Two oblique drill holes are made 2.0 cm apart in a horizontal plane and then connected. The graft is passed superficial to the peroneal tendons and then, from posterior to anterior, through the calcaneus, where it is sutured under tension to periosteum. Any remaining graft may be sutured back onto itself at the fibula or to the talus. Reconstruction is accomplished using 2–0 nonabsorbable suture.

The wound is then irrigated, and the peroneal tendon sheath is closed. The subcutaneous tissues are closed with 3–0 absorbable suture, and the skin is closed with a subcuticular suture. Postoperatively, a dressing splint is initially applied, after which a short-leg cast is used for about 6 weeks, with weight bearing as tolerated. The lower leg is then protected with a pneumatic splint, and the patient is started on an aggressive rehabilitation program. The level of activity allowed progresses over time, with jogging usually allowed within 4 months.

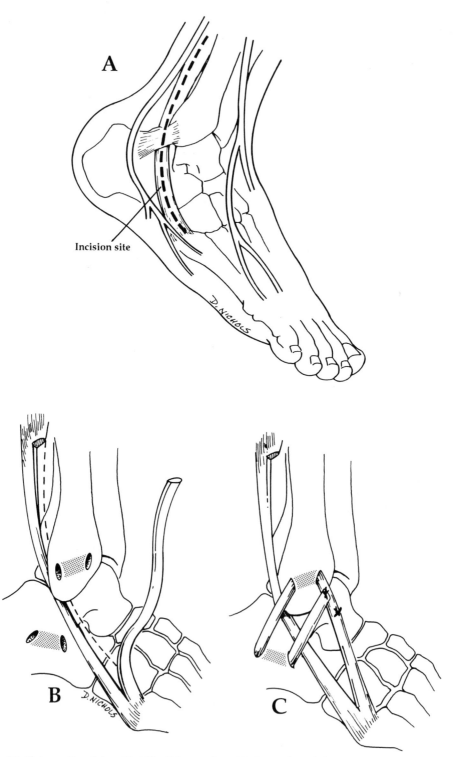

FIGURE 46–13. Chrisman-Snook (modified Elmslie) procedure. (*A*), Posterolateral skin incision. (*B*), The peroneal tendon sheath is split over the peroneus brevis. The anterior one-half of the tendon is detached proximally. (*C*), The tendon is passed first through the fibula from anterior to posterior, then superficial to the peroneal tendons, and finally from posterior to anterior through the calcaneus. It is then sutured back onto itself just anterior to the fibula. The tendon is also sutured to the remnant of the anterior talofibular ligament at the talus.

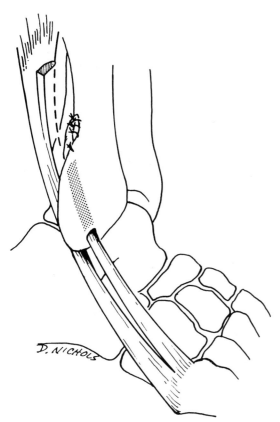

FIGURE 46–14. Modified Evans procedure. The anterior half of the peroneus brevis tendon is passed through a drill hole in the fibula.

Modified Evans Procedure (Fig. 46–14)

An incision is made along the posterior border of the fibular shaft, beginning proximally at the junction of the middle and distal thirds, curving anterior and distal to the lateral malleolus, and ending 5.0 cm distal to its tip. The sural nerve is identified and protected. The peroneal sheath is then divided, and the peroneus brevis tendon is identified and followed to the musculotendinous junction. The tendon is split beginning at the musculotendinous junction, and the anterior half is retracted distally, leaving the attachment at the fifth metatarsal base intact.

A drill hole is made, beginning distally at the anteroinferior tip of the lateral malleolus and emerging 3.0 cm proximally on the posterior edge of the malleolus. Curettes are used to enlarge the holes so that tendon can be relatively easily passed from inferior to superior. The tendon is then sutured under tension to the adjacent soft tissues proximally and

distally, with the ankle in neutral flexion-extension, and slight eversion. After the wound is irrigated, the peroneal tendon sheath is closed. Closure of the subcutaneous tissue and skin is the same as with the Chrisman-Snook procedure, as is the patient's postoperative course.

Watson-Jones Procedure (Fig. 46–15)

The skin incision and soft tissue dissection are identical to those used in the Chrisman-Snook and Evans procedures. The peroneus brevis tendon is cut proximally to preserve as much length as possible. A drill hole is made in the lateral malleolus, beginning posteriorly about 2.5 cm proximal to the tip of the malleolus and extending obliquely, distally, and anteriorly to emerge at the attachment of the anterior talofibular ligament. A second drill hole is made through the neck of the talus, in line with the longitudinal axis of the leg just anterior to the talofibular articulation. The tunnel must be placed far enough medially so that the drill does not break the lateral cortex.

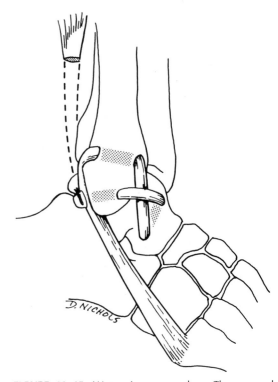

FIGURE 46–15. Watson-Jones procedure. The peroneal tendon is passed posterior to anterior through the fibula, from inferior to superior through the talus, and then back to itself and the lateral surface of the fibula.

It usually is easier to drill superior and inferior tunnels that can be connected.

The proximal end of the tendon is passed through the fibular drill hole from posterior to anterior and then through the talus from inferior to superior. The tendon is brought posteroinferiorly beneath the periosteal slip on the lateral surface of the malleolus and is sutured to itself and periosteum. The closing of the wound and the patient's postoperative course are the same as for the Chrisman-Snook procedure.

SPRAINS OF THE SYNDESMOSIS

Incidence and Mechanism of Injury

Injuries to the ligaments of the tibiofibular syndesmosis are usually associated with ankle fractures. Several reports have discussed sprains without concomitant fractures. Outland suggested that sprains of the syndesmosis were the most serious of all ankle ligament injuries and were as common as lateral ligament sprains.[73] Close demonstrated that diastasis of the tibia and fibula could occur only with rupture of the syndesmosis and either the medial or lateral ligaments.[29] Bröstrom reported that 10 percent of all ankle sprains involved rupture of the anterior tibiofibular ligament and that sometimes the deltoid ligament was simultaneously ruptured secondary to an external rotation injury.[16] Mullins and Sallis believe the true incidence of partial tibiofibular diastasis in recurrent ankle sprains is between 70 and 80 percent.[67]

Classification of Injury

Edwards and DeLee discussed "latent" tibiofibular diastasis, which can be demonstrated only by stress external rotation radiographs, and "frank" tibiofibular diastasis, in which the standard radiographs show abnormal findings.[31] Frank ankle diastasis can be classified into the following types: Type I is straight lateral fibular subluxation, type II is straight lateral fibular subluxation with plastic deformation of the fibula, type III is posterior rotatory subluxation of the fibula and type IV is superior dislocation of the talus (Fig. 46–16).

Diagnosis

A sprain of the syndesmosis should be suspected if the patient's history and the mechanism of injury are not those of the usual inversion injury. For example, this may be the case when a football offensive lineman is stopped and then pushed back on his planted foot, resulting in an eversion–external rotation stress. On physical examination, tenderness over the distal tibiofibular and deltoid ligaments is present and confirms the diagnosis. In a study comprising 1344 ankle sprains, Hopkinson and colleagues reported that the "squeeze test" (Fig. 46–17) indicated syndesmotic injury in 1 percent of cases.[49]

Anteroposterior, lateral, and mortise radiographs of the ankle should be obtained for all patients suspected of having syndesmotic injury. Harper and Keller reported that the width of the tibiofibular "clear space," measured 1.0 cm proximal to the ankle joint on the mortise view, should be less than 6.0 mm (Fig. 46–18).[47] (This measurement is very sensitive to changes in rotation, however, and may need to be compared with that in the contralateral ankle.) If findings on routine radiographs are normal, stress views with external rotation may confirm the diagnosis of syndesmotic injury. Arthrography and radionuclide imaging have also been reported to help demonstrate disruptions of the syndesmosis.[20, 55, 62, 72] Magnetic resonance imaging may prove to be helpful, but its exact role has not yet been determined.

Treatment

The treatment of syndesmotic sprains depends on the severity of the injury and the degree of instability present. Edwards and DeLee recommended 6 weeks of casting for all latent diastases and the rare types III and IV frank diastases if an anatomic reduction could not be obtained and maintained.[31] Other authors have recommended that only those patients with no demonstrable diastases (i.e., incomplete tears) be treated nonoperatively.[38, 49]

Patients in whom a diagnosis of syndesmotic disruption is suspected but who do not demonstrate instability on plain radiographs should undergo stress testing. If no instability is detected, the patient is allowed to bear weight

FIGURE 46–16. Classification of frank tibiofibular diastasis. (From Edwards GS, DeLee JC: Ankle diastasis without fracture. Foot Ankle 4:305–312, 1984. © American Orthopaedic Foot Society 1984.)

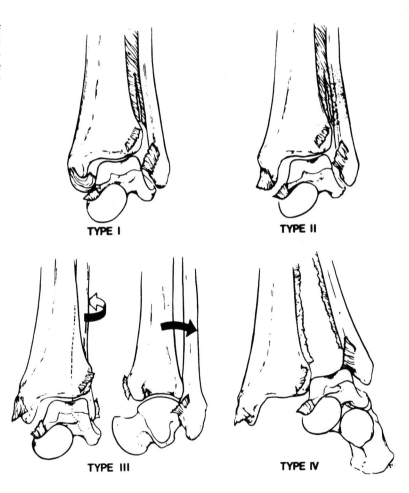

TYPE I TYPE II

TYPE III TYPE IV

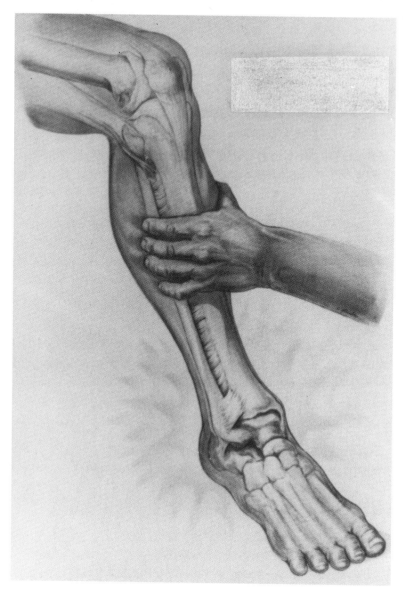

FIGURE 46–17. ''Squeeze test.'' (From Hopkinson WJ, St Pierre P, Ryan JB, Wheeler JH: Syndesmosis sprains of the ankle. Foot Ankle 10:325–330, 1990. © American Orthopaedic Foot and Ankle Society 1990.)

as tolerated using a pneumatic splint and proceeds through a rehabilitation program similar to that for patients with inversion sprains. Patients in whom routine radiographs show normal findings but who demonstrate syndesmotic laxity on stress testing are treated with a long-leg cast for 6 weeks and followed up with frequent radiographs during the first 3 weeks.

For patients in whom acute disruption of the syndesmosis is documented on radiographs or those who develop diastasis after closed treatment, we prefer syndesmotic screw fixation. We believe that stable syndesmotic injuries

occur more frequently than appreciated, and when this diagnosis is made, we emphasize to the athlete and the trainer that a longer recovery period can be expected than that needed following a typical inversion sprain.

Surgical Technique

Fixation of a syndesmotic rupture requires a lateral incision over the distal fibula and open reduction and internal fixation of the tibiofibular joint with a transfibular screw (Fig. 46–19). Reduction should be accomplished

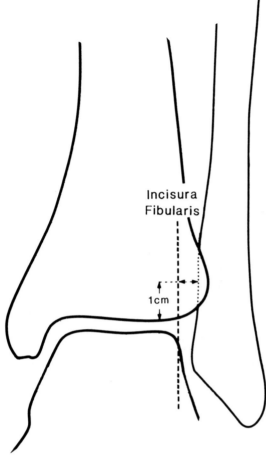

Incisura
Fibularis

1cm

FIGURE 46–18. The tibiofibular "clear space" is widened if it is greater than 6 mm. (From Harper MC, Keller TS: A radiographic evaluation of the tibiofibular syndesmosis. Foot Ankle 10:156–160, 1989. © American Orthopaedic Foot and Ankle Society 1989.)

with the ankle dorsiflexed, remembering that the talus is wider anteriorly and must be accommodated by the ankle mortise. A single 4.5-mm cortical screw is placed parallel and 2.0 cm proximal to the ankle joint. Both cortices of the fibula and one cortex of the tibia are drilled and tapped. Overcompression of the joint is avoided by not overdrilling the fibula and by dorsiflexing the ankle as the screw is tightened. The reduction must be verified by an intraoperative mortise view of the ankle.

The deltoid ligament usually is simultaneously ruptured, but it is repaired only if reduction of the mortise is impeded by the torn ends of the ligament. Any type II frank diastasis, in which plastic deformation of the fibula has

occurred, requires an osteotomy of the fibula to attain anatomic reduction. If desired, a small anterior arthrotomy through the same lateral incision can be performed to inspect the joint surfaces for osteochondral fragments. A suture also can be placed through the torn ends of the anteroinferior tibiofibular ligament if the surgeon desires, although we do not routinely do this.

After the wounds have healed, a postoperative splint is applied for patient comfort, range-of-motion exercises are begun immediately, and protective weight bearing is allowed as tolerated. The screw is removed 8 to 12 weeks after surgery, and the rehabilitation program allows a progressive return to activities. It usually takes 3 to 4 months for the athlete to return to activity after undergoing surgical stabilization of the syndesmosis. Although other physicians have allowed their patients to return to athletic activities with the screw in place, we have no experience with this treatment choice. We do have some concerns, however, of possible adverse effects of this practice on the ankle joint secondary to loss of tibiofibular motion, even after removal of the screw.

MEDIAL LIGAMENT SPRAINS

Isolated tears of the deltoid ligament are rare but can occur secondary to external rotation and abduction of the foot. Usually, a concomitant syndesmotic injury or fibular fracture is noted. It also has been shown that because the deltoid ligament offers significant restraint to internal rotation during axial loading, injuries to it can accompany lateral ligament sprains.[87]

Close[29] and Pankovich and Shivaram[74] described the anatomy of the medial malleolus and the deltoid ligament. The superficial deltoid originates primarily from the anterior colliculus of the medial malleolus, whereas the deep deltoid originates from the posterior colliculus and the intercollicular groove (Fig. 46–20). Avulsion fractures from these areas are often encountered.

Physical examination demonstrates tenderness over the deltoid ligament and, depending on the presence of associated injuries, over the anterior syndesmosis, lateral malleolus, or proximal fibula. Posterior tibial tendon function should be assessed, and ankle joint stabil-

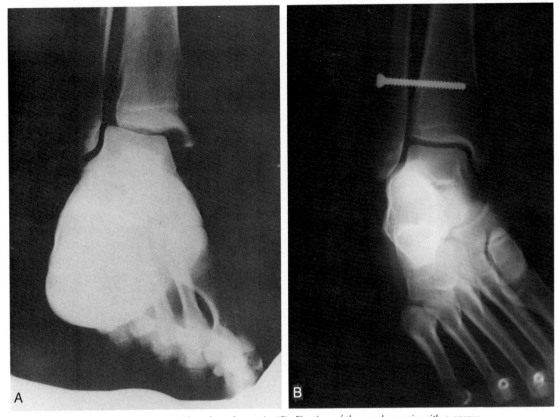

FIGURE 46–19. (*A*), Widened syndesmosis. (*B*), Fixation of the syndesmosis with a screw.

ity documented. Routine radiographs and stress views are helpful in evaluating stability and planning treatment.

Nonoperative treatment with protected mobilization or cast immobilization is used for the rare isolated deltoid rupture or for patients with an associated stable syndesmotic sprains. Surgical treatment for associated unstable syndesmotic ruptures was described previously. The deep deltoid ligament is approached surgically only when its extrication is necessary to reduce the ankle joint.

A 5.0-cm curved incision is made through the skin, subcutaneous tissues, and flexor retinaculum over the posterior tibial tendon, distal to the medial malleolus. After the tendon is retracted and the sheath is incised, the deep deltoid is visualized and repaired. The repair suture should be placed before final fixation of a fibular fracture of the tibiofibular joint and should then be tied at the end of the operation (Fig. 46–21).

OSTEOCHONDRAL LESIONS OF THE TALUS

The terms *osteochondritis dissecans,*[53] *transchondral fractures,*[10] and *osteochondral fractures*[25] have all been used to describe identical talar dome lesions. The confusion in nomenclature reflects the controversial etiology of these lesions, which usually occur in adolescents and young adults. Vascular, hereditary, and hormonal factors have been suggested to predispose patients to the development of these lesions.[24, 46, 91]

The term *osteochondritis dissecans* was originally used by König to describe loose bodies in the knee joint.[58] Kappis used the same term to describe a similar-appearing lesion in the ankle, which he thought resulted from "spontaneous necrosis" of the talar dome.[53] Berndt and Harty, in 1959, convincingly demonstrated that trauma usually is the cause of this condition, and the term *transchondral fractures* was

FIGURE 46–20. The superficial deltoid inserts onto the anterior colliculus of the medial malleolus, and the deep deltoid inserts into the posterior colliculus of the medial malleolus and the intercollicular groove. Nav, navicular; Ta, talus; Ti, tibia.

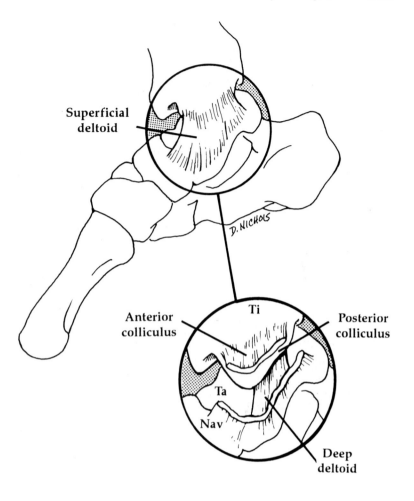

suggested.[10] In combining their clinical and laboratory experience with an extensive review of the literature, Berndt and Harty contributed greatly to our understanding of the etiology and treatment of these lesions. Much of the subsequent literature has corroborated their conclusions.

Lesions tend to be either posteromedial or anterolateral. Posteromedial lesions occur secondary to talar compression against the tibial plafond during ankle plantar flexion and inversion. Anterolateral lesions are caused by talar compression against the lateral malleolus during inversion and dorsiflexion. In a review of the literature, a history of trauma was noted in 98 percent of lateral talar dome lesions and in 70 percent of medial lesions.[34] Concomitant foot and ankle injuries have been found in 28 to 45 percent of these patients.[1, 10, 34] Morphologically, lateral lesions are wafer shaped, whereas medial lesions are cup shaped (Fig.

46–22). Histologically, the lesions appear similar.[25]

Classification of Lesions

Much of the literature categorizes osteochondral lesions based on the radiographic classification of Berndt and Harty (Fig. 46–23), in which a stage I lesion is a compression fracture of subchondral bone, a stage II lesion is a partially detached osteochondral fragment, a stage III lesion is a completely detached osteochondral fragment remaining in the crater, and a stage IV lesion is a displaced osteochondral fragment free within the joint.[10]

However, several problems have been encountered with this classification system. Stage I lesions are hard to identify, stage II and III lesions are difficult to distinguish from each other,[34] and arthroscopic findings do not cor-

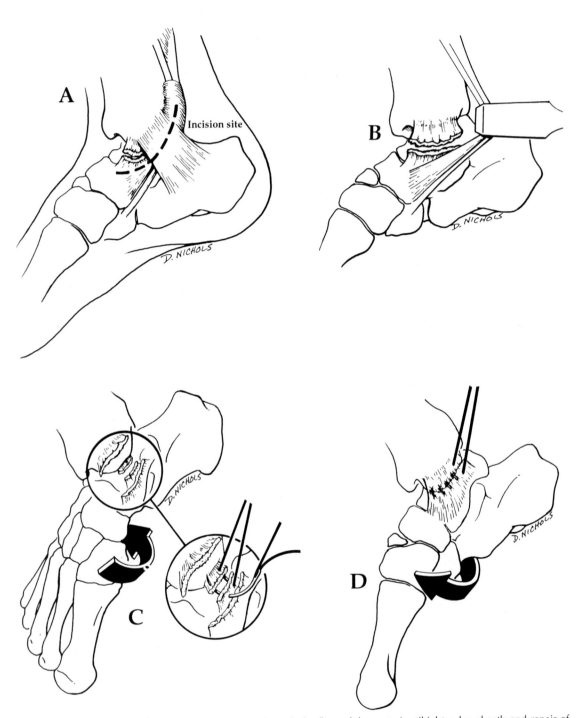

FIGURE 46–21. Repair of the deep deltoid ligament through the floor of the posterior tibial tendon sheath and repair of the superficial deltoid ligament. (*A*), The incision site. (*B*), The tendon is retracted. (*C*), The foot is everted to allow suture of the deep deltoid ligament. (*D*), The superficial deltoid ligament is repaired.

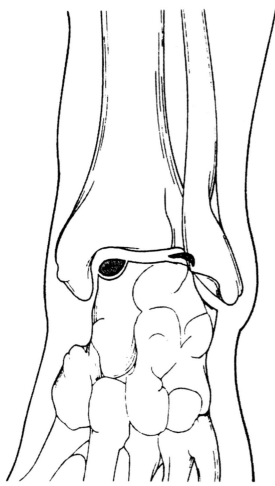

FIGURE 46–22. An anterolateral talar dome lesion is wafer shaped and a posteromedial lesion is cup shaped. (From Canale ST, Belding RH: Osteochondral lesions of the talus. J Bone Joint Surg 62A:97–102, 1980.)

relate with the authors' staging.[78] As a result, Pritsch and colleagues recommended the following arthroscopic grading to help determine the appropriate treatment: grade I has intact, firm, shiny cartilage; grade II has intact, soft, spongy cartilage; and grade III has frayed or deficient cartilage.[78]

Diagnosis

Although talar dome lesions occur in 6.8 to 22 percent of ankle sprains, they are frequently missed on initial examination.[1, 13] Acutely, the signs and symptoms of talar dome lesions are quite similar to those seen in typical ankle sprains, and the diagnosis is made by radiography. Tomograms, computed tomographic scans, and magnetic resonance images are helpful in identifying subtle lesions and in more accurately staging lesions before surgery. Anderson and colleagues recommended using computed tomography to help stage lesions initially seen on plain radiography (Fig. 46–24).[2] They used technetium bone scanning to screen patients with persistent symptoms 6 weeks after an inversion injury; if bone scan findings were positive, a magnetic resonance image was obtained for better delineation of the lesion.

We find magnetic resonance images to be quite helpful in the preoperative evaluation of these lesions. In addition, these images frequently provide useful information about co-existing soft tissue pathology about the ankle, such as impingement lesions, syndesmotic ligament injury, and peroneal tendon pathology. Several other authors are optimistic that magnetic resonance imaging will accurately predict the pathology seen with the various types of osteochondral lesions of the talus, and classification systems are currently being proposed based on magnetic resonance findings.[69]

Individuals with talar dome lesions usually recover partially from their "sprain" but have some persistent symptoms of pain and swelling. Lateral lesions are more frequently associated with chronic symptoms.[25] If the talar dome lesion is displaced, crepitus, catching, or locking can also occur.

Conservative Versus Surgical Treatment

Tremendous controversy exists regarding the appropriate treatment of osteochondral lesions. In a review of 154 cases, Berndt and Harty found overall poor results in 75 percent of those treated conservatively.[10] Flick and Gould also reported poor results in 75 percent when they used short-leg casts for 12 to 18 weeks as nonsurgical treatment.[34] However, although they have reported progression of lesions from stage II to stage IV, they agree with others that a delay in surgery for several months to 1 year does not alter results.[1, 76] Flick and Gould also noted some degeneration of the joint in 50 percent of patients and a propensity for failure of nonoperative treatment in stage III lateral lesions.[34] However, other authors have reported an incidence of

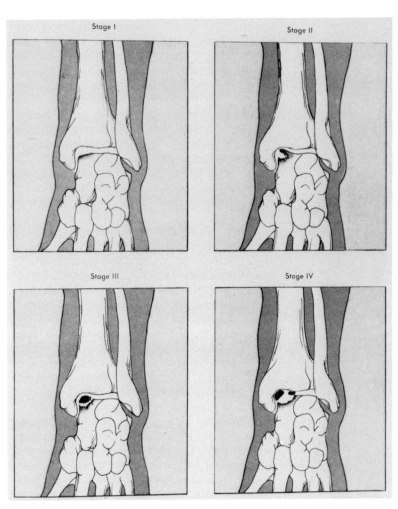

Stage I

Stage II

Stage III

Stage IV

FIGURE 46–23. Classification of osteochondral talar dome lesions according to Berndt and Harty. (From Canale ST, Belding RH: Osteochondral lesions of the talus. J Bone Joint Surg 62A:97–102, 1980.)

degenerative joint disease of less than 20 percent, and in the majority of these cases (95 percent), degenerative changes were noted before treatment.[4]

Canale and Belding concluded that nonoperative treatment was indicated only for stage I, II, and III medial lesions, and they cautioned that 3 to 4 months of casting may be required.[25] Since their report in 1980, immediate surgery has generally been recommended for Berndt and Harty stage III lateral lesions and it has been recommended for all stage IV lesions.[25] Stage III medial lesions are operated on only after initial conservative treatment has failed. Flick and Gould agreed with initial conservative treatment for stage I, II, and III medial lesions and also for stage III lateral lesions, but they believe that surgery was also indicated for stage II lesions that did not respond to a 2- to 3-month trial of casting.[34]

Because radiographic findings do not correlate with surgical findings, we hesitate to operate based solely on radiographic criteria. In time, computed tomography and magnetic resonance imaging may allow more accurate staging of the lesions and thus help to guide treatment. Until then, we consider the duration of the patient's symptoms, the degree of mechanical symptoms (i.e., catching and locking) present, and the goals of the patient in deciding on a conservative or surgical approach.

The presence of symptoms for less than 3 months, the absence of mechanical symptoms, and low athletic demands are relative indications for nonoperative treatment. Conservative treatment with casting and without weight bearing is attempted for 6 weeks in all acute injuries. This is usually followed by another 4 to 6 weeks of casting with weight bearing as

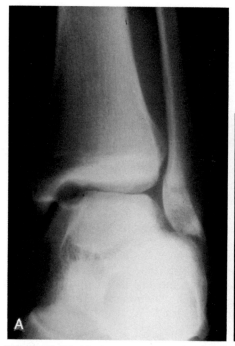
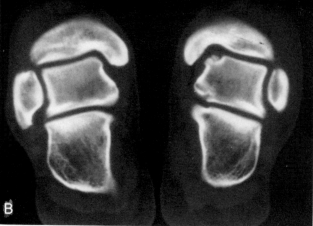

FIGURE 46–24. (A), Anteroposterior radiograph demonstrating a posteromedial talar dome lesion. (B), Coronal section of a computed tomographic scan demonstrating the same lesion.

tolerated. Our relative indications for surgery are the presence of symptoms for longer than 3 months, the presence of mechanical symptoms, and high athletic demands. Otherwise, surgery is performed only when appropriate conservative therapies have failed.

Arthroscopic Treatment

Arthroscopy is of tremendous help in both evaluating and treating talar dome lesions, and it has revolutionized the surgical apjproach to these lesions. Results of arthroscopic treatment have been reported to be good or very good, ranging from 77 to 90 percent of cases.[7, 35, 75, 78] Results of open surgical procedures have also been satisfactory, with long-term follow-up showing good or very good results at 5 years in 88 percent of cases[1] and good results at 11.2 years in 73 percent of cases.[25] However, with current arthroscopic techniques, most lateral and medial lesions can be treated without an open surgical procedure. Rehabilitation and recovery are much faster in these cases, particularly when compared with those open cases requiring medial malleolar osteotomy.

With the arthroscopic grading system, spe-cific treatment plans can be made.[78] Lesions with intact, firm cartilage (grade I) can be treated conservatively, with restriction of patient activities or with casting. Lesions with intact, soft cartilage (grade II) are usually drilled, and the ankle is placed in a non–weight-bearing cast for 6 weeks. Pritsch and colleagues did report that two of their three poor results with grade II lesions occurred in lesions that had been drilled,[78] so perhaps initial curettage is preferable even for grade II lesions. All lesions with frayed cartilage (grade III) demonstrate necrotic bone and fibrous tissue underneath. These require débridement and curettage, followed by the application of soft dressings and the immediate use of range-of-motion and strengthening exercises with weight bearing as tolerated. The patient can expect to return to sports activities within approximately 8 weeks.

Excellent visualization of intra-articular pathology is usually provided by 4.0-mm 30- and 70-degree arthroscopes. A 70-degree arthroscope is most useful for posterior lesions, which also may require use of the smaller, 2.7-mm wide-angle scope, especially if distraction is not performed. We have not found it necessary to use a distraction-type device routinely. Occasionally, however, we have used a calcaneal traction pin that, while distracting the tibiotalar joint, allows dorsiflexion and plantar flexion. Other distraction devices are available using skeletal fixation, and new non-invasive distractors are currently being tested.[45]

We routinely use anteromedial and antero-lateral portals. Medially, the portal is created between the saphenous vein and the anterior tibial tendon, whereas laterally, the portal is made between the medial edge of the lateral malleolus and the lateral edge of the peroneus tertius tendon (Fig. 46–25). Eighteen-gauge needles are inserted at the anteromedial and anterolateral joint lines. Ringer's lactate is injected through one needle, and the egress is observed through the opposite needle. Vertical skin incisions are made anterolaterally, and a small hemostat is used to spread the subcutaneous tissue down to the capsule, thus protecting the superficial peroneal nerve.

For treating lesions located in the medial aspect of the joint, visualization can best be obtained from the anterolateral portals, and working instruments are introduced from the anteromedial portal. The opposite holds true for lateral lesions.

A posterolateral portal is used as an inflow portal and in visualizing posteromedial lesions. It is made just lateral to the Achilles tendon and slightly distal to the ankle joint line (Fig. 46–26). The subcutaneous tissue is spread with a hemostat to avoid the sural nerve. For drilling posteromedial lesions, transmalleolar portals may be made through the medial malleolus 2.0 to 3.0 cm proximal to the joint.[45]

The arthroscope is inserted at a 45-degree angle from lateral to medial, and using intermittent flow through the scope cannula, the needle in the anteromedial portal is identified. The needle is removed, and an outflow cannula through which instruments can be interchanged is inserted. We routinely use a com-

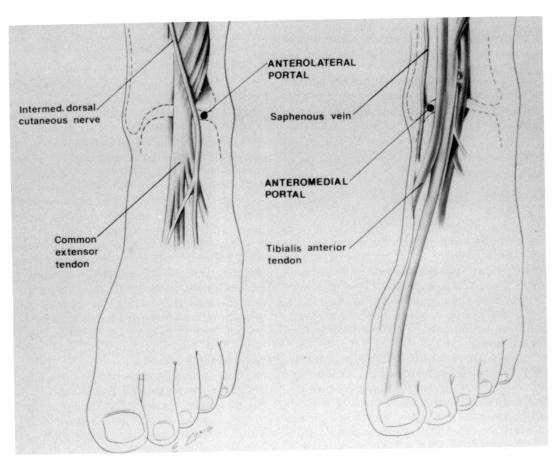

FIGURE 46–25. Anterolateral and anteromedial arthroscopic portals. (From Baker CL, Andrews JR, Ryan JB: Arthroscopic treatment of transchondral talar dome fractures. Arthroscopy 2:82–87, 1986.)

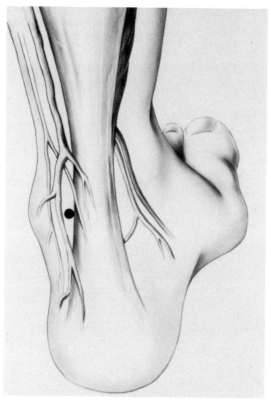

FIGURE 46–26. Posterolateral arthroscopic portal. (Courtesy of James F. Guhl, M.D.)

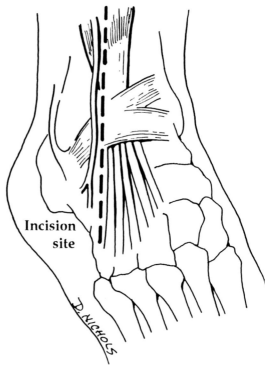

FIGURE 46–27. Anterolateral approach to the ankle for exposure of anterolateral talar dome lesions.

mercial intra-articular pressure monitor cannula, which has been helpful in distending joints with marked synovitis and in minimizing problems caused by bleeding. Many conditions are associated with marked synovitis and synovial hypertrophy, which should be débrided early to allow suitable visualization and decreased operative time. At the conclusion of the procedure, the wounds are closed with a 3–0 nylon suture.

Open Surgery

Open surgical procedures have yielded long-term results comparable to those of arthroscopy, and they are certainly recommended for orthopaedists not efficient with arthroscopy.[1, 25, 75, 78] A well-performed open procedure is always preferable to a poorly performed arthroscopy.

The anterolateral approach to the ankle (made lateral to the extensor digitorum communis tendons, with care taken to identify and protect the superficial peroneal nerve) gives excellent exposure of anterolateral dome lesions (Fig. 46–27). Flick and Gould described one case of a central lateral lesion that required incision of the anterior talofibular ligament along with internal rotation of the talus for exposure.[34] Most lesions also occur posteriorly and require a medial malleolar osteotomy, either the anteromedial incision with notching of the tibia as described by Gould and colleagues[43] or the combined anteromedial and posteromedial approaches described by Thompson and Loomer.[88]

For a medial malleolar osteotomy, an incision is made at the tip of the medial malleolus over the posterior tibial tendon. The malleolus is exposed anteriorly and posteriorly, and a drill hole is placed through the malleolus into the metaphysis of the tibia. The osteotomy is then performed at the level of the ankle joint. The malleolus is retracted distally, the ankle is everted, and the talar dome lesion is identified. The necessary drilling and débridement or curettage are performed, the malleolus is reduced, and two 4.0-mm cancellous screws are inserted (Fig. 46–28). A disadvantage of

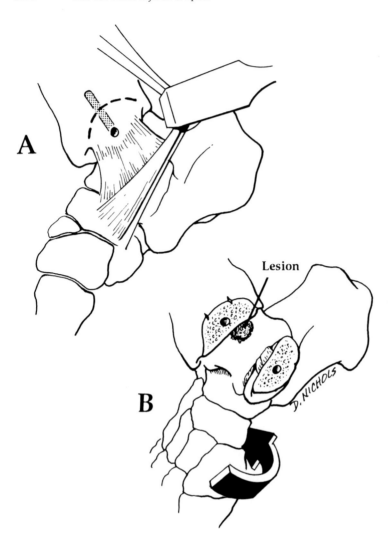

A

B

Lesion

D. NICHOLS

FIGURE 46–28. Medial malleolar osteotomy for exposure of postero-medial talar dome lesions. (*A*), A drill hole is placed through the malleolus. (*B*), The malleolus is retracted distally, and the lesion is identified.

this approach is the 6 weeks of postoperative immobilization needed.

Flick and Gould preferred an anteromedial approach with grooving of the distal tibia to access posteromedial bone lesions (Fig. 46–29).[34] A 5.0-cm incision is made lateral to the anterior tibial tendon at the ankle joint. The anterior tibial tendon sheath is then incised, and the tendon is retracted medially. The arthrotomy is made sharply through the deep portion of the tendon sheath, with coagulation of the anteromedial tarsal artery and vein as necessary. Care is taken to protect the dorsalis pedis artery and deep peroneal nerve, which are lateral to the sheath. With the foot plantarflexed, the anteromedial articular surface of the tibia is grooved with a narrow gouge, usually 4.0 to 5.0 mm wide and 6.0 to 8.0 mm

deep. The lesion is then curetted and drilled. Next, the capsule and deep tendon sheath are closed with a 4–0 absorbable suture. The anterior tibial tendon is anatomically positioned, and the superficial sheath and retinaculum are carefully closed. After the gliding ability of the tendon is checked, the subcutaneous tissue and skin are closed. Postoperatively, patients can begin early active range-of-motion exercises.

Thompson and Loomer described another alternative to the medial malleolus osteotomy.[88] A 10.0-cm curved incision is made posterior to the malleolus, the tissue is dissected to expose the anteromedial capsule, and the capsule is incised to expose the anterior joint (Fig. 46–30). If the lesion cannot be adequately inspected with anterior plantar flexion, another incision is made through the pos-

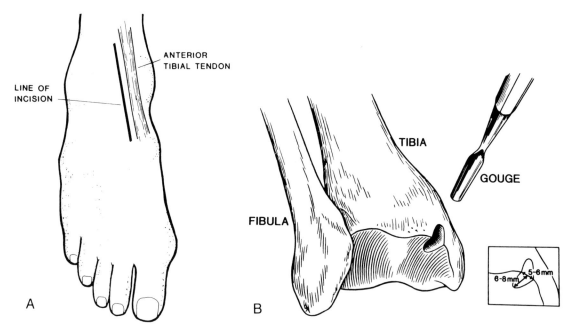

FIGURE 46–29. Alternative approach to posteromedial talar dome lesions with an anteromedial approach (*A*) and grooving of the distal tibia (*B*). (From Flick AB, Gould N: Osteochondritis dissecans of the talus (transchondral fractures of the talus): Review of the literature and new surgical approach for medial dome lesions. Foot Ankle 5:165–185, 1985. © American Orthopaedic Foot and Ankle Society 1985.)

terior tibial tendon sheath, the tendon is retracted anteriorly, and the deep surface of the sheath is incised. The neurovascular structures are gently retracted posteriorly, and with the foot dorsiflexed, the dome of the talus is examined. After appropriate curettage and drilling of the lesion have been performed, the wound is closed, as described earlier. The patient's postoperative course also is the same.

SYNOVIAL IMPINGEMENT LESIONS

In athletes, synovial impingement lesions usually occur secondary to ankle sprains. Wolin and colleagues, in 1950, first reported on nine patients with chronic anterolateral pain following inversion ankle sprains.[92] After conservative treatment had failed, open arthrotomies demonstrated a "mass of hyalinized connective tissue arising from the anteroinferior portion of the talofibular joint capsule and extending into the joint." The authors postulated that the synovial thickening and exudation resulted from injury and that when absorption of this material was incomplete, it became hyalinized and impinged. This condi-

tion may be a reaction to hemarthrosis or to synovial injury.[61]

Synovial impingement lesions, which were previously called meniscoid lesions, are nonspecific. Histologic examination reveals hypertrophic, hyperplastic, hypervascular synovium, with various degrees of fibrosis or scarring.[92] The pathology is usually found anteriorly or anterolaterally between the talus and the lateral malleolus (Fig. 46–31) or at the superior synovial recess of the distal tibiofibular articulation (Fig. 46–32). Soft tissue impingement lesions can occur medially, posteriorly, or from Bassett's ligament, a separate distal fascicle of the anteroinferior tibiofibular ligament.[9] Although less commonly noted in athletes, a more specific synovitis related to rheumatoid arthritis, which is called synovial chondromatosis or pigmented villonodular synovitis, can also be seen in the ankle.

Diagnosis

The diagnosis of anterolateral synovial impingement is most often made by clinical history taking and physical examination. Occasionally, it is suggested by magnetic resonance findings. Typically, the patient describes an

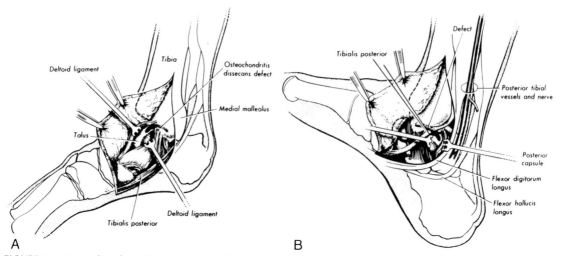

FIGURE 46–30. Another alternative to posteromedial talar dome lesions combining an anteromedial (*A*) and a posteromedial (*B*) capsular incision. (From Thompson JP, Loomer RL: Osteochondral lesions of the talus in a sports medicine clinic. A new radiographic technique and surgical approach. Am J Sports Med 12:460–463, 1984. © 1984, The Williams & Wilkins Company, Baltimore.)

ankle sprain involving the lateral ligaments that failed to respond to conservative treatment. Symptoms usually include pain and intermittent swelling at the anterolateral aspect of the ankle. A sensation of giving way is often present, and popping or catching is occasionally noted.

Localized tenderness over the anterolateral aspect of the ankle is noted on physical examination. Localized swelling in this area is often present. The pain is exacerbated when the ankle is inverted or everted or when the malleolus is compressed. Occasionally, crepitus is demonstrated.

Other lesions with similar presentations must also be included in the differential diagnosis. Lateral joint instability should be ruled out by assessing the anterior drawer, talar tilt, and internal rotation of the ankle. Peroneal tendon pathology, sural or superficial peroneal nerve injury, and fractures of the talar dome or lateral process of the talus must also be considered. Routine ankle radiographs, stress views of the ankle, and either a bone scan or a magnetic resonance image should be obtained to assist in the diagnosis.

Nonsurgical Treatment

An aggressive nonsurgical program should be initiated, and it should be maintained for at least 6 months before arthroscopic surgery

is considered. Strengthening, range-of-motion, and proprioceptive exercises, along with ultrasound, hot or cold therapy, and other modalities, constitute the patient's physical therapy. Nonsteroidal anti-inflammatory drugs are used, and usually one local injection of lidocaine and steroid is given.

Surgery

Surgery is indicated only when all nonsurgical treatments over a 6-month period have failed and a thorough work-up has ruled out other pathologies. The arthroscopic technique is the same as that previously described. We prefer to use a 4.0-mm arthroscope, but a 2.7-mm arthroscope can be helpful, especially if distraction is not used. In most cases, invasive distractors can be avoided. Usually, the anteromedial portal is used for visualization, and the anterolateral portal is used for the shaver and other instruments. Care is taken to avoid all neurovascular structures and overly aggressive débridement of the anterior talofibular ligament.

Postoperatively, the patient's ankle is protected with a bulky compressive dressing for 1 week. The patient then resumes the preoperative physical therapy program. Sports and full activities usually are not resumed for 8 to 12 weeks. Outcome from this procedure generally has been good, with Martin and colleagues[61]

FIGURE 46–31. Lateral gutter of the ankle joint.

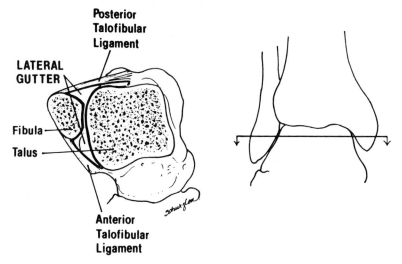

reporting long-term relief of symptoms in 75 percent of cases and Karzel[54] reporting good or excellent results in 84 percent. Complications can include injury to nerves, deep infections, and recurrent symptoms.

IMPINGEMENT EXOSTOSES

Bony impingement lesions of the ankle also occur and include anterior impingement exostoses at the tibia, the talus, or both. Posterior impingement lesions, which are usually associated with an os trigonum, are typically seen in ballet dancers. The reader is referred to the chapter in this text on dancing injuries (Chap-

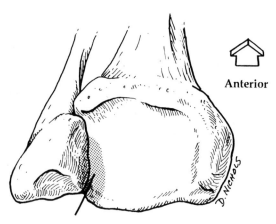

Area of lesion

FIGURE 46–32. Superior synovial recess of the distal tibiofibular articulation in a right ankle.

ter 48), where the subject is extensively covered.

FRACTURES OF THE POSTERIOR PROCESS OF THE TALUS

The posterior process of the talus consists of the medial and lateral tubercles, which are separated by a groove for the flexor hallucis longus tendon. The lateral tubercle, also called Stieda's process, is larger and more posterior than the medial tubercle (Fig. 46–33). Fractures of the lateral tubercle have been called Shepherd's fractures.[83] An os trigonum can resemble a lateral tubercle fracture, especially an old fracture with nonunion in which the sclerosed fracture margins approximate the smooth cortical borders of a typical os trigonum. A bone scan can be helpful in these cases. A separated os trigonum is present in 6.5 percent of the population.[23] Another 42 percent of the population has an elongated lateral tubercle that represents a fused os trigonum. In nearly 60 percent of cases these bones occur bilaterally, and they are usually asymptomatic. Fracture of the medial tubercle is rare, but if present, it is caused by avulsion of the posterior aspect of the deltoid ligament.[27] Even more rare is fracture of the entire posterior process of the talus.[68] When this fracture occurs, the suggested mechanism of injury is maximum plantar flexion of the ankle. Examination often demonstrates painful range of motion of the great toe (flexor hallucis longus tendon). A high index of suspicion,

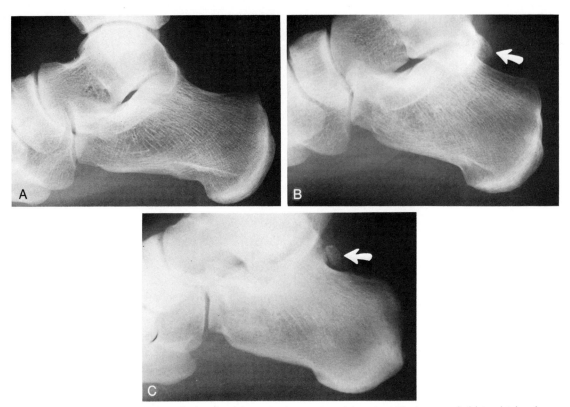

FIGURE 46–33. (*A*), No visible lateral tubercle of the posterior process of the talus. (*B*), An extended lateral tubercle, or Stieda's process. (*C*), The os trigonum.

along with a careful examination, is required to make the diagnosis.

Nonsurgical Treatment

Acute nondisplaced fractures of the talar posterior process are treated with cast immobilization for approximately 6 weeks. Most fractures of the lateral tubercle are nondisplaced or minimally displaced and respond well to casting. Chronic cases involving symptomatic nonunion are initially treated nonsurgically with immobilization and a short-leg walking cast. Strengthening and range-of-motion exercises, along with other physical therapy modalities, are then initiated. If conservative treatment fails, surgery can be considered.

Surgery

Surgery is indicated for acute displaced fractures of the entire posterior process, for which open reduction plus internal fixation is feasible. Otherwise, surgery involves excision of the ununited fragment after conservative treatment has failed. A posterolateral approach is used to excise the lateral tubercle (the technique is described in Chapter 48). Reports suggest that pain usually is relieved and motion is restored following surgical intervention.

COMPLICATIONS AND SALVAGE

Complications can occur after nonsurgical or surgical treatment of ankle injuries and can be particularly devastating to athletes. Significant potential complications include nerve injury, infection, persistent instability, and degenerative joint disease. Treatment and salvage of these conditions include both surgical and nonsurgical protocols.

Nerve injuries are possible with any surgical procedure (arthroscopic or open), and certain nerves are at specific risk during particular procedures: the superficial peroneal nerve during placement of an anterolateral arthroscopic portal and with open anterolateral approaches, the sural nerve during placement of a posterolateral portal and during ankle ligament reconstructions, the saphenous nerve during placement of an anteromedial portal and with anteromedial approaches, and the deep peroneal nerve during arthroscopic débridement because the nerve is located deep to the extensor retinaculum and close to the anterior capsule.

Even those most experienced with the technique report nerve injuries secondary to ankle arthroscopy in 3 to 8 percent of cases.[8, 45, 61] Some of the injuries were temporary, whereas others were permanent. In these cases, salvage usually requires physical therapy programs for desensitization, and it may also necessitate neuroma resection or other procedures.

Reflex sympathetic dystrophy, which can be a complication of either conservatively or surgically treated injuries, has been reported following ankle arthroscopy.[8] Early recognition of this condition is vital because treatment is much more effective if performed early in the disease process. Early treatment consists of physical therapy and encouraging the patient to continue weight bearing and full activity, if possible. Sympathetic blocks, transcutaneous electric nerve stimulator units, steroids, and a number of other medications and modalities also are available, if deemed necessary.

Neurapraxia has been reported to occur at the time of injury in up to 86 percent of patients with grade III ankle sprains.[65] Involvement of the peroneal nerve and posterior tibial nerves is probably secondary to nerve traction trauma. Although rehabilitation can be markedly prolonged, these injuries usually are transient and require only extended physical therapy for treatment.

Of particular concern with ankle arthroscopy is the relatively high incidence of subsequent fistula formation and infection. Infection was noted in 5.6 percent of cases in one series and in 7 percent in another.[45, 61] Several of these were deep infections, with one following a hemarthrosis. Administering preoperative antibiotics, minimizing instrument exchanges, and suturing the portal sites all help to decrease the chances of postoperative infection. If infection occurs, irrigation and débridement, along with antibiotics, are usually required.

Persistent instability following ankle sprains can be either mechanical, as demonstrated by stress testing, or functional, which is often associated with peroneal weakness and loss of proprioception. Lace-up or pneumatic ankle braces, along with strengthening and proprioceptive exercises, are used for treating instability. Late surgical reconstruction is performed if needed. We prefer the anatomic reconstruction described by Broström[19] and modified by Gould and associates[43] and when possible avoid techniques requiring transfer and weakening of the peroneus brevis tendon.[34] Complications are rare following surgical reconstruction, but rerupture or "stretching out" of repairs can occur. The subtalar joint may be unstable after injury to the lateral ligaments and must thus be included in treatment plans.[15] Syndesmotic injuries also can be complicated by instability, diastasis, and degenerative changes if undertreated.[31]

Degenerative joint diseases can result from osteochondral talar dome lesions, posterior process fractures, long-standing lateral ligament instability, and syndesmotic injuries. Canale and Belding noted degeneration of the ankle at follow-up in 50 percent of patients with osteochondral lesions.[25] Most authors, however, agree that delaying surgery for up to 1 year does not alter results or increase the likelihood of degenerative changes.[1, 34, 76] Because fractures of the posterior process of the talus are intra-articular, they can lead to degenerative arthritis. Harrington reported degenerative arthritis associated with chronic lateral ligament instability and recommended reconstruction when early signs of degeneration were noted.[48] After reconstruction, he noted symptomatic improvement and widening of the medial joint space in 14 of 22 patients. Syndesmotic injuries causing diastasis significantly decrease the tibiotalar contact surface area, resulting in degenerative joint disease. Ramsey and Hamilton[78a] demonstrated a 42-percent decrease in the tibiotalar contact surface area with only 1.0 mm of fibular displacement. Ankle braces, nonsteroidal anti-inflammatory drugs, and cortisone injections can be used to treat the symptoms of ankle arthritis. Arthroscopy has been of little value in these cases. The definitive salvage procedure for post-traumatic ankle arthritis is ankle arthrodesis.

References

 1. Alexander AH, Lichtman DM: Surgical treatment of transchondral talar-dome fracture (osteochondritis

dissecans). Long-term follow-up. J Bone Joint Surg 62A:646–652, 1980.

2. Anderson IF, Crichton KJ, Grattan-Smith T, et al: Osteochondral fractures of the dome of the talus. J Bone Joint Surg 71A:1143–1152, 1989.

3. Anderson KJ, LeCocq JF: Operative treatment of injury to the fibular collateral ligament of the ankle. J Bone Joint Surg 36A:825–832, 1954.

4. Angermann P, Jensen P: Osteochondritis dissecans of the talus: Long-term results of surgical treatment. Foot Ankle 10:161–163, 1989.

5. Arciero RA, Shishido NS, Parr TJ: Acute anterolateral compartment syndrome secondary to rupture of the peroneus longus muscle. Am J Sports Med 12:366–367, 1984.

6. Attarian DE, McCrackin HJ, DeVito DP, et al: Biomechanical characteristics of human ankle ligaments. Foot Ankle 6:54–58, 1985.

7. Baker CL, Andrews JR, Ryan JB: Arthroscopic treatment of transchondral talar dome fractures. Arthroscopy 2:82–87, 1986.

8. Barber FA, Click J, Britt BT: Complications of ankle arthroscopy. Foot Ankle 10:263–266, 1990.

9. Bassett FH, Gates HS, Billys JB, et al: Talar impingement by the anteroinferior tibiofibular ligament. A cause of chronic pain in the ankle after inversion sprain. J Bone Joint Surg 72A:55–59, 1990.

10. Berndt AL, Harty M: Transchondral fractures (osteochondritis dissecans) of the talus. J Bone Joint Surg 41A:988–1020, 1959.

11. Black HM, Brand RL, Eichelberger MR: An improved technique for the evaluation of ligamentous injury in severe ankle sprains. Am J Sports Med 6:276–282, 1978.

12. Bleichrodt RP, Kingma LM, Binnendijk B, Klein JP: Injuries of the lateral ankle ligaments: Classification with tenography and arthrography. Radiology 173:347–349, 1989.

13. Bosien WR, Staples OS, Russell SW: Residual disability following acute ankle sprains. J Bone Joint Surg 37A:1237–1243, 1955.

14. Brand RL, Collins MDF, Templeton T: Surgical repair of ruptured lateral ankle ligaments. Am J Sports Med 9:40–43, 1981.

15. Brantigan JW, Pedegana LR, Lippert FG: Instability of the subtalar joint. Diagnosis by stress tomography in three cases. J Bone Joint Surg 59A:321–324, 1977.

16. Broström L: Sprained ankles: I. Anatomic lesions in recent sprains. Acta Chir Scand 128:483–495, 1964.

17. Broström L: Sprained ankles: III. Clinical observations in recent ligament ruptures. Acta Chir Scand 130:560–569, 1965.

18. Broström L: Sprained ankles: VI. Surgical treatment of chronic ligament ruptures. Acta Chir Scand 132:551–565, 1966.

19. Broström L: Sprained ankles: V. Treatment and prognosis in recent ligament ruptures. Acta Chir Scand 132:537–550, 1966.

20. Broström L, Liljedahl SO, Lindvall N: Sprained ankles: II. Arthrographic diagnosis of recent ligament ruptures. Acta Chir Scand 129:485–499, 1965.

21. Broström L, Sundelin P: Sprained ankles: IV. Histologic changes in recent and "chronic" ligament ruptures. Acta Chir Scand 132:248–253, 1966.

22. Bulucu C, Thomas KA, Halvorson TL, Cook SD: Biomechanical evaluation of the anterior drawer test: The contribution of the lateral ankle ligaments. Foot Ankle 11:389–393, 1991.

23. Burman MS, Lapidus PW: The functional disturbances caused by the inconstant bones and sesamoids of the foot. Arch Surg 22:936–975, 1931.

24. Campbell CJ, Ranawat CS: Osteochondritis dissecans: The question of etiology. J Trauma 6:201–221, 1966.

25. Canale ST, Belding RH: Osteochondral lesions of the talus. J Bone Joint Surg 62A:97–102, 1980.

26. Cass JR, Morrey BF: Ankle instability: Current concepts, diagnosis, and treatment. Mayo Clin Proc 59:165–170, 1984.

27. Cedell CA: Rupture of the posterior talotibial ligament with the avulsion of a bone fragment from the talus. Acta Orthop Scand 45:454–461, 1974.

28. Chrisman OD, Snook GA: Reconstruction of lateral ligament tears of the ankle. An experimental study and clinical evaluation of seven patients treated by a new modification of the Elmslie procedure. J Bone Joint Surg 51A:904–912, 1969.

29. Close JR: Some applications of the functional anatomy of the ankle joint. J Bone Joint Surg 38A:761–781, 1956.

30. Cox JS, Hewes TF: "Normal" talar tilt ankle. Clin Orthop 140:37–41, 1979.

31. Edwards GS, DeLee JC: Ankle diastasis without fracture. Foot Ankle 4:305–312, 1984.

32. Evans DL: Recurrent instability of the ankle—a method of surgical treatment. Proc R Soc Med 46:343–344, 1953.

33. Evans GA, Hardcastle P, Frenyo AD: Acute rupture of the lateral ligament of the ankle. To suture or not to suture? J Bone Joint Surg 66B:209–212, 1984.

34. Flick AB, Gould N: Osteochondritis dissecans of the talus (transchondral fractures of the talus): Review of the literature and new surgical approach for medial dome lesions. Foot Ankle 5:165–185, 1985.

35. Frank A, Cohen P, Beaufils P, Lamare J: Arthroscopic treatment of osteochondral lesions of the talar dome. Arthroscopy 5:57–61, 1989.

36. Freeman MAR: Treatment of ruptures of the lateral ligament of the ankle. J Bone Joint Surg 47B:661–668, 1965.

37. Freeman MAR, Dean MRE, Hanham IWF: The etiology and prevention of functional instability of the foot. J Bone Joint Surg 47B:678–685, 1965.

38. Fritschy D: An unusual ankle injury in top skiers. Am J Sports Med 17:282–285, 1986.

39. Fordyce AJW, Horn CV: Arthrography in recent injuries of the ligaments of the ankle. J Bone Joint Surg 54B:116–121, 1972.

40. Funder V, Jørgensen JP, Andersen A, et al: Ruptures of the lateral ligaments of the ankle. Clinical diagnosis. Acta Orthop Scand 53:997–1000, 1982.

41. Garrick JG: The frequency of injury, mechanism of injury, and epidemiology of ankle sprains. Am J Sports Med 5:241–242, 1977.

42. Gauffin H, Tropp H, Odenrick P: Effect of ankle disk training on postural control in patients with functional instability of the ankle joint. Int J Sports Med 9:141–144, 1988.

43. Gould N, Seligson D, Gassman J: Early and late repair of lateral ligaments of the ankle. Foot Ankle 1:84–89, 1980.

44. Grace DL: Lateral ankle ligament injuries. Inversion and anterior stress radiography. Clin Orthop 183:153–159, 1984.

45. Guhl JF: New techniques for arthroscopic surgery of the ankle: Preliminary report. Orthopaedics 9:261–269, 1986.

46. Hanley WB, McKusick VA, Barranco FT: Osteochondritis dissecans with associated malformations in two brothers. A review of familial aspects. J Bone Joint Surg 49A:925, 1967.

47. Harper MC, Keller TS: A radiographic evaluation of the tibiofibular syndesmosis. Foot Ankle 10:156–160, 1989.

48. Harrington KD: Degenerative arthritis of the ankle secondary to long-standing lateral ligament instability. J Bone Joint Surg 61A:354–361, 1979.

49. Hopkinson WJ, St. Pierre P, Ryan JB, Wheeler JH: Syndesmosis sprains of the ankle. Foot Ankle 10:325–330, 1990.

50. Inman VT: The Joints of the Ankle. Baltimore, Williams & Wilkins, 1976.

51. Jackson DW, Ashley RL, Powell JW: Ankle sprains in young athletes. Relation of severity and disability. Clin Orthop 101:201–214, 1974.

52. Kannus P, Renström P: Treatment for acute tears of the lateral ligaments of the ankle. Operation, cast, or early controlled mobilization. J Bone Joint Surg 73A:305–312, 1991.

53. Kappis M: Weitere Beiträge zur traumatish-mechanishen Entschung der "spontanen" Knorpelablosungseon (sogen. Osteochondritis Dissecans). Dtsch Z Chir 171:13–29, 1922.

54. Karzel RP: Arthroscopic treatment of soft tissue lesions in the ankle. *In* Arthroscopic Surgery of the Shoulder and Ankle Update 1991. Course syllabus, Chicago, 1991.

55. Katznelson A, Lin E, Militiano J: Ruptures of the ligaments about the tibiofibular syndesmosis. Injury 15:170–172, 1983.

56. Kelikian H, Kelikian AS: Disorders of the Ankle. Philadelphia, WB Saunders, 1985.

57. Klein J, et al: Operative or conservative treatment of recent rupture of the fibular ligament in the ankle (English abstract). Unfallchirurg 91:154–160, 1988.

58. König F: Veber freie Körper in den Gelenken. Dtsch Z Chir 27:90–109, 1888.

59. Korkala O, Rusanen M, Jokipii P, et al: A prospective study of the treatment of severe tears of the lateral ligament of the ankle. Int Orthop 11:13–17, 1987.

60. Maehlum S, Daljord OA: Acute sports injury in Oslo: A one year study. Br J Sports Med 18:181–185, 1984.

61. Martin DF, Curl WW, Baker CL: Arthroscopic treatment of chronic synovitis of the ankle. Arthroscopy 5:110–114, 1988.

62. Marymont JV, Lynch MA, Henning CE: Acute ligamentous diastasis of the ankle without fracture. Evaluation by radionuclide imaging. Am J Sports Med 14:407–409, 1986.

63. McCluskey GM, Blackburn TA, Lewis T: Prevention of ankle sprains. Am J Sports Med 4:151–157, 1976.

64. McCullough CJ, Burge PD: Rotatory stability of the load-bearing ankle. An experimental study. J Bone Joint Surg 62B:460–464, 1980.

65. Meals RA: Peroneal-nerve palsy complicating ankle sprain. Report of two cases and review of the literature. J Bone Joint Surg 59A:966–968, 1977.

66. Møller-Larsen F, Wethelund JO, Jurik AG, et al: Comparison of three different treatments for ruptured lateral ankle ligaments. Acta Orthop Scand 59:564–566, 1988.

67. Mullins JFP, Sallis JG: Recurrent sprain of the ankle joint with diastasis. J Bone Joint Surg 40B:270–273, 1958.

68. Nasser S, Manoli A: Fracture of the entire posterior process of the talus: A case report. Foot Ankle 10:235–238, 1990.

69. Nelson DW, DiPaola J, Colville M, Schmidgall J: Osteochondritis dissecans of the talus and knee: Prospective comparison of MR and arthroscopic classifications. J Comput Assist Tomogr 14:804–808, 1990.

70. Niedermann B, Andersen A, Andersen SB, et al: Rupture of the lateral ligaments of the ankle: Operation or plaster cast? A prospective study. Acta Orthop Scand 52:579–587, 1981.

71. O'Donoghue DH: Treatment of Injuries to Athletes. Philadelphia, WB Saunders, 1970.

72. Olson RW: Ankle arthrography. Radiol Clin North Am 19:255–268, 1981.

73. Outland T: Sprains and separations of the inferior tibiofibular joint without important fracture. Am J Surg 59:320–329, 1943.

74. Pankovich AM, Shivaram MS: Anatomical basis of variability in injuries of the medial malleolus and the deltoid ligament. I. Anatomical studies. Acta Orthop Scand 50:217–223, 1979.

75. Parisien JS: Arthroscopic treatment of osteochondral lesions of the talus. Am J Sports Med 14:211–217, 1986.

76. Pettine KA, Morrey BF: Osteochondral fractures of the talus. A long-term follow-up. J Bone Joint Surg 69B:89–92, 1987.

77. Prins JG: Diagnosis and treatment of injury to the lateral ligament of the ankle. A comparative clinical study. Acta Chir Scand Suppl 486, 1978.

78. Pritsch M, Horoshovski H, Farine I: Arthroscopic treatment of osteochondral lesions of the talus. J Bone Joint Surg 68A:862–865, 1986.

78a. Ramsey PL, Hamilton W: Changes in tibiotalar area of contact caused by lateral talar shift. J Bone Joint Surg 58A:356–357, 1976.

79. Rubin G, Witten M: The talar-tilt ankle and the fibular collateral ligaments. A method for the determination of talar tilt. J Bone Joint Surg 42A:311–326, 1960.

80. Ruth CJ: The surgical treatment of injuries of the fibular collateral ligaments of the ankle. J Bone Joint Surg 43A:229–239, 1961.

81. Sandelin J: Acute Sports Injuries. A Clinical Epidemiological Study. Dissertation, University of Helsinki, Finland, 1988, pp 1–66.

82. Seligson D, Gassman J, Pope M: Ankle instability: Evaluation of the lateral ligaments. Am J Sports Med 8:39–42, 1980.

83. Shepherd FJ: A hitherto undescribed fracture of the astragalus. J Anat Physiol 18:79–81, 1982.

84. Smith RW, Reischl S: The influence of dorsiflexion in the treatment of severe ankle sprains: An anatomical study. Foot Ankle 9:28–33, 1988.

85. Sommer HM, Arza D: Functional treatment of recent ruptures of the fibular ligament of the ankle. Int Orthop 13:157–160, 1989.

86. Spiegel PK, Staples OS: Arthrography of the ankle joint: Problems in diagnosis of acute lateral ligament injuries. Radiology 114:587–590, 1975.

87. Storemont DM, Morrey BF, An KN, Cass JR: Stability of the loaded ankle. Relation between articular restraint and primary and secondary static restraints. Am J Sports Med 13:295–300, 1985.

88. Thompson JP, Loomer RL: Osteochondral lesions of the talus in a sports medicine clinic. A new radiographic technique and surgical approach. Am J Sports Med 12:460–463, 1984.

89. Van Moppen FI, Van Den Hoogenband CR: Diag-

nostic and Therapeutic Aspects of Inversion Trauma of the Ankle Joint. Thesis, University of Maastricht, Netherlands. Utrecht, Bohn, Scheltema, and Holkema, 1982.

90. Watson-Jones R: Fractures and Joint Injuries, Vol 2, 3rd Ed. Baltimore, Williams & Wilkins, 1944.

91. White J: Osteochondritis dissecans in association with dwarfism. J Bone Joint Surg 39B:261–267, 1957.

92. Wolin I, Glassman F, Sideman S, Levinthal DH: Internal derangement of the talofibular component of the ankle. Surg Gynecol Obstet 91:193–200, 1950.

93. Woo SL-Y, Inoue M, McGurk-Burleson E, Gomez MA: Treatment of medial collateral injury. II: Structure and function of canine knees in response to differing treatment regimens. Am J Sports Med 15:22–29, 1987.

47

Bone and Joint Injuries of the Foot in Athletes

DAVID G. SCOTT
KEVIN P. BLACK

Sports-related bone and joint injuries of the foot have greatly increased over the past several decades as vast numbers of Americans have taken up new forms of recreation and physical conditioning and as professional athletes have strived for ultimate performance. Along with certain sports-specific acute injuries, a wide array of chronic overuse injuries are now recognized. The most common bone and joint problems of the foot seen in athletes include stress fractures, sesamoid problems, fifth metatarsal base fractures, turf toe, hallux rigidus, and avascular necrosis of the second metatarsal head.

STRESS FRACTURES

Stress fractures are among the most common and disabling foot injuries in athletes. Long recognized as a problem in military recruits, these injuries became increasingly prevalent in athletes during the running boom of the 1970s.[52]

Stress fractures result when bones are subjected to repetitive forces that exceed their reparative capabilities.[43] These fractures occur as a result of training errors approximately 70 percent of the time[44] and have been related to biomechanical factors. Athletes with rigid pes cavus feet are at risk for tarsal fractures.[41] Athletes with an abnormal gait, leg length discrepancy, excessive weight, or lower extremity malalignment may be at greater risk for stress fractures.[44]

Stress fractures of the foot are relatively activity specific and account for 22 to 35 percent of all lower extremity stress fractures.[41, 44] Calcaneal fractures are common in military recruits who march in stiff boots on hard surfaces[16] but are rare in athletes. Fifth metatarsal fractures are most commonly seen in football linemen,[64] whereas basketball players have a predilection for navicular fracture.[61] In runners, the metatarsals are the usual site of stress fractures, with the second metatarsal being involved most often (55 percent of cases), followed by the third metatarsal (35 percent) and then by the first, fourth, or fifth metatarsal (10 percent).[44]

Women runners may exhibit a higher rate of stress fracture of the lower extremities than do men on similar training programs. Additionally, when oligomenorrheic or amenorrheic women runners are compared with women runners who have normal menstrual cycles, they have been found to have an increased rate of stress fracture of the lower extremities,[2, 35, 40] have started their serious training years earlier (before or at the time of menarche),[2, 13] have low plasma estradiol levels,[40] and have a high incidence of eating disorders, which may further increase their risk of stress fractures.[2, 14] It has been suggested that in addition to paying particular attention to proper training technique, women may lessen their risk of stress fracture by waiting until maturation of hypothalamic-pituitary hormonal function before initiating serious endurance training, by increasing daily dietary calcium intake to 1500 mg, by correcting any nutritional deficiency or eating disorder, and by taking estrogen replacement therapy (oral contraceptives) if they are oligomenorrheic or amenorrheic.[2, 40]

Two specific metatarsal stress fractures pose treatment or diagnostic difficulties.[25] The Jones fracture, discussed later in this chapter, may progress to delayed union or nonunion if casually treated. Fractures of the base of the second metatarsal involving Lisfranc's joint are seen in female ballet dancers who dance en pointe.[46] These rare injuries present as midfoot pain, are frequently misdiagnosed as sprains, and may require oblique radiographs or bone scans for diagnosis. Linear or computed tomography may be needed to show specific detail of the fracture.

Tarsal stress fractures are more common than previously recognized and take the longest time to diagnose and treat.[41] Of these, stress fractures of the navicular are of particular concern.[27, 53, 59, 61, 62] In the largest series of

navicular fractures, the average time to diagnosis was 7.2 months from the onset of symptoms. More than half of these patients had no fracture visible on initial radiographs, and more than 75 percent of patients who were treated with activity modification or immobilization but continued weight bearing developed recurrent fracture, delayed union, or nonunion.[61]

Stress fractures at the base of the great toe have been described in three athletes.[65] All patients had hallux valgus. Excessive tension of the extensor hallucis longus and adductor hallucis was the proposed cause of the injury. All healed with rest.

Diagnosis

Athletes with stress fractures of the foot present with aching foot pain of insidious onset.[51] At first, the athlete notes the pain following activity. Eventually, the pain occurs during

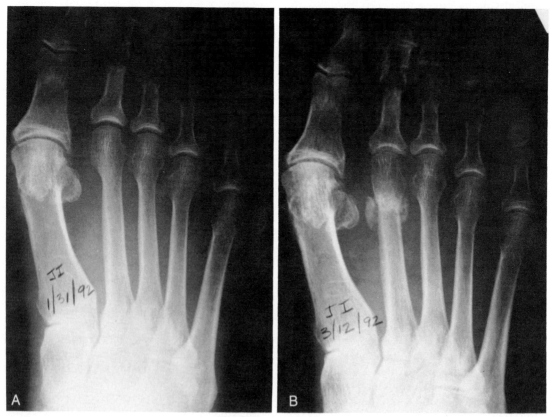

FIGURE 47–1. Left foot anteroposterior radiographs of a 53-year-old woman with aching foot pain. (A), The normal appearance, 4 weeks after she started a daily exercise walking program. (B), Six weeks later, a healing second metatarsal stress fracture is revealed.

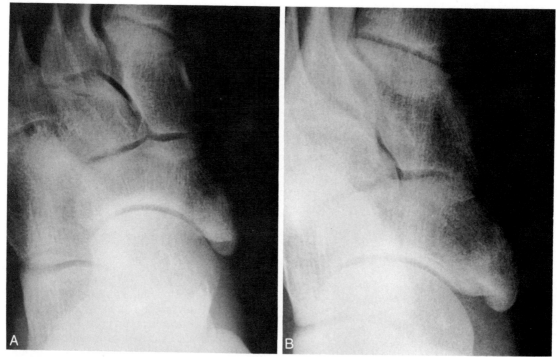

FIGURE 47–2. Anteroposterior radiographs of the tarsal navicular bone. *(A)*, Routine view. *(B)*, View with the foot supinated until the widest aspect of the navicular is visualized.

activity and limits the duration of play.[25] The pain is sharpest during foot impact and may be accompanied by cramping and local soreness. Examination may show local bony tenderness and modest swelling. There is generally no skin discoloration.

The clinical diagnosis of a stress fracture usually can be confirmed with standard anteroposterior, lateral, and oblique radiographs of the foot if the characteristic changes of periosteal new bone, cortical sclerosis, and linear lucency are found[25] (Fig. 47–1). The earliest of these changes may be seen a minimum of 2 weeks after the onset of symptoms, and changes sometimes require up to 3 months to be visible.[40, 62]

The radiographic diagnosis of navicular stress fracture is difficult because the fracture is oriented obliquely off the sagittal plane and frequently is not seen on standard views. Radiographic sensitivity improves greatly if the foot is positioned to obtain an anatomic anteroposterior view of the widest part of the navicular (Fig. 47–2). To do this, the forefoot must be supinated until the first metatarsal head is elevated several centimeters off the x-ray cannister and the x-ray beam is tangential to the talonavicular joint[53] (Fig. 47–3).

If midfoot symptoms persist after conservative treatment and findings on standard radiographs of the navicular remain normal, the diagnosis of navicular stress fracture may be made if a technetium bone scan is focally positive[25, 41, 53] (Fig. 47–4). Magnetic resonance imaging, xeroradiography, and thermography have also been reported to be useful adjuncts

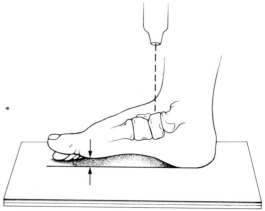

FIGURE 47–3. The position of the foot to obtain a true anteroposterior view of the tarsal navicular. The first metatarsal head is elevated off the film canister approximately 2 cm.

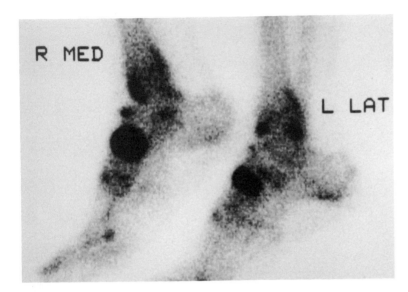

FIGURE 47–4. A bilateral tarsal navicular stress fracture demonstrated by increased uptake on a ^{99m}Tc bone scan.

in making the diagnosis.[44] Bony detail of navicular stress fractures may be demonstrated more clearly with true anteroposterior linear tomography or computed tomography.[53, 61] In our center, we have found computed tomography most helpful (Fig. 47–5).

Treatment

The great majority of stress fractures of the foot can be treated by simple immobilization and subsequent activity modification until symptoms abate.[25, 43] After a gradual return to full activity, cross-training and low-impact activities should be substituted for previous training techniques as possible to minimize the chance of recurrence. Shoe modification, such

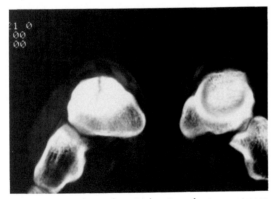

FIGURE 47–5. A tarsal navicular stress fracture not seen on routine radiographs but well illustrated by a midfoot computed tomographic scan.

as heel wedges of shock absorbing material and cushioned inserts, may speed return to training and prevent recurrence.

Nondisplaced complete or incomplete navicular fractures should be treated by immobilization in a non–weight-bearing cast for at least 6 weeks, followed by protected, progressive return to activity.[27, 61] Displaced complete fractures of the navicular bone require open reduction and internal fixation. Navicular nonunions are treated by bone grafting with or without internal fixation.

Second metatarsal base fractures of ballet dancers are treated with non–weight bearing and immobilization for 4 to 6 weeks. This is followed by progressive weight bearing in a short-leg walking cast or molded below-knee thermoplastic orthosis and by a gradual return to dancing over 6 more weeks. Excision of the necrotic second metatarsal base fragment has been reported, with good results in one painful case.[46]

Authors' Preferred Surgical Treatment

For a displaced navicular stress fracture, anatomic open reduction plus internal fixation with lag screws is the preferred treatment.

1. A 4-cm, slightly curved longitudinal incision is centered over the dorsum of the navicular bone just medial to the anterior tibial tendon (Fig. 47–6). The tendon is retracted laterally. The medial dorsal cutaneous nerve is protected at the distal extent of the incision.

5. Postoperatively, the patient is immobilized in a non–weight-bearing cast for 6 weeks or until some healing is shown radiographically. The patient is then protected in a short-leg walking cast or a postoperative shoe with an arch support for 6 weeks while gradually returning to activity. If healing is difficult to prove with standard radiographs, then computed tomographic scanning is helpful in demonstrating bone bridging at the old fracture site.

For established navicular nonunion or for persistent medial midfoot pain with bony sclerosis of the navicular but no demonstrable fracture, corticocancellous inlay bone grafting is preferred. For nonunion, internal fixation is added to increase bone stability after grafting.

1. With the surgical exposure described earlier for acute fractures, the dorsal surface of the tarsal navicular is visualized.

2. A 2.0 × 0.8-cm cortical window is outlined on the dorsal medial navicular, centered on the fracture line. The corners are drilled with a 2.0-mm drill (Fig. 47–8), and the cortex is cut with a small osteotome and removed.

3. All fibrous material and callus between navicular fragments are débrided. Cancellous bone is curetted from the center of the navicular.

4. A similarly sized rectangular corticocancellous graft is harvested from the iliac crest. Additional cancellous bone graft is harvested and packed into the depths of the navicular bone. The corticocancellous inlay graft is

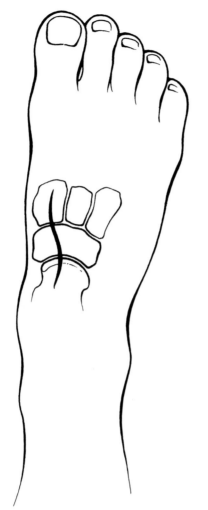

FIGURE 47–6. The skin incision for open reduction and internal fixation of a displaced navicular stress fracture.

2. The capsule of the talonavicular joint, the periosteum of the navicular, and the capsule of the navicular–first cuneiform joint are exposed and split longitudinally through the length of the incision. The periosteum is elevated off the navicular bone until the fracture is seen. Fracture hematoma and fibrous tissue are débrided with a small curette.

3. Anatomic restoration of joint surfaces is mandatory. Fixation is obtained with two parallel cannulated 4.0-mm cancellous screws lagged from medial to lateral across the navicular and perpendicular to the fracture line (Fig. 47–7).

4. The periosteum and subcutaneous tissues are closed with fine absorbable sutures, and the skin is closed with interrupted nylon sutures. A compression dressing is applied.

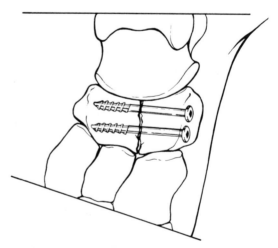

FIGURE 47–7. Internal fixation of a displaced navicular stress fracture obtained with two cancellous lag screws.

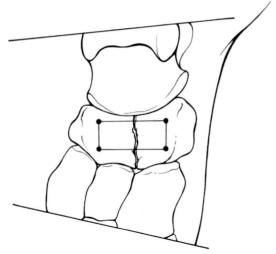

FIGURE 47–8. Removal of a corticocancellous window from the dorsal medial surface of a navicular nonunion in preparation for inlay bone grafting.

tamped snugly into the navicular window, bridging the fracture.

5. Lag screw internal fixation is performed as described for displaced fractures.

6. Closure and postoperative management are identical to that for displaced navicular stress fractures.

Complications

Long-term complications of stress fractures of the foot in athletes are very rare. With proper management, almost all athletes are eventually able to return to vigorous, if not maximum, activity. One reported patient with nonunion of the tarsal navicular developed osteoarthrosis at the navicular articulations.[51] Such arthrosis would require appropriate midtarsal fusions to alleviate pain.

A high index of suspicion, timely diagnosis, and aggressive nonsurgical treatment will minimize delays in healing and the need for surgical intervention.

SESAMOID PROBLEMS

Despite their small size, the sesamoid bones of the metatarsophalangeal joint in the great toe bear heavy, repetitive loads and therefore are vulnerable to the same acute, chronic, and post-traumatic changes as any other bone.[45]

The sesamoids are subjected to up to three times the body weight during normal walking,[63] and they are stressed in tension and bending by the flexor hallucis brevis tendons.[49] This routine stress is magnified by the high forces and impact loading developed during sports activities.

Sesamoid injuries in athletes may be acute or chronic. Acute sesamoid fractures are generally avulsion-type injuries generated through the sesamoid by the plantar first metatarsophalangeal joint complex during forceful push-off. Because of the large forces involved, the fragments may be separated, but the overall mechanism is maintained by the strong medial and lateral investing structures.[45] Acute sesamoid fracture may also occur from direct impact, yielding a widely displaced intra-articular fracture. Such injuries, although rare, may lead to degenerative arthritis of the sesamoid-metatarsal articulation.[45]

Chronic problems of the great toe sesamoid bones in athletes include sesamoiditis (sesamoid chondromalacia and synovitis), stress fracture, avascular necrosis, and osteoarthritis. Avascular necrosis of a sesamoid may occur as a primary problem but is more commonly seen as the late sequela of sesamoid stress fractures.[45] Contusions of small branches of the medial plantar digital nerve beneath the sesamoids result in neuritic pain that mimics sesamoiditis.[50]

Diagnosis

Sesamoiditis presents with the insidious onset of aching pain at the plantar first metatarsophalangeal joint. The pain is accompanied by local swelling and point tenderness beneath one or both of the sesamoids and is worse with weight bearing. The tibial sesamoid is more often affected because it bears more weight during the repetitive impact loading of running and other sports.[26, 45] Great toe dorsiflexion is limited and painful.

The symptoms of sesamoid stress fracture and avascular necrosis are similar to those of sesamoiditis: insidious aching pain following activity.[63] With acute fracture, the onset of pain is abrupt, but the clinical presentation is indistinguishable from that of other sesamoid problems.

Differentiation between sesamoiditis, sesamoid fracture, and avascular necrosis can usu-

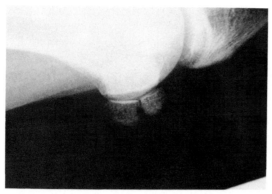

FIGURE 47–9. Lateral view of a tibial sesamoid fracture.

ally be made by standard radiographs, including anteroposterior, lateral (Fig. 47–9), and sesamoid axial views.[34] The axial view is especially helpful in demonstrating avascular necrosis or degenerative narrowing of the sesamoid-metatarsal articulation. Tomograms, magnetic resonance images and computed tomographic scans may help delineate a poorly visualized sesamoid fracture. Bone scanning, although not diagnosis specific, may delineate medial versus lateral sesamoid involvement. As reported by McBryde and Anderson, a significant decrease in pain following a dorsally introduced intra-articular metatarsophalangeal joint lidocaine injection indicates sesamoiditis instead of sesamoid fracture as the painful problem.[45]

Treatment

Treatment of sesamoiditis is aimed at controlling inflammation and altering the provoking activity. For acute painful episodes, intermittent ice application, elevation, the use of nonsteroidal anti-inflammatory medications, and a short period of partial weight bearing using crutches are initiated. When symptoms have improved, progression to full weight bearing is allowed in conjunction with orthotic use. The molded arch orthotic should feature a metatarsal pad proximal to the painful area with relief (indentation or softer material) under the metatarsal head and sesamoids. Injectable steroids are avoided. Ionophoresis, ultrasound, and gentle range-of-motion exercises may be helpful. Patience on the part of the patient and treating physician is required.

If the painful sesamoid is prominent on the axial sesamoid radiograph and there is a tough callus or intractable plantar keratosis directly beneath it on the bottom of the foot, shaving of the plantar sesamoid prominence may be all that is necessary to relieve the symptoms.

For chronic sesamoiditis that has failed to respond to all conservative measures for up to a year, single-sesamoid excision is indicated. Both sesamoids should not be excised to avoid hyperextension of the metatarsophalangeal joint (cock-up toe).[54] Careful preservation of the plantar plate and associated intrinsic tendons, with repair and reefing of the flexor brevis tendon deficit after sesamoid removal, is necessary to prevent hallux valgus or varus.[34]

If the patient has an excessively plantar-flexed first ray, as demonstrated by examination, by Harris mat impressions, and by bilateral foot radiographs, a basilar osteotomy to elevate the first metatarsal head 2 or 3 degrees may be helpful.[34]

Treatment of a nondisplaced acute sesamoid fracture consists of ice application, elevation, limited weight bearing, and the use of nonsteroidal anti-inflammatory drugs, as for the treatment of sesamoiditis. Weight bearing is gradually reinstituted as symptoms disappear. Immobilization in a short-leg walking cast with toe extension for 3 to 6 weeks will prevent metatarsophalangeal dorsiflexion and enforce activity limitations. The rare displaced fracture with two or three main fragments may be treated with bone grafting and immobilization or with excision. A widely displaced comminuted sesamoid fracture is treated with fragment or total sesamoid excision. Full recovery after single-sesamoid surgical excision is expected within 12 weeks for most athletes, although some decrease in hallux push-off force may occur.[34]

In the past, stress fractures of the sesamoids have healed poorly with conservative measures.[63] If symptoms persist after 6 weeks of immobilization and 4 to 6 months of activity modification combined with the use of a stiff-soled rocker-bottom shoe and a weight-relieving total contact shoe insert, surgical treatment is indicated. Surgical options for sesamoid nonunion include sesamoid excision[63] and sesamoid bone grafting.[1] The results of excision are the same as noted previously for acute fractures of the sesamoids. Sesamoid bone grafting yields greater than 90 percent healing[1] and avoids the risk of hallux push-off weakness.

Avascular necrosis of the sesamoid is treated like a sesamoid stress fracture.

Authors' Preferred Surgical Treatment

For chronic sesamoiditis unrelieved by long-term conservative treatment, sesamoid excision is necessary. The tibial sesamoid is excised through a medial incision, and the lateral sesamoid may be reached through a dorsal or plantar incision centered between the first and second metatarsal heads. The plantar incision is a much easier approach but runs the risk of causing a painful plantar callus.[54]

Excision of the tibial sesamoid is performed as follows:

1. A 4-cm longitudinal medial incision just below the midline is made over the first metatarsophalangeal joint (Fig. 47–10). The incision is carefully deepened to the capsule, protecting the plantar digital nerve.

2. The plane between the plantar plate enveloping the sesamoids and the subcutaneous tissues is developed until the tibial sesamoid is well visualized (Fig. 47–11).

3. The periosteum over the tibial sesamoid is incised longitudinally, and the sesamoid is subperiosteally dissected out (Fig. 47–12). Caution is taken to preserve the medial head of the flexor brevis and the abductor hallucis.

4. The defect created by removal of the sesamoid is closed by imbrication of the residual flexor brevis tendon with 4–0 absorbable sutures.

5. After routine skin closure, a compressive bulky dressing is applied.

6. Postoperatively, weight bearing is avoided completely for 2 weeks to allow soft tissue healing and resolution of inflammation. Then the sutures are removed, the patient is placed

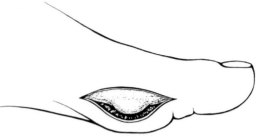

FIGURE 47–11. For tibial sesamoid excision, the sesamoid is exposed through an extra-articular approach.

in a wooden postoperative shoe, and partial weight bearing is allowed for 4 weeks. Next, active and active-assisted stretching exercises with devices such as a TheraBand and full weight bearing are initiated. By 8 weeks, the patient returns to distance walking and easy jogging. Unrestricted activity is allowed 12 weeks after surgery.

For intractable fibular sesamoiditis, the plantar approach to the lateral sesamoid is preferred:

1. A longitudinal 3-cm incision is made between the first and second metatatarsal heads. The plantar crease is followed. Blunt dissection is carried along the septa that separate the whorls of fat down to the lateral aspect of the fibular sesamoid, avoiding the plantar digital nerves and vessels.

2. The fibular sesamoid is shelled out of its investing periosteum through a longitudinal incision. A No. 64 Beaver blade facilitates precise dissection. The lateral head of the flexor brevis and adductor hallucis must be preserved.

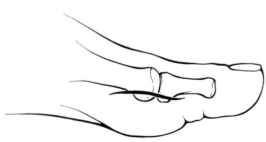

FIGURE 47–10. The plantar medial incision for excision of the tibial sesamoid.

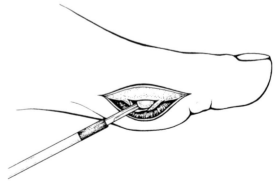

FIGURE 47–12. Subperiosteal exposure of the tibial sesamoid for excision.

3. The defect left by removal of the lateral sesamoid is imbricated with 4–0 absorbable sutures.

4. Closure and postoperative care are identical to that provided for tibial sesamoidectomy.

Bone grafting for sesamoid nonunion is preferred in athletes. In the great majority of cases, the tibial sesamoid is affected. The approach to the tibial sesamoid for bone grafting is identical to that for sesamoidectomy.

1. A curved longitudinal medial incision, just below midline and 3 to 4 cm long, is made directly down to the first metatarsophalangeal capsule.

2. The capsule is split longitudinally and the joint is inspected (Fig. 47–13). If severe chondromalacia of the sesamoid is present, sesamoidectomy is performed.

3. If such articular changes are not present, an extraperiosteal plantar approach is made to the tibial sesamoid between the plantar plate and the subcutaneous tissues.

4. The plantar periosteum over the sesamoid is split longitudinally and elevated carefully. The fibrous areas of nonunion are curetted until clean.

5. The capsule of the medial first metatarsal head is elevated.

6. A 7 × 5-mm rectangular bone window is made with a small osteotome at the medial metatarsal head. Cancellous bone is harvested. The cortical window fragment is replaced in its bed, and the medial capsule is reapproximated tightly with 2–0 nonabsorbable sutures.

7. At the plantar sesamoid, the bone graft is packed into the nonunion defect. The sesamoidal periosteum is closed with 4–0 absorbable sutures.

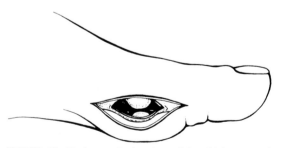

FIGURE 47–13. Intra-articular view of the tibial sesamoid and first metatarsal head obtained to rule out significant chondromalacia before an extra-articular sesamoid approach is made for bone grafting of sesamoid nonunion.

8. After routine skin closure, the foot is kept elevated in a bulky dressing for several days.

9. Postoperatively, the patient remains non–weight bearing with the hallux immobilized for 3 weeks. Then, a short-leg walking cast with toe extension to prevent dorsiflexion of the hallux is applied. At the 8-week interval, a stiff-soled shoe with a medial arch support is prescribed, and active range-of-motion exercises are begun. At 12 weeks after surgery, if tomograms demonstrate bony union, a gradual return to full activity over the next 6 weeks is initiated.

For persistent sesamoid nonunion after grafting or for chronically painful sesamoid osteochondritis (avascular necrosis with fragmentation or joint surface destruction), sesamoid excision as described for sesamoiditis is the preferred surgical treatment.

Complications

Great care is needed during the surgical approaches for sesamoid operations because the delicate plantar digital nerves may be injured, resulting in painful neuromas. Should a painful neuroma occur, exploration of the nerve is indicated.[31] Treatment options include resection of the neuroma with direct repair, resection with nerve grafting, and proximal resection of the neuroma with placement of the nerve stump into a non–weight-bearing bed. Recalcitrant cases may require more imaginative solutions, such as wandering nerve grafting, nerve stump placement into proximal veins, or nerve stump placement into vein conduits.[24] Peripheral nerves in continuity may be treated by other investigational techniques, such as vein wrapping.[18]

Preservation of plantar plate integrity is essential. Hallux varus, hallux valgus, or cock-up toe can result if these structures are violated and not repaired. Late treatment of these deformities may require tendon transfers or metatarsophalangeal joint fusion.[39]

FIFTH METATARSAL BASE FRACTURES

Since Jones first reported on proximal fifth metatarsal fractures in 1902,[28] these fractures have been widely observed in athletes[9, 29, 51, 60] and fall into two distinct groups.[9] The more common metaphyseal styloid avulsion fracture, an inversion injury, heals predictably with minimal treatment.[10] The Jones fracture, a transverse fracture of the proximal fifth metatarsal shaft just distal to the metaphyseal flare, occurs frequently in younger patients, especially early in athletic training.[29] This fracture may cause prolonged disability; up to 25 percent of these fractures go on to nonunion[6, 9] and 67 percent progress to delayed union[29] when conservatively treated.

A simplified classification system for Jones' fractures has been described by Lehman and coworkers.[33] Type I metatarsal base fractures represent the acute Jones fracture with no preexisting history of pain or signs of bone stress. Type II fractures are transverse fractures of the proximal shaft associated with a history of prodromal pain or prior injury and signs of chronic bone stress, such as periosteal thickening, widened fracture line, and some degree of medullary sclerosis. Type III fractures are characterized as recurrently symptomatic and show a widened fracture line, bony periosteal reaction, and complete medullary sclerosis.

The metaphyseal avulsion fracture occurs when sudden ankle inversion stress is strongly resisted by the peroneus brevis.[10] Type I Jones' fractures occur when the equinus foot is loaded heavily along its lateral border,[9] as described by Jones when he himself broke his fifth metatarsal while dancing.[28]

Types II and III fifth metatarsal base fractures are seen most frequently in athletes involved in long distance running, basketball, and other high-impact sports. These injuries are preceded by a prodrome of chronic aching fifth metatarsal pain during or after activity and represent completion of a stress fracture.[10, 33]

Diagnosis

Patients with acute fifth metatarsal base fractures complain of sharp, severe pain at the lateral foot during weight bearing. Examination shows point tenderness at the fifth metatarsal base with mild swelling. Inversion positioning of the plantarflexed foot is strongly resisted by the patient.[29] Anteroposterior and lateral radiographs of the fifth metatarsal are diagnostic (Fig. 47–14).

Treatment

Nondisplaced avulsions of the fifth metatarsal tuberosity can be treated by a short period

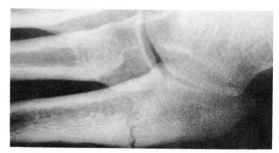

FIGURE 47–14. A type II Jones fracture with thickened cortex and incomplete medullary sclerosis.

of protection with a compressive foot wrap or by wearing a hard shoe while weight bearing on crutches as tolerance allows.[15] If symptoms resolve over 3 to 6 weeks, progression to a normal shoe and gradual return to activity are allowed. If the fracture is markedly displaced, a few weeks of immobilization in a short-leg walking cast may be needed initially to control pain.[10]

Nondisplaced types I or II fifth metatarsal fractures in less active patients should be treated conservatively.[33, 67] Treatment consists of immobilization in a short-leg non–weight-bearing cast for 9 weeks or until the fracture is painless during weight bearing and nontender to palpation. After casting, a molded arch support is provided. Full activity may be resumed 3 to 6 weeks after final casting if the patient remains pain-free and radiographs show continued healing.

Immediate surgery is preferred for the serious amateur or professional athlete to expedite healing and minimize time away from training.[7, 29, 33] Surgery is also indicated for delayed union or nonunion resulting from conservative treatment.[9, 60]

Surgical treatment options for fifth metatarsal fractures include intramedullary compression screw fixation,[29, 33] plate fixation, tension band wiring, reverse slot grafting,[23] and medullary curettage plus open inlay or sliding bone grafting.[9, 60]

Authors' Preferred Surgical Treatment

In athletes, intramedullary screw fixation is the surgical procedure of choice for type I or II fractures and for delayed union or nonunion without complete medullary obliteration because it allows early postoperative weight bearing, promotes rapid healing, and permits the quickest return to sports of all the surgical options.

1. With the patient in the lateral decubitus position, a 2-cm longitudinal incision is extended proximally from the styloid of the fifth metatarsal parallel to the bottom of the foot.

2. The styloid tip is approached directly through the interval between the peroneus longus and the peroneus brevis. The peroneus brevis insertion is split sharply over the tip of the styloid and elevated.

3. A Kirschner wire is inserted across the styloid tip and distally down the medullary canal. Correct wire position is verified by fluoroscopy. To facilitate screw insertion, a sterile marking pen is used to mark the direction of the wire on the skin proximal to the styloid.[33]

4. The wire is removed and the metatarsal is axially drilled, countersunk, tapped, and filled with a 4.5-mm malleolar screw using ASIF technique (Fig. 47–15). The fracture is forcefully compressed. The screw must be long enough so that all threads lie distal to the fracture line. Countersinking the screw decreases the prominence of the screw head postoperatively. A 6.5-mm cancellous screw may be used for very large athletes.

5. The incision is closed routinely, and a compressive dressing is applied.

6. Postoperatively, the patient is treated in a non–weight-bearing cast for 2 to 4 weeks, followed by progressive weight bearing in a hard shoe for an additional 4 weeks. Return to running is allowed when metatarsal tenderness on palpation and pain during vigorous walking are absent.

For type III fractures and established nonunions with complete medullary sclerosis, the preferred surgical procedure is medullary curettage and open inlay bone grafting.

1. With the patient supine with a large bolster under the ipsilateral hip, the base of the fifth metatarsal is approached through a 4-cm dorsolateral incision. Branches of the sural nerve are protected.

2. The periosteum is incised longitudinally through the length of the incision and elevated to expose the fracture.

3. A rectangular cortical window, 2.0 × 0.8 cm and centered at the fracture, is outlined on the fifth metatarsal. The corners are drilled with a 2.0-mm drill (Fig. 47–16), and the cortex is cut with a small osteotome and removed.

4. The sclerotic bone filling the canal on either side of the fracture is curetted until the medullary canal is re-established.

5. A corticocancellous bone graft is taken from the iliac crest and contoured to fit precisely into the window. The graft is snugly tamped into place. A small amount of cancellous graft is added around the metatarsal at the level of the fracture.

6. The periosteum and subcutaneous layers are closed in layers with 4–0 absorbable sutures and the skin is closed with 4–0 nylon sutures. A compression dressing with splints is applied.

7. Postoperatively, the patient is protected for 6 weeks in a non–weight-bearing short-leg cast, followed by progressive weight bearing in a hard shoe for an additional 4 weeks. Healing is verified radiographically. A return to running is allowed when metatarsal tenderness to palpation and pain during vigorous walking are absent.

FIGURE 47–15. Intramedullary screw fixation of a Jones fracture through the proximal tip of the fifth metatarsal styloid.

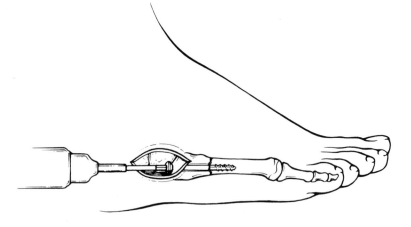

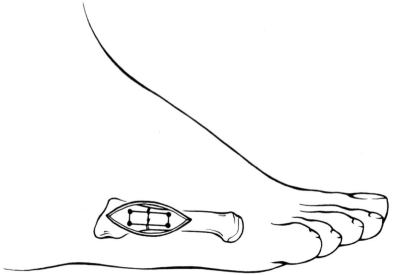

Complications

Intramedullary screw fixation has been associated with intraoperative technical difficulties (e.g., screw breakage and fixation malalignment).[29, 60] Use of much stronger modern screws and careful fluoroscopic verification of pin and screw placement should prevent those problems. Postoperative pain at the screw head prominence and fifth metatarsalgia have been reported.[10, 33] Such complaints can be avoided by countersinking the screw at surgery and by providing the athlete postoperatively with a padded shoe insert that is recessed at the prominent screw site. The symptomatic screw should not be removed until the fracture is well healed and the athlete's competitive season is over.

TURF TOE

Turf toe is an acute or chronic plantar capsular ligament sprain of the first metatarsophalangeal joint and is seen most commonly in football offensive linemen, receivers, and running backs.[55] It is caused by forced hyperextension of the hallux when ball carriers are tackled or offensive linemen push off to block, Turf toe has been associated with hard artificial playing surfaces, flexible soccer-style shoes,[4] and increased ankle dorsiflexion.[55] The severity of turf toe is generally mild, but the condition may be quite severe. In fact, according to one study at a major state university, a football player was four times as likely to miss a game if he had turf toe than if he had sprained his ankle.[8]

Diagnosis

The initial discomfort of turf toe increases over the first 24 hours after injury as the plantar capsular ligament and surrounding tissues become inflamed.[4] The metatarsophalangeal joint is warm, swollen, and diffusely tender, with maximum tenderness located plantarly just proximal to the sesamoids. Passive dorsiflexion is very painful, and the player cannot push off or accelerate when running.

Treatment

For mild cases, treatment consists of ice and elevation for several days, followed by limited activity until the pain abates. Anti-inflammatory agents may be given, and future hallux dorsiflexion is prevented by toe taping or shoe modification (sole stiffening with an extended steel shank and a mild rocker-bottom sole). For severe cases, this regimen is followed after the toe is protected for 2 weeks in a short-leg walking cast with a toe plate. Surgical treatment is not indicated for turf toe.

Complications

Chronic injury of the first metatarsophalangeal joint leads to painful hallux rigidus,[36] and joint motion has been shown to be decreased after turf toe injury.[55] If chronic pain and stiffness result from repetitive turf toe injury, hallux rigidus may ensue and may require surgical treatment to alleviate symptoms.

HALLUX RIGIDUS

Hallux rigidus is a painful condition of the first metatarsophalangeal joint that is characterized by loss of dorsiflexion[57] and by hypertrophic osteoarthritic joint changes. Hallux rigidus has been classified into four etiologic types: hereditary, developmental or post-traumatic, secondary to a systemic arthritic process, and secondary to postoperative deformity.[11]

The onset of hallux rigidus in athletes is seen most commonly during adolescence and early adulthood.[19] It becomes a problem for female ballet dancers late in their careers.[3, 20] It has been attributed to a long first metatarsal,[3] an elevated first metatarsal,[30] metatarsal head abnormalities,[17] abnormal metatarsal-sesamoid articulation,[47] and acute and chronic trauma.[36]

Hallux rigidus presents as intermittent pain and swelling over the first metatarsophalangeal joint. In time, a dorsal spur of the metatarsal head develops, motion decreases, and pain worsens during or after activity. Activities that dorsiflex the metatarsophalangeal joint vigorously are particularly painful. The decreased dorsiflexion leads to minor gait alterations but is rarely debilitating.[22]

Physical findings include thickening of the joint with dorsal prominence, synovitis, tenderness, restricted dorsiflexion of 30 degrees or less,[38] and pain at the extremes of the range of motion. Radiographs reveal varying degrees of degenerative arthritis manifest by joint space narrowing, dorsal lipping and periarticular osteophytes (Fig. 47–17), and enlargement of the articular surfaces.

Treatment

Conservative treatment options consist of nonsteroidal anti-inflammatory medications, toe taping or wearing extended stiff orthoses

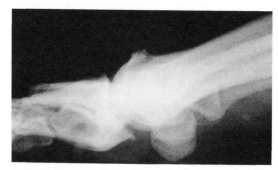

FIGURE 47–17. A first metatarsal head dorsal osteophyte characteristic of hallux rigidus.

to limit joint motion, activity modification, brief periods of protection in a short-leg walking cast with toe extension, and long-term use of shoes with wide toe boxes, stiff soles, and rocker bottoms.

Surgical treatment, especially for adolescents, should be reserved for patients in whom conservative treatment has failed and who have significant disability. Surgical options include cheilectomy, arthrodesis, dorsal wedge osteotomy of the proximal phalanx, Keller's arthroplasty, and implant arthroplasty.[22]

In athletes, the latter two options are poor choices. The Keller arthroplasty can lead to hallux push-off weakness and metatarsophalangeal joint instability. Implant arthroplasty has the potential for silicone synovitis and is not durable enough for heavy use.[58]

Osteotomy of the proximal phalanx may be helpful, especially in hereditary hallux rigidus of adolescents, if the patient retains 30 degrees of plantar flexion at the metatarsophalangeal joint.[32, 48] Osteotomy may be used in conjunction with cheilectomy to redirect more favorably the available arc of motion.[34]

Cheilectomy has been popularized for the treatment of active individuals,[11, 21, 38] with arthrodesis reserved for the patients in whom surgery has failed[34] and those whose joints have severe degenerative changes.[22]

Authors' Preferred Surgical Treatment

For athletes, cheilectomy is the preferred initial surgical procedure.

1. Under tourniquet control, a 5-cm longitudinal incision is centered over the first metatarsophalangeal joint just medial to the extensor hallucis tendon.

2. The extensor is retracted laterally, and cutaneous nerves are protected.

3. The capsule is longitudinally incised and elevated from the metatarsal head and the base of the proximal phalanx. Excessive synovium and loose bony fragments are removed. Osteophytes from the sides and dorsum of the base of the proximal phalanx and from the sides of the metatarsal head are removed with a rongeur.

4. The toe is maximally plantarflexed. With a small oscillating saw or osteotome, cutting from distal to proximal, the dorsal one-third of the metatarsal articular surface is obliquely osteotomized (Fig. 47–18). Rough edges are smoothed with a rongeur.

5. If passive dorsiflexion of at least 60 degrees is not demonstrated, a Freer elevator is passed between the plantar plate and metatarsal head to lyse any sesamoidal adhesions.

6. If adequate dorsiflexion is still not achieved and plantar flexion of 30 degrees is present, a dorsal closing wedge osteotomy of the proximal phalanx is performed. With an oscillating saw, a transverse osteotomy is made in the proximal phalanx 5 mm distal to the articular surface. From the distal fragment, a 2-mm dorsally based wedge of bone is removed. The osteotomy is tightly closed, hinging on the plantar cortex and periosteum. The osteotomy is pinned percutaneously with two smooth 0.045-inch Kirschner wires directed obliquely from distal medial to proximal lateral across the osteotomy site. The pins are cut and capped.

7. The dorsal capsular incision is closed with 4–0 absorbable sutures, and after routine skin closure, a compression foot dressing is applied.

8. Postoperatively, the patient remains non–weight bearing with the foot elevated for several days until the first dressing change. Then, weight bearing as tolerated in a post-

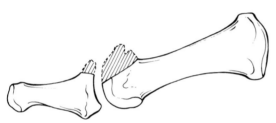

FIGURE 47–18. Lateral view of the first metatarsophalangeal joint showing a portion of the metatarsal head and osteophytes excised during cheilectomy for hallux rigidus.

operative shoe is initiated. Active and passive range-of-motion exercises are started as soon as soft tissue healing has occurred. Pins, if used, are removed after 3 weeks. Improvement in motion and relief of pain are generally seen within 3 months, but it may take 6 months or longer for maximum improvement.

Complications

Persistent first metatarsophalangeal joint pain after cheilectomy that has not improved in 6 months despite shoe stiffening and other conservative measures may be remedied by metatarsophalangeal joint arthrodesis.

AVASCULAR NECROSIS OF THE SECOND METATARSAL HEAD

Avascular necrosis of the second metatarsal head, first described by Freiberg in 1914[12] as a type of metatarsalgia, is a disease of the growing epiphysis that presents in athletes in the second or third decade of life. Repetitive loading of the primary growth center during athletics is hypothesized to cause vascular injury and secondary structural changes.[5]

Diagnosis

Symptoms of second metatarsal head avascular necrosis can vary from mild metatarsalgia that does not limit activity to pronounced second metatarsophalangeal joint pain that is greatly limiting. The pain is generally worse after activity and is accompanied by local tenderness, swelling, and crepitus. Standard radiographs of the forefoot demonstrate flattening and relative sclerosis of the second metatarsal head with peripheral osteophytes and loose articular fragments.

Treatment

Initial treatment consists of activity modification and immobilization in a short-leg walking cast with toe extension. After symptoms have decreased, the joint may be further protected by use of an orthotic with a metatarsal pad and shoes with extended steel shanks and mild rocker bottoms.

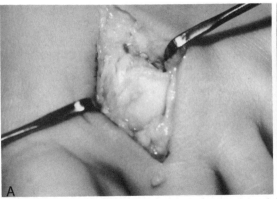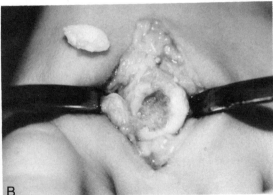

FIGURE 47–19. Exposure of the second metatarsal head for avascular necrosis showing articular irregularity *(A)* and débridement of loose osteochondritic fragments *(B)*.

Surgical treatment is indicated in adults who have persistent pain at the second metatarsophalangeal joint.[37] Surgical management has included resection of the metatarsal head,[12] metatarsal head resection with syndactylization of the second toe to the third toe,[30] and second metatarsal head arthroplasty with removal of excessive bone fragments.[11]

Authors' Preferred Surgical Treatment

Remodeling arthroplasty of the second metatarsal head with removal of all the loose body fragments, as advocated by DuVries[11] is preferred.

1. A 3-cm dorsal longitudinal S-shaped incision is centered over the second metatarsophalangeal joint. The long extensor is retracted laterally, and the joint capsule is split longitudinally.

2. The capsule is elevated sharply from all sides of the metatarsal head. The head is delivered into the wound.

3. Loose bony fragments and osteophytes from the metatarsal head and the proximal phalangeal base are débrided with a small rongeur (Fig. 47–19).

4. The head is trimmed with the rongeur until it is normal in size and contour.

5. The joint is irrigated well and then pinned in retrograde fashion with a 0.062-inch Kirschner wire to prevent joint subluxation during soft tissue healing. The pin is bent, cut off, and capped at the tip of the toe.

6. The capsule is tightly closed with 4–0 absorbable suture.

7. After routine skin closure, a bulky dressing is applied.

8. Postoperatively, a postoperative shoe is worn for 2 weeks, and weight bearing is allowed as tolerated. The pin is then pulled, and progressive activity is initiated. Gradual improvement of second metatarsophalangeal joint symptoms is expected for up to 1 year after surgery.

Complications

Persistent postoperative pain is treated with resection arthroplasty of the base of the proximal phalanx and subtotal syndactylization of the second toe to the third toe.

References

1. Anderson R, McBryde AM: Autogenous home grafting of hallux sesamoid nonunions. Presented at the AOFAS Specialty Day Conference, AAOS Annual Meeting. Anaheim, CA, February 1991.
2. Barrow GW, Subrata S: Menstrual irregularity and stress fractures in collegiate female distance runners. Am J Sports Med 16:209–216, 1988.
3. Bonney G, MacNab I: Hallux valgus and hallux rigidus: A critical survey of operative results. J Bone Joint Surg 34B:366–385, 1952.
4. Bowers KD, Martin RB: Turf-toe: A shoe-surface related football injury. Med Sci Sports 8:81–83, 1976.
5. Braddock GIF: Experimental epiphyseal injury and Freiberg's disease. J Bone Joint Surg 4B:154, 1959.
6. Carp L: Fracture of the fifth metatarsal bone with special reference to delayed union. Ann Surg 86:308–320, 1927.
7. Cass JR: Fractures and dislocations involving the midfoot. *In* Chapman M (Ed): Operative Orthopaedics. Philadelphia, JB Lippincott, 1988.

8. Cohen TP, Arnold JA, Weber DL: Traumatic lesions of the metatarsophalangeal joint of the great toe in athletes. Am J Sports Med 6:326–334, 1978.
9. Dameron TB: Fractures and anatomic variations of the proximal portion of the fifth metatarsal. J Bone Joint Surg 57A:788–792, 1975.
10. DeLee JC: Fractures and dislocations of the foot. In Marin R (Ed): Surgery of the Foot. St. Louis, CV Mosby, 1986.
11. DuVries HL: Surgery of the Foot. St. Louis, CV Mosby, 1978.
12. Freiberg AH: Infraction of the second metatarsal bone—a typical injury. Surg Gynecol Obstet 19:191–193, 1914.
13. Frisch RE, Gotz-Welbergen AV, McArthur JW, et al: Delayed menarche and amenorrhea of college athletes in relation to onset of training. JAMA 246:1559–1563, 1981.
14. Gadpaille WJ, Sanlearn CF, Wagner WW: Athletic amenorrhea, affective disorders and eating disorders. Am J Psychiatry 144:939–942, 1987.
15. Giamestras NJ, Sammarco GH: Fractures and dislocations in the foot. In Rockwood CA, Green DP (Eds): Fractures in Adults. Philadelphia, JB Lippincott, 1975.
16. Gilbert RS, Johnson HA: Stress fractures in military recruits—a review of twelve years experience. Milit Med 131:716–721, 1966.
17. Goodfellow J: Etiology of hallux rigidus. Proc R Soc Med 59:821, 1966.
18. Gould J: Treatment of the painful injured nerve in continuity. In Gilberman RH (Ed): Operative Nerve Repair and Reconstruction. Philadelphia, JB Lippincott, 1991.
19. Gould N, Schneider W, Ashikaga T: Epidemiological survey of foot problems in the continental United States 1978–1979. Foot Ankle 1:8–10, 1980.
20. Hamilton WG: Foot and ankle injuries in dancers. Clin Sports Med 7:148–173, 1988.
21. Hattrup SJ, Johnson KA: Subjective results of hallux rigidus following treatment with cholestectomy. Clin Orthop 226:182–191, 1988.
22. Hawkins BJ, Haddad RJ: Hallux rigidus. Clin Sports Med 7:37–49, 1988.
23. Hens J, Martens M: Surgical treatment of Jones' fractures. Orthop Trauma Surg 109:277–279, 1990.
24. Herndon JH, Hess AV: Neuromas. In Gilberman RH (Ed): Operative Nerve Repair and Reconstruction. Philadelphia, JB Lippincott, 1991.
25. Hershman EB, Mailly T: Stress fractures. Clin Sports Med 9:183–214, 1990.
26. Hulkko A, Orava S, Pellinen P, Puranen J: Stress fractures of the sesamoid bones of the first metatarsophalangeal joint in athletes. Acta Orthop Trauma Surg 104:113–117, 1985.
27. Hunter L: Stress fractures of the tarsal navicular. Am J Sports Med 9:217–219, 1981.
28. Jones R: Fracture of the base of the fifth metatarsal bone by indirect violence. Ann Surg 35:697–700, 1902.
29. Kavanaugh JH, Bower TD, Mann RV: The Jones fractures revisited. J Bone Joint Surg 60A:776–782, 1978.
30. Kelekian H: Hallux valgus, allied deformities of the forefoot and metatarsalgia. Philadelphia, WB Saunders, 1965.
31. Kinzara JE: Sensory nerve neuromas—leading to failed foot surgery. Foot Ankle 7:110–117, 1986.
32. Kessel L, Bonney G: Hallux rigidus in the adolescent. J Bone Joint Surg 40B:668, 1958.
33. Lehman RC, Torg JS, Pavlov H, DeLee JC: Fractures of the base of the fifth metatarsal distal to the tuberosity: A review. Foot Ankle 7:245–252, 1987.
34. Lillich JS, Baxter DE: Common forefoot problems in runners. Foot Ankle 7:149–150, 1986.
35. Lloyd T, Triantafyllou SJ, Baker ER, et al: Women athletes with menstrual irregularity have increased musculoskeletal injuries. Med Sci Sports Exerc 16:343–348, 1984.
36. Mann RA: Hallux rigidus. Instr Course Lect 39:15–21, 1990.
37. Mann RA: Miscellaneous afflictions of the foot. In Mann RA (Ed): Surgery of the Foot. St. Louis, CV Mosby, 1986.
38. Mann RA, Clanton TO: Hallux rigidus: Treatment by cheilectomy. J Bone Joint Surg 70A:400–406, 1988.
39. Mann RA, Coughlin MJ: Hallux valgus and complications of hallux valgus. In Mann RA (Ed): Surgery of the Foot. St. Louis, CV Mosby, 1986.
40. Marcus R, Cann C, Modvig P, et al: Menstrual function and bone mass in elite women distance runners: Endocrine and metabolic features. Ann Intern Med 102:158–163, 1985.
41. Matheson GO, Clement DB, McKenzie DC, et al: Stress fractures in athletes. Am J Sports Med 15:46–56, 1987.
42. McBryde AM: Disorders of the foot and ankle. In Grana WA, Kalenak A (Eds): Clinical Sports Medicine. Philadelphia, WB Saunders, 1991.
43. McBryde AM: Stress fractures in athletes. J Sports Med 5:212–217, 1976.
44. McBryde AM: Stress fractures in runners. Clin Sports Med 4:737–752, 1985.
45. McBryde AM, Anderson RB: Sesamoid foot problems in the athlete. Clin Sports Med 7:51–60, 1988.
46. Micheli LJ, Sohn RS, Solomon R: Stress fractures of the second metatarsal involving Lisfranc's joint in ballet dancers. J Bone Joint Surg 67A:1372–1375, 1985.
47. Miller LF, Arendt J: Deformity of the first metatarsal head due to faulty foot mechanics. J Bone Joint Surg 22:349–353, 1940.
48. Moberg E: A simple operation for hallux rigidus. Clin Orthop 142:55–56, 1979.
49. Morton DJ: Biomechanics of the human foot. Instruct Course Lect 4:92–99, 1944.
50. Murphy PC, Baxter DE: Nerve entrapment of the foot and ankle in runners. Clin Sports Med 4:753, 1985.
51. Orava S, Halkko A: Delayed unions and nonunions of stress fractures in athletes. Am J Sports Med 16:378–382, 1988.
52. Orava S, Puranch J, Ala-ketoala L: Stress fractures caused by physical exercise. Acta Orthop Scand 49:19–27, 1978.
53. Pavlov H, Jorg JS, Freiberger RH: Tarsal navicular stress fractures: Radiographic evaluation. Radiology 148:641–645, 1983.
54. Pfeffinger LL, Mann RA: Sesamoid and accessory bones. In Mann RA (Ed): Surgery of the Foot. St. Louis, CV Mosby, 1986.
55. Rodeo SA, O'Brien S, Warren RF, et al: Turf-toe: An analysis of metatarsophalangeal joint sprains in professional football players. Am J Sports Med 18:280–285, 1990.

56. Scranton PE, Rutkowski R: Anatomic disorders of the first ray: Part II. Disorders of the sesamoids. Clin Orthop 151:256–264, 1980.
57. Shereff MJ, Bejjani FJ, Kummer FJ: Kinematics of the first metatarsophalangeal joint. J Bone Joint Surg 68A:392–398, 1986.
58. Singer KM, Jones DC: Soft tissue conditions of the foot and ankle. *In* Nicholas I, Hershman E (Eds): The Lower Extremity and Spine in Sports Medicine. St. Louis, CV Mosby, 1986.
59. Ting A, King W, Yocum L, et al: Stress fractures of the tarsal navicular in long-distance runners. Clin Sports Med 17:89–101, 1988.
60. Torg JS, Baldini FC, Zelko RR, et al: Fractures of the base of the fifth metatarsal distal to the tuberosity. J Bone Joint Surg 66A:209–214, 1984.
61. Torg JS, Pavlov H, Cooley LH, et al: Stress fractures of the tarsal navicular. J Bone Joint Surg 64A:700–712, 1982.
62. Towne LC, Blazina ME, Cozen LN: Fatigue fractures of the tarsal navicular. J Bone Joint Surg 52A:376–378, 1970.
63. Van Hal ME, Keene JS, Lange TA, Claney WG: Stress fractures of the great toe sesamoids. Ann J Sports Med 10:122–128, 1982.
64. Whiteside JA, Fleagle SB, Kalenak A: Fractures and refractures in intercollegiate athletes. Am J Sports Med 9:369–377, 1981.
65. Yokoe K, Taketomo M: Stress fractures of the proximal phalanx of the great toe. Am J Sports Med 14:240–242, 1986.
66. Zelko RR, Torg JS, Rachun Z: Proximal diaphyseal fractures of the fifth metatarsal—treatment of the fractures and their complications in athletes. Am J Sports Med 7:95–101, 1979.
67. Zogby RG, Baker BE: A review of nonoperative treatment of Jones' fracture. Am J Sports Med 15:304–307, 1987.

MUSCULOTENDINOUS

INJURIES

48

Conditions Seen in Classical Ballet and Modern Dance

WILLIAM G. HAMILTON

A BRIEF PRIMER ON DANCE

Ballet is considered the queen of dance. It had its origins in Renaissance Italy and was brought to France by Catherine Di Medici (1518–1589) when she married Henry II. It flourished in the courts of the French kings in the seventeenth and eighteenth centuries, reaching its pinnacle under Louis XIV at Versailles. Ballet was the natural outgrowth of the arts of the Renaissance gentleman as practiced at court. These arts included court dancing, classical fencing (the five positions of the feet in ballet supposedly were derived from positions used in fencing), and classical horsemanship.

All positions of the feet and poses of the body were codified circa 1680 by Pierre Beauchamps, Louis XIV's ballet master, and these same positions and French terms continue to be used today. The five positions of the feet are fundamental. In all positions, the feet are turned out 180 degrees so that the audience sees a maximum profile, or line. The dancers dance on the balls of their feet on demi-pointe in soft (ballet) shoes or on their toes on full pointe (females only) in toeshoes that contain

a hardened cardboard toe box. Certain positions and movements are basic:

The five positions of the feet (Fig. 48–1A to E):

First position. The heels are together and the feet are turned out 90 degrees from the sagittal plane.
Second position. The feet are shoulder width apart and turned out.
Third position. The feet are turned out and overlapped by 50 percent so that the heel of one foot is next to the instep of the other foot. (This position is rarely used in ballet today.)
Fourth position. The feet are turned out but separated from front to back by about a foot.
Fifth position. The feet are turned out and completely overlapped so that the heel of one foot is next to the toe of the other foot. This position is most commonly used and is also the most difficult to achieve. With poor turnout, the dancer cannot "close in fifth."
Relevé: The movement of the foot from flat up to the ball of the foot (demi-pointe) or onto full toe (full pointe) (Fig. 48–1F).
Plié: The ballet dancer's knee bend. The heel is left on the floor in the demi-plié but

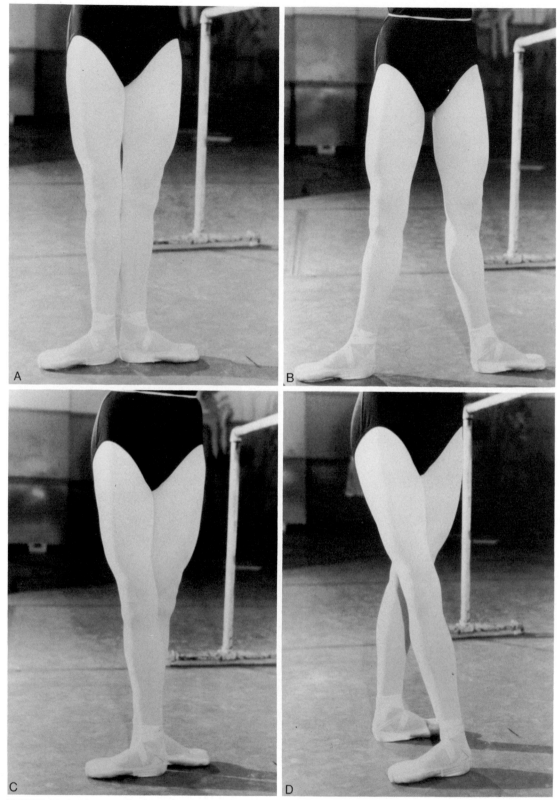

FIGURE 48–1. (A to E), The five positions of the feet. (A), First position. (B), Second position. (C), Third position. (D), Fourth position.

Illustration continued on following page

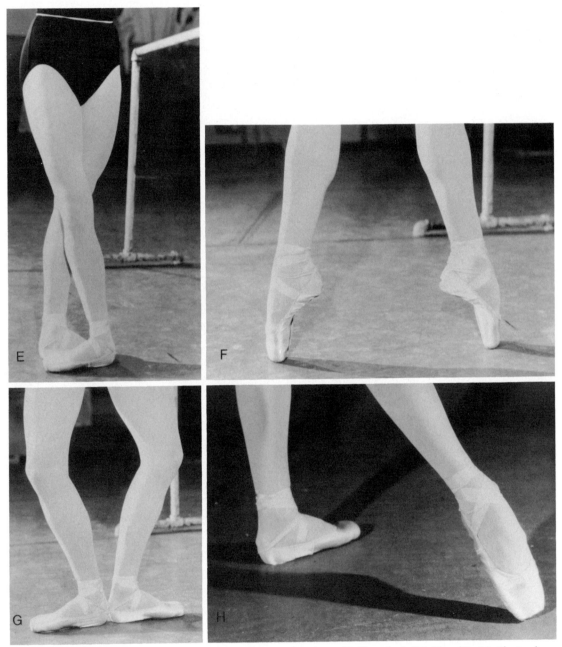

FIGURE 48–1 *Continued* (*E*), Fifth position. (*F* to *L*), Basic movements. (*F*), The relevé. (*G*), The plié. (*H*), The tendu.

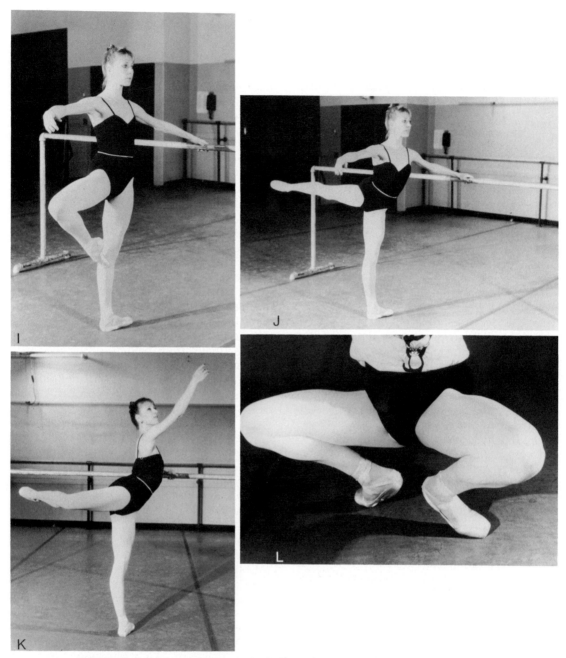

FIGURE 48–1 *Continued* (*I*), The passé. (*J*), The arabesque. (*K*), The attitude. (*L*), Rolling in.

comes off the floor in the deep knee bend, or grand plié (Fig. 48–1*G*).

Tendu: A stretching out of the foot, either forward, sideways, or backward, usually from the first or fifth positions. As the foot moves, the toes are kept close to the floor (Fig. 48–1*H*).

Passé: One foot is moved upward along the inner border of the opposite leg to the level of the knee. The hip remains in the turned-out position (Fig. 48–1*I*).

Developpé: From the passé position, the leg is then extended either forward, backward, or sideways.

Rond de jambe, en l'air, par terre: The foot is moved so that it traces a circle on the ground (par terre) or in the air (en l'air).

Battement: Throwing the leg into the air with the knee in extension.

Arabesque: A pose on one leg while the other leg is extended backward with the knee straight (Fig. 48–1*J*).

Attitude: A position similar to the arabesque, but the knee of the leg behind is bent 90 degrees (Fig. 48–1*K*).

Jeté: A leap forward.

Entrechat six: The dancer jumps off the ground from fifth position and, while in the air, changes the position of the feet from front to back six times (three times with each foot). Many sprained ankles in females occur during this step, especially if the dancer is tired and is able to execute only five and one-half changes while in the air.

Double saut de basque: A flamboyant jump done by male dancers in the style of the Basques. It is a turning step in the air with the leg in the passé position and is a frequent cause of sprained ankles in male dancers.

In proper ballet technique, the knee should remain over the foot when the foot is in the turned-out position and should not move inside of it. This causes excessive rotation in the knee and pronation in the foot ("rolling in") (Fig. 48–1*L*).

MEDIAL ANKLE INJURIES

Posterior Tibial Tendinitis

Posterior tibial tendinitis, so commonly seen in athletes, is rare in dancers—an example of altered kinesiology producing changes in the patterns of injury normally found. Working primarily in the equinus position produces stress on the flexor hallucis longus (FHL) tendon (sometimes called the "Achilles tendon of the foot") as it passes through its pulley behind the medial malleolus. In this position, the posterior tibial tendon is relatively shortened and the subtalar joint is in inversion. In addition, dancers are selected for, and usually have, cavus feet, and these individuals seem less prone to posterior tibial tendinitis. Indeed, more often than not, a dancer diagnosed as having posterior tibial tendinitis will, on careful examination, be found to have FHL tendinitis (dancer's tendinitis) instead.[4, 5]

Medial Sprains of the Ankle

Medial sprains of the ankle are rare because the medial structures are strong and rigid compared with the lateral structures. Persistent symptoms on the medial side may be due to an unrecognized stress fracture of the sustentaculum tali, which can be picked up on a bone scan, or to a localized posteromedial fibrous tarsal coalition. Sprains of the medial ankle do occur, usually from landing off-balance with sudden pronation; again, however this is more likely to produce a sprain of the deltoid ligament than a strain of the posterior tibial tendon.

The sprain usually affects the portion of the ligament that was under tension when the force was applied: the anterior deltoid if the foot was in equinus, the middle deltoid if it was plantigrade, and the posterior portion if the foot was in dorsiflexion (very rare). If a significant injury to the deltoid ligament is found, one must always look for damage to the lateral structures, especially the syndesmosis and proximal fibula.

Isolated injuries to the lateral ankle are common, but isolated injuries to the medial side are rare. An accessory bone, the os subtibiale, may be present in the deep layer of the deltoid, and this bone can be involved in the sprain, becoming symptomatic when it had not been before. An x-ray study should be taken to rule out bone, syndesmosis, or epiphyseal injury.

Recovery is usually uneventful. Occasionally, a trigger point can form in the deltoid, usually around a chip fracture or accessory ossicle. These may require a corticosteroid injection if they do not respond to conservative therapy. Nodules may form on the flexor digitorum longus or posterior tibial tendons following medial strains, but they are usually not symptomatic.

Other Conditions

In the differential diagnosis of medial ankle pain, the physician must keep in mind the possibility of *osteochondritis dissecans* of the talus. This condition usually occurs in the posterior portion of the medial talar dome and the anterior portion of the lateral dome. It can cause vague pains that are hard to localize, and symptoms can be present before the lesion appears on regular x-ray studies. If it is suspected, a bone scan, computed tomographic scan, or magnetic resonance imaging may be indicated.

In dancers, a common cause of pain around the medial malleolus comes from pronating the foot to obtain proper turnout (Fig. 48–1*L*). This produces a chronic strain of the deltoid ligament and is one of many overuse syndromes seen in dancers.

Contusion of the medial prominence of the tarsal navicular can occur. This usually happens when one foot is brought forward past the other, and as they pass, the navicular strikes the medial malleolus of the other ankle. These contusions usually heal with symptomatic treatment. On rare occasions, a fracture of the medial tubercle or disruption of an accessory navicular can occur. If the symptoms warrant, the injury should be treated in a short-leg walking cast or ankle-foot orthosis for 4 to 6 weeks to prevent it from becoming chronic.

Sprains of the spring ligament or the plantar fascia can be mistaken for medial ankle pain, but a careful physical examination should make the diagnosis apparent.

Another cause of medial pain just above the medial malleolus is the *soleus syndrome*.[19] This syndrome presents as chronic pain resembling a shin splint but is too far distal on the posteromedial tibial metaphysis to be a true shin splint. It is caused by an abnormal slip in the origin of the soleus muscle, usually 3 to 6 cm above the medial malleolus. Normally, the tibial origin of the soleus ends at the junction of the middle and distal thirds of the tibia. In this syndrome, the origin continues down the

tibia to just above the medial malleolus. This condition, which is similar to a compartment syndrome, is much more common in athletes who engage in sustained muscular activity than in dancers, whose efforts are usually intermittent. It usually responds to conservative therapy. On rare occasions, subcutaneous release of the tight band may be necessary (Table 48–1).

TABLE 48–1. DIFFERENTIAL DIAGNOSIS OF MEDIAL ANKLE PAIN IN THE DANCER	
FREQUENCY OF OCCURRENCE	**CAUSE OF PAIN**
Most common	Flexor hallucis longus tendinitis
Less common	Deltoid ligament sprain
Rare	Posterior tibial tendinitis
Very rare	Flexor digitorum longus tendinitis
	Soleus syndrome

ANTERIOR ANKLE INJURIES

Dancers are selected for an extreme range of motion in their joints and for cavus feet, which give them maximum plantar flexion of the foot and ankle. Despite this extreme flexibility, they will constantly take the joints of the lower extremity to the limits of their range of motion. The cavus foot has increased plantar flexion but decreased dorsiflexion. For this reason, impingement syndromes of the ankle are very common. Impingement occurs anteromedially and posterolaterally. When motion in the ankle is limited by impingement, dancers, and sometimes dance teachers, will blame the Achilles tendon for the lack of dorsiflexion. They will spend hours trying to stretch the posterior structures of the calf to obtain a better plié when, in reality, no more dorsiflexion is possible in the talocrural joint. (It would not increase even if the Achilles tendon were severed.) The fact often must be explained to the dancer.

Anterior Impingement Syndrome

The most common cause of anterior ankle pain in the dancer is the anterior impingement syndrome.[16, 21] It is typically seen in the older male dancer with cavus feet who has spent his career dancing the "bravura" technique—that is, big jumps and deep pliés. The impingement of the bones, one on the other, stimulates the cambium layer of the periosteum to form the exostoses, like stalactites in a cave. When they form, they limit dorsiflexion, facilitating further impingement resulting in more periosteal stimulation, setting up a repetitive cycle. As the spurs build up, they can break off and become loose bodies (Fig. 48–2).

Diagnosis is made on the basis of the history, physical examination, and x-ray findings. On physical examination, the following signs are usually present:

- Anterior tenderness and thickening of the synovium, often with an effusion
- Palpable osteophytes
- Limited dorsiflexion when compared with the opposite ankle
- A positive "dorsiflexion sign," (i.e., pain with forced dorsiflexion of the ankle with the knee flexed)

A standard lateral x-ray study of the ankle usually shows the spurs. If further information is needed, a lateral view in forced dorsiflexion can be taken.

Conservative treatment consists of making the dancer aware of the problem and having him not "hit bottom" in his plié. Heel lifts will help open up the front of the ankle and relieve the symptoms, but dancers often find them difficult to dance in. Show dancers (on Broadway or in Las Vegas–type shows), who dance in "character shoes," often tolerate heel lifts and orthotics much better than ballet dancers.

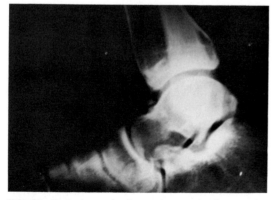

FIGURE 48–2. Loose bodies and spurs in the anterior ankle.

Dancers with loose ankles secondary to repeated ankle sprains also tend to form these impingement spurs. In this situation, consideration should be given to tightening the ankle ligaments at the time of the anterior cleanout, preferably by the Broström-Gould procedure.

If symptoms are disabling, an anterior débridement, either through a small anteromedial incision or through the arthroscope, may be indicated. The anterior impingement syndrome of the ankle usually is one of three types, depending on the location of the exostoses: (1) primarily on the anterior lip of the tibia, (2) primarily on the neck of the talus, or (3) a combination of both.

The first type can be removed easily with the arthroscope. In my opinion, the second and third types are best treated with a small arthrotomy behind the anterior tibial tendon. The open method in these cases is faster and more thorough than arthroscopy. When ankle arthroscopy became popular, I performed many arthroscopic anterior débridements, hoping to facilitate an earlier return to dancing. I found that it took 3 months to return to full dancing with either technique, but the arthroscopic procedures were taking 1 to 1 ½ hours versus 20 to 30 minutes for the open technique. I presently perform the open arthrotomy, except in cases that involve only the anterior lip of the tibia, which I treat arthroscopically.

The physician should always look for an impingement exostosis on the medial shoulder of the talus that impinges against the anterior aspect of the medial malleolus. This spur can be hard to visualize on an x-ray study but can contribute considerably to the symptoms. Dancers undergoing this operation should be warned that although the cleanout is a relatively minor procedure with minimal risk, it may take 3 to 4 months before they regain all of their plié.

Several conditions can mimic the anterior impingement syndrome:

- Osteochondritis dissecans of the talus
- An acute or chronic "high" ankle sprain involving the anterior tibiofibular ligament
- Bassett's ligament, which is an aberrant distal insertion of the anterior talofibular ligament that can cause persistent symptoms[1] (Fig. 48–3)
- Degenerative joint disease of the tibiotalar or talonavicular joints, especially in the early phases when the x-ray findings are subtle

FIGURE 48–3. Bassett's ligament. (From Bassett FH, Gates HS, Billys JB, et al: Talar impingement by the anteroinferior tibiofibular ligament. J Bone Joint Surg 72A:55–59, 1990.)

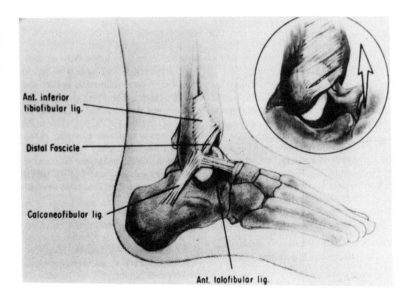

Ant. inferior tibiofibular lig.

Distal Fascicle

Calcaneofibular lig.

Ant. talofibular lig.

- An osteoid osteoma in the tarsal navicular (Fig. 48–4)

These conditions will usually give a characteristic picture on either the x-ray study or the bone scan.

Other Conditions

Anterior tibial, extensor hallucis longus, and extensor digitorum longus tendinitis, like posterior tibial tendinitis, are very rare in dancers. Symptoms in this area are almost always due to ankle impingement. Irritation of the extensor tendons in the anterior extensor retinaculum can occur. This is often due to either a ganglion in the region or tightness in an elastic strap passing over this area. This strap is sewn onto the shoe by the dancer to hold it on (Fig. 48–5). The position of the strap on the dance shoe should be adjusted so that it does not press against the extensor retinaculum if the dancer is having symptoms in that area.

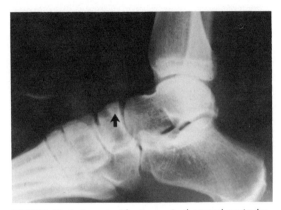

FIGURE 48–4. An osteoid osteoma in the tarsal navicular.

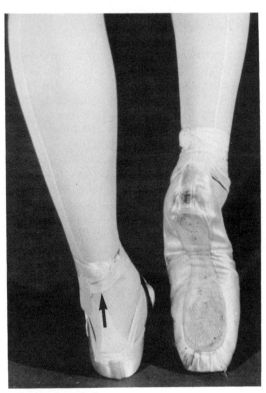

FIGURE 48–5. The elastic strap on a dancer's shoe.

Irritation of the extensor hallucis longus can occur in the region of the medial cuneiform–first metatarsal joint. A bossing, or exostosis, is often found on the dorsum of this joint in older dancers, exactly where this tendon passes over it. Any tight shoe or strap in this area will press the tendon down against the underlying bone and cause pain and irritation. It is rarely necessary to remove this exostosis surgically; instead, the dancer should simply avoid direct pressure on the tendon in the region of the exostosis. Recurrent or recalcitrant symptoms may be an indication for surgery. The surgeon should be extremely careful when operating in this area—incisional neuromas are very common here.

Just distal to this area, in the first web space of the foot, the orthopaedist should be aware of the pseudotumor of the foot. I have seen several young dancers with a slowly enlarging mass that did not transilluminate, had a normal x-ray appearance, and did not yield ganglionic fluid on aspiration. At exploration, enlarged, normal muscle fibers were found attached to the extensor hallucis brevis tendon, extending to the region of the first metatarsophalangeal joint.

LATERAL ANKLE INJURIES

The most common acute injury in dance is the inversion sprain of the ankle.[6] Sprains may occur in any ligament in the foot or ankle, but they most commonly involve the lateral ligament complex of the ankle (the anterior talofibular, the calcaneofibular, and the posterior talofibular ligaments); the anterior tibiofibular ligament; the lateral talocalcaneal ligament; and occasionally, the medial (deltoid) ligament. The posterior talofibular ligament is rarely, if ever, injured.

Other conditions, however, can closely resemble the classic lateral ankle sprain. The exact mechanism of injury may not always be apparent, especially in dancers who may have been in the pointe position when the injury occurred. In this position, many possible combinations of forces are possible. Some of these injuries even occur during a helical or corkscrew movement, exerting both inversion and eversion forces on the ankle at the same time. The physician is well advised to examine the patient carefully for the following conditions that can simulate or accompany a simple sprain:

- A complete tear of the lateral collateral ligaments (actually a medial dislocation of the talus that has spontaneously reduced, or a grade III sprain)
- An injury to the anteroinferior tibiofibular ligament, known as the "high" ankle sprain (more common in pronation and external rotation injuries than during inversions)
- A complete tear of both the distal anterior and posterior tibiofibular ligaments (the syndesmosis) and the interosseous membrane, without fracture of the malleoli but with diastasis of the ankle mortise and occasionally with fracture of the proximal isthmus of the fibula—the Maisonneuve fracture
- A sprain of the subtalar joint with disruption of the calcaneofibular ligament and the lateral talocalcaneal ligament[16]
- A fracture of the base of the fifth metatarsal
- An undisplaced fracture of the lateral malleolus or malleolar epiphysis in a young dancer
- A fracture of the anterior process of the os calcis in the sinus tarsi[13] (Fig. 48–6)
- Subluxation of the cuboid[18]
- A fracture of the posterior lip of the distal tibia or fracture of a trigonal process behind the talus (Shepherd's fracture)[24] (see Fig. 48–11)
- A lateral sprain of the tarsometatarsal (Lisfranc's) joints
- A rupture of the Achilles tendon

Classification and Treatment of Sprains

Ankle sprains are usually classified as grade I, II, or III, depending on the extent of the injury[6] (see Table 48–2).

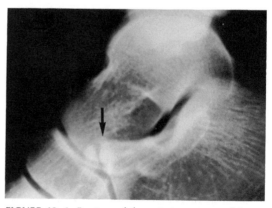

FIGURE 48–6. Fracture of the anterior process of the os calcis.

Grade I sprains are partial tears, usually of the anterior talofibular ligament or occasionally of the anterior tibiofibular ligament, with little or no resultant instability. On physical examination, the drawer sign is negative, and stress films are usually normal. After the initial 48 hours of "RICE" (rest, ice, compression, and elevation), the patient should begin early active use of the limb with a compression bandage, taping, or an Aircast.

Grade II sprains are complete tears, usually of the anterior talofibular ligament, with minimal damage to the calcaneofibular ligament. They produce a moderately positive drawer sign but a normal or minimal talar tilt on the stress film. They often result in some residual instability, although this usually can be controlled by good peroneal strength. Treatment consists of some type of support—either taping, an Aircast, or a walking plaster cast for 3 to 6 weeks—followed by aggressive peroneal rehabilitation.

The grade II sprain is the type of ankle sprain most commonly seen in dancers. It usually occurs when they are on demi-pointe (up on the ball of the foot). In this position, the anterior talofibular ligament is almost vertical—in the position normally taken by the calcaneofibular ligament when the foot is plantigrade—and it is easily torn when an adduction-inversion force is applied. In this position, the calcaneofibular ligament is almost parallel to the floor; it is out of harm's way and is rarely injured.

Grade III sprains are fortunately rare injuries. They consist of a complete rupture of the lateral ligament complex (the anterior talofibular and the calcaneal fibular ligaments). I have never seen a tear of the posterior talofibular ligament and doubt that such a thing exists. This injury results in gross instability. It is actually a spontaneously reduced medial dislocation of the talus. The drawer sign and stress film findings are grossly positive on physical examination and x-ray study (Fig. 48–7). The healing time is long and uncertain (3 to 4 months), and the likelihood of significant permanent laxity of the ligaments is great. Dancers with residual laxity of the lateral ankle ligaments from this injury usually complain more of rotatory instability than of varus instability (i.e., they develop anterolateral rotatory instability of the ankle analogous to ligament injuries of the knee).

For this reason, many orthopaedists, includ-

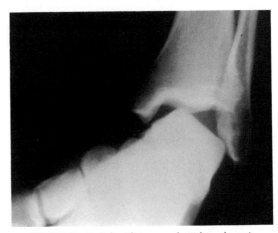

FIGURE 48–7. Talar tilt in a grade III lateral sprain.

ing myself, believe that grade III lateral ankle sprains in *professional* athletes and dancers should be surgically repaired primarily, (within 7 to 10 days of the injury). The repair itself is a simple procedure performed under regional anesthesia with a small incision over the distal fibula (see the Broström-Gould procedure, described later in this chapter). The ligaments are easily identified, as they are within the capsule, similar to the anterior capsule of the shoulder. They are usually avulsed from the fibula rather than torn in their midsubstance, making them easy to reattach. Occasionally, the calcaneofibular ligament is avulsed from the calcaneus rather than from the fibula, making the repair somewhat more difficult. Postoperative immobilization in a short-leg walking cast for 4 weeks is followed by protection in an Aircast and early rehabilitation. Recreational dancers should be treated in a short-leg walking cast or an analogous removable splint for 1 month.

Stress films can be obtained in the office, using a local anesthetic if necessary. I have found, along with other authors, that the drawer sign is as good a gauge of the extent of the injury, as well as a predictor of later dysfunction, as the stress films (Table 48–2).

Rehabilitation

Regardless of the method of treatment, adequate physical therapy and proper rehabilitation are necessary to restore normal use after injury. Restoration of full peroneal strength is

GRADE	ANATOMIC INJURY	PHYSICAL EXAMINATION FINDINGS	X-RAY FINDINGS
I	Partial tear, ATF* or CF†	Negative or 1 + drawer sign	Negative drawer sign Negative talar tilt
II	Torn ATF, intact CF	2 + drawer sign	Positive drawer sign Negative talar tilt
III	Torn ATF, torn CF	3 + drawer sign	Positive drawer sign Positive talar tilt

TABLE 48–2. **WORKING CLASSIFICATION OF ACUTE ANKLE SPRAINS**

*ATF, anterior talofibular ligament.
†CF, calcaneofibular ligament.

essential. Unrecognized peroneal weakness is a common condition in dancers[6] and can be the cause of a myriad of obscure symptoms, such as unexplained swelling and discomfort or poor timing with "beats." Any dancer complaining of these symptoms should be checked for weak peroneals. This is done by having them place their foot in full plantar flexion and in neutral with regard to abduction and adduction (the tendu position) and asking them to hold this position against varus and then valgus stress (Fig. 48–8). A well-conditioned dancer should be able to resist as much force as the examiner can manually apply to the foot in this position. The uninjured side can be checked for comparison, if necessary.

Often, either these dancers have not been adequately rehabilitated, or they have been exercising in the neutral position rather than

in full plantar flexion. (Cybex and other exercise machines are not very good for ankle rehabilitation, as they cannot be placed in full plantar flexion.) I use a home exercise program performed over the end of a sofa or couch, with the dancer on one side using a weight bag in full plantar flexion (Fig. 48–9). Abduction exercises are performed with the ankle supported so that it can only move upward in valgus and the patient can relax the ankle in between lifts. The patient lifts 3 lb, 25 times slowly, morning and evening, increasing the weight in the bag by 3 lb each week to a maximum of 15 lb. When they can lift 15 lb slowly 25 times, they are adequately rehabilitated. I have never seen this method fail to restore normal peroneal strength. However, the symptoms do not always disappear, and if they do not, the physician must look elsewhere

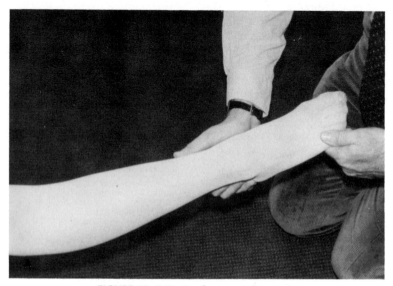

FIGURE 48–8. Testing for peroneal strength.

FIGURE 48–9. Peroneal exercises over the end of a couch.

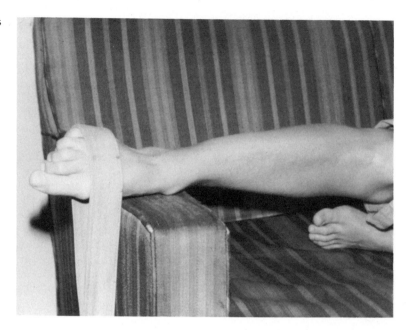

for the problem (when there is doubt, a bone scan is recommended).

Reconstruction

Secondary or delayed ankle ligament reconstruction is occasionally necessary in a dancer but should be considered only after full peroneal strength has been obtained (see previous paragraph) and the dancer is still unable to dance. Often, as previously mentioned, the problem is rotatory instability rather than varus instability. It must be emphasized that reconstruction should be performed only for *functional* difficulties and not simply on the basis of a drawer sign or a positive stress x-ray finding. Many professional dancers dance quite well with loose ankles that are not symptomatic enough to warrant surgical repair.

I strongly believe that the peroneus brevis tendon should not be used for ankle reconstruction in a professional dancer for two reasons. First, the peroneus brevis is too important as a support tendon for dancing on full pointe to be sacrificed. Second, it is not necessary to use it—I have had excellent results using the Broström repair as described by Gould.[2] The procedure is simply a reefing of the anterior talofibular and calcaneofibular ligaments with reattachment to their anatomic locations on the fibula, then sewing the lateral extensor retinaculum over the tip of the fibula

in a pants-over-vest manner to limit inversion. The patient is placed in a short-leg walking cast for 1 month, then taken out for rehabilitation and swimming and protected in a removable Aircast for another 2 to 3 weeks. In 20 professional dancers, this technique has not failed to give an excellent result with full range of motion and strength. Ten years' follow-up of my first case has not revealed any stretching of the repaired ligaments, despite another sprain in the same ankle.[11]

The Broström-Gould Repair for Acute and Chronic Lateral Ankle Instability

The Broström-Gould repair is performed with the patient in the lateral decubitus position. A tourniquet is used, so general, spinal, or epidural anesthesia is needed. A curvilinear incision is made along the anterior border of the distal fibula, stopping at the peroneal tendons. (The sural nerve is just below this area.) The lesser saphenous vein frequently crosses the distal fibula at this level and must usually be divided. The dissection is then carried down to the joint capsule along the anterior border of the lateral malleolus. The lateral portion of the extensor retinaculum is then identified distal to this area. It is dissected off the capsule and mobilized so that it can be pulled over the repair later in the procedure (Fig. 48–10).

Care should be taken when working anterior

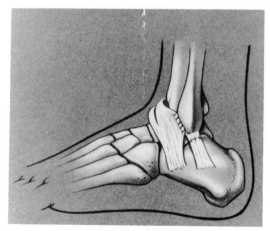

FIGURE 48–10. The Broström-Gould repair. (Drawing by William B. Westwood courtesy of LTI Medica and The Upjohn Company. Copyright 1990 by Learning Technology Incorporated.)

to the malleolus because the lateral branch of the superficial peroneal nerve often lies in this area and can be damaged by dissection or a sharp retractor. The capsule is then divided along the anterior border of the fibula down to the peroneal tendons, leaving a 2- to 3-mm cuff. The anterior talofibular ligament lies within this capsule, much like the anterior glenohumeral ligaments lie within the shoulder. Frequently the ligament can be identified as a thickening in the capsule. The calcaneofibular ligament must then be identified. It lies deep to the peroneal tendons, running obliquely downward and posteriorly to the calcaneus. It is often stretched out and attenuated, or it may be dislodged so that it lies outside the peroneals. If it is in continuity, it is also divided, leaving a cuff at its insertion in the fibula. By leaving a cuff of tissue at the insertion of the ligaments, the surgeon will be able to repair the ligaments in their anatomic locations, thus preserving isometry and an unrestricted range of motion.

The ligaments must now be shortened and repaired. The ankle should be placed in the fully reduced position. The stumps of the ligaments are pulled up, and the redundancy is trimmed off. The ligaments are then sutured to their anatomic locations with 2–0 nonabsorbable sutures, starting with the calcaneofibular ligament (because it is the most difficult to visualize) and then proceeding to the anterior talofibular ligament. At this point, the ankle should be examined for stability and

range of motion. The previously identified lateral extensor mechanism is then pulled over the repair and sutured to the tip of the fibula with 2–0 chromic catgut. This is done for three reasons: it reinforces the repair, limits inversion, and helps correct the subtalar component of the instability. (If the calcaneofibular ligament is attenuated, there is usually some degree of subtalar instability, because the ligament is a stabilizing ligament of the subtalar joint.[16]) A layered closure is then performed with an absorbable subcutaneous suture and Steri-Strips. The patient is placed in plaster splints until the swelling has subsided, and then a short-leg walking cast is worn for 3 to 4 weeks. The cast is removed for swimming, range-of-motion, and isometric peroneal exercises. Unrestricted activities are allowed at 10 to 12 weeks if full peroneal strength is present.

The Sprained Ankle That Does Not Heal

Miscellaneous problems following ankle sprains are not uncommon:

A trigonal process may be fractured (Shepherd's fracture) (Fig. 48–11) at the time of the injury and may continue to be symptomatic after the sprain heals. In such cases, a bone scan is needed.

Dancers will often develop FHL tendinitis or posterior impingement following an ankle sprain, occasionally involving an os trigonum that had previously been asymptomatic.[7, 9] These complications are not always related to the severity of the sprain.

A unique type of posterior impingement may follow grade III sprains with residual

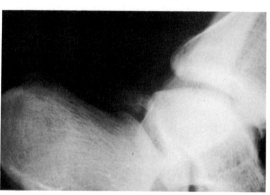

FIGURE 48–11. Shepherd's fracture.

ligamentous laxity. In this condition, the loose anterior talofibular ligament cannot hold the talus under the tibial plafond in the full relevé position, and the talus slips forward, allowing the posterior lip of the tibia to settle down on the os calcis (Fig. 48–12).

If there is looseness in the ankle, an anterior impingement may follow, with osteophyte formation in the anterior tibiotalar joint. This is secondary to rotatory instability and is often opposite the tip of the medial malleolus.

An osteochondral fracture or osteochondritis dissecans may be present.

Problems around the tip of the fibula may persist after the sprain heals and include the following:

- Soft tissue entrapment (the "meniscoid" of the ankle).[27]
- An avulsion fracture of the tip of the fibula.
- A previously asymptomatic accessory ossicle (the os subfibulare).
- An unrecognized fracture of the anterior process of the os calcis. This fracture is an avulsion fracture of the extensor digitorum brevis origin[13] (see Fig. 48–6).
- Damage to the peroneal tendons has been found following sprains. Often the peroneus brevis has longitudinal tears and the tendon becomes enlarged and flattened. This condition usually can be diagnosed by a peroneal tenogram or with a magnetic resonance imaging study.[22]
- A lateral process fracture of the talus.[14]
- The sinus tarsi syndrome.[25]
- Subluxation of the cuboid.[18, 20]

The high ankle sprain of the tibiofibular syndesmosis should be recognized as a different entity from the common ankle sprain seen at the lateral malleolus. This injury represents a partial tear of the anterior tibiofibular ligament in the syndesmosis, usually by pronation and external rotation. It can take an extraordinarily long time to heal and may be associated with an avulsion fracture at the tibial or fibular origin of the ligament—the fragment of Tillaux. Treatment of this injury should be aggressively conservative, and the dancer should be warned at the beginning that symptoms may remain for as long as 3 to 6 months.

There have been cases in which symptoms remained despite the passage of time and conservative therapy. Surgical exploration of these ankles has revealed any of the following states:

- A rent in the ligament with a synovial hernia
- Entrapment of tissue in the syndesmosis
- A Tillaux fragment too small to appear on the x-ray study
- Bassett's ligament, which is a slip of the anteroinferior tibiotalar ligament that inserts so far down on the fibula that it causes irritation of the shoulder of the talus[1]

Acute peroneal dislocation is usually obvious, but chronic peroneal subluxation in dancers can sometimes be difficult to diagnose. This condition should be kept in mind in any dancer with vague but persistent symptoms such as "giving way" in the peroneal area. The technique for repair of recurrent dislocating peroneal tendons is similar to the Broström-Gould procedure, involving taking down the retinaculum, shortening it to its proper length, and reattaching it to its anatomic location on the posterior border of the distal fibula. Afterward, the patient must be kept in a short-leg walking cast for 6 weeks. As usual, postoperative rehabilitation is essential.

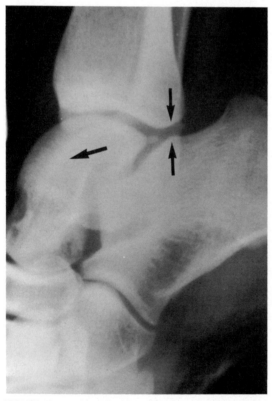

FIGURE 48–12. Posterior impingement secondary to loose ankle ligaments.

POSTERIOR ANKLE INJURIES

Two things separate ballet from other forms of dancing: the 180 degrees of turnout at the hips, and the ballerina dancing on full pointe in a toeshoe. Thus, the full equinus position is essential for proper ballet technique, especially in females. Not only should there be at least 90 degrees of plantar flexion in the foot-ankle complex, but it is also preferable to have 10 to 15 degrees more than that to compensate for the recurvatum usually present in the knee above.

The shape of the dome of the talus can vary considerably from one individual to another. Some are round, like an oil drum, and have excellent motion, both in plantar flexion and dorsiflexion. Others are congenitally flattened and have very limited motion. It is possible that these tali can be molded and improved to some degree if training is begun at an early age, while the bones are growing, but a stiff flatfoot and a flat-domed talus will never achieve the desired amount of motion, and that dancer is far better off choosing a career in some form of dancing other than ballet.

A considerable amount of this dorsiflexion and plantar flexion comes from the subtalar joint and from the basic turned-out position assumed by the dancer. This position of forefoot mild pronation and abduction loosens the subtalar joint and allows maximum motion. This can be seen by comparing a lateral x-ray study in the plantigrade position with one taken during relevé. The subtalar space usually opens considerably when the dancer goes on pointe (Fig. 48–13). Dancers with a tarsal coalition are usually weeded out of ballet early because this condition limits motion in the foot-ankle complex and produces a poor relevé, often before the onset of pain and discomfort. Lack of subtalar motion can be very subtle, for tarsal coalitions can range from solid and bony to cartilaginous or fibrous with moderate loss of motion. These subtle coalitions usually are located posteriorly (often in association with an os trigonum) and are caused by marked fibrosis and thickening of the posterior talocalcaneal ligament complex surrounding the os trigonum or posterior lateral tubercle of the talus.

Early training usually produces a notch in the neck of the talus to accept the anterior lip of the tibia and allow a deep plié (Fig. 48–14). Conversely, some posterior molding may be

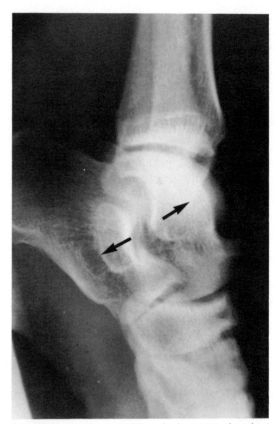

FIGURE 48–13. Opening of the subtalar joint in the relevé.

necessary, especially if an os trigonum or trigonal process is present. In the younger group (ages 13 to 16), posterior ankle pain frequently occurs when an os trigonum is present and full plantar flexion is limited, especially if the other ankle is normal. The symptoms in this situation are usually due to the machinations that the young dancer is going through to force the "bad" ankle to go down as far as the "good"

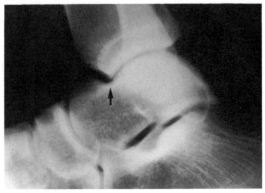

FIGURE 48–14. The notch in the neck of the talus.

TABLE 48–3. SYNDROMES OF POSTERIOR ANKLE PAIN IN DANCERS	
POSTEROMEDIAL CONDITIONS	**POSTEROLATERAL CONDITIONS**
Flexor hallucis longus tendinitis	Posterior impingement (os trigonum syndrome)
Soleus syndrome	Fractured trigonal process (Shepherd's fracture)
Posterior tibial tendinitis	Peroneal tendinitis
Posteromedial fibrous tarsal coalition	Pseudomeniscus syndrome

one. These activities include hooking the toes underneath the piano and levering the forefoot into equinus, sitting on the heels with the foot in full plantar flexion. When the diagnosis has been made, the problem should be explained to the dancer and her family. The symptoms usually subside when the dancer stops forcing the ankle and understands that the lack of motion is due to a bony block and that the ankle cannot go any further down, no matter how hard it is pushed (Table 48–3).

Posterior Impingement Syndrome

The posterior impingement syndrome of the ankle, or talar compression syndrome[7, 15] (Fig. 48–15), is the natural result of full weight bearing in maximum plantar flexion of the ankle in the demi-pointe or full pointe position, especially if an os trigonum or trigonal process is present. It presents as posterolateral pain in the back of the ankle when the posterior lip of the tibia closes against the superior border of the os calcis, as during the tendu, the frappé, the relevé, or leaving the ground in a jump. It can be confirmed on physical examination by tenderness behind the peroneal tendons in back of the lateral malleolus (it is often mistaken for peroneal tendinitis) and by pain with forced passive plantar flexion of the ankle—the plantar flexion sign. The syndrome is often associated with an os trigonum or trigonal process in the back of the ankle. On occasion, the syndrome can be caused by soft tissue entrapment between the posterior lip of the talus and the os calcis. It also can be found in association with lateral ligament laxity.

The posterior aspect of the talus normally has two tubercles: the medial tubercle and the lateral tubercle. Between the two tubercles lies the fibro-osseous tunnel of the FHL tendon. The os trigonum is the ununited lateral tubercle on the posterior aspect of the talus. It is present in 7 to 10 percent of people and has a 50-percent incidence of bilaterality.[3, 8] Most people who have an os trigonum are not aware of its presence, and the posterior impingement syndrome is rare in athletes. In dancers, the os trigonum may or may not be symptomatic, and the degree of the symptoms is not always related to the size of the os trigonum. Large os trigona can be minimally symptomatic, and small ones are sometimes disabling. Usually the symptoms are mild, and on the whole, the os trigonum is more often asymptomatic than symptomatic. Many world-famous ballerinas have asymptomatic os trigona, and they work with them without any trouble. It is important

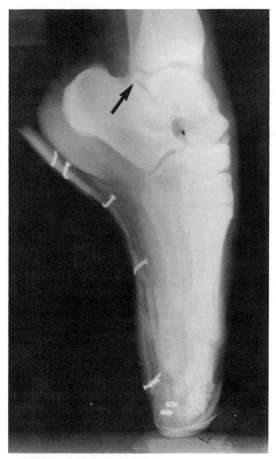

FIGURE 48–15. Posterior impingement on an os trigonum.

to stress this fact to the patient and her parent when discussing the problem, because the condition is frequently overdiagnosed by paramedical practitioners who may recommend surgery unnecessarily, perhaps because of the dramatic appearance of the bone on the x-ray study. It is best seen on a lateral view of the ankle on pointe or in full plantar flexion. The diagnosis can be confirmed if necessary by injecting 0.5 to 0.75 ml of lidocaine (Xylocaine) into the posterior soft tissues behind the peroneal tendons. If the pain is relieved by this small injection, the diagnosis is almost certain.

Treatment of the posterior impingement syndrome should follow an orderly sequence. The first approach, as with tendinitis, is modification of activities (avoid activities that hurt); administration of nonsteroidal anti-inflammatory drugs if the dancer is over age 16; and physical therapy. As noted earlier, if the patient is forcing the foot into equinus to achieve further plantar flexion, she must be instructed not to do this. These patients should be told that it will take a few weeks for the pain to subside, usually as long as they had been dancing with the condition before they began treatment. Thus, if they had been working with the pain for a month, it will often take a month of treatment and reduced activities before they can resume normal activities without discomfort. In cases in which this approach has failed, or the symptoms recur, and the patient is 16 years of age or older, an injection of 0.5 to 0.75 ml of a mixture of a long- and a short-acting corticosteroid can often give dramatic and permanent relief of symptoms. Before the steroid preparation is injected, the diagnosis should be confirmed with a lidocaine injection. If the lidocaine does not relieve the symptoms, there is no point in injecting the steroids. It should be stressed that the os trigonum is not usually a surgical problem; most dancers with an os trigonum do not need to have it removed surgically.

Occasionally, it does cause enough disability to warrant surgical excision, but as with most elective surgery, it is indicated only after the failure of conservative therapy in a serious dancer at least 16 years of age. If the problem is an isolated os trigonum with no medial symptoms, then it can be approached posterolaterally between the FHL tendon and the peroneals (to protect the sural nerve). Not infrequently, there is a combined problem of FHL tendinitis and the os trigonum syndrome.

In these patients, the posteromedial approach is used so that the neurovascular bundle can be isolated and protected. A tenolysis of the FHL tendon and removal of the adjacent os trigonum can then be performed safely.

Other causes of posterior impingement include the following:

• A previously asymptomatic os trigonum may become persistently symptomatic following an ankle sprain owing to disruption of its ligamentous connections and a subtle shift in position.
• Posterior impingement can follow an ankle sprain that stretches out the lateral ligaments that hold the talus under the tibia during the relevé.[9] As the talus slips forward, the posterior lip of the tibia comes to rest on the os calcis (see Fig. 48–12). The treatment for this type of posterior impingement is to tighten the lateral ankle ligaments (preferably by the Broström-Gould technique). If the drawer sign can be corrected, the posterior impingement will usually disappear.
• A posterior pseudomeniscus or plica in the posterior ankle, with or without an os trigonum,[9] can cause the posterior impingement syndrome in the absence of an os trigonum or loose ligaments. Bucket-handle tears have been seen in this structure, causing locking and other mechanical symptoms more often seen in the knee than in the ankle.

In summary, the posterior impingement syndrome consists of posterior or posterolateral ankle pain that occurs during the takeoff in jumping, push-off in running, going down an incline, or the relevé. It is often mistaken for heel pain, Achilles tendinitis, or peroneal tendinitis. It is a common problem in ballet dancers.

Diagnosis is made on the basis of the following:

• The location and nature of the pain
• Tenderness behind the peroneal tendons
• The plantar flexion sign (forced passive plantar flexion mimics the acute pain)

A work-up should include regular x-ray studies, plus a lateral view in full plantar flexion. Tomograms, bone scans and computed tomographic scans may be helpful, but the diagnosis can usually be made without these studies by injecting 1 ml of lidocaine into the trigger point behind the ankle. The patient should then be pain-free; if not, another diagnosis should be considered.

The etiology includes the following factors:

- The os trigonum, present in 7 to 10 percent of people, with a 50-percent incidence of bilaterality
- A trigonal process (Stieda's process, named for Ludwig Stieda, German anatomist, 1837–1918)
- Soft tissue impingement, the posterior pseudomeniscus of the ankle

The differential diagnosis (Table 48–4) includes the following:

- Posterior process fracture; may be a hairline or stress fracture
- FHL tendinitis (dancer's tendinitis)
- Peroneal tendinitis
- Posteromedial localized talocalcaneal coalition
- Osteoid osteoma

Conservative treatment consists of several measures. Acute fracture of the posterior process of the talus, if undisplaced, should be treated with a short-leg walking cast. In the chronic condition, physical therapy modalities (cortisone phonophoresis), low-heeled shoes, and modified activities are indicated. If the pain is relieved by the small injection of lidocaine, the injection of 0.75 ml of cortisone acetate may give dramatic relief.

Operative treatment is indicated when conservative therapy has failed and when the diagnosis has been confirmed with lidocaine. The posterior "cleanout" can be done from either the medial or the lateral side of the Achilles tendon. The lateral approach should be used if the dancer has an isolated posterior impingement without a history of FHL tendinitis or medial difficulties. A medial incision is indicated if the patient has a combined problem of FHL tendinitis and posterior impingement, or if the problem is primarily FHL tendinitis with an incidental os trigonum that the surgeon wishes to remove along with an FHL tenolysis. The medial incision is safer and more utilitarian because the surgeon can work safely on the lateral side from the medial, but it is dangerous to work medially from the lateral side, because the neurovascular bundle cannot be isolated and protected from that side.

Tendinitis of the Flexor Hallucis Longus Tendon

Tendinitis of the FHL tendon behind the medial malleolus of the ankle is so common in dancers that it is known as *dancer's tendinitis*. It is often misdiagnosed as posterior tibial or Achilles tendinitis, but careful examination usually reveals the true diagnosis. The FHL tendon is considered the "Achilles tendon of the foot" for the dancer. It passes through a fibro-osseous tunnel from the posterior aspect of the talus to the level of the sustentaculum tali, like a rope through a pulley. As it passes through this pulley, it can be strained. When strained, rather than moving smoothly in the pulley, it begins to bind. This binding causes irritation and swelling, which in turn causes further binding, irritation, and swelling, setting up the familiar cycle. Because it is swollen and irritated, it binds; and because it binds, it is swollen and irritated. If a nodule or partial tear is present, triggering of the big toe may occur and is known as hallux saltans (Fig. 48–16), or the tendon may become completely frozen in the sheath, causing a pseudo hallux rigidus.

This tendinitis typically responds to the usual conservative measures. Rest is an important component of the therapy so that the chronic cycle just described can be broken. Nonsteroidal anti-inflammatory drugs can help, but they should be used only as part of an overall treatment program, not to mask the pain so that the dancer can continue dancing and ignore the symptoms. As with other tendon problems, steroid injections should be

TABLE 48–4. FLEXOR HALLUCIS LONGUS TENDINITIS VERSUS POSTERIOR IMPINGEMENT	
FLEXOR HALLUCIS LONGUS TENDINITIS	**POSTERIOR IMPINGEMENT**
Posteromedial location	Posterolateral location
Tenderness over the flexor hallucis longus tendon	Tenderness behind the fibula
Pain or triggering with motion of the hallux	Pain with plantar flexion of the ankle
Tomasen's sign[26]	Plantar flexion sign
May be mistaken for posterior tibial tendinitis	May be mistaken for peroneal tendinitis

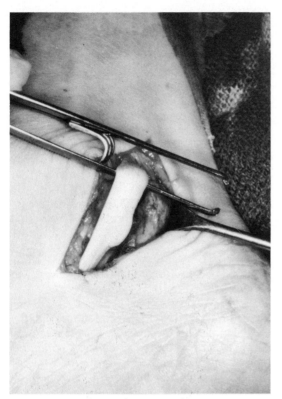

FIGURE 48–16. Hallux saltans. (Note the thickening of the flexor hallucis tendon.)

avoided. On some occasions, in professional or high-level amateur dancers, FHL tendinitis may be recurrent and disabling. In these cases, operative tenolysis may be indicated, but only after the failure of conservative therapy. The situation is similar to de Quervain's stenosing tenosynovitis in the wrist.

FHL tendinitis usually occurs behind the medial malleolus, but it can occasionally be found at Henry's knot under the base of the first metatarsal where the flexor digitorum longus crosses over the FHL, and under the head of the first metatarsal where it passes between the sesamoids. A fibrous subtalar coalition may be present in the posteromedial ankle, mimicking FHL tendinitis or the tarsal tunnel syndrome. This condition should be suspected when there is less than normal subtalar motion on physical examination.

Tenolysis of the Flexor Hallucis Longus and Excision of the Os Trigonum from the Medial Side

This procedure can be performed with the patient supine because dancers usually have increased external rotation of the hip that allows visualization of the posterior ankle from the medial side. A bloodless field is desirable, so I use a tourniquet on the distal thigh over cast padding. For this reason, the procedure cannot be done under local anesthesia or ankle block. A curvilinear incision is made over the neurovascular bundle behind the medial malleolus, beginning just above the superior border of the os calcis and continuing to a line just posterior to the tip of the medial malleolus. This incision should be made carefully! The deep fascia and laciniate ligament in this area are often quite thin. If the incision is made too enthusiastically, the surgeon may be in the midst of the neurovascular bundle before planning to be there. The deep fascia is then divided carefully to avoid damage to the artery and nerve beneath it (Fig. 48–17).

At this point, the surgeon must decide whether to go in front of the bundle or behind it. The posterior approach goes into the variable branches of the nerves to the os calcis. It is safer to go anterior to the bundle. All branches of the tibial nerve at this level go posteriorly, so the safe plane is between the posterior aspect of the medial malleolus and the neurovascular bundle. The bundle can be taken down off the malleolus by blunt dissection. There often are several small vessels here that need to be ligated, but once the bundle is mobilized, it can be held with a blunt retractor, such as a loop or Army-Navy retractor—never with a sharp rake.

The tibial nerve (since there is no anterior tibial nerve, calling it the posterior tibial nerve is redundant) is much larger than one expects: it is usually about the size of a pencil. The surgeon should examine the neurovascular bundle carefully. There are frequent anatomic variations within the tarsal tunnel. Both the nerve and the artery divide into medial and lateral plantar branches as they leave the tarsal canal. It is not unusual for one or both of them to divide above this area, leading to reduplication within the tunnel. There may also be reduplication of the tendons—the flexor hallucis accessorius. With the neurovascular bundle retracted posteriorly, the FHL is easily identified by moving the hallux.

The thin fascia is opened proximally, and a tenolysis is performed by opening the sheath from proximal to distal. Usually it is stenotic and tough, and the FHL can be seen entering it at an acute angle. Care should be taken distally because the FHL tunnel and the nerve

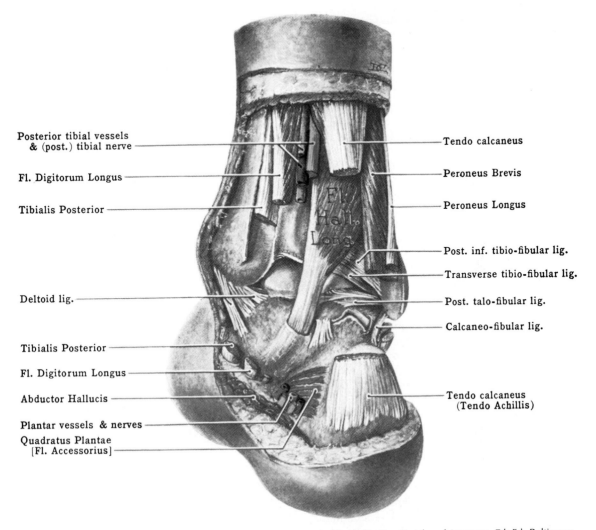

Posterior tibial vessels & (post.) tibial nerve

Fl. Digitorum Longus

Tibialis Posterior

Deltoid lig.

Tibialis Posterior

Fl. Digitorum Longus

Abductor Hallucis

Plantar vessels & nerves
Quadratus Plantae [Fl. Accessorius]

Tendo calcaneus

Peroneus Brevis

Peroneus Longus

Post. inf. tibio-fibular lig.

Transverse tibio-fibular lig.

Post. talo-fibular lig.

Calcaneo-fibular lig.

Tendo calcaneus (Tendo Achillis)

FIGURE 48–17. The posteromedial anatomy of the ankle. (From Anderson JE: Grant's Atlas of Anatomy, 7th Ed. Baltimore, Williams & Wilkins, 1978. © 1978, The Williams & Wilkins Company, Baltimore.)

are quite close together here. As the tenolysis approaches the area of the sustentaculum, it thins out so that there no longer seems to be anything more to divide. The tendon should by retracted with a blunt retractor and inspected for nodules and partial or longitudinal tears. If present, these should be débrided carefully or repaired. At this point, the FHL can be retracted posteriorly with the neurovascular bundle.

The os trigonum or trigonal process will be found just on the lateral side of the FHL tunnel. If the posterior aspect of the talus cannot be visualized, a capsulotomy should be performed. If there is difficulty in visualizing the os trigonum, it helps to identify the superior border of the os calcis, which is the sub-

talar joint, by moving the os calcis into adduction and abduction. The subtalar joint is then dissected from medial to lateral, and this will reveal the os trigonum underneath. Once identified, it can be removed by circumferential dissection.

Care should be taken to stay on the bone when this part of the procedure is performed. This can be somewhat difficult, especially if the os trigonum is quite large. Once it is removed, the posterior ankle joint should be inspected for remnants, bone fragments or loose bodies, soft tissue entrapment, or a large articular facet on the upper surface of the os calcis that articulated with the os trigonum. If this is present, it may need to be removed with a thin osteotome.

The wound is then irrigated, checked for any residual impingement by putting the foot in maximum plantar flexion, and then closed in layers with plain catgut. I usually leave a small Hemovac in place in the wound overnight in case there is excessive bleeding, and I often place the patient in a posterior mold until the wound is healed. Recovery begins with weight bearing as tolerated with crutches and proceeds to swimming and physical therapy. If the tenolysis is done without excision of the os trigonum, the recovery period is about 6 weeks. If the os trigonum is removed along with the tenolysis, the recovery time is 8 to 12 weeks. It is important to get these patients moving early to prevent stiffness. In dancers who have a rather large os trigonum, it is necessary to warn them that, once it is removed, the ankle does not automatically drop down into maximum plantar flexion. They must realize that the bone has been there since they were born, and removing it does not lead to full range of motion immediately. The increased plantar flexion is obtained slowly and can be accompanied by many strange symptoms, both anteriorly and posteriorly, as the soft tissues adjust to the new range of motion.

Excision of the Os Trigonum Using the Lateral Approach

Under anesthesia, the patient is placed in the lateral decubitus position with a pneumatic tourniquet on the leg or thigh over cast padding. (Because dancers have increased external rotation of the hip, it is extremely difficult to perform this operation with the patient in the supine position.) A curvilinear incision is made at the level of the posterior ankle mortise (Fig. 48–18). There is a tendency to make this incision a little too distal. Exposure will be easier if the approach is slightly on the high side. The sural nerve is identified and protected in the subcutaneous tissues. The dissection is carried down in the interval between the peroneal tendons laterally and the muscle belly of the FHL medially. A posterior capsular incision is then made with the ankle in neutral or slight dorsiflexion. The os trigonum or trigonal process (Stieda's process) can be found on the superior surface of the posterior talus just on the lateral side of the FHL tendon. It has attachments on all its sides:

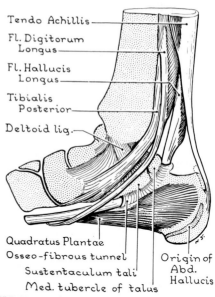

FIGURE 48–18. The posterolateral musculotendinous, ligament, and osseous anatomy of the ankle. (From Anderson JE: Grant's Atlas of Anatomy, 7th Ed. Baltimore, Williams & Wilkins, 1978. © 1978, The Williams & Wilkins Company, Baltimore.)

- Superior: the posterior capsule of the talo-crural joint
- Inferior: the posterior talocalcaneal ligament, at times quite thick and fibrous
- Medial: the FHL tunnel with its sheath
- Lateral: the origin of the posterior talofibular ligament

The bone can be removed by circumferential dissection. The surgeon must be careful not to stray too far medially—the tibial nerve rests on the FHL tunnel. The proximal entrance of this FHL tunnel can be opened if there are muscle fibers attaching distally on the FHL tendon that crowd into the tunnel when the hallux is brought into dorsiflexion (Tomasen's sign). The surgeon should not dissect back here, where there is inadequate visualization; there are branches of the posterior tibial artery here that can begin to bleed. It is important to check for loose bodies; I have found them even in the FHL sheath. The foot should be brought into maximum plantar flexion to look for any residual impingement. At times it is necessary to remove more of the remains of the posterior lateral tubercle. Frequently, there is a facet on the cephalad portion of the os calcis that articulated with the os trigonum, and this can be large enough to impinge against the posterior lip of the tibia after the os trigonum has been removed.

I usually drain the wound with a small Hemovac because a postoperative hematoma will delay recovery and make early motion difficult for the patient. A layered closure is then performed with catgut stitches. I usually close the wound with a running absorbable suture. The patient is placed in a posterior mold until the wound is healed; then weight bearing with crutches is begun. The dancer is encouraged to swim and to progress to barre exercises as tolerated. The average time for a return to full dancing is 2 to 3 months.

References

1. Bassett FH, Gates HS, Billys JB, et al: Talar impingement by the anterior inferior tibiofibular ligament. J Bone Joint Surg 72A:55–59, 1990.
2. Gould N, Seligson D, Gassman J: Early and late repair of the lateral ligament of the ankle. Foot Ankle 1:84–89, 1980.
3. Grant JCB: A Method of Anatomy. Baltimore, Williams & Wilkins, 1958.
4. Hamilton WG: "Dancer's tendinitis" of the FHL tendon. Am Orthop Soc Sports Med, Durango, CO, July 1976.
5. Hamilton WG: Tendinitis about the ankle joint in classical ballet dancers: "Dancer's tendinitis." J Sports Med 5:84, 1977.
6. Hamilton WG: Post traumatic peroneal tendon weakness in classical ballet dancers. Am Orthop Soc Sports Med, Lake Placid, NY, July 1978.
6a. Hamilton WG: Sprained ankles in ballet dancers. Foot Ankle 3:99–102, 1982.
7. Hamilton WG: Stenosing tenosynovitis of the flexor hallucis longus tendon and posterior impingement upon the os trigonum in ballet dancers. Foot Ankle 3:74–80, 1982.
8. Hamilton WG: Surgical anatomy of the foot and ankle. Clin Symp 37, 1985.
9. Hamilton WG: Foot and ankle injuries in dancers. Clin Sports Med 7:143–173, 1988.
10. Hamilton WG, Thompson FM, Snow S: The modified Broström procedure for lateral ankle instability. Foot Ankle 14:1–7, 1993.
11. Hamilton WG, Hamilton LH, Marshall P, et al: A physical profile of the musculoskeletal characteristics of elite professional ballet dancers. Am J Sports Med 20:267–273, 1992.
12. Hamilton WG: Ballet. *In* Reider B (Ed): The School-Age Athlete. Philadelphia, WB Saunders, 1991.
13. Harburn T, Ross H: Avulsion fracture of the anterior calcaneal process. Physician Sports Med 15:73–80, 1987.
14. Hawkins LG: Fractures of the lateral process of the talus. J Bone Joint Surg 52A:991, 1970.
15. Howse AJG: Posterior block of the ankle joint in dancers. Foot Ankle 3:81–84, 1982.
16. Kleiger B: Mechanisms of ankle injury. Orthop Clin North Am 5:127, 1974.
17. Kleiger B: Anterior tibiotalar impingement syndromes in dancers. Foot Ankle 3:69–73, 1982.
18. Marshall PM, Hamilton WG: Subluxation of the cuboid in professional ballet dancers. Am J Sports Med, 20:169–175, 1992.
19. Michael RH, Holder LE: The soleus syndrome. Am J Sports Med 13:87–94, 1985.
20. Newell S, Woodie A: Cuboid syndrome. Physician Sports Med 9:71–76, 1981.
21. Parkes JC, Hamilton WG, Patterson AH, Rawles JG: The anterior impingement syndrome of the ankle. J Trauma 20:895–898, 1980.
22. Sammarco JG, DiRaimondo CV: Chronic peroneus brevis tendon lesions. Foot Ankle 9:163–170, 1989.
23. Quirk R: The talar compression syndrome in dancers. Foot Ankle 3:65–68, 1982.
24. Shepherd FJ: A hitherto undescribed fracture of the astragalus. J Anat Physiol 17:79–81, 1882.
25. Taillard W, Meyer J, Garcia J, Blanco V: The sinus tarsi syndrome. Int Orthop 5:117–130, 1981.
26. Tomasen E: Diseases and Injuries of Ballet Dancers. Denmark, Universitetsforlaget I. Arhus, 1982.
27. Wolin I, Glassman F, Sideman S, Leventhal D: Internal derangement of the talofibular component of the ankle. Surg Gynecol Obstet 91:193–200, 1950.

49

Injuries of the Gastrocnemius-Soleus Complex

ROBERT S. ADELAAR

The gastrocnemius-soleus complex is the prime power source for acceleration and deceleration for lower extremity activities. Lesions or frank tears of this complex cause significant disability. This chapter focuses on the medical and surgical treatment of disorders of the gastrocnemius-soleus complex, with special emphasis on acute and degenerative tears of the distal one-third.

ANATOMY

The medial and lateral heads of the gastrocnemius muscle originate from the posterior femoral condyles and joint at the junction of the proximal and middle thirds with the soleus muscle. The soleus muscle and fascia remain an easily separated entity until joining with the gastrocnemius to form the common tendinous structure that inserts onto the posterior portion of the calcaneus. The tendinous substance varies from person to person, but most often the musculotendinous unit is at the junction of the middle and distal thirds of the gastrocnemius-soleus complex. The distal third is usually tendinous, with a deeper muscle attachment. The plantaris muscle originates in the posterior proximal tibia, and it travels on the medial portion of the Achilles tendon. Ruptures or tears of the plantaris complex can be difficult to differentiate from injuries of the proximal or middle third of the gastrocnemius-soleus complex. This discussion focuses on the musculotendinous unit, which is surrounded by a tendon synovial sheath. This sheath can thicken in disorders of the tendon (Fig. 49–1A).

At the insertion of the Achilles tendon complex into the calcaneus, the medial and lateral portions insert proximally, and the central portion inserts more distally. The very central portion of the Achilles tendon is not attached to the calcaneal tubercle because a retrocalcaneal bursa is present (Fig. 49–1B). This bursa has been described by Frey and colleagues[1] as having the potential of accepting up to 2 cm of arthrographic dye into the bursa, which is in a horseshoe configuration (see Fig. 49–1). This bursa can become pathologic or inflamed when there is an increase in the Phillip-Fowler angle of the posterior calcaneus, which leads to a hatchet-shaped os calcis that can cause impingement to the anterior portions of the Achilles tendon. This condition has been described as Haglund's disorder, or retrocalcaneal bursitis. It is manifested by pump bumps that are aggravated by shoewear.[2]

The other major bursa in the area of the Achilles tendon insertion is the Achilles tendon bursa. This bursa is the most posterior bursal tissue between the Achilles tendon and the skin (see Fig. 49–1A). This bursal tissue allows decreased friction between skin and subcutaneous tissue and the Achilles tendon and can be a source of an inflammatory focus. Inflammation of this bursa needs to be differentiated from retrocalcaneal bursitis; this can be accomplished by palpation or diagnostic injection. The neural structures about the Achilles tendon deserve attention when the anatomy is focused on (Fig. 49–2). The sural nerve is approximately 1 cm from the peroneal

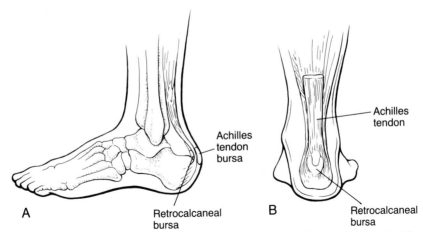

FIGURE 49–1. *(A)*, The bursa and tendon sheath that are associated with the Achilles tendon. The Achilles tendon bursa is between the skin and the tendon, and the retrocalcaneal bursa is between the tendon and the os calcis. *(B)*, An end-down or Harris view of the heel demonstrating that the Achilles tendon inserts medially and laterally but not in the center area where the retrocalcaneal bursa is.

tendon sheath and from the Achilles tendon, and it certainly can be injured during anatomic exposure down to the Achilles tendon or the posterior process of the os calcis, for example in the treatment of a symptomatic os trigonum impingement. With a lateral posterior approach to the Achilles tendon complex, an important landmark is the muscle portion of the flexor hallucis longus. This is draped over the back of the ankle and subtalar capsule and leads to the flexor hallucis longus tendon, which lies between the larger lateral posterior process and the smaller medial posterior process. Nonunions of the lateral posterior process occur in approximately 15 percent of individuals and are usually symptomatic only in performing artists who hold their feet in the equinus position for long periods.

The blood supply of the Achilles tendon area is important. The blood supply of the distal segment is limited to the longitudinal vessels that are within the tendinous substance and sheath. In the middle portion of the gastrocnemius-soleus complex, perforating branches from the interosseous membrane posteriorly supply the muscle in a segmental manner. A distally based soleus flap has a high failure rate because of its poor blood supply from the distal portion of the Achilles tendon going in a retrograde manner to the soleus muscle. The decreased blood supply to the area should make the surgeon aware of appropriate incisions and tension-free closure in this area, which is prone to necrosis because of its limited

blood supply. Because of the high incidence of skin problems, I usually do not make an incision directly over the Achilles tendon.

PATHOLOGIC DISORDERS OF THE GASTROCNEMIUS-SOLEUS COMPLEX

The pathologic disorders that can occur with the Achilles tendon are tenosynovitis or peritendinitis of the Achilles tendon, with inflammation about the tendon with or without the involvement of the sheath. Usually the sheath is involved, and this involvement results in a constricting, stenosing type of tendinitis with compromise to an already-deficient blood supply. Possibly one-fifth to one-third of lesions of the tendons or the sheaths in the foot and ankle involve the Achilles tendon.[3, 4] Irritation to the tendon or sheath can be either inflammatory or mechanical. Inflammatory disorders are most commonly seen with rheumatoid arthritis and more rarely with ulcerative colitis, Reiter's disease, or certain types of bacterial infections such as gonococcal infections.[3] The peroneal tendon sheath is more commonly involved in rheumatoid arthritis than is the Achilles tendon. Inflammatory disorders are not the focus of this discussion, but they certainly should be ruled out before mechanical problems are considered.

Mechanical problems primarily involve overuse disorders; friction from shoeing or from

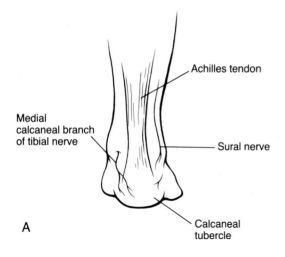

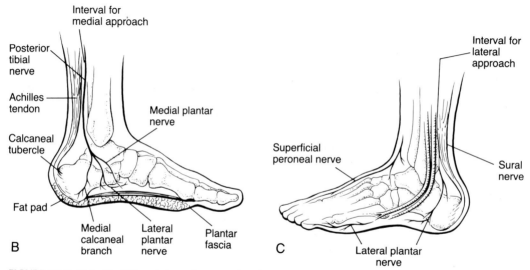

FIGURE 49–2. *(A to C),* Different views demonstrating the innervation around the calcaneus and Achilles tendon.

the adjacent Achilles tendon, as in retrocalcaneal bursitis; or direct injury from athletic stress over and above the limit that the Achilles tendon can tolerate. Mechanical problems of the Achilles tendon itself are relatively common and must be differentiated from retrocalcaneal bursitis, os trigonum impingement, and tenosynovitis of the flexor hallucis longus. Lesions between the tendons and their sheaths (e.g., lipomas or deposition diseases such as in cholesterol, amyloid, and gouty disorders) must also be ruled out and are not a focus of this chapter. Accessory muscles have been rarely reported as a source of mechanical problems.

The prime focus of this chapter is on tears, which may occur spontaneously, associated with underlying connective tissue disorders, but are more commonly due to traumatic or overuse rupture situations. Direct lacerations of the Achilles tendon are not focused on because they should be repaired primarily with the same techniques as when they are found within 6 weeks of the direct laceration. Any direct trauma from blunt objects or from penetrating wounds to the Achilles tendon must be diagnosed appropriately at an early time and treated appropriately, as is discussed in the section on the treatment of spontaneous and overuse ruptures.

Ruptures of the Gastrocnemius-Soleus Complex

Muscle ruptures above the musculotendinous level are fairly common, particularly in younger individuals participating in strenuous athletic events. These muscle tears are usually smaller and heal by benign neglect and avoidance of high-intensity activity. The area of concern in this chapter is the musculotendinous area. This area usually ruptures in younger individuals without pre-existing problems in the area, which usually has an adequate blood supply. Ruptures of the musculotendinous area tend to be in younger, more vigorous athletes who overstress the area beyond the area of the capacity of the muscle (Fig. 49–3*A*). Attritional tears usually occur in older individuals and are commonly in the distal third of the gastrocnemius-soleus complex, concentrated within the distal 2 to 3 cm of the Achilles tendon (Fig. 49–3*B*). These tears are accompanied by discomfort or tightness in the area, known as Achilles tendinitis. The damaged Achilles tendon with compromised circulation can rupture during normal activity with repetitive stresses within the normal upper limits of stress or with unusual or unexpected high forces.

Avulsion fractures of the Achilles tendon usually occur after falls from heights or sudden blows to the back of the heel. Patients with these injuries do not have pre-existing lesions of the Achilles tendon. These avulsions involve a small but fixable portion of the calcaneal tubercle and should be repaired in a bone-to-bone method using rigid fixation techniques (Fig. 49–3*C* and *D*). Therefore, the areas that I stress in the treatment section are the acute musculotendinous rupture, the Achilles tendon degenerative rupture, and the avulsion injury of the distal tubercle of the os calcis (see Fig. 49–3).

Diagnosis of Traumatic Ruptures of the Achilles Tendon

Twenty-five percent of Achilles tendon ruptures are not diagnosed. Most of the injuries occur during events in which there is already maximum contraction of the gastrocnemius-soleus complex, exerting maximum tension forces on the tendon, which is then stressed by an additional sudden tension force. The elastic component of the tendon has already been used up by the initial stretch, and with the additional overload, the system will deform. Certain activities concentrate high stresses in these specific areas. In a tennis serve, with the foot supinated, the knee and ankle are extended; the medial gastrocnemius vigorously contracts to decelerate the force forward. Because this muscle is better anchored to the femur, the tendon tends to rupture at the musculotendinous junction or at the heel insertion. When older individuals stumble or catch the ball of one foot on the edge of a hole, they are stressing an already prestressed Achilles tendon with greater dorsiflexion torque.

To diagnose a ruptured Achilles tendon, the physician must have a high index of suspicion and acutely be able to palpate a defect in the injured foot or to create the defect by dorsiflexion. A simple test was devised by Thompson in which the patient sits down in a chair and the physician grasps the calf distal to the largest part of the calf mass. The calf is squeezed and simultaneously pushed toward the knee. If the complex is intact, the ankle will flex; if the tendon is ruptured, there will be no motion at the ankle.[5] The physician must be careful because weak plantar flexion with a complete Achilles tendon lesion can occur with activity of the peroneals, toe flexors, and tibialis posterior.

Palpation of a defect is the other clinical sign the physician must look for. It is also helpful in making a surgical decision. If a musculotendinous tear is acute and without a great deal of edema, an indurated area or defect can usually be palpated. The physician can also test whether with reasonable plantar flexion the defect will be closed. Similar palpations should be carried out in the Achilles tendon. Therefore, through the clinical examination, the physician should be able to determine the presence of a tear, its location, its relative size, and whether it reduces with plantar flexion.

Magnetic resonance imaging (MRI) is the most sensitive technique for diagnosing Achilles tendon pathology. MRI can detect separation between the ends of the tendon, the extent of the tear, and degeneration in the Achilles tendon. It also can be used to diagnose lesions that may represent a prerupture state, such as degenerative disorders of the Achilles tendon insertion. A sagittal T_1-weighted image demonstrates focal thickening,

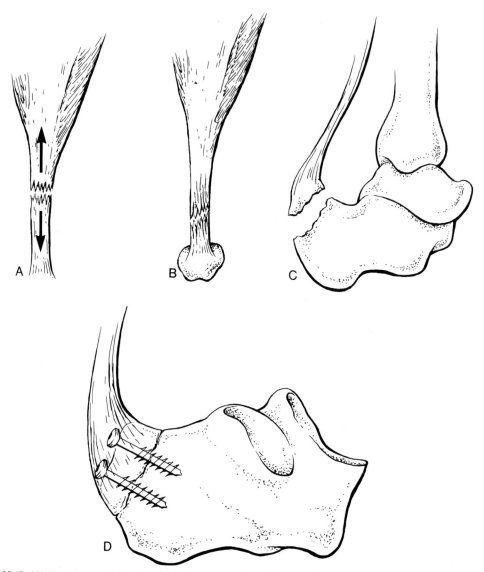

FIGURE 49–3. *(A)*, An anteroposterior view demonstrates musculotendinous tear. *(B)*, An anteroposterior view demonstrates rupture and shredding of the insertion over a 2- to 3-cm segment of the Achilles tendon. This is usually seen in a patient with chronic Achilles tendinitis who finally has a rupture or a partial rupture. *(C)*, A lateral view demonstrates an avulsion fracture of the tubercle of the os calcis. The tendon is intact, and there is a traction injury to the bone. *(D)*, An avulsion fracture of the Achilles tendon is treated by lag screw fixation with at least two screws.

as seen in chronic tendinitis, or focal areas of increased signal intensity over retracted coiled tendon ends, as seen in partial tears.[6]

Ultrasonography has been used for diagnosing Achilles tendon pathology, but it is not as accurate as MRI. Routine radiography of soft tissue detail can be used to look at the amount of edema in the fascial sheath. The most significant advantage of MRI is its ability to image

the internal substance of tendons, and by altering the pulse, the physician can distinguish between hemorrhage, edema, and fibrosis. Injection of arthrographic dye into the tendinous substance can sometimes give some definition to the suspected tear. MRI is most useful in determining the extent of the tear, which is helpful in selecting the appropriate surgical technique if surgery is indicated.

Nonsurgical Treatment

After diagnosis of the musculotendinous or Achilles tendon insertional rupture, the physician must determine whether to treat it by surgical or nonsurgical means. If the palpable defect is large and does not reduce with a mild degree of equinus of the foot, surgery should be performed unless it is contraindicated. If the ends do not come together when the hindfoot is put into equinus, there will be significant fibroblastic replacement at the defect site, which will result in tissue that will yield more easily than normal tissue and will have a higher rerupture rate and prolonged healing time.[7] If there is a question whether the defect is significant, it would be appropriate to obtain an MR image in the appropriate casting position to determine how much deficit still remains. If the Achilles tendon is ruptured in an older person, treatment would tend to be more conservative because the tendon rupture is usually secondary to a period of degeneration and loss of vascular supply. The limited vascular supply will increase healing time and possible complications at the time of surgery. If the Achilles tendon has significant degeneration, as demonstrated by MRI, I would tend to use more conservative treatment in that case to avoid altering an already-diminished blood supply by surgical invasion. Avulsion fractures of the Achilles tendon that are not displaced with some equinus can be treated in a cast. As a rule, these tend not to reduce easily. Percutaneous fixation of the avulsion fractures can also be attempted with some percutaneous Kirschner wires or small cannulated screws under image intensification.

In the patient treated conservatively, a long-leg cast should be applied for the first 4 to 6 weeks. I believe that in the younger person, this treatment may be appropriate for a short time, but I like to place these patients in non–weight-bearing short-leg casts as soon as possible so that some stress is applied to the tendon once the defect has been replaced with fibrous tissues, which do not stretch easily. The sooner tension can be placed through the tear site, the faster will be the healing time and the stronger the tendon. One way to create physiologic tension through the tear site is to place the patient in a short-leg cast and allow him or her non–weight-bearing motion on crutches, with no significant contraction forces. After 6 to 8 weeks in the non–weight-bearing cast, the patient is placed in a series of weight-bearing casts or cast braces with ankle hinges, in which equinus is decreased by tapering the heel pads. In the conservative treatment of these lesions, it is important that the physician not start with a severe equinus of the hindfoot and cause a contracture of the gastrocnemius-soleus complex. The contractures are often more difficult to treat successfully than the original lesion.[8, 9] The cast is usually removed in 3 months, and the patient starts walking with gradually decreasing heel lifts. The patient is not allowed to return to any forceful sports participation for 9 months but can start biking and swimming 4 months after the injury as long as there is no pain at the injury site.

For the closed treatment of an avulsion fracture of the os calcis, weight bearing is delayed until there is evidence of trabeculation at the fracture site. This area may take a long time to heal because the blood supply in the area, which amounts to the old epiphyseal scar, is not as good as that in the rest of the calcaneus. This usually requires approximately 8 weeks without weight bearing, after which a weight-bearing cast is applied and serial changes are made in the heel height using heel pads.

Surgical Treatment

There is still anecdotal controversy over whether to use open treatment, with surgical repair or augmentation, or closed treatment for Achilles tendon tears.[11] The advocates of surgical treatment cite a higher rerupture rate and a lower strength in the Achilles tendon that has been nonsurgically treated.[7] The proponents of conservative treatment state that strength is not a significant factor and that complications occur with open repair of the Achilles tendon.[8, 9] They indicate that the drop in strength is not really significant.[10, 12, 13] Therefore, the age and athletic activity potential of the patient help in making a decision about surgery. The older patient with circulatory difficulty and a pre-existing Achilles tendon lesion would not be a surgical candidate if the lesion came together in a cast or brace. Another alternative to open treatment is percutaneous treatment of Achilles tendon lesions. This treatment is certainly not widely used but has had increasing interest due to its ability to keep the skin and vascular status intact while a percutaneous repair is performed with synthetic suture.[14, 15] This treatment requires a lesion that is not extensive and also one that is primarily in the musculotendinous junction. The use of large needles and meticulous care of the sural and posterior tibial calcaneal nerves are indicated. A Bunnell weave or Kessler suture can be used (Fig. 49–4).

The actual method of surgical repair varies from study to study. My philosophy is not to use the peroneus brevis since because I believe that this important muscle should not be sac-

rificed if at all possible. Therefore, my last choice is to use the peroneus brevis or to split the peroneus brevis for augmentation (Fig. 49–5).[16] The plantaris can be used, if it is large enough. The use of synthetic grafts has also been reported, but they have not been approved by the US Food and Drug Administration.[17] I use a synthetic Mersilene tape that is 5 mm in diameter in a Kessler-type tendon weave (Fig. 49–6), which does not strangulate the tissue as much as the Bunnell weave. Augmentation can be done with fascia lata or a proximal strip of fascia that is turned down.

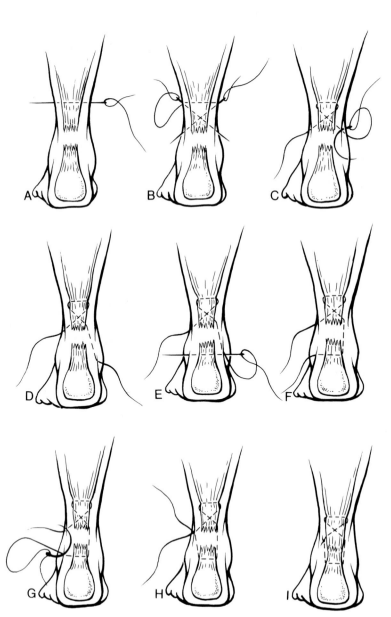

FIGURE 49–4. *(A to I)*, A percutaneous suture technique using a Bunnell-type suture with a nonabsorbable nylon-type material.

FIGURE 49–5. Augmentation of a segmental defect in a musculotendinous tear of the Achilles tendon with a peroneus brevis tendon.

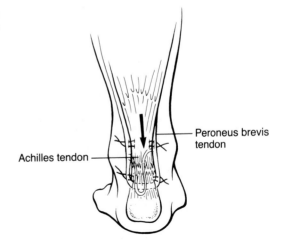

Achilles tendon

Peroneus brevis tendon

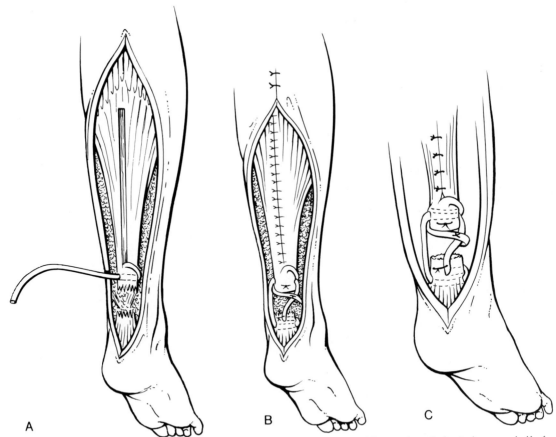

A

B

C

FIGURE 49–6. (A), Augmentation with a plantaris tendon, a proximal strip of fascia (shown), fascia lata, one-half of a peroneus brevis, or synthetic tape. (B), The graft is woven into the proximal and distal segments of the Achilles tendon (Kessler or Bunnell weave). (C), The gap should be filled by graft material and closed as much as possible, but the foot should not be put in severe equinus.

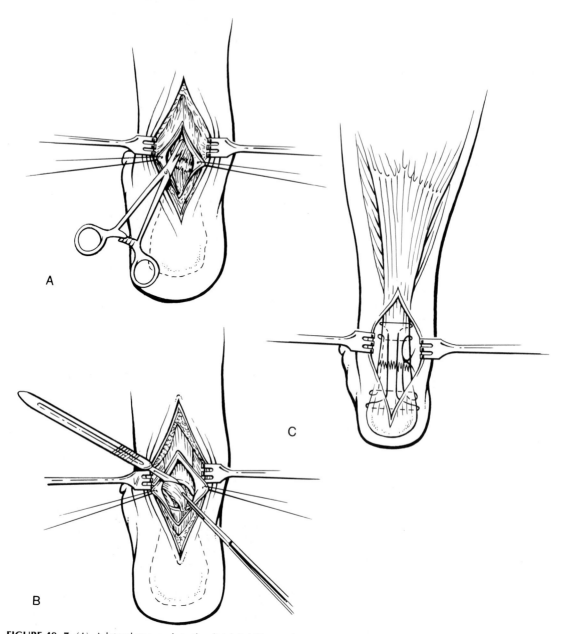

FIGURE 49–7. *(A)*, A lateral approach to the distal Achilles tendon is important. An approach 1 cm lateral to the Achilles tendon in a straight-line fashion will demonstrate the sural nerve in the superior portion of the flap and the flexor hallucis longus in the depth of the wound. This gives good exposure of the Achilles tendon. *(B)*, Degenerated tissue is excised from the exposed tendon ends. *(C)*, A double-loop Kessler-type suture for Achilles tendon repair when there is no significant gap.

Augmentation is still a controversial issue, but if I find a defect that cannot be closed by suture methods or mild equinus, I elect to augment with one of these methods.

When I use a Kessler-type suture, I often use two Kessler sutures—one toward the center of the tendon and one toward the periph-

ery. The suture is placed in either the anterior or the posterior portion of the tendon so as not to compromise the suture material (Fig. 49–7). A No. 1 or 2 Mersilene suture is used. I believe that nonabsorbable sutures should be used because of the prolonged healing time for this tendon.

The incision used is important because it is important to preserve as much blood supply in the area as possible. The medial Achilles tendon approach has been noted to give a significant incidence of wound slough; therefore, the blood supply of the Achilles tendon may be somewhat compromised in the traumatic situation. I therefore make my incision as follows: at the lower part of the Achilles tendon, I go in on the lateral side, trying to avoid the sural nerve and thus leaving the medial complex and its vascular contributories intact. On the lateral side, for the distal third, a nice approach is possible starting approximately 1 cm from the tendon and extending down into the Achilles insertion. Fracture avulsions are treated by direct exposure from the lateral side. In the distal portion, I avoid the medial side particularly because of the branching of the posterior tibial nerve and its medial calcaneal branches. Toward the junction of the middle and distal tendon areas, a medial approach is used. I never use a zig-zag type of incision over the tendon but rather usually use a line that follows Langer's lines or a gentle C-shaped curve.

In the difficult huge or chronic injury in which there is a large gap, a V-Y plasty can be performed, with the realization that advancement of a muscular block of tissue may result in compromise of that segment and also in a great deal of scarring in the postoperative period. These techniques violate more normal portions of the Achilles complex, and I have not used them because there are no studies to show that they are any more effective than autogenous augmentation with other tissue.

Postoperative rehabilitation usually consists of the use of a short-leg cast for 6 weeks without weight bearing, followed by the use of a functional brace on short-leg cast with gradual weight bearing for another 6 weeks. After 3 months, the patient is started on a gradual weight-bearing program with sequential heel lifts. As stated previously, the ultimate strength is usually not achieved until 9 months. Biking, walking, swimming, and weight lifting are allowed from 4 months to 9 months. After 9 months, there is a gradual return to normal activity.

Complications

Complications of lesions of the Achilles tendon complex can fall under errors in judgment and errors in surgical or conservative management. An error in judgment would be the use of closed treatment when open treatment should have been used. This results in weakness and decreased power in the Achilles tendon after conservative treatment. Even after open repair, restoration of completely normal function is not possible. The most serious complication is the wound slough with infection, which is particularly associated with medial incisions. It is usually treated by débridement, wet-to-dry dressings, and a cast with a window. A drain is inserted after all surgical procedures to ensure that no significant hematoma forms. Other complications, involving the use of autogenous tendons, would be ones of donor site morbidity, particularly in the case of the peroneus brevis.

CONCLUSIONS

If a surgical procedure is elected, meticulous technique should be used to obtain the strongest repair (with or without augmentation) without significant compromise to the skin, donor site, and subcutaneous tissue. Whichever method is used, there will be a long period before the ultimate strength of the tendon is reached. Surgical repair is appropriate in the younger, more active adult, and these techniques are outlined in the text. Appropriate patient selection gives the best ultimate outcome. Care must be taken in the postoperative period because the rehabilitation for these injuries is often just as important as the choice of surgical or closed management. A long time is needed to prevent stretch with tension, and these tendons tend to take a long time to reach their ultimate strength. Great care must be taken with the older, heavy patient with a preexisting tendon lesion because good surgical results will be difficult to achieve in this patient. Therefore, when in doubt, the physician should not operate. MRI is helpful in difficult decisions to define the extent of injury and the gap.

References

1. Frey C, Rosenberg Z, Shereff MJ: The retrocalcaneal bursae: Anatomy and bursography. Presented at the American Orthopaedic Foot and Ankle Society Meeting. Las Vegas, NV, February 1986.
2. Keck SW, Kelly PJ: Bursitis of the posterior part of

the heel: Evaluation of 18 patients. J Bone Joint Surg 47A:67, 1965.

3. Mann RA: Traumatic injuries to the soft tissues of the foot and ankle. *In* Mann RA (Ed): Surgery of the Foot, 5th Ed. St. Louis, CV Mosby, 1985, pp 472–499.

4. Lipscomb PR, Kelley PJ: Injuries to the extensor tendon in the distal part of the leg and ankle. J Bone Joint Surg 32A:175, 1950.

5. Thompson TC: A test for rupture of the tendo Achilles. Acta Orthop Scand 32:461, 1962.

6. Panageas E, Greenberg S, Franklin PD, et al: MRI of pathologic conditions of the Achilles tendon. Orthop Rev 19:975–980, 1990.

7. Inglis AE, Scott WM, Sculco TP, Patterson AH: Ruptures of the tendo-Achilles: An objective assessment of surgical and nonsurgical treatment. J Bone Joint Surg 58:990, 1976.

8. Lea RB, Smith L: Nonsurgical treatment of tendo Achilles rupture. J Bone Joint Surg 54:1398, 1972.

9. Stein SR, Levlans CA Jr: Closed treatment of Achilles tendon ruptures. Orthop Clin North Am 7:241, 1976.

10. Keller J, Rasmussen TB: Closed treatment of Achilles tendon rupture. Acta Orthop Scand 55:548–550, 1984.

11. Wilks CA, Woshburg S, Ciaozzo V, Preitlo CA:

Achilles tendon rupture: A review of the literature comparing surgical vs nonsurgical treatment. Clin Orthop 107:156, 1986.

12. Therman H: Operative vs conservative functional treatment of acute Achilles tendon rupture. Presented at the American Orthopaedic Foot and Ankle Society Meeting. Banff, Canada, June 1990.

13. Sjöström M, Fugl-Meyer AR, Wåhlby L: Achilles tendon injury: Plantar flexion strength and structure of soleus muscle after surgical repair. Acta Chir Scand 144:219, 1978.

14. Ma GWC, Griffith TG: Percutaneous repair of acute closed ruptured Achilles tendon. Clin Orthop 128:247, 1977.

15. Hockenbury RT, Johns JC: A biomechanical comparison of open repair versus percutaneous repair of the Achilles tendon defects. Presented at the AAOS Summer Institute. Monterey, CA, 1990.

16. Turco V, Spinella J: Peroneus brevis transfer for Achilles tendon rupture in athletes. Orthop Rev 17:822, 1988.

17. Lynn TA: Repair of the torn Achilles tendon using the plantaris tendon as the reinforcing membrane. J Bone Joint Surg 48:268, 1977.

Index

Note: Page numbers in *italics* refer to illustrations;
page numbers followed by t refer to tables.

987

Vertical talus *(Continued)*
  postoperative period in, 774
  radiologic features of, 767–768, *768–769*
  range of motion of, evaluation of, 767
  surgical treatment of, 770–774
   complications of, 774
   in older child, 774
  in child with myelomeningocele, 822–823, *822–823*
Villonodular synovitis, pigmented, of foot, 250, *250*
Volkmann's contracture, treatment of, 577
Volkmann's fragment, 340, *341*
V-osteotomy, foot deformity correction with, 493, *497–498*
  Ilizarov apparatus used in, 509–510
Vulpius procedure, for equinus deformity, in cerebral palsy patient, 233–234, *234*
V-Y fasciocutaneous flap, 550, 551

Walker, swivel, for foot deformities, in child with myelomeningocele, 818
Walking, peroneal muscle spasms during, in tarsal coalitions, 863
  pistoning during, in equinus deformity, 227, *228*
Walking cast. See *Short-leg cast.*

Wart(s), plantar, 69
Watson-Jones procedure, for lateral ligament sprain, *915*, 915–916
Web plasty, for syndactyly reconstruction, 592, *592*
Web space incision, metatarsophalangeal joint exposure by, 151, *152*
Web space infection, 271–273
  author's preferred surgical approach to, 272, 273
  drainage of, 211, *211*
  treatment of, 271–273, *272*
Wedge osteotomy, dorsal, for lesion under metatarsal head, *73*, 73–74
  technique for, 181
  open, for varus deformity, 234
Wedge resection, of nail margin, matrix, and groove, complications of, 97
  postoperative care in, 96
  technical pitfalls in, 96–97
  technique of, 96, *97*
Whitesides infusion technique, of tissue pressure measurement, 570–573, *571–572*
Winograd procedure, 93
Wire problems, due to Ilizarov distraction osteotomy, 511
Wound(s), classification of, 546–547
  by anatomic site, 546t
  by size, 546t
  closure of, in clubfoot repair, 737–738

Wound(s) *(Continued)*
  coverage options for, 547–549, *548*
  disant pedicle flaps as, 549, 550t
  island pedicle flaps as, 549, 550t
  select free flaps as, 549, 550t
  transpositional flaps as, 549, 549t
  drainage of, in diabetic foot, 215
  persistent, silicone implants and, 133
  infection of, due to clubfoot surgery, 759
  puncture, 273–274, *274*
  author's preferred surgical approach to, 274, *275*
  ulceration of, chronic, *556, 560*

Xanthoma, synovial, 250, *250*

Y-plate, in calcaneal fracture repair, 442

Zadik procedure, for ingrown toenail, 94, *94*
Zig-zag incision, for drainage of web space infection, *272*, 273
Z-plasty, for constriction band syndrome, 610–611
Z-shaped incision, in Girdlestone procedure, 84, *86*